Routledge International Handbook of Psychopathy and Crime

For over two centuries, psychopathy has stood as perhaps the most formidable risk factor for antisocial behavior, crime, and violence. The *Routledge International Handbook of Psychopathy and Crime* presents the state-of-the-art on the full landscape of research on antisocial behavior that employs psychopathy as a central correlate. It is the largest and most comprehensive work of its kind, and includes contributions from renowned scholars from around the world.

Organized into five distinctive sections, this book covers the etiology of psychopathy; the measurement of psychopathy; the association between psychopathy and diverse forms of homicidal and sexual offending, including serial murder, sexual homicide, rape, and child molestation; criminal careers and psychopathy; and the role of psychopathy in criminal justice system supervision, including institutional misconduct, noncompliance, and recidivism.

This book is an essential resource for students and researchers in criminology, psychology, and criminal justice and will be of interest to all those interested in criminal behavior, sexual and violent crime, forensic psychology, and forensic mental health.

Matt DeLisi is Coordinator of Criminal Justice Studies, Professor in the Department of Sociology, and Faculty Affiliate of the Center for the Study of Violence at Iowa State University, USA.

Routledge International Handbook of Psychopathy and Crime

Edited by Matt DeLisi

Routledge
Taylor & Francis Group
LONDON AND NEW YORK

First published 2019
by Routledge
2 Park Square, Milton Park, Abingdon, Oxon OX14 4RN

and by Routledge
52 Vanderbilt Avenue, New York, NY 10017

First issued in paperback 2020

Routledge is an imprint of the Taylor & Francis Group, an informa business

British Library Cataloguing-in-Publication Data
A catalogue record for this book is available from the British Library

Library of Congress Cataloging-in-Publication Data
Names: DeLisi, Matt, editor.
Title: Routledge international handbook of psychopathy and crime / [edited by] Matt Delisi.
Description: Abingdon, Oxon ; New York, NY : Routledge, 2019. | Series: Routledge international handbooks | Includes bibliographical references.
Identifiers: LCCN 2018010297 | ISBN 9781138085169 (hardback) | ISBN 9781315111476 (ebook)
Subjects: LCSH: Criminal psychology. | Criminology. | Forensic psychology. | Criminal justice, Administration of—Psychological aspects.
Classification: LCC HV6080 .R76 2019 | DDC 364.3—dc23
LC record available at https://lccn.loc.gov/2018010297

ISBN 13: 978-0-367-58057-5 (pbk)
ISBN 13: 978-1-138-08516-9 (hbk)

Typeset in Bembo
by Apex CoVantage, LLC

Contents

Figures

Tables

Contributors

Isabel Alberto is a faculty member of psychology and education sciences at the University of Coimbra in Portugal.

Henrik Andershed is Professor of Criminology and Psychology and one of the senior researchers at CAPS – Center for Criminological and Psychosocial Research at Örebro University in Sweden.

Katherine M. Auty is a research associate at the Institute of Criminology at Cambridge University in the United Kingdom.

Michael T. Baglivio is Chief Research Officer at TrueCore Behavioral Solutions in the United States.

Edward D. Barker is Professor in the Department of Psychology, Institute of Psychiatry, Psychology, and Neuroscience at King's College London in the United Kingdom.

Christopher T. Barry is Associate Professor in the Department of Psychology at Washington State University in the United States.

Eric Beauregard is Professor in the School of Criminology at Simon Fraser University in Canada.

Daniel Boduszek is Professor in the Department of Psychology at the University of Huddersfield in the United Kingdom.

Gayle Brewer is Lecturer in the School of Psychology at the University of Liverpool in the United Kingdom.

Melanie Burton is a doctoral candidate in the School of Law at the University of New South Wales in Australia.

Jesse Cale is Senior Lecturer in the School of Social Sciences at the University of New South Wales in Australia.

Jonathan W. Caudill is Associate Professor and Director of the Master of Criminal Justice Program at the University of Colorado, Colorado Springs in the United States.

Luna C. M. Centifanti is Senior Lecturer in the Institute of Psychology, Health, and Society at the University of Liverpool in the United Kingdom.

Heng Choon (Oliver) Chan is Associate Professor in the Department of Criminology at the City University of Hong Kong.

Olivier F. Colins is Assistant Professor in the Department of Child and Adolescent Psychiatry at Leiden University Medical Centre in The Netherlands.

Raymond R. Corrado is Professor in the School of Criminology at Simon Fraser University in Canada and Founding Director of the Incarcerated Serious and Violent Young Offender Study.

Agata Debowska is a faculty member in the Department of Psychology at the University of Sheffield in the United Kingdom.

Matt DeLisi is Coordinator of Criminal Justice Studies, Professor in the Department of Sociology, and Affiliate with the Center for the Study of Violence at Iowa State University in the United States.

David DeMatteo is Associate Professor of Psychology and Law at Drexel University in the United States.

Katie Dhingra is a faculty member in the School of Social, Psychological, and Communication Sciences at Leeds Beckett University in the United Kingdom and Editor-in-Chief of the *Journal of Criminal Psychology*.

Hailey L. Dotterer is a graduate student in the Department of Psychology at the University of Michigan in the United States.

Simon Duff is Deputy Director of Forensic Programmes and Faculty Member of Medicine and Health Sciences at the University of Nottingham in the United Kingdom.

John F. Edens is Professor in the Department of Psychology at Texas A & M University in the United States.

Bethany Edwards is a clinical doctoral student in the Department of Psychology at the University of New Mexico in the United States.

Vincent Egan is Associate Professor of Medicine and Health Sciences and Director of Forensic Psychology Programmes at the University of Nottingham in the United Kingdom.

Kostas Fanti is Assistant Professor in the Department of Psychology and Director of the Developmental Psychopathology Lab at the University of Cyprus.

Bryanna Fox is Assistant Professor in the Department of Criminology at the University of South Florida and former Special Agent with the Federal Bureau of Investigation in the United States.

Yu Gao is Associate Professor in the Department of Psychology at Brooklyn College and the Graduate Center City University of New York in the United States.

Carlo Garofalo is Assistant Professor in the Department of Developmental Psychology at Tilburg University in The Netherlands.

Jeremy G. Gay is a Forensic Psychology Postdoctoral Fellow at Augusta University in the United States.

Steven M. Gillespie is Lecturer in Clinical Psychology in the Department of Psychological Sciences at the University of Liverpool in the United Kingdom.

Amy Hoffmann is a doctoral student in the Department of Psychology at the University of South Florida in the United States.

Kristin M. Holland is a behavioral scientist in the Division of Violence Prevention at the Centers for Disease Control and Prevention in the United States.

Luke W. Hyde is Assistant Professor in the Department of Psychology at the University of Michigan in the United States.

Shayne Jones is Professor in the Department of Criminal Justice at Texas State University in the United States.

Raymond Knight is Professor Emeritus in the Department of Psychology at Brandeis University in the United States.

Sonja Krstic is a researcher in the Department of Psychology at Brandeis University in the United States.

Claire Lankford is a researcher in the Department of Psychology at Drexel University in the United States.

Shichun Ling is a doctoral candidate in the Department of Criminology at the University of Pennsylvania in the United States.

David A. Lishner is Professor in the Department of Psychology at the University of Wisconsin Oshkosh in the United States.

Laura López-Romero is a faculty member in the Department of Clinical Psychology at the University of Santiago de Compostela in Spain.

Nicholas Longré is a postdoctoral associate in the Department of Psychology at Brandeis University in the United States.

Donald R. Lynam is Distinguished Professor in the Department of Psychological Sciences at Purdue University in the United States.

Brandy R. Maynard is Assistant Professor in the School of Social Work at Saint Louis University in the United States.

Evan McCuish is Assistant Professor in the School of Criminology at Simon Fraser University in Canada.

Alan J. Meehan is a graduate student in the Department of Psychology, Institute of Psychiatry, Psychology, and Neuroscience at King's College London in the United Kingdom.

Tina D. Wall Meyers is an endowed postdoctoral fellow in the Department of Psychology at the University of Dayton in the United States.

Joshua D. Miller is Professor in the Department of Psychology at the University of Georgia in the United States.

Laura Murray is a graduate student in the Department of Psychology at the University of Michigan in the United States.

Daniel C. Murrie is Professor in the Department of Psychiatry and Neurobehavioral Sciences at the University of Virginia in the United States.

Craig S. Neumann is Distinguished Research Professor in the Department of Psychology at the University of North Texas in the United States.

Julie R. Odom-Dixon is a graduate student in the Department of Psychology at Washington State University in the United States.

Mark E. Olver is Professor in the Department of Psychology at the University of Saskatchewan in Canada.

Pedro Pechorro is a research associate with the School of Psychology at the University of Minho in Portugal.

Sofia Persson is a doctoral student in the Department of Psychology at Manchester Metropolitan University in the United Kingdom.

Devon Polaschek is Professor in the School of Psychology at the University of Waikato in New Zealand.

Adrian Raine is the Richard Perry University Professor of Criminology, Psychiatry, and Psychology at the University of Pennsylvania in the United States and past President of the Academy of Experimental Criminology.

James V. Ray is Assistant Professor in the Department of Criminal Justice at the University of Central Florida in the United States.

Kylie Reale is a doctoral student in the School of Criminology at Simon Fraser University in Canada.

Dennis E. Reidy is a behavioral scientist in the Division of Violence Prevention at the Centers for Disease Control and Prevention in the United States.

Shari R. Reiter is a doctoral student in the Department of Psychology at Washington State University in the United States.

Carrie Robertson is Assistant Director of Admission and Title IX Administrator at Brandeis University in the United States.

Estrella Romero is a faculty member in the Department of Clinical Psychology at the University of Santiago de Compostela in Spain.

Christopher P. Salas-Wright is Assistant Professor in the School of Social Work at Boston University in the United States.

Martin Sellbom is Associate Professor in the Department of Psychology at the University of Otago in New Zealand.

Mário R. Simões is a faculty member of psychology and education sciences at the University of Coimbra in Portugal.

Marc T. Swogger is Associate Professor in the Department of Psychiatry at the University of Rochester Medical Center in the United States.

Nicholas D. Thomson is Assistant Professor in the Department of Surgery at Virginia Commonwealth University in the United States.

Amanda Trice is Researcher in the Department of Psychiatry and Health Behavior at Augusta University in the United States.

Rebecca Umbach is a doctoral candidate in the Department of Criminology at the University of Pennsylvania in the United States.

Michael G. Vaughn is Professor and Director of the doctoral program in the School of Social Work at Saint Louis University in the United States.

Edelyn Verona is Professor and Director of Clinical Training in the Department of Psychology at University of South Florida in the United States.

Beth A. Visser is Assistant Professor in the Departments of Interdisciplinary Studies and Psychology at Lakehead University Orillia in Canada.

Michael J. Vitacco is Associate Professor in the Department of Psychiatry and Health Behavior at Augusta University in the United States.

Rebecca Waller is Assistant Professor in the Department of Psychology at the University of Pennsylvania in the United States.

Glenn D. Walters is Associate Professor in the Department of Criminal Justice at Kutztown University and previously worked for 27 years as a clinical psychologist in the Federal Bureau of Prisons in the United States.

Henriikka Weir is Assistant Professor in the School of Public Affairs at the University of Colorado, Colorado Springs, in the United States.

Brandon Weiss is a graduate student in the Department of Psychology at the University of Georgia in the United States.

Dominic Willmott is a research fellow in the Department of Psychology at the University of Huddersfield in the United Kingdom.

Stephen C. P. Wong is Adjunct Professor in the Department of Psychology at the University of Saskatchewan in Canada.

Russell Woodfield is a doctoral candidate in the Department of Behavioral and Social Sciences at the University of Huddersfield in the United Kingdom.

Enzo Yaksic is Cofounder of the Atypical Homicide Research Group at Northeastern University in the United States.

Acknowledgments

Routledge is a wonderful publisher to work with, and I want to specifically acknowledge Hannah Catterall, Thomas Sutton, Kerry Boettcher, and everyone behind the scenes for their assistance. A special thank you to the many wonderful contributors for their thought-provoking scholarship.

Part I

Etiology of psychopathy

1

Psychopathy and crime are inextricably linked

Matt DeLisi

Introduction

The human population is marked by extraordinary heterogeneity in terms of behavioral functioning and capacity for norm-violating, antisocial, and violent behavior. Some individuals are exceedingly compliant, self-disciplined, and easy to get along with in terms of their basic nature, characteristics that personality psychologists would recognize as high Conscientiousness and high Agreeableness. These individuals tend to do very well in life and experience success in their family relationships, their school and work careers, and their ability to lead a crime-free life. Most individuals – comprising the bulk of the population – also do fairly well in terms of their ability to get along with others and regulate their conduct. Although they are not as ascetic as the former type of person, they nevertheless are able to regulate their conduct appropriately in most situations and in accordance with societal demands. And a fairly small number of individuals, certainly less than 5 percent of the human population, are generally noncompliant, have difficulty regulating their conduct, and face many hardships due to their unwillingness and incapacity to get along with others (DeLisi, 2005; Vaughn et al., 2011; Vaughn, Salas-Wright, DeLisi, & Maynard, 2014). Indeed, empirical assessment of the most serious, chronic, and violent offending pathways inevitably comports with persons that are also the most psychopathic (Baskin-Sommers & Baskin, 2016; Colins & Vermeiren, 2013; McCuish, Corrado, Hart, & DeLisi, 2015; McCuish, Corrado, Lussier, & Hart, 2014; Vaughn, Howard, & DeLisi, 2008).

When considering the three types of people that were just described, the highly compliant and highly self-regulated, the moderately compliant and generally well-regulated, and the chronically noncompliant and difficult, distinct and significant differences can be observed in terms of their behavioral functioning and in the diverse ways that one's sense of self relates to other people. The highly compliant individual is almost selfless in the way that he or she modulates and controls his or her thoughts, impulses, emotions, and behaviors. Such a person is able to inhibit conduct even in challenging contexts in favor of the greater good. The moderately compliant individual occasionally prioritizes themselves over the greater good. In this way, he or she periodically engages in selfish, self-centered, or narcissistic acts where the benefits of an immediate behavioral choice are selected in favor of a different behavioral choice. Many crimes can be understood from this basic calculation of self-regulation and the self. For instance, drunk driving is an immediate attempt to provide some benefit (e.g., driving home in the comfort of one's own vehicle) as opposed to a costlier alterative (e.g., paying for a taxicab, taking the bus, and thus having to pick up one's vehicle the next day because of one's current intoxicated state). Theft can provide something of value now as opposed to engaging in some delayed (e.g., waiting in line to purchase the item) activity. In both of these examples, drunk driving and theft, consideration is also not given to how the behavior negatively affects other people, whether other motorists that could be placed in danger by the individual's intoxicated driving or the shopkeeper whose livelihood suffers from the lost sale.

In the extreme case, for instance an individual whose entire behavioral repertoire is motivated by impulsive self-interest and virtually absent self-regulation, very serious crimes can occur. Sexual homicide is an example. Here, an offender procures a suitable victim, usually by force, and then sexually abuses and kills the victim. The reasoning or motivation is simple: the person wanted to engage in these behaviors and does not consider the effects on the victim or the victim's surviving family. Certainly more extreme than theft or drunk driving, the focus on the self and one's selfish desires is the driver of the conduct and is nevertheless the same as the mundane criminal acts.

In previous works (DeLisi, 2009, 2016), the current author has suggested that psychopathy is the unified theory of crime because the basic characteristics that comprise the disorder effectively map onto the basic characteristics of antisocial and criminal behavior. To use the aforementioned examples of crime, and as shown in Figure 1.1, antisocial behavior or crime can be understood as a behavioral action that is self-centered, short-sighted, inconsiderate, impulsive, defiant, and mean. Not all of these characteristics must be present to coincide with every criminal act, but these elemental characteristics are at the heart of antisocial conduct, particularly when a multiplicity of these characteristics is present. To illustrate: in isolation, these characteristics can produce negative situations relating to impulsivity (e.g., buying clothing on impulse

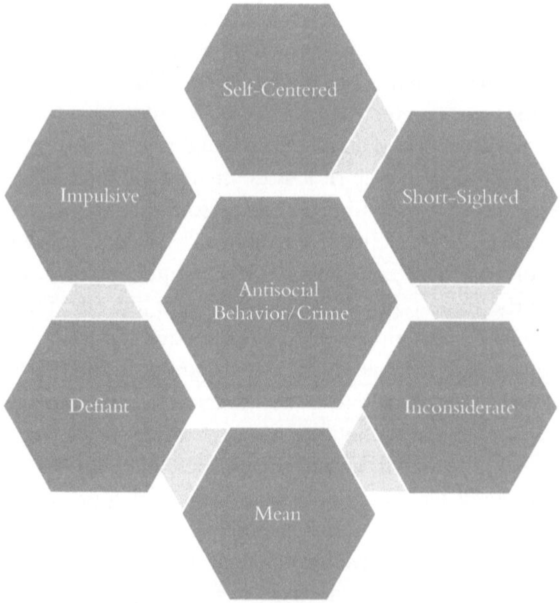

Figure 1.1 Elemental characteristics of antisocial behavior/crime

when one cannot afford it), self-centeredness (e.g., looking out for oneself at the expense of one's friends or family), short-sightedness (e.g., refusing to study for tomorrow's exam because one is tired now), meanness and inconsideration (e.g., making fun of a colleague without thinking of how the teasing negatively affects the target), or defiance (e.g., refusing to follow procedures at work). However, these isolated manifestations of crime characteristics do not necessarily mean that one will commit crime.

But what about when the assorted characteristics of crime are repeatedly apparent in the disposition and behavioral actions of an individual? As shown in Figure 1.2, if one extrapolates the elemental characteristics of crime, the result is effectively a listing of psychopathic traits. The self-centeredness of committing an antisocial act is congruent with the egocentricity, self-centeredness, and pathological narcissism of the psychopath. The short-sightedness of an antisocial act is consistent with the short time horizon, unplanning, and low wherewithal of the psychopath. Inconsideration involved in antisocial conduct is conceptually similar to the antagonistic, inconsiderate, blaming, guiltless, remorseless features of the psychopath. The meanness inherent in victimizing a person or property dovetails with the psychopath's mean, callous, indifferent, and malevolent disposition. Defiant action is matched by the defiance, scheming, and manipulative nature of the psychopath. And impulsivity of crime matches the impulsivity, proneness to boredom, and sensation seeking of the psychopath. Perhaps rivaled by no criminological theory but self-control theory (Gottfredson & Hirschi, 1990), the theory of psychopathy provides the instantiation of the antisocial person.

Psychopathy also maps well onto the most troubling typologies of offenders, such as those that evince chronic, serious, and violent offending trajectories. For example, using the Comprehensive Assessment of Psychopathic Personality (CAPP) framework, Corrado, DeLisi, Hart, and McCuish (2015) suggested that the behavioral and cognitive domains of psychopathy are particularly facilitative of chronic offending, including the traits of impulsivity, disruptiveness,

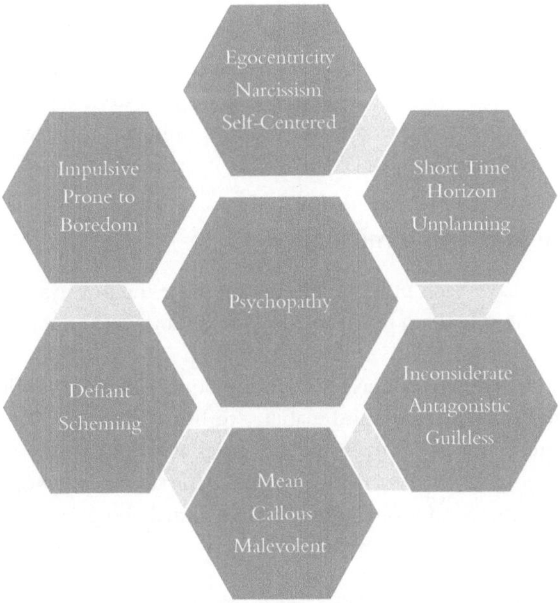

Figure 1.2 Elemental characteristics of psychopathy

aggressiveness, unreliability, restlessness, and the lack of perseverance. Chronic offenders are also theorized to be cognitively intolerant and suspicious of others, unfocused, and lacking plans for the future. They are aimless, disorganized, and prone to a transient lifestyle that also sustains frequent criminal activity and criminal justice system involvement. Serious offenders are theorized to draw most of their negative personality features from the dominance and self domains the CAPP model. For instance, serious offenders are characterized as self-centered, self-entitled, self-aggrandizing, self-justifying, and tend to view themselves as invulnerable and risk-taking. In terms of dominance features, serious offenders are portrayed as domineering, manipulative, antagonistic, insincere, and deceitful. Violent offenders are theorized to derive their traits primarily from the attachment and emotional domains of the CAPP model. Violent offenders are theorized to be remote, cold, cruel, callous, and thoroughly inconsiderate of others and, in terms of their emotional life, are fearless, unconcerned, dark, indifferent, irritable, and unrepentant. These traits allow them to inflict violence on victims without feeling any of the self-sanctioning emotions that inhibit such conduct among non-psychopathic persons.

Psychopathy can be understood as an organizing construct for other foundational correlates of crime. For instance, sex is the most powerful demographic correlate of crime and far exceeds the effects of other important factors, such as age, race, ethnicity, and social class. In a recent study, Gray and Snowden (2016) examined the inter-relationships between sex, psychopathy, and various forms of crime and criminal justice system noncompliance using data from the Partnerships in Care and the MacArthur Risk Assessment Study. Among data from the Partnerships in Care study, males were significantly more superficial, grandiose, remorseless, irresponsible, and antisocial during both adolescence and adulthood. In the MacArthur study, males were significantly more superficial, grandiose, remorseless, unempathic, irresponsible, impulsive, and antisocial during both adolescence and adulthood. On no feature of psychopathy were females more severe than males, suggesting that a simple indexing of psychopathic features is another way to index sex differences in criminal conduct. Irrespective of sex, psychopathy was significantly correlated with reconviction at two time-points and aggression and violence at two time-points.

The current chapter reviews recent criminological research that has focused on the associations between psychopathy and diverse forms of antisocial conduct, crime, and violence. It is noteworthy that no study exists, to my knowledge, that has found that psychopathy was *unrelated* to crime and various aberrant conduct. When considering the diversity of research findings and the diverse forms of antisociality therein, the intimate connection between psychopathy and crime becomes even more clear.

The psychopathy and crime mutuality

Many colorful passages have been published to demonstrate the powerful linkage between psychopathy and crime. The following by Arboleda-Flórez (2007:375) is among my favorites:

> Psychopathic tendencies are noticeable even in young children who later become known for their continuous lawbreaking and inability to live within the rules of society. Psychopaths carry a historical load of reported difficulties at school, in the military and at work, besides police reports and court dockets. Like a hurricane, psychopaths leave a path of broken promises, damage to property, physical or sexual abuse, rape, mayhem, murder and destruction of the dreams of others.

Psychopathy rears its ugly head almost irrespective of context, even when considering mundane behaviors in the workplace such as using a computer. For instance, there is evidence that persons with more psychopathic personality traits are more likely to engage in counterproductive work behaviors that are damaging to their employer (Blickle & Schütte, 2017). Similarly, using an online sample of participants recruited from MTurk, Siegfried-Spellar, Villacís-Vukadinović, and Lynam (2017) examined associations between psychopathy and diverse forms of deviant computer behaviors, including gaining unauthorized access to a network, writing/creating computer viruses, engaging in identity theft or fraud, monitoring network traffic, and website defacement. Using the Elemental Psychopathy Assessment Short Form (EPA–SF), they found significant correlations between total psychopathy scores and all forms of computer crime. The correlation was strongest for total computer crime. In addition, psychopathy had significant inverse correlations with Agreeableness and Conscientiousness and significant positive correlations with total antisocial behavior, violent crime, nonviolent crime, alcohol use, and DUI. In other words, although their focus was on the association between psychopathy and computer crime, it quickly became clear that the construct unfolds to affect generalized involvement in an array of offenses.

There is ample evidence for the psychopathy-generalized offending link. Using data from 103 females selected from forensic settings and 274 females selected from school settings in Portugal, Pechorro, Gonçalves, Andershed, and DeLisi (2017) found that psychopathy was significantly correlated with a broad range of outcomes, including proactive aggression, reactive aggression, violence, alcohol use, drug use, and having an earlier starting delinquent career. More psychopathic juvenile offenders also have an earlier age of onset of antisocial conduct, an earlier age of onset of police contact, and an earlier age of incarceration, in addition to more self-reported delinquency and more severe/serious delinquency (Pechorro, Maroco, Gonçalves, Nunes, & Jesus, 2014). Put another way, the most psychopathic youth will be those that are the most precocious offenders and those whose delinquent activity most quickly activates the discretion of law enforcement and the juvenile court.

Offenders with more extensive psychopathic features have also been shown to recidivate at higher levels, recidivate faster after release from custody, and recidivate with more dangerous crimes than their non-psychopathic peers (Shepherd, Campbell, & Ogloff, 2018; Thomson, Tiihonen, Miettunen, Virkkunen, & Lindberg, 2018), and these relationships have been shown using data from multiple nations. For example, Gretton, Hare, and Catchpole (2004) analyzed data from boys that had been referred to Youth Forensic Psychiatric Services in Canada and followed over a ten-year period. The investigators divided the youth into low, medium, and high grouping based on their scores on the Psychopathy Checklist: Youth Version (PCL: YV). The most psychopathic youth were worse in history of abuse, including physical, sexual, and emotional victimization, prevalence of substance abuse, and Conduct Disorder symptoms. They also had the most collective involvement in violent, nonviolent, and sexual offending. The follow-up results were eye-opening. A gradient was seen in terms of prevalence of recidivism and the adolescent psychopathy profile. One decade after release, 90 percent of the low psychopathy group, 96 percent of the medium psychopathy group, and 97 percent of the high psychopathy group had committed a nonviolent offense. In terms of violent offending, 46 percent of the low psychopathy group, 73 percent of the medium psychopathy group, and 82 percent of the high psychopathy group had recidivated. For sexual crimes, 7 percent of the low psychopathy group, 9 percent of the medium psychopathy group, and 21 percent of the high psychopathy group had recidivated. In additional survival analyses, Gretton et al. (2004) also found that those who had been highly psychopathic during adolescence committed nonviolent and violent crimes faster upon release than their less psychopathic peers.

Deviance beyond violence also shows the mutuality of psychopathic features and antisocial behavior. In terms of substance use and drug offending, psychopathy is overrepresented among drug offenders and contributes to the increased likelihood that drug-abusing criminals will continue to offend and recidivate after contact with the justice system (Vaughn, Salas-Wright, & Reingle-Gonzalez, 2016). Cross-national research has shown that substance-abusing individuals that have more severe addiction problems, including criminal justice system involvement, are also commensurately more likely to exhibit personality profiles that are suffused with psychopathy (Gori et al., 2017). Psychopathy and drug addiction also appear across population subgroups. For instance, Edwards and Verona (2016) found that psychopathy and addiction are interwoven risk factors among women who engage in prostitution and sex work in exchange for drugs. Sellbom and colleagues (2017) examined the psychopathy–drug crime association in four samples of data derived from university, forensic, and correctional settings. Irrespective of the composition of the sample, they found that psychopathy was significantly associated with greater alcohol abuse and substance abuse. As the substance abuse problem intensifies, psychopathy becomes more apparent.

In their study of 91 male prisoners that were convicted of theft, Prospero-Luis and colleagues (2017) found that psychopathic traits were associated not only with reduced expectations of negative outcomes associated with continued criminal offending, but also with increased expectations of positive outcomes associated with recidivism (Próspero-Luis et al., 2017). In other words, property offenders with psychopathy anticipate great upside and little downside to continuing their criminal career. Significant associations between psychopathy and property delinquency have also been found among institutionalized delinquents (DeLisi, Tostlebe, Burgason, Heirigs, & Vaughn, 2017).

Numerous studies have shown that the most violent criminals are often entrenched with psychopathic features. In their study using the Cambridge Study in Delinquent Development, Theobald, Farrington, Coid, and Piquero (2016) found that various features of psychopathy were associated with intimate partner violence, violence occurring outside the home, such as assaults against strangers, and violence across contexts – characterized as generally violent men. The generally violent men were the most psychopathic, suggesting that the condition is a fundamental driver of violent responses and attacks.

Psychopathy is also closely associated with other highly pernicious antisocial features, such as sexual sadism. Using two samples of male sexual offenders, Robertson and Knight (2014) found that psychopathy was significantly correlated with sexual sadism, and across models, the interpersonal, affective, impulsive, and antisocial features were linked with sexual sadism. Psychopathy was significantly correlated with three forms of non-sexual aggression, including unsocialized aggression, juvenile assault, and adult assault and with four sexual crime behaviors, including violence, physical control, sexual behavior, and paraphilia. In fact, the correlations between psychopathy and sexual crime behaviors were larger than correlations between sexual sadism and sexual crime behaviors.

A Federal Bureau of Investigation study of criminals that engage in the sexual trafficking of juveniles revealed that 75 percent of the offenders were clinically psychopathic (Hargreaves-Cormany, Patterson, Muirhead, & the Federal Bureau of Investigation, 2016). In a study of female prisoners, Thomson (2017) reported evidence that women with more psychopathic personality features were significantly likely to engage in drug-related violent crime and non-drug-related violent crime. In a study of male serial homicide offenders, Culhane, Walker, and Hildebrand (2017) found elevated scores on psychopathy that, although not as dramatically high as expected given the severity of the offense, were nevertheless comparable to elevated scores found in other correctional samples. Psychopathy has also been linked to assaults with intent to rape or murder (Reidy, Lilienfeld, Berke, Gentile, & Zeichner, 2016), child molestation (Walters, Knight, Looman, & Abracen, 2016), rape and child molestation (Petruccelli et al., 2017), sexual and non-sexual recidivism (Wijetunga, Nijdam-Jones, Rosenfeld, Martinez, & Cruise, 2017), and animal abuse and sadistic violence (Stupperich & Strack, 2016).

The aversive mien of the psychopathy not only negatively impacts others but also is significantly damaging to the psychopath himself. A study of psychopathic persons in Finland compared them to those in the general population using data from the Finnish National Statistics database (Vaurio, Repo-Tiihonen, Kautiainen, & Tiihonen, 2018). Those that were evaluated as clinically psychopathic had mortality rates that were fivefold higher than those in the general population. Psychopaths not only were more likely to die at a relatively young age, but the manner of their death was also much more likely to be violent compared to those in the general population.

The general public and the criminal justice system take psychopathy very seriously, and perceptions that offenders embody psychopathic traits tend to exacerbate the punitive punishment mood of the general public. For instance, Cox and colleagues (2016) found that jury-eligible community members that were presented with information about a white-collar criminal were more likely to make more severe sentencing recommendations when the offender was characterized as remorseless, refusing to accept responsibility for the crime, and lacking empathy for victims in the crime (Cox, Edens, Rulseh, & Clark, 2016).

Community members are correct to assume that psychopathic offenders are more problematic given that the condition is a robust predictor of multitudinous involvement in the criminal justice system. For instance, Beaver, Boutwell, Barnes, Vaughn, and DeLisi (2017) examined data from the National Longitudinal Study of Adolescent to Adult Health and found that psychopathy was positively associated with ever being arrested, sentenced to probation, and incarcerated. These effects held for the entire sample, for males, and for females. Psychopathic personality features also significantly predicted self-reported delinquency for the entire sample, for males, and for females.

More psychopathic correctional clients are likely to engage in diverse forms of crime and misconduct while in confinement and on supervision in the community, such as probation and parole. In their study of 224 mentally disordered forensic inpatients, for instance, Jeandarme, Pouls, Oei, and Bogaerts (2017) found that psychopathy was associated with a range of problematic behaviors while in treatment. Those who scored high on psychopathy were more likely to engage in therapy-interfering behaviors, including willful noncompliance and dropping out. Psychopathy has been linked to violent prison misconduct (Thomson, Towl, & Centifanti, 2016), disruptive behavior in treatment facilities (Jeandarme, Pouls, Oei, & Bogaerts, 2017), and nonviolent prison misconduct (Thomson et al., 2016). The correctional system evidently serves little deterrent effect to psychopathic offenders.

Conclusion

Three groups, each with differential behavioral functioning, were described in the introduction to this chapter. One small group had exceptional behavioral functioning, the largest group had moderately good behavioral functioning with occasional lapses in conduct that would rise to the level of criminal justice intervention, and another small group – the pathological offending and thus psychopathic group – had severe self-regulation problems and the widespread and interconnected problems that unfold from those self-regulation deficits. These groups were not constructed from thin air but are empirically supported. For example, a study of psychopathy in the general population in England, Wales, and Scotland found that the prevalence of psychopathy was just 0.6 percent and that nearly 71 percent of the population not only was not psychopathic, but also *had zero traits of the disorder* (Coid, Yang, Ullrich, Roberts, & Hare, 2009).

The implications of their finding are important. Most people in the general population function well in terms of their conduct if one merely uses as an indicator an ability to abstain from criminal behavior and thus criminal justice system contact (of course, aside from an occasional traffic offense, which is trivial). Most people are not criminal or antisocial and also, not surprisingly, have personalities that are devoid of psychopathic features. Scores of research studies, some of which were explored in the current chapter, reveal that once one examines increasingly more antisocial trajectories or groupings, one simultaneously increases their exposure to psychopathy. At the right-tail of the offending distribution where life-course-persistent offenders, career criminals, and the severe 5 percent reside, psychopathy is endemic. And when one considers multiple homicide offenders and sexual murderers, psychopathy is a virtual membership requirement.

References

Arboleda-Flórez, J. (2007) 'The psychopath in prison,' in A. R. Felthous & H. Saß (Eds.), *The* international handbook of psychopathic disorders and the law (pp. 373–391), Hoboken, NJ: John Wiley & Sons.

Baskin-Sommers, A. R., and Baskin, D. (2016) 'Psychopathic traits mediate the relationship between exposure to violence and violent juvenile offending,' *Journal of Psychopathology and Behavioral Assessment*, *38*(3):341–349.

Beaver, K. M., Boutwell, B. B., Barnes, J. C., Vaughn, M. G., and DeLisi, M. (2017) 'The association between psychopathic personality traits and criminal justice outcomes: Results from a nationally representative sample of males and females,' *Crime & Delinquency*, *63*(6):708–730.

Blickle, G., and Schütte, N. (2017) 'Trait psychopathy, task performance, and counterproductive work behavior directed toward the organization,' *Personality and Individual Differences*, *109*:225–231.

Coid, J., Yang, M., Ullrich, S., Roberts, A., and Hare, R. D. (2009) 'Prevalence and correlates of psychopathic traits in the household population of Great Britain,' *International Journal of Law and Psychiatry*, *32*(2):65–73.

Colins, O. F., and Vermeiren, R. R. (2013) 'The usefulness of DSM–IV and DSM–5 conduct disorder subtyping in detained adolescents,' *Journal of Nervous and Mental Disease*, *201*(9):736–743.

Corrado, R. R., DeLisi, M., Hart, S. D., and McCuish, E. C. (2015) 'Can the causal mechanisms underlying chronic, serious, and violent offending trajectories be elucidated using the psychopathy construct,' *Journal of Criminal Justice*, *43*(4):251–261.

Cox, J., Edens, J. F., Rulseh, A., and Clark, J. W. (2016) 'Juror perceptions of the interpersonal–affective traits of psychopathy predict sentence severity in a white-collar criminal case,' *Psychology, Crime & Law*, *22*(8):721–740.

Culhane, S. E., Walker, S., and Hildebrand, M. M. (2017) 'Serial homicide perpetrators' self-reported psychopathy and criminal thinking,' *Journal of Police and Criminal Psychology*, in press:1–13.

DeLisi, M. (2005) *Career criminals in society*, Thousand Oaks, CA: Sage.

DeLisi, M. (2009) 'Psychopathy is the unified theory of crime,' *Youth Violence and Juvenile Justice*, 7(3):256–273.

DeLisi, M. (2016) *Psychopathy as unified theory of crime*, New York, NY: Palgrave Macmillan.

DeLisi, M., Tostlebe, J., Burgason, K., Heirigs, M., and Vaughn, M. (2017). 'Self-control versus psychopathy: A head-to-head test of general theories of antisociality,' *Youth Violence and Juvenile Justice*, doi:10.1177/1541204016682998

Edwards, B. G., and Verona, E. (2016) 'Gendered contexts: Psychopathy and drug use in relation to sex work and exchange,' *Journal of Abnormal Psychology*, *125*(4):514–522.

Gori, A., Ponti, L., Tani, F., Iraci Sareri, G., Giannini, M., Meringolo, P., . . ., and Paterniti, R. (2017) 'Psychopathological features in a sample of substance-abusing individuals with criminal history: Towards a definition of a personality prototype of an "Addict with Criminal Conduct",' *Criminal Behaviour and Mental Health*, *27*(4):312–325.

Gottfredson, M. R., and Hirschi, T. (1990) *A general theory of crime*, Stanford, CA: Stanford University Press.

Gray, N. S., and Snowden, R. J. (2016) 'Psychopathy in women: Prediction of criminality and violence in UK and USA psychiatric patients residing in the community,' *Psychiatry Research*, *237*:339–343.

Gretton, H. M., Hare, R. D., and Catchpole, R. E. (2004) 'Psychopathy and offending from adolescence to adulthood: A 10-year follow-up,' *Journal of Consulting and Clinical Psychology*, 72(4):636–645.

Hargreaves-Cormany, H. A., Patterson, T. D., Muirhead, Y. E., and the Federal Bureau of Investigation. (2016) 'A typology of offenders engaging in the sex trafficking of juveniles (STJ): Implications for risk assessment,' *Aggression and Violent Behavior, 30*:40–47.

Jeandarme, I., Pouls, C., Oei, T. I., and Bogaerts, S. (2017) 'Forensic psychiatric patients with comorbid psychopathy: Double trouble?,' *International Journal of Forensic Mental Health, 16*(2):149–160.

McCuish, E. C., Corrado, R. R., Hart, S. D., and DeLisi, M. (2015) 'The role of symptoms of psychopathy in persistent violence over the criminal career into full adulthood,' *Journal of Criminal Justice, 43*(4):345–356.

McCuish, E. C., Corrado, R., Lussier, P., and Hart, S. D. (2014) 'Psychopathic traits and offending trajectories from early adolescence to adulthood,' *Journal of Criminal Justice, 42*(1):66–76.

Pechorro, P., Gonçalves, R. A., Andershed, H., and DeLisi, M. (2017) 'Female psychopathic traits in forensic and school context: Comparing the Antisocial Process Screening Device Self-Report and the Youth Psychopathic Traits Inventory–Short,' *Journal of Psychopathology and Behavioral Assessment, 39*(4):642–656.

Pechorro, P., Maroco, J., Gonçalves, R. A., Nunes, C., and Jesus, S. N. (2014) 'Psychopathic traits and age of crime onset in male juvenile delinquents,' *European Journal of Criminology, 11*(3):288–302.

Petruccelli, I., Barbaranelli, C., Costantino, V., Gherardini, A., Grilli, S., Craparo, G., and D'Urso, G. (2017). 'Moral disengagement and psychopathy: A study on offenders in Italian jails,' *Psychiatry, Psychology and Law, 24*(5):670–681.

Próspero-Luis, J., Moreira, P. S., Paiva, T. O., Teixeira, C. P., Costa, P., and Almeida, P. R. (2017) 'Psychopathy, criminal intentions, and abnormal appraisal of the expected outcomes of theft,' *Legal and Criminological Psychology, 22*(2):314–331.

Reidy, D. E., Lilienfeld, S. O., Berke, D. S., Gentile, B., and Zeichner, A. (2016) 'Psychopathy traits and violent assault among men with and without history of arrest,' *Journal of Interpersonal Violence*, doi:10.1177/0886260516660972

Robertson, C. A., and Knight, R. A. (2014) 'Relating sexual sadism and psychopathy to one another, non-sexual violence, and sexual crime behaviors,' *Aggressive Behavior, 40*(1):12–23.

Seigfried-Spellar, K. C., Villacís-Vukadinović, N., and Lynam, D. R. (2017) 'Computer criminal behavior is related to psychopathy and other antisocial behavior,' *Journal of Criminal Justice, 51*:67–73.

Sellbom, M., Donnelly, K. M., Rock, R. C., Phillips, T. R., and Ben-Porath, Y. S. (2017) 'Examining gender as moderating the association between psychopathy and substance abuse,' *Psychology, Crime & Law, 23*(4):376–390.

Shepherd, S. M., Campbell, R. E., and Ogloff, J. R. (2018) 'Psychopathy, antisocial personality disorder, and reconviction in an Australian sample of forensic patients,' *International Journal of Offender Therapy and Comparative Criminology, 62*(3):609–628.

Stupperich, A., and Strack, M. (2016) 'Among a German sample of forensic patients, previous animal abuse mediates between psychopathy and sadistic actions,' *Journal of Forensic Sciences, 61*(3):699–705.

Theobald, D., Farrington, D. P., Coid, J. W., and Piquero, A. R. (2016) 'Are male perpetrators of intimate partner violence different from convicted violent offenders? Examination of psychopathic traits and life success in males from a community survey,' *Journal of Interpersonal Violence, 31*(9):1687–1718.

Thomson, N. D. (2017) 'An exploratory study of female psychopathy and drug-related violent Crime,' *Journal of Interpersonal Violence*, doi:10.1177/0886260517690876

Thomson, A., Tiihonen, J., Miettunen, J., Virkkunen, M., and Lindberg, N. (2018) 'Firesetting and general criminal recidivism among a consecutive sample of Finnish pretrial male firesetters: A register-based follow-up study,' *Psychiatry Research, 259*:377–384.

Thomson, N. D., Towl, G. J., and Centifanti, L. (2016) 'The habitual female offender inside: How psychopathic traits predict chronic prison violence,' *Law and Human Behavior, 40*(3):257–274.

Vaughn, M. G., DeLisi, M., Gunter, T., Fu, Q., Beaver, K. M., Perron, B. E., and Howard, M. O. (2011) 'The severe 5%: A latent class analysis of the externalizing behavior spectrum in the United States,' *Journal of Criminal Justice, 39*(1):75–80.

Vaughn, M. G., Howard, M. O., and DeLisi, M. (2008) 'Psychopathic personality traits and delinquent careers: An empirical examination,' *International Journal of Law and Psychiatry, 31*(5):407–416.

Vaughn, M. G., Salas-Wright, C. P., DeLisi, M., and Maynard, B. R. (2014) 'Violence and externalizing behavior among youth in the United States: Is there a severe 5%?,' *Youth Violence and Juvenile Justice, 12*(1):3–21.

Vaughn, M. G., Salas-Wright, C. P., and Reingle-Gonzalez, J. M. (2016) 'Addiction and crime: The importance of asymmetry in offending and the life course,' *Journal of Addictive Diseases, 35*(4):213–217.

Vaurio, O., Repo-Tiihonen, E., Kautiainen, H., and Tiihonen, J. (2018) 'Psychopathy and Mortality,' *Journal of Forensic Sciences*, *63*(2):474–477.
Walters, G. D., Knight, R. A., Looman, J., and Abracen, J. (2016) 'Child molestation and psychopathy: A taxometric analysis,' *Journal of Sexual Aggression*, *22*(3):379–393.
Wijetunga, C., Nijdam-Jones, A., Rosenfeld, B., Martinez, R., and Cruise, K. R. (2017) 'Using the Juvenile Sex Offender Assessment Protocol–Revised to assess psychopathy: A preliminary investigation,' *Criminal Justice and Behavior*, doi:10.1177/0093854817745912

2

Tracing the effect of psychopathy on future offending through two layers of proactive criminal thinking

Glenn D. Walters

Introduction

Psychopathy's role in criminal offending has been a source of controversy and confusion from the time of its inception. Some of this can be traced back to Hervey Cleckley's vacillating views on the relationship between psychopathy and crime, a perspective that gradually moved in the direction of greater acceptance of a meaningful connection between criminality and psychopathy in later editions of his landmark book, *The Mask of Sanity* (Cleckley, 1941/1976). By the time the fifth edition of *The Mask of Sanity* had been published, Robert Hare had already begun his work with criminal psychopaths. Unlike Cleckley, Hare displayed no equivocation when it came to gauging the significance of psychopathy for those working with criminal offenders. In fact, he has referred to psychopathy as the "single most important clinical construct in the criminal justice system" (Hare, 1998:99). This perspective has been accepted in many corners but not all. Skeem and Cooke (2010), for instance, argue that crime is a downstream correlate rather than a central component of the psychopathy construct and that Hare's (1996, 1998; Hare & Neumann, 2008) contention that psychopathy and crime are inextricably linked is attributable to the fact that his early studies were conducted nearly exclusively on prison inmates.

In determining the degree to which crime is central to psychopathy and psychopathy is predictive of crime, we need to examine the empirical evidence, and the evidence is reasonably supportive of Hare's (1996, 1998) contention that crime and psychopathy are closely linked and that psychopathy is a strong predictor of future criminal behavior (DeLisi, 2009). Most studies have shown that psychopathy, whether measured with a version of Hare's (2003) Psychopathy Checklist or one of several self-report measures, does a fairly good job of predicting future criminal conduct (Brinkley, Schmitt, Smith, & Newman, 2001; Cale & Lilienfeld, 2006; Frick, Stickle, Dandreaux, Farrell, & Kimonis, 2005; Harris, Rice, & Lalumiére, 2001; Neumann, Schmidt, Carter, Embley, & Hare, 2012; Salekin, Rogers, & Sewell, 1997; Vaughn & DeLisi, 2008; Vaughn, Newhill, DeLisi, Beaver, & Howard, 2008). The results of several studies, however, suggest that psychopathy may not possess incremental validity relative to basic demographic and background variables like age and criminal history (Douglas, Epstein, & Poythress, 2008; Walters, 2012b). Part of the problem may be that the focus of psychopathic theories of crime is on the independent variable (i.e., the stable trait of psychopathy). Examining motivating and mediating factors may not only do a better job of distinguishing between theories of crime, which tend to share many of the same independent variables (Agnew, 1995), but it may also help identify the mechanism that actually links psychopathy to future crime.

In searching for a potential mediator of the psychopathy–offending relationship, we might want to consider a variable like criminal thinking which satisfies many of the criteria of a good mediator (e.g., sufficiently stable to serve as a predictor and sufficiently mutable to serve as an outcome: Bandura, 1986; Wu & Zumbo, 2008). Cross-sectional studies indicate that psychopathy and criminal thinking correlate well in prison inmates (Mandracchia, Gonzalez, Patterson, & Smith, 2015), psychiatric inpatients (Magyar, Carr, Rosenfeld, & Rotter, 2010), and college students (Ragatz, Anderson, Fremouw, & Schwartz, 2011; Riopka, Coupland, & Olver, 2015). Longitudinal studies indicate that criminal thinking is capable of predicting recidivism above and beyond measures of psychopathy like Hare's (2003) Psychopathy Checklist–Revised (PCL–R; Gonsalves, Scalora, & Huss, 2009) and Hart, Cox, and Hare's (1995) Psychopathy Checklist: Screening Version (PCL: SV; Walters, 2009). There has been only one study, to the author's knowledge, conducted on the mediating effect of criminal thinking on the psychopathy–offending relationship. In that study, Walters and DeLisi (2015) determined that proactive (planned, calculated) but not reactive (impulsive, reckless) criminal thinking mediated the psychopathy–violence relationship.

Based on the nonlinear dynamical systems concept of fractals (Williams & Arrigo, 2002), it has been proposed that mediators are capable of mediating other mediators. The mediators-within-mediators conceptualization was first tested in a study by Walters (2016), in which he found that a first-stage mediator (reactive criminal thinking) mediated the past crime–future crime relationship and a second-stage mediator (short-term hostility) mediated reactive criminal thinking. According to the results of a second study, parental acceptance of child delinquency mediated proactive criminal thinking, another common mediating variable in a model that predicted subsequent serious offending (Walters, 2017a). One of the questions raised by these studies is what makes some variables better second-order mediators than other variables. In the Walters (2016) study, for instance, the second-order mediator was shorter in duration than the first-order mediator (past week vs. past six months). In Walters (2017a), the second-order mediator was less stable than the first-order mediator (test–retest r = .40 vs. .52). A third way to differentiate between first- and second-order mediators is to compare a general measure of criminal thinking with a more specific measure. The Moral Disengagement scale (MD: Bandura, Barbaranelli, Caprara, & Pastorelli, 1996) measures three of the four proactive criminal thinking styles (i.e., mollification, entitlement, and power orientation) and was used as a general measure of proactive criminal thinking in the current study. An index of a person's perception of the certainty of punishment as applied to themselves, when inverted, provided a good estimate of the more specific proactive criminal thinking style of superoptimism.

The hypothesis tested in this study predicted that a specific measure of proactive criminal thinking (superoptimism) would successfully mediate a broad measure of proactive criminal thinking (MD), but a broad measure of proactive criminal thinking would not mediate a specific indicator of proactive criminal thinking. Although the current study used the same sample of participants as the previous Walters and DeLisi (2015) study, the two studies differed in four respects. First, the two Psychopathy Checklist: Youth Version (PCL: YV) factor scores served as the independent variables in Walters and DeLisi (2015), whereas the total PCL: YV score served as the independent variable in the current investigation. Second, the dependent variable in Walters and DeLisi (2015) was aggressive criminality, whereas the dependent variable in the present study was total offending. Third, the MD score alone served as the mediator in Walters and

DeLisi (2015); in the current study, both MD and superoptimism served as mediators. Finally, whereas Walters and DeLisi (2015) utilized the first three waves of data from the Pathways study, the current investigation comprised five waves of data. Beyond basic demographic measures (age, race), several other control variables were included in this study – parental socioeconomic status, neighborhood disorder, and low self-control – given research showing that these variables may influence the psychopathy–offending relationship (Lynam, Miller, Vachon, Loeber, & Stouthamer-Loeber, 2009; Vaughn, DeLisi, Beaver, Wright, & Howard, 2007). In addition, certainty of punishment for others was controlled for the purpose of ruling out the possibility that superoptimism was simply tapping a broad deterrence effect (Kleck, 2016).

Method

Participants

The sample for this investigation consisted of all 1,170 male participants from the Pathways to Desistance study (Mulvey, 2012). The 184 girls from the Pathways study were left out of the analyses because of differences in how boys and girls were selected into the Pathways study (i.e., there were significantly more girls with simple drug possession charges than boys). Each participant in the Pathways study had been adjudicated delinquent or convicted of a felony in Maricopa County (Phoenix), Arizona or Philadelphia, Pennsylvania when they were between the ages of 14 and 18. The average age of participants at the time of the baseline interview was 16.05 years (SD = 1.16, range = 14–19), and the ethnic breakdown for the sample was 19.2 percent Caucasian, 42.1 percent African American, 34.0 percent Hispanic, and 4.6 percent other.

Measures

Independent variable

The independent variable for this study was psychopathy as measured by the Psychopathy Checklist: Youth Version (PCL: YV: Forth, Kosson, & Hare, 2003). The PCL: YV is a 20-item checklist designed to assess the interpersonal, affective, lifestyle, and antisocial features of psychopathy. Each item on the PCL: YV is rated on a 3-point scale (0 = does not apply, 1 = applies to a certain extent, 2 = applies). Ratings are based on information obtained in an open-ended interview and a review of available files. Item ratings are then summed to produce a total score, two factor scores, and four facet scores. The total score was the PCL: YV measure used in the current study (range = 0–40). These ratings achieved good internal consistency ($\alpha = .87$) and excellent interrater reliability (ICC = .92) in the Pathways study (Mulvey, 2012).

Dependent variable

The total offending variety score from the Self-Reported Offending scale (SRO: Huizinga, Esbensen, & Weihar, 1991) served as the dependent variable in this study based on prior research showing that variety scores do a better job than frequency scores of assessing criminality (Sweeten, 2012). The total offending variety score was calculated as the ratio of total crime categories the respondent acknowledged engaging in over the past six months to the total number of crime categories available on the SRO (i.e., 22): destroyed/damaged property, set fire, broke in to steal, shoplifted, bought/received/sold stolen property, used check/credit card illegally, stole car or motorcycle, sold marijuana, sold other drugs, carjacked, drove drunk or high, been paid by someone for sex, forced someone to have sex, killed someone, shot someone, shot at someone, took by force with a weapon, took by force without a weapon, beat up someone with serious injury, in a fight, beat someone as part of a gang, and carried a gun. Test–retest reliability for the total offending variety score was moderate over the two-year span between Waves 0 and 4 (r = .30).

Mediator variables

There were two mediator variables included in the present investigation. One was a broad measure of proactive criminal thinking and the other was a narrow measure of proactive criminal thinking. The broad measure of criminal thinking was based on the 32-item Moral Disengagement scale (MD: Bandura et al., 1996). The MD scale assesses three of the four criminal thinking styles that make up proactive criminal thinking (Walters, 2012a): mollification ("Damaging some property is no big deal when you consider that others are beating people up"), entitlement ("It is all right to fight when your group's honor is threatened"), and power orientation ("Slapping and shoving someone is just a way of joking"). The MD scale achieved excellent internal consistency over the first several waves of the Pathways study (α = .90–.92).

Whereas the MD scale assesses three out of the four criminal thinking styles associated with proactive criminal thinking (Walters, 2012a), the second mediator focused on the one proactive criminal thinking style not covered by the MD: namely, superoptimism. The certainty of punishment–self scale from the Indices of Personal and Social Costs and Rewards (Nagin & Paternoster, 1994) was used to measure superoptimism in this study. Participants were asked to rate seven antisocial activities (e.g., fighting, theft) on an 11-point scale (0 = no chance of being caught, 10 = absolute certainty of being caught) as to the perceived likelihood of them being caught and receiving punishment should they engage in the behavior. Scores were reverse scored (multiplied by −1) so that higher scores indicated a lower perceived likelihood of being caught (superoptimism). This scale displayed good internal consistency in the Pathways study (α = .85–.92).

Control variables

There were six control variables included in the present investigation. Three of these variables were basic demographic/background measures: age in years, race (White = 1, Nonwhite = 2), and parental socioeconomic status (SES). Parental SES took into account the educational attainment and occupational status of both parents, with lower scores indicating higher status. The fourth control variable was a measure of neighborhood disorder, encompassing both physical (cigarettes on the street; graffiti on buildings) and psychological (adults fighting or arguing loudly; people using syringes to take drugs) disorder. The neighborhood disorder measure achieved excellent internal consistency in the Pathways study (α = .94). Behavioral problems appearing before age 11 (trouble for cheating, trouble for disturbing class, trouble for being drunk/stoned, trouble for stealing, trouble for fighting) served as a fifth control variable (mean inter-item correlation = .20). A sixth and final control variable was the certainty of punishment–other score, which was scored in the exact same manner as the certainty of punishment–self score except that the question asked about "other kids in the neighborhood" rather than oneself. This variable was added in order to control for general deterrence beliefs.

All of the control variables were measured at baseline (Wave 0) along with precursor measures of each predicted variable. Cole and Maxwell (2003) assert that prior or precursor measures of a predicted variable should be controlled in order to rule out the alternate hypothesis that causal direction goes from the predicted variable to the predictor variable. It is important that these precursor measures be assessed prior to or concurrent with the independent variable so as to reduce the influence of endogenous selection bias and collider effects (Elwert & Winship, 2014). Accordingly, baseline proactive criminal thinking was included as a predictor in the regression equation where Wave 1 proactive criminal thinking served as the outcome; baseline superoptimism was included as a predictor in the regression equation where Wave 2 superoptimism served as the outcome; Wave 1 proactive criminal thinking (to permit evaluation of the PCT-1–PCT-3 path) was included as a predictor in the regression equation where Wave 3 proactive criminal thinking served as the outcome; and baseline total offending was included in the regression equation where Wave 4 total offending served as the outcome. Because time covered by the Wave 4 interview ranged from two to eight months ($M = 5.94$, $SD = 0.99$) time at risk was also included as a control variable.

Procedure

The research design for this study was a fixed-sample multiple mediator panel design, with no overlap between waves. These prospective data were analyzed in a four-equation path analysis using algorithms from *MPlus 5.2* (Muthén & Muthén, 1998–2007). In this analysis, Wave 0 PCL: YV scores served as the independent variable; Wave 1 proactive criminal thinking (MD score) served as the first-stage mediator; Wave 2 superoptimism (certainty of punishment–self) served as the second-stage mediator; Wave 3 proactive criminal thinking (MD score) served as the third-stage mediator; and Wave 4 total offending variety score served as the dependent variable. Normal theory approaches like the Sobel (1982) delta test lack power when it comes to evaluating indirect effect because indirect effects often assume a skewed distribution (Hayes, 2013). Significance was accordingly determined by constructing 95 percent Confidence Intervals from bias-corrected bootstrapped Standard Errors using 5,000 replications. A significant Confidence Interval is one that does not include zero. Research has consistently shown that bootstrapping is superior to normal theory z-tests in modeling the non-normal distribution of indirect effects (MacKinnon, Kisbu-Sakarya, & Gottschall, 2013; Pituch, & Stapleton, 2008).

Kenny's (2013) "failsafe ef" procedure – $(r_{my.x}) \times (sd_{m.x}) \times (sd_{y.x}) / (sd_m) \times (sd_y)$ – was used to conduct sensitivity testing designed to rule out omitted variable bias. The "failsafe ef" yields a coefficient that denotes how strongly an unobserved covariate confounder would need to correlate with the mediator and dependent variable to eliminate a significant coefficient along the *b* path of the indirect effect. Because the "failsafe ef" can only be tested for consecutive path coefficient pairs (i.e., *a* and *b* paths), three separate "failsafe efs" were computed. A second sensitivity test was performed to rule out endogenous selection bias as an explanation for the current results given the fact that conditioning on a precursor measure could create a collider effect (Elwert & Winship, 2014). In this particular sensitivity analysis, all of the baseline precursor measures (PCT-0, Superoptimism-0, and Offending-0) and the one Wave 1 precursor (PCT-1) were removed from the regression and the analyses recomputed.

Missing data

Three-quarters of the participants in this study had complete data on all 14 variables included in the study (76.4 percent). Of the remaining participants, 15.1 percent had missing data on one variable, 4.4 percent had missing data on two variables, and 4.1 percent had missing data on 3 to 7 variables. Four variables had more than 5 percent missing data: PCT-1 (6.9 percent), Superoptimism-2 (8.0 percent), Offending-4 (9.2 percent), and PCT-3 (9.3 percent). All missing data were handled with full information maximum likelihood (FIML). This is a procedure whereby model parameters and Standard Errors are calculated on all non-missing data and then applied to the entire sample. Research indicates that estimates derived from FIML are significantly less biased than those produced by more traditional missing data procedures like simple imputation and listwise deletion (Allison, 2012; Peyre, Leplége, & Coste, 2011).

Results

Descriptive statistics for the 14 study variables are listed in Table 2.1. The inter-correlational matrix from this table indicates that over two-thirds of the 78 zero-order correlations achieved Bonferroni-corrected significance. When each of the regression equations was tested for multicollinearity, there was no evidence of collinearity between any of the predictor variables: Tolerance = .547–.963; Variance Inflation Factor = 1.039–1.829.

The results of the main path analysis revealed that each of the coefficients on the four pathways connecting psychopathy to offending by way of general proactive criminal thinking and superoptimism were significant (see Table 2.2 and Figure 2.1). The indirect effect running from PCT-1 to superoptimism-2 to PCT-3, as well as the indirect effects running from PCT-1 to PCT-3 and from superoptimism-2 to PCT-3, also achieved significance (see Table 2.3).

When the two mediators were switched, so that proactive criminal thinking mediated superoptimism, two of the path coefficients were no longer significant (see Figure 2.2), and none of the indirect effects, including the one running from the PCL to Superoptimism-1 to PCT-2 to Superoptimism-3 to Offending-4 (Estimate = 0.0000017, 95 percent Confidence Interval = −0.0000004, 0.0000146), achieved significance.

The sensitivity of the significant PCL → PCT-1 → Superoptimism-2 → PCT-3 → Offending-4 pathway to omitted variable bias was tested using Kenny's "failsafe ef" procedure. Results indicated that an unobserved covariate confounder would need to correlate .13 with PCT-1 and Superoptimism-2, controlling for the PCL and PCT-1 in the case of the latter, to completely eliminate the significant PCT-1 → Superoptimism-2 path. Likewise, a confounding variable would need to correlate .08 with Superoptimism-2 and PCT-3, controlling for PCT-1 and Superoptimism-2 in the case of the latter, to abolish the significant Superoptimism-2 → PCT-3 relationship and .27 with PCT-3 and Offending-4, controlling for Superoptimism-2 and PCT-3 in the case of the latter, to bring the significant PCT-3 → Offending-4 coefficient down to zero.

The sensitivity of the significant PCL → PCT-1 → Superoptimism-2 → PCT-3 → Offending-4 pathway to endogenous selection bias was tested by conducting the analyses after the baseline and Wave 1 precursors had been removed from their respective regression equations. The results indicated that all four path coefficients ($p < .001$) and the overall indirect effect (Estimate = 0.000108, 95 percent Confidence Interval = 0.000035, 0.000270) remained significant.

Discussion

The current study builds on the previous Walters and DeLisi (2015) investigation, in which it was demonstrated that general proactive criminal thinking, as measured by the MD scale, mediated the relationship between Factors 1 and 2 of the PCL: YV and violent offending. Using this same sample of participants, the total PCL: YV score instead of the two PCL: YV factor scores, the total offending variety score instead of the aggressive offending variety score, and a multiple serial mediation design that encompasses three rather than one mediator, it was noted that

Table 2.1 Descriptive statistics and correlations for the 14 independent, dependent, mediator, and control variables

Variable	*n*	*M*	*SD*	*Range*	*2*	*3*	*4*	*5*	*6*	*7*	*8*	*9*	*10*	*11*	*12*	*13*	*14*
1 Age	1170	16.05	1.16	14–19	.06	–.06	.06	–.04	.10	.13*	.16*	.14*	.00	.02	–.02	.01	–.01
2 Race	1170	1.81	0.39	1–2		.22*	.19*	–.04	.06	–.01	.10*	.13*	.03	.08	.03	–.07	–.04
3 SES	1164	51.66	12.37	11–77			.13*	–.04	–.04	–.02	–.06	–.02	.07	.07	.07	.01	–.06
4 Neighborhood	1168	2.35	0.74	1–4				.12*	.14*	.20*	.16*	.15*	.14*	.11*	.10	.14*	.13*
5 Low self-control	1170	1.60	1.19	0–5					.06	.32*	.10	.09	.21*	.30*	.12*	.26*	.25*
6 Certainty–other	1168	5.45	2.25	0–10						.15*	.62*	.29*	.09	.07	.07	.13*	.14*
7 PCL: YV	1123	16.12	7.77	0–39							.27*	.23*	.32*	.29*	.19*	.44*	.22*
8 Superoptimism-0	1168	5.12	2.88	0–10								.42*	.23*	.15*	.13*	.24*	.18*
9 Superoptimism-2	1074	5.08	2.88	0–10									.21*	.20*	.18*	.18*	.14*
10 Proactive-0	1167	1.63	0.35	1–3										.59*	.48*	.30*	.20*
11 Proactive-1	1090	1.59	0.36	1–3											.55*	.25*	.20*
12 Proactive-3	1057	1.52	0.38	1–3												.16*	.26*
13 Offending-0	1167	0.16	0.16	0–.91													.30*
14 Offending-4	1060	0.07	0.11	0–.86													

Note. Variable = variables included in the current study; *n* = number of participants with non-missing data; *M* = mean; *SD* = standard deviation; Range = range of scores in the current sample; Age = chronological age in years measured at baseline (Wave 0); Race = 1 (White) or 2 (Nonwhite); SES = parental socioeconomic status measured at Wave 0; Neighborhood = neighborhood disorder measured at Wave 0; Low Self-Control = count of early onset behavioral problems measured at Wave 0; Certainty–other = certainty of punishment for others measured at Wave 0 (score inverted for correlations); PCL: SV = total score on the Psychopathy Checklist: Youth Version measured at Wave 0; Superoptimism-0 = certainty of punishment for self at Wave 0 (score inverted for correlations); Superoptimism-2 = certainty of punishment for self at Wave 2 (score inverted for correlations); Proactive-0 = proactive criminal thinking measured with the moral disengagement scale at Wave 0; Proactive-1 = proactive criminal thinking measured with the moral disengagement scale at Wave 1; Proactive-3 = proactive criminal thinking measured with the moral disengagement scale at Wave 3; Offending-0 = total offending variety score at Wave 0; Offending-4 = total offending variety score at Wave 4.

*p < .00064 (Bonferroni-corrected alpha level; .05 / 78 correlations).

Table 2.2 Maximum likelihood path analysis of the pathway running from psychopathy to offending

Predictor	*b(95% CI)*	*β*	*t*	*p*
Proactive-1 (outcome)				
PCL: YV	0.005(0.002, 0.007)	0.102	3.55	< .001
Age	0.000(−0.016, 0.016)	0.001	0.02	.980
Race	0.067(0.024, 0.112)	0.072	3.04	.002
SES	0.000(−0.001, 0.001)	0.006	0.20	.839
Neighborhood	−0.007(−0.036, 0.022)	−0.014	−0.47	.641
Low self-control	0.020(0.002, 0.038)	0.064	2.16	.031
Certainty–other	0.000(−0.009, 0.008)	−0.002	−0.06	.953
Proactive-0	0.558(0.493, 0.620)	0.538	16.95	< .001
Superoptimism-2 (outcome)				
Proactive-1	0.852(0.403, 1.297)	0.108	3.71	< .001
Age	0.165(0.037, 0.299)	0.066	2.42	.016
Race	0.510(0.126, 0.870)	0.070	2.66	.008
SES	−0.002(−0.012, 0.007)	−0.010	−0.35	.728
Neighborhood	0.173(−0.042, 0.392)	0.044	1.56	.118
Low self-control	0.009(−0.130, 0.153)	0.004	0.12	.902
Certainty–other	0.057(−0.049, 0.152)	0.044	1.11	.269
PCL: YV	0.034(0.012, 0.056)	0.093	3.08	.002
Superoptimism-0	0.325(0.243, 0.407)	0.326	7.70	< .001
Proactive-3 (outcome)				
Superoptimism-2	0.012(0.005, 0.019)	0.092	3.19	.001
Age	−0.013(−0.028, 0.004)	−0.039	−1.57	.116
Race	−0.036(−0.087, 0.010)	−0.038	−1.46	.145
SES	0.000(−0.002, 0.002)	0.012	0.33	.742
Neighborhood	0.023(−0.005, 0.054)	0.046	1.54	.124
Low self-control	−0.001(−0.020, 0.018)	−0.002	−0.09	.930
Certainty–other	0.000(−0.009, 0.009)	0.001	0.09	.929
PCL: YV	0.001(−0.002, 0.004)	0.019	0.62	.537
Proactive-1	0.540(0.468, 0.612)	0.524	14.83	< .001
Offending-4 (outcome)				
Proactive-3	0.056(0.028, 0.087)	0.184	3.74	< .001
Age	−0.002(−0.008, 0.003)	−0.024	−0.88	.381
Race	−0.011(−0.029, 0.006)	−0.038	−1.23	.217
SES	0.000(−0.001, 0.000)	−0.055	−2.02	.043
Neighborhood	0.009(−0.001, 0.019)	0.059	1.75	.080
Low self-control	0.014(0.008, 0.020)	0.144	4.26	< .001
Certainty–other	0.003(0.001, 0.006)	0.066	2.38	.017
PCL: YV	0.000(−0.001, 0.001)	0.025	0.77	.443
Superoptimism-2	0.001(−0.001, 0.004)	0.037	1.29	.197
Proactive-1	0.002(−0.025, 0.030)	0.007	0.15	.881
Offending-0	0.136(0.067, 0.213)	0.186	3.60	< .001
Time at risk	0.009(0.003, 0.016)	0.079	2.65	.008

Note. Proactive-1 (outcome) = regression equation with proactive criminal thinking measured at Wave 1 as the outcome measure; Superoptimism-2 (outcome) = regression equation with superoptimism measured at Wave 2 as the outcome measure; Proactive-3 = regression equation with proactive criminal thinking measured at Wave 3 as the outcome measure; Offending-4 (outcome) = regression equation with total offending variety score measure at Wave 4 as the outcome measure; Age = chronological age in years measured at Wave 0; Race = 1 (White) or 2 (Nonwhite); SES = parental socioeconomic status measured at Wave 0; Neighborhood = neighborhood disorder measured at

Table 2.2 (Continued)

Wave 0; Low self-control = count of early onset behavioral problems measured at Wave 0; Certainty–other = certainty of punishment for others measured at Wave 0 (score inverted for correlations); PCL: SV = total score on the Psychopathy Checklist: Youth Version measured at Wave 0; Superoptimism-0 = certainty of punishment for self at Wave 0 (score inverted for correlations); Superoptimism-2 = certainty of punishment for self at Wave 2 (score inverted for correlations); Proactive-0 = proactive criminal thinking measured with the moral disengagement scale at Wave 0; Proactive-1 = proactive criminal thinking measured with the moral disengagement scale at Wave 1; Proactive-3 = proactive criminal thinking measured with the moral disengagement scale at Wave 3; Offending-0 = total offending variety score at Wave 0; b(95% CI) = unstandardized coefficient and the lower and upper limits of the 95% Confidence Interval for the unstandardized coefficient (in parentheses); β = standardized coefficient; *t* = asymptotic *t*-test; *p* = significance level of the asymptotic *t*-test; *N* = 1170.

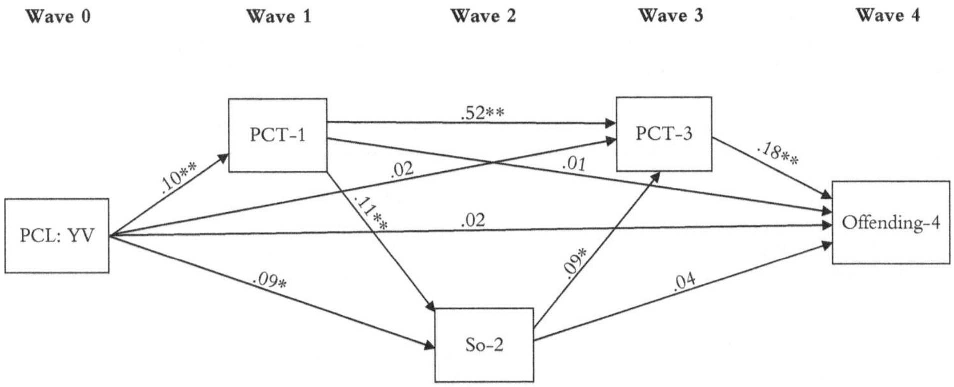

Figure 2.1 Maximum likelihood path analysis of Wave 1 proactive criminal thinking, Wave 2 superoptimism, and Wave 3 proactive criminal thinking as mediators of the PCL: YV–offending relationship

Note. Standardized beta coefficients are reported; PCL: YV = Psychopathy Checklist: Youth Version; PCT-1 = proactive criminal thinking measured at Wave 1; So-2 = superoptimism measured at Wave 2; PCT-3 = proactive criminal thinking measured at Wave 3; Offending-4 = total offending variety score measured at Wave 4; control and precursor variables are not shown.

*p < .05; **p < .001.

three consecutive mediators (general proactive criminal thinking, followed by superoptimism, followed by general proactive criminal thinking) displayed a significant layered indirect effect as part of a five-variable pathway. Non-mediated general proactive criminal thinking (PCL-0 → PCT-1 → Offending-4; PCL-0 → PCT-3 → Offending-4) and a reversed three-mediator pathway (superoptimism, followed by proactive criminal thinking, followed by superoptimism) failed to achieve significant indirect effects. The two-layered mediating effect obtained in the current study supports the nonlinear dynamical systems theory concept of fractals (Williams & Arrigo, 2002) and the lifestyle concept of mediators-within-mediators (Walters, 2016).

The current study was the third to examine the mediators-within-mediators theorem. In the first study to examine this theorem, Walters (2016) distinguished between first- (reactive criminal thinking) and second- (hostile feelings) order mediators by measuring the two mediators over different time frames: six months for reactive criminal thinking and one week for hostile feelings. In the second study, Walters (2017a) distinguished between first- (proactive criminal thinking) and second- (perceptions of parental acceptance of child delinquency) order mediators by using a second-order mediator that was less stable than the first-order mediator. Because less stable mediators are more malleable than more stable mediators, they make better

Table 2.3 Total, direct, and indirect effects for the pathway running from psychopathy to offending

Pathways	*BCBCI*		
	Estimate	*Lower*	*Upper*
PCL: YV → Total offending			
Total effect	0.005021	−0.002194	0.012118
Direct effect	0.002788	−0.004546	0.009860
Total indirect effect	0.002233	0.000633	0.004272
Specific indirect effects			
PCL → PCT-1 → Off-4	0.000078	−0.000940	0.001281
PCL → PCT-3 → Off-4	0.000407	−0.000824	0.001882
PCL → So-2 → Off-4	0.000394	−0.000123	0.001306
PCL → PCT-1→ PCT-3 → Off-4	0.001110	0.000461	0.002221
PCL → PCT-1 → So-2 → Off-4	0.000046	−0.000012	0.000169
PCL → So-2 → PCT-3 → Off-4	0.000177	0.000047	0.000474
PCL → PCT-1 → So-2 → PCT-3 → Off-4	0.000021	0.000006	0.000063

Note. PCL: YV/PCL = Psychopathy Checklist: Youth Version measured at baseline (Wave 0); PCT-1 = proactive criminal thinking measured at Wave 1; PCT-3 = proactive criminal thinking measured at Wave 3; So-2 = superoptimism measured at Wave 2; Off-4 = total offending variety score measured at Wave 4; BCBCI = bias-corrected bootstrapped 95% Confidence Interval (b = 5,000); Estimate = unstandardized point estimate; Lower = lower boundary of the 95% Confidence Interval; Upper = upper boundary of the 95% Confidence Interval; *N* = 1170.

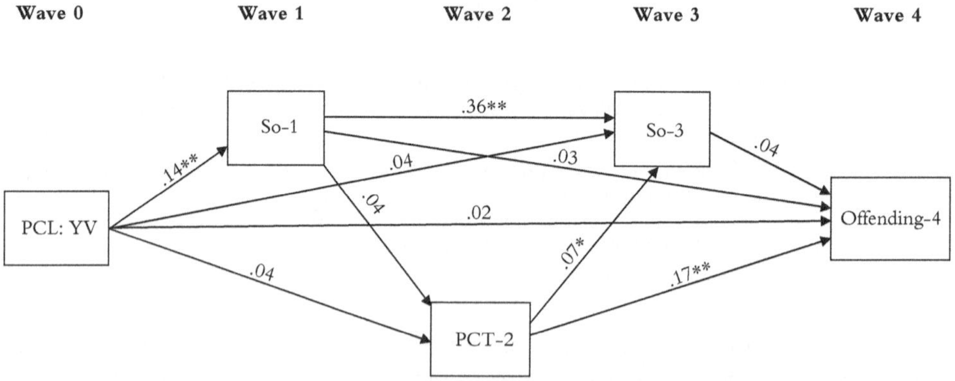

Figure 2.2 Maximum likelihood path analysis of Wave 1 superoptimism, Wave 2 proactive criminal thinking, and Wave 3 superoptimism as mediators of the PCL: YV–offending relationship

Note. Standardized beta coefficients are reported; PCL: YV = Psychopathy Checklist: Youth Version; So-1 = superoptimism measured at Wave 1; PCT-2 = proactive criminal thinking measured at Wave 2; So-3 = superoptimism measured at Wave 3; Offending-4 = total offending variety score measured at Wave 4; control and precursor variables are not shown.

*p < .05; **p < .001.

second-order mediators than more stable mediators (Wu & Zumbo, 2008). In the current study, a broader, more general, and more stable measure of proactive criminal thinking served as the first-order mediator, and a narrow, more specific, and less stable measure, superoptimism, served as the second-order mediator. Methodologically, then, a layered or mediator-within-mediators indirect effect requires a first-order mediator that is broader, more stable, and has a longer duration than the second-order mediator, whereas a second-order mediator should be narrower, less stable, and have a shorter duration.

There are several theoretical implications to the present findings. First, these results suggest that psychopathy may have an indirect rather than a direct effect on offending behavior. Although the direct effect of psychopathy on offending in the current study was non-significant, thereby suggesting full mediation, researchers no longer consider the difference between full and partial mediation to be especially meaningful. All mediation, it has been argued, is partial mediation (Rucker, Preacher, Tormala, & Petty, 2011). Because of suppressor effects (Preacher, 2015), multiple parallel mediation (Hayes, 2013), and total and direct effect that have less power to reject the null hypothesis than the indirect effect (Kenny & Judd, 2014), total and direct effects are often underestimated. Still, given that the only outcome predicted by the direct effect of psychopathy was Wave 1 general proactive criminal thinking, the impact of psychopathy on crime may require mediation by cognitive variables. A second theoretical implication of the current study is that it tests the notion that psychopathy is of major consequence when it comes to predicting offending behavior. DeLisi (2009), in fact, argues that psychopathy is the ideal foundation for a unified theory of crime. Like other leading theories of crime, however, the principal focus of psychopathy theories of crime is on the more distal independent variable (e.g., Agnew, 1992; Akers, 1998; Gottfredson & Hirschi, 1990; Moffitt, 1993). Because many of these theories, including psychopathic theories of crime, share many of the same independent variables, Agnew (1995) advises that innovative methodologies be used evaluate the more proximal motivational processes that do a better job of distinguishing between theoretical models in criminology. In the current investigation, the motivational processes were the first- and second-order mediators and the methodology was causal mediation analysis.

There are several reasons why we might want to focus on motivational and mediational variables instead of an independent variable like psychopathy. As previously stated, it makes more sense to employ motivational and mediational variables when it comes to testing criminological theories than it is to rely on independent variables that frequently overlap between theories. Another reason is that motivational and mediational variables offer better targets for intervention and prevention than psychopathy. Whereas the traditional view that psychopathy is unamenable to change (Hare, 2003) is no longer considered valid (Polaschek, 2014; Salekin, Worley, & Grimes, 2010), psychopathy is a stable trait that changes slowly (van Baardewijk, Vermeiren, Stegge, & Doreleijers, 2011). If, as the results of the current investigation suggest, a good portion of the effect of psychopathy on delinquency and crime is the result of intervening cognitive variables like general proactive criminal thinking and more specific facets of proactive criminal thinking like superoptimism, then it may be possible to target these thinking patterns and styles with cognitive behavior therapy (Walters, 2017b). Moreover, if it turns out that the more specific features of criminal thinking are capable of mediating the broader aspects of criminal thinking, as superoptimism did in the current study, then it may be advisable to focus our attention on the more specific facets of proactive and reactive criminal thinking when working with offenders. The principals used to challenge and change general irrational beliefs should provide a means of addressing the general and specific criminal thinking styles that appear to underpin the psychopathy–offending relationship (Tafrate & Mitchell, 2014).

The principal limitation of this study is the use of proxy measures to assess the two mediator variables, general proactive criminal thinking and superoptimism. The Psychological Inventory of Criminal Thinking Styles (PICTS: Walters, 1995) is the instrument upon which the proactive–reactive criminal thinking distinction was originally based. Unfortunately, the PICTS was not administered as part of the Pathways study and so proxy measures had to be found. The MD scale served as a proxy measure for general proactive criminal thinking given item content that covers three of the four thinking styles that make up proactive criminal thinking (mollification, entitlement, and power orientation). In addition, scores on the MD scale have been found to correlate to a moderately high degree with the PICTS Proactive Criminal Thinking (PCT) score. A reverse-scored certainty of punishment for antisocial behavior index served as the proxy measure for superoptimism. Given that the assessment was based on risk to self rather than risk to other people, certainty of punishment was assessed in the current study as a perceptual rather than objective phenomenon. Research, in fact, suggests that even when certainty of punishment is assessed as risk to others, the process is more properly interpreted as perceptual rather than objective (Kleck, 2016). External validity could also be raised as a limitation of this study in that only male participants were examined, given that the female subsample for the Pathways study was too small to base meaningful subanalyses on and the selection criteria for inclusion in the Pathways study differed across gender, making simple drug possession charges twice as common in female participants as in male participants.

If, in fact, the mediators-within-mediators effect observed in the current and previous studies (Walters, 2016, 2017a) is a true case of self-similarity or fractal geometry, then we would expect each mediator to be mediated into infinity. This would be impossible to demonstrate, however, using current methodologies. With increased complexity comes increased sensitivity to the effects of less-than-perfect measurement on an indirect effect (Cole & Preacher, 2014). In addition, with an increase in the number of serial mediators comes a corresponding decrease in the fidelity of one's results, not unlike what occurs when connections are added to an electrical circuit (Preacher, 2015). The introduction of nuisance covariance and the loss of fidelity that occurs when multiple serial mediators are examined in a standard mediation path analysis will make it difficult to test the mediators-within-mediators theorem beyond three or four serial mediators. This is the second time a five-variable, three-serial mediator model has been tested, although in the previous study (Walters, 2016), only the indirect effect was evaluated (i.e., there were no direct effects of prior variables on subsequent variables). In the current study, a significant indirect effect was obtained even though all possible pathways were included in the analysis. With the development of new methodologies and more precise and reliable measures, it may eventually be possible to test the fractal nature of multiple-layered mediating variables beyond three or four serial mediators and determine whether the mediators-within-mediators concept represents a genuine fractal. After all, just because we cannot observe a phenomenon does not mean that the phenomenon does not exist.

References

Agnew, R. (1992) 'Foundation for a general strain theory of crime and delinquency,' *Criminology*, *30*:47–87.

Agnew, R. (1995) 'Testing the leading crime theories: An alternative strategy focusing on motivational processes,' *Journal of Research in Crime & Delinquency*, *32*:363–398.

Akers, R. L. (1998) *Social learning and social structure: A general theory of crime and deviance*, Boston, MA: Northeastern University Press.

Allison, P. D. (2012) 'Handling missing data by maximum likelihood,' *SAS Global Forum 2012* (Paper 312–2012), Cary, NC: SAS Institute.

Bandura, A. (1986) *Social foundations of thought and action: A social cognitive theory*, Englewood Cliffs, NJ: Prentice-Hall.

Bandura, A., Barbarnelli, C., Caprara, G. V., and Pastorelli, C. (1996) 'Mechanisms of moral disengagement in the exercise of moral agency,' *Journal of Personality and Social Psychology*, 71:364–374.

Brinkley, C. A., Schmitt, W. A., Smith, S. S., and Newman, J. P. (2001) 'Construct validation of a self-report psychopathy scale: Does Levenson's self-report psychopathy scale measure the same constructs as Hare's Psychopathy Checklist–Revised?,' *Personality and Individual Differences*, *31*:1021–1038.

Cale, E. M., and Lilienfeld, S. O. (2006) 'Psychopathy factors and the risk for aggressive behavior: A test of the "threatened egotism" hypothesis,' *Law and Human Behavior, 30*:51–74.

Cleckley, H. (1976) *The mask of sanity* (5th ed.), St. Louis, MO: Mosby. (Original work published 1941)

Cole, D. A., and Maxwell, S. E. (2003) 'Testing mediational models with longitudinal data: Questions and tips in the use of structural equation modeling,' *Journal of Abnormal Psychology, 112*:558–577.

Cole, D. A., and Preacher, K. J. (2014) 'Manifest variable path analysis: Potentially serious and misleading consequences due to uncorrected measurement error,' *Psychological Methods, 19*:300–315.

DeLisi, M. (2009) 'Psychopathy is the unified theory of crime,' *Youth Violence and Juvenile Justice*, 7:256–273.

Douglas, K. S., Epstein, M. E., and Poythress, N. G. (2008) 'Criminal recidivism among juvenile offenders: Testing the incremental and predictive validity of three measures of psychopathic features,' *Law and Human Behavior, 32*:423–438.

Elwert, F., and Winship, C. (2014) 'Endogenous selection bias: The problem of conditioning on a collider variable,' *Annual Review of Sociology, 40*:31–53.

Forth, A. E., Kosson, D., and Hare, R. D. (2003) *Psychopathy Checklist: Youth Version technical manual*, Toronto, ON: Multi-Health Systems.

Frick, P. J., Stickle, T. R., Dandreaux, D. M., Farrell, J. M., and Kimonis, E. R. (2005) 'Callous–unemotional traits in predicting the severity and stability of conduct problems and delinquency,' *Journal of Abnormal Child Psychology, 33*:471–487.

Gonsalves, V. M., Scalora, M. J., and Huss, M. T. (2009) 'Prediction of recidivism using the Psychopathy Checklist–Revised and the Psychological Inventory of Criminal Thinking Styles,' *Criminal Justice and Behavior, 36*:741–756.

Gottfredson, M. R., and Hirschi, T. (1990) *A general theory of crime*, Stanford, CA: Stanford University Press.

Hare, R. D. (1996) 'Psychopathy: A clinical construct whose time has come,' *Criminal Justice and Behavior, 23*:25–54.

Hare, R. D. (1998) 'The Hare PCL–R: Some issues concerning its use and misuse,' *Legal and Criminological Psychology, 3*:99–119.

Hare, R. D. (2003) *The Hare Psychopathy Checklist–Revised manual* (2nd ed.), Toronto, ON: Multi-Health Systems.

Hare, R. D., and Neumann, C. S. (2008) 'Psychopath as a clinical and empirical construct,' *Annual Review of Clinical Psychology, 4*:217–246.

Harris, G. T., Rice, M. E., and Lalumiére, M. (2001) 'Criminal violence: The roles of psychopathy, neurodevelopmental insults, and antisocial parenting,' *Criminal Justice and Behavior, 28*:402–426.

Hart, S. D., Cox, D. N., and Hare, R. D. (1995) *Manual for the Psychopathy Checklist: Screening Version (PCL: SV)*, Toronto, ON: Multi-Health Systems.

Hayes, A. F. (2013) *Introduction to mediation, moderation, and conditional process analysis: A regression-based approach*, New York, NY: Guilford.

Huizinga, D., Esbensen, F., and Weihar, A. (1991) 'Are there multiple paths to delinquency?,' *Journal of Criminal Law and Criminology, 82*:83–118.

Kenny, D. A. (2013) *Mediation: Sensitivity analysis* [webinar]. Retrieved from http://davidakenny.net/webinars/Mediation/Sensitivity/Sensitivity.html

Kenny, D. A., and Judd, C. M. (2014) 'Power anomalies in testing mediation,' *Psychological Science, 25*:334–339.

Kleck, G. (2016) 'Objective risks and individual perceptions of those risks,' *Criminology and Public Policy, 15*:767–775.

Lynam, D. R., Miller, D. J., Vachon, D., Loeber, R., and Stouthamer-Loeber, M. (2009) 'Psychopathy in adolescence predicts official reports of offending in adulthood,' *Youth Violence and Juvenile Justice*, 7:189–207.

MacKinnon, D. P., Kisbu-Sakarya, Y., and Gottschall, A. C. (2013) 'Developments in mediation analysis,' in T. D. Little (Ed.), *The Oxford handbook of quantitative methods* (Vol. 2, pp. 338–360), New York, NY: Oxford University Press.

Magyar, M., Carr, W. A., Rosenfeld, B., and Rotter, M. (2010) 'An exploration of the relationship between criminal cognitions and psychopathy in a civil psychiatric sample,' *International Journal of Offender Therapy and Comparative Criminology, 54*:865–877.

Mandracchia, J. T., Gonzalez, R. A., Patterson, K. L., and Smith, P. N. (2015) 'Psychopathy and criminogenic thinking in adult male prisoners,' *Journal of Contemporary Criminal Justice, 31*:409–425.

Moffitt, T. E. (1993) 'Adolescence-limited and life-course-persistent antisocial behavior: A developmental taxonomy,' *Psychological Review, 100*:674–701.

Mulvey, E. P. (2012, November) *The Pathways to Desistance study: Design and methods.* Paper presented at the American Society of Criminology Annual Meeting, Chicago, IL. Retrieved June 3, 2013 from http://citation.allacademic.com/meta/p574246_index.html

Muthén, B., and Muthén, L. (1998–2007) *Mplus user's guide* (5th ed.), Los Angeles, CA: Muthén and Muthén.

Nagin, D. S., and Paternoster, R. (1994) 'Personal capital and social control: The deterrence implications of individual differences in criminal offending,' *Criminology, 32*:581–606.

Neumann, C. S., Schmidt, D. S., Carter, R. C., Embley, I., and Hare, R. D. (2012) 'Psychopathic traits in females and males across the globe,' *Behavioral Sciences & the Law, 30*:557–574.

Peyre, H., Leplége, A., and Coste, J. (2011) 'Missing data methods for dealing with missing items in quality of life questionnaires: A comparison by simulation of personal mean score, full information maximum likelihood, multiple imputation, and hot deck techniques applied to the SF–36 in the French 2003 decennial health survey,' *Quality of Life Research, 20*:287–300.

Pituch, K. A., and Stapleton, L. M. (2008) 'The performance of methods to test upper-level mediation in the presence of nonnormal data,' *Multivariate Behavioral Research, 43*:237–267.

Polaschek, D. L. L. (2014) 'Adult criminals with psychopathy: Common beliefs about treatability and change have little empirical support,' *Psychological Science, 23*:296–301.

Preacher, K. J. (2015) 'Advances in mediation analysis: A survey and synthesis of new developments,' *Annual Review of Psychology, 66*:825–852.

Ragatz, L. L., Anderson, R. J., Fremouw, W., and Schwartz, R. (2011) 'Criminal thinking patterns, aggression styles, and the psychopathic traits of late high school bullies and bully–victims,' *Aggressive Behavior, 37*:145–160.

Riopka, S. J., Coupland, R. B. A., and Olver, M. E. (2015) 'Self-reported psychopathy and its association with criminal cognition and antisocial behavior in a sample of university undergraduates,' *Canadian Journal of Behavioural Science, 47*:216–225.

Rucker, D. D., Preacher, K. J., Tormala, Z. L., and Petty, R. E. (2011) 'Mediation analysis in social psychology: Current practices and new recommendations,' *Social and Personality Psychology Compass, 5*:359–371.

Salekin, R. T., Rogers, R., and Sewell, K. W. (1997) 'Construct validity of psychopathy in a female offender sample: A multitrait–multimethod evaluation,' *Journal of Abnormal Psychology, 106*:576–585.

Salekin, R. T., Worley, C., and Grimes, R. D. (2010) 'Treatment of psychopathy: A review and brief introduction to the mental model approach for psychopathy,' *Behavioral Sciences and the Law, 28*:235–266.

Skeem, J. L., and Cooke, D. J. (2010) 'Is criminal behavior a central component of psychopathy? Conceptual directions for resolving the debate,' *Psychological Assessment, 22*:433–445.

Sobel, M. (1982) 'Asymptotic confidence intervals for indirect effects in structural equation models,' *Sociological Methods, 13*:290–312.

Sweeten, G. (2012) 'Scaling criminal offending,' *Journal of Quantitative Criminology, 28*:533–557.

Tafrate, R. C., and Mitchell, D. (Eds.) (2014) *Forensic CBT: A handbook for clinical practice*, Chichester: Wiley.

van Baardewijk, Y., Vermiren, R., Stegge, H., and Doreleijers, T. (2011) 'Self-reported psychopathic traits in children: Their stability and concurrent and prospective association with conduct problems and aggression,' *Journal of Psychopathology and Behavioral Assessment, 33*:236–245.

Vaughn, M. G., and DeLisi, M. (2008) 'Were Wolfgang's chronic offenders psychopaths? On the convergent validity of psychopathy and career criminality,' *Journal of Criminal Justice, 36*:33–42.

Vaughn, M. G., DeLisi, M., Beaver, K., Wright, J. P., and Howard, M. O. (2007) 'Toward a psychopathology of self-control theory: The importance of narcissistic traits,' *Behavioral Sciences and the Law, 25*:803–821.

Vaughn, M. G., Newhill, C. E., DeLisi, M., Beaver, K. M., and Howard, M. O. (2008) 'An investigation of psychopathic features among delinquent girls: Violence, theft, and drug abuse,' *Youth Violence and Juvenile Justice, 6*:240–255.

Walters, G. D. (1995) 'The Psychological Inventory of Criminal Thinking Styles: Part I. Reliability and initial validity,' *Criminal Justice and Behavior, 22*:307–325.

Walters, G. D. (2009) 'The Psychological Inventory of Criminal Thinking Styles and Psychopathy Checklist: Screening Version as incrementally valid predictors of recidivism,' *Law and Human Behavior, 33*:497–505.

Walters, G. D. (2012a) *Crime in a psychological context: From career criminals to criminal careers*, Thousand Oaks, CA: Sage.

Walters, G. D. (2012b) 'Psychopathy and crime: Testing the incremental validity of PCL–R-measured psychopathy as a predictor of general and violent recidivism,' *Law and Human Behavior, 36*:404–412.

Walters, G. D. (2016) Mediating the mediator: The indirect effect of short-term hostility on the past reactive criminal thinking–future reactive criminal thinking relationship, Manuscript submitted for publication.
Walters, G. D. (2017a) Mediating proactive criminal thinking with perceived parental acceptance of child delinquency: Testing the fractal nature of criminal development, Manuscript submitted for publication.
Walters, G. D. (2017b) 'Effect of a brief cognitive behavioural intervention on criminal thinking and prison misconduct in male inmates: Variable-oriented and person-oriented analyses,' *Criminal Behaviour and Mental Health*, *27*(5):457–469.
Walters, G. D., and DeLisi, M. (2015) 'Psychopathy and violence: Does antisocial cognition mediate the relationship between the PCL: YV factor scores and violent offending?,' *Law and Human Behavior*, *39*:350–359.
Williams, C. R., and Arrigo, B. A. (2002) *Law, psychology, and justice: Chaos theory and the new disorder*, Albany, NY: SUNY Press.
Wu, A. D., and Zumbo, B. D. (2008) 'Understanding and using mediators and moderators,' *Social Indicators Research*, *87*:367–392.

3

Structural models of personality and psychopathy

Donald R. Lynam and Joshua D. Miller

Introduction

We work with a simple definition of personality: personality refers to an individual's characteristic pattern of thinking, feeling, and acting. Although simple, this definition has many implications. Personality is internal; it refers to characteristics that reside within the individual. Personality has broad effects; it is manifested in how individuals think, feel, get along with others, and behave. Personality accounts for stable behavior patterns across time and situations. It is our contention that psychopathy can be understood as a particular personality pattern.

Although we might say it most explicitly, the idea of psychopathy as a personality configuration is not new. All classic descriptions of psychopathy reference personality traits (Miller & Lynam, 2015). Personality runs throughout Cleckley's seminal descriptions in *The Mask of Sanity* (1941/1988). Based on his work with psychopathic individuals, Cleckley offered 16 criteria for psychopathy. At least ten of these are obvious personality traits: superficial charm and good "intelligence," absence of "nervousness," unreliability, untruthfulness and insincerity, lack of remorse or shame, poor judgment and failure to learn by experience, pathologic egocentricity and incapacity for love, general poverty in major affective reactions, unresponsiveness in general interpersonal relations, and failure to follow any life plan. The remaining six criteria reference more specific behaviors or states, many of which are likely influenced by personality dispositions (e.g., inadequately motivated antisocial behavior, suicide rarely carried out, and sex life impersonal, trivial, and poorly integrated).

Drawing on and expanding Cleckley's description, Hare's model of psychopathy – Psychopathy Checklist–Revised (PCL–R; Hare, 2003) – identifies 20 constructs as central to psychopathy. These 20 constructs collapse into four more specific facets. The interpersonal facet includes glibness/superficial charm, grandiose sense of self-worth, pathological lying, and conning/manipulative. The affective facet is made up of lack of remorse/guilt, shallow affect, callous/lack of empathy, and failure to accept responsibility. The erratic lifestyle facet includes need for stimulation/proneness to boredom, parasitic lifestyle, lack of realistic long-term goals, impulsivity, and irresponsibility. The antisocial behavior facet is composed of poor behavioral controls, early behavioral problems, juvenile delinquency, revocation of conditional release, and criminal versatility. Only four of these fail to directly reference personality – early behavioral problems, juvenile delinquency, revocation of conditional release, and criminal versatility.

Structural models of personality

We believe that psychopathy is personality. Specifically, we believe that psychopathy is a particular personality configuration. To demonstrate this, we utilize the Five Factor Model of Personality (FFM) – one of several structural models of personality that might be employed. In general, structural models use multiple dimensions or superfactors to organize the vast array of personality traits (Wiggins & Pincus, 1992). They share fundamental assumptions: (1) traits are the basic building blocks, (2) there are a finite number of traits, and (3) traits provide full coverage of human personality. There are multiple benefits to using these models to understand clinical or criminological constructs. First, these models were developed in research efforts to identify and organize the primary building blocks of personality. Traits from these models are based in the science of personality and not in the minds of psychopathy observers and theorists. Second, because these models were identified in basic science efforts and not in efforts to predict specific criteria, problems with predictor–criterion overlap are minimized. Third, each of these models has been widely used and well validated in various kinds of research.

Several structural models have been examined in relation to psychopathy, including Eysenck's Psychoticism, Extraversion, and Neuroticism (PEN) model, Tellegen's three-factor model, and the FFM/Big Five. Eysenck's PEN model includes factors of Neuroticism, Extraversion, and Psychoticism (Eysenck & Eysenck, 1970): Neuroticism entails emotional stability and adjustment; Extraversion reflects traits related to sociability and agency; and Psychoticism encompasses egocentricity, (lack of) interpersonal warmth, (lack of) empathy, and impulsiveness. Tellegen's (1985) model also posits three basic dimensions: Positive Emotionality, which refers to the tendency to be positively engaged with others and the world; Negative Emotionality, which reflects an individual's tendency to experience negative emotions (e.g., fear, anxiety, and anger) and his or her tendency to break down under stress; and Constraint, which assesses an individual's ability to control impulses, act deliberately, avoid potentially dangerous situations, and endorse traditional values and standards.

The FFM was derived from studies of the English language undertaken to identify the domains of personality functioning most important in describing oneself and others (Digman, 1990; John & Srivastava, 1999; Wiggins & Pincus, 1992). This lexical research emphasized five broad domains, identified as Extraversion, Agreeableness, Conscientiousness, Neuroticism, and Openness to Experience (John & Srivastava, 1999). Extraversion entails an individual's proneness to positive emotions and sociability. Agreeableness is concerned with an individual's interpersonal relationships and strategies; people high in Agreeableness tend to be trusting, straightforward, and empathic, whereas those who score low tend to be manipulative, arrogant, and unconcerned about others. Conscientiousness relates to the "control of impulses," as well as to the ability to plan, organize, and complete behavioral tasks. The domain of Neuroticism entails emotional adjustment and stability. The fifth domain, Openness to Experience, refers to an individual's interest in culture and the preference for and interest in experiencing and exploring new activities, ideas, and emotions. Each of these five broad domains can be further divided into finer-grained facets or components. Costa and McCrae (1995a) proposed six facets within each domain on the basis of their research with the NEO Personality Inventory–Revised (NEO PI–R; Costa & McCrae, 1992). For example, they parse the domain of Agreeableness (vs. Antagonism) into more specific facets of trust (vs. suspicion), straightforwardness (vs. deception), altruism (vs. exploitation), compliance (vs. aggression), modesty (vs. arrogance), and tender-mindedness (vs. tough-mindedness). The domains and facets of the FFM, along with sample items, are given in Table 3.1 from one particular instantiation – the International Personality Item Pool – Neuroticism, Extraversion, and Openness to Experience IPIP–NEO (Maples, Guan, Carter, & Miller, 2014).

Despite being derived independently and including different numbers of basic traits, there is substantial agreement across the models. All include explicit representations of the "Big

Table 3.1 FFM domains and facets with example items from the IPIP–NEO

Domain/Facet	*Descriptors from IPIP–NEO*
Neuroticism (vs. Emotional Stability)	
N1: Anxiety	+ Am afraid of many things – Am relaxed most of the time
N2: Angry Hostility	+ Lose my temper – Am not easily annoyed
N3: Depression	+ Dislike myself – Seldom feel blue
N4: Self-Consciousness	+ Am afraid to draw attention to myself – Am not easily embarrassed
N5: Impulsiveness	+ Do things I later regret – Am able to control my cravings
N6: Vulnerability	+ Become overwhelmed by events – Am calm in tense situations
Extraversion (vs. Introversion)	
E1: Warmth	+ Make friends easily – Often feel uncomfortable around others
E2: Gregariousness	+ Enjoy being part of a group – Want to be left alone
E3: Assertiveness	+ Take control of things – Don't like to draw attention to myself
E4: Activity	+ Am always on the go – Like a leisurely lifestyle
E5: Excitement-Seeking	+ Am willing to try anything once – Would never go hang gliding or bungee jumping
E6: Positive emotions	+ Look at the bright side of life – Am not easily amused
Openness (vs. closedness) to experience	
O1: Fantasy	+ Love to daydream – Have difficulty imagining things
O2: Aesthetics	+ Believe in the importance of art – Do not like art
O3: Feelings	+ Experience my emotions intensely – Am not easily affected by my emotions
O4: Actions	+ Prefer variety to routine – Don't like the idea of change
O5: Ideas	+ Enjoy thinking about things – Avoid difficult reading material
O6: Values	+ Believe there is no absolute right and wrong – Believe laws should be strictly enforced

Domain/Facet	*Descriptors from IPIP–NEO*
Agreeableness (vs. Antagonism)	
A1: Trust	+ Believe that others have good intentions – Suspect hidden motives in others
A2: Straightforwardness	+ Stick to the rules – Use others for my own ends
A3: Altruism	+ Am concerned about others – Am indifferent to the feelings of others
A4: Compliance	+ Hate to seem pushy – Get back at others
A5: Modesty	+ Consider myself an average person – Believe that I am better than others
A6: Tender-Mindedness	+ Feel sympathy for those who are worse off – Believe people should fend for themselves
Conscientiousness (vs. Disorder/Dyscontrol)	
C1: Competence	+ Know how to get things done – Have little to contribute
C2: Order	+ Want everything to be "just right" – Often forget to put things back in their place
C3: Dutifulness	+ Try to follow the rules – Break my promises
C4: Achievement-Striving	+ Do more than what's expected of me – Put little time and effort into my work
C5: Self-Discipline	+ Carry out my plans – Need a push to get started
C6: Deliberation	+ Choose my words with care – Jump into things without thinking

Two" – Extraversion (Positive Emotionality) and Neuroticism (Negative Emotionality). Additionally, the FFM and Tellegen's model both contain dimensions related to control of impulses and orientation to convention – Conscientiousness from the FFM and Constraint from Tellegen's model. Eysenck's model does include Conscientiousness, although not as a unique and single factor: research indicates that Eysenck's Psychoticism dimension can be considered a blend of low Conscientiousness and low Agreeableness (Costa & McCrae, 1995b). All models also include Agreeableness. In Eysenck's model, it is a component of the Psychoticism dimension. In Tellegen's model, it is represented primarily by subscales of the Negative Emotionality dimension (i.e., aggression and alienation). Thus, these structural models are far from discrepant with one another. In fact, Watson, Clark, and Harkness (1994:24) have argued that

> the Big Three and Big Five models define a common "Big Four" space in which (a) two traits are equivalent (Neuroticism and Extraversion), (b) the third Big Three dimension (Constraint or Psychoticism) represents some combination of two Big Five factors (Conscientiousness and Agreeableness), and (c) the final Big Five trait (Openness, or imagination) is excluded.

They go on to label the Big Four as Neuroticism (or Negative Emotionality), Extraversion (or Positive Emotionality), Conscientiousness (or Constraint), and Agreeableness.

The Five Factor Model and psychopathy

In what follows, we use the FFM as the organizing structure to integrate various findings on psychopathy and personality. Our preference for the use of the FFM is driven by several factors. First, the FFM was derived from the natural language, ensuring that important aspects of personality are represented (John & Srivastava, 1999). Second, the FFM provides an extensive and comprehensive lexicon of 30 facets versus the 11 subscales of the Multidimensional Personality Questionnaire (MPQ) or the three factors of the PEN model. Third, the FFM, at both the domain and facet levels, enjoys considerable empirical support in the form of convergent and discriminant validation across self, peer, and spouse ratings (Costa & McCrae, 1988), temporal stability (Roberts & DelVecchio, 2000), cross-cultural support (Church, 2001; McCrae, Martin, & Costa, 2005), and behavior genetics (Yamagata et al., 2006). The FFM is the model of choice for both individual studies and meta-analytic reviews on the relations between basic personality traits and critical outcomes, including academic achievement (Poropat, 2009), work performance (Barrick & Mount, 1991) and satisfaction (Judge, Heller, & Mount, 2002), leadership (Judge, Bono, Ilies, & Gerhardt, 2002), physical (Bogg & Roberts, 2004) and psychological health (Malouff, Thorsteinsson, & Schutte, 2005; Samuel & Widiger, 2008), subjective well-being (DeNeve & Cooper, 1998), and relationship satisfaction (Malouff, Thorsteinsson, Schutte, Bhullar, & Rooke, 2010). With regard to behavioral outcomes of most relevance to psychopathy, the FFM has also been used to meta-analytically characterize the relations between personality and antisocial behavior (Jones, Miller, & Lynam, 2011; Miller & Lynam, 2001), substance use and abuse (Kotov et al., 2011), and risky sexual behavior (Hoyle, Fejfar, & Miller, 2000).

Fourth, in addition to the research base supporting the FFM, there is a substantial research base emanating from this model. Researchers have used the FFM to study the development and continuity of personality over time (e.g., Caspi, Roberts, & Shiner, 2005; De Clerq & De Fruyt, 2012; Tackett et al., 2012), as well as the levels of these traits as a function of gender, age, and culture (e.g., Allik & McCrae, 2004; Schmitt, Realo, Voracek, & Allik, 2008; Soto & John, 2012). Similarly, the FFM framework has been used to study the processes underlying and outcomes attributable to specific personality domains, such as the basic processes underlying Agreeableness. For example, Robinson, Meier, and Wilkowski have used a basic science approach to examine the way in which (dis)agreeable individuals interpret interpersonal and contextual cues and behave in more or less adaptive ways (Meier, Robinson, & Wilkowski, 2006, 2007; Robinson, Wilkowski, Meier, Moeller, & Fetterman, 2012). Meier and colleagues (2006) found that individuals high in Agreeableness were less susceptible to aggression-related cues and more likely to activate prosocial thoughts in response to such cues than were individuals low in Agreeableness. Roberts and colleagues have worked to delineate the basic composition (e.g., Roberts, Chernyshenko, Stark, & Goldberg, 2005), correlates (e.g., Roberts, Jackson, Burger, & Trautwein, 2009), and consequences of Conscientiousness (e.g., Bogg & Roberts, 2004). DeYoung has systematically explored the broad domain of Openness/intellect, specifying its relation to cognitive ability (DeYoung, Quilty, Peterson, & Gray, 2014), describing its broad outlines (DeYoung, 2015), and identifying its sources (DeYoung, Peterson, & Higgins, 2005) and biological underpinnings (DeYoung et al., 2011). There are also multiple programs of research aimed at the basic processes underlying the facet-level traits within the FFM, including the work of Whiteside and Lynam (2001) on diverse personality pathways to impulsive behavior. Understanding psychopathy from the perspective of the FFM allows this large body of basic research to inform theorizing on assessment, etiology, course, and treatment.

Fifth, and perhaps most important, substantial research exists on personality and psychopathy employing the FFM framework. Expert ratings of prototypical cases of psychopathy have been conducted using the FFM (Miller, Lynam, Widiger, & Leukefeld, 2001). Similarly, the FFM has been used as a tool to translate prominent psychopathy assessments into a basic trait perspective (Widiger & Lynam, 1998). Empirically, the FFM has been examined in relation to all major psychopathy instruments (see meta-analyses by Decuyper, De Pauw, De Fruyt, De Bolle, & De Clerq, 2009; Lilienfeld, Watts, Smith, Berg, & Latzman, 2015; Lynam & Derefinko, 2006). In their recent meta-analysis, O'Boyle, Forsyth, Banks, Story, and White (2015) identified between 76 and 86 studies that reported on relations between one or more of the Big Five dimensions and one or more psychopathy instruments.

The advantages of the FFM in conceptualizing, assessing, and diagnosing personality disorders (PDs) are such that this approach has been included in the two most prominent psychiatric nosologies, the Diagnostic and Statistical Manual of Mental Disorders–5th edition (DSM–5; APA, 2013) and the International Classification of Diseases–11th edition (ICD–11; see Tyrer, 2013). For example, the DSM–5 Personality and Personality Disorder Work Group proposed a model in which PDs are diagnosed on the basis of personality-related impairment in self and interpersonal functioning, as well as elevated scores on one or more traits from a pathological trait version of the FFM. Although the new approach did not replace the traditional approach in DSM–5, it was placed in Section III on "emerging measures and models" and may become the predominant or only approach in future iterations.

Meta-analysis

Conceptualizing psychopathy from the FFM involves identifying the FFM traits that characterize it. One of the most compelling approaches involves correlating explicit measures of psychopathy with measures of the FFM. The logic of this approach is straightforward. Multiple psychopathy assessments have been derived from various conceptualizations and using divergent approaches; looking across these conceptions allows points of agreement to emerge and idiosyncratic aspects to be blunted. In their meta-analyses of the relations between elements of the Dark Triad (i.e., psychopathy, narcissism, and Machiavellianism) and the domains (i.e., higher-order factors) and facets of the FFM, O'Boyle and colleagues (2015) identified between 76 and 86 studies (with *N*s ranging from 23,216 to 25,465) reporting on the relations between at least one FFM domain and one psychopathy measure.

At the domain level, psychopathy is characterized by very low scores on Agreeableness (corrected $r = -.53$) and moderately low scores on Conscientiousness (corrected $r = -.39$); effect sizes were statistically significant but very small for Neuroticism (corrected $r = .06$), Extraversion (corrected $r = .05$), and Openness to experience (corrected $r = .05$). These results are consistent with earlier meta-analyses by Lynam and Derefinko (2006), Decuyper and colleagues (2009), and Lilienfeld and colleagues (2015). Lilienfeld and colleagues found that PCL-assessed psychopathy was most strongly related to Agreeableness ($r = -.32$) and Conscientiousness ($r = -.14$), and unrelated to Neuroticism ($r = .06$), Extraversion ($r = .02$), and Openness ($r = .01$).

More relevant to our purposes, however, O'Boyle and colleagues (2015) also meta-analyzed between 11 and 19 studies (with *N*s ranging from 2,267 to 4,733) that reported on the relations between at least one of 30 facets of the FFM and psychopathy. Corrected, average correlations are reported in the second column of Table 3.2. As with the domain-level analyses, facet-level analyses highlight the role of traits from Agreeableness and Conscientiousness and reveal mixed relations for Neuroticism (e.g., high anger and impulsiveness) and Extraversion (e.g., low warmth; high excitement seeking). Taking any facet with an absolute correlation greater than or equal to .25 as characteristic, 14 FFM facets describe the psychopathic individual. The psychopathic person is low in all facets of Agreeableness; he/she is distrustful, lying and manipulative,

Table 3.2 FFM profiles of psychopathy derived using different approaches

NEO PI–R	*O'Boyle et al.*	*W & L transl.*	*Expert*
N1: Anxiety	–.03	.00	**1.47**
N2: Angry Hostility	**.37**	**1.00**	3.87
N3: Depression	.10	**–1.00**	**1.40**
N4: Self-Consciousness	–.01	.00	**1.07**
N5: Impulsiveness	**.39**	**1.00**	**4.53**
N6: Vulnerability	.08	.00	**1.47**
E1: Warmth	–.24	**–1.00**	**1.73**
E2: Gregariousness	.00	.00	3.67
E3: Assertiveness	.09	.00	**4.47**
E4: Activity	.06	.00	3.67
E5: Excitement Seeking	**.28**	**1.00**	**4.73**
E6: Positive Emotions	–.17	**–1.00**	2.53
O1: Fantasy	.09	.00	3.07
O2: Aesthetics	–.04	.00	2.33
O3: Feelings	–.07	.00	**1.80**
O4: Actions	.09	.00	**4.27**
O5: Ideas	.04	.00	3.53
O6: Values	.06	.00	2.87
A1: Trust	**–.35**	.00	**1.73**
A2: Straightforwardness	**–.56**	**–2.00**	**1.13**
A3: Altruism	**–.40**	**–2.00**	**1.33**
A4: Compliance	**–.47**	**–2.00**	**1.33**
A5: Modesty	**–.25**	**–2.00**	**1.00**
A6: Tendermindedness	**–.36**	**–2.00**	**1.27**
C1: Competence	–.23	.00	**4.20**
C2: Order	**–.25**	.00	2.60
C3: Dutifulness	**–.41**	**–2.00**	**1.20**
C4: Achievement-Striving	**–.26**	**–2.00**	3.07
C5: Self-discipline	**–.31**	**–2.00**	**1.87**
C6: Deliberation	**–.46**	**–2.00**	**1.60**
	Similarity indices		
Translation	.84		
Experts	.67	.67	

selfish, oppositional, immodest, and callous. He/she is low on five of six Conscientiousness facets, described as disorganized, unreliable, unmotivated, unrestrained, and rash. Finally, he/she is high in angry hostility, impulsiveness, and excitement seeking.

Other approaches

This empirically derived FFM description agrees well with other available descriptions. Widiger and Lynam (1998) "translated" the PCL–R into the language of the FFM. Beginning with narrative descriptions of the 20 PCL–R items, Widiger and Lynam identified NEO PI–R facets that captured the content of the descriptions. The third column in Table 3.2 provides the FFM profile from this exercise, in which scores of 0 are assigned to facets that did not appear in any item translation (e.g., anxiety), scores of +1 (high) or −1 (low) are given to facets that appear in the translation of only one PCL–R item (e.g., angry hostility), and scores of +2 (high) or −2 (low) are given to facets that appear in the translation of more than one item. From this PCL–R-based profile, psychopathic individuals are viewed as being low in: depression from the domain of Neuroticism; warmth and positive emotions from Extraversion; all facets of Agreeableness except trust; and four of six facets of Conscientiousness (dutifulness, achievement-striving, self-discipline, and deliberation). Additionally, psychopathic individuals are rated as somewhat high in angry hostility and impulsiveness from the Neuroticism domain and high in excitement seeking from Extraversion. No facets from the domain of Openness characterized psychopathy.

In yet a third approach, Miller, Lynam, Widiger, and Leukefeld (2001) invited psychopathy experts to describe the personality of the prototypic Cleckley psychopath using the language of the FFM. Miller et al. (2001) wrote to 21 psychopathy researchers and asked each to "rate the prototypical, classic Cleckley psychopath" on each of 30 bipolar scales which corresponded to the 30 facets of the FFM. For example, to assess the facet of straightforwardness (a facet of Agreeableness), experts were asked "to what extent is the male psychopath honest, genuine, and sincere versus deceptive and manipulative?" Response choices ranged from 1 (extremely low) to 5 (extremely high). Fifteen experts returned the ratings. Aggregating the ratings across experts served to bring out the aspects on which experts agree and blunt the idiosyncratic elements of each description. The experts' mean ratings for each of the facets are given in the fourth column of Table 3.2. Taking any facet with an average rating less than 2 or greater than 4 as characteristic, the prototypical psychopathic individual is low in anxiety, depression, self-consciousness, and vulnerability from Neuroticism; low in warmth from Extraversion; low in openness to feelings from Openness; low in all facets of Agreeableness; and low in dutifulness, self-discipline, and deliberation from Conscientiousness. The prototypical psychopathic individual is also high in impulsiveness from Neuroticism; assertiveness and excitement seeking from Extraversion; openness to actions from Openness; and competence from Conscientiousness – a finding likely due to asking experts to report how the psychopathic person sees himself.

There is general agreement on the FFM description of the psychopathic individual across the three different approaches, as can be seen in the similarity indices at the bottom of the table. The psychopathic individual is low in all facets of Agreeableness and most facets of Conscientiousness. He/she is also high in two other facets dealing with impulsivity: impulsiveness from Neuroticism (referencing difficulty resisting cravings) and Excitement-seeking from Extraversion. There is also some suggestion that the psychopathic person is rather high in angry hostility and low in depression. In sum, across approaches there is a clear consensual trait description of the psychopathic person.

Using the FFM to assess psychopathy

In addition to demonstrating a consistent and robust FFM profile of psychopathy, research shows that psychopathy can be assessed using the FFM. If the nomological network that surrounds explicit assessments of psychopathy can be recreated by FFM-assessed indices of psychopathy, then the argument that psychopathy is these traits is strengthened. Results from multiple studies (Derefinko & Lynam, 2006; Miller et al., 2001; Miller, Jones, & Lynam, 2011; Ross, Benning, Patrick, Thompson, & Thurston, 2009) show high convergence between FFM-assessed psychopathy and explicit indices of psychopathy, including the Levenson Self-Report Psychopathy scale (LSRP; Levenson, Keihl, & Fitzpatrick, 1995), Hare Self-Report Psychopathy Scale (SRP–III; Williams, Paulhus, & Hare, 2007), the Psychopathic Personality Inventory–Revised (PPI–R; Lilienfeld & Widows, 2005), and the Youth Psychopathic Traits Inventory (YPI; Andershed, Ker, Stattin, & Levander, 2002). Using the original data from Lynam, Gaughan, Miller, Miller, Mullins-Sweatt, and Widiger (2011) for the PPI, SRP, and LSRP, from Sherman, Lynam, and Heyde (2013) for the YPI, and from Few, Miller, and Lynam (2013) for DSM–5, Lynam and Miller (2015) examined the convergent correlations between these five psychopathy scales and FFM psychopathy scores computed from the NEO PI–R; these convergent correlations ranged from .63 for the YPI to .72 for the PPI with an average of .66. Additionally, across samples of undergraduates (Miller & Lynam, 2003), community participants (Miller et al., 2011; Miller et al., 2001), and drug abusers (Derefinko & Lynam, 2007), relations of FFM psychopathy scores to external criteria (e.g., antisocial behavior, aggression, substance use, and other forms of psychopathology) mirror those found when explicit assessments of psychopathy are used.

More recently, two studies have examined the outcomes of an FFM-based psychopathy measure in a nationally representative sample of over 15,000 men and women. In the first, Beaver et al. (2014) examined the relations between FFM-assessed psychopathy and a variety of health outcomes. These authors found that higher scores on FFM-assessed psychopathy were associated with significant reductions in general health and significant increases in chronic diseases and neurological disorders. Specifically, higher scores on FFM-assessed psychopathy were associated with increased odds of diabetes, high blood pressure, high cholesterol, and an assortment of neurological disorders. These results held generally across men and women. More recently, Beaver, Boutwell, Barnes, Vaughn, and DeLisi (2017) examined the relations between an FFM-based psychopathy assessment and criminal justice outcomes. After controlling for gender, age, and race, Beaver et al. found that FFM-psychopathy had a statistically significant and positive effect on the odds of being arrested, incarcerated, and sentenced to probation and on the level of self-reported delinquency. These results held for both men and women.

In an alternative approach, Lynam et al. (2011) developed an explicit assessment of psychopathy built on the FFM – the Elemental Psychopathy Assessment (EPA). This was done in response to concerns that instruments developed in the general population to assess personality in that population (e.g., the NEO PI–R) may not be optimal for assessing pathological personality traits. In creating the EPA, Lynam et al. used the basic structure of the FFM to build new scales that remain tied to basic personality science yet better assess the more pathological ends of basic trait dimensions (see Lynam, 2012). For the EPA, Lynam et al. (2011) began with a consensus profile of psychopathy (Lynam & Widiger, 2007a) that included 18 traits. All six facets from Agreeableness were included (trust, straightforwardness, altruism, compliance, modesty, tender-mindedness), as were the six facets of Neuroticism, although some represented high levels (i.e., angry hostility and impulsiveness) whereas others reflected low levels (i.e., anxiety, depression, self-consciousness, and vulnerability). Three facets from Conscientiousness were also included (i.e., dutifulness, self-discipline, and deliberation), along with three facets from Extraversion representing, like the facets from Neuroticism, both high (i.e., assertiveness and excitement seeking) and low levels of Extraversion (i.e., warmth). We will only note that the EPA shows good reliability, good convergence with other extant psychopathy scales, and good predictive utility. Importantly, these characteristics are maintained in the 18-item, super short form of the EPA (Collison, Miller, Gaughan, Widiger, & Lynam, 2016) developed specifically for use in criminology where large, broad survey assessments are the norm and assessment space is at a premium.

Advantages to understanding psychopathy using the FFM

There are a number of advantages to understanding psychopathy as a constellation of traits from the FFM that derive from the breadth and articulation of the FFM itself and the enormous research base that supports it. We detail these advantage below; one is specific to criminology, whereas others are more general.

Criminology-specific issue

The strong theoretical and empirical overlap between psychopathy and criminal and antisocial behavior (e.g., Hare, 1999) has led to increased interest in psychopathy within the field of criminology (e.g., Polaschek & Daly, 2013). DeLisi (2009) has even argued that psychopathy should be considered the unified theory of crime because of its embodiment of the "pejorative essence of antisocial behavior" as well as its ability to accommodate both dimensional and categorical conceptualizations of antisocial behavior across diverse populations. Research has shown that psychopathy may be useful in identifying the prolific but small group of offenders identified as "career criminals" (Wolfgang, Figlio, & Sellin, 1972; Tracy, Wolfgang, & Figlio, 1990; Hare, 1999). Vaughn and DeLisi (2008) found that psychopathic traits nearly doubled the total explanatory power for career criminality when demographic and mental health variables had been taken into account. In addition, psychopathic traits demonstrated 70–88 percent accuracy when predicting career criminal membership.

A long-standing objection to using psychopathy to understand the etiology of criminal behaviors has been that some measures include explicit assessments of antisocial and other externalizing behaviors. Such predictor–criterion overlap leads to a potential tautology in which one measure of antisocial behavior is used to predict another measure of antisocial behavior. This is certainly true of the most widely used psychopathy measure in forensic research – Hare's Psychopathy Checklist–Revised (PCL–R; Hare, 1991, 2003). The PCL–R consists of 20 items that are rated by an interviewer following an interview and a review of records. Several items explicitly assess antisocial behavior – early behavior problems, juvenile delinquency, revocation of conditional release, and criminal versatility. Several more items instruct the interviewer to rely on certain types of antisocial behavior when making a rating; for example, interviewers are instructed to look for criminal charges for fraud and embezzlement in rating Conning/Manipulative or for charges and convictions that involve spontaneous and unprovoked violence to rate Poor Behavioral Controls. This problem with predictor–criterion overlap is also present for the self-report scales that are based on the conception of psychopathy inherent in the PCL–R, including the commonly used Self-Report Psychopathy Scale (SRP; Hare, 1985; SRP–II; Paulhus, Neumann, & Hare, in press), which includes four subscales, one of which, antisocial, is assessed by reference to explicitly antisocial acts. This problem is also present in the more recently developed Triarchic Psychopathy Measure (TriPM; Patrick, 2010), which is based on a three-factor conceptualization of psychopathy that includes Boldness, Meanness, and disinhibition. Unfortunately, multiple disinhibition items reference frankly antisocial behavior (e.g., "I have robbed someone" and "I have stolen something out of a vehicle").

This problem does not exist with psychopathy measures that use the elements of the Five Factor Model, including the NEO PI–R (Costa & McCrae, 1992) and the International Personality Item Pool NEO–120 (Maples et al., 2014). These are basic personality inventories that ask about characteristic ways of thinking, feeling, and acting and do not reference explicitly antisocial acts. Similarly, predictor–criterion overlap is absent in all versions of the Elemental Psychopathy Assessment (EPA; Lynam et al., 2011; EPA Short Form; Lynam et al., 2013; EPA Super Short Form; Collison et al., 2016); Table 3.3 provides the items from the super short form of the EPA.

Issues related to psychopathy

Understanding psychopathy as a collection of traits from a general model of personality also has implications for the study of psychopathy generally. These advantages include, among others,

Table 3.3 Items from the EPA super short form

Subscale	*Item*
Antagonism factor	
Arrogance	I deserve special treatment
Coldness	I care a lot about my relationships with others. (R)
Callousness	Feeling sorry for others is a sign of weakness.
Distrust	When someone does something nice for me, I wonder what they want from me.
Disobliged	People would say I am reliable and dependable. (R)
Impersistence	I quit things pretty easily.
Manipulative	I could make a living as a con artist.
Self-centered	I have more important things to worry about than other people's feelings.
Disinhibition factor	
Anger	My temper has gotten me into trouble.
Opposition	I am known as a bit of a rebel.
Rashness	"Act first, think later" describes me well.
Thrill-seeking	I like doing things that are risky or dangerous.
Urgency	When I am upset, I will do things that I later regret.
Emotional Stability factor	
Unconcern	I am a bit of a worrier. (R)
Self-contentment	I am not the type to depressed about things I've done wrong.
Invulnerable	I remain cool, calm, and collected when things get stressful.
Dominance	I often emerge as the leader in a group.
Self-assured	I am pretty comfortable when meeting new people.

Note. Respondents are instructed: "The following statements deal with how you think, feel, and act. Please read each item carefully and fill in the bubble on the bubble sheet that best corresponds to your agreement or disagreement. If you disagree strongly blacken 1, if you disagree a little blacken 2, if you neither agree nor disagree blacken 3, if you agree a little blacken 4, and if you strongly agree blacken 5. There are no right or wrong answers, and you need not be an expert to complete this questionnaire." (R) indicates that an item is reverse-scored.

accounting for the factor structures of various inventories, making sense of available epidemiological data pertaining to psychopathy and antisocial behavior, and interpreting the putative etiologically relevant deficits associated with psychopathy.

Factor structures of psychopathy inventories

The FFM can be used to understand the factor structures of various established inventories of psychopathy. Items/subscales cohere with one another and factors correlate with each other to the extent that they assess similar FFM traits, and they diverge to the extent that the traits they assess are different. The PCL–R serves as an excellent example. The FFM translation of the PCL–R shows that Factor 1 is mostly a measure of low Agreeableness, whereas Factor 2 is a measure of low Agreeableness and low Conscientiousness, with some aspects measuring low and high elements of Neuroticism and Extraversion (Widiger & Lynam, 1998). The factors correlate highly because both assess Agreeableness but are not isomorphic because Factor 2 also includes a substantial amount of Conscientiousness. Similar patterns have been found using the two factors of the Child Psychopathy Scale (CPS; Lynam et al., 2005), the three factors of the Youth Psychopathy Traits Inventory (YPI; Sherman, Lynam, & Heyde, 2013), the two factors of the

Levenson Self-Report Psychopathy scales, and the four factors of the Self-Report Psychopathy scale (SRP; Lynam & Miller, 2015). In each of these cases, low Agreeableness suffused all subscales and accounted for much of the subscale overlap within a given inventory. Subscales were distinguished from each other by their differential relations to Conscientiousness, Neuroticism, and Extraversion.

In the case of measures including subscales that do not share variance with one another, the FFM serves to explain this phenomenon as well. For example, the Psychopathic Personality Inventory (PPI; Lilienfeld & Andrews, 1996; Revised version: Lilienfeld & Widows, 2005) includes two higher-order factors – Self-Centered Impulsivity (SCI) and Fearless Dominance (FD). FD is unrelated to SCI, most other indicators of psychopathy, and antisocial behavior, but is positively related to a variety of positive outcomes (Lynam & Miller, 2012). This state of affairs is easily understood when viewed through the lens of the FFM. Almost all indicators of psychopathy are suffused with low Agreeableness and low Conscientiousness; these are the basic building blocks of psychopathy (Lynam, & Miller, 2015). The SCI factor of the PPI is similarly infused and bears the expected relations to antisocial behavior. FD, however, primarily assesses low Neuroticism and high Extraversion; it is unrelated or slightly positive to Agreeableness and Conscientiousness. Thus, it is unrelated to its PPI counterpart (i.e., SCI), most other measures of psychopathy, and antisocial behavior. The case is similar for Patrick, Fowles, and Krueger's (2009) Triarchic Psychopathy Measure (TriPM), which posits that psychopathy consists of three components: Meanness, Boldness, and disinhibition. As with the PPI, however, the TriPM lacks a general positive manifold in that Meanness and disinhibition are highly positively correlated with one another but uncorrelated with Boldness. Boldness appears to be another indicator of FD, uncorrelated with most measures of psychopathy and antisocial outcomes but highly correlated with FD and salubrious outcomes (Miller, Lamkin, Maples-Keller, & Lynam, 2016). Again, the FFM provides a compelling explanation. The strongest correlates of Meanness and disinhibition are Agreeableness ($r = -.82$ for Meanness and $-.40$ for disinhibition) and Conscientiousness ($r = -.36$ for Meanness and $-.62$ for disinhibition), but the strongest correlates of Boldness are Neuroticism ($r = -.73$), Extraversion ($r = .70$), and Conscientiousness ($r = +.40$). Thus, Meanness and disinhibition are highly correlated with one another but uncorrelated with Boldness.

The epidemiology of psychopathy

Understanding psychopathy using traits from the FFM provides a parsimonious and compelling explanation for many of the epidemiological facts that surround psychopathy, specifically its relations to other personality disorders and its distribution across gender and age. This explanation makes use of the vast empirical literature on the FFM, which provides the FFM coordinates for all PDs, gender differences in each of the facets, and the relations between age and mean trait levels.

In terms of comorbidity, psychopathy and other PDs should be comorbid to the extent that they assess similar traits. Lynam and Derefinko (2006) generated correlations between the FFM profiles for psychopathy and the other PDs, providing a comorbidity estimate for psychopathy with each PD. Some PDs were predicted to be highly comorbid with psychopathy, whereas others were predicted to very distinct. For example, psychopathy and antisocial PD should be highly comorbid (i.e., predicted $r = .88$) as both are characterized by low scores on all facets of Agreeableness, several facets of Conscientiousness, anxiousness, and self-consciousness, and high scores on impulsiveness, assertiveness, and excitement seeking. In contrast, psychopathy should not co-occur with dependent PD (i.e., predicted $r = -.84$) as they are characterized by opposite poles of the Agreeableness facets, several Neuroticism facets (i.e., anxiousness, self-consciousness, and vulnerability), and two facets of Extraversion (i.e., assertiveness and excitement seeking). When compared to meta-analytically derived comorbidities, the predicted comorbidities aligned very well.

With regard to gender differences, Lynam and Miller (2015), extending work by Lynam and Widiger (2007b), used what is known about gender differences in FFM traits to predict gender differences in personality disorders, including psychopathy. Sex differences are predicted to be large for PDs that are characterized by FFM facets exhibiting large sex differences. For example, men score lower than women on all facets of Agreeableness, anxiousness, self-consciousness, and vulnerability; both Antisocial Personality Disorder (ASPD) and psychopathy are characterized by low scores on all of these facets as well. Thus, ASPD and psychopathy were predicted to be more common among men than women. In contrast, dependent personality disorder (DPD) is characterized by high scores on anxiety, self-consciousness, vulnerability, trust, compliance, and modesty; women score higher than men on each of these facets. Thus, DPD was expected to be more common among women than among men. These FFM-based estimates were then compared to empirical results from studies of sex-differences in the PDs. Across the PDs, the estimated differences were quite similar to the observed differences.

Using similar logic, Vachon et al. (2013) examined the ability of the FFM to account for age-related changes in psychopathy assessed via the PCL–R (Hare, 2003). These authors posited that the prevalence of psychopathy will change across the life course in synchrony with normative changes in the FFM traits underlying psychopathy. Normative changes in absolute levels of the traits that comprise psychopathy were obtained from a large sample of adolescents and adults (McCrae et al., 2005). Using FFM profiles of overall psychopathy, Factor 1, Factor 2, and antisocial PD as a comparison, the authors used the normative information on trait changes to make specific predictions about changes in psychopathy across the life course. These predicted changes were compared to prevalence estimates based on the explicit assessment of psychopathy in a forensic setting. Results demonstrated that the FFM trait information (1) predicted the rate of decline for psychopathy over the life span, (2) discriminated the decline of psychopathy from that of a similar disorder, Antisocial Personality Disorder, and (3) accurately predicted the differential decline of two psychopathy factors.

Possible etiologically relevant deficits

Much research in psychopathy is aimed at identifying *the* core deficit underlying the disorder. Many candidate deficits have been proposed; unfortunately, these various deficits are not easily subsumed under a single construct. This is exactly the state of affairs expected if psychopathy were a constellation of diverse traits from a general model of personality; different researchers are focusing on different elements or domains of the larger psychopathy–personality profile. Several theories suggest that psychopathy is rooted in deficient fear conditioning (Lykken, 1995; Patrick, 1994), which has been related to the broad domain of negative affectivity; in contrast to deficient fear conditioning, Newman's (1998) response modulation model is focused on a different area of functioning. Newman has offered that psychopaths have a difficult time suspending a reward-based response set in order to assimilate feedback from the environment. This deficit is more likely to be linked to aspects of psychopathy related to impulse control – impulsiveness, excitement seeking, and facets from Conscientiousness. Still other researchers have focused on deficits in empathic responding as a core deficit of psychopathy (Blair, 2001). These deficits in empathy would seem to align fairly straightforwardly with low Agreeableness.

Conclusion

Not only is there a tremendous research base supporting the FFM, but there is also a tremendous research base emanating from it. Understanding psychopathy from this framework allows this massive body of basic research to be brought to bear on psychopathy to inform assessment, etiology, course, and treatment. Multiple researchers are studying the development and continuity of FFM traits over time (e.g., Caspi et al., 2005; De Clercq & De Fruyt, 2012). Other researchers study the processes underlying and outcomes attributable to specific domains within the FFM. Several researchers are studying the basic processes underlying Agreeableness (e.g., Meier et al., 2006; Graziano & Tobin, 2002) and Conscientiousness (e.g., Roberts et al., 2005). Others are examining negative affective traits, including anxiety, depression, and shame or guilt, and how these emotions relate to behavior (e.g., Beer, Heerey, Keltner, Scabini, & Knight, 2003). To the extent that psychopathy can be connected to this vast literature, this empirical literature can be leveraged to increase our understanding of psychopathy.

References

Allik, J., and McCrae, R. R. (2004) 'Toward a geography of personality traits: Patterns of profiles across 36 cultures,' *Journal of Cross-Cultural Psychology*, *35*:13–28.

American Psychiatric Association. (2013) *Diagnostic and Statistical Manual of Mental Disorders* (5th ed.), Washington, DC: American Psychiatric Association.

Andershed, H., Ker, M., Stattin, H., and Levander, S. (2002) 'Psychopathic traits in non-referred youths: A new assessment tool,' in E. Blaauw & L. Sheridan (Eds.), *Psychopaths: Current international perspectives* (pp. 131–158), The Hague: Elsevier.

Barrick, M. R., and Mount, M. K. (1991) 'The big five personality dimensions and job performance: A meta-analysis,' *Personnel Psychology*, *44*:1–26.

Beaver, K. M., Boutwell, B. B., Barnes, J. C., Vaughn, M. G., and DeLisi, M. (2017) 'The association between psychopathic traits and criminal justice involvement: Results from a nationally representative sample of males and females,' *Crime & Delinquency*, *63*:708–730.

Beaver, K. M., Nedelec, J. I., de Silva Costa, C., Poersch, A. P., Stelmach, M. C., Freddi, M. C., . . ., and Boccio, C. (2014) 'The association between psychopathic personality traits and health-related outcomes,' *Journal of Criminal Justice*, *42*:399–407.

Beer, J. S., Heerey, E. A., Keltner, D., Scabini, D., and Knight, R. T. (2003) 'The regulatory function of self-conscious emotion: Insights from patients with orbitofrontal damage,' *Journal of Personality and Social Psychology*, *85*:594–604.

Blair, R. J. R. (2001) 'Neurocognitive models of aggression, the antisocial personality disorders and psychopathy,' *Journal of Neurology, Neurosurgery, and Psychiatry*, *71*:727–731.

Bogg, T., and Roberts, B. W. (2004) 'Conscientiousness and health-related behaviors: A meta-analysis of the leading behavioral contributors to mortality,' *Psychological Bulletin*, *130*:887–919.

Caspi, A., Roberts, B. W., and Shiner, R. L. (2005) 'Personality development: Stability and change,' *Annual Review of Psychology*, *56*:453–484.

Church, T. A. (2001) 'Personality measurement in cross-cultural perspective,' *Journal of Personality*, *69*:979–1006.

Cleckley, H. (1941/1988) *The mask of sanity*, St. Louis, MO: Mosby.

Collison, K. L., Miller, J. D., Gaughan, E. T., Widiger, T. A., and Lynam, D. R. (2016) 'Development and validation of the super-short form of the Elemental Psychopathy Assessment,' *Journal of Criminal Justice*, *47*:143–150.

Costa, P. T., and McCrae, R. R. (1988) 'Personality in adulthood: A six-year longitudinal of self-reports and spouse ratings on the NEO Personality Inventory,' *Journal of Personality and Social Psychology*, *54*:853–863.

Costa, P. T., and McCrae, R. R. (1992) *Revised NEO Personality Inventory (NEO PIR) and the NEO Five-Factor Inventory (NEOFFI) professional manual*, Odessa, FL: PAR.

Costa, P. T., and McCrae, R. R. (1995a) 'Domains and facets: Hierarchical personality assessment using the revised NEO personality inventory,' *Journal of Personality Assessment*, *64*:21–50.

Costa, P. T., and McCrae, R. R. (1995b) 'Primary traits of Eysenck's P-E-N model: Three- and five-factor solutions,' *Journal of Personality and Social Psychology*, *69*:308–317.

De Clercq, B., and De Fruyt, F. (2012) 'A five-factor model framework for understanding childhood personality disorder antecedents,' *Journal of Personality, 80*:1534–1563.

Decuyper, M., De Pauw, S., De Fruyt, F., De Bolle, M., and De Clerq, B. J. (2009) 'A meta-analysis of psychopathy-, antisocial PD- and FFM associations,' *European Journal of Personality, 23*:531–565.

DeLisi, M. (2009) 'Psychopathy is the unified theory of crime,' *Youth Violence and Juvenile Justice*, 7:256–273.

DeNeve, K. M., and Cooper, H. (1998) 'The happy personality: A meta-analysis of 137 personality traits and subjective well-being,' *Psychological Bulletin, 124*:197–229.

Derefinko, K. J., and Lynam, D. R. (2006) 'Convergence and divergence among self-report psychopathy measures: A personality-based approach,' *Journal of Personality Disorders, 20*:261–28.

Derefinko, K. J., and Lynam, D. R. (2007) 'Using the FFM to conceptualize psychopathy: A test using a drug abusing sample,' *Journal of Personality Disorders, 21*:638–656.

DeYoung, C. G. (2015) 'Openness/intellect: A dimension of personality reflecting cognitive exploration,' in M. Mikulincer, P. R. Shaver, M. L. Cooper, & R. J. Larsen (Eds.), *APA handbook of personality and social psychology, Vol. 4: Personality processes and individual differences* (pp. 369–399), Washington, DC: American Psychological Association.

DeYoung, C. G., Cicchetti, D., Rogosch, F. A., Gray, J. R., Eastman, M., and Grigorenko, E. L. (2011) 'Sources of cognitive exploration: Genetic variation in the prefrontal dopamine system predicts Openness/Intellect,' *Journal of Research in Personality, 45*:364–371.

DeYoung, C. G., Peterson, J. B., and Higgins, D. M. (2005) 'Sources of Openness/Intellect: Cognitive and neuropsychological correlates of the fifth factor of personality,' *Journal of Personality, 73*:825–858.

DeYoung, C. G., Quilty, L. C., Peterson, J. B., and Gray, J. R. (2014) 'Openness to experience, intellect, and cognitive ability,' *Journal of Personality Assessment, 96*:46–52.

Digman, J. (1990) 'Personality structure: Emergence of the five factor model,' *Annual Review of Psychology, 41*:417–440.

Eysenck, S. G., and Eysenck, H. J. (1970) 'Crime and personality: An empirical study of the three-factor theory,' *British Journal of Criminology, 10*:225–239.

Few, L. R., Miller, J. D., and Lynam, D. R. (2013) 'An examination of the factor structure of the Elemental Psychopathy Assessment,' *Personality Disorders: Theory, Research, and Treatment, 4*:247–253.

Graziano, W. G., and Tobin, R. (2002) 'Agreeableness: Dimension of personality or social desirability artifact?,' *Journal of Personality, 70*:695–727.

Hare, R. D. (1985) 'Comparison of procedures for the assessment of psychopathy,' *Journal of Consulting and Clinical Psychology, 53*:7–16.

Hare, R. D. (1991) *Manual for the Psychopathy Checklist–Revised*, Toronto, ON: Multi-Health Systems.

Hare, R. D. (1999) 'Psychopathy as a risk factor for violence,' *Psychiatric Quarterly, 70*:181–197.

Hare, R. D. (2003) *The Hare Psychopathy Checklist–Revised* (2nd ed.), Toronto, ON: Multi-Health Systems, Inc.

Hoyle, R. H., Fejfar, M. C., and Miller, J. D. (2000) 'Personality and sexual risk taking: A quantitative review,' *Journal of Personality, 68*:1203–1231.

John, O. P., and Srivastava, S. (1999) 'The big five trait taxonomy: History, measurement, and theoretical perspectives,' in L. A. Pervin & O. P. John (Eds.), *Handbook of personality* (pp. 102–138), New York, NY: Guilford.

Jones, S. E., Miller, J. D., and Lynam, D. R. (2011) 'Personality, antisocial behavior, and aggression: A meta-analytic review,' *Journal of Criminal Justice, 39*:329–337.

Judge, T. A., Bono, J. E., Ilies, R., and Gerhardt, M. W. (2002) 'Personality and leadership: A qualitative and quantitative review,' *Journal of Applied Psychology, 87*:765–78.

Judge, T. A., Heller, D., and Mount, M. K. (2002) 'Five-factor model of personality and job satisfaction: A meta-analysis,' *Journal of Applied Psychology, 87*:530–541.

Kotov, R., Gamez, W., Schmidt, F., and Watson, D. (2010) 'Linking "big" personality traits to anxiety, depressive, and substance use disorders: A meta-analysis,' *Psychological Bulletin, 136*:768–821.

Levenson, M., Kiehl, K., and Fitzpatrick, C. (1995) 'Assessing psychopathic attributes in a non-institutionalized population,' *Journal of Personality and Social Psychology, 68*:151–158.

Lilienfeld, S. O., and Andrews, B. P. (1996) 'Development and preliminary validation of a self-report measure of psychopathic personality traits in noncriminal populations,' *Journal of Personality Assessment, 66*:488–524.

Lilienfeld, S. O., Watts, A. L., Smith, S. F., Berg, J. M., and Latzman, R. D. (2015) 'Psychopathy deconstructed and reconstructed: Identifying and assembling the Personality building blocks of Cleckley's chimera,' *Journal of Personality, 83*(6):593–610.

Lilienfeld, S. O., and Widows, M. R. (2005) *Professional Manual for the Psychopathic Personality Inventory–Revised*, Lutz, FL: Psychological Assessment Resources.

Lykken, D. T. (1995) *The antisocial personalities*, Hillsdale, NJ: Erlbaum.

Lynam, D. R. (2012) 'Assessment of maladaptive variants of Five-Factor Model traits,' *Journal of Personality*, *80*:1593–1613.

Lynam, D. R., Caspi, A., Moffitt, T. E., Raine, A., Loeber, R., and Stouthamer-Loeber, M. (2005) 'Adolescent psychopathy and the Big Five: Results from two samples,' *Journal of Abnormal Child Psychology*, *33*:431–443.

Lynam, D. R., and Derefinko, K. J. (2006) 'Psychopathy and Personality,' in C. J. Patrick (Ed.), *Handbook of the psychopathy* (pp. 133–155), New York, NY: Guilford Press.

Lynam, D., Gaughan, E., Miller, J., Miller, D., Mullins-Sweatt, S., and Widiger, T. (2011) 'Assessing the basic traits associated with psychopathy: Development and validation of the Elemental Psychopathy Assessment,' *Psychological Assessment*, *23*:108–124.

Lynam, D. R., and Miller, J. D. (2012) 'Fearless dominance and psychopathy: A response to Lilienfeld et al.,' *Personality Disorders: Theory, Research, and Treatment*, *3*:341–353.

Lynam, D. R., and Miller, J. D. (2015) 'Psychopathy from a basic trait perspective: The utility of a five-factor model approach,' *Journal of Personality*, *83*(6):611–626.

Lynam, D. R., Sherman, E. D., Samuel, D., Miller, J. D., Few, L. R., and Widiger, T. A. (2013) 'Development of a short form of the Elemental Psychopathy Assessment,' *Assessment*, *20*:659–669.

Lynam, D. R., and Widiger, T. A. (2007a) 'Using a general model of personality to identify the basic elements of psychopathy,' *Journal of Personality Disorders*, *21*:160–178.

Lynam, D. R., and Widiger, T. A. (2007b) 'Using a general model of personality to understand sex differences in the personality disorders,' *Journal of Personality Disorders*, *21*:583–602.

Malouff, J. M., Thorsteinsson, E. B., and Schutte, N. S. (2005) 'The relationship between the five-factor model of personality and symptoms of clinical disorders: A meta-analysis,' *Journal of Psychopathology and Behavioral Assessment*, *27*:101–114.

Malouff, J. M., Thorsteinsson, E. B., Schutte, N. S., Bhullar, N., and Rooke, S. E. (2010) 'The five-factor model of personality and relationship satisfaction of intimate partners: A meta-analysis,' *Journal of Research in Personality*, *44*:124–127.

Maples, J. L., Guan, L., Carter, N. T., and Miller, J. D. (2014) 'A test of the International Personality Item Pool representation of the Revised NEO Personality Inventory and development of a 120-item IPIP-based measure of the five-factor model,' *Psychological Assessment*, *26*:1070–1084.

McCrae, R. R., Martin, T. A., and Costa, P. T., Jr. (2005) 'Age trends and age norms for the NEO Personality Inventory-3 in adolescents and adults,' *Assessment*, *12*:363–373.

Meier, B., Robinson, M., and Wilkowski, B. M. (2006) 'Turning the other cheek: Agreeableness and the regulation of aggression-related primes,' *Psychological Science*, *17*:136–142.

Meier, B., Robinson, M., and Wilkowski, B. M. (2007) 'Aggressive primes activate hostile information in memory: Who is most susceptible?,' *Basic and Applied Social Psychology*, *29*:23–34.

Miller, J. D., Gaughan, E. T., Maples, J., Gentile, B., Lynam, D. R., and Widiger, T. A. (2011) 'Examining the construct validity of the Elemental Psychopathy Assessment,' *Assessment*, *18*:106–114.

Miller, J. D., Jones, S. E., and Lynam, D. R. (2011) 'Psychopathic traits from the perspective of self and informant reports: Is there evidence for a lack of insight?,' *Journal of Abnormal Psychology*, *120*:758–764.

Miller, J. D., Lamkin, J., Maples-Keller, J. L., and Lynam, D. R. (2016) 'Viewing the triarchic model of psychopathy through general personality and expert-based lenses,' *Personality Disorders: Theory, Research, and Treatment*, 7:247–258.

Miller, J. D., and Lynam, D. R. (2001) 'Structural models of personality and their relation to antisocial behavior: A meta-analytic review,' *Criminology*, *39*:765–792.

Miller, J. D., and Lynam, D. R. (2003) 'Psychopathy and the Five Factor Model of personality: A replication and extension,' *Journal of Personality Assessment*, *81*:168–178.

Miller, J. D., and Lynam, D. R. (2015) 'Understanding psychopathy using the basic elements of personality,' *Social and Personality Psychology Compass*, *9*:223–237.

Miller, J., Lynam, D., Widiger, T., and Leukefeld, C. (2001) 'Personality disorders as extreme variants of common personality dimensions: Can the five factor model adequately represent psychopathy?,' *Journal of Personality*, *69*:253–276.

Newman, J. P. (1998) 'Psychopathy: An information processing perspective,' in D. J. Cooke, A. E. Forth, & R. D. Hare (Eds.), *Psychopathy: Theory, research, and implications for society* (pp. 81–104), London: Kluwer Academic Press.

O'Boyle, E. H., Forsyth, D. R., Banks, G. C., Story, P. A., and White, C. D. (2015) 'A meta-analytic test of redundancy and relative importance of the dark triad and five-factor model of personality,' *Journal of Personality, 83*(6):644–664.

Patrick, C. J. (1994) 'Emotion and psychopathy: Startling new insights,' *Psychophysiology, 31*:319–33.

Patrick, C. J. (2010) *Triarchic psychopathy measure (TriPM)*. Retrieved from www.phenxtoolkit.org/index.php?pageLink_browse.protocoldetails&id_121601

Patrick, C. J., Fowles, D. C., and Krueger, R. F. (2009) 'Triarchic conceptualization of psychopathy: Developmental origins of disinhibition, boldness, and meanness,' *Development and Psychopathology, 21*:913–938.

Paulhus, D. L., Neumann, C. S., and Hare, R. D. (in press) *Manual for the Hare self-report psychopathy scale*, Toronto, ON: Multi-Health Systems.

Polaschek, D. L. L., and Daly, T. E. (2013) 'Treatment and psychopathy in forensic settings,' *Aggression and Violent Behavior, 18*:592–603.

Poropat, A. E. (2009) 'A meta-analysis of the five-factor model of personality and academic performance,' *Psychological Bulletin, 135*:322–338.

Roberts, B. W., Chernyshenko, O. S., Stark, S., and Goldberg, L. R. (2005) 'The structure of conscientiousness: An empirical investigation based on seven major personality questionnaires,' *Personnel Psychology, 58*:103–139.

Roberts, B. W., and DelVecchio, W. F. (2000) 'The rank-order consistency of personality traits from childhood to old age: A quantitative review of longitudinal studies,' *Psychological Bulletin, 126*:3–25.

Roberts, B. W., Jackson, J. J., Burger, J., and Trautwein, U. (2009) 'Conscientiousness and externalizing psychopathology: Overlap, developmental patterns, and etiology of two-related constructs,' *Development and Psychopathology, 21*:871–888.

Robinson, M. D., Wilkowski, B. M., Meier, B. P., Moeller, S. K., and Fetterman, A. K. (2012) 'Counting to ten milliseconds: Low-anger, but not high-anger, individuals pause following negative evaluations,' *Cognition and Emotion, 26*:261–281.

Ross, S. R., Benning, S. D., Patrick, C. J., Thompson, A., and Thurston, A. (2009) 'Factors of the Psychopathic Personality Inventory criterion-related validity and relationship to the BIS/BAS and five-factor models of personality,' *Assessment, 16*:71–87.

Samuel, D. B., and Widiger, T. A. (2008) 'A meta-analytic review of the relationships between the five-factor model and DSMIV–TR personality disorders: A facet level analysis,' *Clinical Psychology Review, 28*:1326–1342.

Schmitt, D. P., Realo, A., Voracek, M., and Allik, J. (2008) 'Why can't a man be more like a woman? Sex differences in big five personality traits across 55 cultures,' *Journal of Personality and Social Psychology, 94*:168–182.

Sherman, E., Lynam, D., and Heyde, B. (2013) 'Agreeableness accounts for the factor structure of the Youth Psychopathic Traits Inventory,' *Journal of Personality Disorders, 44*:1–19.

Soto, C. J., and John, O. P. (2012) 'Development of big five domains and facets in adulthood: Mean-level age trends and broadly versus narrowly acting mechanisms,' *Journal of Personality, 80*:881–914.

Tackett, J., Slobodskaya, H., Mar, R., Deal, J., Halverson, C., Baker, S., . . ., and Besevegis, E. (2012) 'The hierarchical structure of childhood personality in five countries: Continuity from early childhood to early adolescence,' *Journal of Personality, 80*:847–879.

Tellegen, A. (1985) 'Structures of mood and personality and their relevance to assessing anxiety with an emphasis on self-report,' in A. H. Tuma & J. D. Maser (Eds.), *Anxiety and the anxiety disorders* (pp. 681–706), Hillsdale, NJ: Erlbaum.

Tracy, P. E., Wolfgang, M. E., and Figlio, R. M. (1990) *Delinquency careers in two birth cohorts*, New York, NY: Plenum.

Tyrer, P. (2013) 'The classification of personality disorders in ICD11: Implications for forensic psychiatry,' *Criminal Behaviour and Mental Health, 23*:1–5.

Vachon, D. D., Lynam, D. R., Widiger, T. A., Miller, J. D., McCrae, R. R., and Costa, P. T. (2013) 'Using basic traits to predict personality disorder prevalence across the lifespan: The example of psychopathy,' *Psychological Science, 24*:698–705.

Vaughn, M. G., and DeLisi, M. (2008) 'Were Wolfgang's chronic offenders psychopaths? On the convergent validity between psychopathy and career criminality,' *Journal of Criminal Justice, 36*:33–42.

Watson, D., Clark, L. A., and Harkness, A. R. (1994) 'Structures of personality and their relevance to psychopathology,' *Journal of Abnormal Psychology, 103*:18–31.

Weiss, B., Miller, J. D., and Lynam, D. R. (in press) The elemental psychopathy assessment.

Whiteside, S. P., and Lynam, D. R. (2001) 'The Five Factor Model and impulsivity: Using a structural model of personality to understand impulsivity,' *Personality and Individual Differences*, *30*:669–689.

Widiger, T. A., and Lynam, D. R. (1998) 'Psychopathy and the five-factor model of personality,' in T. Millon, E. Simonsen, M. BirketSmith, & R. D. Davis (Eds.), *Psychopathy: Antisocial, criminal, and violent behavior* (pp. 171–187), New York, NY: Guilford Press.

Wiggins, J. S., and Pincus, A. L. (1992) 'Personality: Structure and assessment,' *Annual Review of Psychology*, *43*:473–504.

Williams, K., Paulhus, D., and Hare, R. (2007) 'Capturing the four factor structure of psychopathy in college students via self-report,' *Journal of Personality Assessment*, *88*:205–219.

Wolfgang, M. E., Figlio, R. M., and Sellin, T. (1972) *Delinquency in a birth cohort*, Chicago, IL: University of Chicago Press.

Yamagata, S., Suzuki, A., Ando, J., Ono, Y., Kijima, N., Yoshimura, K., and Jang, K. (2006) 'Is the genetic structure of human personality universal? A cross-cultural twin study from North America, Europe, and Asia,' *Journal of Personality and Social Psychology*, *90*:987–998.

4

Psychopathy and empathy

Michael J. Vitacco, David A. Lishner, Jeremy G. Gay, and Amanda Trice

Introduction

The construct of psychopathy has long been linked to deficits in empathy. In fact, deficits of empathy are considered a cardinal characteristic of the construct of psychopathy. From its earliest conceptions, such deficits were considered fundamental to the core of psychopathy. Cleckley (1941), considered one of the originators of the current construct of psychopathy, developed the first criteria for the classification of psychopathy. In his seminal book *The Mask of Sanity*, he listed 16 criteria he posited were part of psychopathy. Of these, several are linked to specific empathy deficits. For example, deficits of remorse or shame, pathological egocentricity and incapacity for love, general poverty in major affective reactions, unresponsiveness in general interpersonal reactions, and sex life that is impersonal, trivial, and poorly integrated all could be conceptualized as arising, at least in part, from deficits in empathy.

Early conceptualizations of psychopathy have given way to newer, more empirically informed models of psychopathy. However, deficits in empathy and the presence of callousness/unemotional (CU) have remained key components of all models. For instance, Hare's (1979) early work that formed the basis for the Psychopathy Checklist (PCL) integrated lack of empathy and callousness in a state-of-the-art assessment tool for evaluating psychopathy. Other instruments of psychopathy have followed suit. For example, Lilienfeld and colleagues developed the original and revised Psychopathic Personality Inventory (PPI; Lilienfeld & Andrews, 1996; Lilienfeld & Widows, 2005). The PPI–R contains a scale named Coldheartedness that includes items with content that refers to a diminished capacity for empathy and a lack of emotional responsivity to others. Additionally, a more recent model of psychopathy referred to as the Triarchic Psychopathy Model consists of three factors, one of which (Meanness) can be conceptualized as involving deficiency in the capacity for empathy and callousness toward others (Patrick, Fowles, & Krueger, 2009). An important consideration moving forward is that callousness/unemotional traits seems to capture a range of traits (of which one or more forms of empathy impairment may be included). Some of the youth measures of callous traits seem to include a subset of traits that measure a general sense of apathy toward events in general, not just impoverished social emotionality toward others. The Psychopathy Checklist–Revised (PCL–R) and Self-Report Psychopathy scale (SRP) seem to assess callousness as impoverished social emotionality toward others, and the PPI seems to assess callousness (i.e., Coldheartedness) as low empathy. Clinicians and researchers must be mindful of what measure they are using and how CU is defined.

In Blair's (2005a, 2005b) neurobiological model of psychopathy, he suggests that psychopathy involves deficits in affect recognition and experience. These deficits pertain particularly to the recognition and experience of negative states in others, which can be interpreted as a form of empathy deficiency. Indeed, based on the conceptual linkage between psychopathy and empathy as well as his interpretation of empirical and clinical research regarding brain dysfunction and emotional processing among those high in psychopathy, Soderstrom (2003) referred to psychopathy as a disorder of empathy. The fundamental description of empathy deficits in psychopathy has been a focus of considerable research, and much of it will be discussed in this chapter.

As noted, all major theoretical formulations of psychopathy include some reference to empathic deficits. These formulations have, in turn, informed measurement. This background forms the foundation for this specialty chapter focusing on the relationship between empathy and psychopathy. In considering this relationship, this chapter will take a developmental perspective that delineates findings with both youth and adults. As part of this developmental approach, various measurement strategies will be reviewed with consideration of how they measure and incorporate empathy deficits. Definitions of empathy also will be explored, some of which have been virtually ignored by many psychopathy researchers. Such restrictions may have led to a restricted view of the linkage between psychopathy and empathy. Specificity and clarity on these constructs are required, especially as psychopathy has increasingly made its way into the legal arena (see Farahany, 2016; Vitacco, Erickson, & Lishner, 2013; Gazzaniga, 2011; Morse, 2008; Litton, 2007).

What is empathy?

It is important to realize that many definitions of empathy exist in the literature. As such, it is necessary to be specific as to the particular type of empathy deficit being described. The most basic definition of empathy provided by the Oxford dictionary (Empathy, 2017) is the "ability to understand and share the feelings of another." However, empathy is complex and involves multiple aspects. As noted by Batson (2009, 2011), empathy can be viewed as consisting of eight distinct but related phenomena. These phenomena in include the following: (1) accurately identifying what another person is thinking or feeling; (2) imagining what another person is feeling; (3) imagining how oneself would feel in the place of another; (4) aesthetically projecting oneself into the state of another individual or object; (5) feeling the same emotion as another; (6) feeling other-oriented concern for another; (7) feeling personally distressed by another's negative situation; and (8) matching the behavioral posture of another. When considering the relationship between empathy impairments and psychopathy, it is necessary to fully unpack the concept of empathy into its distinct parts in order to obtain a more coherent and nuanced understanding of this relationship. In fact, it may very well be that psychopathy is related to some empathy impairments but not others.

Broad discussions of empathy, although helpful in framing the discussion, often fail to pinpoint specific deficits or definitions. A prime and broad example is considering differences between cognitive and affective empathy (Buck, Powers, & Hull, 2017). Many clinicians fail to accurately differentiate between these two global categories of empathy, even though they are quite distinct. Specifically, cognitive empathy refers to the attempt or ability to understand what someone is thinking or feeling (Eisenberg & Miller, 1987; Kohler, 1929). This can be measured by being able to accurately indicate what another is feeling (e.g., Ickes 1993). In contrast, affective empathy describes affective processes of emotionally reacting to or feeling what another is experiencing (Baron-Cohen & Wheelwright, 2004; Blair, 2005a, 2005b). But even the broader conceptualization of cognitive and affective empathy may be further subdivided into many of the concepts of empathy noted previously. Thus, as much as possible, an effort will be made to clarify the exact nature of the empathic deficits examined in the cited studies. Hopefully, this will allow a fuller and more nuanced discussion of psychopathy constructs associated with empathy, which will facilitate a deeper appreciation of the complex relationship between psychopathy and empathy.

What is psychopathy?

When considering the construct of psychopathy, one of the most widely used and simplistic definitions was written by Hare (1996:26) and adopted by the Society for the Scientific Study of Psychopathy. According to this definition, psychopathy is a

> constellation of traits that comprises affective features, interpersonal features, as well as impulsive and antisocial behaviors. The affective features include lack of guilt, empathy, and deep emotional attachments to others; the interpersonal features include narcissism and superficial charm; and the impulsive and antisocial behaviors include dishonesty, manipulativeness, and reckless risk-taking.

That said, one of the most contentious areas in the field of psychopathy over the last decade has been the debate over the adequacy of this proposed structure (Cooke & Mickie, 2001; Hare, 2003). This debate goes well beyond the scope of this chapter. Nonetheless, as noted previously, virtually all models of psychopathy include a component that features callousness and impairments in empathy.

Psychopathy, empathy, and Conduct Disorder in youth

Like their adult counterparts, theories of youth psychopathy have highlighted cognitive and affective empathy deficits as an essential aspect of psychopathy (Brouns et al., 2013). These deficits are commonly linked to the presence of CU personality characteristics (Frick, 2004, 2009; Frick, Cornell, Barry, Bodin, & Dane, 2003). To that end, the measurement of CU traits has been incorporated into youth measures of psychopathy. Instruments such as the Psychopathy Checklist: Youth Version (PCL: YV; Forth, Kosson, & Hare, 2003), Antisocial Processing Screening Device (APSD; Frick & Hare, 2001), Inventory of Callous Unemotional Traits (ICU; Frick, 2004), and the Youth Psychopathic Traits Inventory (YPI; Andershed, Kerr, Stattin, & Levander, 2002) all highlight empathy deficiency and the presence of CU as part of the core of psychopathy. Clinically, the presence of psychopathic traits has significant behavioral and treatment ramifications, especially the presence of CU traits (Salekin, Worley, & Grimes, 2010).

The most widely researched instrument available for measuring psychopathic traits in youth is the PCL: YV (Forth, Kosson, & Hare, 2003; Cauffman, Kimonis, Dmitrieva, & Monahan, 2009). The PCL: YV consists of four distinct yet related facets. These facets include interpersonal, affective, lifestyle, and antisocial behavior (Neumann, Kosson, Forth, & Hare, 2006). With regards to empathy, the affective facet is related to empathic deficits and includes items related to CU traits, shallow affect, and not accepting responsibility for their behavior (Forth, Kosson, & Hare, 2003). In considering the affective facet, the PCL: YV manual provides a description of what an evaluator should consider when scoring this facet, which involves looking for evidence of the behavior across life domains. For example, it is necessary to consider if the adolescent manifests the behavior at home and school or if the lack of empathy is confined to very limited circumstance (e.g., interactions with a particular teacher). Notably, Kosson and colleagues (Kosson, Cyterski, Steuerwald, Neumann, & Walker-Matthews, 2002) have indicated the PCL: YV represents a coherent syndrome, similar to psychopathic traits manifested in adulthood. Yet, it is also key to understand that the empathic deficits evidenced in adolescents high on psychopathy should not be considered life-long. Instead, these deficits should be considered part of a distinct developmental phase (Seagrave & Grisso, 2002; Vitacco, Salekin, & Rogers, 2010).

In the most recent iteration of the Diagnostic and Statistical Manual of Mental Disorders by the American Psychiatric Association (APA, 2013), Conduct Disorder is described as a "repetitive and persistent pattern of behavior in which the basic rights of others or major age-appropriate societal norms or rules are violated" (p. 469). Fifteen specific behaviors are considered consistent with the disorder. A change to the diagnosis of Conduct Disorder from previous DSM editions is the addition of specifiers. Most germane to this chapter is the specifier "callous–lack of empathy." Specifically, the callous–lack of empathy specifier includes the following definition: "Disregards and is unconcerned about the feelings of others. The individual is described as cold and uncaring" (APA, 2013:470).

Certainly, as noted above, lack of empathy is found in both a formal diagnosis of Conduct Disorder and within items related to psychopathy. However, in order to more fully understand the relationship among these two constructs, we must turn to several studies that have relied on experimental paradigms to explore empathic deficits in youth as a function of psychopathic traits, as well as some research that evaluates behavioral indices of low empathy.

Experimental paradigms: psychopathy and empathy in youth

In addition to measurement, multiple studies have addressed the relationship between psychopathic traits and empathy through the use of experimental paradigms. In an influential study, Dadds and colleagues (2006) evaluated the ability of children and adolescents to recognize fear in others. Notably, differential findings were found for youth with antisocial behavior compared to youth with CU traits. Youth with antisocial behavior tended to "oversee hostility" compared to youth with CU traits, who present with significant deficits observing fear in people's faces. The authors attributed the lack of ability to recognize fear to the amygdala, which is an area of the brain widely implicated in psychopathy research and reduced sensitivity to understanding and identifying others' pain responses (Marsh et al., 2013). Several studies have examined the influence of CU traits on attachment issues with insightful results. For example, Dadds, Jambrak, Pasalich, Hawes, and Brennan (2011) found boys with higher levels of CU traits had deficits in eye contact toward their parents. To that end, Han, Alders, Greening, Neufeld, and Mitchell (2012) used functional magnetic resonance imaging (fMRI) to study brain activation responding to fearful stimuli. The findings implicate the amygdala in these empathy tasks; specifically, individuals with higher levels of CU traits showed less activity in the amygdala and prefrontal cortex.

The exact implication of this brain-connection to empathy remains unknown, but it may be shown in manifestations of violent behavior. For instance, one study found adolescents with higher levels of CU traits who engaged in violence were more likely to significantly injure their victim compared to adolescents with lower levels of CU traits (Vitacco, Caldwell, Van Rybroek, & Gabel, 2007). Yet, there other differences manifested as a function of CU traits, including the engagement of instrumental aggression. Instrumental aggression or violence is considered cold-blooded, planned, goal-directed, and provoking in nature (see Cornell et al., 1996). Multiple studies have demonstrated that higher levels of CU and interpersonal traits associated with psychopathy tend to engage in higher levels of instrumental violence (Blair, 2001; Vitacco, Neumann, & Caldwell, 2010). As shown by Flight and Forth (2007), who studied 51 incarcerated adolescents, psychopathy, especially the personality traits, were associated with instrumental violence. What is empirically unclear but would be expected based on the assumed relation between psychopathy and empathy deficiency is that higher tendency to engage in instrumental aggression and violence among those high in psychopathy is due, at least in part, to deficiency in empathy. Specifically, reduced ability to feel distress or compassion for others results in lower inhibition of aggressive tendencies and the degree of violence one is willing to inflict on others. These findings and their important implications highlight the importance of seeking to understand the implications of callousness and its link to empathy deficiency on violence typology.

Beyond violence, there have been differences in aggressive cognition and affect experienced by adolescents depending on their level of CU traits. Pardini, Lochman, and Frick (2003:366) reported that the presence of CU traits was associated with having more positive associations with aggression and less focus on negative aspects of violence. The authors described this as a "specific social information-processing pattern," but such descriptions are also consistent with potential deficits in cognitive empathy, such that those high in psychopathy may not consider how aggression or violence impacts the experiences of others. Clinicians must also consider how diagnostic issues interact with CU traits. For example, Pijper et al. (2016) discovered deficits in affective empathy were associated with diagnoses of oppositional defiant disorder or Conduct Disorder. However, boys with autism spectrum disorder manifested deficits in cognitive, not affective, empathy. Other research by Pasalich and colleagues (Pasalich, Waschbusch, Dadds, & Hawes, 2014) found similar results in a clinic-referred sample of boys whereby Conduct Disorder and symptoms of autism were both clearly associated with deficits in cognitive empathy, but not clearly associated with deficits in affective empathy. Specifically, they found a larger negative relationship between CU traits and affective empathy in individuals with higher levels of autism spectrum symptoms (see Blair, 2010; Jones, Happe, Gilbert, Burnett, & Viding, 2010). In a longitudinal study, Brouns and colleagues (2013) studied a community sample of 126 females and 107 males to evaluate the association between cognitive empathy and psychopathy. As expected, psychopathy was associated with lower ratings of cognitive empathy.

A final issue worth considering is how CU traits are related to pathogeneses of psychopathy and the potential development of effective treatments. To date, the treatment of psychopathic traits in youth has received significant clinical and scholarly resources. Despite some documented treatment successes with adolescent offenders high in psychopathic traits, the results from these studies have been limited given lack of cross-validation and minimal attempts to evaluate generalizability of the findings. Moreover, the exact underpinnings of how treatment improves adolescent behavior has not been well elucidated. It is likely that changing contingencies in a highly regulated and structured environment is insufficient to long-term meaningful change in less regulated and unstable environments.

The research presented in this section related to empathy and psychopathy in youth is multifaceted. Effective treatments will likely need to mirror the complexity of development. In other words, it would not be sufficient to implement a one size fits all approach to treatment with youth manifesting antisocial behavior with concomitant CU traits. We are encouraging researchers to continue to develop tasks to study empathy in youth, as well as to be specific on the type of empathy being studied.

Another consideration for clinicians dealing with youth who lack empathy is what to do with them and how to most effectively manage them. Although there have been suggestions that youth who lack empathy are poor treatment candidates, strong empirical evidence exists to indicate there is reason to be optimistic concerning prognosis (Salekin, 2002). As reported by White and Frick (2010), fewer conduct problems, effective parenting, and higher standards of living all predicted a decrease of callousness (lack of empathy) over time. Moreover, intensive treatment has also shown success in minimizing the effect of lacking empathy (Caldwell, Skeem, Salekin, & Van Rybroek, 2006). Additional discussion will occur in the final section of this chapter on future directions

Antisocial Personality Disorder, empathy, and psychopathy in adulthood

Research with adults has focused on the intersection of psychopathy and Antisocial Personality Disorder. Typically, it has been noted that they are two distinct constructs with significant overlap. In classic research, Meloy and Gacono (1998) found only about 33 percent of inmates who were diagnosed with Antisocial Personality Disorder (ASPD) met criteria for psychopathy. Darke, Kaye, and Finlay-Jones (1998) found similar results in a sample of 200 inmates enrolled in a methadone treatment program. In their sample, they found 30 out of 32 individuals who scored high in the psychopathic range on the PCL–R also met criteria for ASPD. However, only 11 percent of individuals meeting criteria for ASPD met comorbid criteria for PCL–R-based psychopathy. Certainly, this demonstrates the importance of the personality-based items of psychopathy, including lack of empathy, in differentiating psychopathy from ASPD. This is exemplified by considering the DSM–5 (APA, 2013), which includes seven criteria for ASPD, three of which must be present to qualify for the diagnosis. Of the seven, only one deals with deficiency in empathy. Unlike its Conduct Disorder counterpart, there is no specific subtype dealing with lacking empathy. Notably, the only mention of psychopathy regarding DSM–5 ASPD references similar syndromes associated with "a pervasive pattern of disregard for, and violation of, the rights of others that begins in childhood or early adolescence and continues into adulthood" (APA, 2013:659).

The lack of inclusion and differentiation in the ASPD diagnosis for individuals with deficits in empathy is a limiting issue for the diagnosis. We suggest that, similar to Conduct Disorder, subsequent versions of the DSM would be well served to include a psychopathic variant with a focus on deficiency in empathic capacities. Research has shown critical differences between individuals with traits associated with psychopathy (e.g., callousness and lack of empathy) and ASPD without those traits. For instance, several meta-analyses have found moderate to large effect sizes between violence and criminal behavior as a function of psychopathy (Leistico, Salekin, DeCoster, & Rogers, 2008; Salekin, Rogers, & Sewell, 1996), with Factor 2 (facets 3 and 4) having a larger association with violent behavior compared with Factor 1 (facets 1 and 2). However, similar to adolescents, the situation changes when the outcome is instrumental aggression.

In a seminal study, Woodworth and Porter (2002) evaluated psychopathic traits and crime characteristics of 125 Canadian offenders convicted of homicide. As reported in the study, the homicides of individuals higher in psychopathy were more instrumental. As the authors reported, the

> results indicate that the PCL–R factor scores were differentially related to the instrumentality of homicides. Specifically, Factor 1 scores accounted for much more of the variance associated with the instrumentality of homicides, whereas Factor 2 scores did not contribute to this dimension.
>
> *(Woodworth & Porter, 2002, p. 443)*

As such, understanding the violence of individuals with psychopathic traits requires understanding that individuals with higher levels of interpersonal and affective traits may engage in different types of violence than individuals lower on these traits. In contrast, individuals who have Antisocial Personality Disorder without Factor 1 traits of psychopathy will primarily engage in reactive violence, the most common form of violent behavior (Cornell et al., 1996).

Experimental paradigms: psychopathy and empathy in adults

Experimental and correlational designs also have been used to advance knowledge on the relationship between psychopathy and empathy. Brook and Kosson (2013) applied a laboratory instrument of empathy in sample of 103 incarcerated adults to examine cognitive empathy. Results showed psychopathy was negatively related to accurately identifying emotional states in others. The inability to have a cognitive awareness of emotions in others is seemingly a hallmark of individuals with higher levels of the affective facet.

Lishner and colleagues (Lishner, Hong, Jiang, Vitacco, & Neumann, 2015; Lishner et al., 2012) noted a number of studies that report evidence of negative association between measures of psychopathy and measures purported to asses affective empathy. However, they also noted that many of these studies relied on indirect measures of affective empathy that can be interpreted as assessing other constructs besides empathy. For instance, much of the evidence of associations between self-report measures of psychopathy and self-report measures of dispositional empathy may arise in part or in whole due to common source method biases shared between the two types of measures (see Podsakoff, Mackenzie, Lee, & Podsakoff, 2003). Indeed, when Lishner et al. (2015) tested the "empathy-impairment hypothesis" in two large samples of undergraduate students using direct but covert measures of empathy designed to mitigate the influence of common source method biases, they found evidence that only psychopathic callousness was related to lower change in affect empathy for those in need.

Various affective recognition studies have been applied to adults, often considering the impact of psychopathy on people's abilities. In fact, a recent meta-analysis conducted by Wilson, Juodis, and Porter (2011), which relied on 22 non-overlapping studies with a total of 1,387 individuals, found psychopathy to be related to left amygdala dysfunction in evaluating and accurately determining emotions in others' faces. However, it is not just recognizing facial affect where deficits are manifested. Verona, Curtin, Patrick, Bradley, and Lang (2004) evaluated physiological reactions to sounds as a function of psychopathy in a group of 68 incarcerated individuals. In this study, individuals with higher Factor 1 scores on the PCL–R demonstrated decreased skin conductance to both unpleasant and pleasant sounds. They hypothesized that offenders high on Factor 1 would present with clear deficits in their emotional response.

This aforementioned research highlights a greater body of research describing how psychopathy is associated with lack of response to distress cues. Decety, Skelly, and Kiehl (2013) used an MRI to scan brains while individuals were viewing images of being harmed and in pain. They found that levels of psychopathy were related to brain activation, and higher levels of psychopathy predicted less brain activation in areas of the brain associated with empathic responses. Certainly, this research has implications for how individuals with higher levels of psychopathy empathize with others in pain. This is consistent with a study by Blair and colleagues (Blair, Jones, Clark, & Smith, 1997), who found individuals higher on psychopathy had reduced electrodermal responses to distress cues, but no differences to threatening or neutral stimuli.

The final study we will discuss in this section highlights the importance of moving beyond self-report to evaluate empathy. Through the use of skin conductance responses (SCR), Pfabigan, Sailer, and Lamm (2015) found differences as a function of psychopathy in offenders and controls with higher levels of psychopathy having lower responses to SCR. This result is consistent with previous research, discussed in this chapter, demonstrating lower levels of correlates associated with empathy as a function of psychopathy. However, results of self-report emotional responses were noteworthy. When compared to controls, inmates classified as high psychopathy responded to self-report measures consistent with controls, even in light of clear SCR differences. In coming full circle, this is what Cleckley (1941) referred to when he authored *The Mask of Sanity* – despite clear deficits in both affect regulation and emotion identification, individuals with high levels of psychopathy strive to appear normal and hide their lack of empathy. Or, as Hare (1993) stated in his book *Without Conscience*, psychopaths may know the words, but not the music.

Future directions

This chapter has focused on the relationship between psychopathy and empathy, both in terms of developmental aspects and how empathy deficiency may manifest behaviorally. A review of extant research indicates several research areas that are worth pursuing. There also remains a need for clinical applications that more fully and effectively treat individuals who are low in empathic capacities. The following are provided as areas that appear most undeveloped or offer the greatest potential to advance understanding of the role of empathy deficits as a function of psychopathy.

1 The use of experimental paradigms to evaluate the relationship between correlates of empathy (e.g., helping behavior) and psychopathy. For instance, Beussink, Hackney, and Vitacco (2017) found college students higher in callousness were less likely to assist someone in need of help. However, some of the unwillingness to help could be mitigated by using techniques to improve cognitive empathy. Results from experimental paradigms have had positive implications for both researchers and clinicians looking to better understand how lacking empathy can be related to antisocial behavior.
2 New, empirically supported treatment strategies are needed, specifically to deal with offenders with low empathy. To date, only one true treatment manual (Wong & Hare, 2005) has been developed and marketed to deal with offenders with low empathy. There have been some other reported treatment successes with juvenile offenders possessing psychopathic traits (Caldwell et al., 2006). However, these treatment successes have not been cross-validated, and the treatments are not manualized, although the goal of subsequent research is the development of systematic techniques to work with low empathy offenders. Moreover, this research needs to generalize across samples.
3 To date, physiological research has been central to understanding deficits associated with low empathy offenders (Shirtcliff et al., 2009). This targeted research has found clear evidence of physiological markers associated with high levels of callousness. Such research is useful to understanding developmental trajectories of psychopathic traits, such as callousness. However, little research directly examines the extent to which physiological makers of callousness reflect corresponding deficits in empathy.
4 Research has shed light on the effects of low empathy and callousness, traits of psychopathy on violent behavior, with clear links between callousness and instrumental violence in both adolescents and adults (Woodworth & Porter, 2002). This research identifies key aspects of antisocial behavior that may be associated with empathy deficiency, although clear empirical evidence is lacking. As such, an area ripe for future research would be to examine the extent to which the link between callousness and instrumental aggression and violence can be linked to corresponding deficiencies in various forms of empathy.

5 The fifth recommendation for advancing the inter-relationship between psychopathy and empathy is expanding resources in neuroscience devoted to their study. Recent advances in fMRI technology have led to insights into empathic deficits with individuals high in psychopathic traits. For instance, Decety, Chen, Harlenski, and Kiel (2013) demonstrated specific brain areas associated with deficits of empathy as a function of psychopathy using an fMRI. This application of imaging studies to experimental paradigms focusing on empathy may provide useful information for moving the discussion forward and increasing understanding of common brain areas associated with both constructs. Future research would be well served to continue to use advanced imaging techniques to add to the literature on psychopathy and empathic behavior.

6 The final recommendation in this section is recognizing that researchers must continue to expand both populations and contexts that have been previously understudied. Some examples of these areas include white collar crime, with a specific emphasis on so-called successful psychopathy (Hall & Benning, 2006; Lilienfeld et al., 2015; Steinert, Lishner, Vitacco, & Hong, 2017). Moreover, continuing to evaluate the relationship between psychopathy and empathy in community-based or even college students is needed. The continued movement away from non-clinical/non-incarcerated samples is a profitable approach to developing nuanced understanding of this relationship.

Conclusions

This chapter explored some of the ideas surrounding the notion that psychopathy is linked to significant deficits in affective and cognitive empathy. As evidenced by the information presented in this chapter, these deficits are clear in both adolescents and adults, notably with regard to psychopathic callousness. Evidence is found in both clinical and community samples, and the association may have real world consequences in the form of more injury and instrumental violence. However, the field of empathy, as it relates to psychopathy, has been buttressed by experimental paradigms and imaging techniques allowing for advanced study of brain areas and neural connections associated with empathy and empathic behaviors. Future research will continue to bring forth new developments regarding this relationship, and eventually, empirically supported treatments may be developed to more effectively work with high psychopathy individuals to improve their empathy and reduce future problematic behaviors.

References

American Psychiatric Association. (2013) *Diagnostic and statistical manual of mental disorders* (5th ed.), Arlington, VA: American Psychiatric Publishing.

Andershed, H., Kerr, M., Stattin, H., and Levander, S. (2002) 'Psychopathic traits in non-referred youths: A new assessment tool,' in E. Blauuw & L. Sheridan (Eds.), *Psychopaths: Current international perspectives* (pp. 131–158), The Hague: Elsevier.

Baron-Cohen, S., and Wheelwright, S. (2004) 'The empathy quotient: An investigation of adults with Asperger syndrome or high functioning autism, and normal sex differences,' *Journal of Autism and Developmental Disorders*, *34*(2):163–175.

Batson, C. D. (2009) 'These things called empathy: Eight related but distinct phenomena,' in J. Decety & W. Ickes (Eds.), *The social neuroscience of empathy* (pp. 3–15), Cambridge, MA: MIT Press.

Batson, C. D. (2011) *Altruism in humans*, New York, NY: Oxford University Press.

Beussink, C. N., Hackney, A. A., and Vitacco, M. J. (2017) 'The effects of perspective taking on empathy-related responses for college students higher in callous traits,' *Personality and Individual Differences*, *11*:986–991.

Blair, R. J. R. (2001) 'Neurocognitive models of aggression, the antisocial personality disorders, and psychopathy,' *Journal of Neurology, Neurosurgery and Psychiatry*, *71*(6):727–731.

Blair, R. J. R. (2005a) 'Responding to the emotions of others: Dissociating forms of empathy through the study of typical and psychiatric populations,' *Consciousness and Cognition*, *14*(4):698–718.

Blair, R. J. R. (2005b) 'The neurobiology of antisocial behavior and psychopathy,' in A. Easton & N. J. Emery (Eds.), *The cognitive neuroscience of social behavior*, New York, NY: Psychology Press.

Blair, R. J. R. (2010) 'Psychopathy, frustration, and reactive aggression: The role of ventromedial prefrontal cortex,' *British Journal of Psychology*, *101*:383–399.Blair, R. J. R, Jones, L., Clark, F., and Smith, M. (1997) 'The psychopathic individual: A lack of responsiveness to distress cues?,' *Psychophysiology*, *34*(2):192–198.

Blair, K. S., Richell, R. A., Mitchell, D. V., Leonard, A., Morton, J., and Blair, R. J. R. (2006) 'They know the words, but not the music: Affective and semantic priming in individuals with psychopathy,' *Biological Psychology*, *73*(2):114–123.

Brook, M., and Kosson, D. S. (2013) 'Impaired cognitive empathy in criminal psychopathy: Evidence from a laboratory measure of empathic accuracy,' *Journal of Abnormal Psychology*, *122*(1):156–166.

Brouns, B. J., de Wied, M. A., Keijsers, L., Branje, S., van Goozen, S. M., and Meeus, W. J. (2013) 'Concurrent and prospective effects of psychopathic traits on affective and cognitive empathy in a community sample of late adolescents,' *Journal of Child Psychology and Psychiatry*, *54*(9):969–976.

Buck, R., Powers, S. R., and Hull, K. S. (2017) 'Measuring emotional and cognitive empathy using dynamic, naturalistic, and spontaneous emotion displays,' *Emotion*, *17*(7):1120–1136.

Caldwell, M., Skeem, J., Salekin, R., and Van Rybroek, G. (2006) 'Treatment response of adolescent offenders with psychopathy features: A 2-year follow-up,' *Criminal Justice and Behavior*, *33*(5):571–596.

Cauffman, E., Kimonis, E. R., Dmitrieva, J., and Monahan, K. C. (2009) 'A multimethod assessment of juvenile psychopathy: Comparing the predictive utility of the PCL: YV, YPI, and NEO PRI,' *Psychological Assessment*, *21*(4):528–542.

Cleckley, H. M. (1941) *The mask of sanity*, St. Louis, MO: Mosby.

Cooke, D. J., and Michie, C. (2001) 'Refining the construct of psychopathy: Towards a hierarchical model,' *Psychological Assessment*, *13*(2):171–188.

Cornell, D. G., Warren, J., Hawk, G., Stafford, E., Oram, G., and Pine, D. (1996) 'Psychopathy in instrumental and reactive violent offenders,' *Journal of Consulting and Clinical Psychology*, *64*(4):783–790.

Dadds, M. R., Jambrak, J., Pasalich, D., Hawes, D. J., and Brennan, J. (2011) 'Impaired attention to the eyes of attachment figures and the developmental origins of psychopathy,' *Journal of Child Psychology and Psychiatry, and Allied Disciplines*, *52*(3):238–245.

Dadds, M., Perry, Y., Hawes, D., Merz, S., Riddell, A., Haines, D., . . ., and Abeygunawardane, A. (2006) 'Attention to the eyes and fear-recognition deficits in child psychopathy,' *The British Journal of Psychiatry*, *189*(3):280–281.

Darke, S., Kaye, S., and Finlay-Jones, R. (1998) 'Antisocial Personality Disorder, psychopathy, and injecting heroin use,' *Drug and Alcohol Dependence*, *52*(1):63–69.

Decety, J., Chen, C., Harenski, C., and Kiehl, K. A. (2013) 'An fMRI study of affective perspective taking in individuals with psychopathy: Imagining another in pain does not evoke empathy,' *Frontiers in Human Neuroscience*, 7:1–12.

Decety, J., Skelly, L., and Kiehl, K. (2013) 'Brain response to empathy-eliciting scenarios involving pain in incarcerated individuals with psychopathy,' *JAMA Psychiatry*, *70*(6):638–645.

Eisenberg, N., and Miller, P. A. (1987) 'The relation of empathy to prosocial and related behaviors,' *Psychological Bulletin*, *101*(1):91–119.

Empathy. (2017) In *Oxfordictionaries.com*. Retrieved December 20, 2017 from https://en.oxforddictionaries.com/definition/empathy

Farahany, N. A. (2016) 'Use of neuroimaging in the courtroom,' *Annual Review of Neuroscience*, *39*:1–20.

Flight, J. I., and Forth, A. E. (2007) 'Instrumentally violent youths: The roles of psychopathic traits, empathy, and attachment,' *Criminal Justice and Behavior*, 34(6):739–751.

Forth, A., Kosson, D., and Hare, R. (2003) *The Hare Psychopathy Checklist: Youth Version, Technical Manual*, New York, NY: Multi-Health Systems, Inc.

Frick, P. J. (2004) *The Inventory of Callous–Unemotional Traits*, New Orleans, LA: University of New Orleans.

Frick, P. J. (2009) 'Extending the construct of psychopathy to youth: Implications for understanding, diagnosing, and treating antisocial children and adolescents,' *Canadian Journal of Psychiatry*, *54*:803–812. Frick, P. J., Cornell, A. H., Barry, C. T., Bodin, S. D., and Dane, H. E. (2003) 'Callous–unemotional

traits and conduct problems in the prediction of conduct problem severity, aggression, and self-report of delinquency,' *Journal of Abnormal Child Psychology, 31*(4):457–470.
Frick, P. J., and Hare, R. D. (2001) *Antisocial processes screening device*, Toronto, ON: Multi-Health Systems.
Gazzaniga, M. (2011) 'Neuroscience in the courtroom,' *Scientific American, 304*:54–59.
Hall, J. R., and Benning, S. D. (2006) 'The "Successful" psychopath: Adaptive and subclinical manifestations of psychopathy in the general population,' in C. J. Patrick (Ed.), *Handbook of psychopathy* (pp. 459–478), New York, NY: Guilford.
Han, T., Alders, G. L., Greening, S. G., Neufeld, R. J., and Mitchell, D. V. (2012) 'Do fearful eyes activate empathy-related brain regions in individuals with callous traits?,' *Social Cognitive & Affective Neuroscience*, 7(8):958–968.Hare, R. D. (1979) 'Psychopathy and laterality of cerebral function,' *Journal of Abnormal Psychology, 88*(6):605–610.
Hare, R. D. (1993) *Without conscience: The disturbing worm of the psychopaths around us*, New York, NY: Pocket Books.
Hare, R. D. (1996) 'Psychopathy: A clinical construct whose time has come,' *Criminal Justice and Behavior, 23*(1):25–54.
Hare, R. D. (2003) *Manual for the Psychopathy Checklist–Revised* (2nd ed.), Toronto, ON: Multi-Health Systems.
Ickes, W. (1993) 'Empathic accuracy,' *Journal of Personality, 61*:587–610.
Jones, A. P., Happe, F. G., Gilbert, F., Burnett, S., and Viding, E. (2010) 'Feeling, caring, knowing: Different types of empathy deficit in boys with psychopathic tendencies and autism spectrum disorder,' *Journal of Child Psychology and Psychiatry, 51*(11):1188–1197.
Kohler, W. (1929) *Gestalt psychology*, New York, NY: Liveright.
Kosson, D. S., Cyterski, T. D., Steuerwald, B. L., Neumann, C. S., and Walker-Matthews, S. (2002) 'The reliability and validity of the Psychopathy Checklist: Youth Version (PCL: YV) in nonincarcerated adolescent males,' *Psychological Assessment, 14*(1):97–109.
Leistico, A. M., Salekin, R., DeCoster, J., and Rogers, R. (2008) 'A large-scale meta-analysis relating the Hare measures of psychopathy to antisocial conduct,' *Law and Human Behavior, 32*:28–45.
Lilienfeld, S. O., and Andrews, B. P. (1996) 'Development and preliminary validation of a self-report measure of psychopathic personality traits in noncriminal population,' *Journal of Personality Assessment, 66*(3):488–524.
Lilienfeld, S. O., and Widows, M. R. (2005) *Psychopathic Personality Inventory–Revised*, Lutz, FL: Psychological Assessment Resources, Inc.
Lishner, D. A., Hong, P. Y., Jiang, L., Vitacco, M. J., and Neumann, C. S. (2015) 'Psychopathy, narcissism, and borderline personality: A critical test of the affective empathy-impairment hypothesis,' *Personality and Individual Differences, 86*:257–265.
Lishner, D. A., Vitacco, M. J., Hong, P. Y., Mosely, J., Miska, K., and Stocks, E. L. (2012) 'Evaluating the relation between psychopathy and affective empathy: Two preliminary studies,' *International Journal of Offender Therapy and Comparative Criminology, 56*:1161–1181.
Litton, P. (2007) 'Responsibility status of the psychopath: On moral reasoning and rational self-governance,' *Rutgers Law Journal, 39*:349–392.
Marsh, A. A., Finger, E. C., Fowler, K. A., Adalio, C. J., Jurkowitz, I. N., Schechter, J. C., . . ., and Blair, R. J. R. (2013) 'Empathic responsiveness in amygdala and anterior cingulate cortex in youths with psychopathic traits,' *Journal of Child Psychology and Psychiatry, and Allied Disciplines, 54*(8):900–910.
Meloy, J., and Gacono, C. (1998) 'The internal world of the psychopath,' in T. Millon, E. Simonsen, M. Birket-Smith, & R. Davis (Eds.), *Psychopathy: Antisocial, Criminal, and Violent Behavior* (pp. 95–109), New York, NY: Guilford Press.
Morse, S. J. (2008) 'Psychopathy and criminal responsibility,' *Neuroethics, 1*:205–212.
Neumann, C. S., Kosson, D. S., Forth, A. E., and Hare, R. D. (2006) 'Factor structure of the Hare Psychopathy Checklist: Youth Version (PCL: YV) in incarcerated adolescents,' *Psychological Assessment, 18*:142–154.
Pardini, D. A., Lochman, J. E., and Frick, P. J. (2003) 'Callous/unemotional traits and social–cognitive processes in adjudicated youths,' *Journal of the American Academy of Child and Adolescent Psychiatry, 42*:364–371.
Pasalich, D., Waschbusch, D., Dadds, M., and Hawes, D. (2014) 'Emotion socialization style in parents of children with callous–unemotional traits,' *Child Psychiatry and Human Development, 45*(2):229–242.
Patrick, C. J., Fowles, D. C., and Krueger, R. F. (2009) 'Triarchic conceptualization of psychopathy: Developmental origins of disinhibition, boldness, and meanness,' *Development & Psychopathology, 21*(3):913–938.

Pfabigan, D. M., Sailer, U., and Lamm, C. (2015) 'Size does matter! Perceptual stimulus properties affect event-related potentials during feedback processing,' *Psychophysiology*, *52*(9):1238–1247.

Pijper, J., de Wied, M., van Rijn, S., van Goozen, S., Swaab, H., and Meeus, W. (2016) 'Callous unemotional traits, autism spectrum disorder symptoms and empathy in boys with oppositional defiant disorder or conduct disorder,' *Psychiatry Research*, *245*:340–345.

Podsakoff, P. M., Mackenzie, S. B., Lee, J., and Podsakoff, N. P. (2003) 'Common method biases in behavioral research: A critical review of the literature and recommended remedies,' *Journal of Applied Psychology*, *88*:879–903.

Salekin, R. T. (2002) 'Psychopathy and therapeutic pessimism. Clinical lore or clinical reality?,' *Clinical Psychology Review*, *22*:79–112.

Salekin, R. T., Rogers, R., and Sewell, K. W. (1996) 'A review and meta-analysis of the Psychopathy Checklist and Psychopathy Checklist–Revised: Predictive validity of dangerousness,' *Clinical Psychology: Science and Practice*, *3*(3):203–215.

Salekin, R. T., Worley, C., and Grimes, R. D. (2010) 'Treatment of psychopathy: A review and brief introduction to the mental model approach for psychopathy,' *Behavioral Sciences & the Law*, *28*:235–266.

Seagrave, D., and Grisso, T. (2002) 'Adolescent development and the measurement of juvenile psychopathy,' *Law and Human Behavior*, *26*(2):219–239.

Shirtcliff, E. A., Vitacco, M. J., Graf, A. R., Gostisha, A. J., Merz, J. L., and Zahn-Waxler, C. (2009) 'Neurobiology of empathy and callousness: Implications for the development of antisocial behavior,' *Behavioral Sciences and the Law*, *27*(2):137–171.

Society for the Scientific Study of Psychopathy. (2016) Retrieved December 26, 2017 from www.psychopathysociety.org/en/

Soderstrom, H. (2003) 'Psychopathy as a disorder of empathy,' *European Child & Adolescent Psychiatry*, *12*(5):249–252.

Steinert, S. W., Lishner, D. A., Vitacco, M. J., and Hong, P. Y. (2017) 'Conceptualizing successful psychopathy: An elaboration of the moderated-expression model,' *Aggression and Violent Behavior*, *36*:44–51.

Verona, E., Curtin, J. J., Patrick, C. J., Bradley, M. M., and Lang, P. J. (2004) 'Psychopathy and physiological response to emotionally evocative sounds,' *Journal of Abnormal Psychology*, *113*(1):99–108.

Vitacco, M. J., Caldwell, M. F., Van Rybroek, G. J., and Gabel, J. (2007) 'Psychopathy and behavioral correlates of victim injury in serious juvenile offenders,' *Aggressive Behavior*, *33*(6):537–544.

Vitacco, M. J., Erickson, S., and Lishner, D. (2013) 'Comment: Holding psychopaths morally and criminally culpable,' *Emotion Review*, *5*:423–425.

Vitacco, M. J., Neumann, C. S., and Caldwell, M. F. (2010) 'Predicting antisocial behavior in high-risk male adolescents: Contributions of psychopathy and instrumental violence,' *Criminal Justice and Behavior*, *37*(8):833–846.

Vitacco, M. J., Salekin, R. T., and Rogers, R. (2010) 'Forensic issues for child and adolescent psychopathy,' in R. T. Salekin & D. R. Lynam (Eds.), *Handbook of Child and Adolescent Psychopathy* (pp. 374–397), New York, NY: Guilford Press.

White, S., and Frick, P. (2010) 'Callous–unemotional traits and their importance to causal models of severe antisocial behavior in youth,' in R. T. Salekin & D. R. Lynam (Eds.), *Handbook of child and adolescent psychopathy* (pp. 135–155), New York, NY: Guilford Press.

Wilson, K., Juodis, M., and Porter, S. (2011) 'Fear and loathing in psychopaths: A meta-analytic investigation of the facial affect recognition deficit,' *Criminal Justice and Behavior*, *38*(7):659–668.

Wong, S., and Hare, R. D. (2005) *Guidelines for a Psychopathy Treatment Program*, Toronto, ON: Multi-Health Systems.

Woodworth, M., and Porter, S. (2002) 'In cold blood: Characteristics of criminal homicides as a function of psychopathy,' *Journal of Abnormal Psychology*, *111*(3):436–445.

5

Psychopathy and emotion regulation

Taking stock and moving forward

Carlo Garofalo and Craig S. Neumann

Introduction

Emotion regulation (ER) refers to the processes responsible for monitoring, evaluating, and modifying emotional experience to attain desired emotional states in the service of adaptive behavior (Gross, 1998, 2015; Thompson, 1994). From a clinical standpoint, a contemporary conceptualization defines ER in terms of six related components: (1) emotional acceptance; (2) attention to and awareness for emotions; (3) emotional clarity; (4) ability to engage in goal-directed behavior under intense emotional arousal; (5) ability to refrain from impulsive behavior under intense emotional arousal; and (6) ability to rely on a range of ER strategies that are effective in a given context (Gratz & Roemer, 2004). Difficulties in each of these domains are indicative of emotion dysregulation, which in turn is considered a hallmark of psychopathology (Fernandez, Jazaieri, & Gross, 2016; Aldao & Nolen-Hoeksema, 2010; Kring & Sloan, 2009). Although problems in ER have been linked to personality pathology (Carpenter & Trull, 2013; Dimaggio et al., 2017; Livesley, Dimaggio, & Clarkin, 2016), Conduct Disorder (Frick & Morris, 2004), and aggression (Davidson, Putnam, & Larson, 2000; Garofalo, Velotti, & Zavattini, 2017; Roberton, Daffern, & Bucks, 2012), research on ER and psychopathy has been limited until recently. Given that psychopathy involves fundamental personality pathology (i.e., disturbances in self and interpersonal functioning) and is strongly linked to aggression, empirical demonstration of the relevance of ER in psychopathy would further our understanding of the nature and development of this personality disorder. Such a demonstration could help elucidate possible mechanisms linking psychopathy and dissocial behavior, and to identify possible treatment targets for psychopathic individuals (e.g., maladaptive ER). Here, we first review the concept of ER, clarifying definitional issues. Then, we review historical and contemporary theories on the links between psychopathy and ER. Finally, we take stock of existing empirical findings and proffer a conceptual integration for the role of ER in psychopathy.

Emotion regulation: definitional issues and operationalization

Among the potential advantages of a multidimensional conceptualization of ER is the possibility of examining the dissociable nature of each dimension to elucidate if specific dimensions might be related to distinct forms of psychopathology (Gratz & Roemer, 2004). Yet, the preponderance of empirical evidence suggests that impairments in specific ER dimensions are more likely to reflect a broader underlying difficulty (i.e., emotion dysregulation). In particular, the different ER dimensions demonstrate weak discriminant validity, indicating that impairments across domains covary substantially, and thus it appears that ER disturbances vary by degree (i.e., low to high) rather than in kind (for a recent review, see John & Eng, 2014). This perspective has also been corroborated from a person-centered perspective. Specifically, using latent profile analysis in our current research (Garofalo, Neumann, & Kosson, 2017; Garofalo, Neumann, Kosson, & Velotti, 2018; Garofalo, Neumann, & Velotti, 2017), we have found across different ER measures and different populations (e.g., student, community, and offender samples) that individuals can be best subtyped in terms of different levels of ER skills across domains, rather than based on different constellations of ER difficulties (i.e., showing problems in some but not other ER domains).

Another critical issue in ER research concerns the jingle-jangle fallacy as it pertains to the operationalization of the ER construct. For instance, there can be confusion between the concept of emotional intelligence versus ER. Indeed, the concept of emotional intelligence has attracted heated controversies because of inconsistencies in its definition and operationalization across theoretical frameworks and assessment methods (Mayer, Salovey, & Caruso, 2008; Matthews, Roberts, & Zeidner, 2004; Locke, 2005; MacCann, Joseph, Newman, & Roberts, 2014). More specifically, some scholars adopt a broader definition of emotional intelligence, which includes concepts like assertiveness, impulsivity, relational capacities, self-esteem, self-motivation, empathy, happiness, and optimism (Petrides, 2009). However, when it does not include these more extended (and perhaps peripheral) concepts, measures of emotional intelligence appear to tap into the same dimensions that characterize contemporary definitions of ER (e.g., emotional awareness, clarity, and modulation; Gratz & Roemer, 2004; Salovey, Mayer, Goldman, Turvey, & Palfai, 1995), rather than representing a standalone construct. Thus, in the present chapter we consistently use the term ER for ease of discussion and sake of clarity.

In operationalizing the construct of ER, investigators often distinguish between ER ability (i.e., state) versus trait ER (Mayer, Salovey, & Caruso, 2002; Pérez, Petrides, & Furnham, 2005; Petrides & Furnham, 2001). ER ability, which is strongly associated with IQ, is an index of the potential capacity for ER, rather than assessing the typical expression and effectiveness of ER in daily life (i.e., trait ER). That is, ER ability is assessed explicitly by asking participants to complete "performance" tasks while focusing on the emotional content of hypothetical social interactions (Mayer et al., 2002). This can introduce a potential confound in relation to psychopathy, because research has documented that the emotional dysfunctions found in psychopathic individuals can be temporarily diminished when their attention is explicitly directed toward target emotional stimuli (Baskin-Sommers, Curtin, & Newman, 2011; Newman, Curtin, Bertsch, & Baskin-Sommers, 2010). In contrast, trait ER entails individual propensities in each ER domain as they naturally manifest in everyday life, which are typically assessed via self-report questionnaires (Salovey et al., 1995; Gross, 2013; Gratz & Roemer, 2004). Additionally, while ER ability includes competences related to emotions in others (e.g., emotion recognition) and social skills more generally, trait ER typically refers in large part to *intra*personal aspects of ER, which are the focus of the present chapter.

Psychopathy and emotion regulation: theoretical perspectives

Despite being one of the most intensively researched forms of personality pathology, and one that has long attracted the interest of clinical, personality, and forensic investigators (DeLisi, 2009;

Hare, 1996; Miller, Gaughan, & Pryor, 2008; Hare & Neumann, 2008), there are still substantive controversies regarding the nomological network of psychopathy (Verschuere et al., 2017). One of the most recent debates involves the relevance of Fearless Dominance(FD)/Boldness within the construct of psychopathy (Lilienfeld et al., 2012; Miller & Lynam, 2012; Crego & Widiger, 2015). While the broader debate regarding FD and psychopathy goes beyond the scope of the present chapter, an element that is germane to this chapter concerns the link between psychopathic traits and ER. That is, FD includes traits alternatively referred to as Stress Immunity or emotional stability (Patrick, Fowles, & Krueger, 2009; Lilienfeld & Widows, 2005; Sorman et al., 2016; Lynam et al., 2011), which tap into some aspects of the broader ER construct. As such, some conceptualizations of psychopathy appear to already embed in the psychopathy construct the notion of superior ER skills, at least in terms of adaptive functioning in short-term interpersonal situations (Lilienfeld et al., 2015; Patrick, 2011). Thus, the FD perspective departs from most conceptualizations of psychopathy which hold that it involves personality disturbance and maladaptive functioning (Hare, Neumann, & Mokros, in press). In this section, we review historical and contemporary perspectives that have addressed the link (or lack thereof) between psychopathy and ER difficulties, beginning with perspectives on the emotional experiences of psychopathic individuals.

Do psychopathic individuals feel emotions?

Before examining the relation between psychopathy and ER, it is helpful to discuss the issue of the emotional experiences of psychopathic individuals, a traditional topic of popular speculation and investigation (e.g., the cold, unfeeling psychopath). In general, equating the experience of certain emotions with emotion dysregulation may not be warranted (Tamir & Gross, 2011; Garofalo & Velotti, 2017). Moreover, the incapacity to experience a broad range of emotions in appropriate contexts is generally related with poorer ER (Werner & Gross, 2009). However, if psychopathy were characterized by a complete absence of emotional experience, this would make it difficult to examine and interpret findings on ER and psychopathy. One of Cleckley's (1941/1988:338) criteria for psychopathy was "general poverty in major affective reactions." Elaborating on Cleckley's description, some authors have argued that a genetically influenced inability to experience (negative) emotions lies at the core of psychopathy and is consequential for the development of its affective features (Fowles & Dindo, 2009; Cooke, Michie, Hart, & Clark, 2004; Patrick et al., 2009; Patrick, Bradley, & Lang, 1993; Blair, Peschardt, Budhani, Mitchell, & Pine, 2006; Frick & White, 2008; Lykken, 1995). This conceptualization has fueled the popular, but incorrect, belief that individuals with high levels of psychopathy are fundamentally devoid of emotions (Baskin-Sommers, 2017; Helfgott, 2008) and in turn do not need to engage in ER efforts (Dargis, Newman, & Koenigs, 2016; Long, Felton, Lilienfeld, & Lejuez, 2014; Patrick et al., 2009; Patrick and Zempolich, 1998). Yet, from the description that Cleckley (1941/1988:348) provided of this same criterion, it is evident that he did not consider psychopathic individuals to be devoid of emotions. For example, he described that

> vexation, spite, quick and labile flashes of quasi-affection, peevish resentment, shallow moods of self-pity, puerile attitudes of vanity, and absurd and showy poses of indignation are all within his emotional scale and are freely sounded as the circumstances of life play upon him.

Therefore, it appears that Cleckley describes abnormalities in the *type* of emotions that are experienced and expressed, as well as in the limited range of the emotional repertoire that psychopathic individuals experience. He clarified that psychopathic individuals become vexed and fret rather than experiencing grievance or sorrow, and connected the reduced range, maturity, and depth of feelings to an incapacity for object love, rather than describing a complete absence of emotions (Cleckley, 1941/1988). Notably, a limited range of emotional experiences and a rigid tendency to turn grievance into vexation appear consistent with impairments in at least some of the domains described in the definition of ER. Other, partly overlapping perspectives on psychopathy posited more specific deficiencies in the experience of fear and sadness (Blair et al., 2006; Lykken, 1995; Patrick et al., 2009). Yet, recent reviews and meta-analyses have indicated that the notion that psychopathy is related to an absence of (some) negative emotions is not supported by empirical evidence (Hoppenbrouwers, Bulten, & Brazil, 2016; Derefinko, 2015; Kosson, Vitacco, Swogger, & Steuerwald, 2016; Brook, Brieman, & Kosson, 2013; Jackson, Neumann, & Vitacco, 2007). Actually, among children (Cardinale & Marsh, 2017), youth (Salekin, Neumann, Leistico, & Zalot, 2004), and young adult (Colins, Fanti, Salekin, & Andershed, 2016) samples, psychopathic traits tend to be associated with increased levels of negative emotions. In adults, psychopathy seems largely unrelated to fear, anxiety, and sadness, but positively related to Anger, and negatively related to happiness (Hoppenbrouwers et al., 2016). There is also evidence of dysregulation in basic behavioral systems associated with positive and negative emotion across cultures (Hoppenbrouwers, Neumann, Lewis, & Johansson, 2015).

Overall, historical and contemporary descriptions of psychopathy seem to agree regarding dysfunctions in the experience of certain emotions (i.e., long-circuited, mature, and social emotions), rather than negative emotions *tout court* (for a review, see Hoppenbrouwers et al., 2016). With respect to investigators who hold some psychopathic traits are linked with adaptive functioning, they also posit that negative emotions are related only to the behavioral traits of psychopathy, because of their overlap with externalizing psychopathology, whereas the Interpersonal/Affective features (operationalized in terms of FD) that are considered unique to psychopathy are supposedly related to lower levels of negative emotional experience (Hicks & Patrick, 2006; Fowles & Dindo, 2009; Patrick et al., 2009). Recently, some scholars have proffered more nuanced views on the emotional experience related to psychopathy by parsing the broader construct of negative emotionality in narrow-band emotion families (Tellegen & Waller, 2008), as well as disentangling the theoretically central features of psychopathy into separate interpersonal and affective components (Hare & Neumann, 2005). In this context, it appears that psychopathy – including its affective features – might be related to lower levels of self-directed negative emotions, but greater levels of other-directed negative emotions (Benning, 2013; Lynam & Widiger, 2007; Meloy, 1988), and especially anger (Jackson et al., 2007; Hoppenbrouwers et al., 2016; Kosson et al., 2016). In sum, early theoretical formulations and empirical evidence highlight that psychopathy is associated with disturbances in emotional experience, as opposed to absence of emotion, and the pattern of findings appear consistent with difficulties in ER.

An historical journey into the relations between psychopathy and emotion regulation

If psychopathy is not related to the *complete absence* of emotional experiences, and in contrast there is good evidence for the presence of certain negative emotions, it stands to reason that individual differences in ER may be related to psychopathic traits. Nevertheless, the decision by some investigators to consider traits related to FD/Boldness (including emotional stability/Stress Immunity) as an important part of the psychopathy construct was based largely on an interpretation of Cleckley's (1941/1988) writings, specifically four of Cleckley's (1941/1988) 16 criteria for psychopathy – i.e., superficial charm and good intelligence; absence of delusions and other signs of irrational thinking; absence of nervousness or psychoneurotic manifestations; and suicide rarely carried out (Patrick et al., 2009). In particular, the criterion "absence of nervousness or psychoneurotic manifestations" seems the most intimately linked to the contemporary concept of ER. Cleckley described this criterion in terms of absence of anxiousness and worry. Besides the fact that an exclusive reliance on Cleckley's (1941/1988) original description "would be a rather dogmatic scholasticism" (Crego & Widiger, 2015:7), some investigators have pointed out that the context in which Cleckley saw his psychopathic patients may have had an influence and may explain the differences with other early descriptions of psychopathy (Neumann, Johansson, & Hare, 2013). That is, it is plausible that psychopathic patients were likely viewed as less neurotic (and by extension emotionally dysregulated) *relative to* the typical patients in the same institutions where Cleckley worked (e.g., suffering from psychosis or mood disorders), rather than in *absolute* terms (Vize, Lynam, Lamkin, Miller, & Pardini, 2016). Accordingly, Cleckley (1941/1988) went on to say that psychopathic individuals seemed free from psychoneurotic manifestations to the same extent as the general run of humanity, in turn leaving open the possibility of individual differences in ER among psychopathic individuals. Notably, in his description of the criterion "absence of nervousness or psychoneurotic manifestations," Cleckley (1941/1988:340) added that

> it is true he [the psychopath] may become vexed and restless when held in jails or psychiatric hospitals. This impatience seems related to his inability to realize the need or justification for his being restrained. What tension or uneasiness of this sort he may show seems provoked entirely by external circumstances, never by feelings of guilt, remorse, or intrapersonal insecurity.

Therefore, here again Cleckley seemed to refer more to the origins of emotional tension rather than to its complete absence, in line with his description of the emotional experiences of psychopathic patients.

Other early accounts of psychopathy placed less emphasis on the purported absence of worry and anxiety and related emotional stability (for a review, see Hoppenbrouwers et al., 2016). In one of the first descriptions of psychopathy ("*manie sans delire*" [mania without delusion]), a common characteristic of the patients described by Pinel (1806) was the presence of violent, *uncontrolled emotions* (Werlinder, 1978). Moreover, Karpman (1948), Arieti (1963), and McCord and McCord (1964) all agreed that individuals with psychopathy experience simple – short-circuited – emotions like tension, worry, and frustration related to current situations (but not long-term consequences). Specifically, Arieti (1963:302) posited that an *emotional immaturity* makes psychopaths "act at the spur of the moment, which relieves any tension they may experience," suggesting that impulsive behavior enacted by psychopathic individuals may represent a maladaptive effort to regulate emotions (i.e., negative urgency). In addition, McCord and McCord (1964) postulated that psychopaths were "*prone* [emphasis ours] to tension and frustration and experience intense but transitory emotions" (Hoppenbrouwers et al., 2016:4), which is one of the defining features of emotion dysregulation (Carpenter & Trull, 2013). Interestingly, an early review of historical descriptions of psychopathic personality found general agreement among scholars in considering emotional instability and low frustration tolerance (both intimately linked to emotion dysregulation; Carpenter & Trull, 2013) among the defining features of psychopathy (Albert, Brigante, & Chase, 1959).

Competing contemporary views on psychopathy and emotion regulation

An explicit reference to a lack of emotional stability remains in the Comprehensive Assessment of Psychopathic Personality (CAPP) model (Cooke, Hart, Logan, & Michie, 2012), but other contemporary conceptualizations diverge in the emphasis placed on emotion dysregulation (or, by contrast, emotional stability) in relation to psychopathic traits. Also, other scholars, in light of the lack of empirical support for a complete absence of emotional experience in psychopathy, have argued that individuals with psychopathic traits do feel emotions, but have difficulty regulating them (Baskin-Sommers, Stuppy-Sullivan, & Buckholtz, 2016; Harenski & Kiehl, 2010). Baskin-Sommers, Stuppy-Sullivan, and Buckholtz (2016) found that individuals with psychopathic traits showed normal reactivity to regret-inducing stimuli during a decision-making laboratory task but failed to adjust their behavior accordingly. This finding suggests that psychopathic individuals have difficulties using the information contained in an emotional experience to guide their behavior, which is considered an important component of adaptive ER (Werner & Gross, 2009; Gratz & Roemer, 2004). Harenski and Kiehl (2010), in contrast, argued that it is a low tolerance for frustration that triggers emotion dysregulation in psychopathic individuals. A similar perspective was also advanced by Gacono and Meloy (1994) from a psychodynamic perspective. Although these perspectives did not elaborate further on the role of ER in psychopathy, they do acknowledge the possibility that psychopathic individuals may have trouble regulating emotions, as is generally the case for other forms of personality pathology. In their *Guidelines for a psychopathy treatment program*, Wong and Hare (2005:12) posited that "anger and emotional management programs may be inappropriate with psychopaths for whom violence is clearly instrumental and not motivated by anger or other emotional states." However, when describing the specific treatment targets for psychopathic patients, they also clarified that one such target concerns "dysfunctional emotions and lack of emotional control," explaining that a focus on poor anger control and mismanagement of negative affect (such as Anger, resentment, and jealousy) might be appropriate for treating psychopathic offenders, especially those who engage in violent and aggressive behavior that are both instrumental and reactive. In addition, Wong and Hare (2005:14) also asserted that decision-making choices in psychopaths can be "compromised by high arousal levels (resentment/anger)." Overall, while research is needed to examine if affective arousal and emotion dysregulation play a role in the violent behavior enacted by psychopathic individuals, it is interesting to note that the potential relevance of ER in psychopathy is acknowledged for risk assessment and clinical purposes.

These perspectives, which highlighted dysfunctional aspects of ER, had in common a focus on the overarching syndrome of psychopathy. However, initial factor analytic research based on the Psychopathy Checklist (PCL) and its progeny (e.g., PCL–R; Hare, 2003) identified two factors underlying the psychopathy syndrome: one encompassing the interpersonal and affective features of psychopathy (Factor 1) and one encompassing the lifestyle and antisocial features (Factor 2). In relation to this conceptualization of psychopathy, the response modulation (RM) theory of psychopathy attempted to link impairments in specific ER domains with certain psychopathic features. In particular, the Interpersonal/Affective traits of psychopathy were hypothetically tied to poor attention to emotions (i.e., lack of emotional awareness and clarity), in turn explaining the reduced emotional reactivity linked to these traits. In contrast, lifestyle–antisocial traits were hypothesized to be related to problems in modulating emotions and behavior when upset (Patterson & Newman, 1993; Malterer, Glass, & Newman, 2008). As mentioned previously, however, whether specific components of trait ER are empirically dissociable and can be selectively impaired while other components remain intact is a notion that is still wanting in empirical support. In addition, a related postulate of the RM theory of psychopathy is that the reduced reactivity to negative emotional stimuli (and fear-inducing stimuli, in particular) in psychopathic individuals is qualified by attentional and motivational mechanisms. That is, psychopathic individuals do not show reduced emotional reactivity when their attention is directed to the emotional stimulus or when the emotional stimulus is motivationally salient (Baskin-Sommers et al., 2013; Newman et al., 2010). From this perspective, ER efforts could only be enacted in some circumstances, and only in those circumstances would it be possible for investigators to examine the effectiveness of these efforts.

The alternative FD/Boldness perspective, developed in the context of the dual-pathway model of psychopathy (Fowles & Dindo, 2009), proposed that emotion dysregulation may have opposite relations to distinct psychopathic trait domains. In line with hypotheses on the experience of negative emotions, some scholars have argued that problems in ER were exclusively related to behavioral (i.e., antisocial–lifestyle, corresponding to the earlier Factor 2 of the PCL–R) traits of psychopathy, because they are associated with externalizing symptoms and general psychological distress. Conversely, this model assumed that the Interpersonal/Affective traits of psychopathy (i.e., PCL–R Factor 1) were associated with intact ER, largely based on inverse associations between the unique variance in PCL–R Factor 1 and low levels of negative emotionality and internalizing symptoms (Fowles & Dindo, 2009; Hicks & Patrick, 2006; Long et al., 2014). Based on these considerations, these authors did not consider the construct of ER important for the development and manifestation of psychopathy.

Both these models (RM and FD/Boldness) were based on the earlier two-factor conceptualization of the PCL–R. As mentioned previously, however, while recent conceptualizations of psychopathy differ in the number and characteristics of the dimensions underlying psychopathic personality, they do agree in parsing interpersonal and affective traits into separate components (Neumann, Hare, & Pardini, 2015; Neumann, Schmitt, Carter, Embley, & Hare, 2012; Hare & Neumann, 2008; Neumann, Hare, & Newman, 2007; Sellbom, Cooke, & Hart, 2015; Cooke & Michie, 2001; Patrick et al., 2009; Lynam et al., 2011). Notably, studies that have adopted these conceptualizations have shown that the interpersonal and affective traits of psychopathy show differential associations with external correlates that are conceptually linked to ER. Indeed, these studies have provided emerging evidence for a positive link between affective traits of psychopathy and both negative emotionality (e.g., other-directed negative emotions; Benning, 2013; Benning, Patrick, Hicks, Blonigen, & Krueger, 2003; Lynam & Widiger, 2007; Jackson et al., 2007; Lishner et al., 2012) and general psychological distress (e.g., anxiety, depression; Colins, Fanti, Salekin, & Andershed, 2016; Neumann & Pardini, 2014). Other studies have shown that the interpersonal and affective components of psychopathy had differential associations with IQ (Salekin, Neumann, Leistico, & Zalot, 2004), executive functioning (EF) (Baskin-Sommers et al., 2015), and the behavioral inhibition and activation (BIS/BAS) systems (Hoppenbrouwers et al., 2015). Across these studies, the PCL–R interpersonal facet had positive associations with IQ and EF, while the affective factor was negatively related to IQ, EF, and BIS activity. These findings are in line with Hare's (1998:117) proposal that "psychopathy is associated with anomalies in cortical/subcortical structures and functional circuits responsible for the integration of cognition, affect, and behavior" and suggest that interpersonal and affective psychopathic traits may have distinct relations with ER as well (Bridgett, Oddi, Laake, Murdock, & Bachmann, 2013). Interestingly, in the recently developed triarchic model of psychopathy, Patrick et al. (2009) identified negative affectivity, poor effortful control, and poor ER (i.e., "difficult temperament") as developmental precursors of Meanness and disinhibition (akin to the affective and behavioral traits of PCL–R-assessed psychopathy, respectively), but not Boldness/FD, that capture interpersonal functioning. Thus, based on theory and empirical results, it seems important to examine the role of ER both in relation to overall levels of psychopathy and in relation to specific features of the broader psychopathy construct.

Psychopathy and emotion regulation: the state of empirical knowledge

When the experts disagree: prototypicality of emotion (dys)regulation for psychopathy

Studies that have investigated what features are prototypical of psychopathy in the eyes of experts and laypeople alike can also provide conceptual reasons to examine empirically the potential links between psychopathy and ER. When 15 psychopathy researchers from the United States rated the prototypical psychopath in terms of the five-factor model of personality, there was consensus for the inclusion in this profile of the low vulnerability facet of Neuroticism (Miller, Lynam, Widiger, & Leukefeld, 2001), which can be considered an index of intact or superior ER and seems aligned with the lack of psychoneurotic manifestations described by Cleckley. Similarly, Cooke and collaborators asked experts (e.g., researchers, mental health professionals) and laypersons to rate the extent to which each of the 33 traits included in the CAPP (Cooke et al., 2012) were prototypical of psychopathy on a 1 to 7 scale, considering average ratings ≥ 5 as indicative of prototypicality. This set of investigations has clear relevance for the present chapter in light of the inclusion in the CAPP of the item "lacks emotional stability," which "reflects problems with mood regulation, such as the tendency to experience shallow, labile emotions." Across four studies, the ratings of the *lacks emotional stability* item ranged between 4.74 (*SD* = 1.72) and 5.85 (*SD* = 1.30), thus placing the item at the edge of the prototypicality cut-off (Sorman et al., 2014; Kreis, Cooke, Michie, Hoff, & Logan, 2012; Florez et al., 2015; Hoff, Rypdal, Mykletun, & Cooke, 2012).

Examining the prototypicality of the item "emotional stability" as part of the Boldness construct, Sorman et al. (2016) found that only forensic mental health practitioners, but not probation officers and laypersons, rated emotional stability as prototypical of psychopathy. As noted previously, it could be that in the eyes of experts that are in contact with patients often presenting major psychiatric disorders, the *relatively* less disturbed and dramatic emotional manifestations of psychopathic patients is what stands out. Notably, also for forensic mental health practitioners, emotional stability was the least prototypical item within the Boldness construct. Likewise, Miller, Lamkin, Maples-Keller, and Lynam (2016) found that, although Boldness was associated with experts' prototypical ratings of Cleckley's description of psychopathy, it was not related to a meta-analytically derived profile of psychopathy based on the five-factor model. Moreover, researchers rated Boldness as significantly less prototypical of psychopathy compared to the other two domains of the triarchic model, Meanness and disinhibition (Miller, Lamkin, Maples-Keller, & Lynam, 2016). Overall, it appears that there is little agreement regarding the relevance of emotional (in)stability for the construct of psychopathy, and this is also reflected in the content of several widely used psychopathy measures.

The role of emotion regulation items in psychopathy measures

Based on theory-driven positions (mainly derived from Cleckley's writings) and expert consensus, items tapping on Stress Immunity/low nervousness were included in several psychopathy measures, including the first versions of the Psychopathy Checklist (PCL) and Self-Report

Psychopathy (SRP) scale (Patrick, 2006). However, these items were later dropped from the PCL, SRP, and other psychopathy measures (e.g., Minnesota Temperament Inventory-derived measure of Cleckley's criteria) due to their lack of construct validity, their poor performances in factor analyses, and their inconsistency in discriminating psychopathic patients in forensic populations (Hare & Neumann, 2008). For instance, in an early empirical analysis of Cleckley's 16 criteria, the item–total correlation for "absence of nervousness or other psychoneurotic manifestations" was only 0.05, indicating that it was unrelated to the construct measured by the total scale (Hare, 2003; Hare & Neumann, 2008).

As discussed, other psychopathy measures have retained scales that assess largely adaptive traits (e.g., FD/Boldness), including Stress Immunity. For example, the Triarchic Psychopathy Measure (TriPM) includes both emotion dysregulation (disinhibition domain) and the Boldness dimension of emotional stability (Patrick & Drislane, 2015; Patrick et al., 2009).[1] The current chapter does not aim to contribute directly to the debate about the presence of adaptive features in the construct and measurement of psychopathy. Nevertheless, an inspection of studies on the internal structure of such measures can help elucidate relations between psychopathic traits and ER. A chief example is the Stress Immunity scale of the Psychopathic Personality Inventory (PPI) and its derivatives (Lilienfeld & Widows, 2005). Notably, this scale has demonstrated weak or null correlations with the PPI total score and correlates negatively with other PPI scales, showing that most of the subscales that make up the Self-Centered Impulsivity (SCI) factor of the PPI are negatively related to Stress Immunity (Donahue, McClure, & Moon, 2014; Long et al., 2014; Benning et al., 2003; Neumann, Malterer, & Newman, 2008; Neumann, Uzieblo, Crombez, & Hare, 2013; Visser, Ashton, & Pozzebon, 2012). Accordingly, a recent meta-analytic factor analysis ($N > 19{,}000$) of PPI lower-order scales revealed that most PPI–SCI scales were robustly and negatively related to Stress Immunity (Ruchensky et al., 2017), which suggests that the bulk of psychopathic traits are associated with poorer ER.

A recent item response theory study also showed that the Boldness scale of the TriPM may include a sub-dimension measuring emotional stability (Shou, Sellbom, & Xu, 2017). These emotional stability items were found to capture individuals within a normal range of the latent trait and to reflect a blend of adaptive and maladaptive traits, as opposed to what was found for Meanness and disinhibition factors, which had greater precision at the positive end of the latent distribution, indicating that they capture maladaptive traits and are better able to discriminate between individuals with high and low levels of psychopathy. Recently, the CAPP model was refined to align with the triarchic conceptualization of psychopathy. Sellbom et al. (2015) documented adequate fit for a bi-factor model which included a general psychopathy factor and three bi-factors akin to Boldness, Meanness, and disinhibition. Interestingly, the "lacks emotional stability" item had a negative loading on the Boldness factor but positive loading on the general psychopathy factor, suggesting that if Boldness included emotional stability as theoretically expected, overall levels of psychopathy were partly defined by a lack of emotional stability.

Based in part on clinical expert ratings of the prototypical psychopath, an emotional stability scale was also included in the Elemental Psychopathy Assessment (EPA; Lynam et al., 2011) in order to "examine which elements are most central, which are peripheral, and which are unnecessary to the construct of psychopathy" (p. 5). Recent studies have shown that the emotional stability scale of the EPA correlated only weakly or non-significantly with other measures of psychopathy and with external criteria traditionally related to psychopathy (Collison, Miller, Gaughan, Widiger, & Lynam, 2016). Further, a network analysis of the EPA scales has revealed that one of the central nodes in the EPA–psychopathy network (i.e., one of the subscales with stronger associations with most of the other subscales in the network) was the invulnerability subscale of the emotional stability scale, but with negative sign, suggesting that one of the central features of psychopathy was low invulnerability (Carnovale, Carlson, Lynam, & Miller, 2017). This finding is partly consistent with a recent network analysis of the PCL–R, which revealed that the poor behavioral controls item (which includes poor Anger control) was a moderately central node in the PCL–R network across three samples (Verschuere et al., 2017). In sum, there is now emerging evidence that questions the role of the FD/Boldness construct as a whole and especially its Stress Immunity/emotional stability subdomains, and more importantly, this evidence suggests that disturbances in ER are likely very relevant to our understanding of psychopathy.

Insights from studies on emotional functioning

While the experts disagree, the empirical findings on the links between psychopathy and ER are beginning to become clearer. Some indirect evidence that psychopathic individuals may show problems in ER emerges from the long tradition of studies that have provided evidence for broad deficits in emotional processing related to psychopathy (Brook et al., 2013). Notably, emotional processing and ER are tightly linked throughout development (Dennis, Malone, & Chen, 2009) and share common neurobiological mechanisms (Reidy et al., 2017); therefore, it is reasonable that impairments in emotional processing and ER might also co-occur in the context of psychopathy. For instance, one function of emotional processing is to provide the individual with knowledge of the self and its impact on others, which in turn can guide emotion regulatory efforts, including the ability to modulate emotional arousal and corresponding behavior (Gratz & Roemer, 2004; Gross, 2014).

As discussed previously, there is evidence that challenges the notion of psychopathic "incapacity" to experience emotions. At the same time, blunted emotional reactivity traditionally linked to psychopathy (Cleckley, 1941/1988; Lykken, 1995) has been interpreted as tentative evidence that psychopathic individuals may exert cognitive or emotional regulation processes in an effort to minimize the negative impact of aversive stimuli (Shane & Peterson, 2004). From this perspective, such minimization of negative emotional responses could contribute to a hypo-reactivity to aversive information often seen in psychopathic individuals. Notably, previous research has documented that while these minimization strategies can be effective in the short-term by reducing negative affective responses, they are also associated with a variety of maladaptive outcomes, such as reduced fear-potentiated startle, impaired detection of pain-inducing stimuli, and inferior passive avoidance learning (Shane & Peterson, 2004). This perspective appears consistent with the possibility that individuals with psychopathic traits make chronic use of mechanisms of emotional suppression (Nentjes, Bernstein, Meijer, Arntz, & Wiers, 2016; Casey, Rogers, Burns, & Yiend, 2013; Hare, 1978; Albert et al., 1959), a maladaptive ER strategy that is linked to a plethora of negative outcomes, including trait emotion dysregulation and aggression (Gross & John, 2003; Roberton et al., 2012; Roberton, Daffern, & Bucks, 2014).

Another group of studies has used physiological and neurobiological indices to assess aspects related to ER and yielded mixed findings. Among youth, psychopathic traits have shown robust associations with abnormal autonomic reactivity that are considered indices of ER processes (i.e., patterns of sympathetic and parasympathetic activation; Munoz, Frick, Kimonis, & Aucoin, 2008; Munoz Centifanti, Kimonis, Frick, & Aucoin, 2013). Further, forensic patients with psychopathic traits showed increased cardiovascular response during an ER task, although no significant differences occurred on self-report ability to experience or suppress emotions between high and low psychopathic individuals (Casey et al., 2013). In contrast, a recent investigation did not find any significant group differences between high-psychopathic forensic patients, low-psychopathic forensic patients, and healthy controls on self-report, physiological, and facial expressive indices of emotion experience when participants were instructed to either express or suppress an emotion after a laboratory induction technique (Nentjes et al., 2016). That is, psychopathic offenders appear able to increase their emotional reactions when explicitly asked to do so (Nentjes et al., 2016; Meffert, Gazzola, den Boer, Bartels, & Keysers, 2013). Likewise, a recent study with undergraduate students reported that, despite reduced emotional activation in conditions of passive viewing, individuals with high levels of psychopathic traits (compared to a low-psychopathy group) did not show expected deficiencies in brain activation when instructed to regulate (i.e., increase/decrease) their emotional reaction to negative emotional stimuli. Further, participants in the high-psychopathy group self-reported greater emotional activation than low-psychopathy participants after being instructed to decrease their emotional response, suggesting that the regulatory efforts of individuals with high levels of psychopathic traits were not successful (Ellis, Schroeder, Patrick, & Moser, 2017).[2]

Taken together, these studies suggest that psychopathic individuals do show emotional reactivity, at least to some extent, and have some capacity to engage in efforts to modify their emotional response and associated behavior. Yet, these efforts can go awry, at least for some psychopathic individuals or in some contexts, and in particular, psychopathic individuals seem to be better able at increasing their emotional reactions rather than decreasing them. However, all of the above studies explicitly asked participants to engage in some form of ER. In so doing, these studies are valuable for examining the potential capacity for ER engagement, but unfortunately, they did not test the regular use and effectiveness of ER in everyday life.

Review of empirical studies on the association between emotion regulation and psychopathy

Emotion regulation ability

Studies that have examined associations between psychopathy and ER using ability measures of ER/emotional intelligence (i.e., the Mayer–Salovey–Caruso Emotional Intelligence Test, MSCEIT; Mayer et al., 2002) have revealed a negative association between overall levels of psychopathy and ER ability, as evidenced by a recent meta-analysis (Megias, Gomez-Leal, Gutierrez-Cobo, Cabello, & Fernandez-Berrocal, 2018). Across studies, these associations were strikingly consistent for the antisocial–lifestyle factor of psychopathy, but less so for the Interpersonal/Affective traits (e.g., Vidal, Skeem, & Camp, 2010; Ermer, Kahn, Salovey, & Kiehl, 2012; Howe, Falkenbach, & Massey, 2014; Visser, Bay, Cook, & Myburgh, 2010; Lishner, Swim, Hong, & Vitacco, 2011).[3] Interestingly, some of these studies showed that, by and large, psychopathy was related to widespread impairments in ER that spanned across the different components assessed in the ER task adopted (Lishner et al., 2011), in line with the possibility that the different ER components reflect a global ER disturbance rather than selected impairments. Studies examining ER ability, however, can only provide a partial view regarding the possibility that psychopathic individuals experience trait-like impairments in ER. Additionally, Megias et al.'s (2018) meta-analytic work showed important differences across studies depending on which measure of psychopathy was used, an issue that is also reflected in studies that have investigated relations between psychopathy and trait ER.

Trait emotion regulation

Studies based on Hare's (2003) PCL–R conceptualization have consistently shown that both the Interpersonal/Affective and the antisocial–lifestyle traits of psychopathy were related to poorer

ER across different populations (i.e., community and offender samples) and different assessment methods (i.e., self-report and clinician-rated), with relatively larger effect sizes for antisocial–lifestyle psychopathic traits (Grieve & Mahar, 2010; Malterer et al., 2008; Ali, Amorim, & Chamorro-Premuzic, 2009; Miller, Gentile, Wilson, Pryor, & Campbell, 2010). Also, across these ER studies, and consistent with those on ER ability, a pattern of select impairments in ER components related to psychopathy did not emerge. Instead, the results reveal that widespread difficulties across ER domains are associated with psychopathic traits. In contrast, studies that have used the Psychopathic Personality Inventory–Revised (PPI–R; Lilienfeld & Widows, 2005) have found significant links between the PPI–R Self-Centered Impulsivity (SCI; akin to antisocial–lifestyle features) scale and poorer ER, whereas the PPI–R FD factor (which reflects a different operationalization of the Interpersonal/Affective traits of psychopathy compared to the PCL–R) was associated with better ER (Long et al., 2014; Donahue et al., 2014; Watts et al., 2016). Lastly, across these studies, ER had inconsistent associations with PPI–R Coldheartedness scale (Long et al., 2014; Watts et al., 2016), which assesses callous affective traits. In terms of total scores, however, all these studies reported significant associations between overall levels of psychopathy and impairments in ER. Interestingly, some of the studies above reviewed have shown that the relations between psychopathic traits and poor ER – both ability and trait-like – could not be accounted for by general levels of negative affect or IQ (Donahue et al., 2014; Megias et al., 2018).

Notably, those few studies that have adopted a more nuanced perspective, by parsing PCL–R-based Factor 1 and PPI–R FD in narrower components that separate interpersonal and affective traits, have provided more consistent evidence across studies and psychopathy instruments. Specifically, ER difficulties were positively related to affective traits (i.e., PCL–R affective, PPI fearlessness and – to a lesser extent – PPI Coldheartedness; see Watts et al., 2016) and negatively related or unrelated to interpersonal traits of psychopathy (i.e., PCL–R interpersonal, PPI–R Stress Immunity, and Social Potency; Donahue et al., 2014; Vidal et al., 2010; Garofalo, Neumann, Kosson et al., 2018; Garofalo, Neumann et al., 2017; Garofalo, Neumann, & Velotti, 2017). In our current work (Garofalo, Neumann, Kosson et al., 2018; Garofalo et al., 2017a; Garofalo, Neumann, & Velotti, 2017; Garofalo, Neumann, Zeigler-Hill et al., 2018), we found that this pattern of associations was strikingly robust. First, it extended across different measures of psychopathy (e.g., PCL–R, SRP, PPI–R, TriPM) and across different populations (e.g., undergraduate students, community, offenders) from different countries (United States, Italy, Netherlands). Second, it was evident from both latent variable- and person-centered perspectives (i.e., in Structural Equation Modeling and Latent Profile Analyses, respectively). Third, this pattern was robust when we controlled for a variety of possible confounds, such as: negative affect, general psychological distress, narcissism and Machiavellianism, intelligence, age, and gender.

Conclusion

Overall, it appears that the current state of knowledge points to a significant association between overall levels of psychopathy and ER difficulties. These difficulties are likely to span across several overlapping ER domains, including emotional non-acceptance, poor emotional awareness and clarity, access to limited repertoire of effective ER strategies, difficulties engaging in goal-directed behavior when upset (i.e., poor distress tolerance), and difficulties inhibiting impulsive behavior under emotional arousal (i.e., negative urgency). This pattern seems generally consistent with historical and contemporary conceptualizations of psychopathy reviewed. The fact that more overt features of psychopathy (i.e., behavioral) are strongly related to emotion dysregulation is also in line with the different contemporary perspectives reviewed earlier (e.g., Patterson & Newman, 1993; Patrick et al., 2009). However, existing research extended beyond theoretical expectations by showing that the ER disturbances linked to psychopathy are widespread and not limited to specific ER components, and also that these disturbances are not merely the reflection of general externalizing psychopathology or negative emotionality.

Perhaps more importantly, the extant body of research emphasizes the importance of parsing interpersonal and affective traits of psychopathy in separate components, in order to achieve a more precise picture of the nomological network surrounding psychopathy and its components. Consistent with previous research on cognitive functioning and psychopathy (e.g., Baskin-Sommers et al., 2015; Salekin et al., 2004; Vitacco et al., 2005), current knowledge suggests that there may be interesting differential associations between interpersonal and affective psychopathic traits and ER. Specifically, the interpersonal traits of psychopathy tend to be related to better ER, just as it is related to better cognitive functioning. In contrast, the affective traits of psychopathy were robustly linked to poorer ER (as they are linked with poorer cognitive functioning), with strength comparable to the links between ER and behavioral traits of psychopathy. The association between affective traits of psychopathy and poorer ER is also consistent with reduced emotional processing and the use of maladaptive emotion regulation strategies (e.g., suppression) that have been linked to the affective features of psychopathy. The fact that not only behavioral traits of psychopathy but also the theoretically central affective features of psychopathy are strongly related to ER can have notable implications for theory and research on psychopathic personality. Together with the increasing body of findings linking negative emotions – and Anger in particular – with the affective traits of psychopathy, these findings call for an integration of the proverbial affective shallowness considered part and parcel of the psychopathy construct, with the possibility that certain emotional experiences and their (dys) regulation are central for the psychopathic personality.

The association between interpersonal features of psychopathy and better ER (and cognitive functioning) might provide a partial explanation for their links with indices of short-term adaptive functioning (e.g., Lilienfeld et al., 2016; Patrick et al., 2009). However, it is important to note that these features alone are not sufficient to indicate the presence of psychopathy (Lilienfeld et al., 2012; Lynam & Miller, 2012). Thus, these associations should be considered in light of the overall pattern of associations that characterizes psychopathy as related to poorer ER. From this point of view, the Stress Immunity/emotional stability component that is included in some conceptualizations of psychopathy (i.e., as part of Boldness/FD) can co-exist conceptually with a general pattern of emotion dysregulation related to psychopathy. Indeed, if the adaptive side of these features has been related to short-term interpersonal functioning (Lilienfeld et al., 2015; Patrick, 2011) or to a relative resilience against anxiety and internalizing psychopathology (Lilienfeld et al., 2012), neither of these characteristics exclude the possibility that individuals with psychopathic traits may also manifest ER difficulties. Crego and Widiger (2015) have convincingly articulated that – if Stress Immunity is related to psychopathy – it should entail a maladaptive absence of stress reactivity, including a lack of inhibition of maladaptive behavior. For instance, individuals with psychopathic traits may not show problems in ER in social contexts when they are trying to manipulate or dominate others. However, to the extent they are not affected by or do not care about signs of distress that their relational partners may show, this is evidence of a fundamental disturbance in self–other dynamics, perhaps due to early attachment problems (Meloy, 1997). In addition, individuals with elevated psychopathic traits may apparently not show ER disturbances in dangerous contexts, whereas most people would normally experience some sort of distress, because of deficient threat-detection (Hoppenbrouwers et al., 2016) or because they do not care about the long-term consequences of their actions, as opposed to deficient affective experience. Notably, the interpersonal traits of psychopathy have shown unique predictive effects for increased costs for society, especially in terms of crimes committed (DeLisi et al., 2018), suggesting that these traits can be "adaptive" and contribute to successful (short-term) outcomes for some psychopathic individuals. Still, these traits are nevertheless maladaptive for society at large and likely unsuccessful in the long-term for those who consistently rely on conning and deception in a society that operates in terms of trusting and genuine relations (Neumann et al., 2007).

The fact that in certain circumstances psychopathic individuals appear to keep their emotions in check does not necessarily exclude the possibility that individuals with psychopathic traits can manifest ER difficulties in other circumstances, for example in response to the experience of Anger or frustration, or when their social–interpersonal goals are thwarted. Actually, global maladaptive ER dysfunction can manifest in different forms, beyond the inability to change an emotional response in the desired way. Maladaptive ER also occurs when the long-term costs of an emotional response (or lack thereof) outweigh its short-term functionality, when ER strategies are applied in a rigid fashion that hinders long-term adaptive functioning, or when attempts to down-regulate emotional responses result in maladaptive secondary emotional responses (Werner & Gross, 2009). Considering these various possibilities, it seems clear that research on ER and psychopathy is still in its infancy, and that several testable hypotheses can be delineated to guide future research in this area. For instance, questions unanswered include what ER strategies psychopathic individuals tend to use and to what extent these are effective, and what the short- and long-term consequences of ER are for psychopathic individuals.

Future research should build on the current state of the art, which suggests that ER problems are evident in psychopathy and are more relevant and specific than previously acknowledged. Future research can also elucidate similarities and differences in ER, comparing psychopathy with other forms of personality pathology. Also, a fruitful approach might involve examining associations of ER disturbances with cognitive functioning, early temperament, and basic personality dispositions (Lynam & Miller, 2015; DeLisi & Vaughn, 2015). A promising avenue for future studies could also be one that integrates insights from motivational science as it applies to self- and emotion-regulation (Tamir & Millgram, 2017; Tamir, 2016; Tamir, Bigman, Rhodes, Salerno, & Schreier, 2015; Gross, 2015). There is evidence that psychopathic traits are related to Antagonism (i.e., low affiliation; Glenn, Efferson, Iyer, & Graham, 2017; Meloy, 1988; Neumann et al., 2007), deficit in threat detection (Hoppenbrouwers et al., 2016), and in the defensive motivational system (Patrick et al., 2009; Fowles & Dindo, 2009). Therefore, it is reasonable to speculate that abnormal motivational processes may impact on the experience and regulation of emotions in psychopathic individuals. For instance, psychopathic individuals may have different desired emotional states (i.e., emotion goals, or what people *want* to feel), which in turn provide the direction for ER efforts. If psychopathic individuals are motivated to feel anger (Spantidaki-Kyriazi, Bogaerts, & Garofalo, 2017), for instance, it would not be surprising that they do not down-regulate anger when it occurs, and they may actually engage in ER to increase their anger experiences. In addition to providing a potential explanation for the emotional experience of psychopathic individuals, a motivational perspective could help explain why, among psychopathic individuals, ER can appear intact in certain contexts but nevertheless be impaired in other contexts. For example, in contexts in which an antagonistic motivation is not activated, psychopathic individuals may show reduced emotional reactivity and may not engage in ER, and in this context possible ER difficulties may not be evident. In contrast, in situations where such antagonistic motivation is activated or challenged by external circumstances (e.g., frustrated reward pursuit), psychopathic individuals may be required to engage in ER efforts and manifest possible difficulties in regulating emotions. That is, ER difficulties may emerge only in conditions that are motivationally salient for individuals with psychopathic traits.

Furthermore, the association between ER difficulties and psychopathy, and in particular the differential associations that interpersonal and affective traits have with ER, may point to distinct etiological pathways that contribute to the development of psychopathy and warrant further investigation. As mentioned above, for instance, the triarchic model of psychopathy posits that early ER difficulties represent a developmental precursor of the affective, but not interpersonal, features of psychopathy (Patrick et al., 2009), an assumption that seems worth testing. An intriguing possibility that is also worth pursuing is to understand whether early callous traits contribute to increased emotion dysregulation throughout development, and whether early ER difficulties increase affective callousing, or whether a pattern of reciprocal influences over time more aptly describe the development of psychopathic traits (Hoppenbrouwers et al., 2015; Viding & McCrory, 2017). From a developmental perspective, affective callousness seen in adult individuals with psychopathic traits could be the result of ineffective ways to down-regulate negative affect (Hoppenbrouwers et al., 2015; Shane & Peterson, 2004), at least for some psychopathic individuals. Accordingly, a recent study found that emotion dysregulation in children aged 8–14 years predicted increased callousness four years later (De Caluwe, Decuyper, & De Clercq, 2013), and previous research has shown that increased autonomic arousal and skin conductance at age 3 predicted elevated psychopathy scores 25 years later (Glenn, Raine, Venables, & Mednick, 2007). Yet, this possibility will need to be synthesized with evidence that some children show calloused affect at very early age (Viding & McCrory, 2017; Frick, Ray, Thornton, & Kahn, 2014; Kimonis et al., 2016; Centifanti, Meins, & Fernyhough, 2016), a synthesis that appears only possible to achieve with studies that start as early as possible, and ideally during pregnancy or at birth (Tremblay, Vitaro, & Cote, 2018).

Another area of potential extensions concerns the relevance of ER to explain some of the correlates of psychopathic personality. For example, future research may investigate whether emotion dysregulation mediates some of the associations between psychopathic traits, externalizing behavior, and antagonistic interpersonal orientation (Long et al., 2014; Harenski & Kiehl, 2010; Lynam & Miller, 2015; Neumann et al., 2007). In light of its relevance for risk assessment and treatment of psychopathic offenders, future studies should clarify whether the potential mediating role of emotion dysregulation is limited to reactive forms of violence or can also provide a partial explanation for violent behavior that is more instrumental in nature. Alternatively, future research may try to elucidate whether emotion dysregulation moderates some of these relations, such that they can be strengthened or buffered based on individual differences in ER. Importantly, incremental knowledge on the relevance of ER for the construct of psychopathy may prove invaluable to refine prevention and treatment programs by providing concrete targets of intervention that may be protective for the development of psychopathic traits or reduce their maladaptive manifestations.

Notes

1 This choice was based on the argument that psychopathy may be a compound of unrelated – or even negatively related – traits (Lilienfeld, 2013). Tests of the viability of this model have examined the incremental or interactive effects of these traits in predicting relevant outcomes and have so far produced mixed findings (Gatner et al., 2016; Lilienfeld et al., 2012; Lynam and Miller, 2012; Miller and Lynam, 2012; Vize et al., 2016). Because these studies have focused on the broader domain of FD/boldness – rather than on ER in particular – they do not have direct relevance for the present chapter. As such, we did not address this issue in the interest of space considerations.

2 It should be noted, however, that the psychopathy groups in this study were based on boldness scores only, which alone are not sufficient indicators of psychopathic personality (Crego and Widiger, 2015; Lilienfeld et al., 2012; Lynam and Miller, 2012).

3 Of note, in the Vidal et al. 2010 study, the negative association between the PPI–R total score and ER ability only approached significance ($r = -.14, p = .06$). However, when items explicitly measuring Stress Immunity (which is in itself an index of superior ER, e.g., "I function well under stress") were removed from the PPI–R total score, the negative association between overall psychopathy and ER reached statistical significance ($r = -.21, p < .001$; Vidal et al., 2010). This seems interesting to note, as embedding items capturing good ER in psychopathy scales may obscure associations between these scales and external indices of ER.

References

Albert, R. S., Brigante, T. R., and Chase, M. (1959) 'The psychopathic personality: A content analysis of the concept,' *The Journal of General Psychology*, *60*:17–28.

Aldao, A., and Nolen-Hoeksema, S. (2010) 'Specificity of cognitive emotion regulation strategies: A transdiagnostic examination,' *Behaviour Research and Therapy*, *48*:974–983.

Ali, F., Amorim, I. S., and Chamorro-Premuzic, T. (2009) 'Empathy deficits and trait emotional intelligence in psychopathy and Machiavellianism,' *Personality and Individual Differences*, *47*:758–762.

Arieti, S. (1963) 'Psychopathic personality: Some views on its psychopathology and psychodynamics,' *Comprehensive Psychiatry*, *4*:301–312.

Baskin-Sommers, A. R. (2017) 'Psychopaths have feelings: Can they learn how to use them?,' *Aeon* [Online]. Retrieved July 22, 2017 from https://aeon.co/ideas/psychopaths-have-feelings-can-they-learn-how-to-use-them.

Baskin-Sommers, A. R., Brazil, I. A., Ryan, J., Kohlenberg, N. J., Neumann, C. S., and Newman, J. P. (2015) 'Mapping the association of global executive functioning onto diverse measures of psychopathic traits,' *Personal Disorders*, *6*:336–346.

Baskin-Sommers, A. R., Curtin, J. J., and Newman, J. P. (2011) 'Specifying the attentional selection that moderates the fearlessness of psychopathic offenders,' *Psychological Science*, *22*:226–234.

Baskin-Sommers, A. R., Curtin, J. J., and Newman, J. P. (2013) 'Emotion-modulated startle in psychopathy: Clarifying familiar effects,' *Journal of Abnormal Psychology*, *122*:458–468.

Baskin-Sommers, A. R., Stuppy-Sullivan, A. M., and Buckholtz, J. (2016) 'Psychopathic individuals exhibit but do not avoid regret during counterfactual decision making,' *Proceedings of the National Academy of Sciences of the United States of America*, *113*:14438–14443.

Benning, S. D. (2013) 'Heterogeneity in content and psychopathies: Comment on Marcus et al.,' *Personality Disorders – Theory Research and Treatment*, *4*:83–84.

Benning, S. D., Patrick, C. J., Hicks, B. M., Blonigen, D. M., and Krueger, R. F. (2003) 'Factor structure of the psychopathic personality inventory: Validity and implications for clinical assessment,' *Psychological Assessment*, *15*:340–350.

Blair, R. J. R., Peschardt, K. S., Budhani, S., Mitchell, D. G., and Pine, D. S. (2006) 'The development of psychopathy,' *Journal of Child Psychology and Psychiatry*, *47*:262–276.

Bridgett, D. J., Oddi, K. B., Laake, L. M., Murdock, K. W., and Bachmann, M. N. (2013) 'Integrating and differentiating aspects of self-regulation: Effortful control, executive functioning, and links to negative affectivity,' *Emotion*, *13*:47–63.

Brook, M., Brieman, C. L., and Kosson, D. S. (2013) 'Emotion processing in Psychopathy Checklist-assessed psychopathy: A review of the literature,' *Clinical Psychology Review*, *33*:979–995.

Cardinale, E. M., and Marsh, A. A. (2017) 'The reliability and validity of the inventory of Callous unemotional traits: A meta-analytic review,' *Assessment*:1073191117747392.

Carnovale, M., Carlson, E. N., Lynam, D., and Miller, J. D. (2017) 'What are the central features of psychopathy? A network analysis approach to understanding the structure of psychopathy,' *Biennial Conference of the Association for Research in Personality*, Sacramento, CA.

Carpenter, R. W., and Trull, T. J. (2013) 'Components of emotion dysregulation in borderline personality disorder: A review,' *Current Psychiatry Reports*, *15*:335.

Casey, H., Rogers, R. D., Burns, T., and Yiend, J. (2013) 'Emotion regulation in psychopathy,' *Biological Psychology*, *92*:541–548.

Centifanti, L. C., Meins, E., and Fernyhough, C. (2016) 'Callous–unemotional traits and impulsivity: Distinct longitudinal relations with mind-mindedness and understanding of others,' *Journal of Child Psychology and Psychiatry*, *57*:9.

Cleckley, H. (1941/1988) *The mask of sanity*, St. Louis, MO: Mosby.

Colins, O. F., Fanti, K., Salekin, R. T., and Andershed, H. (2016) 'Psychopathic personality in the general population: Differences and similarities across gender,' *Journal of Personality Disorders*, *31*(1):49.
Collison, K. L., Miller, J. D., Gaughan, E. T., Widiger, T. A., and Lynam, D. R. (2016) 'Development and validation of the super-short form of the Elemental Psychopathy Assessment,' *Journal of Criminal Justice*, *47*:143–150.
Cooke, D. J., Hart, S. D., Logan, C., and Michie, C. (2012) 'Explicating the construct of psychopathy: Development and validation of a conceptual model, the Comprehensive Assessment of Psychopathic Personality (CAPP),' *International Journal of Forensic Mental Health*, *11*:242–252.
Cooke, D. J., and Michie, C. (2001) 'Refining the construct of psychopathy: Towards a hierarchical model,' *Psychological Assessment*, *13*:171–188.
Cooke, D. J., Michie, C., Hart, S. D., and Clark, D. A. (2004) 'Reconstructing psychopathy: Clarifying the significance of antisocial and socially deviant behavior in the diagnosis of psychopathic personality disorder,' *Journal of Personality Disorders*, *18*:337–357.
Crego, C., and Widiger, T. A. (2015) 'Psychopathy and the DSM,' *Journal of Personality*, *83*:665–677.
Dargis, M., Newman, J., and Koenigs, M. (2016) 'Clarifying the link between childhood abuse history and psychopathic traits in adult criminal offenders,' *Personal Disorders*, 7:221–228 Davidson, R. J., Putnam, K. M., and Larson, C. L. (2000) 'Dysfunction in the neural circuitry of emotion regulation – A possible prelude to violence,' *Science*, *289*:591–594.
De Caluwe, E., Decuyper, M., and De Clercq, B. (2013) 'The child behavior checklist dysregulation profile predicts adolescent DSM-5 pathological personality traits 4 years later,' *European Child & Adolescent Psychiatry*, *22*:401–411.
DeLisi, M. (2009) 'Psychopathy is the unified theory of crime,' *Youth Violence and Juvenile Justice*, 7:256–273.
DeLisi, M., Reidy, D. E., Heirigs, M. H., Tostlebe, J. J., and Vaughn, M. G. (2018) 'Psychopathic costs: A monetization study of the fiscal toll of psychopathy features among institutionalized delinquents,' *Journal of Criminal Psychology*, *8*:112–124
DeLisi, M., and Vaughn, M. G. (2015) 'Ingredients for criminality require genes, temperament, and psychopathic personality,' *Journal of Criminal Justice*, *43*:290–294.
Dennis, T. A., Malone, M. M., and Chen, C. C. (2009) 'Emotional face processing and emotion regulation in children: An ERP study,' *Developmental Neuropsychology*, *34*:85–102.
Derefinko, K. J. (2015) 'Psychopathy and low anxiety: Meta-analytic evidence for the absence of inhibition, not affect,' *Journal of Personality*, *83*:693–709.
Dimaggio, G., Popolo, R., Montano, A., Velotti, P., Perrini, F., Buonocore, L., . . ., and Salvatore, G. (2017) 'Emotion dysregulation, symptoms, and interpersonal problems as independent predictors of a broad range of personality disorders in an outpatient sample,' *Psychology and Psychotherapy: Theory, Research and Practice*, *90*(4):586–599.
Donahue, J. J., McClure, K. S., and Moon, S. M. (2014) 'The relationship between emotion regulation difficulties and psychopathic personality characteristics,' *Personality Disorders*, *5*:186–194.
Ellis, J. D., Schroeder, H. S., Patrick, C., and Moser, J. S. (2017) 'Emotional reactivity and regulation in individuals with psychopathic traits: Evidence for a disconnect between neurophysiology and self-report,' *Psychophysiology*, *54*(10):1574–1585.
Ermer, E., Kahn, R. E., Salovey, P., and Kiehl, K. A. (2012) 'Emotional intelligence in incarcerated men with psychopathic traits,' *Journal of Personality and Social Psychology*, *103*:194–204.
Fernandez, K. C., Jazaieri, H., and Gross, J. J. (2016) 'Emotion regulation: A transdiagnostic perspective on a new RDoC domain,' *Cognitive Therapy and Research*, *40*:426–440.
Florez, G., Casas, A., Kreis, M. K. F., Forti, L., Martinez, J., Fernandez, J., . . ., and Cooke, D. J. (2015) 'A prototypicality validation of the comprehensive assessment of psychopathic personality (CAPP) model Spanish Version,' *Journal of Personality Disorders*, *29*:707–718.
Fowles, D. C., and Dindo, L. (2009) 'Temperament and psychopathy: A dual-pathway model,' *Current Directions in Psychological Science*, *18*:179–183.
Frick, P. J., and Morris, A. S. (2004) 'Temperament and developmental pathways to conduct problems,' *Journal of Clinical Child and Adolescent Psychology*, *33*:54–68.
Frick, P. J., Ray, J. V., Thornton, L. C., and Kahn, R. E. (2014) 'Annual research review: A developmental psychopathology approach to understanding callous-unemotional traits in children and adolescents with serious conduct problems,' *Journal of Child Psychology and Psychiatry*, *55*:532–548.
Frick, P. J., and White, S. F. (2008) 'Research review: The importance of callous-unemotional traits for developmental models of aggressive and antisocial behavior,' *Journal of Child Psychology and Psychiatry*, *49*:359–375.

Gacono, C. B., and Meloy, J. R. (1994) *The Rorschach assessment of aggressive and psychopathic personalities*, New York, NY: Routledge.
Garofalo, C., and Velotti, P. (2017) 'Negative emotionality and aggression in violent offenders: The moderating role of emotion dysregulation,' *Journal of Criminal Justice*, *51*:9–16.
Garofalo, C., Neumann, C. S., and Kosson, D. S. (2017) Psychopathic traits and emotion regulation. 7th biennial meeting of the Society for the Scientific Study of Psychopathy (SSSP 2017), Antwerp, BE.
Garofalo, C., Neumann, C. S., and Velotti, P. (2017) 'Difficulties in emotion regulation and psychopathic traits in violent offenders.' Paper under review.
Garofalo, C., Velotti, P., and Zavattini, G. C. (2017) 'Emotion regulation and aggression: The incremental contribution of alexithymia, impulsivity, and emotion dysregulation facets,' *Psychology of Violence* [Online].
Garofalo, C., Neumann, C. S., Kosson, D., and Velotti, P. (2018) 'Psychopathy and emotion dysregulation: More than meets the eye.' Paper under review.
Garofalo, C., Neumann, C. S., Zeigler-Hill, V., and Meloy, J. R. (2018) 'Spiteful and contemptuous: A new look at the emotional experiences related to psychopathic traits.' Paper under review.
Gatner, D. T., Douglas, K. S., and Hart, S. D. (2016) 'Examining the incremental and interactive effects of boldness with meanness and disinhibition within the triarchic model of psychopathy,' *Personality Disorders: Theory, Research, and Treatment*, 7:259–268.
Glenn, A. L., Efferson, L. M., Iyer, R., and Graham, J. (2017) 'Values, goals, and motivations associated with psychopathy,' *Journal of Social and Clinical Psychology*, *36*:108–125.
Glenn, A. L., Raine, A., Venables, P. H., and Mednick, S. A. (2007) 'Early temperamental and psychophysiological precursors of adult psychopathic personality,' *Journal of Abnormal Psychology*, *116*:508–518.
Gratz, K. L., and Roemer, L. (2004) 'Multidimensional assessment of emotion regulation and dysregulation: Development, factor structure, and initial validation of the difficulties in emotion regulation scale,' *Journal of Psychopathology and Behavioral Assessment*, *26*:41–54.
Grieve, R., and Mahar, D. (2010) 'The emotional manipulation–psychopathy nexus: Relationships with emotional intelligence, alexithymia and ethical position,' *Personality and Individual Differences*, *48*:945–950.
Gross, J. J. (1998) 'The emerging field of emotion regulation: An integrative review,' *Review of General Psychology*, *2*:271–299.
Gross, J. J. (2013) 'Emotion regulation: Taking stock and moving forward,' *Emotion*, *13*:359–365.
Gross, J. J. (2014) 'Emotion regulation: Conceptual and empirical foundations,' in J. J. Gross (Ed.), *Handbook of emotion regulation* (2nd ed.), New York, NY: The Guilford Press.
Gross, J. J. (2015) 'Emotion regulation: Current status and future prospects,' *Psychological Inquiry*, *26*:1–26.
Gross, J. J., and John, O. P. (2003) 'Individual differences in two emotion regulation processes: Implications for affect, relationships, and well-being,' *Journal of Personality and Social Psychology*, *85*:348–362.
Hare, R. D. (1978) 'Electrodermal and cardiovascular correlates of psychopathy,' in R. D. Hare & D. Schalling (Eds.), *Psychopathic behavior: Approaches to research*, New York, NY: Wiley.
Hare, R. D. (1996) 'Psychopathy: A clinical construct whose time has come,' *Criminal Justice and Behavior*, *23*:25–54.
Hare, R. D. (1998) 'The Hare PCL–R: Some issues concerning its use and misuse,' *Legal and Criminological Psychology*, *3*:99–119.
Hare, R. D. (2003) *Manual for the Psychopathy Checklist–Revised*, Toronto, ON: Multi-Health System.
Hare, R. D., and Neumann, C. S. (2005) 'Structural models of psychopathy,' *Current Psychiatry Reports*, 7:57–64.
Hare, R. D., and Neumann, C. S. (2008) 'Psychopathy as a clinical and empirical construct,' *Annual Review of Clinical Psychology*, *4*:217–246.
Hare, R. D., Neumann, C. S., and Mokros, A. (in press) 'The PCL–R assessment of psychopathy: Development, structural properties, and new directions,' in C. Patrick (Ed.), *Handbook of psychopathy* (2nd ed.), New York, NY: Guilford Press.
Harenski, C., and Kiehl, K. A. (2010) 'Reactive aggression in psychopathy and the role of frustration: Susceptibility, experience, and control,' *British Journal of Psychology*, *101*:6.
Helfgott, J. B. (2008) *Criminal behavior: Theories, typologies and criminal justice*, Thousand Oaks, CA: Sage.
Hicks, B. M., and Patrick, C. J. (2006) 'Psychopathy and negative emotionality: Analyses of suppressor effects reveal distinct relations with emotional distress, fearfulness, and anger–hostility,' *Journal of Abnormal Psychology*, *115*:276–287.
Hoff, H. A., Rypdal, K., Mykletun, A., and Cooke, D. J. (2012) 'A prototypicality validation of the comprehensive assessment of psychopathic personality model (CAPP),' *Journal of Personality Disorders*, *26*:414–427.

Hoppenbrouwers, S. S., Bulten, B. H., and Brazil, I. A. (2016) 'Parsing fear: A reassessment of the evidence for fear deficits in psychopathy,' *Psychological Bulletin*, *142*:573–600.
Hoppenbrouwers, S. S., Neumann, C. S., Lewis, J., and Johansson, P. (2015) 'A latent variable analysis of the Psychopathy Checklist–Revised and behavioral inhibition system/behavioral activation system factors in North American and Swedish offenders,' *Personality Disorders*, *6*:251–260.
Howe, J., Falkenbach, D., and Massey, C. (2014) 'The relationship among psychopathy, emotional intelligence, and professional success in finance,' *International Journal of Forensic Mental Health*, *13*:337–347.
Jackson, R. L., Neumann, C. S., and Vitacco, M. J. (2007) 'Impulsivity, anger, and psychopathy: The moderating effect of ethnicity,' *Journal of Personality Disorders*, *21*:289–304.
John, O. P., and Eng, J. (2014) 'Three approaches to individual differences in affect regulation: Conceptualization, measures, and findings,' in J. J. Gross (Ed.), *Handbook of emotion regulation* (2nd ed.), New York, NY: The Guilford Press.
Karpman, B. (1948) 'The myth of the psychopathic personality,' *American Journal of Psychiatry*, *104*:523–534.
Kimonis, E. R., Fanti, K. A., Anastassiou-Hadjicharalambous, X., Mertan, B., Goulter, N., and Katsimicha, E. (2016) 'Can callous–unemotional traits be reliably measured in preschoolers?, *Journal of Abnormal Child Psychology*, *44*:625–638.
Kosson, D. S., Vitacco, M. J., Swogger, M. T., and Steuerwald, B. L. (2016). 'Emotional experiences of the psychopath,' in C. B. Gacono (Ed.) *The clinical and forensic assessment of psychopathy: A practitioner's guide* (2nd ed.), New York, NY: Routledge.
Kreis, M. K. F., Cooke, D. J., Michie, C., Hoff, H. A., and Logan, C. (2012) 'The comprehensive assessment of psychopathic personality (CAPP): Content validation using prototypical analysis,' *Journal of Personality Disorders*, *26*:402–413.
Kring, A. M., and Sloan, D. M. (2009) *Emotion regulation and psychopathology. A transdiagnostic approach to etiology and treatment*, New York, NY, Guilford Press.
Lilienfeld, S. O., Patrick, C. J., Benning, S. D., Berg, J., Sellbom, M., and Edens, J. F. (2012) 'The role of fearless dominance in psychopathy: Confusions, controversies, and clarifications,' *Personality Disorders*, *3*:327–340.
Lilienfeld, S. O., Smith, S. F., Sauvigne, K. C., Patrick, C. J., Drislane, L. E., Latzman, R. D., and Krueger, R. F. (2016) 'Is boldness relevant to psychopathic personality? Meta-analytic relations with non-Psychopathy Checklist-based measures of psychopathy,' *Psychological Assessment*, *28*:1172–1185.
Lilienfeld, S. O., Watts, A. L., Francis Smith, S., Berg, J. M., and Latzman, R. D. (2015) 'Psychopathy deconstructed and reconstructed: Identifying and assembling the personality building blocks of Cleckley's Chimera,' *Journal of Personality*, *83*:593–610.
Lilienfeld, S. O., and Widows, M. (2005) *Psychopathic Personality Inventory–Revised, professional manual*, Lutz, FL: Psychological Assessment Resources.
Lishner, D. A., Swim, E. R., Hong, P. Y., and Vitacco, M. J. (2011) 'Psychopathy and ability emotional intelligence: Widespread or limited association among facets?,' *Personality and Individual Differences*, *50*:1029–1033.
Lishner, D. A., Vitacco, M. J., Hong, P. Y., Mosley, J., Miska, K., and Stocks, E. L. (2012) Evaluating the relation between psychopathy and affective empathy: Two preliminary studies,' *International Journal of Offender Therapy and Comparative Criminology*, *56*:1161–1181.
Livesley, J., Dimaggio, G., and Clarkin, J. F. (Eds.) (2016) *Integrated treatment for personality disorder: A modular approach*, New York, NY: Guilford Press.
Locke, E. A. (2005) 'Why emotional intelligence is an invalid concept,' *Journal of Organizational Behavior*, *26*:425–431.
Long, K., Felton, J. W., Lilienfeld, S. O., and Lejuez, C. W. (2014) 'The role of emotion regulation in the relations between psychopathy factors and impulsive and premeditated aggression,' *Personality Disorders*, *5*:390–396.
Lykken, D. T. (1995) *The antisocial personalities*, Hillsdale, NJ, Erlbaum.
Lynam, D. R., Gaughan, E. T., Miller, J. D., Miller, D. J., Mullins-Sweatt, S., and Widiger, T. A. (2011) 'Assessing the basic traits associated with psychopathy: Development and validation of the elemental psychopathy assessment,' *Psychological Assessment*, *23*:108–124.
Lynam, D. R., and Miller, J. D. (2012) @Fearless dominance and psychopathy: A response to Lilienfeld et al.,' *Personality Disorders: Theory, Research, and Treatment*, *3*:341–353.
Lynam, D. R., and Miller, J. D. (2015) 'Psychopathy from a basic trait perspective: The utility of a five-factor model approach,' *Journal of Personality*, *83*:611–626.

Lynam, D. R., and Widiger, T. A. (2007) 'Using a general model of personality to identify the basic elements of psychopathy,' *Journal of Personality Disorders*, *21*:160–178.
Lilienfeld, S. O. (2013) 'Is psychopathy a syndrome: Commentary on Marcus, Fulton, and Edens,' *Personality Disorders: Theory, Research, and Treatment*, *4*:85–86.
MacCann, C., Joseph, D. L., Newman, D. A., and Roberts, R. D. (2014) 'Emotional intelligence is a second-stratum factor of intelligence: Evidence from hierarchical and bifactor models,' *Emotion*, *14*:358–374.
Malterer, M. B., Glass, S. J., and Newman, J. P. (2008) 'Psychopathy and trait emotional intelligence,' *Personality and Individual Differences*, *44*:735–745.
Matthews, G., Roberts, R. D., and Zeidner, M. (2004) 'Seven myths about emotional intelligence,' *Psychological Inquiry*, *15*:179–196.
Mayer, J., Salovey, P., and Caruso, D. R. (2002) *Mayer–Salovey–Caruso Emotional Intelligence Test (MSCEIT): User's manual*, Toronto, ON: Multi-Health Systems.
Mayer, J., Salovey, P., and Caruso, D. R. (2008) 'Emotional intelligence – New ability or eclectic traits?,' *American Psychologist*, *63*:503–517.
McCord, W., and McCord, J. (1964) *The psychopath: An essay on the criminal mind*, Princeton, NJ: Van Nostrand.
Meffert, H., Gazzola, V., den Boer, J. A., Bartels, A. A., and Keysers, C. (2013) 'Reduced spontaneous but relatively normal deliberate vicarious representations in psychopathy,' *Brain*, *136*:2550–2562.
Megias, A., Gomez-Leal, R., Gutierrez-Cobo, M. J., Cabello, R., and Fernandez-Berrocal, P. (2018) 'The relationship between trait psychopathy and emotional intelligence: A meta-analytic review,' *Neuroscience & Biobehavioral Review*, *84*:198–203.
Meloy, J. R. (1988) *The psychopathic mind: Origins, dynamics, and treatment*, Northvale, NJ: Jason Aronson.
Meloy, J. R. (1997) *Violent attachments*, Lanham, MD: Jason Aronson.
Miller, J. D., Dir, A., Gentile, B., Wilson, L., Pryor, L. R., and Campbell, W. K. (2010) 'Searching for a vulnerable dark triad: Comparing Factor 2 psychopathy, vulnerable narcissism, and borderline personality disorder,' *Journal of Personality*, *78*:1529–1564.
Miller, J. D., Gaughan, E. T., and Pryor, L. R. (2008) 'The Levenson self-report psychopathy scale an examination of the personality traits and disorders associated with the LSRP factors,' *Assessment*, *15*:450–463.
Miller, J. D., Lamkin, J., Maples-Keller, J. L., and Lynam, D. R. (2016) 'Viewing the triarchic model of psychopathy through general personality and expert-based lenses,' *Personality Disorders–Theory Research and Treatment*, 7:247–258.
Miller, J. D., and Lynam, D. R. (2012) 'An examination of the Psychopathic Personality Inventory's nomological network: A meta-analytic review,' *Personality Disorders*, *3*:305–326.
Miller, J. D., Lynam, D. R., Widiger, T. A., and Leukefeld, C. (2001) 'Personality disorders as extreme variants of common personality dimensions: Can the Five-Factor Model adequately represent psychopathy?,' *Journal of Personality*, *69*:253–276.
Munoz Centifanti, L. C., Kimonis, E. R., Frick, P. J., and Aucoin, K. J. (2013) 'Emotional reactivity and the association between psychopathy-linked narcissism and aggression in detained adolescent boys,' *Development and Psychopathology*, *25*:473–485.
Munoz, L. C., Frick, P. J., Kimonis, E. R., and Aucoin, K. J. (2008) 'Types of aggression, responsiveness to provocation, and callous–unemotional traits in detained adolescents,' *Journal of Abnormal Child Psychology*, *36*:15–28.
Nentjes, L., Bernstein, D. P., Meijer, E., Arntz, A., and Wiers, R. W. (2016) 'The mask of sanity: Facial expressive, self-reported, and physiological consequences of emotion regulation in psychopathic offenders,' *Journal of Personality Disorders*, *30*(6):828.
Neumann, C. S., and Pardini, D. (2014) 'Factor structure and construct validity of the self-report psychopathy (SRP) scale and the youth psychopathic traits inventory (YPI) in young men,' *Journal of Personality Disorders*, *28*:419–433.
Neumann, C. S., Hare, R. D., and Newman, J. P. (2007) 'The super-ordinate nature of the Psychopathy Checklist–revised,' *Journal of Personality Disorders*, *21*:102–117.
Neumann, C. S., Hare, R. D., and Pardini, D. A. (2015) 'Antisociality and the construct of psychopathy: Data from across the globe,' *Journal of Personality*, *83*:678–692.
Neumann, C. S., Johansson, P. T., and Hare, R. D. (2013) 'The Psychopathy Checklist–Revised (PCL–R), low anxiety, and fearlessness: A structural equation modeling analysis,' *Personality Disorders*, *4*:129–137.
Neumann, C. S., Malterer, M. B., and Newman, J. P. (2008) 'Factor structure of the Psychopathic Personality Inventory (PPI): Findings from a large incarcerated sample,' *Psychological Assessment*, *20*:169–174.

Neumann, C. S., Schmitt, D. S., Carter, R., Embley, I., and Hare, R. D. (2012) 'Psychopathic traits in females and males across the globe,' *Behavioral Science and the Law*, *30*:557–574.
Neumann, C. S., Uzieblo, K., Crombez, G., and Hare, R. D. (2013) 'Understanding the Psychopathic Personality Inventory (PPI) in terms of the unidimensionality, orthogonality, and construct validity of PPI–I and –II,' *Personality Disorders*, *4*:77–79.
Newman, J. P., Curtin, J. J., Bertsch, J. D., and Baskin-Sommers, A. R. (2010) 'Attention moderates the fearlessness of psychopathic offenders,' *Biological Psychiatry*, *67*:66–70.
Patrick, C. J. (Ed.) (2006) *Handbook of psychopathy*, New York, NY: Guilford Press.
Patrick, C. J. (2011) *The two faces of psychopathic personality*, Montreal, QC: Society for the Scientific Study of Psychopathy.
Patrick, C. J., Bradley, M. M., and Lang, P. J. (1993) 'Emotion in the criminal psychopath – Startle reflex modulation,' *Journal of Abnormal Psychology*, *102*:82–92.
Patrick, C. J., and Drislane, L. E. (2015) 'Triarchic model of psychopathy: Origins, operationalizations, and observed linkages with personality and general psychopathology,' *Journal of Personality*, *83*:627–643.
Patrick, C. J., Fowles, D. C., and Krueger, R. F. (2009) 'Triarchic conceptualization of psychopathy: Developmental origins of disinhibition, boldness, and meanness,' *Development and Psychopathology*, *21*:913–938.
Patrick, C. J., and Zempolich, K. A. (1998) 'Emotion and aggression in the psychopathic personality,' *Aggression and Violent Behavior*, *3*:303–338.
Patterson, C. M., and Newman, J. (1993) 'Reflectivity and learning from aversive events: Toward a psychological mechanism for the syndromes of disinhibition,' *Psychological Review*, *100*:716–736.
Pérez, J. C., Petrides, K. V., and Furnham, A. (2005) 'Measuring trait emotional intelligence,' in R. Schulze & R. D. Roberts (Eds.), *International handbook of emotional intelligence* (pp. 181–201), Cambridge, MA: Hogrefe & Huber.
Petrides, K. V. (2009) *Technical manual for the Trait Emotional Intelligence Questionnaires (TEIQue)*, London: London Psychometric Laboratory.
Petrides, K. V., and Furnham, A. (2001) 'Trait emotional intelligence: Psychometric investigation with reference to established trait taxonomies,' *European Journal of Personality*, *15*:425–448.
Pinel, P. (1806) *A treatise on insanity*, London: Messers Cadell & Davies, Strand.
Reidy, D. E., Krusemark, E., Kosson, D. S., Kearns, M. C., Smith-Darden, J., and Kiehl, K. A. (2017) 'The development of severe and chronic violence among youth: The role of psychopathic traits and reward processing,' *Child Psychiatry & Human Development*, *48*:967–982.
Roberton, T., Daffern, M., and Bucks, R. S. (2012) 'Emotion regulation and aggression,' *Aggression and Violent Behavior*, *17*:72–82.
Roberton, T., Daffern, M., and Bucks, R. S. (2014) 'Maladaptive emotion regulation and aggression in adult offenders,' *Psychology, Crime & Law*, *20*:933–954.
Ruchensky, J. R., Edens, J. F., Corker, K. S., Donnellan, M. B., Witt, E. A., and Blonigen, D. (2017) 'Evaluating the structure of psychopathic personality traits: A meta-analysis of the Psychopathic Personality Inventory,' *Psychological Assessment*.
Salekin, R. T., Neumann, C. S., Leistico, A. M., and Zalot, A. A. (2004) 'Psychopathy in youth and intelligence: An investigation of Cleckley's hypothesis,' *Journal of Clinical Child & Adolescent Psychology*, *33*:731–742.
Salovey, P., Mayer, J. D., Goldman, S. L., Turvey, C., and Palfai, T. (1995) 'Emotional attention, clarity and repair: Exploring emotional intelligence using the trait meta-mood scale,' in J. Pennebaker (Ed.), *Emotion, disclosure and health* (pp. 125–154), Washington, DC: American Psychological Association.
Sellbom, M., Cooke, D. J., and Hart, S. D. (2015) 'Construct validity of the comprehensive assessment of psychopathic personality (CAPP) concept map: Getting closer to the core of psychopathy,' *International Journal of Forensic Mental Health*, *14*:172–180.
Shane, M. S., and Peterson, J. B. (2004) 'Defensive copers show a deficit in passive avoidance learning on Newman's go/no-go task: Implications for self-deception and socialization,' *Journal of Personality*, *72*:939–966.
Shou, Y., Sellbom, M., and Xu, J. (2017) 'Psychometric properties of the triarchic psychopathy measure: An item response theory approach,' *Personality Disorders: Theory, Research, and Treatment*.
Sorman, K., Edens, J. F., Smith, S. T., Clark, J. W., Kristiansson, M., and Svensson, O. (2016) 'Boldness and its relation to psychopathic personality: Prototypicality analyses among forensic mental health, criminal justice, and layperson raters,' *Law and Human Behavior*, *40*:337–349.
Sorman, K., Edens, J. F., Smith, S. T., Svensson, O., Howner, K., Kristiansson, M., and Fischer, H. (2014) 'Forensic mental health professionals' perceptions of psychopathy: A prototypicality analysis

of the comprehensive assessment of psychopathic personality in Sweden,' *Law and Human Behavior*, *38*:405–417.

Spantidaki-Kyriazi, F., Bogaerts, S., and Garofalo, C. (2017) Emotion goals and psychopathic personality traits in non-clinical samples. *7th biennial meeting of the Society for the Scientific Study of Psychopathy (SSSP 2017)*, Antwerp, BE.

Tamir, M. (2016) 'Why do people regulate their emotions? A taxonomy of motives in emotion regulation,' *Personality and Social Psychology Review*, *20*:199–222.

Tamir, M., Bigman, Y. E., Rhodes, E., Salerno, J., and Schreier, J. (2015) 'An expectancy-value model of emotion regulation: Implications for motivation, emotional experience, and decision making,' *Emotion*, *15*:90–103.

Tamir, M., and Gross, J. J. (2011) Beyond pleasure and pain? 'Emotion regulation and positive psychology,' in K. Sheldon, T. B. Kashdan, & M. F. Steger (Eds.), *Designing positive psychology: Taking stock and moving forward* (pp. 89–100), Oxford: Oxford University Press.

Tamir, M., and Millgram, Y. (2017) 'Motivated emotion regulation: Principles, lessons, and implications of a motivational analysis of emotion regulation,' in A. J. Elliot (Ed.), *Advanced in motivation science*, New York, NY: Academic Press.

Tellegen, A., and Waller, N. G. (2008) 'Exploring personality through test construction: Development of the Multidimensional Personality Questionnaire,' in G. J. Boyle, G. Matthews, & D. H. Aklofske (Eds.), *The SAGE handbook of personality theory and assessment, Vol 2: Personality measurement and testing* (pp. 261–292), Thousand Oaks, CA: Sage Publications.

Thompson, R. A. (1994) 'Emotion regulation: A theme in search of definition,' *Monographs of the Society for Research in Child Development*, *59*:28.

Tremblay, R. E., Vitaro, F., and Cote, S. M. (2018) 'Chronic physical aggression: A bio–psycho–social model for the next generation of preventive interventions,' *Annual Review of Psychology*, *69*:383–407.

Verschuere, B., van Ghesel Grothe, S., Waldorp, L., Watts, A., Lilienfeld, S., Edens, J. F., . . ., and Noordhof, A. (2017) 'What features of psychopathy might be central? A network analysis of the Psychopathy Checklist–Revised (PCL–R) in three large samples,' *Journal of Abnormal Psychology*.

Vidal, S., Skeem, J., and Camp, J. (2010) 'Emotional intelligence: Painting different paths for low-anxious and high-anxious psychopathic variants,' *Law and Human Behavior*, *34*:150–163.

Viding, E., and McCrory, E. J. (2017) 'Understanding the development of psychopathy: Progress and challenges,' *Psychological Medicine*:1–12.

Visser, B. A., Ashton, M. C., and Pozzebon, J. A. (2012) 'Is low anxiety part of the psychopathy construct?,' *Journal of Personality*, *80*:725–747.

Visser, B. A., Bay, D., Cook, G. L., and Myburgh, J. (2010) 'Psychopathic and antisocial, but not emotionally intelligent,' *Personality and Individual Differences*, *48*:644–648.

Vitacco, M. J., Neumann, C. S., and Jackson, R. L. (2005) 'Testing a four-factor model of psychopathy and its association with ethnicity, gender, intelligence, and violence,' *Journal of Consulting and Clinical Psychology*, *73*:466–476.

Vize, C. E., Lynam, D. R., Lamkin, J., Miller, J. D., and Pardini, D. (2016) 'Identifying essential features of juvenile psychopathy in the prediction of later antisocial behavior: Is there an additive, synergistic, or curvilinear role for fearless dominance?,' *Clinical Psychological Science*, *4*:572–590.

Watts, A. L., Salekin, R. T., Harrison, N., Clark, A., Waldman, I. D., Vitacco, M. J., and Lilienfeld, S. O. (2016) 'Psychopathy: Relations with three conceptions of intelligence,' *Personality Disorders*, 7(3):269.

Werlinder, H. (1978) *Psychopathy: A history of the concepts: Analysis of the origin and development of a family of concepts in psychopathology*, Uppsala, SE: University Uppsala.

Werner, K., and Gross, J. J. (2009) 'Emotion regulation and psychopathology: A conceptual framework,' in A. M. Kring & D. M. Sloan (Eds.), *Emotion regulation and psychopathology: A transdiagnostic approach to etiology and treatment* (pp. 13–37), New York, NY: Guilford Press.

Wong, S., and Hare, R. D. (2005) *Guidelines for a Psychopathy Treatment Program*, Toronto, ON: Multi-Health System.

6

Callous–unemotional traits

Relevance and implications for juvenile justice

James V. Ray and Tina D. Wall Myers

Introduction

Psychopathy is a multidimensional personality disorder that characterizes individuals who have an arrogant and deceitful interpersonal style (e.g., conning, manipulative, and narcissistic), are devoid of emotional affect (e.g., callous, remorseless, and uncaring toward others), and have antisocial behavioral styles (e.g., impulsive, unreliable, and criminal involvement; Hare, 2003). An extensive body of research has amassed regarding the construct of psychopathy among adults, particularly addressing its utility in criminal justice settings (Wong & Olver, 2015). This body of research has largely focused on the predictive utility of the psychopathy construct in terms of risk for reoffending, institutional maladjustment, and treatment amenability (Hare, 1998). In general, the research supports the predictive validity of psychopathy assessment instruments regarding these outcomes (Gendreau, Little, & Goggin, 1996). This has led to an increased use of psychopathy assessment tools, such as the Psychopathy Checklist–Revised (PCL–R; Hare, 2003), to inform criminal justice decision-making such as level of security, sentencing, and likelihood of reoffending (Serin, Brown, & De Wolf, 2015).

Given its utility among adults, it is not surprising that researchers and practitioners have begun to extend its use to juveniles and juvenile justice settings. One approach to extending psychopathy downward to youth focuses on the affective components of psychopathy, referred to more commonly as callous–unemotional (CU) traits (Frick & White, 2008). Although other approaches have been taken to extend psychopathy to youth (e.g., Lynam, 1996), CU traits have gained considerable traction as a precursor to adult psychopathy (Frick & White, 2008). To date, an extensive body of research has shown that CU traits are an important construct for identifying a subgroup of youth who have unique etiologies underlying their antisocial behavior and who have particularly severe and persistent patterns of delinquency (Frick, Ray, Thornton, & Kahn, 2014).

Given that CU traits identify a subgroup of antisocial youth, the identification of such youth has important implications for juvenile justice under the Risk–Needs–Responsivity (RNR; Andrews, Bonta, & Wormith, 2006) framework, which focuses on tailored treatment that targets the heterogeneous array of factors that contribute to juveniles' antisocial behavior. Specifically, given this subgroup of youth is responsible for a large amount of serious delinquent behavior, particularly violent behavior, identification of such youth is important from a delinquency reduction standpoint. Additionally, given the unique etiological factors associated with this subgroup's antisocial behavior, it is important to consider such factors so that interventions can be effectively tailored to the individual's criminogenic needs and learning style. However, it is also important to consider the issues that surround diagnosing youth with CU traits, and psychopathy more generally, in the juvenile justice system (e.g., Edens & Vincent, 2008; Seagrave & Grisso, 2002). Based on the extensive body of research regarding the conceptualization, stability, and unique correlates of CU traits, we propose that CU traits can be useful for juvenile risk assessment and treatment. We also highlight limitations and concerns regarding the assessment of CU traits within the juvenile justice system.

Review of research on CU traits

Conceptualization and measurement of CU traits

CU traits have been conceptualized as affective deficits comprising a lack of guilt and remorse, a lack of concern for the feelings and rights of others, shallow or superficial expression of emotions, and a lack of concern regarding performance on important activities (Frick, 2009). These traits have been tied to the conceptualization of the construct that emerged from research with the PCL–R (Hare, 2003). As such, the assessment of CU traits was previously reliant on using facet scores of broader measures of global psychopathy, such as facets from the Psychopathy Checklist–Youth Version (PCL: YV; Forth, Kosson, & Hare, 2003), Antisocial Process Screening Device (APSD; Frick & Hare, 2001), Child Psychopathy Scale (CPS; Lynam, 1997), and Youth Psychopathic Traits Inventory (YPI; Andershed, Kerr, Stattin, & Levander, 2002). However, the few items specifically assessing CU traits, the limited range in response options, and the negatively skewed ratings of CU traits in most samples resulted in these measures having significant psychometric limitations for assessing CU traits (see Frick & Ray, 2015 for a review). To overcome limitations of assessing CU traits as part of the broader construct of psychopathy, the Inventory of Callous Unemotional Traits (ICU; Kimonis et al., 2008) was developed.

The content of the ICU was based on the four items on the APSD that most consistently loaded on the callous–unemotional dimension across samples (Frick, Bodin, & Barry, 2000). To form the items on the ICU, six items (three positively and three negatively worded items) were developed to assess a similar content to each of the four core traits, resulting in a 24-item scale available in self-, parent-, and teacher-report formats. Importantly, several studies have tested the construct validity of the ICU using factor analyses and reported that the best fitting model tends to be one specifying a general CU factor and three sub-factors: callousness (a lack of empathy and remorse), uncaring (an uncaring attitude about performance on tasks and other's feelings), and unemotional (deficient emotional affect). This structure has been supported in samples of children and adolescents of various ages (Essau, Sasagawa, & Frick, 2006; Ezpeleta, de la Osa, Granero, Penelo, & Domenech, 2013) and across multiple language translations (Ciucci, Baroncelli, Franchi, Golmaryami, & Frick, 2014; Essau et al., 2006; Ezpeleta et al., 2013; Fanti, Frick, & Georgiou, 2009; Kimonis et al., 2008). Further, this factor structure has been invariant across boys and girls (Essau et al., 2006; Ciucci et al., 2014) and across rating formats (Roose, Bijttebier, Decoene, Claes, & Frick, 2010). Additionally, the total score of the ICU shows acceptable internal consistency (Cronbach's alpha range between .77 and .89), and similar correlations with antisocial behavior and other emotional and cognitive characteristics have been reported in studies using other measures of CU traits (Frick et al., 2014). However, the available research also highlights several significant limitations of the ICU scale (see Hawes et al., 2014; Waller et al., 2014 for reviews).

Stability of callous–unemotional traits

There is now considerable evidence to suggest that CU traits are relatively stable from late childhood to early adolescence, but with substantial variability in the level of stability. Specifically, CU traits across childhood and adolescence was found to have a mean stability coefficient of .59 (ranging from .27 to .84) and intraclass correlations (ICCs) ranging from .44 to .74 (Barker & Salekin, 2012; Barry, Barry, Deming, & Lochman, 2008; Muñoz & Frick, 2007; Obradović, Pardini, Long, & Loeber, 2007; Pardini, Lochman, & Powell, 2007; van Baardewijk, Vermeiren, Stegge, & Doreleijers, 2011). With respect to younger children, four studies evaluated stability using parent ratings of CU traits. Stability estimates ranged from .41 to .84, with a mean of .58, over a period of six months to two years (Dadds, Fraser, Frost, & Hawes, 2005; Hawes & Dadds, 2007; Waller et al., 2012; Willoughby, Waschbusch, Moore, & Propper, 2011).

These traits have also proven to be relatively stable from adolescence to adulthood. Specifically, Forsman, Lichtenstein, Andershed, and Larsson (2008) reported that the stability of CU traits from ages 16 to 19 years (n = 1,467) was $r = .43$ and $r = .54$ (both $p < .05$) for boys and girls respectively. In a somewhat older sample, Blonigen, Hicks, Kruger, Patrick, and Iacono (2006) reported a stability of $r = .60$ ($p < .001$) from ages 17 to 24 (n = 1,252). Two studies found significant stability of CU traits over somewhat longer periods from childhood into early adulthood. Burke, Loeber, and Lahey (2007) reported that both parent- and teacher-rated CU traits assessed at ages 7 to 12 in a sample of clinic-referred boys ($n = 177$) were significantly associated with clinician-rated CU traits at ages 18 and 19. Also, Lynam, Caspi, Moffitt, Loeber, and Stouthamer-Loeber (2007) reported that self-report of psychopathic traits, which included CU traits, at age 13 ($n = 250$) was significantly associated ($r = .31$, $p < .001$) with clinician ratings of psychopathic traits (again including CU traits) at age 24.

The greatest influence on the strength of stability, besides length of follow-up (i.e., longer follow-up periods accounted for lower stability estimates), was the type of reporter used to assess CU traits. Parent ratings of CU traits tended to be more stable over time than either self-report (Munoz & Frick, 2007) or teacher reports (Barry et al., 2008; Obradovic et al., 2007). For example, Munoz and Frick (2007) compared the three-year stability of parent and youth self-report ratings of CU traits in a sample of high-risk community sample of boys ($n = 91$) and found very high stability for parent ratings ($r = .71$, $p < .01$) and moderate stability for self-report ratings ($r = .48$, $p < .01$). Obradovic et al. (2007) reported relatively high rates of stability for parent report of CU traits ($r = .50$, $p < .001$) over a nine-year period and lower level of stability for teacher ratings ($r = .27$, $p < .001$) in a community sample of boys ($n = 503$).

Further, several studies support the role of genetic factors in the stability of CU traits (Blonigen, Hicks, Kruger, Patrick, & Iacono, 2006; Fontaine, Rijsdijk, McCrory, & Viding, 2010; Forsman, Lichtenstein, Andershed, & Larsson, 2008). For example, Blonigen et al. (2006) found that genetic factors were responsible for a larger proportion of the variance (58 percent) in the stability of CU traits compared to non-shared and shared environmental factors. Forsman et al. (2008) also found that cross-twin stability was higher among monozygotic twins ($r = .31$, $p < .05$) compared to dizygotic twins ($r = .05$ and .15 for boys and girls, respectively, p = n.s.) from ages 16 to 19. Research also suggests that variance in stability is due partially to environmental factors. One such factor that has been consistently documented as being associated with more stable patterns of CU traits is dysfunctional parenting. For example, Waller et al. (2012) found that harsh parenting (e.g., physical and verbal punishment) predicted subsequent CU traits measured one year later after controlling for prior CU traits. Frick, Kimonis, Dandreaux, and Farrell (2003) found that both low positive parenting (e.g., parental involvement and positive reinforcement) and high levels of harsh and inconsistent parenting were associated with more stable patterns of CU traits in a community sample of children (n = 98) across four years. Finally, Pardini and Loeber (2008) reported that poor parent–child communication (e.g., arguing, insulting) predicted high and stable patterns of CU traits across adolescence (ages 14 to 18 years of age) in a community sample of youth (n = 506).

CU traits mark a subgroup of antisocial youth

Research has indicated that within youth with antisocial behavior, CU traits mark a distinct and important subgroup of children and adolescents with distinct biological, cognitive, emotional, and social characteristics that implicate different causal processes leading to their antisocial behavior (Frick et al., 2014). First, the genetic and environmental contributions to early onset serious behavioral problems seem to differ between those with and without elevated CU traits. For those youth with elevated CU traits, research suggests that serious behavioral problems may have considerably greater genetic influences than those of youth with normative levels of CU traits (Viding, Blair, Moffitt, & Plomin, 2005). In turn, research has suggested that because of their temperamental styles, youth with CU traits invoke poor parenting styles (e.g., harsh and inconsistent parenting; Waller et al., 2013) that might preclude more effective forms of parenting. That is, more authoritative parenting styles that incorporate both warmth and supervision are most important for reducing delinquent outcomes (Steinberg, Munts, Lamborn, & Dornbusch, 1991). Research has suggested that it is the warmth aspect of parenting that has the greatest influence on the development of antisocial behavior among youth with CU traits (Waller et al., 2013). Second, and consistent with research on psychopathy in adults, youth with serious behavioral problems and CU traits show abnormalities in the way they process punishment cues. Specifically, CU traits have a reward-dominant response style in which they demonstrate an insensitivity to punishment cues in tasks in which an increasing ratio of punishment to reward occurs for responses (Fisher & Blair, 1998; Frick et al., 2003). Also, when different punishment schedules are compared, youth with behavior problems and high levels of CU traits respond more poorly to gradual punishment schedules compared to youth with behavior problems but normative levels of CU traits (Blair, Colledge, & Mitchell, 2001). Furthermore, several studies have shown that youth with elevated CU traits have unique cognitive styles and are more likely to hold more deviant attitudes, including viewing the use of aggression as a more acceptable means for obtaining goals, Blame Externalization, and identifying dominance and retaliation as important goals of social conflict (Chabrol, van Leeuwen, Rodgers, & Gibbs, 2011; Pardini, Lochman, & Frick, 2003; Stickle, Kirkpatrick, & Brush, 2009). Third, children and adolescents with serious behavioral problems and elevated CU traits show reduced responding to signs of fear and distress in others. This attenuated emotional responsiveness has been found when assessed through self-report measures of physiological arousal (Marsh et al., 2011), cognitive tasks assessing attentional orienting to emotional pictures (Kimonis, Frick, Fazekas, & Loney, 2006), psychophysiological responses to emotionally evocative films (de Wied, van Boxtel, Matthys, & Meeus, 2012), and amygdala responses to fearful faces (Viding et al., 2012). In contrast, children and adolescents with serious behavioral problems but without elevated CU traits show an enhanced emotional response to fear and distress in others (Kimonis et al., 2006; Viding et al., 2012). Finally, another consistent finding for children and adolescents with high levels of CU traits is that these youth often associate with delinquent and antisocial peers, and this level of deviant peer association appears to be higher than what is found for children and adolescents with behavioral problem but with normative levels of CU traits (Kimonis, Frick, & Barry, 2004; Muñoz, Frick, Kimonis, & Aucoin, 2008; Pardini & Loeber, 2008). Additionally, these youths tend to have strong influence on the antisocial behavior of their peers (Kerr, Van Zalk, & Stattin, 2012; Thornton et al., 2015).

Given these unique etiological factors and correlates of CU traits, CU traits are an important construct for use within the juvenile justice system. Antisocial youth who show elevated levels of CU traits often show a severe, persistent, and violent pattern of aggressive and delinquent behavior (Kruh, Frick, & Clements, 2005; Lawing, Frick, & Cruise, 2010). Besides more severe aggression, their aggression is more likely to be instrumental (i.e., for personal gain or dominance) and premeditated compared to other children and adolescents with severe behavioral problems (Frick, Cornell, Barry, Bodin, & Dane, 2003; Kruh et al., 2005; Lawing et al., 2010; Marsee & Frick, 2007). Further, CU traits are associated with an earlier onset of severe behavioral problems (Dandreaux & Frick, 2009; Silverthorn, Frick, & Reynolds, 2001), as well as shorter times to both nonviolent and violent recidivism (Brandt, Kennedy, Patrick, & Curtin, 1997; Catchpole & Gretton, 2003; Lawing et al., 2010). Among justice-involved adolescents, CU traits also predict more frequent and more varied delinquent acts (Ray, Thornton, Frick, Steinberg, & Cauffman, 2016).

Additionally, these youths are also more likely to show antisocial behavioral problems that continue through adolescence and into adulthood (Burke, Loeber, & Lahey, 2007; Byrd, Loeber, & Pardini, 2012). For example, Byrd et al. (2012) conducted a longitudinal study which demonstrated that CU traits at age 7 predicted violent and criminal behavior at age 25, even after controlling for childhood Conduct Disorder, Attention-Deficit/Hyperactivity Disorder, and Oppositional Defiant Disorder. Further, youth with elevated CU traits have also accounted for a disproportionate number of police contact (Christian, Frick, Hill, Tyler, & Frazer, 1997; Frick, Stickle, Dandreaux, Farrell, & Kimonis, 2005), as well as earlier age at first charge (Bauer, Whitman, & Kosson, 2011). For example, Frick et al. (2005) conducted a four-year longitudinal study with elementary and middle school aged children and found that those children with conduct problems and elevated CU traits accounted for more than 50 percent of the police contacts as reported by parents. Within adolescents in the juvenile justice system, the estimated percentages of youth with elevated CU traits have ranged from 13 to 36 percent (Caputo, Frick, & Brodsky, 1999; Corrado, Vincent, Hart, & Cohen, 2004; Gretton, Hare, & Catchpole, 2004).

CU traits and juvenile risk and needs assessment

We now turn our discussion to the utility of CU traits for juvenile justice as it applies to the principles of the RNR framework (Andrews et al., 2006). Thus, it is necessary to describe the principles of the RNR framework. The "risk" principle of the RNR framework refers to the notion that juvenile justice practitioners can determine the probability that an offender will reoffend. In turn, the level of service that a youth receives should be consistent with their level of risk – higher risk equals more intensive intervention/supervision. The "needs" principle highlights the variety and specific needs of individual youth that are necessary for targeted responses to delinquency. The needs principle refers to those factors that, if treated, will have a reduction effect on delinquent outcomes (i.e., criminogenic needs). The "responsivity" principle focuses on maximizing the efficacy of interventions by considering the specific circumstances and learning styles of youth that may impact treatment implementation (Vincent, Guy, Fusco, & Gershenson, 2012). We argue that because of their unique etiologies it is important to identify youth with CU traits for each of these principles of the RNR framework. That is, in addition to their association with violent and persistent patterns of offending, CU traits may moderate the effectiveness of interventions traditionally utilized for youth and may be helpful in terms of matching youth with the most suitable interventions that will have the highest likelihood of resulting in positive change.

CU traits and the risk principle

Adolescence encapsulates a period of development where, for most youth, risky behavior is relatively normative, although short-lived (Moffitt, 1993). However, there is a small subset of youth whose delinquent behavior is quite pervasive and extends from adolescence into adulthood (e.g., Cohen, 1998; Moffitt, 1993). Therefore, youth who encounter the juvenile justice system are a heterogenous group in terms of their risk for future offending. Risk assessment has become integral to identifying juvenile offenders most likely to reoffend. This approach has the benefit of maximizing juvenile justice responses by targeting efforts on those most likely to recidivate and cause societal harm (Schmidt & Campbell, 2011 – see Schwalbe, 2007 for a review of risk assessment). Because psychopathy has been linked to a particularly severe and violent pattern of offending (Cornell et al., 1996), risk assessment instruments often incorporate the psychopathy construct into summary risk levels (Edens & Vincent, 2008). As a matter of fact, the PCL: YV has been consistently, albeit modestly, predictive of recidivism (Edens, Skeem, Cruise, & Cauffman, 2001). Some have argued, however, that it is the behavioral features (i.e., criminal/delinquent involvement) that drive its predictive utility (Edens & Vincent, 2008) and not necessarily the features unique to the psychopathy construct (i.e., affective/interpersonal features). While this might be the case, the behavioral features incorporated in the PCL tools are not unique to psychopathy and, therefore, do not accurately identify those most likely to have psychopathic traits as adults. On the other hand, CU traits have extensive empirical support as an early precursor for psychopathic traits (Frick et al., 2014), making their incorporation into risk assessment crucial for identifying this subgroup of youth.

The predictive utility of CU traits is evident from the extensive research, which has consistently found that youth with elevated levels of CU traits engage in more serious, violent, and persistent antisocial behavior (see review earlier and Frick et al., 2014). In addition to this well-established association between CU traits and antisocial behavior, research has also identified CU traits as a predictor of recidivism. In a recent meta-analysis, Asscher et al. (2011) found CU traits to be a significant predictor of general recidivism ($k = 10$; too few studies examined the effect of violent recidivism), albeit the effect was fairly weak ($r = .18$). Despite this weak effect, research has shown that this association persists even when controlling for other known risk factors. For instance, Kruh et al. (2005) found that even after controlling for demographic characteristics and scores on the Violence Risk Appraisal Guide–Easily Scored Version (VRAG–ESV; Webster, Harris, Rice, Cormier, & Quinsey, 1994), CU traits continued to be associated with history of self-reported violence among a sample of juveniles whose cases were transferred to the adult criminal justice system. More recently, Kimonis, Kennealy, and Goulter (2016) examined if CU traits assessed using the ICU were predictive of recidivism even when controlling for other important risk factors among a sample of incarcerated male juvenile offenders. Specifically, they found that scores on the ICU were predictive of less time between discharge and being charged with a new violent offense even when controlling for levels of aggressive-antisocial behavior.

While we do not dismiss the fact that more research is needed that examines the ability of CU traits to predict recidivism, the research to date is fairly convincing of the unique predictive utility of measures that capture CU traits such as the ICU (Frick et al., 2014). In terms of the risk principle of the RNR model, self-report instruments of CU traits (e.g., ICU) may best be utilized as a screening instrument to identify youth who would then receive a more thorough assessment for psychopathic traits. This approach would serve to reduce the amount of time and resources required by structured assessments (e.g., PCL: YV), reducing the burden on juvenile justice practitioners while increasing the effectiveness of risk assessment.

CU traits and the need principle

Andrews et al. (2006) distinguish between static and dynamic risk factors. Static factors are those that are related to delinquency but do not change (e.g., offense history, gender, age of first contact with the law, parental criminality). Because static risk factors are unlikely to be changed, they are, therefore, not ideal targets of interventions aimed to reduce offending. Dynamic factors, on the other hand, are those that are changeable (e.g., delinquent peer association, antisocial attitudes, personality traits, disruptive behavior problems, poor school performance) and have been identified as "criminogenic needs" factors. Because of their potential to change, dynamic factors typically serve as targets of intervention strategies. We suggest that CU traits are an important need factor for two reasons. First, because of the unique risk factors that have been found to underscore the delinquency of youth with elevated levels of CU traits, identifying youth with CU traits is integral to tailoring treatment to their specific needs. Interventions should be aimed to address the unique risk factors associated with CU traits. Second, to the extent that CU traits are malleable and factors contributing to their malleability can be identified, CU traits themselves may serve as an effective target for treatment.

Research has consistently found that youth with CU traits have higher levels of a number of traditionally established dynamic risk factors (Frick et al., 2014). For example, and as discussed previously, youth with elevated CU traits have unique cognitive styles consisting of more deviant attitudes (Chabrol et al., 2011; Pardini et al., 2003; Stickle et al., 2009), higher levels of deviant peer association (Kimonis et al., 2004; Muñoz et al., 2008; Pardini & Loeber, 2008), and temperaments that evoke poor parenting styles, which are a few of the contextual and individual risk factors reflected in many risk assessment tools. These factors, consistently found among youth with CU traits, are also important criminogenic needs factors that are often targets of multi-systemic interventions designed for justice-involved youth. To the extent that interventions can effectively alter delinquent outcomes, it is important to identify youth with CU traits as candidates for intensive multi-systemic treatment programs given their unique array of dynamic risk factors. White, Frick, Lawing, and Bauer (2013) found that among a sample of juvenile justice-involved youth, Functional Family Therapy (FFT) resulted in greater reductions in social, emotional, and behavioral outcomes (including recidivism) for those with elevated scores on the ICU compared to those without elevated scores. These findings suggest that interventions available in the juvenile justice system can effectively reduce antisocial outcomes for youth with CU traits. However, it is important to consider CU traits as a treatment target themselves. Although there is some evidence that CU traits are fairly stable (Frick & Ray, 2015), research utilizing a person-centered approach to modeling CU traits over time suggests that they may not be immutable for *all* youth – even those high on CU traits (Fontaine et al., 2010). Although more research is needed to identify the specific factors that result in reductions of CU traits themselves, this research suggests the possibility that treatment efforts that attempt to alter levels of CU traits themselves may be effective.

The existing research clearly suggests that tailored treatment approaches that target the unique characteristics of this group (e.g., reward dominance, lack of empathy) may effectively reduce the frequency and severity of their delinquent behavior and may even have a reduction effect on the level of CU traits themselves (Frick et al., 2014). For example, among a sample of serious offenders with elevated CU traits, intensive treatment that focused on their reward-dominant response style, self-interest, and low empathy effectively reduced two-year recidivism rates (Caldwell, Skeem, Salekin, & Van Rybroek, 2006). Although little research exists examining the effect of treatment on levels of CU traits themselves, the few studies that exist suggest that intensive parent-training programs that occur early in development have been shown to result in significant reductions in CU traits from pre- to post-treatment (Hawes & Dadds, 2007; McDonald, Dodson, Rosenfield, & Jouriles, 2011; Somech & Elizur, 2012). Because these treatment effects have been found in young children (ages 3–9), these treatment efforts may be outside the purview of the juvenile justice system. However, one study has found that Multi-Systemic Therapy (MST) significantly reduced CU traits among a sample of adolescents (ages 13–17) who were involved in the juvenile justice system (Butler, Baruch, Hickey, & Fonagy, 2011). In terms of the needs principle, therefore, the inclusion of CU traits in risk and needs assessment instruments would be a useful and necessary treatment target in order to reduce recidivism. This is the case due to the unique set of emotional, cognitive, and behavioral correlates of CU traits that are also typically considered in needs assessment as well as identifying justice-involved youth to receive intensive forms of treatment (e.g., FFT, MST) that have been found to reduce antisocial outcomes among youth with elevated CU traits and levels of CU traits themselves.

CU traits and the responsivity principle

The responsivity principle refers to factors that may not be associated with antisocial outcomes (i.e., non-criminogenic factors) but that impact one's ability and motivation to adhere to a particular treatment program. Andrews et al. (2006) identified two sub-principles of the responsivity principle: the relationship principle and the structuring principle. The relationship principle refers to establishing a positive working climate for clients that fosters positive rapport and treatment effectiveness. The structuring principle focuses on the notion that treatment should be tailored to the learning styles of youth to enhance treatment effectiveness. There is considerable evidence to suggest that meeting these two principles may be an exceptional challenge among youth with CU traits. That is, high levels of CU traits among justice-involved youth may hinder the ability of juvenile justice practitioners to create a positive treatment climate, and such youth may require a unique approach to treatment that capitalizes on their unique characteristics.

In terms of the relationship principle, because of their poor social functioning (Haas, Becker, Epstein, & Frick, 2017), positive expectancies regarding the use of aggression (Pardini & Byrd, 2012), and general influence on peers (Kerr et al., 2012; Thornton et al., 2015), youth with elevated CU traits may be less responsive and more disruptive during treatment. For instance, research has found that adolescents involved in the juvenile justice system with elevated levels of CU traits show lower levels of participation in treatment and poorer adjustment to institutional settings (Falkenbach, Poythress, & Heidi, 2003; Gretton, McBride, Hare, & O'Shaughnessy, 2001; Spain, Douglas, Poythress, & Epstein, 2004). Research has also found that youth with CU traits receiving psychiatric treatment in a secure facility had a longer length of stay and were more likely to receive disciplinary action (e.g., physical restraint, involuntary seclusion) while in treatment (Stellwagen & Kerig, 2010a, 2010b). Although no studies to date have examined how youth with CU traits in group-treatment settings might impact the effectiveness of treatment on peers, research linking CU traits to antisocial influence of peers (e.g., Kerr et al., 2012; Thornton et al., 2015) suggests that combining such youth in group-treatment settings may result in poorer treatment outcomes.

Regarding the structuring principle and tailoring treatment to the unique needs of youth, interventions that have been shown to be effective at reducing negative behavioral outcomes among youth with CU traits tend to incorporate treatment components that account for their unique motivational styles (e.g., reward-dominant response style; Frick et al., 2014). Thus, punishment-oriented interventions that are ubiquitous in the juvenile justice system may have limited efficacy when applied to youth with CU traits. Alternatively, effective treatment strategies among youth with CU traits attempt to capitalize on their reward-oriented learning styles and incorporate components that teach perspective-taking and learning to read and interpret others' emotions (Caldwell et al., 2006; Hawes, Price, & Dadds, 2014). These positive effects for treatment have emerged even when comparing treatment programs (e.g., parent training) with and without such components (Frick et al., 2014). Unique treatment efforts that target youth with CU traits also consider the underlying neurocognitive deficits of youth with CU traits and how these hinder normal developmental processes in conscience and empathy development (Hawes et al., 2014). For instance, treatment that emphasizes attention to the eyes and face of others and trains youth to recognize distress cues may have positive effects on the development of empathy among youth with CU traits (Dadds et al., 2014).

Together, this body of research suggests that, because of their underlying disposition, youth with CU traits may have particularly poor responsivity to treatment. However, in line with the relationship and structuring principles, interventions that attempt to address the unique characteristics of youth with elevated CU traits, particularly social learning-based treatment that is tailored to the unique learning styles of youth with CU traits (Hawes et al., 2014), will enhance treatment efficacy and, in turn, be more effective in reducing antisocial outcomes for this subgroup of antisocial youth.

Concerns regarding the use of CU traits in juvenile justice

While in the current chapter we argue for the inclusion of assessments of CU traits in risk assessment tools to identify those justice-involved youth most at risk for recidivism and to tailor treatment efforts to their specific needs, there are several concerns regarding the diagnosis of youth with CU traits that are particularly salient in a juvenile justice setting. The most common concern regarding the use of CU traits (or psychopathy more generally) in juvenile justice decision-making is the negative stigma that might come with such diagnoses (Edens, Mowle, Clark, & Magyar, 2017). That is, it is possible that decisions made by legal actors working in the juvenile justice system are influenced by a CU diagnosis – that they will be more likely to view such youth as culpable, unamenable to treatment, and to require harsher sanctions.

Given the large concern, there has been a considerable amount of research on this topic (Edens, Magyar, & Cox, 2013), although only a few studies have examined the effects of diagnostic labels on juveniles. These studies have typically used vignettes describing scenarios in which adolescents committed similar crimes, but the descriptions varied as to whether various antisocial labels (e.g., "psychopath," "Conduct Disorder," description of psychopathic traits) or no labels were included and were then presented to various juvenile court actors: judges (Jones & Cauffman, 2008), probation officers (Vidal & Skeem, 2007), and clinicians working in the juvenile justice system (Rockett et al., 2007). This research generally finds that such labels are associated with more negative perceptions of such youth in terms of treatment amenability and harsher dispositions compared to scenarios in which no diagnosis was provided. However, these associations tend to disappear or become weaker when comparing among different antisocial labels. Research has, however, found that the decisions of juvenile court actors might be more influenced by the descriptors associated with psychopathic diagnoses than the label itself. For instance, Murrie, Boccaccini, McCoy, and Cornell (2007) found that when judges were presented with psychopathic criteria (e.g., lacking remorse/guilt, manipulative, callous), they were more punitive in their decisions. While this does not directly assess the impact of a CU trait diagnosis, it does suggest that the core features of psychopathy have a unique effect on decision-making. In the only study to directly examine the influence of a CU trait diagnosis, Edens et al. (2017) examined the influence of the recently introduced Limited Prosocial Emotions (LPE) specifier for Conduct Disorder on a number of legal outcomes. Among a sample of potential jurors, they found that participants were more punitive toward youth with either a psychopathy or LPE diagnosis compared to those with no diagnosis or a Conduct Disorder only diagnosis. However, no differences emerged between the psychopathy and LPE diagnosis.

Another concern regarding the use of CU traits for juvenile justice decision-making concerns the ability to accurately identify these characteristics. There is concern that because characteristics that define CU traits are somewhat normative among youth, it may be hard to accurately diagnose youth with CU traits, particularly in adversarial legal settings (Edens et al., 2013). However, measurement of CU traits has advanced in recent years and, as previously mentioned, the ICU has been found to be an accurate measure for predicting recidivism among juvenile justice-involved populations (Kimonis et al., 2016). Nonetheless, it is necessary for researchers to design measures specifically for use in forensic and juvenile justice settings. Frick (2013) recently developed the Clinical Assessment of Prosocial Emotions (CAPE) to help aid clinicians in the diagnosis of the LPE specifier. While promising, research evaluating the CAPE in diagnosing youth with Conduct Disorder with the LPE specifier is needed along with its utility among juvenile justice-involved populations.

One final concern is the stability of CU traits. If CU traits identify antisocial youth who are most likely to have psychopathic traits as adults, diagnosis of CU traits may then be used to determine which youth will be less amenable to treatment and are a greater threat to society. The juvenile court may, in turn, respond to such youth with harsher sanctions (e.g., longer sentences, secure placement, transfer to the adult court). Such decisions rely on the notion that these traits are stable across developmental periods. While research has suggested some degree of stability for CU traits that is comparable to other personality traits even among younger children, stability estimates also suggest that there is still a considerable degree of change in levels of CU traits across adolescence (see Frick et al., 2014 for a review). This research suggests that for some youth, CU traits are not indicative of whether they will have psychopathic traits as adults. Additionally, this body of research suggests that youth with elevated CU traits are not untreatable. From a juvenile justice perspective, basing decisions that can have lasting influences on youth (e.g., juvenile transfer) on a CU diagnosis should be considered with caution.

Conclusion

In sum, given the large amount of research that has accumulated regarding CU traits and identifying a subgroup of antisocial youth, it is our perspective that CU traits have an important role in the RNR model. The unique factors underlying the antisocial behavior of youth with CU traits makes diagnosis an important factor to be considered for predicting those youth that are most at risk for reoffending and tailoring treatment to their specific needs. It is important, however, that practitioners take precaution when using such diagnoses for decision-making and that research continues to develop and enhance clinical measures specifically geared toward informing such decisions. It is our recommendation that the diagnosis of CU traits should be used to aid decision-making when such diagnoses are accompanied by broader risk assessment tools. That is, such decisions should not be made solely on the diagnosis of CU traits, but decision-makers should instead consider the entirety of the social history of each youth. It is also critical that practitioners consider the current state of the research when CU traits are used to inform juvenile justice decisions. With that being said, more research on CU traits and their implications for juvenile justice are necessary to help inform such decisions.

References

Andershed, H., Kerr, M., Stattin, H., and Levander, S. (2002) 'Psychopathic traits in non-referred youths: A new assessment tool,' in E. Blauuw & L. Sheridan (Eds.), *Psychopaths: Current international perspectives* (pp. 131–158), The Hague: Elsevier.

Andrews, D. A., Bonta, J., and Wormith, J. S. (2006) 'The recent past and near future of risk and/or need assessment,' *Crime & Delinquency*, *52*:7–27.

Asscher, J. J., van Vugt, E. S., Stams, G. J. J., Deković, M., Eichelsheim, V. I., and Yousfi, S. (2011) 'The relationship between juvenile psychopathic traits, delinquency and (violent) recidivism: A meta-analysis,' *Journal of Child Psychology and Psychiatry*, *52*:1134–1143.

Barker, E. D., and Salekin, R. T. (2012) 'Irritable oppositional defiance and callous unemotional traits: Is the association partially explained by peer victimization?,' *Journal of Child Psychology and Psychiatry*, *53*:1167–1175.

Barry, T. D., Barry, C. T., Deming, A. M., and Lochman, J. E. (2008) 'Stability of psychopathic characteristics in childhood: The influence of social relationships,' *Criminal Justice and Behavior*, *35*:244–262.

Bauer, D. L., Whitman, L. A., and Kosson, D. S. (2011) 'Reliability and construct validity of Psychopathy Checklist: Youth Version scores among incarcerated adolescent girls,' *Criminal Justice and Behavior*, *38*:965–987.

Blair, R. J. R., Colledge, E., and Mitchell, D. G. V. (2001) 'Somatic markers and response reversal: Is there orbitofrontal cortex dysfunction in boys with psychopathic tendencies,' *Journal of Abnormal Child Psychology*, *29*:499–511.

Blonigen, D. M., Hicks, B. M., Kruger, R. F., Patrick, C. P., and Iacono, W. G. (2006) 'Continuity and change in psychopathic traits as measured via normal-range personality: A longitudinal-biometric study,' *Journal of Abnormal Psychology*, *115*:85–95.

Brandt, J. R., Kennedy, W. A., Patrick, C. J., and Curtin, J. J. (1997) 'Assessment of psychopathy in a population of incarcerated adolescent offenders,' *Psychological Assessment*, *9*:429–435.

Burke, J. D., Loeber, R., and Lahey, B. B. (2007) 'Adolescent conduct disorder and interpersonal callousness as predictors of psychopathy in young adults,' *Journal of Clinical Child and Adolescent Psychology*, *36*:334–346.

Butler, S., Baruch, G., Hickey, N., and Fonagy, P. (2011) 'A randomized controlled trial of multisystemic therapy and a statutory therapeutic intervention for young offenders,' *Journal of the American Academy of Child & Adolescent Psychiatry*, *50*:1220–1235.

Byrd, A. L., Loeber, R., and Pardini, D. A. (2012) 'Understanding desisting and persisting forms of delinquency: The unique contributions of disruptive behavior disorders and interpersonal callousness,' *Journal of Child Psychology and Psychiatry*, *53*:371–380.

Caldwell, M., Skeem, J., Salekin, R., and Van Rybroek, G. (2006) 'Treatment response of adolescent offenders with psychopathy features: A 2-year follow-up,' *Criminal Justice and Behavior*, *33*:571–596.

Caputo, A. A., Frick, P. J., and Brodsky, S. L. (1999) 'Family violence and juvenile sex offending: The potential mediating role of psychopathic traits and negative attitudes toward women,' *Criminal Justice and Behavior*, *26*:338–356.

Catchpole, R. E. H., and Gretton, H. M. (2003) 'The predictive validity of risk assessment with violent young offenders: A 1-year examination of criminal outcome,' *Criminal Justice and Behavior*, *30*:688–708.

Chabrol, H., van Leeuwen, N., Rodgers, R. F., and Gibbs, J. C. (2011) 'Relations between self-serving cognitive distortions, psychopathic traits, and antisocial behavior in a non-clinical sample of adolescents,' *Personality and Individual Differences*, *51*:887–892.

Christian, R. E., Frick, P. J., Hill, N. L., Tyler, L., and Frazer, D. R. (1997) 'Psychopathy and conduct problems in children: Implications for subtyping children with conduct problems,' *Journal of the American Academy of Child and Adolescent Psychiatry*, *36*:233–241.

Ciucci, E., Baroncelli, A., Franchi, M., Golmaryami, F. N., and Frick, P. J. (2014) 'The association between callous–unemotional traits and behavioral and academic adjustment in children: Further validation of the Inventory of Callous–Unemotional Traits,' *Journal of Psychopathology and Behavioral Assessment*, *36*:189–200.

Cohen, M. A. (1998) 'The monetary value of saving a high-risk youth,' *Journal of Quantitative Criminology*, *14*:5–33.

Cornell, D. G., Warren, J., Hawk, G., Stafford, E., Oram, G., and Pine, D. (1996) 'Psychopathy in instrumental and reactive violent offenders,' *Journal of Consulting and Clinical Psychology*, *64*:783–790.

Corrado, R. R., Vincent, G. M., Hart, S. D., and Cohen, I. M. (2004) 'Predictive validity of the Psychopathy checklist: Youth version for general and violent recidivism,' *Behavioral Sciences and the Law*, *22*:5–22.

Dadds, M. R., Allen, J. L., McGregor, K., Woolgar, M., Viding, E., and Scott, S. (2014) 'Callous-unemotional traits in children and mechanisms of impaired eye contact during expressions of love: A treatment target?,' *Journal of Child Psychology and Psychiatry*, *55*:771–780.

Dadds, M. R., Fraser, J., Frost, A., and Hawes, D. J. (2005) 'Disentangling the underlying dimensions of psychopathy and conduct problems in childhood: A community study,' *Journal of Consulting and Clinical Psychology*, *73*:400–410.

Dandreaux, D. M., and Frick, P. J. (2009) 'Developmental pathways to conduct problems: A further test of the childhood and adolescent-onset distinction,' *Journal of Abnormal Child Psychology*, *37*:375–385.

de Wied, M., van Boxtel, A., Matthys, W., and Meeus, W. (2012) 'Verbal, facial and autonomic responses to empathy-eliciting film clips by disruptive male adolescents with high versus low callous–unemotional traits,' *Journal of Abnormal Child Psychology*, *40*:211–223.

Edens, J. F., Magyar, M. S., and Cox, J. (2013) 'Taking psychopathy measures "out of the lab" and into the legal system: Some practical concerns,' in K. Kiehl & W. Sinnott-Armstrong (Eds.), *Handbook of Psychopathy and Law*. New York, NY: Oxford University Press.

Edens, J. F., Mowle, E. N., Clark, J. W., and Magyar, M. S. (2017) '"A Psychopath by Any Other Name?": Juror perceptions of the DSM-5 "Limited Prosocial Emotions" specifier,' *Journal of Personality Disorders*, *31*:90–109.

Edens, J. F., Skeem, J. L., Cruise, K. R., and Cauffman, E. (2001) 'Assessment of "juvenile psychopathy" and its association with violence: A critical review,' *Behavioral Sciences & the Law*, *19*:53–80.

Edens, J. F., and Vincent, G. M. (2008) 'Juvenile psychopathy: A clinical construct in need of restraint?,' *Journal of Forensic Psychology Practice*, *8*:186–197.

Essau, C. A., Sasagawa, S., and Frick, P. J. (2006) 'Callous–unemotional traits in adolescents,' *Assessment*, *20*:1–16.

Ezpeleta, L., de la Osa, N., Granero, R., Penelo, E., and Domenech, J. M. (2013) 'Inventory of callous–unemotional traits in a community sample of preschoolers,' *Journal of Clinical Child & Adolescent Psychology*, *42*:91–105.

Falkenbach, D. M., Poythress, N. G., and Heide, K. M. (2003) 'Psychopathic features in a juvenile diversion population: Reliability and predictive validity of two self-report measures,' *Behavioral Sciences & the Law*, *21*:787–805.

Fanti, K. A., Frick, P. J., and Georgiou, S. (2009) 'Linking callous–unemotional traits to instrumental and non-instrumental forms of aggression,' *Journal of Psychopathology and Behavioral Assessment*, *31*:285–298.

Fisher, L., and Blair, R. J. R. (1998) 'Cognitive impairment and its relationship to psychopathic tendencies in children with emotional and behavioral difficulties,' *Journal of Abnormal Child Psychology*, *26*:511–519.

Fontaine, N. M. G., Rijsdijk, F. V., McCrory, E. J. P., and Viding, E. (2010) 'Etiology of different developmental trajectories of callous–unemotional traits,' *Journal of the American Academy of Child & Adolescent Psychiatry*, *49*:656–664.

Forsman, M., Lichtenstein, P., Andershed, H., and Larsson, H. (2008) 'Genetic effects explain the stability of psychopathic personality from mid- to late adolescence,' *Journal of Abnormal Psychology*, *117*:606–617.

Forth, A. E., Hart, S. D., and Hare, R. D. (1990) 'Assessment of psychopathy in male young offenders,' *Psychological Assessment: A Journal of Consulting and Clinical Psychology*, *2*(3):342–344.

Forth, A. E., Kosson, D. S., and Hare, R. D. (2003). *Hare Psychopathy Checklist: Youth Version*. Toronto, ON: Multi-Health Systems.

Frick, P. J. (2009) 'Extending the construct of psychopathy to youths: Implications for understanding, diagnosing, and treating antisocial children and adolescents,' *Canadian Journal of Psychiatry*, *12*:803–812.

Frick, P. J. (2013) *Clinical assessment of prosocial emotions: Version 1.1 (CAPE 1.1)*, University of New Orleans.

Frick, P. J., Bodin, S. D., and Barry, C. T. (2000) 'Psychopathic traits and conduct problems in community and clinic-referred samples of children: Further development of the psychopathy screening device,' *Psychological Assessment*, *12*:382–393.

Frick, P. J., Cornell, A. H., Barry, C. T., Bodin, S. D., and Dane, H. A. (2003) 'Callous–unemotional traits and conduct problems in the prediction of conduct problem severity, aggression, and self-report of delinquency,' *Journal of Abnormal Child Psychology*, *31*:457–470.

Frick, P. J., and Hare, R. D. (2001) *The antisocial process screening device*, Toronto, ON: Multi-Health Systems.

Frick, P. J., Kimonis, E. R., Dandreaux, D. M., and Farrell, J. M. (2003) 'The 4 year stability of psychopathic traits in non-referred youth,' *Behavioral Sciences and the Law*, *21*:713–736.

Frick, P. J., and Ray, J. V. (2015) 'Evaluating callous–unemotional traits as a personality construct,' *Journal of Personality*, *83*:710–722.

Frick, P. J., Ray, J. V., Thornton, L. C., and Kahn, R. E. (2014) 'Can callous–unemotional traits enhance the understanding, diagnosis, and treatment of serious conduct problems in children and adolescents? A comprehensive review,' *Psychological Bulletin*, *140*:1–57.

Frick, P. J., Stickle, T. R., Dandreaux, D. M., Farrell, J. M., and Kimonis, E. R. (2005) 'Callous–unemotional traits in predicting the severity and stability of conduct problems and delinquency,' *Journal of Abnormal Child Psychology*, *33*(4):471–487.

Frick, P. J., and White, S. F. (2008) 'The importance of callous–unemotional traits for the development of aggressive and antisocial behavior,' *Journal of Child Psychology and Psychiatry*, *49*:359–375.

Gendreau, P., Little, T., and Goggin, C. (1996) 'A meta-analysis of the predictors of adult offender recidivism: What works!,' *Criminology*, *34*(4):575–608.

Gretton, H. M., Hare, R. D., and Catchpole, R. E. H. (2004) 'Psychopathy and offending from adolescence to adulthood: A 10-year follow-up,' *Journal of Consulting and Clinical Psychology*, *72*:636–645.

Gretton, H. M., McBride, M., Hare, R. D., O'Shaughnessy, R., and Kumka, G. (2001) 'Psychopathy and recidivism in adolescent sex offenders,' *Criminal Justice and Behavior*, *28*:427–449.

Haas, S. M., Becker, S. P., Epstein, J. N., and Frick, P. J. (2017) 'Callous–unemotional traits are uniquely associated with poorer peer functioning in school-aged children,' *Journal of Abnormal Child Psychology*, in press:1–13.

Hare, R. D. (1998) 'Psychopaths and their nature: Implications for the mental health and criminal justice systems,' in D. J. Cooke, A. E. Forth, & R. D. Hare (Eds.), *Psychopathy: Antisocial, criminal, and violent behavior* (pp. 188–212). Boston, MA: Kluwer Academic Publishers.

Hare, R. D. (2003) *The Psychopathy Checklist–Revised manual* (2nd ed.), Toronto, ON: Multi-Health Systems.

Hawes, S. W., Byrd, A. L., Henderson, C. E., Gazda, R. L., Burke, J. D., Loeber, R., and Pardini, D. A. (2014) 'Refining the parent-reported inventory of callous–unemotional traits in boys with conduct problems,' *Psychological Assessment*, *26*:256–266.

Hawes, D. J., and Dadds, M. R. (2007) 'Stability and malleability of callous–unemotional traits during treatment for childhood conduct problems,' *Journal of Clinical Child and Adolescent Psychology*, *36*:347–355.

Hawes, D. J., Price, M. J., and Dadds, M. R. (2014) 'Callous–unemotional traits and the treatment of conduct problems in childhood and adolescence: A comprehensive review,' *Clinical Child and Family Psychology Review*, *17*:248–267.

Jones, S., and Cauffman, E. (2008) 'Juvenile psychopathy and judicial decision making: An empirical analysis of an ethical dilemma,' *Behavioral Sciences & the Law*, *26*:151–165.

Kerr, M., Van Zalk, M., and Stattin, H. (2012) 'Psychopathic traits moderate peer influence on adolescent delinquency,' *Journal of Child Psychology and Psychiatry*, *53*:826–835.

Kimonis, E. R., Frick, P. J., and Barry, C. T. (2004) 'Callous–unemotional traits and delinquent peer affiliation,' *Journal of Consulting and Clinical Psychology*, *72*:956–964.

Kimonis, E. R., Frick, P. J., Fazekas, H., and Loney, B. R. (2006) 'Psychopathic traits, aggression, and the processing of emotional stimuli in non-referred children,' *Behavioral Sciences and the Law*, *24*:21–37.

Kimonis, E. R., Frick, P. J., Skeem, J. L., Marsee, M. A., Cruise, K., Munoz, L. C., . . ., and Morris, A. S. (2008) 'Assessing callous–unemotional traits in adolescent offenders: Validation of the inventory of callous–unemotional traits,' *International Journal of Law and Psychiatry*, *31*:241–252.

Kimonis, E. R., Kennealy, P. J., and Goulter, N. (2016) 'Does the self-report Inventory of Callous–Unemotional Traits predict recidivism?,' *Psychological Assessment*, *28*:1616–1623.

Kruh, I. P., Frick, J. P., and Clements, C. B. (2005) 'Historical and personality correlates to the violence patterns of juveniles tried as adults,' *Criminal Justice and Behavior*, *32*(1):69–96.

Lawing, K., Frick, P. J., and Cruise, K. R. (2010) 'Differences in offending patterns between adolescent sex offenders high or low in callous–unemotional traits,' *Psychological Assessment*, *22*(2):298–305.

Lynam, D. R. (1996) 'Early identification of chronic offenders: Who is the fledgling psychopath?,' *Psychological Bulletin*, *120*:209–234.

Lynam, D. R. (1997) 'Pursuing the psychopath: Capturing the fledgling psychopath in a nomological net,' *Journal of Abnormal Psychology*, *106*(3):425–438.

Lynam, D. R., Caspi, A., Moffitt, T. E., Loeber, R., and Stouthamer-Loeber, M. (2007) 'Longitudinal evidence that psychopathy scores in early adolescence predict adult psychopathy,' *Journal of Abnormal Psychology*, *116*:155–165.

Marsee, M. A., and Frick, P. J. (2007) 'Exploring the cognitive and emotional correlates of proactive and reactive aggression in a sample of detained girls,' *Journal of Abnormal Child Psychology*, *35*:969–981.

Marsh, A. A., Finger, E. C., Schechter, J. C., Jurkowitz, I. T. N., Reid, M. E., and Blair, R. J. R. (2011) 'Adolescents with psychopathic traits report reductions in physiological responses to fear,' *Journal of Child Psychology and Psychiatry*, *52*:838–841.

McDonald, R., Dodson, M. C., Rosenfield, D., and Jouriles, E. N. (2011) 'Effects of a parenting intervention on features of psychopathy in children,' *Journal of Abnormal Child Psychology*, *39*:1013–1023.

Moffitt, T. E. (1993) 'Adolescence-limited and life-course-persistent antisocial behavior: A developmental taxonomy,' *Psychological Review*, *100*:674–701.

Muñoz. L. C., and Frick, P. J. (2007) 'The reliability, stability, and predictive utility of the self-report version of the Antisocial Process Screening Device,' *Scandinavian Journal of Psychology*, *48*:299–312.

Munoz, L. C., Frick, P. J., Kimonis, E. R., and Aucoin, K. J. (2008) 'Verbal ability and delinquency: Testing the moderating role of psychopathic traits,' *Journal of Child Psychology and Psychiatry*, *49*(4):414–421.

Murrie, D. C., Boccaccini, M. T., McCoy, W., and Cornell, D. G. (2007) 'Diagnostic labeling in juvenile court: How do descriptions of psychopathy and conduct disorder influence judges?,' *Journal of Clinical Child and Adolescent Psychology*, *36*:228–241.

Obradovic, J., Pardini, D. A., Long, J. D., and Loeber, R. (2007) 'Measuring interpersonal callousness in boys from childhood to adolescence: An examination of longitudinal invariance and temporal stability,' *Journal of Clinical Child and Adolescent Psychology*, *36*:276–292.

Pardini, D. A., and Byrd, A. L. (2012) 'Perceptions of aggressive conflicts and others' distress in children with callous-unemotional traits: "I'll show you who's boss, even if you suffer and I get in trouble",' *Journal of Child Psychology and Psychiatry*, *53*:283–291.

Pardini, D. A., Lochman, J. E., and Frick, P. J. (2003) 'Callous/unemotional traits and social–cognitive processes in adjudicated youths,' *Journal of the American Academy of Child & Adolescent Psychiatry*, *42*:364–371.

Pardini, D. A., Lochman, J. E., and Powell, N. (2007) 'The development of callous–unemotional traits and antisocial behavior in children: Are there shared and/or unique predictors?,' *Journal of Clinical Child and Adolescent Psychology*, *36*:319–333.

Pardini, D. A., and Loeber, R. (2008) 'Interpersonal callousness trajectories across adolescence: Early social influences and adult outcomes,' *Criminal Justice and Behavior*, *35*:173–196.

Ray, J. V., Thornton, L. C., Frick, P. J., Steinberg, L., and Cauffman, E. (2016) 'Impulse control and callous–unemotional traits distinguish patterns of delinquency and substance use in justice involved adolescents: Examining the moderating role of neighborhood context,' *Journal of Abnormal Child Psychology*, *44*:599–611.

Rockett, J. L., Murrie, D. C., and Boccaccini, M. T. (2007) 'Diagnostic labeling in juvenile justice settings: Do psychopathy and conduct disorder findings influence clinicians?,' *Psychological Services*, *4*:107–122.

Roose, A., Bijttebier, P., Decoene, S., Claes, L., and Frick, P. J. (2010) 'Assessing the affective features of psychopathy in adolescence: A further validation of the Inventory of Callous and Unemotional traits,' *Assessment*, *17*:44–57.

Schmidt, F., Campbell, M. A., and Houlding, C. (2011) 'Comparative analyses of the YLS/CMI, SAVRY, and PCL: YV in adolescent offenders: A 10-year follow-up into adulthood,' *Youth Violence and Juvenile Justice*, *9*:23–42.

Schwalbe, C. S. (2007) 'Risk assessment for juvenile justice: A meta-analysis,' *Law and Human Behavior*, *31*:449–460.

Seagrave, D., and Grisso, T. (2002) 'Adolescent development and the measurement of juvenile psychopathy,' *Law and Human Behavior*, *26*:219–239.

Serin, R. C., Brown, S. L., and De Wolf, A. H. (2015) 'The clinical use of the Hare Psychopathy Checklist–Revised (PCL–R),' in C. B. Gacono (Ed.), *The Clinical and Forensic Assessment of Psychopathy: A Practitioner's Guide* (pp. 293–310). New York, NY: Routledge.

Silverthorn, P., Frick, P. J., and Reynolds, R. (2001) 'Timing of onset and correlates of severe conduct problems in adjudicated girls and boys,' *Journal of Psychopathology and Behavioral Assessment*, *23*:171–181.

Somech, L. Y., and Elizur, Y. (2012) 'Promoting self-regulation and cooperation in pre-kindergarten children with conduct problems: A randomized controlled trial,' *Journal of the American Academy of Child & Adolescent Psychiatry*, *51*:412–422.

Spain, S. E., Douglas, K. S., Poythress, N. G., and Epstein, M. (2004) 'The relationship between psychopathic features, violence and treatment outcome: The comparison of three youth measures of psychopathic features,' *Behavioral Sciences & the Law*, *22*:85–102.

Steinberg, L., Mounts, N. S., Lamborn, S. D., and Dornbusch, S. M. (1991) 'Authoritative parenting and adolescent adjustment across varied ecological niches,' *Journal of Research on Adolescence*, *1*:19–36.

Stellwagen, K. K., and Kerig, P. K. (2010a) 'Relation of callous–unemotional traits to length of stay among youth hospitalized at a state psychiatric inpatient facility,' *Child Psychiatry & Human Development*, *41*:251–261.

Stellwagen, K. K., and Kerig, P. K. (2010b) 'Relating callous–unemotional traits to physically restrictive treatment measures among child psychiatric inpatients,' *Journal of Child and Family Studies*, *19*:588–595.

Stickle, T. R., Kirkpatrick, N. M., and Brush, L. N. (2009) 'Callous–unemotional traits and social information processing: Multiple risk-factor models for understanding aggressive behavior in antisocial youth,' *Law and Human Behavior*, *33*:515–529.

Thornton, L. C., Frick, P. J., Shulman, E. P., Ray, J. V., Steinberg, L., and Cauffman, E. (2015) 'Callous–unemotional traits and adolescents' role in group crime,' *Law and Human Behavior*, *39*:368–377.

Van Baardewijk, Y., Vermeiren, R., Stegge, H., and Doreleijers, T. (2011) 'Self-report psychopathic traits in children: Their stability and concurrent and prospective association with conduct problems and aggression,' *Journal of Psychopathology and Behavioral Assessment*, *33*:236–245.

Vidal, S., and Skeem, J. L. (2007) 'Effect of psychopathy, abuse, and ethnicity on juvenile probation officers' decision-making and supervision strategies,' *Law and Human Behavior*, *31*:479–498.

Viding, E., Blair, R. J. R., Moffitt, T. E., and Plomin, R. (2005) 'Evidence for substantial genetic risk for psychopathy in 7-year-olds,' *Journal of Child Psychology and Psychiatry*, *46*:592–597.

Viding, E., Sebastian, C. L., Dadds, M. R., Lockwood, P. L., Cecil, C. A. M., De Brito, S. A., and McCrory, E. J. (2012) 'Amygdala response to preattentive masked fear in children with conduct problems: The role of callous–unemotional traits,' *American Journal of Psychiatry*, *169*:1109–1116.

Vincent, G. M., Guy, L. S., Fusco, S. L., and Gershenson, B. G. (2012) 'Field reliability of the SAVRY with juvenile probation officers: Implications for training,' *Law and Human Behavior*, *36*:225–236.

Waller, R., Gardner, F., and Hyde, L. W. (2013) 'What are the associations between parenting, callous – unemotional traits, and antisocial behavior in youth? A systematic review of evidence,' *Clinical Psychology Review*, *33*:593–608.

Waller, R., Gardner, F., Hyde, L. W., Shaw, D. S., Dishion, T. J., and Wilson, M. N. (2012) 'Do harsh and positive parenting predict parent reports of deceitful–callous behavior in early childhood?,' *Journal of Child Psychology and Psychiatry*, *53*:946–953.

Waller, R., Wright, A. G., Shaw, D. S., Gardner, F., Dishion, T. J., Wilson, M. N., and Hyde, L. W. (2014) 'Factor Structure and Construct Validity of the Parent-Reported Inventory of Callous–unemotional traits among high-risk 9-year-olds,' *Assessment*, Advance online publication.

Webster, C. D., Harris, G. T., Rice, M. E., Cormier, C., and Quinsey, V. L. (1994) *The violence prediction scheme: Assessing dangerousness in high risk men*, Toronto, ON: University of Toronto Centre of Criminology.

White, S. F., Frick, P. J., Lawing, K., and Bauer, D. (2013) 'Callous–unemotional traits and response to Functional Family Therapy in adolescent offenders,' *Behavioral Sciences & the Law*, *31*:271–285.

Willoughby, M. T., Waschbusch, D. A., Moore, G. A., and Propper, C. B. (2011) 'Using the ASEBA to screen for callous unemotional traits in early childhood: Factor structure, temporal, stability, and utility,' *Journal of Psychopathology and Behavioral Assessment*, *33*:19–30.

Wong, S. C., and Olver, M. E. (2015) 'Risk reduction treatment of psychopathy and applications to mentally disordered offenders,' *CNS Spectrums*, *20*:303–310.

7

Neurogenetics approaches to understanding psychopathy

Laura Murray, Hailey L. Dotterer, Rebecca Waller, and Luke W. Hyde

Introduction

Psychopathy is a disorder defined by problematic personality traits, including lack of remorse or guilt, interpersonal manipulation, callousness, impulsivity, and antisocial behaviors such as aggression and rule breaking (Hare, 1991). Psychopathy confers tremendous emotional and financial costs to victims, families, and society (McCollister, French, & Fang, 2010). Thus, considerable research has focused on understanding the measurement, etiology, and treatment of psychopathy (Hare & Neumann, 2008; Skeem, Polaschek, Patrick, & Lilienfeld, 2011). Despite this work, there are few examples of lasting effective treatment or prevention programs for psychopathy, perhaps due to remaining questions regarding the etiology of the disorder (see Salekin, 2002). Examining the etiology of psychopathy can provide clues as to how these harmful behaviors emerge and help to identify underlying mechanisms of psychopathy that can be targeted in treatment. Given that many theories on the etiology of psychopathy have emphasized the contributions of biology (e.g., neurobiology, genes) in conferring risk for psychopathy (Blair, 2005; Gao & Raine, 2010; Raine, 2008), researchers have begun to utilize neuroimaging to identify brain abnormalities that are associated with psychopathic traits.

Neuroimaging studies of psychopathy have primarily focused on brain regions associated with the behavioral deficits assumed to be critical to the psychopathy construct. Psychopathy has been linked to lower emotional response to distress and threat, greater impulsivity and risk-taking, and deficits in attentional allocation (Hare & Neumann, 2008; Kosson & Newman, 1986; Skeem et al., 2011). As such, researchers have examined activation of brain regions involved in socioemotional processes (e.g., amygdala, orbitofrontal cortex, anterior cingulate cortex; Blair, 2010, 2007a), reward (e.g., striatum; Buckholtz et al., 2010), attention, and inhibitory control (e.g., dorsolateral prefrontal cortex, inferior frontal gyrus; Hoppenbrouwers et al., 2013; Rodman et al., 2016). The findings of this research thus have identified specific neural and behavioral correlates of psychopathy, including socioemotional, reward, and cognitive (i.e., attentional, inhibitory control) processes that may be amenable to targeted treatments (e.g., Baskin-Sommers, Curtin, & Newman, 2015).

Although an understanding of the neural correlates of psychopathy and broader antisocial behavior (AB) are important for understanding etiology, to understand the developmental etiology of psychopathy we must also understand how these neural differences develop. Given that previous research has found psychopathy to be heritable (e.g., 30–50 percent; Beaver, Barnes, May, & Schwartz, 2011; Beaver, Vaughn, DeLisi, Barnes, & Boutwell, 2012; Blair, Peschardt, Budhani, Mitchell, & Pine, 2006; Moffitt, 2005), researchers have attempted to identify genes that could contribute to the development of psychopathy (e.g., Viding et al., 2010). However, studies have also found environmental influences, such as harsh parenting and neighborhood disadvantage, to be associated with the emergence of psychopathy or early risk markers for psychopathy (i.e., Callous–Unemotional or CU traits; Farrington, Ullrich, & Salekin, 2010; Waller, Gardner, & Hyde, 2013). Indeed, research on gene-by-environment (G × E) interactions suggests that brain function and subsequent behavior may develop through the interplay of genetic risk and experience. A neurogenetics approach offers the ability to integrate across multiple levels of analysis to probe mechanisms by which biological vulnerability and environmental experience interact to predict brain dysfunction and the resulting individual variability in complex behavior (e.g., psychopathy; Hyde, Bogdan, & Hariri, 2011).

The goal of this chapter is to provide an overview of the current state of the literature on the neurogenetics of psychopathy and, to a lesser extent, broader AB. First, we briefly define neurogenetics and highlight its utility in understanding the etiological mechanisms of psychopathy. Second, we identify key neural mechanisms linked to emotional and behavioral deficits that characterize psychopathy, which may differentiate psychopathy from broader AB. Third, we discuss additional risk factors (i.e., genetic variation, environment) associated with psychopathy, including the evidence from studies that have begun to examine the interplay of these factors (e.g., G × E interaction models, neurogenetics pathways) in the development of psychopathy and AB more broadly. Finally, to motivate future research in this emerging field, we provide an imaging gene-by-environment (IG × E) interaction model of psychopathy that integrates current research on genetic and environmental influences on psychopathy and AB via brain function.

What is neurogenetics?

Neurogenetics approaches originated with imaging genetics studies that sought to link variability in genetic background to variability in brain structure or function (Hariri, 2009; Hariri, Drabant, & Weinberger, 2006). The goal of these early studies was to understand how variability in genes, particularly those in neurotransmitter systems, shapes neural structure or reactivity, which in turn should increase the risk for psychopathology and influence the expression of complex behavior. To better understand significant associations found between genetic variability, brain, and behavior, researchers began examining the brain as a plausible mechanism through which genes influence complex behavior (Fakra et al., 2009). This imaging genetics approach offers several advantages. First, by examining variability in genes with known functions, these studies leverage knowledge from animal models about how variability in specific genes might affect downstream proteins and neurotransmitter levels, thus providing a detailed molecular account of how genes influence behavior. Second, imaging genetics studies further establish underlying molecular mechanisms by incorporating other complementary techniques, including positron emission tomography (PET) imaging (to measure neurotransmitter binding; e.g., Fisher, Meltzer, Ziolko, Price, & Hariri, 2006) and pharmacological functional magnetic resonance imaging (to directly manipulate neurotransmitter levels; e.g., Bigos et al., 2008). This broad approach, which we refer to as neurogenetics, examines the pathways from genes to behavior via detailed molecular mechanisms that shape brain structure and function. One recent addition to neurogenetics is an examination of the role of the environment within pathways, as environmental experiences likely shape neurodevelopment and interact with genetic background to impact the brain (Bogdan, Williamson, & Hariri, 2012; Hyde, 2015; White et al., 2012). A growing number of studies have shown that variability in brain structure and function are correlated with various complex behaviors and forms of psychopathology. Thus, neurogenetics approaches have emerged as even more critical, because they may help us to understand how variation in neural functioning develops and contributes to psychopathological outcomes. In the case of psychopathy, a neurogenetics approach can help us to understand how neural correlates of psychopathy emerge and, ultimately, how to treat and prevent the development of this dangerous and costly disorder at multiple levels.

What is psychopathy?

Psychopathy encompasses a variety of personality traits and behavioral features, including AB. Psychopathic traits include grandiosity and superficial charm, manipulativeness, lack of remorse, shallow affect, impulsivity, irresponsibility, and poor behavioral control. To isolate more specific etiological mechanisms of psychopathy, researchers typically examine two separate factors consisting of: (1) traits related to interpersonal and affective domains such as grandiosity and lack of remorse (i.e., Factor 1); and (2) traits related to general sensation seeking, impulsivity, low behavioral control, behavioral problems, and criminality (i.e., Factor 2; Hare & Neumann, 2008). In general, Factor 2 traits are more strongly correlated with externalizing behaviors such as disinhibition and substance abuse (Venables & Patrick, 2012), which capture a broad latent trait common to psychopathy, AB, Attention-Deficit/Hyperactivity Disorder (ADHD), and substance use disorders (Krueger et al., 2002; Krueger, Markon, Patrick, Benning, & Kramer, 2007; Patrick et al., 2013). Among youth, CU traits have been used to identify individuals who display similar affective features to adult psychopathy (i.e., Factor 1) and who therefore may be at risk for developing psychopathy (Frick & White, 2008). Studies often delineate neural correlates for CU traits versus AB or neural correlates of antisocial youth high versus low on CU traits, in the same way that many studies of adults separate between correlates of Factor 1 and Factor 2 psychopathic traits. Identifying etiological and behavioral mechanisms that may (or may not) be specific to psychopathy (or Factor 1) rather than AB (or Factor 2) is a continued goal within this work (Hare & Neumann, 2010; Skeem & Cooke, 2010), though note that Factor 1 and 2 are highly correlated and both are necessary for the diagnosis of psychopathy.

Studies have found the most consistent behavioral deficits in those high on psychopathy to be in affective processing, reward sensitivity, and attention (Hamilton, Hiatt Racer, & Newman, 2015). First, individuals high on psychopathy (especially Factor 1) often appear under-reactive to emotional stimuli, most consistently to distress or threat. For example, individuals high in psychopathic traits demonstrate reduced startle responses to aversive stimuli (Patrick, Bradley, & Lang, 1993). Individuals with psychopathy may not appropriately learn to associate these cues with a negative aversive response and thus persist in aggressive and harmful behaviors (Blair, 2017). Second, psychopathy (especially Factor 2) is associated with impulsive and risky behaviors, which have been hypothesized to emerge from an overactive reward system and an underactive punishment system (Newman, MacCoon, Vaughn, & Sadeh, 2005; Quay, 1993). Accordingly, individuals high on Factor 2 psychopathy may perseverate on previously rewarded stimuli that are now punished (e.g., poor performance on response reversal tasks; Budhani & Blair, 2005; Budhani, Richell, & Blair, 2006). Third, psychopathic traits have been associated with impaired attention. Specifically, Factor 1 has been linked to increased attention to specific cues related to goal attainment (i.e., hyper-focus on relevant cues, able to ignore irrelevant cues), while Factor 2 psychopathy has been associated with impaired attention and increased distractibility (i.e., inability to ignore irrelevant cues; Baskin-Sommers, Zeier, & Newman, 2009; Sadeh & Verona, 2008). Taken together, compared to those low on psychopathy, those high on psychopathy may respond less to affective stimuli, learn less from punishment and emotion, be impulsive, and have difficulty modulating their attention in ways that lead to normative behavior. Neuroimaging has the potential to identify neural mechanisms of these behavioral deficits and to better understand the biological etiology of psychopathy (Blair, 2015).

Neural correlates of psychopathy

There has been rapid growth in the use of neuroimaging techniques to better understand biological mechanisms underpinning behavioral and personality traits specific to psychopathy. Neuroimaging studies can be divided into those using functional magnetic resonance imaging (fMRI) to assess brain activity, structural methods (i.e., sMRI) to assess brain structure, and connectivity methods to assess structural and functional connections between brain regions. Functional connectivity (e.g., psychophysiological interactions; PPI) is measured by examining correlated neural activity between brain regions. Structural connectivity is measured by examining the integrity of white matter tracts that connect brain regions by using diffusion tensor imaging (i.e., DTI). Connectivity approaches can establish how regions function as networks; that is, they look for disrupted connections (due either to structural or functional impairments) that may impact system-level functioning and psychological processes key to psychopathy. Studies using these neuroimaging techniques have identified brain regions implicated in adult psychopathy and youth CU traits, particularly those related to deficits in socioemotional processing, reward processing, attention, and inhibitory control (Blair, Veroude, & Buitelaar, 2016). Note that we constrain our overview to studies using MRI approaches, though many other neuroimaging approaches (e.g., PET, electroencephalogram or EEG) have been used effectively to understand psychopathy (e.g., Raine et al., 1998; Venables, Hall, Yancey, & Patrick, 2015).

Functional neuroimaging

Socioemotional processing

Psychopathy is consistently associated with behavioral deficits in socioemotional processing, including emotion recognition, regulation, and empathy, making these processes key targets for neuroimaging research (Blair, 2017). One overarching theory of psychopathy is that it stems, in part, from fearlessness that emerges from low automatic affective response to threat and distress (Blair, Mitchell, & Blair, 2005; Blair et al., 2002). Research focusing on socioemotional processing in psychopathy using fMRI has primarily focused on corticolimbic regions, including the amygdala, that are involved in emotion processing and affective decision-making (Carré, Hyde, Neumann, Viding, & Hariri, 2013; Contreras-Rodríguez et al., 2014; Dotterer, Hyde, Swartz, Hariri, & Williamson, 2017; Hyde, Shaw, Murray et al., 2016; Kiehl et al., 2001; Viding et al., 2012). The amygdala is responsible for processing salient emotional stimuli, generating affective responses, fear conditioning/learning, and threat detection (LeDoux, 1995), making it a key target for research in psychopathy. Individuals high on psychopathic traits and youth high on CU traits appear to have diminished amygdala reactivity to emotional stimuli (i.e., fearful faces), which may in turn contribute to deficits in empathy (Blair, 2010, 2015; Hyde, Shaw, & Hariri, 2013). For example, decreased amygdala reactivity has been found among criminal psychopaths in tasks contrasting emotional to neutral phrases (Kiehl et al., 2001) and when viewing sad and fearful (Blair, 2005) as well as angry and fearful (Contreras-Rodríguez et al., 2014) facial expressions.

Notably, amygdala function may be one mechanism by which individuals with psychopathy differ from those high on AB only. For example, among youth with conduct problems, those with high CU traits had reduced amygdala reactivity to fearful faces, whereas those with low CU traits had increased amygdala reactivity (Viding et al., 2012). Similarly, in a sample of community adults, Hyde and colleagues (2014) found that Factor 1 psychopathic traits were linked to lower negative emotionality and lower amygdala reactivity, whereas Factor 2 psychopathic traits were linked to higher negative emotionality and greater amygdala reactivity to emotional faces (Hyde et al., 2014). Similar associations were also reported in youth with CU traits compared to youth with ADHD (Marsh & Blair, 2008). These studies suggest that amygdala reactivity during affective processing, particularly neural and behavioral response to distress in others (i.e., fear; Blair, 2005), may distinguish individuals high on AB (but not psychopathy) from individuals with psychopathy (Carré et al., 2013). However, see Hyde and colleagues (2016) and Dotterer and colleagues (2017) for notable studies that did not replicate this effect in community samples.

In addition to facial emotion processing, reduced amygdala reactivity has also been reported for those high on psychopathy in other tasks involving socioemotional processing. For example, psychopathy was linked to reduced amygdala reactivity when making judgments about the severity of moral transgressions (Harenski, Harenski, Shane, & Kiehl, 2010) and when making emotional moral decisions (e.g., deciding whether to harm a child to save numerous people; Glenn, Raine, & Schug, 2009). Together, current research suggests that those with psychopathic traits may persist in aggressive behaviors due to their diminished amygdala reactivity and lack of aversive response to signals of distress in others or moral transgressions. In contrast, those high on AB without psychopathy generally display amygdala hypersensitivity to emotional stimuli, which may lead to emotionally dysregulated reactive aggression (Waller, Dotterer, Murray, & Hyde, in press).

Psychopathy has also been linked to abnormal functioning in other brain regions implicated in affective and socioemotional processing, including the orbitofrontal cortex/ventromedial prefrontal cortex (OFC/vmPFC), anterior cingulate cortex (ACC), and insula. The OFC is responsible for the representation of affective stimuli, emotional responding, and inhibitory control (Blair, 2007b; Damasio, Grabowski, Frank, Galaburda, & Damasio, 1994). Individuals high on psychopathy have demonstrated reduced OFC activation while viewing aversive cues (Decety, Chen, Harenski, & Kiehl, 2013) and happy and sad facial expressions (Decety, Skelly, Yoder, & Kiehl, 2014) as well as during an emotional memory task (Kiehl et al., 2001). Psychopathy was also linked to reduced OFC and amygdala reactivity to pictures of moral transgressions compared to non-psychopaths (Harenski et al., 2010), and Factor 1 psychopathic traits were related to reduced medial prefrontal cortex response during emotional moral decision-making (i.e., harming others; Glenn et al., 2009). Thus, reduced OFC/vmPFC function may contribute to decreased reactivity to distress in others, which in turn may contribute to aggressive behaviors (Blair, 2008, 2003).

The ACC plays an important role in socioemotional processing due to its involvement in error monitoring, affective response, and response modulation (Botvinick, Cohen, & Carter, 2004; Etkin, Egner, & Kalisch, 2011). The insula plays an important role in interoception and sensory integration (Critchley, Wiens, Rotshtein, Öhman, & Dolan, 2004). Together with the ACC, the insula is involved in the processing of pain in the self and in others (Medford & Critchley, 2010). In youth, CU traits have been linked to decreased ACC and anterior insula reactivity to images of others' pain (Lockwood et al., 2013; Michalska, Zeffiro, & Decety, 2016). Furthermore, several studies have reported decreased ACC reactivity among criminal psychopaths during tasks assessing empathy (Meffert, Gazzola, den Boer, Bartels, & Keysers, 2013), while viewing emotionally salient scenes (Müller et al., 2003), and while viewing painful facial expressions (Decety et al., 2013). Reduced ACC and insula activity may therefore contribute to decreased reactivity to others' pain, resulting in decreased empathy and fewer prosocial behaviors.

In sum, fMRI studies using tasks related to socioemotional processing suggest that psychopathy is associated with reduced emotional response to signals of distress (i.e., fear) in others that likely stems from neural dysfunction across many corticolimbic structures important for the representation of emotion and pain in others, and in behavior change in response to aversive stimuli (Waller et al., in press).

Reward, attention, and inhibitory control

Psychopathy has also been characterized by deficits in processing of rewards and punishments (i.e., perseverating on rewards despite continued punishment), impairments in attention allocation, and poor behavioral control that leads to risky decision-making (Newman, Patterson, & Kosson, 1987; Newman, Widom, & Nathan, 1985). Neuroimaging research on these behaviors has primarily implicated areas in the prefrontal cortex that are responsible for inhibitory/cognitive control and decision-making (e.g., dorsolateral prefrontal cortex; dlPFC), and regions within the dopaminergic reward system (e.g., ventral striatum) that play an important role in the valuation of rewards and reward-related decision-making (Buckholtz et al., 2010; White et al., 2013).

Psychopathy is associated with a persistent pattern of reward-seeking behavior, suggesting that psychopaths have a reward-dominant style due to hypersensitivity to rewards (or hyposensitivity to punishments). The ventral striatum has been a primary target of this line of research due to its role in the valuation, anticipation, and consumption of reward (Heekeren et al., 2007). Indeed, several studies in community samples (and one that compared community and incarcerated samples) have identified positive associations between Factor 2, but not Factor 1, psychopathic traits and neural response to reward in the ventral striatum (Bjork, Chen, & Hommer, 2012; Buckholtz et al., 2010; Carré et al., 2013; Geurts et al., 2016; Murray, Shaw, Forbes, & Hyde, 2017). This research generally suggests that psychopathy, at least the Factor 2 traits characteristic of broader AB and externalizing, are characterized by hypersensitivity to reward.

Attention and executive functioning may additionally distinguish psychopathy from AB. Factor 1 psychopathic traits have been associated with improved attentional control, whereas Factor 2 psychopathic traits have been linked to reduced attentional control during behavioral tasks (Baskin-Sommers, Brazil, Ryan, Kohlenberg et al., 2015; Baskin-Sommers, Zeier, & Newman, 2009). For example, those high on Factor 1 psychopathic traits display less interference (i.e., better performance) on Stroop tasks than those high on Factor 2 psychopathic traits (for a review of attentional differences between psychopathy and externalizing, see Baskin-Sommers & Newman, 2013). It is also possible that differences in the allocation of attention in psychopathy (i.e., early attention bottleneck) may underlie socioemotional deficits in psychopathy (Baskin-Sommers, Curtin, & Newman, 2011). Specifically, individuals with psychopathic traits may be limited in their ability to process emotionally salient information when it is peripheral to goal-directed behavior. For instance, Larson and colleagues (2013) found that individuals high on psychopathy only displayed decreased amygdala reactivity to threat when threat cues were presented after individuals were already engaged in a different goal-directed task (i.e., early alternative goal focus condition). Furthermore, individuals high on psychopathy also displayed increased recruitment of the lateral prefrontal cortex during this early alternative goal focus condition. Importantly, this increased prefrontal neural reactivity completely mediated the association between psychopathy and decreased amygdala activation to threat cues (Larson et al., 2013). Moreover, increased frontoparietal activity (including the inferior frontal gyrus and dlPFC) has also been observed in incarcerated offenders high in psychopathy during non-affective executive function tasks that probe interference suppression and response inhibition (Rodman et al., 2016). In contrast, self-reported externalizing behavior was linked to reduced activity in the dlPFC during response inhibition (Rodman et al., 2016). The authors also reported that inferior frontal gyrus activity was negatively correlated with inhibition and attentional switching on a Stroop task. Thus, frontoparietal activity during attentional tasks may be one mechanism by which psychopathy diverges from AB (Rodman et al., 2016). Together, these findings support the notion that psychopathy is associated with impaired attentional flexibility (i.e. "attentional bottleneck") relative to individuals with low psychopathy, with some evidence suggesting that reduced attention may contribute to impairments in emotional processing.

Structural and connectivity neuroimaging

Structural MRI

Structural MRI allows researchers to study individual- and group-based differences in brain structure and thus identify structural differences in brain regions that are associated with psychopathy. Structural MRI investigations of psychopathy highlight structural differences (i.e., grey matter volume) in many of the same brain regions emphasized in the functional literature. A meta-analysis of 12 studies established links between psychopathy and reduced grey matter volume in brain regions including OFC, dlPFC, and ACC (Yang & Raine, 2009). Psychopathy has also been linked to lower grey matter volume in the amygdala in adults (Pardini, Raine, Erickson, & Loeber, 2014) and in youth high on CU traits (Cohn et al., 2016). Lower grey matter volume has also been found in the hippocampus, OFC, temporal pole, and posterior cingulate for both adults (Ermer, Cope, Nyalakanti, Calhoun, & Kiehl, 2012) and incarcerated youth with psychopathic traits (Ermer, Cope, Nyalakanti, Calhoun, & Kiehl, 2013). Finally, psychopathy has also been linked to greater grey matter volume in the striatum (Glenn, Raine, Yaralian, & Yang, 2010; Korponay et al., 2017). Lower volume in regions such as the OFC, ACC, and amygdala, but greater volume in the striatum, mirrors the specific functional activation patterns often observed in these regions within psychopathy. Specifically, lower volume in brain regions associated with socioemotional processes may contribute to the decreased activation of these regions, whereas greater volume in reward-related regions such as the striatum may contribute to increased activation. Thus, similar to the findings of functional neuroimaging studies, psychopathy is associated with structural aberrations in brain regions that may underlie impaired affective processing, attention and executive function deficits, and increased reward-driven behavior.

Connectivity

Structural connectivity within the brain can be examined using diffusion tensor imaging (DTI). DTI measures the diffusion of water molecules along neurons to index the integrity of white-matter (i.e., myelinated axon) connections between brain regions (Assaf & Pasternak, 2008). Thus, DTI provides a physical measure of how efficiently brain regions are communicating and may help to identify neural networks of dysfunction in psychopathy. DTI studies of psychopathy have focused on the uncinate fasciculus, a white-matter tract that connects the amygdala and the OFC, two regions that are functionally and structurally implicated in psychopathy (Blair, 2007b). Results from a recent systematic review suggest that psychopathy and AB among adults are associated with reduced integrity of a wide range of white-matter tracts, including the uncinate fasciculus as well as the corpus callosum, cingulum, and superior longitudinal fasciculus (Waller, Dotterer, Murray, Maxwell, & Hyde, 2017). However, most of the DTI studies in this area investigated structural differences in groups high on both AB and psychopathy compared to healthy controls, making it difficult to determine whether results are specific to psychopathy or common to both AB and psychopathy. In one study that did compare incarcerated offenders (i.e., all high on AB) with and without psychopathy, psychopathy was found to be uniquely associated with reduced uncinate fasciculus integrity (Motzkin, Newman, Kiehl, & Koenigs, 2011). Together with sMRI and fMRI findings of psychopathy, this study highlights that psychopathy appears to be linked to specific amygdala and OFC deficits and, potentially, the connections between these areas (Blair et al., 2005; Blair, 2003).

Functional connectivity analyses can be used to identify correlated activity between brain regions (O'Reilly, Woolrich, Behrens, Smith, & Johansen-Berg, 2012). Functional connectivity analyses aid the understanding of the neural mechanisms of psychopathy by identifying networks of altered communication either during rest (i.e., resting state functional connectivity) or during a task (i.e., task-based functional connectivity). Adults with psychopathy have demonstrated decreased functional connectivity between the amygdala, visual cortex, and prefrontal cortex during an emotional face-matching task (Contreras-Rodríguez et al., 2014), between the medial dorsal prefrontal cortex and amygdala, insula, hypothalamus, and posterior cingulate at rest (Contreras-Rodríguez et al., 2015), and between the amygdala and OFC during a perspective-taking task (Decety et al., 2013). Similarly, decreased functional connectivity between the amygdala and OFC was found in youth with psychopathic traits during a moral judgment task (Marsh et al., 2011) and between the amygdala, ACC, and insula when observing harm directed to others (Yoder, Lahey, & Decety, 2016). These findings suggest that reduced functional connectivity between the amygdala and various areas of the prefrontal cortex may contribute to dysfunctional processing of emotionally salient cues and may potentially lead to increased aggression and decreased empathy in psychopathy. Finally, similar to fMRI findings during reward processing, Factor 2 psychopathic traits in adult inmates were linked to increased functional connectivity between the striatum and the midbrain, the striatum and the dlPFC (Korponay et al., 2017), and the striatum and the dorsomedial prefrontal cortex (dmPFC; Geurts et al., 2016). As such, increased connectivity within the corticostriatal network may lead those high on psychopathy to perseverate on risky reward-seeking behavior. Taken together, the decreased functional connectivity within socioemotional brain regions but increased functional connectivity between reward-related brain regions mirrors findings from the other neuroimaging modalities (i.e., task-related fMRI, sMRI, DTI), which bolsters the notion that psychopathy is characterized by diminished emotional responses via under-reactive socioemotional networks but increased reward-seeking and risk-taking via over-reactive reward networks.

Summary

In summary, Factor 1 psychopathic traits are correlated with differences in (and between) brain regions associated with socioemotional processing, including the amygdala, OFC, insula, and ACC. Across functional, structural, and connectivity analyses, the amygdala has been established as an important region to the etiology of psychopathy, likely due to its role in emotional responding, learning, and threat detection. Reduced amygdala reactivity to distress is one of the most-studied neural correlates of psychopathy, with a potentially divergent pattern of activity compared to AB. Furthermore, altered structural and functional connectivity between the amygdala and the prefrontal cortex (especially the OFC/vmPFC) have also been identified in those high on psychopathy and may contribute to deficits in socioemotional functioning (e.g., affective decision-making, aversive conditioning to cues of distress). Factor 2 traits that overlap with broader conceptualizations of AB, and include reward-dominance and impulsivity, appear to arise from altered structure and function in the OFC, dlPFC, and ventral striatum, which are regions that are critical for attention, reward valuation, and decision-making. Together, these findings suggest that psychopathy likely arises from dysfunction in a network of regions critical to socioemotional processing, reward sensitivity, and attention (Kiehl et al., 2001). The next step is to understand how these individual differences in neural reactivity within psychopathy arise.

Genetics and psychopathy

Although neuroimaging research has greatly informed our current understanding of psychopathy, the source of these differences in brain structure and function associated with psychopathy is largely unknown. Examining genetic factors that contribute to the neural mechanisms characteristic of psychopathy could help to explain the development of psychopathy. Indeed, twin studies have found a variety of personality traits and cognitive processes to be at least moderately heritable (e.g., 40–70 percent; Plomin, Owen, & McGuffin, 1994), including psychopathy (e.g., 30–50 percent; Beaver et al., 2011; Beaver et al., 2012; Blair et al., 2006; Moffitt, 2005). Based on previous neuroimaging research, genes that influence neurotransmission within implicated brain regions, such as the amygdala and OFC, could be key risk factors for psychopathy. Genetic variation that results in alterations to neurotransmitter pathways may contribute to differences in structure or activation in neural regions that have high levels of these neurotransmitters, which may, in turn, contribute to behavioral deficits associated with psychopathy (Hariri, 2009; Hariri et al., 2006).

Genetic variation can occur within regions of the genome that have multiple versions represented by different alleles (i.e., common genetic polymorphisms), including change in a single nucleotide polymorphism (i.e., SNP) or varying numbers of base pairs (i.e., variable number of tandem repeats polymorphisms; VNTR). These polymorphisms can then affect the transcription of a gene and the structure of the resulting translated protein, resulting in divergent patterns of neurotransmission within the synapse (Hariri, 2009; Hariri et al., 2006; Moffitt, 2005). Molecular genetic studies of constructs related to psychopathy, including aggression, violence, and AB, have focused on genetic variation related to dopaminergic and serotonergic pathways due to their role in emotion, reward, and learning, which are processes that are often impaired in psychopathy and AB (Yildirim & Derksen, 2013).

Although there is a growing body of research regarding specific candidate genes implicated in AB, as summarized in previous reviews (e.g., Fernàndez-Castillo & Cormand, 2016; Gunter, Vaughn, & Philibert, 2010; Hyde, 2015; Waller, Dotterer, & Hyde, 2015), there have not been any genome-wide studies of adult psychopathy. Moreover, a genome-wide study of children failed to identify any genes that were significantly associated with CU traits (Viding et al., 2010). Indeed, only five studies to date have found associations between specific variations in genes and psychopathic traits. These studies reported associations between psychopathy and genes involved in the metabolism of dopamine and serotonin (e.g., MAOA, COMT; Fowler et al., 2009), serotonin transporters (e.g., 5-HTTLPR; Herman et al., 2011; Sadeh, Javdani, & Verona, 2013), and dopamine receptors (e.g., DRD2; Ponce et al., 2008, DRD2 & DRD4; Wu & Barnes, 2013).

In one of the first studies on this topic, a study of older adolescents found a significant association between psychopathic traits and the low-activity variant (i.e., two and three repeat) of the MAOA gene (i.e., Monoamine Oxidase A; Fowler et al., 2009). MAOA is involved in the catabolism of monoamines, including dopamine and serotonin. The low-activity variant (i.e., MAOA-L) has been associated with increased amygdala reactivity and decreased regulation of the amygdala by the PFC, which could underlie AB or behaviors related to Factor 2 psychopathy (Meyer-Lindenberg et al., 2006). Within the same sample, Fowler and colleagues (2009) also reported a significant association between psychopathy and the homozygous valine (val/val) genotype of the Val158Met polymorphism of the COMT gene (catechol-o-methyltransferase), which has been linked to the metabolism of dopamine specifically affecting the prefrontal regions, including the dlPFC (Egan et al., 2001).

Second, two studies have reported an association between psychopathy and the long allele of a common polymorphism in the promotor region of the serotonin transporter gene (SLC6A4) (Herman et al., 2011; Sadeh et al., 2010). Although the *short* allele of 5-HTTLPR (serotonin-transporter-linked polymorphic region) has been connected across many studies to greater risk for anxiety and depression (Clarke, Flint, Attwood, & Munafo, 2010; Sen, Burmeister, & Ghosh, 2004), researchers have posited that the *long* allele of 5-HTTLPR may relate to reduced stress reactivity due to its association with reduced amygdala reactivity (e.g., Heinz et al., 2005). As such, Glenn has suggested that the long allele could be a risk factor for psychopathy, as lower affect and fearlessness may be linked to the long allele and is certainly relevant to psychopathy (Glenn, 2011). Finally, two studies reported associations between variation in dopamine receptors and psychopathic traits. In a community sample of adults, psychopathic traits were associated with the long repeat variant (i.e., seven or more) of a 48 base pair VNTR on DRD4 (i.e., dopamine receptor, type 4), which is believed to result in altered receptor activity and thus increased levels of dopamine (Wu & Barnes, 2013). Within the same study, the minor variant A1 allele (versus A2) of DRD2 (i.e., dopamine receptor, type 2) was also associated with psychopathic traits (Wu & Barnes, 2013), while a separate study found an interaction between DRD2 and DRD4 that predicted AB (Beaver et al., 2007).

Additional research on CU traits in youth has focused on serotonin pathways based on the notion that reduced serotonin neurotransmission may lead to reduced amygdala reactivity and decreased stress responses (Moul, Killcross, & Dadds, 2012). Studies have found associations between CU traits and variability in genes coding for serotonin receptors (e.g., HTR2A, HTR1B; Moul, Dobson-Stone, Brennan, Hawes, & Dadds, 2013), methylation of serotonin receptors (e.g., 1B; Moul, Dobson-Stone, Brennan, Hawes, & Dadds, 2015), and serotonin transporters (e.g., 5-HTTLPR; Sadeh et al., 2010). In addition, CU traits have been associated with variations in the prolactin receptor gene (e.g., PRLR; Hirata et al., 2016), the oxytocin gene (e.g., OXT; Beitchman et al., 2012; Dadds et al., 2014b), and the oxytocin receptor gene (e.g., OXTR; Beitchman et al., 2012; Dadds et al., 2014a; Dadds et al., 2014b), as oxytocin and prolactin hormones have been associated with attachment, which is thought to be disrupted in CU traits (Turner et al., 2002). These genes may be particularly important as children with CU traits are more likely to experience and provoke poorer quality parent–child relationships, including disrupted attachment and less parental warmth (Pasalich, Dadds, Hawes, & Brennan, 2012; Waller et al., 2013; Waller et al., 2014). However, similar to the previously reviewed studies on adult psychopathic traits, the evidence for each of these candidate genes typically stems from a single study (or at best, two), and none of these candidate genes have been consistently associated with CU traits. Moreover, many of these studies have very small samples, promoting concerns about replication.

In summary, there is limited research directly linking genetic variation to psychopathic traits. The five existing studies in adults vary in sample type, including age range and population (e.g., comorbid ADHD, criminal, alcoholism, community) and often utilize small sample sizes, which likely contribute to small effect sizes. However, given that no single gene is likely to exist that specifically translates to risk for a complex construct like psychopathy, it is not surprising that studies rarely find significant direct associations between a single SNP and psychopathy. As a result, studies have begun to examine genetic risk in combination with additional factors previously implicated in psychopathy, such as the influence of environmental experience.

Gene-by-environment interactions in psychopathy

Environmental influences

A variety of environmental factors have been shown to influence the development of psychopathy, including parenting and maltreatment (Farrington et al., 2010). Specifically, psychopathic and CU traits have been associated with low parental warmth and harsh parenting (Hyde, Waller, Trentacosta et al., 2016; Salekin & Lochman, 2008; Waller et al., 2013; Waller, Shaw, Forbes, & Hyde, 2015), maternal psychopathology (e.g., Barker, Oliver, Viding, Salekin, & Maughan, 2011), parental substance use (e.g., Fowler et al., 2009), child abuse and neglect (e.g., Gao, Raine, Chan, Venables, & Mednick, 2010; Krischer & Sevecke, 2008; Weiler & Widom, 1996), parental conflict (Farrington et al., 2010), parental criminality (Farrington, 2000; Hyde, Waller, Trentacosta et al., 2016), and low income (Farrington, 2000; Frick, Kimonis, Dandreaux, & Farell, 2003). However, it is important to note that despite the large body of work supporting the role of environmental risk factors, many children exposed to these factors do not develop psychopathy (Farrington et al., 2010). Moreover, twin studies of psychopathy have found that genetic factors contribute important variance over and above environmental factors (Rhee & Waldman, 2002; Taylor, Loney, Bobadilla, Iacono, & McGue, 2003). Thus, it seems likely that certain genes may make some children more susceptible to harsh environments, further emphasizing the need for research that examines multiple risk factors for psychopathy. Indeed, a large body of work now emphasizes the important influence of environmental factors on gene expression (e.g., epigenetics; Meaney, 2010). A Gene × Environment (G × E) interaction indicates that the effect of an environmental experience on an outcome is conditional on genetics (Moffitt, 2005). Although researchers have been less successful in linking genes directly to psychopathy, there are some results from G × E interaction studies of psychopathy to suggest that genetic risk may be associated with psychopathy via interactions with environmental risk. Findings from a recent study of adopted children (age 3) support the notion that genes and environments interact in the development of psychopathy. Within an adoption model that can parse genetic from non-heritable environmental influence, Hyde and colleagues (2016) found that severe biological parent AB predicted child CU traits even though the biological parents had spent an average of only two days with the child before adoption, indicating a genetic pathway to CU traits. On the other hand, greater positive adoptive parenting predicted lower CU traits, indicating non-heritable environmental effects. Moreover, these two influences interacted such that for children with very positive adoptive parents, there was no relationship between their biological risk and CU traits. Though this approach cannot identify specific genes that are associated with psychopathy, CU traits, or brain structure and function, it does provide compelling evidence that genes and experiences interact in the development of early risk for CU traits and subsequent psychopathy.

G × E interaction models of psychopathy

Three studies have tested for G × E interactions in CU traits and psychopathy using candidate molecular genetic approaches. Sadeh and colleagues (2013) found significant associations between genetic variants and psychopathy in adult male offenders (e.g., the 5-HTTLPR long allele and the Factor 1 psychopathy; MAOA-L and Factor 2 psychopathy). Interestingly, the authors did not find evidence for a G × E interaction, as these genetic associations were not moderated by childhood maltreatment. In contrast, Sadeh and colleagues (2010) found that adolescents who had lower socioeconomic status (SES) and were homozygous long (l/l) genotype of 5-HTTLPR had higher levels of callous–unemotional and narcissistic features, but this association was not present for adolescents with higher SES. Finally, Willoughby and colleagues (2013) found that harsh-intrusive parenting in infancy was more strongly associated with the development of CU traits at age 3 for children with a methionine allele of the brain-derived neurotrophic factor gene (BDNF), a gene involved in neural plasticity that has previously been implicated in fear conditioning (Hajcak et al., 2009). Thus, there is some evidence that genetic effects may be magnified in harsh contexts, though the evidence for psychopathy, specifically, is fairly weak with little research testing these questions. This sparse literature is surprising given the multitude of studies linking G × E interactions to other forms of psychopathology, including depression (Karg, Burmeister, Shedden, & Sen, 2011; Risch et al., 2009) and ADHD (Nikolas & Burt, 2010). In fact, as described later, there has been much attention paid to G × E interactions in the development of AB, particularly with regard to MAOA × context interactions (Byrd & Manuck, 2014; Waller, Dotterer et al., 2015).

Thus, although there is a growing body of research documenting neural correlates of psychopathy, there are no current studies of the neurogenetics (i.e., genetics and neural correlates) of psychopathy, likely because there is so little gene–psychopathy or G × E interaction–psychopathy work. This lack of literature stands in contrast to the more voluminous neurogenetics literature related to internalizing disorders such as depression (Hariri, 2009; Hyde, Swartz, Waller, & Hariri, 2016; Sacchet, Foland-Ross, & Gotlib, 2016) or other psychopathologies such as schizophrenia (Lancaster, Doherty, Linden, & Hall, 2016). Given the limited research on psychopathy using a neurogenetics approach, few conclusions can be drawn about how genetic, neural, and environmental risks might interact in or mediate risk for psychopathy. Although the few existing G × E interaction studies of psychopathy provide some preliminary support for the usefulness of integrating a variety of factors to better understand psychopathy, the state of the current literature emphasizes the need for additional research that incorporates neuroimaging along with genetic variation and environmental risk.

Though the literature is still building with regards to neurogenetic models of psychopathy, there has been more research examining the integration of genetic, neural, and environmental factors in relation to AB. Given the overlap between psychopathy and AB, the results of this work could be used to inform similar designs in the study of psychopathy. We review this work next in an effort to suggest future directions for the study of AB and psychopathy.

Imaging gene–environment interactions linked to antisocial behavior

Gene–brain–behavior pathways

AB has been more consistently associated with variation in specific genes, and researchers have now begun to examine potential gene–brain–behavior pathways using previously identified neural correlates of AB. The majority of human research on the neurogenetics of AB has focused on genetic variation in MAOA. A meta-analysis of 31 studies found that AB was significantly associated with MAOA-L (Ficks & Waldman, 2014).

Building on these gene-behavior studies, three innovative studies have examined associations between MAOA and brain function and thus can provide evidence for a hypothesized gene–brain pathway to AB (Buckholtz et al., 2008; Kolla et al., 2016; Meyer-Lindenberg et al., 2006). First, in a community sample, Meyer-Lindenberg and colleagues (2006) found that MAOA-L carriers had decreased cingulate, insula, hypothalamus, and amygdala volumes compared to MAOA-H carriers. They also reported a gene-by-sex interaction whereby MAOA-L was associated with increased OFC volume, but only in men. MAOA-L was also linked to greater amygdala reactivity and reduced OFC, cingulate, and insula activity during tasks probing affective processing (fearful and angry face matching; memory for negative stimuli) and inhibitory control (i.e., no-go flanker task; Buckholtz & Meyer-Lindenberg, 2008; Meyer-Lindenberg et al., 2006). Second, linking these gene–brain associations to outcomes related to AB, Buckholtz and colleagues (2008) found that male MAOA-L carriers had greater harm avoidance and less reward dependence than MAOA-H carriers, and found that this association was mediated by amygdala–vmPFC functional connectivity. This study thus suggests that MAOA-L carriers may have deficient regulation of the amygdala by the cingulate, potentially leading to amygdala hyper-reactivity and reactive aggression. Third, in a study using PET imaging and fMRI, Kolla and colleagues (2016) reported that lower striatal MAOA availability was linked to reduced functional connectivity between the ventral striatum and the dmPFC, and greater functional connectivity between the ventral striatum and the right hippocampus in male offenders with Antisocial Personality Disorder who were high on psychopathic traits. Furthermore, less functional connectivity between the ventral striatum and dmPFC and between the ventral striatum and right hippocampus were associated with greater self-reported impulsivity but not overall psychopathy scores (Kolla et al., 2016). This finding suggests that impulsivity related to AB and psychopathy may be related to lower MAOA availability and reduced functional coupling between the ventral striatum and regulatory prefrontal regions. Together, the results of these studies highlight a potential pathway in which MAOA-L genotype is linked to disruptions in corticolimbic and corticostriatal circuitry (e.g., amygdala, OFC, cingulate, insula, ventral striatum, dmPFC) that lead to disruptions in affective processing and reward, which may in turn contribute to greater emotion dysregulation, reactive aggression, impulsivity, and potentially AB. Though this hypothesis has not been tested in a single study, these results help to demonstrate the ways in which a neurogenetics approach leveraging imaging genetics, PET imaging, and the neuroimaging literature related to AB can inform a multilevel model of AB from gene to neurotransmitter to brain to behavior.

Beyond MAOA, Waller and colleagues (2016) investigated associations between the oxytocin receptor (OXTR) and AB, due to the important role that oxytocin plays in social behavior (Kumsta & Heinrichs, 2013). Specifically, Waller and colleagues (2016) found that among young adult men, the TT genotype of OXTR was linked to increased right amygdala reactivity to angry facial expressions, and increased amygdala reactivity was related to self-reported AB (though not CU traits). This study is one of the first to model and demonstrate evidence of a gene–brain–behavior pathway between OXTR, amygdala reactivity, and AB.

G × E interactions predicting AB

In one of the first G × E interaction studies of complex behavior, Caspi and colleagues (2002) found that MAOA-L was associated with adult AB, but only among individuals who had experienced childhood maltreatment (Caspi et al., 2002). Many studies have tested this association, and in a recent meta-analysis, Byrd and Manuck (2014) found evidence that this interaction is important in the prediction of AB. Specifically, they reported that maltreatment was robustly linked to AB in males with the MAOA-L genotype and weakly associated with females with the MAOA-H genotype (Byrd & Manuck, 2014). Beyond MAOA, genetic variation in dopamine and serotonin receptor and/or transporter expression has also been linked to AB in the context of harsh environments. For example, Barnes and Jacobs (2013) reported a G × E interaction between dopamine risk index (number of risky alleles across DAT1, DRD2, and DRD4 genes) and exposure to neighborhood disadvantage and violent crime that predicted greater levels of violent crime (Barnes & Jacobs, 2013). G × E interactions between the short allele 5-HTTLPR and chronic stress (Conway et al., 2012), and negative parenting and the 9-repeat VNTR polymorphism of DAT1 (Lahey et al., 2011), also predicted greater AB. These studies highlight the role of interactions between genetic variation in dopamine and serotonin neurotransmitter systems and environmental context in predicting violence and AB (for a review of all G × E interaction studies of AB to date, see Waller, Dotterer, & Hyde, 2015).

IG × E interaction

We have previously outlined an "Imaging Gene–Environment Interaction" framework that can be used to integrate the study of genetic, neural, and environmental risk factors that interact to contribute to psychopathy (IG × E interaction; Hyde et al., 2011; Hyde, Swartz, Waller, & Hariri, 2015). An IG × E interaction approach incorporates pathways through which genes, environments, and the brain interact to predict behavior and risk for psychopathology (Bogdan, Hyde, & Hariri, 2013; Hyde et al., 2011). Specifically, G × E interactions are proposed to predict behavior and psychopathology via brain structure and function. Thus, an IG × E interaction framework includes paths representing the main effects of genetic risk (Figure 7.1, path d) and environmental risk (Figure 7.1, path b) as well as G × E interactions (Figure 7.1, path c) that predict neural functioning. Differences in neural functioning are then posited to influence intermediate behavior phenotypes (e.g., affective processing), which in turn predict the key outcome of interest (e.g., psychopathy; Figure 7.1, pathway e). In this way, IG × E interaction models incorporate the influence of the environment into neurogenetics models that specify molecular mechanisms through which genes influence brain and behavior.

Despite considerable evidence supporting the impact of genes and environment on neural function and on AB, very few studies have formally tested these associations in a full IG × E interaction model. MAOA is a promising target for IG × E interaction studies of AB due to: (1) strong evidence linking both MAOA and environmental stress to later AB (e.g., Caspi et al., 2002; Kim-Cohen et al., 2006) and (2) findings linking MAOA to neural abnormalities (e.g., Buckholtz & Meyer-Lindenberg, 2008; Meyer-Lindenberg et al., 2006). Animal models also have helped to establish that early life stress impacts MAOA expression, brain function, and later aggressive behavior. For example, Marques and colleagues (2013) found that rats that were exposed to stress during puberty displayed increased MAOA and 5-HTT prefrontal cortex mRNA expression. These rats were also more aggressive and had elevated and sustained amygdala responses, as well as decreased amygdala–OFC coupling during encounters with other rats. Notably, MAOA inhibitor treatment reversed the enhanced aggression induced by pubertal stress (Marquez et al., 2013). This example provides a promising model for a potential neurogenetic and environmental mechanism in the etiology of AB.

Among humans, Holz and colleagues used an IG × E interaction approach to investigate interactions of MAOA, early life stress, and gender on brain reactivity during tasks probing emotional processing and inhibitory control (Holz et al., 2014). The authors reported that MAOA-L, early life stress, and male gender interacted to predict increased amygdala reactivity to fearful and angry faces, which in turn predicted aggressive behavior. These results were among the first to demonstrate a three-way interaction of gender × MAOA × environmental stress predicting both brain reactivity and aggression (Holz et al., 2014). This study provides further

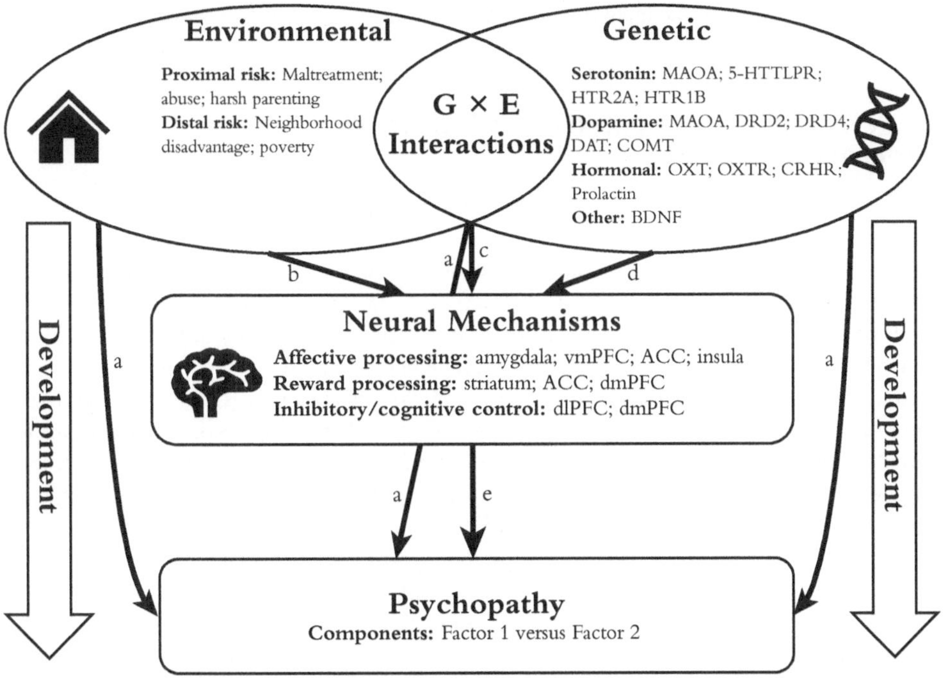

Figure 7.1 IG × E interaction model of psychopathy

A preliminary hypothetical model outlining potential targets for future IG × E interaction studies examining the development of psychopathy. Relationships of the variables are shown for more traditional G × E interaction and imaging genetics paths, as well as new paths possible in IG × E interaction studies. The "a" paths model direct effects of genes, environments, and G × E interaction relationships on psychopathy; "b" paths show direct effects of the environment on neural functioning; "c → e" paths model gene–environment interactions predicting behavior via neural functioning; "d → e" paths model traditional neurogenetics links. We highlight gene variants, environmental factors, and neural mechanisms that have been identified in traditional G × E interaction and neurogenetics investigations of psychopathy, and thus are primary targets for future IG × E interaction studies.

evidence that MAOA and early life stress interactions, and associated corticolimbic dysfunction, may contribute to AB.

In a study examining stress-related pathways to AB in a low-income sample of boys, Gard and colleagues (2017) found that harsh parenting and neighborhood impoverishment at age 2 was associated with AB at age 20 via increased amygdala reactivity to emotional faces in early adulthood. Further, the relationship between harsh parenting (but not neighborhood impoverishment) and AB via amygdala reactivity was moderated by genetic variation in the corticotropin releasing hormone receptor (CRHR) gene, which is involved in the hypothalamic–pituitary–adrenocortical (HPA) axis stress response (Gard et al., 2017). These results indicated that youth with a specific variant in the gene were more sensitive to the neurobehavioral effects of harsh parenting and provide an excellent model for how early experience shapes the developing brain and risk for AB, but potentially more strongly among those with specific genetic variants.

Together, these two preliminary IG × E interaction studies indicate that both genetic (MAOA; CRHR) and environmental (early life stress, harsh parenting) factors influence increased amygdala reactivity and subsequent AB. Drawing on this literature, we propose an IG × E interaction model of psychopathy to facilitate the continued use of such approaches in application to psychopathic traits specifically.

Future directions: a proposed IG × E interaction model of psychopathy

In lieu of empirical evidence from formal IG × E interaction studies of psychopathy, we present a summary of potentially important variables in each domain (i.e., genes, environment, brain) and how they could interact to predict psychopathy based on research to date. This summary provides a testable model of multiple IG × E interaction pathways to understanding psychopathy (Figure 7.1). In this model, proximal and/or distal environmental risk interacts with genetic vulnerability (e.g., candidate gene SNPs, cumulative genetic risk scores) to alter brain structure or function in key brain regions/circuits responsible for affective processing, reward sensitivity, attention, and inhibitory control (Figure 7.1, pathway c). Disruptions to one or more of these neural circuits are then proposed to contribute to psychopathy (Figure 7.1, pathway e). Importantly, our model also includes development, as harsh environments such as maltreatment, harsh parenting, and poverty may exhibit varying effects on brain and behavior at different points in development (i.e., developmental sensitive periods), and individuals may persist or desist from AB and psychopathy throughout development (Dodge & Pettit, 2003).

Based on behavioral genetic, G × E interaction, and neurogenetic research, future IG × E interaction studies of psychopathy are likely to focus on genetic risk in the monoamine systems, as the monoamine systems have been most reliably associated with neural functioning in AB (i.e., corticolimbic, striatal circuitry) and traits associated with psychopathy (i.e., aggression, impulsivity). Although no genes have been consistently directly associated with psychopathy, MAOA is a potential target for this research due to the association between MAOA-L and AB. As such, it is important to emphasize that MAOA cannot be considered a "psychopathic gene," but a factor that confers risk for altered brain function, which may lead to increased risk for behaviors characteristic of AB and/or psychopathy under certain environmental conditions. One point that should be noted is that in most G × E interaction studies or other neurogenetics studies, the environment/context is often the most robust and strongest predictor of AB and other outcomes.

One pathway through which MAOA may influence the development of psychopathy might be interactions between MAOA-L (in men) and early life stress (i.e., maltreatment). The combination of these two factors may lead individuals to have greater amygdala reactivity to signals of distress, decreased amygdala–prefrontal cortex connectivity, and decreased ACC reactivity during performance monitoring. This altered neural circuitry may contribute to greater levels of reactive aggression and reduced utilization of important feedback information to guide individuals towards more appropriate behaviors. These deficits may contribute to the patterns of harmful behavior (i.e., rule-breaking, aggression) observed with psychopathy. On the other hand, this pathway may be more important in understanding behaviors composing Factor 2 of psychopathy, and thus may not be specific to psychopathy, but rather to AB broadly (hence the need for greater attention to Factor 1-specific risk factors at the environmental, neural, and genetic level).

Furthermore, psychopathy has also been characterized by excessive reward-seeking behavior. Due to its role in dopamine expression in the ventral striatum, MAOA-L may also influence behavioral manifestations of psychopathy via reducing functional connectivity between limbic-motivational centers (i.e., ventral striatum) and prefrontal regulatory regions, thus increasing impulsivity. However, at this point, it is unclear whether gender moderates these relationships, or whether environmental experience may alter the relationship between MAOA, ventral striatum–PFC connectivity, and Factor 2 psychopathic traits. In addition, MAOA appears to be linked to reactive forms of aggression, which is strongly linked to AB as well as psychopathy. Thus, future research should examine the extent to which MAOA × early life stress interactions uniquely predict psychopathy versus AB.

In addition to MAOA, other genetic factors may also contribute to the development of psychopathy via their effect on amygdala functioning. Variants of CRHR and OXTR genes involved in stress response and social affiliative behaviors have been associated with increases in amygdala reactivity (Gard et al., 2017; Waller et al., 2016) and subsequent AB. One of these studies (Gard et al., 2017) has also highlighted the importance and specificity of harsh parenting (versus neighborhood disadvantage) on associations between CRHR, amygdala reactivity, and AB. Finally, the short allele of 5-HTTLPR has been associated with increased amygdala reactivity (Hariri et al., 2005) and may contribute to reactive aggression. However, the long allele of 5-HTTLPR may be protective from the development of depression after childhood maltreatment (Caspi et al., 2003), though possibly risky for the development of CU traits/ psychopathy (Sadeh et al., 2010).

In addition to testing these models, future research must consider several important questions. First, while IG × E interaction models will likely greatly advance our understanding of psychopathy, it is highly unlikely that *one* environmental condition interacts with *one* genetic polymorphism to predict behavior via the brain. It is more likely that multiple environments (G × E × E) or multiple genes (G × G × E) interact to confer increased risk for psychopathology (Hyde et al., 2015; Waller, Dotterer, & Hyde, 2015). Second, researchers must select appropriate samples that have sufficient power to detect significant effects and at the same time are representative of the individuals who engage in antisocial and psychopathic behaviors rather than being merely "convenient" (e.g., undergraduates; Falk et al., 2013). For example, psychopathic traits in undergraduate samples may tap maladaptive but not necessarily harmful components of psychopathy (e.g., risk-taking, unemotionality). Studies using these populations may be unable to assess more severe forms of callousness, manipulation, lack of remorse, and violence that characterize psychopathy within incarcerated samples. Relatedly, neuroimaging research rarely considers sample diversity, including racial and ethnic differences. Demographic factors including race, as well as sex and SES, have been differentially associated with neural functioning in AB (e.g., Hyde, Shaw, Murray et al., 2016), and are likely important moderators of IG × E interaction models of AB and psychopathy (Baskin-Sommers, Newman, Sathasivam, & Curtin, 2011; Lorenz & Newman, 2002; Thornquist & Zuckerman, 1995). Third, considerable research supports the notion that AB with or without psychopathic traits is characterized by unique genetic risk, neural function, structure, connectivity, and behavioral phenotypes (e.g., hypo- versus hyper-emotional reactivity). As such, research that directly parses the unique variance of these constructs using either dimension or group-based analyses will be of great benefit to the field. Finally, it will be important to consider associations derived from IG × E interaction models through a developmental psychopathology lens. Indeed, very few studies have considered the role of development in the neurobiological etiology of psychopathy (Hyde et al., 2011; Waller and Hyde, 2017). For example, environmental stressors may have a greater impact on brain function, and thus result in greater risk for AB, during certain periods in development (i.e., developmental sensitive periods). Further, identifying genetic, environmental, or neural predictors of desistence from or resilience to (i.e., differential susceptibility) AB over time may potentially inform novel treatment approaches.

Conclusion

Integrative neurogenetics approaches emphasize the complex interactions between genetic risk, environmental experience, neural structure and function, and the development of psychopathology. Although the application of neurogenetics to psychopathy remains novel, several candidate genes and environmental factors have already been linked to altered function in key neural circuits implicated in psychopathy and AB. Testing these factors within IG × E interaction models will greatly advance our understanding of the neural etiology of these constructs and aid in the classification, prediction, and treatment of psychopathy.

References

Assaf, Y., and Pasternak, O. (2008) 'Diffusion tensor imaging (DTI)-based white matter mapping in brain research: A review,' *Journal of Molecular Neuroscience, 34*:51–61.

Barker, E. D., Oliver, B. R., Viding, E., Salekin, R. T., and Maughan, B. (2011) 'The impact of prenatal maternal risk, fearless temperament and early parenting on adolescent callous-unemotional traits: A 14-year longitudinal investigation,' *Journal of Child Psychology and Psychiatry, 52*:878–888.

Barnes, J., and Jacobs, B. A. (2013) 'Genetic risk for violent behavior and environmental exposure to disadvantage and violent crime: The case for gene–environment interaction,' *Journal of Interpersonal Violence, 28*:92–120.

Baskin-Sommers, A. R., Brazil, I. A., Ryan, J., Kohlenberg, N. J., Neumann, C. S., and Newman, J. P. (2015) 'Mapping the association of global executive functioning onto diverse measures of psychopathic traits,' *Personality Disorders: Theory, Research, and Treatment, 6*:336–346.

Baskin-Sommers, A. R., Curtin, J. J., and Newman, J. P. (2011) 'Specifying the attentional selection that moderates the fearlessness of psychopathic offenders,' *Psychological Science, 22*:226–234.

Baskin-Sommers, A. R., Curtin, J. J., and Newman, J. P. (2015) 'Altering the cognitive–affective dysfunctions of psychopathic and externalizing offender subtypes with cognitive remediation,' *Clinical Psychological Science, 3*:45–57.

Baskin-Sommers, A. R., and Newman, J. P. (2013) 'Differentiating the cognition–emotion interactions that characterize psychopathy versus externalizing,' *Handbook of cognition and emotion*, 501–520.

Baskin-Sommers, A. R., Newman, J. P., Sathasivam, N., and Curtin, J. J. (2011) 'Evaluating the generalizability of a fear deficit in psychopathic African American offenders,' *Journal of Abnormal Psychology, 120*:71–78.

Baskin-Sommers, A. R., Zeier, J. D., and Newman, J. P. (2009) 'Self-reported attentional control differentiates the major factors of psychopathy,' *Personality and Individual Differences, 47*:626–630.

Beaver, K. M., Barnes, J., May, J. S., and Schwartz, J. A. (2011) 'Psychopathic personality traits, genetic risk, and gene–environment correlations,' *Criminal Justice and Behavior, 38*:896–912.

Beaver, K. M., Vaughn, M. G., DeLisi, M., Barnes, J., and Boutwell, B. B. (2012) 'The neuropsychological underpinnings to psychopathic personality traits in a nationally representative and longitudinal sample,' *Psychiatric Quarterly, 83*:145–159.

Beaver, K. M., Wright, J. P., DeLisi, M., Walsh, A., Vaughn, M. G., Boisvert, D., and Vaske, J. (2007) 'A gene × gene interaction between DRD2 and DRD4 is associated with conduct disorder and antisocial behavior in males,' *Behavioral and Brain Functions, 3*:30.

Beitchman, J. H., Zai, C. C., Muir, K., Berall, L., Nowrouzi, B., Choi, E., and Kennedy, J. L. (2012) 'Childhood aggression, callous–unemotional traits and oxytocin genes,' *European Child & Adolescent Psychiatry, 21*:125–132.

Bigos, K. L., Pollock, B. G., Aizenstein, H. J., Fisher, P. M., Bies, R. R., and Hariri, A. R. (2008) 'Acute 5-HT reuptake blockade potentiates human amygdala reactivity,' *Neuropsychopharmacology: Official publication of the American College of Neuropsychopharmacology, 33*:3221.

Bjork, J. M., Chen, G., and Hommer, D. W. (2012) 'Psychopathic tendencies and mesolimbic recruitment by cues for instrumental and passively obtained rewards,' *Biological Psychology, 89*:408–415.

Blair, J., Mitchell, D., and Blair, K. (2005) *The psychopath: Emotion and the brain*, Oxford: Blackwell Publishing.

Blair, R. J. R. (2003) 'Neurobiological basis of psychopathy,' *The British Journal of Psychiatry, 182*:5–7.

Blair, R. J. R. (2005) 'Applying a cognitive neuroscience perspective to the disorder of psychopathy,' *Development and Psychopathology, 17*:865–891.

Blair, R. J. R. (2007a) 'The amygdala and ventromedial prefrontal cortex in morality and psychopathy,' *Trends in Cognitive Sciences*, *11*:387–392.

Blair, R. J. R. (2007b) 'Dysfunctions of medial and lateral orbitofrontal cortex in psychopathy,' *Annals of the New York Academy of Sciences*, *1121*:461–479.

Blair, R. J. R. (2008) 'The amygdala and ventromedial prefrontal cortex: Functional contributions and dysfunction in psychopathy,' *Philosophical Transactions of the Royal Society of London B: Biological Sciences*, *363*:2557–2565.

Blair, R. J. R. (2010) 'Neuroimaging of psychopathy and antisocial behavior: A targeted review,' *Current Psychiatry Reports*, *12*:76–82.

Blair, R. J. R. (2015) 'Psychopathic traits from an RDoC perspective,' *Current Opinion in Neurobiology*, *30*:79–84.

Blair, R. J. R. (2017) 'Emotion-based learning systems and the development of morality,' *Cognition*, epub ahead of print.

Blair, R. J. R., Mitchell, D. G., Richell, R. A., Kelly, S., Leonard, A., Newman, C., and Scott, S. K. (2002) 'Turning a deaf ear to fear: Impaired recognition of vocal affect in psychopathic individuals,' *Journal of Abnormal Psychology*, *111*:682.

Blair, R. J. R., Peschardt, K. S., Budhani, S., Mitchell, D. G., and Pine, D. S. (2006) 'The development of psychopathy,' *Journal of Child Psychology and Psychiatry*, *47*:262–276.

Blair, R. J. R., Veroude, K., and Buitelaar, J. K. (2016) 'Neuro-cognitive system dysfunction and symptom sets: A review of fMRI studies in youth with conduct problems,' *Neuroscience & Biobehavioral Reviews*, in press

Bogdan, R., Hyde, L., and Hariri, A. (2013) 'A neurogenetics approach to understanding individual differences in brain, behavior, and risk for psychopathology,' *Molecular Psychiatry*, *18*:288–299.

Bogdan, R., Williamson, D. E., and Hariri, A. R. (2012) 'Mineralocorticoid receptor Iso/Val (rs5522) genotype moderates the association between previous childhood emotional neglect and amygdala reactivity,' *American Journal of Psychiatry*, *169*:515–522.

Botvinick, M. M., Cohen, J. D., and Carter, C. S. (2004) 'Conflict monitoring and anterior cingulate cortex: An update,' *Trends in Cognitive Sciences*, *8*:539–546.

Buckholtz, J., Callicott, J., Kolachana, B., Hariri, A., Goldberg, T., Genderson, M., . . . and Meyer-Lindenberg, A. (2008) 'Genetic variation in MAOA modulates ventromedial prefrontal circuitry mediating individual differences in human personality,' *Molecular Psychiatry*, *13*:313–324.

Buckholtz, J. W., and Meyer-Lindenberg, A. (2008) 'MAOA and the neurogenetic architecture of human aggression,' *Trends in Neurosciences*, *31*:120–129.

Buckholtz, J. W., Treadway, M. T., Cowan, R. L., Woodward, N. D., Benning, S. D., Li, R., . . ., and Zald, D. H. (2010) 'Mesolimbic dopamine reward system hypersensitivity in individuals with psychopathic traits,' *Nature Neuroscience*, *13*:419–21.

Budhani, S., and Blair, R. J. R. (2005) 'Response reversal and children with psychopathic tendencies: Success is a function of salience of contingency change,' *Journal of Child Psychology and Psychiatry*, *46*:972–981.

Budhani, S., Richell, R. A., and Blair, R. J. R. (2006) 'Impaired reversal but intact acquisition: Probabilistic response reversal deficits in adult individuals with psychopathy,' *Journal of Abnormal Psychology*, *115*:552.

Byrd, A. L., and Manuck, S. B. (2014) 'MAOA, childhood maltreatment, and antisocial behavior: Meta-analysis of a gene–environment interaction,' *Biological Psychiatry*, *75*:9–17.

Carré, J. M., Hyde, L. W., Neumann, C. S., Viding, E., and Hariri, A. R. (2013) 'The neural signatures of distinct psychopathic traits,' *Social Neuroscience*, *8*:122–135.

Caspi, A., McClay, J., Moffitt, T. E., Mill, J., Martin, J., Craig, I. W., . . ., and Poulton, R. (2002) 'Role of genotype in the cycle of violence in maltreated children,' *Science*, *297*:851–854.

Caspi, A., Sugden, K., Moffitt, T. E., Taylor, A., Craig, I. W., Harrington, H., . . ., and Braithwaite, A. (2003) 'Influence of life stress on depression: Moderation by a polymorphism in the 5-HTT gene,' *Science*, *301*:386–389.

Clarke, H., Flint, J., Attwood, A., and Munafo, M. (2010) 'Association of the 5-HTTLPR genotype and unipolar depression: A meta-analysis,' *Psychological Medicine*, *40*:1767–1778.

Cohn, M. D., Viding, E., McCrory, E., Pape, L., van den Brink, W., Doreleijers, T. A., . . ., and Popma, A. (2016) 'Regional grey matter volume and concentration in at-risk adolescents: Untangling associations with callous–unemotional traits and conduct disorder symptoms,' *Psychiatry Research: Neuroimaging*, *254*:180–187.

Contreras-Rodríguez, O., Pujol, J., Batalla, I., Harrison, B. J., Bosque, J., Ibern-Regàs, I., . . ., and López-Solà, M. (2014) 'Disrupted neural processing of emotional faces in psychopathy,' *Social Cognitive and Affective Neuroscience*, *9*:505–512.

Contreras-Rodríguez, O., Pujol, J., Batalla, I., Harrison, B. J., Soriano-Mas, C., Deus, J., . . ., and Hernández-Ribas, R. (2015) 'Functional connectivity bias in the prefrontal cortex of psychopaths,' *Biological Psychiatry*, *78*:647–655.

Conway, C. C., Keenan-Miller, D., Hammen, C., Lind, P. A., Najman, J. M., and Brennan, P. A. (2012) 'Coaction of stress and serotonin transporter genotype in predicting aggression at the transition to adulthood,' *Journal of Clinical Child & Adolescent Psychology*, *41*:53–63.

Critchley, H. D., Wiens, S., Rotshtein, P., Öhman, A., and Dolan, R. J. (2004) 'Neural systems supporting interoceptive awareness,' *Nature Neuroscience*, 7:189–195.

Dadds, M. R., Moul, C., Cauchi, A., Dobson-Stone, C., Hawes, D. J., Brennan, J., . . ., and Ebstein, R. E. (2014a) 'Methylation of the oxytocin receptor gene and oxytocin blood levels in the development of psychopathy,' *Development and Psychopathology*, *26*:33–40.

Dadds, M. R., Moul, C., Cauchi, A., Dobson-Stone, C., Hawes, D. J., Brennan, J., . . ., and Ebstein, R. E. (2014b) 'Polymorphisms in the oxytocin receptor gene are associated with the development of psychopathy,' *Development and Psychopathology*, *26*:21–31.

Damasio, H., Grabowski, T., Frank, R., Galaburda, A. M., and Damasio, A. R. (1994) 'The return of Phineas Gage: Clues about the brain from the skull of a famous patient,' *Science*, *264*:1102–1105.

Decety, J., Chen, C., Harenski, C., and Kiehl, K. A. (2013) 'An fMRI study of affective perspective taking in individuals with psychopathy: Imagining another in pain does not evoke empathy,' *Frontiers in Human Neuroscience*, 7:1–12.

Decety, J., Skelly, L., Yoder, K. J., and Kiehl, K. A. (2014) 'Neural processing of dynamic emotional facial expressions in psychopaths,' *Social Neuroscience*, *9*:36–49.

Dodge, K. A., and Pettit, G. S. (2003) 'A biopsychosocial model of the development of chronic conduct problems in adolescence,' *Developmental Psychology*, *39*:349–371.

Dotterer, H. L., Hyde, L. W., Swartz, J. R., Hariri, A. R., and Williamson, D. E. (2017) 'Amygdala reactivity predicts adolescent antisocial behavior but not callous–unemotional traits,' *Developmental Cognitive Neuroscience*, *24*:84–92.

Egan, M. F., Goldberg, T. E., Kolachana, B. S., Callicott, J. H., Mazzanti, C. M., Straub, R. E., Goldman, D., and Weinberger, D. R. (2001) 'Effect of COMT Val108/158 Met genotype on frontal lobe function and risk for schizophrenia,' *Proceedings of the National Academy of Sciences*, *98*:6917–6922.

Ermer, E., Cope, L. M., Nyalakanti, P. K., Calhoun, V. D., and Kiehl, K. A. (2012) 'Aberrant paralimbic gray matter in criminal psychopathy,' *Journal of Abnormal Psychology*, *121*:649.

Ermer, E., Cope, L. M., Nyalakanti, P. K., Calhoun, V. D., and Kiehl, K. A. (2013) 'Aberrant paralimbic gray matter in incarcerated male adolescents with psychopathic traits,' *Journal of the American Academy of Child & Adolescent Psychiatry*, *52*:94–103.

Etkin, A., Egner, T., and Kalisch, R. (2011) 'Emotional processing in anterior cingulate and medial prefrontal cortex,' *Trends in Cognitive Sciences*, *15*:85–93.

Fakra, E., Hyde, L. W., Gorka, A., Fisher, P. M., Muñoz, K. E., Kimak, M., . . ., and Hariri, A. R. (2009) 'Effects of HTR1A C (−1019) G on amygdala reactivity and trait anxiety,' *Archives of General Psychiatry*, *66*:33–40.

Falk, E. B., Hyde, L. W., Mitchell, C., Faul, J., Gonzalez, R., Heitzeg, M. M., . . ., and Maslowsky, J. (2013) 'What is a representative brain? Neuroscience meets population science,' *Proceedings of the National Academy of Sciences*, *110*:17615–17622.

Farrington, D. P. (2000) 'Psychosocial predictors of adult antisocial personality and adult convictions,' *Behavioral Sciences & the Law*, *18*:605–622.

Farrington, D. P., Ullrich, S., and Salekin, R. T. (2010) 'Environmental influences on child and adolescent psychopathy,' in R. T. Salekin & D. R. Lynam (Eds.), *Handbook of child and adolescent psychopathy*, New York, NY: Guilford Press.

Fernàndez-Castillo, N., and Cormand, B. (2016) 'Aggressive behavior in humans: Genes and pathways identified through association studies,' *American Journal of Medical Genetics Part B: Neuropsychiatric Genetics*, *171*:676–696.

Ficks, C. A., and Waldman, I. D. (2014) 'Candidate genes for aggression and antisocial behavior: A meta-analysis of association studies of the 5HTTLPR and MAOA-uVNTR,' *Behavior Genetics*, *44*:427–444.

Fisher, P., Meltzer, C., Ziolko, S., Price, J., and Hariri, A. (2006) 'Capacity for 5-HT1A-mediated autoregulation predicts amygdala reactivity,' *Nature Neuroscience*, *9*:1362.

Fowler, T., Langley, K., Rice, F., van den Bree, M. B., Ross, K., Wilkinson, L. S., . . ., and Thapar, A. (2009) 'Psychopathy trait scores in adolescents with childhood ADHD: The contribution of genotypes affecting MAOA, 5HTT and COMT activity,' *Psychiatric Genetics*, *19*:312–319.

Frick, P. J., Kimonis, E. R., Dandreaux, D. M., and Farell, J. M. (2003) 'The 4 year stability of psychopathic traits in non-referred youth,' *Behavioral Sciences & the Law*, *21*:713–736.

Frick, P. J., and White, S. F. (2008) 'Research review: The importance of callous–unemotional traits for developmental models of aggressive and antisocial behavior,' *Journal of Child Psychology and Psychiatry*, *49*:359–75.

Gao, Y., and Raine, A. (2010) 'Successful and unsuccessful psychopaths: A neurobiological model,' *Behavioral Sciences & the Law*, *28*:194–210.

Gao, Y., Raine, A., Chan, F., Venables, P. H., and Mednick, S. A. (2010) 'Early maternal and paternal bonding, childhood physical abuse and adult psychopathic personality,' *Psychological Medicine*, *40*:1007–1016.

Gard, A. M., Waller, R., Shaw, D. S., Forbes, E. E., Hariri, A. R., and Hyde, L. W. (2017) 'The long reach of early adversity: Parenting, stress, and neural pathways to antisocial behavior in adulthood,' *Biological Psychiatry: Cognitive Neuroscience and Neuroimaging*, *2*(7):582–590.

Geurts, D. E., von Borries, K., Volman, I., Bulten, B. H., Cools, R., and Verkes, R.-J. (2016) 'Neural connectivity during reward expectation dissociates psychopathic criminals from noncriminal individuals with high impulsive/antisocial psychopathic traits,' *Social Cognitive and Affective Neuroscience*, *11*:1326–1334.

Glenn, A. L. (2011) 'The other allele: Exploring the long allele of the serotonin transporter gene as a potential risk factor for psychopathy: A review of the parallels in findings,' *Neuroscience & Biobehavioral Reviews*, *35*:612–620.

Glenn, A. L., Raine, A., and Schug, R. A. (2009) 'The neural correlates of moral decision-making in psychopathy,' *Molecular Psychiatry*, *14*:5–6.

Glenn, A. L., Raine, A., Yaralian, P. S., and Yang, Y. (2010) 'Increased volume of the striatum in psychopathic individuals,' *Biological Psychiatry*, *67*:52–58.

Gunter, T. D., Vaughn, M. G., and Philibert, R. A. (2010) 'Behavioral genetics in antisocial spectrum disorders and psychopathy: A review of the recent literature,' *Behavioral Sciences & the Law*, *28*:148–173.

Hajcak, G., Castille, C., Olvet, D., Dunning, J., Roohi, J., and Hatchwell, E. (2009) 'Genetic variation in brain-derived neurotrophic factor and human fear conditioning,' *Genes, Brain and Behavior*, *8*:80–85.

Hamilton, R. K., Hiatt Racer, K., and Newman, J. P. (2015) 'Impaired integration in psychopathy: A unified theory of psychopathic dysfunction,' *Psychological Review*, *122*:770.

Hare, R. D. (1991) *The Hare Psychopathy Checklist–Revised*, Toronto, ON: Multi-Health Systems.

Hare, R. D., and Neumann, C. S. (2008) 'Psychopathy as a clinical and empirical construct,' *Annual Review of Clinical Psychology*, *4*:217–246.

Hare, R. D., and Neumann, C. S. (2010) 'The role of antisociality in the psychopathy construct: Comment on Skeem and Cooke (2010),' *Psychological Assessment*, *22*:446–454.

Harenski, C. L., Harenski, K. A., Shane, M. S., and Kiehl, K. A. (2010) 'Aberrant neural processing of moral violations in criminal psychopaths,' *Journal of Abnormal Psychology*, *119*:863.

Hariri, A. R. (2009) 'The neurobiology of individual differences in complex behavioral traits,' *Annual Review of Neuroscience*, *32*.

Hariri, A. R., Drabant, E. M., Munoz, K. E., Kolachana, B. S., Mattay, V. S., Egan, M. F., and Weinberger, D. R. (2005) 'A susceptibility gene for affective disorders and the response of the human amygdala,' *Archives of General Psychiatry*, *62*:146–152.

Hariri, A. R., Drabant, E. M., and Weinberger, D. R. (2006) 'Imaging genetics: Perspectives from studies of genetically driven variation in serotonin function and corticolimbic affective processing,' *Biological Psychiatry*, *59*:888–897.

Heekeren, H. R., Wartenburger, I., Marschner, A., Mell, T., Villringer, A., and Reischies, F. M. (2007) 'Role of ventral striatum in reward-based decision making,' *Neuroreport*, *18*:951–955.

Heinz, A., Braus, D. F., Smolka, M. N., Wrase, J., Puls, I., Hermann, D., . . ., and Schumann, G. (2005) 'Amygdala–prefrontal coupling depends on a genetic variation of the serotonin transporter,' *Nature Neuroscience*, *8*:20–21.

Herman, A. I., Conner, T. S., Anton, R. F., Gelernter, J., Kranzler, H. R., and Covault, J. (2011) 'Variation in the gene encoding the serotonin transporter is associated with a measure of sociopathy in alcoholics,' *Addiction Biology*, *16*:124–132.

Hirata, Y., Zai, C. C., Nowrouzi, B., Shaikh, S. A., Kennedy, J. L., and Beitchman, J. H. (2016) 'Possible association between the prolactin receptor gene and callous–unemotional traits among aggressive children,' *Psychiatric Genetics*, *26*:48–51.

Holz, N., Boecker, R., Buchmann, A. F., Blomeyer, D., Baumeister, S., Hohmann, S., . . ., and Witt, S. H. (2014) 'Evidence for a sex-dependent MAOA × childhood stress interaction in the neural circuitry of aggression,' *Cerebral Cortex*, *26*:904–914.

Hoppenbrouwers, S. S., De Jesus, D. R., Stirpe, T., Fitzgerald, P. B., Voineskos, A. N., Schutter, D. J., and Daskalakis, Z. J. (2013) 'Inhibitory deficits in the dorsolateral prefrontal cortex in psychopathic offenders,' *Cortex*, *49*:1377–1385.

Hyde, L., Swartz, J. R., Waller, R., and Hariri, A. (2016) 'Neurogenetics approaches to mapping pathways in developmental psychopathology,' in D. Cicchetti (Ed.), *Developmental Psychopathology*, New York, NY: Wiley.

Hyde, L. W. (2015) 'Developmental psychopathology in an era of molecular genetics and neuroimaging: A developmental neurogenetics approach,' *Development and Psychopathology*, *27*:587–613.

Hyde, L. W., Bogdan, R., and Hariri, A. R. (2011) 'Understanding risk for psychopathology through imaging gene–environment interactions,' *Trends in Cognitive Sciences*, *15*:417–427.

Hyde, L. W., Byrd, A. L., Votruba-Drzal, E., Hariri, A. R., and Manuck, S. B. (2014) 'Amygdala reactivity and negative emotionality: Divergent correlates of antisocial personality and psychopathy traits in a community sample,' *Journal of Abnormal Psychology*, *123*:214–224.

Hyde, L. W., Shaw, D. S., and Hariri, A. R. (2013) 'Understanding youth antisocial behavior using neuroscience through a developmental psychopathology lens: Review, integration, and directions for research,' *Developmental Review*, *33*:168–223.

Hyde, L. W., Shaw, D. S., Murray, L., Gard, A., Hariri, A. R., and Forbes, E. E. (2016) 'Dissecting the role of amygdala reactivity in antisocial behavior in a sample of young, low-income, urban men,' *Clinical Psychological Science*, *4*:527–544.

Hyde, L. W., Swartz, J. R., Waller, R., and Hariri, A. R. (2015) 'Neurogenetics approaches to mapping pathways in developmental psychopathology,' in D. Cicchetti (ed.), *Developmental Psychopathology* (pp. 688–742). Hoboken, NJ: John Wiley & Sons.

Hyde, L. W., Waller, R., Trentacosta, C. J., Shaw, D. S., Neiderhiser, J. M., Ganiban, J. M., . . ., and Leve, L. D. (2016) 'Heritable and nonheritable pathways to early callous–unemotional behaviors,' *American Journal of Psychiatry*, *173*:903–910.

Karg, K., Burmeister, M., Shedden, K., and Sen, S. (2011) 'The serotonin transporter promoter variant (5-HTTLPR), stress, and depression meta-analysis revisited: Evidence of genetic moderation,' *Archives of General Psychiatry*, *68*:444–454.

Kiehl, K. A., Smith, A. M., Hare, R. D., Mendrek, A., Forster, B. B., Brink, J., and Liddle, P. F. (2001) 'Limbic abnormalities in affective processing by criminal psychopaths as revealed by functional magnetic resonance imaging,' *Biological Psychiatry*, *50*:677–684.

Kim-Cohen, J., Caspi, A., Taylor, A., Williams, B., Newcombe, R., Craig, I. W., and Moffitt, T. E. (2006) 'MAOA, maltreatment, and gene–environment interaction predicting children's mental health: New evidence and a meta-analysis,' *Molecular Psychiatry*, *11*:903–913.

Kolla, N. J., Dunlop, K., Downar, J., Links, P., Bagby, R. M., Wilson, A. A., . . ., and Meyer, J. H. (2016) 'Association of ventral striatum monoamine oxidase-A binding and functional connectivity in antisocial personality disorder with high impulsivity: A positron emission tomography and functional magnetic resonance imaging study,' *European Neuropsychopharmacology*, *26*:777–786.

Korponay, C., Pujara, M., Deming, P., Philippi, C., Decety, J., Kosson, D. S., . . ., and Koenigs, M. (2017) 'Impulsive–antisocial dimension of psychopathy linked to enlargement and abnormal functional connectivity of the striatum,' *Biological Psychiatry: Cognitive Neuroscience and Neuroimaging*, *2*:149–157.

Kosson, D. S., and Newman, J. P. (1986) 'Psychopathy and the allocation of attentional capacity in a divided-attention situation,' *Journal of Abnormal Psychology*, *95*:257.

Krischer, M. K., and Sevecke, K. (2008) 'Early traumatization and psychopathy in female and male juvenile offenders,' *International Journal of Law and Psychiatry*, *31*:253–262.

Krueger, R. F., Hicks, B. M., Patrick, C. J., Carlson, S. R., Iacono, W. G., and McGue, M. (2002) 'Etiologic connections among substance dependence, antisocial behavior and personality: Modeling the externalizing spectrum,' *Journal of Abnormal Psychology*, *111*:411.

Krueger, R. F., Markon, K. E., Patrick, C. J., Benning, S. D., and Kramer, M. D. (2007) 'Linking antisocial behavior, substance use, and personality: An integrative quantitative model of the adult externalizing spectrum,' *Journal of Abnormal Psychology*, *116*:645.

Kumsta, R., and Heinrichs, M. (2013) 'Oxytocin, stress and social behavior: Neurogenetics of the human oxytocin system,' *Current Opinion in Neurobiology*, *23*:11–16.

Lahey, B. B., Rathouz, P. J., Lee, S. S., Chronis-Tuscano, A., Pelham, W. E., Waldman, I. D., and Cook, E. H. (2011) 'Interactions between early parenting and a polymorphism of the child's dopamine transporter gene in predicting future child conduct disorder symptoms,' *Journal of Abnormal Psychology*, *120*:33.

Lancaster, T. M., Doherty, J. L., Linden, D. E., and Hall, J. (2016) 'Imaging genetics of Schizophrenia,' in K. L. Bigos, A. Hariri, & D. R., Weinberger (Eds.), *Neuroimaging genetics: Principles and practices* (pp. 187–208), New York, NY: Oxford University Press.

Larson, C. L., Baskin-Sommers, A. R., Stout, D. M., Balderston, N. L., Curtin, J. J., Schultz, D. H., . . ., and Newman, J. P. (2013) 'The interplay of attention and emotion: Top-down attention modulates amygdala activation in psychopathy,' *Cognitive, Affective, & Behavioral Neuroscience*, *13*:757–770.

LeDoux, J. E. (1995) 'Emotion: Clues from the brain,' *Annual Review of Psychology*, *46*:209–235.

Lockwood, P. L., Sebastian, C. L., McCrory, E. J., Hyde, Z. H., Gu, X., De Brito, S. A., and Viding, E. (2013) 'Association of callous traits with reduced neural response to others' pain in children with conduct problems,' *Current Biology*, *23*:901–905.

Lorenz, A. R., and Newman, J. P. (2002) 'Do emotion and information processing deficiencies found in Caucasian psychopaths generalize to African-American psychopaths?,' *Personality and Individual Differences*, *32*:1077–1086.

Marquez, C., Poirier, G. L., Cordero, M. I., Larsen, M. H., Groner, A., Marquis, J., . . ., and Sandi, C. (2013) 'Peripuberty stress leads to abnormal aggression, altered amygdala and orbitofrontal reactivity and increased prefrontal MAOA gene expression,' *Translational Psychiatry*, *3*:e216.

Marsh, A. A., and Blair, R. J. R. (2008) 'Deficits in facial affect recognition among antisocial populations: A meta-analysis,' *Neuroscience & Biobehavioral Reviews*, *32*:454–465.

Marsh, A. A., Finger, E. C., Fowler, K. A., Jurkowitz, I. T., Schechter, J. C., Henry, H. Y., . . ., and Blair, R. (2011) 'Reduced amygdala–orbitofrontal connectivity during moral judgments in youths with disruptive behavior disorders and psychopathic traits,' *Psychiatry Research: Neuroimaging*, *194*:279–286.

McCollister, K. E., French, M. T., and Fang, H. (2010) 'The cost of crime to society: New crime-specific estimates for policy and program evaluation,' *Drug and Alcohol Dependence*, *108*:98–109.

Meaney, M. J. (2010) 'Epigenetics and the biological definition of gene × environment interactions,' *Child Development*, *81*:41–79.

Medford, N., and Critchley, H. D. (2010) 'Conjoint activity of anterior insular and anterior cingulate cortex: Awareness and response,' *Brain Structure and Function*, *214*:535–549.

Meffert, H., Gazzola, V., den Boer, J. A., Bartels, A. A., and Keysers, C. (2013) 'Reduced spontaneous but relatively normal deliberate vicarious representations in psychopathy,' *Brain*, *136*:2550–2562.

Meyer-Lindenberg, A., Buckholtz, J. W., Kolachana, B., Hariri, A. R., Pezawas, L., Blasi, G., . . ., and Callicott, J. H. (2006) 'Neural mechanisms of genetic risk for impulsivity and violence in humans,' *Proceedings of the National Academy of Sciences*, *103*:6269–6274.

Michalska, K. J., Zeffiro, T. A., and Decety, J. (2016) 'Brain response to viewing others being harmed in children with conduct disorder symptoms,' *Journal of Child Psychology and Psychiatry*, *57*:510–519.

Moffitt, T. E. (2005) 'The new look of behavioral genetics in developmental psychopathology: Gene–environment interplay in antisocial behaviors,' *Psychological Bulletin*, *131*:533.

Motzkin, J. C., Newman, J. P., Kiehl, K. A., and Koenigs, M. (2011) 'Reduced prefrontal connectivity in psychopathy,' *Journal of Neuroscience*, *31*:17348–17357.

Moul, C., Dobson-Stone, C., Brennan, J., Hawes, D., and Dadds, M. (2013) 'An exploration of the serotonin system in antisocial boys with high levels of callous–unemotional traits,' *PLoS One*, *8*:e56619.

Moul, C., Dobson-Stone, C., Brennan, J., Hawes, D. J., and Dadds, M. R. (2015) 'Serotonin 1B receptor gene (HTR1B) methylation as a risk factor for callous–unemotional traits in antisocial boys,' *PLoS One*, *10*:e0126903.

Moul, C., Killcross, S., and Dadds, M. R. (2012) 'A model of differential amygdala activation in psychopathy,' *Psychological Review*, *119*:789–806.

Müller, J. L., Sommer, M., Wagner, V., Lange, K., Taschler, H., Röder, C. H., Schuierer, G., Klein, H. E., and Hajak, G. (2003) 'Abnormalities in emotion processing within cortical and subcortical regions in criminal psychopaths: Evidence from a functional magnetic resonance imaging study using pictures with emotional content,' *Biological Psychiatry*, *54*:152–162.

Murray, L., Shaw, D. S., Forbes, E. E., and Hyde, L. W. (2017) 'Reward-related neural correlates of antisocial behavior and callous–unemotional traits in young men,' *Biological Psychiatry: Cognitive Neuroscience and Neuroimaging*, *2*:346–354.

Newman, J. P., MacCoon, D. G., Vaughn, L. J., and Sadeh, N. (2005) 'Validating a distinction between primary and secondary psychopathy with measures of Gray's BIS and BAS constructs,' *Journal of Abnormal Psychology*, *114*:319.

Newman, J. P., Patterson, C. M., and Kosson, D. S. (1987) 'Response perseveration in psychopaths,' *Journal of Abnormal Psychology*, *96*:145.

Newman, J. P., Widom, C. S., and Nathan, S. (1985) 'Passive avoidance in syndromes of disinhibition: Psychopathy and extraversion,' *Journal of Personality and Social Psychology*, *48*:1316.

Nikolas, M. A., and Burt, S. A. (2010) 'Genetic and environmental influences on ADHD symptom dimensions of inattention and hyperactivity: A meta-analysis,' *Journal of Abnormal Psychology*, *119*(1):1.

O'Reilly, J. X., Woolrich, M. W., Behrens, T. E., Smith, S. M., and Johansen-Berg, H. (2012) 'Tools of the trade: Psychophysiological interactions and functional connectivity,' *Social Cognitive and Affective Neuroscience*, 7:604–609.

Pardini, D. A., Raine, A., Erickson, K., and Loeber, R. (2014) 'Lower amygdala volume in men is associated with childhood aggression, early psychopathic traits, and future violence,' *Biological Psychiatry*, *75*:73–80.

Pasalich, D. S., Dadds, M. R., Hawes, D. J., and Brennan, J. (2012) 'Attachment and callous-unemotional traits in children with early-onset conduct problems,' *Journal of Child Psychology and Psychiatry*, *53*:838–845.

Patrick, C. J., Bradley, M. M., and Lang, P. J. (1993) 'Emotion in the criminal psychopath: Startle reflex modulation,' *Journal of Abnormal Psychology*, *102*:82.

Patrick, C. J., Venables, N. C., Yancey, J. R., Hicks, B. M., Nelson, L. D., and Kramer, M. D. (2013) 'A construct-network approach to bridging diagnostic and physiological domains: Application to assessment of externalizing psychopathology,' *Journal of Abnormal Psychology*, *122*:902–916.

Plomin, R., Owen, M. J., and McGuffin, P. (1994) 'The genetic basis of complex human behaviors,' *Science*, *264*(5166):1733–1739.

Ponce, G., Hoenicka, J., Jimenez-Arriero, M., Rodriguez-Jimenez, R., Aragüés, M., Martin-Sune, N., . . ., and Palomo, T. (2008) 'DRD2 and ANKK1 genotype in alcohol-dependent patients with psychopathic traits: Association and interaction study,' *The British Journal of Psychiatry*, *193*:121–125.

Quay, H. C. (1993) 'The psychobiology of undersocialized aggressive conduct disorder: A theoretical perspective,' *Development and Psychopathology*, *5*:165–180.

Raine, A. (2008) 'From genes to brain to antisocial behavior,' *Current Directions in Psychological Science*, *17*:323–328.

Raine, A., Meloy, J. R., Bihrle, S., Stoddard, J., LaCasse, L., and Buchsbaum, M. S. (1998) 'Reduced prefrontal and increased subcortical brain functioning assessed using positron emission tomography in predatory and affective murderers,' *Behavioral Sciences & the Law*, *16*:319–332.

Rhee, S. H., and Waldman, I. D. (2002) 'Genetic and environmental influences on antisocial behavior: A meta-analysis of twin and adoption studies,' *Psychological Bulletin*, *128*:490.

Risch, N., Herrell, R., Lehner, T., Liang, K.-Y., Eaves, L., Hoh, J., . . ., and Merikangas, K. R. (2009) 'Interaction between the serotonin transporter gene (5-HTTLPR), stressful life events, and risk of depression: A meta-analysis,' *JAMA*, *301*:2462–2471.

Rodman, A. M., Kastman, E. K., Dorfman, H. M., Baskin-Sommers, A. R., Kiehl, K. A., Newman, J. P., and Buckholtz, J. W. (2016) 'Selective mapping of psychopathy and externalizing to dissociable circuits for inhibitory self-control,' *Clinical Psychological Science*, *4*:559–571.

Sacchet, M. D., Foland-Ross, L. C., and Gotlib, I. H. (2016) 'Imaging genetics of depression,' in K. L. Bigos, A. Hariri, & D. R. Weinberger (Eds.), *Neuroimaging genetics: Principles and practices* (pp. 210–236), New York, NY: Oxford University Press.

Sadeh, N., Javdani, S., Jackson, J. J., Reynolds, E. K., Potenza, M. N., Gelernter, J., . . ., and Verona, E. (2010) 'Serotonin transporter gene associations with psychopathic traits in youth vary as a function of socioeconomic resources,' *Journal of Abnormal Psychology*, *119*:604.

Sadeh, N., Javdani, S., and Verona, E. (2013) 'Analysis of monoaminergic genes, childhood abuse, and dimensions of psychopathy,' *Journal of Abnormal Psychology*, *122*:167.

Sadeh, N., and Verona, E. (2008) 'Psychopathic personality traits associated with abnormal selective attention and impaired cognitive control,' *Neuropsychology*, *22*:669.

Salekin, R. T. (2002) 'Psychopathy and therapeutic pessimism: Clinical lore or clinical reality?,' *Clinical Psychology Review*, *22*:79–112.

Salekin, R. T., and Lochman, J. E. (2008) 'Child and adolescent psychopathy: The search for protective factors,' *Criminal Justice and Behavior*, *35*:159–172.

Sen, S., Burmeister, M., and Ghosh, D. (2004) 'Meta-analysis of the association between a serotonin transporter promoter polymorphism (5-HTTLPR) and anxiety-related personality traits,' *American Journal of Medical Genetics Part B: Neuropsychiatric Genetics*, *127*:85–89.

Skeem, J. L., and Cooke, D. J. (2010) 'Is criminal behavior a central component of psychopathy? Conceptual directions for resolving the debate,' *Psychological Assessment*, *22*:433.

Skeem, J. L., Polaschek, D. L. L., Patrick, C. J., and Lilienfeld, S. O. (2011) 'Psychopathic personality: Bridging the gap between scientific evidence and public policy,' *Psychological Science in the Public Interest*, *12*:95–162.

Taylor, J., Loney, B. R., Bobadilla, L., Iacono, W. G., and McGue, M. (2003) 'Genetic and environmental influences on psychopathy trait dimensions in a community sample of male twins,' *Journal of Abnormal Child Psychology*, *31*:633–645.

Thornquist, M. H., and Zuckerman, M. (1995) 'Psychopathy, passive-avoidance learning and basic dimensions of personality,' *Personality and Individual Differences*, *19*:525–534.

Turner, R. A., Altemus, M., Yip, D. N., Kupferman, E., Fletcher, D., Bostrom, A., . . ., and Amico, J. A. (2002) 'Effects of emotion on oxytocin, prolactin, and ACTH in women,' *Stress*, *5*:269–276.

Venables, N. C., Hall, J. R., Yancey, J. R., and Patrick, C. J. (2015) 'Factors of psychopathy and electrocortical response to emotional pictures: Further evidence for a two-process theory,' *Journal of Abnormal Psychology*, *124*:319.

Venables, N. C., and Patrick, C. J. (2012) 'Validity of the Externalizing Spectrum Inventory in a criminal offender sample: Relations with disinhibitory psychopathology, personality, and psychopathic features,' *Psychological Assessment*, *24*:88–100.

Viding, E., Hanscombe, K. B., Curtis, C. J., Davis, O. S., Meaburn, E. L., and Plomin, R. (2010) 'In search of genes associated with risk for psychopathic tendencies in children: A two-stage genome-wide association study of pooled DNA,' *Journal of Child Psychology and Psychiatry*, *51*:780–788.

Viding, E., Sebastian, C. L., Dadds, M. R., Lockwood, P. L., Cecil, C. A., De Brito, S. A., and McCrory, E. J. (2012) 'Amygdala response to preattentive masked fear in children with conduct problems: The role of callous–unemotional traits,' *American Journal of Psychiatry*, *160*:1109–1116.

Waller, R., Corral-Frías, N. S., Vannucci, B., Bogdan, R., Knodt, A. R., Hariri, A. R., and Hyde, L. W. (2016) 'An oxytocin receptor polymorphism predicts amygdala reactivity and antisocial behavior in men,' *Social Cognitive and Affective Neuroscience*, *11*:1218–1226.

Waller, R., Dotterer, H. L., and Hyde, L. W. (2015) 'An imaging gene by environment interaction (IG × E) approach to understanding youth antisocial behavior,' *Emerging Trends in the Social and Behavioral Sciences: An Interdisciplinary, Searchable, and Linkable Resource.*

Waller, R., Dotterer, H. L., Murray, L., and Hyde, L. W. (in press) 'Neural substrates of youth and adult antisocial behavior,' in A. T. Vazsonyi, D. J. Flannery, & M. DeLisi (Eds.), *The Cambridge Handbook of Violent Behavior and Aggression* (2nd ed.).New York, NY: Cambridge University Press.

Waller, R., Dotterer, H. L., Murray, L., Maxwell, A. M., and Hyde, L. W. (2017) 'White-matter tract abnormalities and antisocial behavior: A systematic review of diffusion tensor imaging studies across development,' *NeuroImage: Clinical*, *14*:201–215

Waller, R., Gardner, F., and Hyde, L. W. (2013) 'What are the associations between parenting, callous–unemotional traits, and antisocial behavior in youth? A systematic review of evidence,' *Clinical Psychology Review*, *33*:593–608.

Waller, R., Gardner, F., Viding, E., Shaw, D. S., Dishion, T. J., Wilson, M. N., and Hyde, L. W. (2014) 'Bidirectional associations between parental warmth, callous unemotional behavior, and behavior problems in high-risk preschoolers,' *Journal of Abnormal Child Psychology*, *42*:1275–1285.

Waller, R., and Hyde, L. W. (2017) 'Callous–unemotional behaviors in early childhood: Measurement, meaning, and the influence of parenting,' *Child Development Perspectives*, *11*:120–126.

Waller, R., Shaw, D. S., Forbes, E. E., and Hyde, L. W. (2015) 'Understanding early contextual and parental risk factors for the development of limited prosocial emotions,' *Journal of Abnormal Child Psychology*, *43*:1025–1039.

Weiler, B. L., and Widom, C. S. (1996) 'Psychopathy and violent behaviour in abused and neglected young adults,' *Criminal Behaviour and Mental Health*, *6*:253–271.

White, M. G., Bogdan, R., Fisher, P. M., Munoz, K., Williamson, D. E., and Hariri, A. R. (2012) 'FKBP5 and emotional neglect interact to predict individual differences in amygdala reactivity,' *Genes, Brain and Behavior*, *11*:869–878.

White, S. F., Pope, K., Sinclair, S., Fowler, K. A., Brislin, S. J., Williams, W. C., . . ., and Blair, R. J. R. (2013) 'Disrupted expected value and prediction error signaling in youths with disruptive behavior disorders during a passive avoidance task,' *American Journal of Psychiatry*, *170*:315–323.

Willoughby, M. T., Mills-Koonce, R., Propper, C. B., and Waschbusch, D. A. (2013) 'Observed parenting behaviors interact with a polymorphism of the brain-derived neurotrophic factor gene to predict the emergence of oppositional defiant and callous–unemotional behaviors at age 3 years,' *Development and Psychopathology*, *25*:903–917.

Wu, T., and Barnes, J. (2013) 'Two dopamine receptor genes (DRD2 and DRD4) predict psychopathic personality traits in a sample of American adults,' *Journal of Criminal Justice*, *41*:188–195.
Yang, Y., and Raine, A. (2009) 'Prefrontal structural and functional brain imaging findings in antisocial, violent, and psychopathic individuals: A meta-analysis,' *Psychiatry Research: Neuroimaging*, *174*:81–88.
Yildirim, B. O., and Derksen, J. J. (2013) 'Systematic review, structural analysis, and new theoretical perspectives on the role of serotonin and associated genes in the etiology of psychopathy and sociopathy,' *Neuroscience & Biobehavioral Reviews*, *37*:1254–1296.
Yoder, K. J., Lahey, B. B., and Decety, J. (2016) 'Callous traits in children with and without conduct problems predict reduced connectivity when viewing harm to others,' *Scientific Reports*, *6*:20216.

8
The neural basis of psychopathy

Shichun Ling, Rebecca Umbach, and Adrian Raine

Introduction

Psychopathy is a personality disorder characterized by a constellation of interpersonal, affective, and lifestyle impairments as well as persistent antisocial behavior throughout the lifespan. Despite lack of official recognition by the *Diagnostic and Statistical Manual of Mental Disorders* (*5th Edition*; DSM–5; American Psychiatric Association, 2013), the construct of psychopathy has long been operationalized and studied (Millon, Simonsen, & Birket-Smith, 1998). The revised Psychopathy Checklist (PCL–R; Hare, 2003), a 20-item measure of psychopathy administered by a trained clinician, is considered the "gold standard" of psychopathy assessments. Each PCL–R item is rated on a 3-point scale (0 = does not apply/is not characteristic, 1 = applies to some extent/is somewhat characteristic, 2 = definitely applies/is definitely characteristic) based upon a semi-structured interview and a review of the individual's file records and history. The PCL–R provides an overall assessment of psychopathy (Total Psychopathy), the scores of which can range from 0 to 40; the traditional cut-off score for psychopathy is 30 and above. However, this overall assessment can be broken down into two main factors, which can be decomposed into two facets each, all comprised of specific PCL–R items, as shown in Figure 8.1.

Despite the interest and wealth of literature on psychopathic individuals, the neural basis of psychopathy is not well understood. However, advances in neuroimaging methods have allowed researchers to examine biological mechanisms that could contribute to or underlie abnormalities found in psychopathic individuals. In particular, researchers are now able to examine brain structure and function as an avenue to improving the understanding of psychopathy in a non-invasive manner.

Magnetic resonance imaging (MRI) is a common neuroimaging technique used to study a variety of disorders. It is a safe, non-invasive, non-radioactive method and, relevant to this chapter, can reveal structural and functional aberrations of the brain. In structural MRI (sMRI), the relaxation time of protons in water molecules is measured. Magnetic fields within the MRI scanner force hydrogen protons to line up; then, radio waves are used to knock the protons out of line. After the radio waves stop emitting, protons fall back into line and, while doing so, emit resonance signals that are picked up by the MRI machine. Structural MRI is generally based on data from T1 scans, which can provide measures of gray matter volume, thickness, and density/

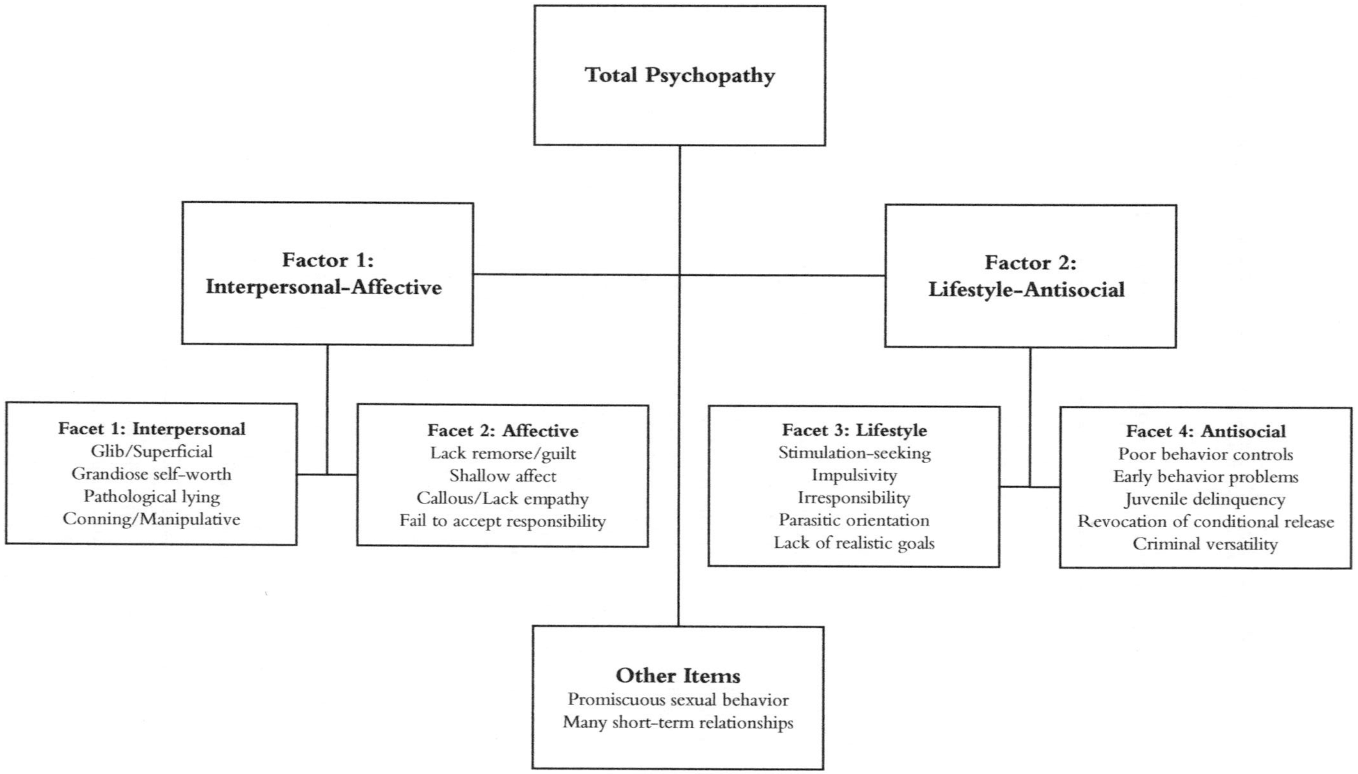

Figure 8.1 PCL–R assessment diagram

concentration. Another type of scan that provides structural brain data is diffusion tensor imaging (DTI), which assesses microstructural integrity of white matter tracts (Pierpaoli & Basser, 1996) and reflects structural connectivity between brain regions. DTI can provide measures of fractional anisotropy (FA) and streamlines (SLs). FA is an indirect measure of white matter integrity and can assess connectivity, or efficiency thereof, between brain areas, while streamlines can be used as a surrogate measure of tract volume.

In functional MRI (fMRI), the concentration of oxygen in the blood in the brain is measured. This is often referred to as BOLD (blood oxygen level dependent) activity. There are two types of functional imaging studies. The first is resting state functional MRI (rsfMRI) or resting state functional connectivity MRI (rs-fcMRI). Studies using rsfMRI/rs-fcMRI measure the degree of spontaneously correlated BOLD activity between brain regions while the subject is at rest (i.e., no task demands). The second type of fMRI study is task-related or event-related fMRI. Task-/Event-related fMRI results reflect the activation of certain brain areas to a specific stimulus *relative to* another condition. For example, in fMRI, observed brain activation associated with a smiling face might be compared to observed brain activation associated with a neutral face. By contrasting (through subtraction) the activation during the smiling face period with the activation during the neutral face period, experimenters are better able to infer what brain areas might be specifically related to the phenomenon of observing a smile, while removing any brain regions that might be involved in other processes common to both the smiling and neutral conditions (e.g., brain activation related to attention, face recognition, etc.). Because task-dependent fMRI results are based upon contrasts, it is important to have the conditions matched as similarly as possible on all features (e.g., face shape, skin tone, background, etc.) except for the feature of interest (smiling v. neutral). fMRI also allows for the study of functional connectivity, which measures interregional relationships. While functional connectivity analyses only examine which regions are coupled and do not explain how they are associated (i.e., no causal inference), they can provide insights into patterns of coupling and differences in coupling patterns between groups (Friston, 2011). However, to determine how one region influences another, analyses of experimental changes using effective connectivity (e.g., psychophysiological interactions [PPI], Granger causality analysis [GCA], dynamic causal modeling [DCM]) methods are needed.

This review covers prior reviews and empirical reports of human neuroimaging findings associated specifically with adult psychopathy using magnetic resonance imaging methods. As such, there are three important related areas of research that are omitted in this review. First, this review will not discuss the neural correlates associated with general antisocial behavior, subtypes of antisocial behavior such as violence (Raine, Buchsbaum, & LaCasse, 1997) or pathological lying (Yang et al., 2005a), nor Antisocial Personality Disorder (Raine, in press). Although the DSM–5 diagnosis of Antisocial Personality Disorder (ASPD) is strongly related to psychopathy, these constructs are not one and the same. Whereas approximately 90 percent of psychopaths meet the diagnostic criteria for Antisocial Personality Disorder, only 25–30 percent of individuals with Antisocial Personality Disorder can be considered psychopathic (DeLisi, 2016). Moreover, there may be neural differences between individuals diagnosed with Antisocial Personality Disorder with and without comorbid psychopathy; whereas antisocial individuals with psychopathy exhibit reduced gray matter in the anterior rostral prefrontal cortex and temporal poles, those without do not show these structural deficits (Gregory et al., 2012). These findings suggest there may be important differences between the psychopathy and antisociality constructs that are worth considering. However, this issue goes beyond the scope of this chapter.

The second area of research this review omits is the relevant area of research in relation to children and adolescents. This chapter will be limited to those studies using adult subjects (i.e., subjects aged 18 and older), recruited either from community or forensic populations. The DSM–5 has recently added a specifier of "callous–unemotional" to the diagnosis of Conduct Disorder (the childhood form of ASPD), and multiple studies have looked at brain functioning in youth with callous–unemotional traits (e.g., Marsh et al., 2008; Viding et al., 2012). Although the study of callous–unemotional traits is important and understanding the relationship between childhood psychopathic-like traits and adult psychopathy warrants attention, this relationship is far from direct and is accordingly beyond the scope of this chapter (Barry et al., 2000; Blair, 2013b; Frick, Ray, Thornton, & Kahn, 2014; Frick & White, 2008).

Lastly, this chapter will focus on structural and functional brain findings associated with psychopathy using magnetic resonance imaging (MRI) methods. As such, this chapter will not examine more granular aspects such as neurotransmitters (e.g., dopamine) within specific brain regions or the effects of hormones (e.g., testosterone) on the brain, nor will it focus on other neuroscientific methods (e.g., EEG/ERP, MEG, TMS, tDCS, CT, or PET/SPECT).

This chapter thus aims to provide a selective review of brain structural and functional imaging studies on adult psychopathy. The most robust brain regions implicated in psychopathy will be reviewed and discussed in depth. In particular, this chapter will focus on the ventromedial prefrontal cortex/orbitofrontal cortex (VMPFC/OFC), amygdala, and striatum. Importantly, although a clinical diagnosis of psychopathy based upon the PCL–R requires a score of 30 or above for diagnosis, this chapter will include those studies that study psychopathy from a more holistic or dimensional view. Additionally, although the PCL–R is designed and validated for use in offender populations (both adult and adolescent), it has been extended for use in community samples. We include those studies where relevant, in keeping with a more dimensional conception of psychopathy. Ultimately, we suggest that the socioemotional and behavioral impairments observed in psychopathy may reflect dysfunction of the VMPFC/OFC, amygdala, and striatum in particular. Together, these three regions may contribute to the behavioral disinhibition and poor representation of expected values (VMPFC/OFC), emotional dysfunction and low avoidance of aversive consequences (amygdala), and heightened reward sensitivity and impaired decision-making (striatum). As such, we offer a prefrontal-amygdala-striatal model of impairment in psychopathy.

Brain regions

Prefrontal cortex

The prefrontal cortex (PFC) has been a key brain area implicated in psychopathy. This region is associated with a variety of executive functions that are generally found to be impaired in antisocial and psychopathic individuals (Morgan & Lilienfeld, 2000). Although there are multiple areas of the PFC that have been implicated in the etiology of psychopathy, this chapter will focus on the ventromedial prefrontal/orbitofrontal cortex (VMPFC/OFC). While OFC is a structural delineation and the VMPFC is a functional delineation, there is enough overlap that these terms are often used interchangeably. In this chapter, we will also use these terms interchangeably.

Ventromedial prefrontal/orbitofrontal cortex

Lesions of the ventromedial/orbitofrontal cortex (VMPFC/OFC) have revealed the crucial role this brain region plays in the development of psychopathy. Perhaps the first and best-known evidence of the importance of the VMPFC/OFC in psychopathy was the case of Phineas Gage, a railroad construction foreman who had an iron rod blown through his head in a freak excavation accident which selectively damaged the prefrontal cortex (Harlow, 1868). Although Gage survived the experience, his personality was permanently altered, and he began exhibiting psychopathic-like behavior (Koenigs, 2012). A number of other case studies involving lesions in the ventral prefrontal cortex have provided further support that damage and dysfunction in this brain region can lead to pseudopsychopathy or acquired psychopathy (Blumer & Benson, 1975; Damasio, 1994), which reflect psychopathic-like personality and behavioral changes but are thought to stem from an environmental trauma that resulted in a brain injury. A variety of neuroimaging methods have since been used to examine how prefrontal cortex and functioning relates to psychopathy.

Structural magnetic resonance imaging (sMRI) studies have demonstrated a negative relationship between psychopathy and prefrontal volume (de Oliveira-Souza et al., 2008; Müller et al., 2008; Weber, Habel, Amunts, & Schneider, 2008) and thickness (Ly et al., 2012; Yang et al., 2012). Although there are other regions of the PFC that have been implicated in psychopathy, we discuss here the studies specifically related to the VMPFC/OFC.

Psychopathic individuals have demonstrated gray matter reductions in the OFC, among other fronto-polar regions, and the degree of structural abnormality is associated with the Interpersonal/Affective (i.e., PCL–R Factor 1) dimension of psychopathy (de Oliveira-Souza et al., 2008). Consistent with this, Ermer, Cope, Nyalakanti, Calhoun, and Kiehl (2012) found that increased total PCL–R psychopathy scores were associated with decreased gray matter volume and gray matter concentration in the VMPFC/OFC in a study of 254 incarcerated adult males. The integrity of the uncinate fasciculus (UF; a major white matter tract connecting the PFC with subcortical structures) has also been found to be reduced in psychopathic individuals. Craig et al. (2009) found reduced fractional anisotropy (FA), an indirect measure of white matter integrity, in the UF in psychopathic individuals compared to age- and IQ-matched non-psychiatric controls as well as psychiatric controls with a history of drug abuse and institutionalization. Moreover, based upon analyses of tract-specific mean group differences in FA, this result was found to be specific to the VMPFC/OFC–amygdala network, with no differences in the inferior longitudinal fasciculus (IFL) or inferior fronto-occipital fasciculus (IFOF) tracts. Consistent with these findings, Motzkin, Newman, Kiehl, and Koenigs (2011) found that psychopathic individuals had reduced integrity in the right UF. At least one study, however, found no difference in VMPFC volumes between controls and individuals with ASPD and high psychopathy (Bertsch et al., 2013).

In addition to reduced gray and white matter volumes, psychopathic individuals exhibit reduced cortical thickness. Yang, Raine, Colletti, Toga, and Narr (2009) found reduced cortical thickness in the right VMPFC among other PFC areas in psychopathic adult males compared to non-psychopathic adult males after controlling for age, gender, and substance abuse. Additionally, Yang, Raine, Colletti, Toga, and Narr (2011) found higher correlations between increased response perseveration (a behavioral pattern involving the inappropriate repetition of a particular response despite the absence or cessation of reward) and reduced cortical thickness in the OFC and anterior temporal regions in psychopathic individuals compared to controls. Although response perseveration has been found to be a selective impairment in executive function in psychopathic individuals (Newman, Patterson, & Kosson, 1987), Yang et al.'s (2011) study provided preliminary evidence of how frontotemporal structural deficits could contribute to neurocognitive impairment with perseveration in psychopathic individuals.

In addition to reduced volume, psychopathic individuals have also demonstrated reduced functioning. In healthy individuals, the prefrontal cortex has been implicated in a variety of social, moral, emotional, and cognitive processes. The VMPFC/OFC in particular has been thought to be important in decision-making processes, especially with regard to integrating potential decision outcomes with goals and emotional states (Damasio, 1994; Grabenhorst & Rolls, 2011; O'Doherty, 2011). This concept is captured by the somatic marker hypothesis posited by Damasio (1994). The somatic marker hypothesis suggests that decision-making is partially influenced by conscious and non-conscious "markers" or signals that arise from bioregulatory emotional processes in response to external stimuli. A somatic marker has been termed as a "gut feeling" (Damasio, 1994:173). Damage to the VMPFC/OFC and other brain structures involved in the representation and regulation of body states may result in an inability to experience these signals, which could predispose to psychopathic behavior by disrupting decision-making processes that facilitate socially appropriate behavior (Bechara, Damasio, Damasio, & Lee, 1999).

Consistent with the notion of VMPFC/OFC impairment in psychopathy, psychopathic individuals exhibit similar poor decision-making patterns as patients with VMPFC/OFC lesions (Koenigs, Kruepke, & Newman, 2010). Psychopathy, particularly facet 2 (affective), has been associated with reduced activation in the medial PFC and amygdala during moral dilemmas (Glenn, Raine, & Schug, 2009). The VMPFC has been posited to be important in moral judgment because it is necessary for the experience of prosocial moral sentiments (Moll & de Oliveira-Souza, 2007). Damage to the VMPFC has been associated with more utilitarian decision-making for dilemmas involving personal (i.e., involving direct physical harm) actions (Koenigs et al., 2007). Similarly, psychopathic individuals are also likely to endorse more utilitarian decision-making (Koenigs, Kruepke, Zeier, & Newman, 2012).

During rest, psychopathic individuals show reduced functional connectivity between the anterior VMPFC and the right amygdala compared to non-psychopathic controls (Motzkin, Newman, Kiehl, & Koenigs, 2011). In task-dependent fMRI studies, psychopathic individuals have shown reduced OFC activation during fear conditioning (Birbaumer et al., 2005) and reduced moral/non-moral distinctions in the VMPFC compared to non-psychopathic individuals (Harenski, Harenski, Shane, & Kiehl, 2010). When observing pain and distress cues expressed by others, psychopathic individuals also exhibit reduced VMPFC/OFC activation compared to antisocial controls (Decety, Skelly, & Kiehl, 2013) and during perception of fear, sadness, happiness, and pain expressions (Decety, Skelly, Yoder, & Kiehl, 2014). These types of VMPFC/OFC deficits may contribute to response preservation (in spite of potentially aversive or negative consequences) and utilitarian decision-making in individuals with psychopathy.

Amygdala

Emotional deficits are a characteristic feature of psychopathy. Such deficits are thought to reflect dysfunction of the amygdala, given that this limbic region of the brain is involved in a variety of affective processes. Importantly, the amygdala is crucially implicated in stimulus reinforcement learning and thus the development of both fear and empathy. Amygdala functioning has been argued to be particularly important for fear conditioning, which may serve to avoid actions that might harm others (Blair, 2007b). An impaired amygdala may disrupt the ability to form stimulus-reinforcement associations, which could result in a lack of deterrence for engaging in harmful behavior (Glenn & Raine, 2009). This neural impairment, which could result in an inability to anticipate negative consequences associated with socially unacceptable behavior (i.e., "fearlessness"), is thought to contribute to the heightened level of instrumental or proactive aggression exhibited by psychopathic individuals (Glenn & Raine, 2009).

Finally, the amygdala is implicated in emotion and affective recognition. Accordingly, psychopaths are often suggested to have emotion recognition deficits, particularly regarding negative emotions (e.g., fear, sadness; Blair et al., 2004). This, in turn, contributes to the lack of affective empathy characteristic of psychopathy.

Reduced amygdala volume has been associated with an early onset of psychopathic traits (Pardini, Raine, Erickson, & Loeber, 2014). Psychopathic individuals tend to exhibit reduced amygdala volumes bilaterally, with a 17.1 percent reduction for left amygdala volume and 18.9 percent reduction for right amygdala volume (Yang, Raine, Narr, Colletti, & Toga, 2009). Moreover, these deformities were localized to the basolateral, lateral, cortical, and central nuclei of the amygdala (Yang, Raine, Narr et al., 2009). Similarly, Ermer et al. (2012) found total PCL–R to be negatively associated with grey matter volume of the amygdala bilaterally. Reduced amygdala volume has also been associated with increased total psychopathic traits in a sample of individuals from the community (i.e., a non-forensic sample), although reductions were isolated to the left amygdala (Vieira, Ferreira-Santos, Almeida, Barbosa, Marques-Teixeira, & Marsh, 2015).

Psychopathy has been found to be generally associated with reduced amygdala function during the processing of emotional stimuli (Kiehl et al., 2001). Using an experiment that required participants to remember neutral and negative words, Kiehl et al. (2001) found that controls, as expected, demonstrated more activity in the limbic region in response to the negative words than in response to the neutral words. These differences were not observed in the criminal psychopaths. Similarly, in a fear conditioning task, male psychopaths showed significantly less activity in the left amygdala and other parts of the front-limbic system compared to healthy controls (Birbaumer et al., 2005). A different task employed by Harenski, Kim, and Hamann (2009) asked participants to view unpleasant images. They found amygdala activity to be negatively correlated with scores on the Coldheartedness subscale of the Psychopathic Personality Inventory (PPI). This amygdala dysfunction is thought to contribute particularly to poor affective processing and recognition, as opposed to prosopagnosia. Gordon, Baird, and End (2004) examined this predicted impairment using an affect and identity recognition task and found that individuals scoring highly on the PPI demonstrated less bilateral amygdala (and frontal) activity in response to the affect recognition task, compared to individuals scoring low on the PPI. This difference was not seen in the identity recognition task. These functional abnormalities are also seen in community samples. In a task of moral decision-making (Glenn, Raine, & Schug, 2009), psychopathy scores of community participants were associated with reduced activity in the left amygdala. Hyde, Byrd, Votruba-Drzal, Hariri, and Manuck (2014) found higher psychopathy scores to be associated with reduced amygdala reactivity to emotional faces.

One exception to this pattern is seen in Schultz, Balderston, Baskin-Sommers, Larson, and Helmstetter (2016). They also examined the proposed "fearlessness" of psychopathic individuals using a Pavlovian fear conditioning task. However, unlike Birbaumer et al. (2005), Schultz et al. (2016) found greater amygdala activity in psychopaths as compared to matched controls. Interestingly, this was particularly true of primary psychopaths and was interpreted as suggesting that the low fear model is applicable specifically to secondary psychopathy. However, primary psychopaths have previously been found to exhibit low levels of anxiety and secondary psychopaths tend to exhibit high levels of anxiety (Skeem, Johansson, Andershed, Kerr, & Louden, 2007), while in the Schultz et al. (2016) study, the primary psychopaths exhibited response patterns similar to the high-anxiety control group and the secondary psychopaths exhibited patterns similar to the low-anxiety control group. These seemingly contradictory results should inspire further research. Nevertheless, structural and functional amygdala deficits have been suggested to be an essential trait of psychopathy due to the well-supported relationship between the amygdala and two constructs: fear conditioning and empathy. Distinguishing these deficits is an important step in trying to identify potential strategies to ameliorate them (e.g., Dadds et al., 2006).

Striatum

The striatum is a subcortical region of the brain that consists of the ventral striatum (nucleus accumbens) and the dorsal striatum (caudate, putamin, and globus pallidus). This region, particularly the ventral striatum, has been associated with reward-seeking and impulsive behavior (Delgado, 2007). The striatum has also been a region implicated in both the Interpersonal/ Affective and impulsive/antisocial features of psychopathy (Glenn & Yang, 2012).

There has been evidence of striatal volume abnormalities associated with psychopathy. One study examining structural abnormalities found a 13 percent smaller nucleus accumbens volume compared to controls (Boccardi et al., 2013). However, Boccardi et al. (2013) acknowledged that their study lacked a control group matched on confounding variables known to be associated with brain morphology (e.g., age, substance use). The majority of studies, however, have reported increases in striatal volume in psychopathic individuals. For example, a 9.6 percent increase in striatal (caudate, putamen, globus pallidus) volume was found in psychopathic individuals compared to controls matched for age, sex, ethnicity, and substance dependence (Glenn, Raine, Yaralian, & Yang, 2010). Similarly, volumes of the caudate and nucleus accumbens were found to be positively associated with total psychopathy scores (Schiffer et al., 2011). Consistent with these findings, Cope et al. (2012) found increased striatal (caudate nucleus and putamen) volume was associated with severity of psychopathy. Finally, using a large sample (n = 127) of adult male inmates, Kopornay et al. (2017) found PCL–R total scores and Factor 2 scores to be associated with increased volume throughout the striatum, particularly in the nucleus accumbens and putamen bilaterally, and larger striatal subnuclei volumes.

There have been functional differences found between psychopathic and non-psychopathic individuals as well. Impulsive/antisocial features of psychopathy have been associated with amphetamine-induced dopamine release in the ventral striatum, specifically during anticipation of a monetary reward but not during the receipt of the reward (Buckholtz et al., 2010). In contrast to positively valenced reward stimuli, reduced ventral striatal activity was found in psychopathic offenders in response to negatively valenced stimuli compared to non-psychopathic offenders and non-criminal controls (Kiehl et al., 2001). Korponay et al. (2017) found Factor 2 PCL–R scores to be associated with aberrant connectivity between the striatum and other brain areas, including the dorsolateral prefrontal cortex and the ventral midbrain. Glenn and Yang (2012) hypothesized that striatal abnormalities associated with psychopathy may in part be dependent upon context (e.g., increased for positive stimuli, decreased for negative stimuli), though this was not tested. Altogether, striatal abnormalities may reflect the aberrant reward processing observed in psychopathic individuals.

Model of neural dysfunction in psychopathy

Several neuroanatomical models have been proposed to psychopathy. Two prominent models are the violence-inhibition mechanism (VIM) deficit hypothesis (Blair, 1995) and the paralimbic dysfunction hypothesis (Kiehl, 2006). In Blair's (1995) VIM deficit model, the VIM is a behavioral inhibitor posited to mediate the suppression of aggressive behavior in the context of distress signals. Thus, distress cues, interpreted to indicate submission, would normally lead to an inhibition of aggressive behavior. However, in psychopathic individuals, distress cues do not elicit a response of reduced aggression because such individuals may lack this behavioral inhibitor. Blair's model implicates the VMPFC/OFC and amygdala as key regions of impairment in psychopathy (Blair, 2008). On the other hand, Kiehl's (2006) model implicates more brain structures than Blair's (1995, 2008) and includes the amygdala, insula, hippocampus, orbital frontal cortex, ventral striatum, anterior and posterior cingulate cortices, and superior temporal cortex.

We discuss a triumvirate model of psychopathy, which is in line with the three main brain areas (VMPFC/OFC, amygdala, and striatum) stressed by Blair (Blair, 2013a) and reduces the number of regions included in Kiehl's (2006) model, some of which have not been implicated in psychopathy. The interconnectedness of the prefrontal cortex, amygdala, and striatum may contribute to a deeper understanding of the underlying mechanisms of psychopathy (see Seara-Cardoso & Viding, 2014 for review). These core regions converge on key features of psychopathy (Blair, 2007b, 2013b): behavioral disinhibition and poor representation of expected values (prefrontal), emotional dysfunction and low avoidance of aversive consequences (amygdala), and heightened reward sensitivity and impaired decision-making (striatum). As such, we suggest a prefrontal-amygdala-striatal model of impairment in psychopathy.

The ability to regulate emotional states and behavioral impulses is dependent upon this triumvirate of structures. The organization of these structures facilitates emotional learning through classical and instrumental learning processes that link affect and emotion with behavior (Tottenham & Galvan, 2016). Blunted fear conditioning, a well-replicated correlate of psychopathy, is thought to reflect impairments in the amygdala. This has been supported by studies of patients with both unilateral and bilateral amygdala lesions failing to show a conditioned response to a reinforced conditioned stimulus (Bechara et al., 1995; LaBar, LeDoux, Spencer, & Phelps, 1995). As such, the amygdala is important in forming stimulus-reinforcement associations for both rewards and punishments (Blair, 2008). Such associations are important in developing moral emotions such as empathy, guilt, and remorse. Without learning these associations, individuals such as psychopaths may be undeterred from engaging in antisocial behavior (Glenn & Raine, 2009). Working in conjunction with the amygdala, the VMPFC/OFC is important in the representation of reinforcement expectancies and subsequent decision-making processes (Blair, 2008). Dysfunction in this region can lead to poor decision-making and inappropriate behavior because individuals may be unable to properly anticipate consequences, as theorized in the somatic marker hypothesis (Damasio, 1994). Lastly, the striatum may contribute to the pleasure-driven motivations of psychopathic individuals.

Psychopathy is partially characterized by approach, reward-driven behavior that is disinhibited and relatively insensitive to the threat of punishment for antisocial behaviors. Disruption to the prefrontal-amygdala-striatal system in a way that minimizes sensitivity to punishment and maximizes reward sensitivity could result in the disinhibited, reward-seeking antisocial behavior of psychopathic individuals.

Limitations and future directions

Given methodological restrictions and costs associated with magnetic resonance imaging methods, many of the aforementioned studies have small sample sizes. Accordingly, when studies report null findings, it is possible that they are simply underpowered to detect significant differences. Dolan, Deakin, Roberts, and Anderson (2002) found no significant differences in frontal volume between a forensic sample of personality disordered inmates (including psychopaths) and staff members (used as healthy controls), but there were only 18 inmates and 19 staff members included in the study. Future studies should consider conducting power analyses to determine an appropriate sample size for a particular expected effect size.

Many studies on psychopathy also tend to rely on forensic samples (e.g., prisoners). In particular, much of the literature on psychopathy has focused on incarcerated males; thus, it is unclear how generalizable the neuroimaging results are to other psychopathic subgroups such as females or non-incarcerated individuals. One psychopathy subgroup differentiation has been between "successful" (those who have not been caught and/or convicted) and "unsuccessful" (those who have been caught and/or convicted) psychopaths. In a study comparing 16 unsuccessful psychopaths, 10 successful psychopaths, and 27 controls, unsuccessful psychopaths exhibited reduced gray matter volume and cortical thickness/surface shape in the orbitofrontal cortex, middle frontal cortex, and amygdala (Yang, Raine, Colletti, Toga, & Narr, 2010). However, successful psychopaths did not differ from controls. Unsuccessful psychopaths, but not successful psychopaths, exhibited a 22.3 percent reduction in prefrontal gray matter volume compared to healthy controls (Yang et al., 2005b). Additionally, unsuccessful psychopaths show an exaggerated structural hippocampal asymmetry (R > L) compared to successful psychopaths and control subjects (Raine et al., 2004). Similar to divergent findings of structural impairments in "successful" versus "unsuccessful" psychopaths (Yang, Raine, Colletti, Toga, & Narr, 2010). Gao and Raine (2010) proposed a neurobiological model whereby "successful" psychopaths exhibit intact prefrontal functioning, whereas "unsuccessful" psychopaths exhibit impaired prefrontal functioning. In addition to the differentiation of "successful" and "unsuccessful" psychopaths, there has been some evidence of differences between "primary" versus "secondary" psychopathy (Skeem, Poythress, Edens, Lilienfeld, & Cale, 2003). Such findings indicate that the manifestation of psychopathic symptoms and the severity of such symptoms is not homogenous across individuals. Although forensic samples likely yield higher rates of psychopathy and perhaps more severe forms of psychopathy, it is nevertheless important to investigate the generalizability of psychopathy findings in forensic samples to community samples of psychopathy, as well as other subgroups of psychopaths (e.g., male v. female).

Additionally, although we focus predominantly on studies that used Hare's revised Psychopathy Checklist (PCL–R), there are other assessments of psychopathy. These include interview-based or observer ratings of psychopathy such as Comprehensive Assessment of Psychopathic Personality (CAPP; Cooke, Hart, & Logan, 2005) as well as self-report measures of psychopathy such as Levenson's Primary and Secondary Psychopathy Scales (LPSP; Levenson, Kiehl, & Fitzpatrick, 1995), the Self-Report Psychopathy Scale II (SRP–II; Hare, Harpur, & Hemphill, 1989), the Psychopathic Personality Inventory–Revised (PPI–R; Lilienfeld & Widows, 2005) or Short Form (PPI–SF; Tonnaer, Cima, Sijtsma, Uzieblo, & Lilienfeld, 2013), and the Triarchic Psychopathy Measure (TriPM; Patrick, 2010). Researchers should carefully weigh the benefits and disadvantages of using observer- v. self-report measures of psychopathy and may consider using observer-report measures to supplement self-report measures or vice versa. Future research should also consider whether to use a categorical or dimensional measure of psychopathy, and clarify whether findings pertain to psychopathy *per se* or variation in certain characteristics (Koenigs, Baskin-Sommers, Zeier, & Newman, 2011).

In addition to the methodological limitations of these studies, there are also methodological limitations to using MRI. While structural and functional MRI methods have good spatial localization (~1 mm for sMRI and ~3 mm for fMRI), they both suffer from poor temporal resolution. Thus, there are some important caveats that need to be acknowledged when discussing the interpretation of neuroimaging results. For structural MRI studies, temporal order is difficult to determine, and such results should not be used to make causal claims. Lesion studies can provide some evidence of the functional importance of a certain brain area; however, lesion studies are based on some degree on the notion of functional specialization and are unable to address potential compensatory brain mechanisms (Ward, 2012). For functional MRI studies, even with manipulation, determining temporal order can be a challenge. Additionally, there are usually one of two inferences made, each with its own limitations. The first inference is forward inference (Henson, 2005), where a brain region or brain activity is inferred to be associated with the observed behavior of a given experimental condition. Forward inference is theory-dependent, and results based upon this approach may be misleading (Henson, 2005), especially if the theory of interest does not make predictions about brain activity (Heit, 2015). Additionally, differences in experimental tasks may contribute to differences in brain activity patterns, and thus the resulting observed differences may not reflect processing differences but rather differences in the content being processed (Heit, 2015). The second inference is reverse inference (Aguirre, 2003; Poldrack, 2006), where activation of a brain region is observed and the underlying cognitive or psychological process is inferred. However, reasoning backwards from observed brain activity to a specific cognitive process can be misleading because brain areas often have more than one function. These assumptions are important to consider when conducting MRI studies in general, and future studies may consider supplementing MRI assessments with other neuroimaging methods to address these limitations.

There are also practical restrictions to acknowledge. Although this chapter discussed the three most robust brain regions associated with psychopathy, there are other brain regions that have been implicated. These include the superior temporal cortex and dorsal anterior cingulate cortex (Kiehl, 2006) as well as the dorsomedial prefrontal cortex (Bertsch et al., 2013). However, given that these have not been supported by neuropsychological findings (Blair, 2006) or have not consistently been found, these were not considered robust neural correlates of psychopathy. However, future studies may consider examining these other regions, as they may provide clinically relevant information. For example, in a study aiming to distinguish psychopathic individuals from healthy controls based upon gray matter quantification and pattern recognition methods, the superior temporal sulcus/gyrus bilaterally was found to be the region containing the most relevant information to distinguish the two groups (Sato et al., 2011).

Lastly, although we have identified the VMPFC/OFC, amygdala, and striatum as the core regions implicated in psychopathy, it is unclear how much of these dysfunctions overlap with Antisocial Personality Disorder and other clinical conditions. One potential neural difference between psychopathic individuals and those with Antisocial Personality Disorder is amygdala reactivity to threat. Whereas higher psychopathy scores have been associated with *lower* amygdala reactivity to emotional faces, higher Antisocial Personality Disorder scores have been associated with *higher* amygdala reactivity to emotional faces, after adjusting for overlapping variance between psychopathy and Antisocial Personality Disorder (Hyde, Byrd, Votruba-Drzal, Hariri, & Manuck, 2014). Accurately differentiating between psychopathy and other disorders can yield important clinical implications and provide insight into potential treatment avenues. However, more research is warranted before such distinctions can be accurately made.

Conclusion

Although the neural basis of psychopathy has not been fully disseminated, the current body of evidence suggests there are impairments in cognitive, affective, and reward regions of the brain. Increased striatal volume and function may reflect the heightened reward sensitivity exhibited by psychopaths. The decreased volume and function of the amygdala may be related to their blunted emotional experience and impaired fear conditioning. The reduced volume and function of the prefrontal cortex, particularly in the VMPFC/OFC, could contribute to their poor decision-making. Altogether, the fronto-amygdala-striatal impairments observed in psychopathic individuals align with their disinhibited, reward-driven, and callous–unemotional behavior.

References

Aguirre, G. K. (2003) 'Functional imaging in behavioral neurology and cognitive Neuropsychology,' in T. E. Feinberg & M. J. Farah (Eds.), *Behavioral neurology and cognitive neuropsychology*, New York, NY: McGraw-Hill.

American Psychiatric Association. (2013) *Diagnostic and statistical manual of mental disorders: DSM–5*, Washington, DC: American Psychiatric Association.

Barry, C. T., Frick, P. J., DeShazo, T. M., McCoy, M., Ellis, M., and Loney, B. R. (2000) 'The importance of callous–unemotional traits for extending the concept of psychopathy to children,' *Journal of Abnormal Psychology*, *109*:335–340.

Bechara, A., Damasio, H., Damasio, A. R., and Lee, G. P. (1999) 'Different contributions of the human amygdala and ventromedial prefrontal cortex to decision-making,' *Journal of Neuroscience*, *19*:5473–5481.

Bechara, A., Tranel, D., Damasio, H., Adolphs, R., Rockland, C., and Damasio, A. R. (1995) 'Double dissociation of conditioning and declarative knowledge relative to the amygdala and hippocampus in humans,' *Science*, *269*:1115–1118.

Bertsch, K., Grothe, M., Prehn, K., Vohs, K., Berger, C., Hauenstein, K., . . ., and Herpertz, S. C. (2013) 'Brain volumes differ between diagnostic groups of violent criminal offenders,' *European Archives of Psychiatry and Clinical Neuroscience*, *263*:593–606.

Birbaumer, N., Veit, R., Lotze, M., Erb, M., Hermann, C., Grodd, W., and Flor, H. (2005) 'Deficient fear conditioning in psychopathy: A functional magnetic resonance imaging study,' *Archives of General Psychiatry*, *62*:799–805.

Blair, R. J. R. (1995) 'A cognitive developmental approach to morality: Investigating the Psychopathy,' *Cognition*, *57*:1–29.

Blair, R. J. R. (2006) 'The emergence of psychopathy: Implications for the neuropsychological approach to developmental disorders,' *Cognition*, *101*:414–442.

Blair, R. J. R. (2007a) 'Dysfunctions of medial and lateral orbitofrontal cortex in psychopathy,' *Annals of the New York Academy of Sciences*, *1121*:461–479.

Blair, R. J. R. (2007b) 'The amygdala and ventromedial prefrontal cortex in morality and Psychopathy,' *Trends in Cognitive Sciences*, *11*:387–392.

Blair, R. J. R. (2008) 'The amygdala and ventromedial prefrontal cortex: Functional contributions and dysfunction in psychopathy,' *Philosophical Transactions of the Royal Society B: Biological Sciences*, *363*:2557–2565.

Blair, R. J. R. (2013a) 'Psychopathy: Cognitive and neural dysfunction,' *Dialogues in Clinical Neuroscience*, *15*, 181–190.

Blair, R. J. R. (2013b) 'The neurobiology of psychopathic traits in youths,' *Nature Reviews Neuroscience*, *14*:786–799.

Blair, R. J. R., Mitchell, D. G. V., Peschardt, K. S., Colledge, E., Leonard, R. A., Shine, J. H., . . ., and Perrett, D. I. (2004) 'Reduced sensitivity to others' fearful expressions in psychopathic individuals,' *Personality and Individual Differences*, *37*(6):1111–1122.

Blumer, D., and Benson, D. F. (1975) 'Personality changes with frontal and temporal lesions,' in D. F. Benson & D. Blumer (Eds.), *Psychiatric aspects of neurological disease*, New York, NY: Stratton.

Boccardi, M., Bocchetta, M., Aronen, H. J., Repo-Tiihonen, E., Vaurio, O., Thompson, P. M., . . ., and Frisoni, G. B. (2013) 'Atypical nucleus accumbens morphology in psychopathy: Another limbic piece in the puzzle,' *International Journal of Law & Psychiatry*, *36*:157–167.

Buckholtz, J. W., Treadway, M. T., Cowan, R. L., Woodward, N. D., Benning, S. D., Li, R., . . ., and Zald, D. H. (2010) 'Mesolimbic dopamine reward system hypersensitivity in individuals with psychopathic traits,' *Nature Neuroscience*, *13*:419–421.

Cooke, D., Hart, S., and Logan, C. (2005) *Comprehensive Assessment of Psychopathic Personality Disorder: Institutional Rating Scale, Version 1.1*. [Unpublished manual].

Cope, L. M., Shane, M. S., Segall, J. M., Nyalakanti, P. K., Stevens, M. C., Pearlson, G. D., Calhoun, V. D., and Kiehl, K. A. (2012) 'Examining the effect of psychopathic traits in gray matter volume in a community substance abuse sample,' *Psychiatry Research*, *204*:91–100.

Craig, M. C., Catani, M., Deeley, Q., Latham, R., Daly, E., Kanaan, R., Picchioni, M., McGuire, P. K., Fahy, T., and Murphy, D. G. (2009) 'Altered connections on the road to psychopathy,' *Molecular Psychiatry*, *14*:946–953.

Dadds, M. R., Perry, Y., Hawes, D. J., Merz, S., Riddell, A. C., Haines, D. J., Solak, E., and Abeygunawardane, A. I. (2006) 'Attention to the eyes and fear-recognition deficits in child psychopathy,' *The British Journal of Psychiatry*, *189*:280–281.

Damasio, A. R. (1994) *Descartes' error*, New York, NY: Putnam.

de Oliveira-Souza, R., Hare, R. D., Bramati, I. E., Garrido, G. J., Ignácio, F. A., Tovar-Moll, F., and Moll, J. (2008) 'Psychopathy as a disorder of the moral brain: Fronto-temporo-limbic grey matter reductions demonstrated by voxel-based morphometry,' *Neuroimage*, *40*:1202–1213.

Decety, J., Skelly, L. R., and Kiehl, K. A. (2013) 'Brain response to empathy-eliciting scenarios involving pain in incarcerated individuals with psychopathy,' *JAMA Psychiatry*, *70*:638–645.

Decety, J., Skelly, L., Yoder, K. J., and Kiehl, K. A. (2014) 'Neural processing of dynamic emotional facial expressions in psychopaths,' *Social Neuroscience*, *9*:36–49.

Delgado, M. R. (2007) 'Reward-related responses in the human striatum,' *Annals of the New York Academy of Sciences*, *1104*:70–88.

DeLisi, M. (2016) *Psychopathy as unified theory of crime*, New York, NY: Palgrave Macmillan.

Dolan, M. C., Deakin, J. F. W., Roberts, N., and Anderson, I. M. (2002) 'Quantitative frontal and temporal structural MRI studies in personality-disordered offenders and control subjects,' *Psychiatry Research: Neuroimaging*, *116*:133–149.

Ermer, E., Cope, L. M., Nyalakanti, P. K., Calhoun, V. D., and Kiehl, K. A. (2012) 'Aberrant paralimbic gray matter in criminal psychopathy,' *Journal of Abnormal Psychology*, *121*(3):649–656.Frick, P. J., Ray, J. V., Thornton, L. C., and Kahn, R. E. (2014) 'Can callous–unemotional traits enhance the understanding, diagnosis, and treatment of serious conduct problems in children and adolescents? A comprehensive review,' *Psychological Bulletin*, *140*:1–57.

Frick, P. J., and White, S. F. (2008) 'The importance of callous–unemotional traits for developmental models of aggressive and antisocial behavior,' *Journal of Child Psychology and Psychiatry*, *49*:359–375.

Friston, K. J. (2011) 'Functional and effective connectivity,' *Brain Connect*, *1*:13–36.

Gao, Y., and Raine, A. (2010) 'Successful and unsuccessful psychopaths: A neurobiological model,' *Behavioral Sciences & the Law*, *28*:194–210.

Glenn, A. L., and Raine, A. (2009) 'Psychopathy and instrumental aggression: Evolutionary, neurobiological, and legal perspectives,' *International Journal of Law and Psychiatry*, *32*:253–258.

Glenn, A. L., Raine, A., and Schug, R. A. (2009) 'The neural correlates of moral decision- making in psychopathy,' *Molecular Psychiatry*, *14*:5–6.

Glenn, A. L., Raine, A., Yaralian, P. S., and Yang, Y. (2010) 'Increased volume of the striatum in psychopathic individuals,' *Biological Psychiatry*, *67*:52–58.

Glenn, A. L., and Yang, Y. (2012) 'The potential role of the striatum in antisocial behaviour and Psychopathy,' *Biological Psychiatry*, *72*.817–822.

Gordon, H. L., Baird, A. A., and End, A. (2004) 'Functional differences among those high and low on a trait measure of psychopathy,' *Biological Psychiatry*, *56*:516–521.

Grabenhorst, F. & Rolls, E. T. (2011) 'Value, pleasure and choice in the ventral prefrontal cortex,' *Trends in Cognitive Sciences*, *15*, 56–67.

Gregory, S., Ffytche, D., Simmons, A., Kumari, V., Howard, M., Hodgins, S., and Blackwood, N. (2012) 'The antisocial brain: Psychopathy matters,' *Archives of General Psychiatry*, *69*:962–972.

Hare, R. D. (2003) *Manual for the Revised Psychopathy Checklist* (2nd ed.), Toronto, ON: Multi-Health Systems.

Hare, R. D., Harpur, T. J., and Hemphill, J. F. (1989) *Scoring pamphlet for the Self-Report Psychopathy scale: SRP–II*, Burnaby, BC: Simon Fraser University [Unpublished manuscript].

Harenski, C. L., Harenski, K. A., Shane, M. S., and Kiehl, K. A. (2010) 'Aberrant neural processing of moral violations in criminal psychopaths,' *Journal of Abnormal Psychology*, *119*:863–874.

Harenski, C. L., Kim, S. H., and Hamann, S. (2009) 'Neuroticism and psychopathy predict brain activation during moral and non-moral emotion regulation,' *Cognitive, Affective, & Behavioral Neuroscience*, *9*(1):1–15.

Harlow, J. M. (1868) 'Recovery from the passage of an iron bar through the head,' *Publications of the Massachusetts Medical Society*, *2*:327–47.

Heit, E. (2015) 'Brain imaging, forward inference, and theories of reasoning,' *Frontiers in Human Neuroscience*, *8*:1056–1061.

Henson, R. (2005) 'What can functional neuroimaging tell the experimental psychologist?,' *The Quarterly Journal of Experimental Psychology Section A*, *58*:193–233.

Hyde, L. W., Byrd, A. L., Votruba-Drzal, E., Hariri, A. R., and Manuck, S. B. (2014) 'Amygdala reactivity and negative emotionality: Divergent correlates of antisocial personality and psychopathy traits in a community sample,' *Journal of Abnormal Psychology*, *123*(1):214–224.

Kiehl, K. A. (2006) 'A cognitive neuroscience perspective on psychopathy: Evidence for paralimbic system dysfunction,' *Psychiatry Research*, *142*:107–128.

Kiehl, K. A., Smith, A. M., Hare, R. D., Mendrek, A., Forster, B. B., Brink, J., and Liddle, P. F. (2001) 'Limbic abnormalities in affective processing by criminal psychopaths as revealed by functional magnetic resonance imaging,' *Biological Psychiatry*, *50*:677–684.

Koenigs, M. (2012) 'The role of prefrontal cortex in psychopathy,' *Reviews in the Neurosciences*, *23*:253–262.

Koenigs, M., Baskin-Sommers, A., Zeier, J., and Newman, J. P. (2011) 'Investigating the neural correlates of psychopathy: A critical review,' *Molecular Psychiatry*, *16*:792–799.

Koenigs, M., Kruepke, M., and Neuman, J. P. (2010) 'Economic decision-making in psychopathy: A comparison with ventromedial prefrontal lesion patients,' *Neuropsychologia*, *48*:2198–2204.

Koenigs, M., Kruepke, M., Zeier, J., and Newman, J. P. (2012) 'Utilitarian moral judgment in Psychopathy,' *Social, Cognitive, and Affective Neuroscience*, 7:708–712.

Koenigs, M., Young, L., Adolphs, R., Tranel, D., Cushman, F., Hauser, M., and Damasio, A. (2007) 'Damage to the prefrontal cortex increases utilitarian moral judgements,' *Nature*, *446*:908–911.

Korponay, C., Pujara, M., Deming, P., Philippi, C., Decety, J., Kosson, D. S., . . ., and Koenigs, M. (2017) 'Impulsive–antisocial dimension of psychopathy linked to enlargement and abnormal functional connectivity of the striatum,' *Biological Psychiatry: Cognitive Neuroscience and Neuroimaging*, *2*(2):149–157.

LaBar, K. S., LeDoux, J. E., Spencer, D. D., and Phelps, E. A. (1995) 'Impaired fear conditioning following unilateral temporal lobectomy in humans,' *Journal of Neuroscience*, *15*:6846–6855.

Levenson, M. R., Kiehl, K. A., and Fitzpatrick, C. M. (1995) 'Assessing psychopathic attributes in a noninstitutional population,' *Journal of Personality and Social Psychology*, *68*:151–158.

Lilienfeld, S. O., and Widows, M. R. (2005) *Professional manual for the Psychopathic Personality Inventory–Revised (PPI–R)*, Lutz, FL: Psychological Assessment Resources.

Ly, M., Motzkin, J. C., Philippi, C. L., Kirk, G. R., Newman, J. P., Kiehl, K. A., and Koenigs, M. (2012) 'Cortical thinning in psychopathy,' *American Journal of Psychiatry*, *169*:743–749.

Marsh, A. A., Finger, E. C., Mitchell, D. G., Reid, M. E., Sims, C., Kosson, D. S., . . ., and Blair, R. J. R. (2008) 'Reduced amygdala response to fearful expressions in children and adolescents with callous-unemotional traits and disruptive behavior disorders,' *American Journal of Psychiatry*, *165*:712–720.

Millon, T., Simonsen, E., and Birket-Smith, M. (1998) 'Historical conceptions of psychopathy in the United States and Europe,' in T. Millon, E. Simonsen, M. Birket-Smith, & R. D. Davis (Eds.), *Psychopathy, Antisocial, Criminal and Violent Behavior*, New York, NY: Guilford Press.

Moll, J., and de Oliveira-Souza, R. (2007) 'Moral judgments, emotions and the utilitarian brain,' *Trends in Cognitive Sciences*, *11*:319–321.

Morgan, A. B., and Lilienfeld, S. O. (2000) 'A meta-analytic review of the relation between antisocial behavior and neuropsychological measures of executive function,' *Clinical Psychology Review*, *20*:113–136.

Motzkin, J. C., Newman, J. P., Kiehl, K. A., and Koenigs, M. (2011) 'Reduced prefrontal connectivity in psychopathy,' *Journal of Neuroscience*, *31*:17348–17357.

Müller, J. L., Gänßbauer, S., Sommer, M., Döhnel, K., Weber, T., Schmidt-Wilcke, T., and Hajak, G. (2008) 'Gray matter changes in right superior temporal gyrus in criminal psychopaths: Evidence from voxel-based morphometry,' *Psychiatry Research: Neuroimaging*, *163*(3):213–222.

Newman, J. P., Patterson, C. M., and Kosson, D. S. (1987) 'Response perseveration in Psychopaths,' *Journal of Abnormal Psychology*, *96*:145–148.

O'Doherty, J. P. (2011) 'Contributions of the ventromedial prefrontal cortex to goal-directed action selection,' *Annals of the New York Academy of Sciences*, *1239*:118–29.

Pardini, D. A., Raine, A., Erickson, K., and Loeber, R. (2014) 'Lower amygdala volume in men is associated with childhood aggression, early psychopathic traits, and future violence,' *Biological Psychiatry*, *75*:73–80.

Patrick, C. J. (2010) Operationalizing the Triarchic Conceptualization of Psychopathy: Preliminary Description of Brief Scales for Assessment of Boldness, Meanness, and Disinhibition, Tallahassee, FL: Florida State University [Unpublished test manual].

Pierpaoli, C., and Basser, P. J. (1996) 'Toward a quantitative assessment of diffusion anisotropy,' *Magnetic Resonance in Medicine*, *36*:893–906.

Poldrack, R. A. (2006) 'Can cognitive processes be inferred from neuroimaging data?,' *Trends in Cognitive Sciences*, *10*:59–63.

Raine, A. (in press) 'Antisocial personality as a neurodevelopmental disorder,' *Annual Review of Clinical Psychology*, in press.

Raine, A., Buchsbaum, M., and LaCasse, L. (1997) 'Brain abnormalities in murderers indicated by positron emission tomography,' *Biological Psychiatry*, *42*:495–508.

Raine, A., Ishikawa, S. S., Arce, E., Lencz, T., Knuth, K. H., Bihrle, S., . . ., and Colletti, P. (2004) 'Hippocampal structural asymmetry in unsuccessful psychopaths,' *Biological Psychiatry*, *55*:185–191.

Sato, J. R., de Oliveira-Souza, R., Thomaz, C. E., Basilio, R., Bramati, I. E., Amaro Jr., E., . . ., and Moll, J. (2011) 'Identification of psychopathic individuals using pattern classification of MRI images,' *Social Neuroscience, 6*:1–13.Schiffer, B., Muller, B. W., Scherbaum, N., Hodgins, S., Forsting, M., Wiltfang, J., Gizewski, E. R., and Leygraf, N. (2011) 'Disentangling structural brain alterations associated with violent behavior from those associated with substance use disorders,' *Archives of General Psychiatry, 68*:1039–1049.

Schultz, D. H., Balderston, N. L., Baskin-Sommers, A. R., Larson, C. L., and Helmstetter, F. J. (2016) 'Psychopaths show enhanced amygdala activation during fear conditioning,' *Frontiers in Psychology*, 7:348–353.

Seara-Cardoso, A., and Viding, E. (2014) 'Functional neuroscience of psychopathic personality in adults,' *Journal of Personality, 83*:723–737.

Skeem, J., Johansson, P., Andershed, H., Kerr, M., and Louden, J. E. (2007) 'Two subtypes of psychopathic violent offenders that parallel primary and secondary variants,' *Journal of Abnormal Psychology, 116*:395–409.

Skeem, J. L., Poythress, N., Edens, J. F., Lilienfeld, S. O., and Cale, E. M. (2003) 'Psychopathic personality or personalities? Exploring potential variants of psychopathy and their implications for risk assessment,' *Aggression and Violent Behavior, 8*:513–546.

Tonnaer, F., Cima, M., Sijtsma, K., Uzieblo, K., and Lilienfeld, S. O. (2013) 'Screening for psychopathy: Validation of the Psychopathic Personality Inventory–Short Form with reference scores,' *Journal of Psychopathology and Behavioral Assessment, 35*:153–161.

Tottenham, N., and Galván, A. (2016) 'Stress and the adolescent brain: Amygdala-prefrontal cortex circuitry and ventral striatum as developmental targets,' *Neuroscience & Biobehavioral Reviews*, 70:217–227.

Viding, E., Sebastian, C. L., Dadds, M. R., Lockwood, P. L., Cecil, C. A., De Brito, S. A., and McCrory, E. J. (2012) 'Amygdala response to preattentive masked ear in children with conduct problems: The role of callous–unemotional traits,' *American Journal of Psychiatry, 169*:1109–1116.

Vieira, J. B., Ferreira-Santos, F., Almeida, P. R., Barbosa, F., Marques-Teizeira, J., and Marsh, A. A. (2015) 'Psychopathic traits are associated with cortical and subcortical volume alterations in healthy individuals,' *Social, Cognitive, and Affective Neuroscience, 10*:1693–1704.

Ward, J. (2012) *The student's guide to social neuroscience*, New York, NY: Psychology Press.

Weber, S., Habel, U., Amunts, K., and Schneider, F. (2008) 'Structural brain abnormalities in psychopaths: A review,' *Behavioral Sciences and the Law, 26*:7–28.

Yang, Y., Raine, A., Lencz, T., Bihrle, S., LaCasse, L., and Colletti, P. (2005a) 'Prefrontal white matter in pathological liars,' *British Journal of Psychiatry, 187*:320–325.

Yang, Y., Raine, A., Lencz, T., Bihrle, S., LaCasse, L., and Colletti, P. (2005b) 'Volume reduction in prefrontal gray matter in unsuccessful criminal psychopaths,' *Biological Psychiatry, 57*:1103–1108.

Yang, Y., Raine, A., Colletti, P., Toga, A. W., and Narr, K. L. (2009) 'Abnormal temporal and prefrontal cortical gray matter thinning in psychopaths,' *Molecular Psychiatry, 14*:561–563.

Yang, Y., Raine, A., Colletti, P., Toga, A. W., and Narr, K. L. (2010) 'Morphological alterations in the prefrontal cortex and the amygdala in unsuccessful psychopaths,' *Journal of Abnormal Psychology, 119*:546–554.

Yang, Y., Raine, A., Colletti, P., Toga, A. W., and Narr, K. L. (2011) 'Abnormal structural correlates of response perseveration in individuals with psychopathy,' *Journal of Neuropsychiatry and Clinical Neurosciences, 23*:107–110.

Yang, Y., Raine, A., Joshi, A. A., Joshi, S., Chang, Y. T., Schug, R. A., . . . & Narr, K. L. (2012). 'Frontal information flow and connectivity in psychopathy,' *The British Journal of Psychiatry, 201*:408–409.

Yang, Y., Raine, A., Narr, K. L., Colletti, P., and Toga, A. W. (2009) 'Localization of deformations within the amygdala in individuals with psychopathy,' *Archives of General Psychiatry, 66*:986–994.

9
The intergenerational transmission of psychopathy

Katherine M. Auty

Introduction

The familial nature of criminal offending has been demonstrated by several prospective longitudinal studies (Farrington, Barnes, & Lambert, 1996; Frick & Loney, 2002; Moffitt & Caspi, 2003; Rowe & Farrington, 1997; Thornberry, Freeman-Gallant, Lizotte, Krohn, & Smith, 2003). These studies have also advanced knowledge on the causes and correlates of antisocial behavior and criminal offending. However, the question remains whether the psychopathic personality traits that often accompany persistent and violent criminal behavior are also transmitted from parents to their children. This chapter reviews evidence for intergenerational continuities in psychopathic traits. It also investigates the environmental mechanisms that may help explain the intergenerational transmission of psychopathy.

Studies of psychopathy in adults and children suggest that psychopathic traits are moderately heritable (Larsson, Andershed, & Lichtenstein, 2006; Taylor, Loney, Bobadilla, Iacono, & McGue, 2003); however, environmental factors, such as socioeconomic status, neighborhood characteristics (Brooks-Gunn, Duncan, Klebanov, & Sealand, 1993), or parenting practices could also mediate the association between parental and offspring psychopathy. Overall, research suffers from a lack of clarity over whether there could be intergenerational transmission of psychopathy due to transmission of the criminal behavioral elements or whether the personality features are also transmitted. The focus of this chapter is to examine this in more detail. This chapter also presents analyses from the Cambridge Study in Delinquent Development (CSDD; Farrington, 2003) that look at the transmission of psychopathy from one generation to the next. It is the first study to relate the psychopathy of fathers to the psychopathy of their adult offspring. This analysis also examines whether the effect of the fathers' psychopathy on offspring psychopathy differs according to the gender of the offspring and whether the effect of the father's psychopathy varies according to the amount of time he spent living in the family home when the child was growing up.

Psychopathy

Psychopathy is a form of personality disorder originally described by Cleckley in *The Mask of Sanity* (1941/1982). It can be distinguished from other personality disorders by its primary symptoms. It is agreed (Cooke & Michie, 2001) that there are at least three major clusters of symptoms: an arrogant interpersonal style; a deficient affective experience; and an impulsive behavioral style. An individual who is psychopathic will have symptoms in all three domains. A fourth symptom cluster, antisocial behavior, has been suggested, but there is some debate in the literature as to whether antisocial behavior is a genuine symptom of psychopathy or whether it is the behavioral outcome of the other three personality symptoms (Cooke, Michie, Hart, & Clark, 2004).

The Hare Psychopathy Checklist is considered to be the "gold standard" for the measurement of psychopathy and has been described by some as 'state of the art' for both clinical and research purposes (Conoley & Impara, 1995). The Psychopathy Checklists (PCLs) are symptom construct rating scales. They have multiple items that are rated by an observer and each item reflects a symptom or characteristic of the disorder. They are subjective, as they require the rater to make a judgment about the individual's functioning. The items are designed to be assessed using all available information. This will usually include direct information obtained from a personal interview, behavioral observations, and indirect information from reviewing the individual's case history, and further information is often obtained from other informants (Hemphill & Hart, 2003). The Psychopathy Checklist–Revised (PCL–R) was published in its revised form in 2003 (Hare, 2003) and the Screening Version (PCL: SV), which was designed for use outside forensic settings, was published in 1995 (Hart, Cox, & Hare, 1995). The reliability of the PCL–R and the PCL: SV are well established as measures of psychopathy (Acheson, 2005; Hare & Neumann, 2008).

Factor analysis has highlighted the importance of the different components of psychopathy. Originally, a two-factor model of the PCL–R was presented (Harpur, Hare, & Hakstian, 1989). Factor 1 captured the personality elements, such as "selfishness, remorseless, and exploitative use of others," and Factor 2 indexed the behavioral features: a "chronically unstable and antisocial life-style." Subsequent work by Cooke and Michie (2001) has produced a three-factor model, which deletes four items that previously loaded onto the antisocial behavior factor. The resulting solution includes the factors interpersonal, affective, and lifestyle. Most recently, Hare (2003) has presented a revised, four-factor solution, which decomposes the original two factors into four facets: interpersonal and affective (personality facets) and lifestyle and antisocial behavior (behavioral facets). Importantly, this four-factor solution reinstates the antisocial behavior items removed from the three-factor solution. There is debate over whether antisocial behavior is an integral facet of psychopathy (Hare & Neumann, 2006) or if antisocial behavior is more accurately described as the outcome of all the other psychopathic personality traits (Cooke, Michie, Hart, & Clark, 2004). This debate is ongoing (Hare & Neumann, 2010; Skeem & Cooke, 2010). The majority of studies that attempt to analyze PCL: SV scores by decomposing the scores usually examine the two factors (for example, see Farrington, Ullrich, & Salekin, 2010). The 12 PCL: SV symptoms are subdivided into two factors and four facets.

Two early conceptualizations of psychopathy can be distinguished from each other. The first focused on the interpersonal and affective personality traits of psychopathy and was influenced by the work of Cleckley (1941/1982), Karpman (1948), and the McCords (1964). They saw personality traits such as superficial charm, dishonesty, and callous disregard for others as central to the concept of psychopathy. The second approach was influenced by the work of Robins (1966), who saw persistent and severe antisocial behavior as an essential feature of the disorder. The omission of the personality features from the diagnostic criteria for Antisocial Personality Disorder in the Diagnostic and Statistical Manual of Mental Disorders, fourth edition (DSM–IV) (American Psychiatric Association, 1994) was the impetus for Hare to develop his own diagnostic tool, which became the Hare Psychopathy Checklist.

Etiology of psychopathy

The specific etiology of psychopathy is unknown; however, the family environment as a causal factor is often dismissed.

> Many adolescents go off track because of a poor social environment – abusive parents, poverty, lack of job opportunities, bad companions – but the psychopath seems off track from the start. Again: Why? Unfortunately, the forces that produce a psychopath are still obscure to researchers.
>
> *(Hare, 1999:165)*

Several researchers have drawn a distinction between primary and secondary psychopathy (Poythress & Skeem, 2006), although Karpman (1941) originally made the distinction. Primary and secondary psychopathy are thought to have very different etiology. Primary psychopathy is thought to have its origins in genetic vulnerabilities, while secondary psychopathy is thought to be caused by environmental risk factors that are specific and unique to each individual. These risk factors trigger a vulnerability, which increases the likelihood of the young person developing psychopathy (Keyes, Legrand, Iacono, & McGue, 2008; Patrick, 2006). There is some research to support this; Frick and White (2008) delineated a low callous–unemotional (CU) type, characterized by low emotional reactivity and low fearfulness, which might make certain children less sensitive to the socialization attempts of parent, and also an impulsive conduct-problem (I-CP) type, where parenting and socioeconomic factors might be more relevant as etiological mechanisms.

Etiological theories of psychopathy

While the etiology of psychopathy may be unknown, several theories have been proposed. First, Lykken (1957) has suggested that psychopathy could be the result of the inability to experience fear. This fearlessness means that it is not possible for psychopaths to "learn to avoid antisocial behaviors and to inhibit forbidden impulses, through punishment and the conditioned fear it leaves behind" (Lykken, 1995:135). Second, Hare (1993, 1996) has asserted that psychopaths are emotionally under-aroused and experience a generalized deficit in the processing of emotional stimuli. They do not incorporate emotions into their planning or day-to-day interactions. Fearlessness and lack of anxiety are two of the consequences of this hypo-emotionality. This could explain findings from research into abnormalities in the linguistic and emotional functioning of psychopaths (Hare, 1993, 1996; Hart & Hare, 1996). Third, Newman has stated that he does not believe that psychopathy is a generalized affective deficit; he views it as a cognitive disturbance (Newman & Wallace, 1993; Newman & Wallace, 1993; Patterson & Newman, 1993). He believes that when psychopaths are presented with competing cues for reward and punishment, they *over-focus* on cues for reward and *ignore* cues for punishment. Therefore, they tend to selectively do things of benefit to themselves and ignore warnings that their actions could have negative consequences (Newman & Wallace, 1993).

Three explanations have been offered to explain these deficits in affective and/or cognitive processing. First, Blair (2007, 2009) has suggested that there may be a problem with the functioning of the amygdala in the brains of psychopaths. The amygdala "enables the individual to learn the goodness and badness of objects and actions" (Blair, 2007:289), and in psychopaths this learning is impaired, making them much more difficult to socialize. Second, Raine and colleagues (Raine, Lencz, Bihrle, LaCasse, & Colletti, 2000) found that there were structural deficits in the prefrontal cortex of antisocial, violent people with psychopathic-like behavior that were living in the community. They have suggested that these deficits could possibly explain antisocial behavior, as psychopaths experience poor fear conditioning, are less responsive to criticism, and are less receptive to socializing punishments. They are also less able to regulate arousal, which leads to sensation seeking behavior, and they are less able to reason effectively, leading to impulsive and reckless behavior. Finally, Widiger (1998) has disputed the idea that psychopathy is caused by a brain abnormality. He conceptualizes psychopathy as an extreme variation of normal personality traits. Psychopaths are individuals who, due to their behavioral genetics, are extremely low on Neuroticism, consciousness, Agreeableness, and openness to experience (Miller, Lyman, Widiger, & Leukefeld, 2001). While there has been a considerable amount of research into the biological and neurocognitive causes of psychopathy, social factors that may influence its development have been largely neglected (Farrington, 2006; Herpertz & Sass, 2000).

The intergenerational transmission of psychopathy

Only one prospective longitudinal study has investigated the relationship between the psychopathy of parents and the psychopathy of their offspring in adulthood. The male participants of the Cambridge Study in Delinquent Development and their biological children were assessed for psychopathy using the PCL: SV. The original male participants are referred to as G2 (generation 2) and their biological children as G3 (generation 3). The fathers' data was linked to their male and female offspring, producing 243 father–son dyads and 235 father–daughter dyads. Auty, Farrington, & Coid (2015) found a strong relationship between the total PCL: SV score of the fathers and those of both their male and female offspring; however, the relationship for females appeared to be weaker. When the relationship between the fathers and their offspring's PCL: SV factor scores were examined, the results for males showed that the personality features of psychopathy (Factor 1) and the behavioral aspects (Factor 2) were both strongly transmitted.

An interesting finding was observed in the results for female offspring. The results for females revealed a strong relationship between the fathers and the female offspring's Factor 2 score, but a weaker relationship was observed for the Factor 1 scores. This finding was explored further using moderated multiple regression analysis, where an interaction term (Gender × Psychopathy Score) was included into the model to see if the effect of the father's psychopathy varies according to the gender of the offspring (Auty, 2013). The results revealed that the effect of the fathers' psychopathy was significantly greater on the psychopathy of the male offspring compared to the female offspring; significant interactions were detected for total PCL: SV scores, Factor 1 scores, and the interaction term for Factor 2 was weakly significant. Without genetic measures, we cannot know how much of the relationship reflects shared genetic risk and how much of it reflects the impact of environmental risk factors on offspring psychopathy.

The final analysis did not find any evidence that the father's presence in the home modified the effect of the fathers' psychopathy on the male offspring's psychopathy. No significant interactions were found for total PCL: SV scores, Factor 1 scores, or Factor 2 scores. From this, we can conclude that psychopathy is strongly transmitted from fathers to male offspring, and as it does not appear to be affected by the father's presence in the home, it is likely that this finding reflects strong underlying genetic factors. The results for females however, showed that the effect of the fathers' Factor 2 score on his female offspring's Factor 2 score decreased as his presence in the home increased. No similar finding was discovered for Factor 1.

It would appear that females do not imitate their father's antisocial behavior. There could also be protective factors that explain why females do not express their antisociality in behaviors that are more commonly associated with men that are captured by the PCL: SV, such as fighting. Or it could suggest that the effect of the father's antisocial behavior on female offspring is somewhat neutralized when it is in the context of a happy and stable marriage. There are also some studies of the relationship between maternal psychopathic traits and callous–unemotional (CU) traits in their children. In a cross-sectional study, Loney, Huntenburg, Counts-Allen and Schmeelk (2007) provide evidence of the intergenerational continuity of maternal psychopathic features, as measured by the Levenson Self-Report Psychopathy Scale (Levenson, Kiehl, & Fitzpatrick, 1995) and callous–unemotional (CU) traits in their children, as assessed by the Antisocial Processing Screening Device (Frick & Hare, 2001). In a non-referred sample of 83 children (38 males and 45 females – mean age 10.4), they found a significant association between maternal affective features of psychopathy and CU traits in their child ($r = 0.22$; $p = < 0.05$). A weaker relationship was found for the interpersonal features of psychopathy in the mother and the child, which did not reach conventional levels of statistical significance.

The findings from studies of small samples are limited as they make it difficult to examine the differential effects of parental psychopathy on male and female offspring. The reliance on self-report psychopathy measures is also a matter of concern. They are considered inappropriate for use in capturing the construct of psychopathy, as deceitfulness is one of the symptoms of psychopathy and psychopathic individuals often lack personal insight. Several studies have found evidence to support this, with Harpur, Hare, and Hakstian (1989) finding that several self-report measures of psychopathy had very small correlations with PCL Factor 1. Although more recently self-report psychopathy measures have shown improved internal consistency and construct validity, their ability to capture the core features of psychopathy is a matter of ongoing debate (Lilienfeld & Fowler, 2007). Some studies have shown that psychopathic traits are quite stable from adolescence to adulthood (Lynam, Caspi, Moffitt, Loeber, & Stouthamer-Loeber, 2007), and research showing that psychopathic traits tend to be relatively stable over time (Frick, Kimonis, Dandreaux, & Farell, 2003) indicates it is possible that some children will grow out of psychopathy. Therefore, it is important to examine transmission to adult offspring where traits will be relatively stable.

A Finnish study found that high levels of parental psychopathy was related to the criminal prosecutions of offspring. Repo-Tiihonen et al. (2010) examined a sample of 179 people (132 males and 47 females), who had been prosecuted for committing a homicide. A file-based PCL–R was completed for each parent and their total score was categorized as low (0–19, 100 offenders), medium (20–29, 45 offenders) or high (30–40, 34 offenders). The criminal prosecutions of their children were investigated to see if there were any significant differences in the offending behavior of the offspring of the parents in the low, medium, and high psychopathy groups. The strongest association the study found was between a father's high psychopathy and their son's prosecution for vandalism. The authors explain that this could be due to genetic transmission of physiological vulnerabilities or impulsive temperament, impulsivity being a key feature of psychopathy. A number of other interesting findings are noted; the proportion of homicide offenders with children that had committed offenses against the person was higher in the high psychopathy group, compared to the low and medium groups ($p = 0.007$). The children of those in the high psychopathy group were prosecuted for their first criminal offense at a younger age than the lower psychopathy group. The parental psychopathy scores are further decomposed into the two factors: Factor 1, Interpersonal/Affective, and Factor 2, social deviance. Associations between their offspring's criminal offending were then re-investigated. Only two weak correlations were found: one between the parents' Factor 2 and the number of offenses against the person committed by their child and another between the parent's Factor 2 score and the early age of their child at first conviction. No such associations were found for Factor 1, suggesting that the psychopathic personality features of parents do not predict the criminal behavior of their offspring.

A further study of maternal prenatal risks (psychopathology, criminality, and substance misuse), the child's fearlessness (at age 2), and parenting (at age 4) as predictors of the child's conduct problems (CP) and CU traits at age 13 was conducted in a sample of 6,673 mothers and children, who were participants in the Avon Longitudinal Study of Parents and Children (ALSPAC). The findings revealed that the mother's prenatal risks increased the child's fearless temperament and their CP and CU. A relationship was also found between the child's fearlessness at age 2 and higher levels of CP and CU at age 13, while controlling for the mother's prenatal risks and parenting. In boys, fearlessness was expressed as a diminished response to punishment cues, while in females it was expressed as uninhibited behavior when faced with new situations or strangers. The authors consider that these finding may support evidence that expressions of antisocial behavior are quite different in girls and boys with CU (Barker, Oliver, Viding, Salekin, & Maughan, 2011).

An important moderator of the effects of the parent's behavior is the amount of time the child is exposed to the parent. Jaffee, Moffitt, Caspi, and Taylor (2003) found that for the offspring of fathers who engaged in low levels of antisocial behavior, the less time he lived in the family home, the more conduct problems the offspring had. However, fathers with high levels of antisocial behavior who lived in the family home predicted poor behavioral outcomes for their children. These children suffer two disadvantages; increased genetic risk of Antisocial Personality Disorder and being raised in a home environment that is not conducive to successful child rearing. Similarly, Lamb (1997) has argued that the amount of time fathers invest in child care is less closely associated with child outcomes than the *quality* of fathers' involvement with their children. Furthermore, intergenerational relationships may be closer among same-sex pairs, as offspring may be more strongly influenced by the parent that is most similar to themselves, and several studies have found that parents have the greatest impact on the negative behaviors of same-sex children through their negative parenting (Deater-Deckard & Dodge, 1997; Koestner, Zuroff, & Powers, 1991).

Psychosocial risk factors as mechanisms of the intergenerational transmission of psychopathy

While much is known about the family backgrounds of juvenile and violent offenders, relatively little is known about the family backgrounds of those with psychopathy. Most studies have focused on biological and genetic factors and neglected social and family factors (Farrington, Ullrich, & Salekin, 2010; Herpertz & Sass, 2000). The degree to which family environmental factors could influence offspring psychopathy is a matter of some debate. It is likely that both genetic and environmental factors explain its development in childhood and adolescence and its persistence into adulthood. It is now often suggested that an interaction between biological factors and environmental factors could be responsible (Farrington et al., 2010; Hare, 1993; Lykken, 1995), while previously, others had maintained that biological and environmental factors operated separately (Cloninger, Reich, & Guze, 1978; Lynam, 1996, 1997).

There are general reservations in the literature over the importance of environmental factors in psychopathy. From Cleckley's (1941/1982) observations we can see that although the family life of his patients appeared to be unproblematic on the surface, he nevertheless seemed to suspect that certain features of the parent–child relationship could be related in some way to psychopathy, but he did not specify how.

> In the patients presented here, social service reports and all ordinary information usually indicated normal and helpful family attitudes and general environments. The families themselves often impressed the examiner as good, healthy, wise, and eminently well-adjusted

> people whose children were particularly fortunate because of what they could offer as parents. When opportunities arose, as they sometimes did, to learn more of matters inward, subtle, and deeply personal, the observer was occasionally led to suspect that even in these apparently superior parents there were attitudes, frustrations, emotional confusions, and deficiencies that might have played a masked but crucially adverse role in the infinite complexities and paradoxes of parent–child relationships.
>
> *(Cleckley, 1941/1982:411)*

Hare (1993) has maintained that the influence of family factors on psychopathy is quite limited.

> The picture that emerges from clinical experience and research is far from clear on this matter. On balance, however, I can find no convincing evidence that psychopathy is the direct result of early social or environmental factors.
>
> *(Hare, 1993:206)*

Hare does, however, acknowledge that although childhood abuse and neglect have a detrimental impact on child development, these do not have a causal role in the etiology of psychopathy. He emphasizes the interplay between biological and social factors:

> Social factors and parenting practices help to shape the behavioral expression of the disorder, but have less effect on the individual's inability to feel empathy or to develop a conscience. No amount of social conditioning will by itself generate a capacity for caring about other or a powerful sense of right and wrong.
>
> *(Hare, 1993:211)*

Lykken (1995) also advocates an interactive approach, where biological factors interact with deficiencies in parenting to produce sociopathy. Children with high levels of fearlessness and impulsivity who are not parented adequately are led to "insecure attachment bonding that forecasts low levels of empathy, compliance, cooperation and self-control" (Lykken, 1995:213), while "emphasizing pride rather than punishment, constructive rather than antisocial risk taking, the potential delinquent can grow up to be a hero rather than a hood, a leader rather than a psychopath" (p. 86). However, parents of extremely aggressive children often fail to implement skillful parenting; possibly for genetic or environmental reasons, the parents are poorly equipped to parent a particularly difficult child.

The inclusion of items measuring antisocial behavior in the Psychopathy Checklist has meant that when evaluating evidence on possible causal risk factors, it is difficult to distinguish between those factors associated with antisocial behavior (for which there is quite a lot of evidence) and those factors associated with psychopathic personality traits (for which there is much less evidence). For this reason, the relationships between family risk factors and psychopathy have been examined in the CSDD by looking at Factor 1 (the personality traits) and Factor 2 (the behavioral characteristics) separately. These findings will be reviewed first. The chapter will then review findings from other studies that have examined social and environmental factors associated with psychopathy.

Findings from the Cambridge Study in Delinquent Development

As previously described, 304 of the G2 males were assessed for psychopathy between 1999 and 2004, when they were approximately age 48 (Farrington, 2006, 2007). Findings from the analysis of the data from the G2 males revealed that the prevalence of psychopathy in this community sample of adult males was very low; only two men scored 16 or more (considered a high score in a community sample), indicating probable psychopathy (Hart et al., 1995). Only 33 men had a score of 10 or more (11 percent); all but one was convicted (97 percent), and almost half (45 percent) were chronic offenders.

Farrington et al. (2010) investigated 25 childhood risk factors (measured at ages 8–10) to see which of them were unique predictors of PCL: SV Factor 1 and Factor 2 at age 48. The most important predictors of high Factor 1 scores were found to be a convicted father, coming from a family with low income, high impulsivity, an uninvolved father, low popularity, and low intelligence/achievement. For Factor 2, the most important predictors of high scores were found to be parental conflict, a disrupted family, a depressed mother, a young mother, large family size, and poor parental supervision. A weakly significant interaction was found between the risk factors large family size and a depressed mother. In families where both of these risk factors were present, 43 percent of boys had high Factor 2 scores.

The CSDD has also examined the relationship between the psychopathy of the G2 men and their outcomes in later life. Ullrich, Farrington and Coid (2008) looked at whether some psychopathic traits may be related to measures of life success. A principal components analysis of the measures used to indicate life success found two factors: "status and wealth," with the items social class, income, number of rooms in home, supervision of others in job, and home ownership; and "successful intimate relationships," with the items living in a relationship and stability and quality of relationship. Scores of life success for each domain were then created by adding up the scores of the observed variables. The scores of the two domains of life success were then related to the four facets of psychopathy: interpersonal, affective, lifestyle, and antisocial. The results revealed that high scores on the affective facet were negatively related to both "status and wealth" and "successful intimate relationships."

High scores on the lifestyle and antisocial facets were also negatively related to "status and wealth," but had no relationship with "successful intimate relationships." The authors concluded that none of the psychopathic personality traits are an asset in achieving life success; the interpersonal facet in particular had no relationship with either dimension of life success, and the other facets were all negatively related to one or both dimensions of life success.

Findings from other studies

Deficiencies in parenting have been regarded as key to the development of psychopathic personality for some time. McCord and McCord (1964) hypothesized that there were three pathways to psychopathy, and in each one parental rejection featured substantially. They proposed that parental rejection in combination with neurological damage, a psychopathic or antisocial parent, and a lack of parental supervision could combine to create a cold, unemotional, detached, callous personality.

There are very few longitudinal studies that look at the mechanisms underlying the transmission of parental psychopathy to adult offspring. Auty, Farrington, and Coid (2015) looked at ten psychosocial risk factors: accommodation problems (two or more of: not a home owner, poor home conditions, and more than two addresses in the past 5 years); cohabitation problems (three or more of: not living with a partner, not married or cohabiting for five years or more, divorced in the past five years, and not getting on well with his partner); employment problems (three or more of: currently unemployed, low occupational class, low wages, and unemployed for more than nine months in the past five years); alcohol misuse (three or more of: driving while under the influence of alcohol, a heavy drinker, a binge drinker, and a problem-drinking (Ewing,

1984) score of two or more); drug use (any illegal drug in the past five years); teenage father (at the birth of first child); large family (father living with four or more children); disrupted family (father left the family home before the child's sixteenth birthday); poor supervision (parents never knew where their child was going when they went out before age 16); harsh discipline (parents hit their children with an implement as a form of discipline). The selection of psychosocial risk factors was based on previous CSDD analyses conducted on the G2 males that found these factors to be important predictors of delinquency: 26 antisocial personalities at age 32 (Farrington, 2000); and PCL: SV scores at age 48 (Farrington, 2006).

The study found that all of the family risk factors had a significant relationship with either the male or the female offspring's Factor 1 or Factor 2 score. Some of the strongest effects were found for the male offspring; poor supervision had a strong relationship with Factor 1 and Factor 2 scores, as did the father's drug use, accommodation problems, and employment problems. For female offspring, poor supervision was also related to both high Factor 1 and Factor 2 scores. For females, the impact of the family risk factors appeared to be weaker.

These relationships can be compared to the findings from Farrington et al. (2010), which related the psychosocial risk factors of the G2 fathers (the previous to their PCL: SV scores). The main similarity is that poor supervision was an independent predictor of Factor 2 PCL: SV scores for the G2 males; it also significantly predicted high Factor 2 scores for both the male and female offspring in this study. A convicted father was an independent predictor of G2 Factor 1 scores and the G3 offsprings' own convicted father had a relationship with their Factor 1 scores. A disrupted family was another independent predictor of the Factor 2 scores of the G2 males and was significantly related to the Factor scores of their offspring.

One interesting difference is that a large family was an independent predictor of the G2 males Factor 2 score but was unrelated to the Factor 2 scores of either the male or the female offspring. It was, however, related to the Factor 1 score of the male offspring. This could possibly be explained by the comparatively more affluent upbringing of the G3 offspring, mainly in the suburbs of south London where, although family size might have been large, that upbringing was perhaps not always accompanied by household overcrowding. Previous findings from the CSDD showed that large family size didn't predict delinquency for boys in least crowded conditions (those with two or more rooms than there were children) (West & Farrington, 1973).

Gender differences in the effect of the family risk factors on the factor scores of the male and female offspring were explored using a series of interactions. The family risk factors that were found to interact with gender when predicting Factor 1 scores to have a more severe impact on male offspring were the fathers' accommodation problems, teenage father, and poor supervision. These variables all differentially impacted boys compared to girls when predicting Factor 1 scores. The family risk factors that interacted with gender when predicting Factor 2 scores and that had a more severe impact on male offspring were the fathers' accommodation problems, employment problems, drug use, and poor supervision. These variables differentially impacted males compared to females when predicting Factor 2 scores.

These findings can also be compared to the findings from the Dunedin Multidisciplinary Health and Development Study (Moffitt, Caspi, Rutter, & Silva, 2001), which studied sex differences in the development of antisocial behavior in young people. They found that some of the family risk factors they examined had a stronger effect on the boys' antisocial behavior compared to the girls'. The family risk factors that were important in predicting boys' antisocial behavior in their study were inconsistent discipline, conflict in the home, multiple changes in caregiver, many family moves, and being raised in a single parent home; and boys who experienced these risk factors were at much greater risk of becoming involved in antisocial behavior than girls who were exposed to the same risks. Although it is difficult to directly compare findings from two studies, which have measured family risk factors slightly differently, it appears that many disruptive processes in the home related to different areas of family functioning – socioeconomic (moving house several times possibly due to financial problems), poor parenting (discipline and supervision), and characteristics of the parent (teenager at the birth of his first child) – all influence psychopathic personality and behavior of offspring.

Moffitt, Caspi, Rutter, and Silva (2001) concluded that the antisocial behavior of females is subject to the same causal processes as males, although they concede that female antisocial behavior is much less likely to be caused by neuro-developmental factors, such as neurocognitive deficits, under-controlled temperament, and hyperactivity, compared to males. Social factors are just as likely to cause antisocial behavior in females as in males, because they are both subject to risk factors for it; however, teenage females are more likely to have prosocial friendships with peers.

However, the Loney et al. (2007) study that found evidence of the intergenerational continuity of maternal psychopathic features also investigated parenting dysfunction, parental hostility/interpersonal insensitivity, and child impulsivity as potential mediators of the relationship between maternal and child CU traits. Parenting dysfunction was defined as "overly harsh, inconsistent or uninvolved parenting characterized by excessive power assertions, low warmth and poor monitoring and supervisions" (Loney et al., 2007:15). The only variable that satisfied Barron and Kenny's (1986) requirements of mediation was parenting dysfunction. In fact, their analysis suggested that parenting dysfunction fully mediated the relationship between maternal affective features of psychopathy and the CU traits in their children. Although the Loney et al. (2007) study has proposed that parenting dysfunction may impact the development of CU traits, the authors concede that it is also possible that child CU traits induce parenting dysfunction across time.

Harris, Rice, and Lalumiè (2001) found that antisocial parents (determined using a composite measure including parental criminality, alcoholism, and abuse and neglect of children) related to high psychopathy in a forensic sample. In a sample of 868 male patients at a forensic psychiatric hospital, Harris et al. (2001) used structural equation modeling to relate latent constructs: neurodevelopmental damage, antisocial parenting, and psychopathy to criminal violence. Most relevant to this study, they found that antisocial parenting was related to neurodevelopmental changes and psychopathy but was not directly related to criminal violence. They proposed that psychopathy could be viewed as "an evolved life history strategy" (p. 402) and that in contrast to views that propose that childhood abuse and neglect cause psychological damage and subsequent psychopathy, from a life history perspective they suggest that negative childhood events may be the "environmental signals that initiate a violent, condition-dependent psychopathic life strategy" (p. 419).

In a sample of 225 male federal prison inmates, Patrick, Zempolich, and Levenston (1997) related three family background variables (coming from a single parent family, the father's occupational status, and childhood abuse history) to PCL–R scores. Four diagnostic groups were created based on their Factor 1 and Factor 2 scores, for example: psychopathic (high scores on both factors), antisocial (high score on Factor 2 but low score on Factor 1), detached (high score for Factor 1 and a low score for Factor 2), and non-psychopathic (low scores on both factors). A negative association was found between total psychopathy scores and emotionally detached prisoners, indicating that this group was less likely to come from a single-parent family. The father's occupational status had a significant positive relationship with the emotionally detached prisoners, controlling for antisociality, suggesting that this group came from more financially privileged backgrounds. Childhood abuse had a significant relationship only with the overall psychopathy scores, suggesting that those with high psychopathy scores were much more likely to have a history of childhood abuse than those with low scores.

The authors conclude those offenders who are antisocial but not psychopathic are more likely to come from single parent families and financially disadvantaged backgrounds. In contrast, those who have psychopathic personality features but lower levels of serious criminal offending are more likely to come from intact families and financially secure backgrounds. A history of childhood abuse separated psychopathic offenders from other offenders, and the authors suggest three explanations for this. First, that child abuse contributes to criminal and psychopathic tendencies; second, that children who are difficult elicit negative responses from parents; or third, that psychopathic individuals are likely to have parents with similar features, of which child maltreatment is one of many antisocial behaviors.

Findings from the Pittsburgh Youth Study, a longitudinal study of 1,517 inner-city boys that began in 1987 by selecting boys from three different grades from state schools, Lynam, Loeber, and Stouthamer-Loeber (2008) found that family socioeconomic status (based on parental education and occupation) interacted with psychopathy in early adolescence to predict psychopathy scores on facets 2 and 3. They find their results to be consistent with Raine's (2002) social push hypothesis, which argues that biological influences are more likely to be seen in benign environments, because in malignant environments, "the social causes of crime camouflage the biological contribution" (p. 314). Boys who had high juvenile psychopathy scores also had high scores in young adulthood, regardless of the status of their moderators. The most important changes concerned the boys with low juvenile psychopathy; those who grew up in a wealthy family, had less antisocial peers, and experienced less physical punishment continued to have low psychopathy scores into young adulthood. Those boys who had low juvenile psychopathy scores and also possessed these risk factors had increased psychopathy scores in adulthood.

Marshall and Cooke (1999) compared the childhood circumstances of 50 criminal psychopaths to 55 criminal non-psychopaths to see if any adverse circumstances distinguished the two groups. They found that there were differences in several of the childhood variables, particularly inconsistent discipline and supervision as well as in school achievement and perceptions of school. Factor analysis of the childhood variables revealed two factors they describe as familial dynamics and societal influences. Stepwise multiple regressions showed that only the familial dynamics factor was related to Factor 1 of the PCL–R, but both familial dynamics and societal influences were related to Factor 2 of the PCL–R. The authors suggest the results demonstrate a differential effect, with family factors being more closely associated with psychopathic personality traits and social factors being more closely associated with the antisocial behavioral component. Further quadratic analyses also suggested that individuals with low or medium PCL–R scores are strongly influenced by family factors, but those with high scores are less influenced by them.

Weiler and Widom (1996) compared 652 males and females who had substantiated histories of abuse or neglect in childhood to a matched control group (n = 489) to see if those who had been abused were more likely to be psychopathic in young adulthood. Psychopathy was measured using the PCL–R. They found that, controlling for demographic variables, there was a significant relationship between childhood abuse or neglect and psychopathic symptoms in early adulthood. After their criminal history was taken into account, this significant relationship was still present in both male and female samples. They also found for their sample that childhood abuse did not have a relationship with violent offending (both official and self-reported) when PCL–R scores were taken into account. They suggest that the relationship between childhood abuse and violent offending could be mediated through psychopathy.

In a Swedish study, Lang, af Klinteberg, and Alm (2002) studied 199 males (95 of these from a matched control group) from an urban area in Stockholm. They were assessed using the PCL between the ages of 32 and 40. Information on their history of childhood abuse and neglect was gathered from official records and interviews with the study participant and their parent. PCL scores were divided into low, medium, and high groups; childhood abuse and neglect were divided into low and high groups. Results showed that high levels of childhood victimization were related to high PCL scores and higher levels of violent behavior; however, further analysis revealed another "type," which included those who had experienced low victimization, high levels of violence, and high PCL scores, suggesting a strong relationship between psychopathy and violence from some individuals, regardless of childhood abuse. Lang et al. (2002) contrast their work with Weiler and Widom (1996) and alternatively propose that the relationship between childhood abuse and psychopathy in adulthood is possibly mediated by psychosocial factors.

The studies here suffer from several limitations. First, many studies of psychopathy are restricted by fairly small sample sizes. Second, much of the research that has been done using the Psychopathy Checklist has been with prison or forensic samples; far fewer community samples have been examined, and findings from high-risk populations are not easily generalizable. Third, the majority of studies have looked at solely at males; very few samples including females have been examined. Fourth, most studies are only able to study the influence of a few family risk factors. This analysis is fortunate in that it is possible to examine a broad range of family factors to attempt to explain the intergenerational transmission of psychopathy. Fifth, many studies that examine the role of family factors are limited by their cross-sectional design. If the family risk factors are assessed at the same time as psychopathy, any relationships will be correlational, as causality cannot be established definitively without longitudinal data.

Furthermore, some studies are limited by their reliance on self-report psychopathy measures. As deceitfulness is one of the symptoms of psychopathy, self-report measures are unlikely to be able to capture the construct of psychopathy. Also, some studies that have used the Psychopathy Checklist have scored it solely on the basis of file data. This is disadvantageous as it may be difficult to assess the interpersonal traits without a face-to-face interview. Finally, several studies have had to prorate Psychopathy Checklist scores due to incomplete information. Fortunately, the data in the Cambridge Study dataset are quite complete and no scores were prorated.

It is important to look at the intergenerational transmission of psychopathy to adult offspring, as studies of the developmental aspects of psychopathic traits find evidence for change and continuity. Stability in psychopathic personality from childhood to adulthood has been shown by Lynam et al. (2007), yet Blonigen, Hicks, Krueger, Patrick, and Iacono (2006) and Fontaine, Rijsdijk, McCrory, and Viding (2010) demonstrate that psychopathic traits are subject to change over time. This finding is important as it suggests the possibility that environmental factors could account for some of these changes. Accurate identification of family risk factors could be informative in designing preventative interventions.

Limitations

Hare's Psychopathy Checklist was developed with male forensic patients and prisoners; although the applicability of the construct of psychopathy to women has been a topic of concern in the literature, it has received little systematic investigation. Studies of gender differences in male and female prisoners using the PCL have found that psychopathy is invariant across gender. More recently, the issue of gender differences has been investigated by Kreis and Cook (2011). Using a recently developed measure of psychopathy, the Comprehensive Assessment of Psychopathic Personality (CAPP), they undertake a prototypicality study, with the aim of discovering if there are gender differences in the construct of psychopathy and content validity of the CAPP across gender. They asked 132 mental health professionals to rate 42 symptoms (33 from the CAPP and nine miscellaneous) according to whether they thought they were more prototypical of psychopathy in men, women, or both genders. The results showed that in a general sense the construct of psychopathy in women was similar to that in males; however, some gender differences were noted. For example, three symptoms were rated as more prototypical of psychopathy in women; lacks emotional stability, unstable self-concept, and manipulative; however, Kreis notes that they were not found to be specific to any gender.

The G2 males and the G3 offspring were assessed for psychopathy at quite different ages. The G2 males were approximately 48 years old, but the age range of the G3 at assessment was much wider (they were aged from 18 years and 1 month to 38 years and 8 months). A further possible limitation could be that the psychopathic traits in the G2 male sample have declined as they have got older, and studies such as the one by Harpur and Hare (1994) have found that Factor 2 scores decreased with age (although this could be a result of decreased criminality rather than a change in personality traits). My analysis has attempted to compensate for this by scoring the Factor 2 items by using supplementary information from the official criminal records held by the study for all participants, as these records give information on all convictions in their lifetime.

The analysis was also limited by the way the child's exposure to the father was measured. This variable indicated how many years up to the age of 16 the father had spent living with that child. It did not tell us anything about the nature or quality of the relationship between the father and the child. Furthermore, in most cases, a father who is not living in the family home will still have some contact with his children. Some studies have argued that the amount of time fathers invest in child care is less closely associated with child outcomes than the quality of fathers' involvement with their children (Lamb, 1997).

Instances of psychopathy above the recommended diagnostic threshold are very rare in community samples such as this one, particularly among females. This problem was resolved by examining psychopathy as a dimensional construct; however, it could be the case that intergenerational relationships could be very different at the far end of the scale. Therefore, intergenerational continuities in psychopathic personality need to be studied in other samples to see if these results are replicated.

PCL: SV Factor 1 and 2 are known to be moderately correlated with each other. This analysis did not control for the potential influence of the father's other factor score. This was because of concerns as to the extent to which another factor could be considered a confounder, and this is an unresolved issue. Analysis that considers the influence of the fathers' and the sons' other factors is outside the scope of this chapter but could be the subject of further work.

Auty and colleagues' (2015) mediation analyses showed that the fathers' employment problems were the only significant mediator of the transmission of Factor 1 scores for male and female offspring and Factor 2 scores for female offspring. The transmission of the fathers' Factor 2 scores to male offspring was mediated by both the fathers' drug use and their accommodation problems. Genetic factors are thought to play a large role in the etiology of psychopathic personality features, so the finding that the transmission of the fathers' Factor 1 score is mediated via environmental risk factors is particularly interesting, as these findings seem to suggest that the intergenerational transmission of psychopathy is driven by the fathers' risk factors and not so much by parenting factors. Of course, it is also possible that the fathers' risk factors cause them to be poor parents. It could be that psychopathic fathers are not able to use their psychopathic personality features to their advantage in the workplace (i.e. adaptively), which results in their poor employment record, which causes economic hardship for the family and tension at home, and thus children who are exposed to this environment have more psychopathic features in adulthood. It is also likely that unemployed fathers would spend more time in the home, and this could also contribute, as this would mean increased exposure to children. It is interesting that the same family risk factor (employment problems) mediates the transmission of psychopathic personality (Factor 1) for male and females; this could suggest that the same processes are occurring for male and female offspring.

Findings here could suggest a gene–environment correlation (rGE) (Jaffee & Price, 2007). Psychopathy is thought to be moderately heritable. So in this study, the G2 fathers who carry the genes for psychopathy would exhibit the personality and behavioral features that are characteristic of psychopathy and therefore score highly on the PCL: SV, and the G2 fathers who are not genetically predisposed to psychopathy would not. Because those who are genetically predisposed to psychopathy are more likely to be psychopathic, and because they tend to have unstable employment and relationship histories, misuse substances, and therefore experience many of the family risk factors, the genes for psychopathy are likely to be correlated with the family risk factors.

Conclusion

Future research would benefit from studying the parent–child relationship as bidirectional. The majority of studies reviewed here study unidirectional relationships. The child's temperament will affect how a parent reacts to them, and this could explain how poor parenting has been shown to be a significant predictor of psychopathy but not a mediator. The conclusions of studies reviewed here are of course dependent on the variables included in each study, and the possibility always exists that other unmeasured factors could have been important. There can be tautological issues when examining which family factors are related to psychopathy, as many of the family factors are actually part of the construct of psychopathy and will be taken into account by the assessor. The same goes for individual factors or constitutional measures such as impulsivity.

Future studies should also attempt to resolve some of the issues regarding the temporal ordering of mediator variables by using data that has been collected before the offspring's psychopathy has been assessed; however, this often not possible to do, especially for parenting variables risk factors that are often retrospectively measured. Furthermore, the Hare Psychopathy Checklist claims to measure the lifetime presence of the disorder. This is conceptually problematic when trying to establish temporal precedence of risk factors in mediation models, as if psychopathy is measured in the parents in mid-adulthood, we have to make the assumption that it has been present in that form since early adulthood.

Future longitudinal research would benefit greatly from new measures of psychopathy that are currently being developed, such as the Comprehensive Assessment of Psychopathic Personality (CAPP) (Kreis, Cooke, Michie, Hoff, & Logan, 2012). These new measures have the key advantage of being sensitive to changes in psychopathy over time. This new measure has particular relevance for the study of the influence of family risk factors, as using this measure would make it possible to study longitudinal changes in psychopathic personality disorder and the role of family risk factors in these changes. It would also make it possible to evaluate treatment interventions for psychopathy.

References

Acheson, S. K. (2005) 'Review of the Hare Psychopathy Checklist–Revised,' in R. A. Spies & B. S. Plake (Eds.), *The sixteenth mental measurements yearbook* (2nd ed., pp. 429–431), Lincoln, NE: Buros Institute of Mental Measurements.

American Psychiatric Association. (1994) *Diagnostic and statistical manual of mental disorders* (4th ed.), New York, NY: APA Press.

Auty, K. M. (2013) *Family factors and the intergenerational transmission of psychopathy, personality disorders and criminal offending* (Unpublished doctoral dissertation), Queen Mary, University of London, London, UK.

Auty, K. M., Farrington, D. P., and Coid, J. W. (2015) 'Intergenerational transmission of psychopathy and mediation via psychosocial risk factors,' *The British Journal of Psychiatry, 206*(1):26–31.

Barker, E. D., Oliver, B. R., Viding, E., Salekin, R. T., and Maughan, B. (2011) 'The impact of prenatal maternal risk, fearless temperament and early parenting on adolescent callous–unemotional traits: A 14-year longitudinal investigation,' *Journal of Child Psychology and Psychiatry, 52*(8):878–888.

Baron, R. M., and Kenny, D. A. (1986) 'The moderator–mediator variable distinction in social psychological research: Conceptual, strategic, and statistical considerations,' *Journal of Personality and Social Psychology, 51*(6):1173–1182.

Blair, R. J. R. (2007) 'The amygdala and ventromedial prefrontal cortex in morality and psychopathy,' *Trends in Cognitive Sciences, 11*(9):387–392.

Blair, R. J. R. (2009) 'The amygdala and ventromedial prefrontal cortex: Functional contributions and dysfunction in psychopathy,' in S. Hodgins, E. Viding, & A. Plodowski (Eds.), *The neurobiological basis of violence: Science and rehabilitation* (pp. 123–136), Oxford: Oxford University Press.

Blonigen, D. M., Hicks, B. M., Krueger, R. F., Patrick, C. J., and Iacono, W. G. (2006) 'Continuity and change in psychopathic traits as measured via normal-range personality: A longitudinal-biometric study,' *Journal of Abnormal Psychology, 115*(1):85–95.

Brooks-Gunn, J., Duncan, G. J., Klebanov, P. K., and Sealand, N. (1993) 'Do neighborhoods influence child and adolescent development?,' *American Journal of Sociology, 99*(2):353–395.

Cleckley, H. (1941/1982) *The mask of sanity: An attempt to clarify some issues about the so-called psychopathic personality* (5th ed.), St. Louis, MO: Mosby-Year Book Inc.

Cloninger, C. R., Reich, T., and Guze, S. B. (1978) 'Genetic-environmental interactions and antisocial behavior,' in R. D. Hare & D. Schalling (Eds.), *Psychopathic behavior: Approaches to research* (pp. 225–237), Chichester: Wiley.

Conoley, J. C., and Impara, J. C. (Eds.) (1995) *The twelfth mental measurements year book*, Lincoln, NE: Buros Institute of Mental Measurements.

Cooke, D. J., and Michie, C. (2001) 'Refining the construct of psychopathy: Towards a hierarchical model,' *Psychological Assessment, 13*(2):171–188.

Cooke, D. J., Michie, C., Hart, S. D., and Clark, D. A. (2004) 'Reconstructing psychopathy: Clarifying the significance of antisocial and socially deviant behavior in the diagnosis of psychopathic personality disorder,' *Journal of Personality Disorders, 18*(4):337–357.

Deater-Deckard, K., and Dodge, K. (1997) 'Externalizing behavior problems and discipline revisited: Nonlinear effects and variation by culture, context, and gender,' *Psychological Inquiry, 8*(3):161–175.

Ewing, J. A. (1984) 'Detecting alcoholism,' *JAMA, 252*(14):1905–1907.

Farrington, D. P. (2000) 'Psychosocial predictors of adult antisocial personality and adult convictions,' *Behavioral Sciences & the Law, 18*(5):605–622.

Farrington, D. P. (2003) 'Key results from the first 40 years of the Cambridge Study in Delinquent Development,' in T. P. Thornberry & M. D. Krohn (Eds.), *Taking stock of delinquency: An overview of findings from contemporary longitudinal studies* (pp. 137–183.), New York, NY: Kluwer/Plenum.

Farrington, D. P. (2006) 'Family background and psychopathy,' in C. J. Patrick (Ed.), *Handbook of psychopathy* (pp. 229–250), New York, NY: Guilford Press.

Farrington, D. P. (2007) 'Social origins of psychopathy,' in A. R. Felthous & H. Sass (Eds.), *International handbook on psychopathic disorders and the law: Vol. 1. Diagnosis and treatment* (pp. 319–334), New York, NY: Wiley.

Farrington, D. P., Barnes, G. C., and Lambert, S. (1996) 'The concentration of offending in families,' *Legal and Criminological Psychology, 1*(1):47–63.

Farrington, D. P., Ullrich, S., and Salekin, R. T. (2010) 'Environmental influences on child and adolescent psychopathy,' in R. T. Salekin & D. R. Lynam (Eds.), *Handbook of child and adolescent psychopathy* (pp. 202–230), New York, NY: Guilford.

Fontaine, N. M. G., Rijsdijk, F. V., McCrory, E. J. P., and Viding, E. (2010) 'Etiology of different developmental trajectories of callous–unemotional traits,' *Journal of the American Academy of Child & Adolescent Psychiatry, 49*(7):656–664.

Frick, P. J., and Hare, R. D. (2001) *The Antisocial Process Screening Device (ASPD)*, Toronto, ON: Multi Health Systems.

Frick, P. J., Kimonis, E. R., Dandreaux, D. M., and Farell, J. M. (2003) 'The 4-year stability of psychopathic traits in non-referred youth,' *Behavioral Sciences & the Law, 21*(6):713–736.

Frick, P. J., and Loney, B. R. (2002) 'Understanding the association between parents and child antisocial behavior,' in R. J. McMahon & R. D. Peters (Eds.), *The effects of parental dysfunction on children*, New York, NY: Kluwer Academic/Plenum Publishers.

Frick, P. J., and White, S. F. (2008) 'Research review: The importance of callous–unemotional traits for developmental models of aggressive and antisocial behavior,' *Journal of Child Psychology and Psychiatry*, *49*:359–375.

Hare, R. D. (1993) *Without conscience: The disturbing world of the psychopaths among us*, New York, NY: Simon & Schuster.

Hare, R. D. (1996) 'Psychopathy: A clinical construct whose time has come,' *Criminal Justice and Behavior*, *23*(1):25–54.

Hare, R. D. (1999) *Without conscience: The disturbing world of the psychopaths among us*, New York, NY: Guilford Press.

Hare, R. D. (2003) *Manual of the Psychopathy Checklist–Revised* (2nd ed.), Toronto, ON: Multi- Health Systems.

Hare, R. D., and Neumann, C. S. (2006) 'The PCL–R assessment of psychopathy: Development, structural properties and new directions,' in C. J. Patrick (Ed.), *Handbook of Psychopathy*, New York, NY: Guildford Press.

Hare, R. D., and Neumann, C. S. (2008) 'Psychopathy as a clinical and empirical construct,' *Annual Review of Clinical Psychology*, *4*(1):217–246.

Hare, R. D., and Neumann, C. S. (2010) 'The role of antisociality in the psychopathy construct: Comment on Skeem and Cooke (2010),' *Psychological Assessment*, *22*(2):446–454.

Harpur, T. J., and Hare, R. D. (1994) 'Assessment of psychopathy as a function of age,' *Journal of Abnormal Psychology*, *103*(4):604–609.

Harpur, T. J., Hare, R. D., and Hakstian, A. R. (1989) 'Two-factor conceptualization of psychopathy: Construct validity and assessment implications,' *Psychological Assessment*, *1*(1):6–17.

Harris, G. T., Rice, M. E., and Lalumière, M. (2001) 'Criminal violence: The roles of psychopathy, neurodevelopmental insults, and antisocial parenting,' *Criminal Justice and Behavior*, *28*(4):402–426.

Hart, S. D., Cox, D. J., and Hare, R. D. (1995) *Manual for the Psychopathy Checklist: Screening Version (PCL:SV)*, Toronto, ON: Multi-Health Systems.

Hart, S. D., and Hare, R. D. (1996) 'Psychopathy and antisocial personality disorder,' *Current Opinion in Psychiatry*, *9*(2):129–132.

Hemphill, J. F., and Hart, S. D. (2003) 'Forensic and clinical issues in their assessment of psychopathy,' in M. Goldstein (Ed.), *Comprehensive Handbook of Psychology* (Vol. 11, pp. 87–107), New York, NY: Wiley.

Herpertz, S. C., and Sass, H. (2000) 'Emotional deficiency and psychopathy,' *Behavioral Sciences & the Law*, *18*(5):567–580.

Jaffee, S. R., Moffitt, T. E., Caspi, A., and Taylor, A. (2003) 'Life with (or without) father: The benefits of living with two biological parents depend on the father's antisocial behavior,' *Child Development*, *74*(1):109–126.

Jaffee, S. R., and Price, T. S. (2007) 'Gene–environment correlations: A review of the evidence and implications for prevention of mental illness,' *Molecular Psychiatry*, *12*(5):432–442.

Karpman, B. (1941) 'On the need for separating psychopathy into two distinct clinical types: Symptomatic and idiopathic,' *Journal of Criminology and Psychopathology*, *3*:112–137.

Karpman, B. (1948) 'The myth of the psychopathic personality,' *American Journal of Psychiatry*, *104*(9):523–534.

Keyes, P. D. M., Legrand, P. D. L., Iacono, P. D. W., and McGue, P. D. M. (2008) 'Parental smoking and adolescent problem behavior: An adoption study of general and specific effects,' *American Journal of Psychiatry*, *165*(10):1338–1344.

Koestner, R., Zuroff, D., and Powers, T. (1991) 'Family origins of adolescent self-criticism and its continuity into adulthood,' *Journal of Abnormal Psychology*, *100*(2):191–197.

Kreis, M. K. F., and Cooke, D. J. (2011) 'Capturing the psychopathic female: A prototypicality analysis of the Comprehensive Assessment of Psychopathic Personality (CAPP) across gender,' *Behavioral Sciences & the Law*, *29*(5):634–648.

Kreis, M. K. F., Cooke, D. J., Michie, C., Hoff, H. A., and Logan, C. (2012) 'The Comprehensive Assessment of Psychopathic Personality (CAPP): Content validation using prototypical analysis,' *Journal of Personality Disorders*, *26*:402–413.

Lamb, M. E. (1997) 'Fathers and child development: An introductory overview and guide,' in M. E. Lamb (Ed.), *The role of the father in child development* (3rd ed., pp. 1–18), New York, NY: Wiley.

Lang, S., af Klinteberg, B., and Alm, P. O. (2002) 'Adult psychopathy and violent behavior in males with early neglect and abuse,' *Acta Psychiatrica Scandinavica*, *106*(Suppl. 412):93–100.
Larsson, H., Andershed, H., and Lichtenstein, P. (2006) 'A genetic factor explains most of the variation in the psychopathic personality,' *Journal of Abnormal Psychology*, *115*(2):221–230.
Levenson, M. R., Kiehl, K. A., and Fitzpatrick, C. M. (1995) 'Assessing psychopathic attributes in a noninstitutionalized population,' *Journal of Personality and Social Psychology*, *68*(1):151–158.
Lilienfeld, S. O., and Fowler, K. A. (2007) 'The self-report assessment of psychopathy: Problems, pitfalls, and promises,' in C. J. Patrick (Ed.), *Handbook of psychopathy* (pp. 107–132), New York, NY: Guilford Press.
Loney, B. R., Huntenburg, A., Counts-Allan, C., and Schmeelk, K. M. (2007) 'A preliminary examination of the intergenerational continuity of maternal psychopathic features,' *Aggressive Behavior*, *33*(1):14–25.
Lykken, D. T. (1957) 'A study of anxiety in the sociopathic personality,' *The Journal of Abnormal and Social Psychology*, 55(1):6–10.
Lykken, D. T. (1995) *The antisocial personalities*, Hillsdale, NJ: Erlbaum.
Lynam, D. R. (1996) 'Early identification of chronic offenders: Who is the fledgling psychopath?' *Psychological Bulletin*, *120*(2):209–234.
Lynam, D. R. (1997) 'Pursuing the psychopath: Capturing the fledgling psychopath in a nomological net,' *Journal of Abnormal Psychology*, *106*(3):425–438.
Lynam, D. R., Caspi, A., Moffitt, T. E., Loeber, R., and Stouthamer-Loeber, M. (2007) 'Longitudinal evidence that psychopathy scores in early adolescence predict adult psychopathy,' *Journal of Abnormal Psychology*, *116*(1):155–165.
Lynam, D. R., Loeber, R., and Stouthamer-Loeber, M. (2008) 'The stability of psychopathy from adolescence into adulthood: The search for moderators,' *Criminal Justice and Behavior*, *35*(2):228–243.
Marshall, L. A., and Cooke, D. J. (1999) 'The childhood experiences of psychopaths: A retrospective study of familial and social factors,' *Journal of Personality Disorders*, *13*(3):211–225.
McCord, W., and McCord, J. (1964) *The psychopath: An essay on the criminal mind*, Princeton, NJ: Van Nostrand.
Miller, J. D., Lyman, D. R., Widiger, T. A., and Leukefeld, C. (2001) 'Personality disorders as extreme variants of common personality dimensions: Can the Five Factor Model adequately represent psychopathy?' *Journal of Personality*, *69*(2):253–276.
Moffitt, T. E., and Caspi, A. (2003) 'Preventing the intergenerational continuity of antisocial behavior: Implications of partner violence,' in D. P. Farrington & J. W. Coid (Eds.), *Early prevention of adult antisocial behavior* (pp. 109–129), Cambridge: Cambridge University Press.
Moffitt, T. E., Caspi, A., Rutter, M., and Silva, P. A. (2001) *Sex differences in antisocial behavior: Conduct disorder, delinquency, and violence in the Dunedin Longitudinal Study*, Cambridge: Cambridge University Press.
Newman, J. P., and Wallace, J. F. (1993) 'Diverse pathways to deficient self-regulation: Implications for disinhibitory psychopathology in children,' *Clinical Psychological Review*, *13*(8):699–720.
Patrick, C. J. (Ed.). (2006) *Handbook of psychopathy*, New York, NY: Guilford Press.
Patrick, C. J., Zempolich, K. A., and Levenston, G. K. (1997) 'Emotionality and violent behavior in psychopaths: A biosocial analysis,' in A. Raine, A. Brennan, & B. R. Mednick (Eds.), *Biosocial bases of violence* (pp. 145–161), New York, NY: Plenum Press.
Patterson, C. M., and Newman, J. P. (1993) 'Reflectivity and learning from aversive events: Toward a psychological mechanism for the syndromes of disinhibition,' *Psychological Review*, *100*(4):716–736.
Poythress, N. G., and Skeem, J. (2006) 'Disaggregating psychopathy: Where and how to look for subtypes,' in C. J. Patrick (Ed.), *Handbook of psychopathy* (pp. 172–192), New York, NY: Guilford Press.
Raine, A. (2002) 'Biosocial studies of antisocial and violent behavior in children and adults: A review,' *Journal of Abnormal Child Psychology*, *30*(4):311–326.
Raine, A., Lencz, T., Bihrle, S., LaCasse, L., and Colletti, P. (2000) 'Reduced prefrontal gray matter volume and reduced autonomic activity in antisocial personality disorder,' *Archives of General Psychiatry*, *57*(2):119–127.
Repo-Tiihonen, E., Tiihonen, J., Lindberg, N., Weizmann-Henelius, G., Putkonen, H., and Häkkänen, H. (2010) 'The intergenerational cycle of criminality–association with psychopathy,' *Journal of Forensic Sciences*, *55*(1):116–120.
Robins, L. N. (1966). *Deviant children grown up*, Baltimore, MD: Williams & Wilkins.
Rowe, D. C., and Farrington, D. P. (1997) 'The familial transmission of criminal convictions,' *Criminology*, *35*(1):177–202.
Skeem, J. L., and Cooke, D. J. (2010) 'Is criminal behavior a central component of psychopathy? Conceptual directions for resolving the debate,' *Psychological Assessment*, *22*(2):433–445.

Taylor, J., Loney, B. R., Bobadilla, L., Iacono, W. G., and McGue, M. (2003) 'Genetic and environmental influences on psychopathy trait dimensions in a community sample of male twins,' *Journal of Abnormal Child Psychology*, *31*(6):633–645.

Thornberry, T. P., Freeman-Gallant, A., Lizotte, A. J., Krohn, M. D., and Smith, C. A. (2003). 'Linked lives: The intergenerational transmission of antisocial behavior,' *Journal of Abnormal Child Psychology*, *31*(2):171–184.

Ullrich, S., Farrington, D. P., and Coid, J. W. (2008) 'Psychopathic personality traits and life- success,' *Personality and Individual Differences*, *44*(5):1162–1171.

Weiler, B. L., and Widom, C. S. (1996) 'Psychopathy and violent behavior in abused and neglected young adults,' *Criminal Behavior and Mental Health*, *6*(3):253–271.

West, D. J., and Farrington, D. P. (1973) *Who Becomes Delinquent?* London: Heinemann.

Widiger, T. (1998) 'Psychopathy and normal personality,' in D. J. Cooke, A. Forth, & R. D. Hare (Eds.), *Psychopathy: Theory, research, and implications for society* (pp. 47–68.), Dordrecht: Kluwer.

10

Neurological profiles of psychopathy

A neurodevelopmental perspective

Yu Gao

Introduction

Increasing evidence has shown brain structural and functional abnormalities in psychopathy. The search for the neurobiological basis of psychopathy began more than 150 years ago, when a railway construction worker, Phineas Gage, suffered severe damage to the prefrontal cortex and subsequently developed a radical change in his personality and became psychopathic-like (Damasio, 1994). Cleckley's book, *The Mask of Sanity*, provided the first and classic description and interpretation of psychopathy and theorized that this form of personality disorder may be due to a biological deficit (Cleckley, 1941, 1988). The aim of this chapter is to present neurobiological evidence for a disruption in the cortical and subcortical areas in people with psychopathy. Key findings from neurological and brain imaging studies will be outlined and discussed in the context of psychopathy as a disorder with a neurodevelopmental basis.

Early evidence implicating the frontal cortex in psychopathy has come from neurological studies that focused on patients who have brain damage due to trauma by an external force or an internal disease. These patients with trauma, a tumor, or neurodegenerative disease have subsequently demonstrated psychopathic traits. For example, damage to the ventromedial prefrontal cortex has been found to result in psychopathic-like characteristics and has thus been referred to as "acquired psychopathy" (Eslinger & Damasio, 1985). A few cases have been reported, including Phineas Gage and the patient E.V.R. (Granacher & Fozdar, 2007). Common features following damage to the frontal lobe in these cases include lack of empathy, difficulties with emotion regulation, impulsivity, disinhibited behavior, poor planning, and blunted emotions. When making moral judgments, people with ventromedial prefrontal cortex damage, compared to control subjects, have been found to be more likely to endorse actions that involve highly emotionally aversive harm. This suggests that the ventromedial prefrontal cortex mediates emotions that are important for certain types of moral judgment (Koenigs et al., 2007).

People with frontotemporal dementia, a progressive neurodegenerative disorder that involves the frontal lobes, temporal lobes, or both, have also shown signs of psychopathic traits, such as frequent violations of social norms, a lack of empathy, loss of insight for the consequences of their behavior and its effect on others, and a failure to respond to the needs of others. Similar to those of people with ventromedial prefrontal cortex damage described previously (Koenigs et al., 2007), people with frontotemporal dementia have also been found to demonstrate more utilitarian moral decision-making to hypothetical scenarios (Mendez, Anderson, & Shapira, 2005).

The idea that psychopathy may represent a neurodevelopmental deficit is supported by evidence that when brain impairments occur early in life, psychopathic-like effects appear to be even more pronounced. For example, patients who incurred damage to the ventromedial prefrontal cortex before the age of 16 months developed irresponsible and criminal behavior, abusive behavior towards others, and a lack of empathy or remorse (Anderson, Bechara, Damasio, Tranel, & Damasio, 1999). These antisocial characteristics and behaviors were more severe than those observed in patients who suffered damage in adulthood. It has been suggested that intact functioning of the ventromedial prefrontal cortex is important for moral development. Therefore, when this region is damaged very early in life, the process of moral socialization may be disrupted. Indeed, the study found that these people exhibited an immature stage of moral reasoning (Anderson et al., 1999).

Although damage to any specific brain region does not entirely replicate the disorder of psychopathy, studies of people with neurological impairments are useful in helping to understand the result of impaired functioning of certain brain regions that may be implicated in psychopathy. In particular, the study of patients who have incurred brain damage very early in life may be especially useful, as it demonstrates how deficits in brain functioning may impair social and moral development in the individual. Future research, particularly in child patients with brain damage, may be helpful in gaining a more precise understanding of the specific impairments that result from abnormal functioning in specific regions.

Brain imaging

As the fastest moving area of research in psychopathy, brain imaging studies have enabled us to directly examine the brains of psychopaths, inform treatment strategies, and improve our understanding of how genes and environment lead to the development of psychopathy. Brain imaging findings, for the most part, have been able to confirm what has been hypothesized based on psychophysiological, neuropsychological, and behavioral data regarding the brain regions that are implicated in psychopathy. Although widespread regions have been implicated in psychopathy, the amygdala and ventromedial/orbitofrontal cortex are the two regions most consistently associated with psychopathy.

Disruption in the prefrontal cortex, including the orbitofrontal, ventromedial prefrontal, and the cingulate cortex, has been linked to psychopathy. These regions are crucial in decision-making, behavioral control, and emotional regulation, and deficits in these regions may contribute to features such as impulsivity and impaired moral judgment in psychopaths. Studies have also implicated regions beyond the prefrontal cortex. The medial temporal regions, particularly the amygdala and hippocampus, are critical for emotional processing, and thus when impaired predispose to a shallow affect and lack of empathy in psychopaths.

Structural brain imaging

Recent developments in brain imaging techniques have allowed researchers to understand *in vivo* the structural brain correlates of psychopathy using structural (sMRI) or anatomical magnetic resonance imaging (aMRI) and diffusion tensor imaging (DTI). Magnetic resonance imaging (MRI) is based on the principle that atoms in the human brain are like small bar magnets that possess magnetic charge in random orientations. When immersed in a strong magnetic field, the nuclei of these atoms tend to align and reach an equilibrium state. A radiofrequency electromagnetic field is then briefly introduced to excite the atoms and induce a transient phase coherence among the nuclei that creates a signal, which can be detected by the MRI scanner receiver. Several different types of scans can be conducted using MRI to examine different aspects of brain structure and function.

Structural brain imaging scans, sometimes referred to as aMRI or sMRI, are designed to gain a very clear, overall picture of brain structure. These scans are usually 4–8 minutes, and images are collected to assess the volume and shape (morphometry) of different brain regions. Initially, trained researchers would manually trace the brain regions following a previously validated protocol. In recent years, approaches using fully automated or semi-automated algorithms, including Voxel-based morphometry (VBM), tensor-based morphometry (TBM), and FreeSurfer, have been used to identify morphological changes in psychopaths. In addition to brain volume, VBM and TBM can also be used to assess gray matter concentration and shape of a region, respectively.

Most structural brain imaging studies have focused on the prefrontal cortex, and findings suggest that psychopaths exhibit impairments in this region. For example, significant prefrontal grey matter volume reductions have been found in patients with Antisocial Personality Disorder who also scored high on psychopathy (Raine, Lencz, Bihrle, Lacasse, & Colletti, 2000). Similarly, significant prefrontal grey reductions have been found in criminal psychopaths compared to control subjects (Yang et al., 2005), and their grey matter is also thinner (Yang, Raine, Colletti, Toga, & Narr, 2009). Studies using VBM have also found reduced grey matter volume in the prefrontal cortex in psychopaths (Müller et al., 2008; de Oliveira-Souza et al., 2008). For example, reduced gray matter volume in the medial prefrontal cortex has been observed in violent offenders with psychopathic traits compared to violent offenders without psychopathic traits and non-offenders (Gregory et al., 2012). Overall, prefrontal deficits have been argued to contribute to the poor decision-making, emotional dysregulation, and impaired moral judgment in psychopathic people.

Evidence linking structural impairments in brain regions beyond the prefrontal cortex with psychopathy has also been found. For example, reduced posterior hippocampus volumes have been found in antisocial alcoholics with high psychopathy scores (Laakso et al., 2001). Psychopaths also show volume reductions in the bilateral amygdala, particularly the basolateral and superficial nuclei groups (Yang, Raine, Colletti, Toga, & Narr, 2010). These regions play a central role in fear conditioning, and deficits in the processing of fear are a well-replicated correlate of psychopathic and antisocial behavior (Gao, Raine, Venables, Dawson, & Mednick, 2010; Veit et al., 2013; Birbaumer et al., 2005). In another study, reduced regional gray matter in the orbitofrontal cortex, parahippocampal, amygdala, hippocampus, temporal pole, and posterior cingulate were found in criminal psychopaths (Ermer et al., 2012). Reduced cortical thickness and gray matter concentrations in the temporal lobes were found in criminal offenders with psychopathy compared to healthy non-criminal individuals (Howner et al., 2012; Müller et al., 2008). Additionally, another study reported significant increased callosal white matter volume, increased callosal length, and increased functional interhemispheric connectivity in psychopaths (Raine et al., 2003). Callosal volume was significantly related to the Deficient Affect factor of psychopathy, and to a lesser extent the Impulsive–Irresponsible factor, but not the Arrogant–Deceptive factor. Another study found a 9.6 percent increase in the volume of the striatum (consisting of the caudate, putamen, nucleus accumbens, and globus pallidus) of psychopathic individuals (Glenn, Raine, Yaralian, & Yang, 2010). Overall, these findings indicate that brain structural abnormalities, particularly in the amygdala, hippocampus, striatum, and corpus callosum, may contribute to the emotional deficits found in psychopaths.

By separating psychopaths with criminal convictions (unsuccessful psychopaths) from those without convictions (successful psychopaths), researchers have found structural deficits specifically to unsuccessful psychopaths. For example, an exaggerated anterior hippocampal volume asymmetry (right greater than left) has been found in unsuccessful psychopaths but not in successful psychopaths or controls (Raine et al., 2004). The same group of unsuccessful (but not successful) psychopaths also showed a significant 18 to 23 percent reduction in the prefrontal grey matter volume (Yang et al., 2005). Findings suggest that neuropathological characteristics such as abnormal hippocampal asymmetry and reduced prefrontal grey matter volume may contribute to the emotional dysregulation and poor fear conditioning in unsuccessful psychopaths and consequently render these people less sensitive to environmental cues predicting danger and capture.

Diffusion tensor imaging (DTI) is a relatively new MRI technique that studies the integrity of white matter structures. Because of the myelin sheath, water diffusion in axonal fibers exhibits an anisotropic feature, that is, the water diffusion is faster along the axial direction (parallel to the fiber) and slower in the radial direction (perpendicular to the fiber). DTI calculates the water diffusion vector in each voxel and quantifies diffusive values such as fractional anisotropy (FA), mean diffusivity (MD), axial diffusivity (AD), and radial diffusivity (RD). Examining these values in psychopathy may help to precisely pinpoint the nature of diffusion differences and thus microstructural white-matter differences.

Overall greater diffusivity or poor integrity across a range of white-matter tracts has been reported in adults with psychopathic traits (Hoppenbrouwers et al., 2013; Craig et al., 2009; Sobhani, Baker, Martins, Tuvblad, & Aziz-Zadeh, 2015; Sundram et al., 2012; Sethi et al., 2015). For example, compared to incarcerated males without psychopathy, those with psychopathy showed reduced FA in the right uncinate fasciculus (the major white matter tract connecting ventral frontal and limbic regions including amygdala), enabling microstructural deficits to be uniquely linked to psychopathy (Motzkin, Newman, Kiehl, & Koenigs, 2011). In a large study of 147 incarcerated criminal offenders, psychopathy, in particular the interpersonal features, was found to be associated with reduced FA in the right (but not left) uncinate fasciculus (Wolf et al., 2015).

Finally, Yang et al. (2012) tested topological characteristics of the entire whole brain anatomical network and found that psychopaths had altered interregional connectivity patterns in the frontal network, and that bilateral superior frontal cortices were identified as information flow control hubs. In contrast, the network hubs were bilateral inferior frontal and medial orbitofrontal cortices for the controls, suggesting that disturbed structural connectivity, particularly within the frontal and associated areas, may play a crucial role in psychopathy (Yang et al., 2012). Reduced connectivity between the cortical and subcortical regions may indicate that emotion-related information from the amygdala that signals cues of risk, threat, or harm to others may not be able to reach cortical areas in order to inform decision-making, resulting in the callousness, lack of empathy, risk taking, and instrumental aggression observed in psychopathy. In addition, cortical regions may be less able to send inhibitory signals to subcortical regions, resulting in deficits in emotion regulation and inhibition (Glenn & Raine, 2014).

Functional brain imaging

Functional MRI (fMRI) is a type of MRI scans that measures changes in brain activity during a task. In fMRI studies, researchers acquire images of changing blood flow in the brain by measuring changes in the blood-oxygen-level-dependent (BOLD) signal, and larger changes in BOLD signal indicate more neural activities in that region. A number of fMRI studies have been conducted to study psychopathy, and overall psychopaths show abnormal activation in the frontal–temporal circuit (Yang & Raine, 2009). For example, in an fMRI study using a semantic task, criminal psychopaths failed to show the appropriate neural differentiation between abstract and concrete stimuli in the right superior temporal gyrus, left ventrolateral prefrontal cortex, middle temporal cortex, and anterior cingulate cortex (Kiehl et al., 2004). Using affective pictures as stimuli, several other fMRI studies have reported abnormal affect-related activation in the dorsolateral prefrontal cortex, ventrolateral prefrontal cortex, anterior and posterior cingulate cortex, amygdala, hippocampus, and parahippocampus gyrus in psychopaths (Gordon, Baird, & End, 2004; Kiehl et al. 2001; Veit et al., 2002). Finally, in a task involving the gain or loss of money, increased levels of psychopathy have been associated with increased left striatal activity following rewards, compared to losses (Pujara, Motzkin, Newman, Kiehl, & Koenigs, 2014).

Studies have also found atypical brain activation in psychopathic individuals when they make moral judgments. In moral decision-making tasks, individuals are required to make utilitarian (e.g., sacrificing life for the greater good) or "nonutilitarian" moral decisions (e.g., prohibiting a loss of life even though more lives could be saved) (Greene, Nystrom, Engell, Darley, & Cohen, 2004). People with higher interpersonal factor of psychopathy demonstrated reduced functioning in regions previously implicated in moral decision-making (that is, the medial prefrontal cortex, posterior cingulate, angular gyrus, and amygdala), providing initial evidence of reduced functioning in psychopaths in regions that may be critical to behaving morally (Glenn, Raine, & Schug, 2009). In addition, although psychopaths made similar moral judgments to controls behaviorally, they showed more activity in the dorsolateral prefrontal cortex when making those judgments. The amygdala is thought to respond to the emotional aspects of the moral dilemmas, whereas the dorsolateral prefrontal cortex is involved in cognitive processing. This finding suggests that psychopathic individuals may be relying less on emotion and more on purely cognitive processes when making moral judgments (Glenn et al., 2009). In another study, individuals with higher psychopathic traits were shown to have deficits in identifying behaviors that cause fear, which in turn was associated with their higher likelihood of judging these behaviors as morally acceptable. In addition, whole-brain fMRI data suggested that reduced activity in the right amygdala during judgments of fear-provoking statements might contribute to their willingness to cause fear in others (Marsh & Cardinale, 2012).

Researchers have used the ultimatum game (a simple, economic strategy situation between two people) to examine how psychopathic traits affect social functioning and the ability to make adaptive decisions in social interactions. In one study, college students with higher psychopathic traits showed higher likelihood to accept unfair offers, as well as reduced activity in the right amygdala to unfair offers compared to fair offers regardless of the presence of punishment. Moreover, the amygdala dysfunction in psychopathic individuals was associated with reduced functional connectivity with areas including the striatum. The authors argued that an insensitive amygdala might disrupt appropriate evaluation of the affective significance of social stimuli, which on one hand leads to their violation of social norms, and on the other hand may contribute to their less maladaptive aggression in an unfair context (Osumi et al., 2012). Using the same paradigm, another study suggested that distinct patterns of brain activation might be involved when high and low psychopathic individuals are making economic decisions in the ultimatum game. Specifically, in individuals with higher psychopathic traits, acceptance of unfair offers was associated with ventromedial prefrontal cortex activity, whereas in those with lower psychopathic traits acceptance of unfair offers was associated with dorsolateral prefrontal cortex activity (Vieira et al., 2013).

In addition to fMRI, other imaging methods have been used to assess functional abnormalities in psychopathy. Functional near-infrared spectroscopy (fNIRS) is a non-invasive optical imaging technique that detects optical property changes of cerebral cortex based on the different absorption characteristics of oxygenated and de-oxygenated hemoglobin. Compared to MRI and other imaging modalities, fNIRS works with a portable device to allow more flexibility in subject setup and is less sensitive to head motion. Although it has lower spatial resolution and measure activity that is limited to the cortical surface, prior work indicates strong correlation between the BOLD signal measured with fMRI and the oxygenated hemoglobin changes measured with fNIRS (Irani, Platek, Bunce, Ruocco, & Chute, 2007). Two fNIRS studies have been conducted to examine the neurobiological correlates of psychopathic or CU traits. In one study, adults with high CU traits showed similar medial prefrontal cortex oxygenated hemoglobin activity to positive and negative films, while the low CU individuals showed more pronounced prefrontal activation to positive than to negative materials (Fanti, Panayiotou, Lombardo, & Kyranides, 2016). In a recent study with college students who had no prior history of mild traumatic brain injury, higher scores in the affective facet of psychopathy were associated with reduced frontal activation during a visual sustained attention task and rest conditions, whereas higher levels of impulsivity were associated with increased activation during rest conditions in the same area; no such relationships were found in those with brain injury history (Gao, Wu & Li, under review). These findings provide further evidence that frontal cortex functioning abnormalities may underline psychopathic traits and highlight the importance of assessing for prior head injury due to its potential moderating effect.

Magnetic resonance spectroscopy (MRS) is used to determine the concentration of a variety of metabolites in the brain and can be implemented in the MRI scanner. The metabolites are considered to reflect the viability of neurons, and the main metabolites of interest include N-acetyl aspartate (NAA), creatine (Cr), and choline (Cho). Although it has been more often used in studies of neurodegenerative diseases, tumors, stroke, or epilepsy, MRS has also been used to study psychopathy and Antisocial Personality Disorder. In a group of military conscripts with high psychopathy scores, Antisocial Personality Disorder diagnosis, and serious violent crimes, a reduced ratio of NAA/Cr in the anterior cingulate cortex, indicating decreased neuronal integrity, was associated with higher levels of psychopathy and the Interpersonal/Affective factor in particular (Basoglu et al., 2008).

Finally, another technique, single photon emission computed tomography (SPECT), has been used to examine the amount of regional cerebral blood flow in brain regions in psychopathic and antisocial individuals. In one study, researchers found significant negative correlations between psychopathy scores (particularly the interpersonal factor) and frontal and temporal perfusion in violent offenders (Soderstrom et al., 2002).

Neurodevelopmental perspective

There have been an increasing number of brain imaging studies on psychopathic-like children and adolescents in recent years. Overall, evidence has suggested that structural and functional deficits in youths with psychopathic tendencies were similar to those reported in adult psychopaths. For example, in a large sample ($N = 108$) of adolescents from the community, researchers found that higher psychopathic scores were associated with thinner cortex in the middle frontal gyrus and thicker cortex in the superior temporal gyrus, middle temporal gyrus, and parahippocampal gyrus, suggesting that abnormal cortical thickness may reflect delayed brain maturation in subclinical psychopathy (Yang et al., 2015b). Decreased white matter concentration has also been found in adolescent boys with psychopathic tendencies (De Brito et al., 2011), in line with findings of white matter abnormalities in the fronto-temporal areas in adult psychopaths (Tiihonen et al., 2008; Craig et al., 2009). Using the same sample, researchers have found that psychopathic-like boys had increased gray matter concentration compared to the normal controls (De Brito et al., 2009), and that variation in gray matter concentration may reflect genetic vulnerability for psychopathic traits (Rijsdijk et al., 2010). Finally, increased striatal volume has been observed in adolescents with psychopathic tendencies (Yang et al., 2015), replicating findings of stratum enlargement in psychopathic adults (Glenn et al., 2010).

Abnormal integrity in white matters have also been found in youths with psychopathic or callous–unemotional (CU) traits, although findings are more mixed compared to adult populations (Waller, Dotterer, Murray, Maxwell, & Hyde, 2017). For example, higher FA in the uncinate fasciculus has been associated with higher psychopathic and CU traits (Pape et al., 2015; Sarkar et al., 2013) and lower CU traits (Breeden, Cardinale, Lozier, Vanmeter, & Marsh, 2015). In contrast, such relationships between psychopathic traits and the FA in the same tract were not found in other studies (Finger et al., 2012; Zhang et al., 2014). Taken together, although further studies are needed to clarify the specific abnormalities in youths with psychopathic tendencies, atypical white and gray matter in childhood may be a result of aberrant brain maturation and suggests that psychopathy is a neurodevelopmental disorder.

Functionally, abnormalities in frontal and limbic regions have also been found in youths with psychopathic tendencies. For example, abnormal ventromedial prefrontal cortex function was found in children and adolescents with CU traits and disruptive behavior disorders in a reversal learning task (Finger et al., 2008). A later study using a passive avoidance learning task revealed that antisocial youths with psychopathic traits showed decreased activation in the ventromedial prefrontal cortex to rewards relative to healthy controls, with no notable differences in response to punished errors (Finger et al., 2011). In addition, psychopathic or CU traits in children with disruptive behavior are consistently linked to disrupted functioning of the amygdala, particularly reduced responses to socio-affective cues such as fearful expressions (Marsh et al., 2008; Jones, Laurens, Herba, Barker, & Viding, 2009; Viding et al., 2012; White et al., 2012), which in turn may mediate the increase in proactive, or goal directed, aggression observed in youths with CU traits (Lozier, Cardinale, Vanmeter, & Marsh, 2014).

Perhaps the strongest evidence supporting the speculation that the condition of psychopathy may in part be a result of neurodevelopmental abnormalities comes from studies linking cavum septum pellucidum (CSP) and psychopathy. In one study, adults with a large CSP, a marker of prenatal limbic and septal neural maldevelopment, were found to have higher levels of psychopathy and Antisocial Personality Disorder (Raine, Lee, Yang, & Colletti, 2010). Another study later replicated these findings and reported a large CSP to be associated with high levels of psychopathic traits in youth (White et al., 2013), further indicating an early neurodevelopmental basis to psychopathy.

Conclusion

Overall, neurological and brain imaging studies have suggested that: (1) the orbitofrontal, ventromedial prefrontal, and the cingulate cortex are crucial in decision-making, behavioral control, and emotional regulation, and that deficits in these regions may contribute to features such as impulsivity and impaired moral judgment in psychopaths; (2) the medial temporal regions, particularly the amygdala and hippocampus, are critical for emotional processing, and thus when impaired predispose to a shallow affect and lack of empathy in psychopaths; and (3) microstructural deficits in the white tract that connects ventral frontal and limbic regions including amygdala may partly contribute to the functional abnormalities in psychopathy.

Although some strong initial evidence has been presented suggesting brain abnormalities in psychopaths, inconsistencies among findings raise several important questions, and future studies are needed to shed light on these issues. For example, are brain impairments restricted to a particular subgroup of psychopaths, specifically criminal (unsuccessful) psychopaths? Furthermore, it is important for future work to incorporate larger samples of male and female participants to investigate the potential influence of sex in the relationships between psychopathy and neurobiology, given that meaningful comparisons between sexes were not allowed in most of the studies due to limited sample size or imbalanced enrollment between the two sex groups.

A growing body of evidence indicates that different dimensions or facets of psychopathic traits may have distinct etiologies and developmental pathways. A dimension/facet-based approach holds the promise of breaking down the complexity of the psychopathy construct and obtaining greater understanding of psychopathic sub-features. More importantly, several findings have demonstrated the presence of suppression effects among the dimensions of psychopathic traits in relation to various neurobiological, psychological, or behavioral correlates (Gao et al., 2018; Anderson, Stanford, Wan, & Young, 2011; Hicks & Patrick, 2006; López, Poy, Patrick, & Moltó, 2013). Suppression effects suggest that when the multifaceted constructs embedded within a single instrument have opposing relations to a criterion variable, to increase their predictive power they should be assessed separately from one another (Hicks & Patrick, 2006). Accordingly, dimensions of psychopathy are more predictive only after accounting for their overlapping variance. For example, when the facets of psychopathy (e.g., interpersonal, affective, lifestyle, and antisocial) were included in one model to predict brain activities, amygdala reactivity to fearful facial expressions was found to be negatively associated with the interpersonal facet of psychopathy, whereas amygdala reactivity to angry facial expressions was positively associated with the lifestyle facet (Carré, Hyde, Neumann, Viding, & Hariri, 2013). This issue becomes more relevant in research on subclinical psychopathy because both psychopathic traits and the correlates are continuous measures. Future studies should test potential suppressor effects by entering multiple dimensions of psychopathy simultaneously when predicting outcome variables.

Similar suppression effects have also been found between psychopathy and antisocial personality disorder (ASPD). For example, after controlling for psychopathy, high ASPD scores have been associated with greater amygdala reactivity and negative emotionality, whereas, after controlling for ASPD scores, psychopaths show the opposite pattern of reduced amygdala functioning and emotional blunting (Hyde, Byrd, Votruba-Drzal, Hariri, & Manuck, 2014). It has been argued that cold-hearted psychopathic individuals (e.g., primary psychopathy) may engage in callous and calculated aggressive behaviors and have reduced brain reactivity, whereas impulsive and hot-blooded aggressive individuals (e.g., secondary psychopathy) may show increased brain activation to emotional stimuli (Glenn & Raine, 2014). It has been argued that psychopathy and ASPD are two related but different constructs, and that psychopathy should be included in future revisions of the Diagnostic and Statistical Manual (DSM) as a specifier for the diagnosis of ASPD, as the presence of absence of psychopathy in ASPD may distinguish different forms of this disorder (Raine, 2018). Future studies focusing on the interaction between ASPD and psychopathy could shed light on this issue.

Although it is clearly difficult to conduct longitudinal studies on psychopathy, examining the development of neurobiological measures for psychopathic traits from an early age is crucial to furthering our knowledge on etiology and testing a neurodevelopmental hypothesis of psychopathy. This knowledge also helps us answer questions including whether brain deficits lead to the development of psychopathy, or whether a psychopathic lifestyle renders these people more prone to brain dysfunction. Furthermore, continued efforts to identify and assess psychopathic-like children and adolescents using prospective longitudinal designs could have potentially important implications for the prevention and management of adult psychopathy. If psychopathic traits and serious offending are, in part, neurodevelopmentally determined, successful prevention and intervention efforts would be most effective if they begin in early childhood, infancy, or even prenatally.

References

Anderson, S. W., Bechara, A., Damasio, H., Tranel, D., and Damasio, A. R. (1999) 'Impairment of social and moral behavior related to early damage in human prefrontal cortex,' *Nature Neuroscience, 2*:1032.

Anderson, N. E., Stanford, M. S., Wan, L., and Young, K. A. (2011) 'High psychopathic trait females exhibit reduced startle potentiation and increased P3 amplitude,' *Behavioral Sciences and the Law, 29*:649–666.

Basoglu, C., Semiz, U., Oner, O., Gunay, H., Ebrinc, S., Cetin, M., . . ., and Sonmez, G. (2008) 'A magnetic resonance spectroscopy study of antisocial behaviour disorder, psychopathy and violent crime among military conscripts,' *Acta Neuropsychiatrica, 20*:72–77.

Birbaumer, N., Veit, R., Lotze, M., Erb, M., Hermann, C., Grodd, W., and Flor, H. (2005) 'Deficient fear conditioning in psychopathy,' *Archives of General Psychiatry, 62*:799–805.

Breeden, A. L., Cardinale, E. M., Lozier, L. M., Vanmeter, J. W., and Marsh, A. A. (2015) 'Callous–unemotional traits drive reduced white-matter integrity in youths with conduct problems,' *Psychological Medicine, 45*:3033–3046.

Carré, J. M., Hyde, L. W., Neumann, C. S., Viding, E., and Hariri, A. R. (2013) 'The neural signatures of distinct psychopathic traits,' *Social Neuroscience, 8*:122–135.

Cleckley, H. C. (1941) *The mask of sanity*, St. Louis, MO, Mosby.

Cleckley, H. C. (1988) *The mask of sanity*, St. Louis, MO, Mosby.

Craig, M. C., Catani, M., Deeley, Q., Latham, R., Daly, E., Kanaan, R., . . ., and Murphy, D. G. (2009) 'Altered connections on the road to psychopathy,' *Molecular Psychiatry, 14*:946–953.

Damasio, A. R. (1994) *Descartes' error: Emotion, reason, and the human brain*, New York, NY: Grosset/Putnam.

De Brito, S. A., Mechelli, A., Wilke, M., Laurens, K. R., Jones, A. P., Barker, G. J., . . ., and Viding, E. (2009) 'Size matters: Increased grey matter in boys with conduct problems and callous–unemotional traits,' *Brain, 132*:843–852.

De Brito, S. A., McCrory, E. J., Mechelli, A., Wilke, M., Jones, A. P., Hodgins, S., and Viding, E. (2011) 'Small, but not perfectly formed: decreased white matter concentration in boys with psychopathic tendencies,' *Molecular Psychiatry, 16*:476–477.

De Oliveira-Souza, R., Hare, R. D., Bramati, I. E., Garrido, G. J., Ignácio, F. A., Tovar-Moll, F. & Moll, J. (2008) 'Psychopathy as a disorder of the moral brain: Fronto-temporo-limbic grey matter reductions demonstrated by voxel-based morphometry,' *Neuroimage, 40*:1202–1213.

Ermer, E., Cope, L. M., Nyalakanti, P. K., Calhoun, V. D., and Kiehl, K. A. (2012) 'Aberrant paralimbic gray matter in criminal psychopathy,' *Journal of Abnormal Psychology, 121*:649–658.

Eslinger, P. J., and Damasio, A. R. (1985) 'Severe disturbance of higher cognition after bilateral frontal lobe ablation: Patient EVR,' *Neurology, 35*:1731–1741.

Fanti, K. A., Panayiotou, G., Lombardo, M. V., and Kyranides, M. N. (2016) 'Unemotional on all counts: Evidence of reduced affective responses in individuals with high callous–unemotional traits across emotion systems and valences,' *Social Neuroscience, 11*:72–87.

Finger, E. C., Marsh, A. A., Blair, K. S., Majestic, C., Evangelou, I., Gupta, K., . . ., and Fowler, K. A. (2012) 'Impaired functional but preserved structural connectivity in limbic white matter tracts in youth with conduct disorder or oppositional defiant disorder plus psychopathic traits,' *Psychiatry Research: Neuroimaging, 202*:239–244.

Finger, E. C., Marsh, A. A., Blair, K. S., Reid, M. E., Sims, C., Ng, P., . . ., and Blair, R. J. R. (2011) 'Disrupted reinforcement signaling in the orbitofrontal cortex and caudate in youths with conduct disorder or oppositional defiant disorder and a high level of psychopathic traits,' *American Journal of Psychiatry, 168*:152–162.

Finger, E. C., Marsh, A. A., Mitchell, D. G. V., Reid, M. E., Sims, C., Budhani, S., . . ., and Leibenluft, E. (2008) 'Abnormal ventromedial prefrontal cortex function in children with psychopathic traits during reversal learning,' *Archives of General Psychiatry, 65*:586–594.

Gao, Y., Raine, A., Venables, P. H., Dawson, M. E., and Mednick, S. A. (2010) 'Association of poor childhood fear conditioning and adult crime,' *American Journal of Psychiatry, 167*:56–60.

Gao, Y., Wu, Z, and Li, X. (under review) *Association between psychopathy and MFG functioning in adults with and without TBI: An fNIRSs study.*

Gao, Y., Zhang, W., Eisenbarth, H., Fung, A. L. U., Lu, M., Raine, A., . . ., and Li, X. (2018) 'P3 amplitude and psychopathic traits in youths: Distinct contributions of the grandiose–manipulative and daring–impulsivity traits,' *Personality and Individual Differences, 120*:87–94.

Glenn, A. L., and Raine, A. (2014) *Psychopathy: An introduction to biological findings and their implications*, New York, NY: NYU Press.

Glenn, A. L., Raine, A., and Schug, R. A. (2009) 'The neural correlates of moral decision-making in psychopathy' *Molecular Psychiatry, 14*:5–6.

Glenn, A. L., Raine, A., Yaralian, P. S., and Yang, Y. (2010) 'Increased volume of the striatum in psychopathic individuals,' *Biological Psychiatry, 67*:52–58.

Gordon, H. L., Baird, A. A., and End, A. (2004) 'Functional differences among those high and low on a trait measure of psychopathy,' *Biological Psychiatry, 56*:516–521.

Granacher, R. P., and Fozdar, M. A. (2007) 'Acquired psychopathy and the assessment of traumatic brain injury' *The International Handbook of Psychopathic Disorders and the Law, 1*:237–250.

Greene, J. D., Nystrom, L. E., Engell, A. D., Darley, J. M., and Cohen, J. D. (2004) 'The neural bases of cognitive conflict and control in moral judgment,' *Neuron, 44*:389–400.

Gregory, S., Simmons, A., Kumari, V., Howard, M., Hodgins, S., and Blackwood, N. (2012) 'The antisocial brain: Psychopathy matters: A structural MRI investigation of antisocial male violent offenders,' *Archives of General Psychiatry, 69*:962–972.

Hicks, B. M., and Patrick, C. J. (2006) 'Psychopathy and negative emotionality: Analyses of suppressor effects reveal distinct relations with emotional distress, fearfulness, and anger–hostility,' *Journal of Abnormal Psychology, 115*:276–287.

Hoppenbrouwers, S. S., Nazeri, A., De Jesus, D. R., Stirpe, T., Felsky, D., Schutter, D. J., . . ., and Voineskos, A. N. (2013) 'White matter deficits in psychopathic offenders and correlation with factor structure,' *PLoS One, 8*:e72375.

Howner, K., Eskildsen, S. F., Fischer, H., Dierks, T., Wahlund, L.-O., Jonsson, T., . . ., and Kristiansson, M. (2012) 'Thinner cortex in the frontal lobes in mentally disordered offenders,' *Psychiatry Research: Neuroimaging, 203*:126–131.

Hyde, L. W., Byrd, A. L., Votruba-Drzal, E., Hariri, A. R., and Manuck, S. B. (2014). 'Amygdala reactivity and negative emotionality: Divergent correlates of antisocial personality and psychopathy traits in a community sample,' *Journal of Abnormal Psychology, 123*:214.

Irani, F., Platek, S. M., Bunce, S., Ruocco, A. C., and Chute, D. (2007) 'Functional near infrared spectroscopy (fNIRS): An emerging neuroimaging technology with important applications for the study of brain disorders,' *The Clinical Neuropsychologist, 21*:9–37.

Jones, A. P., Laurens, K. R., Herba, C. M., Barker, G. J., and Viding, E. (2009) 'Amygdala hypoactivity to fearful faces in boys with conduct problems and callous–unemotional traits,' *American Journal of Psychiatry, 166*:95–102.

Kiehl, K. A., Smith, A. M., Hare, R. D., Forster, B. B., Brink, J., and Liddle, P. F. (2001) 'Limbic abnormalities in affective processing by criminal psychopaths as revealed by functional magnetic resonance imaging,' *Biological Psychiatry, 50*:677–684.

Kiehl, K. A., Smith, A. M., Mendrek, A., Forster, B. B., Hare, R. D., and Liddle, P. F. (2004) 'Temporal lobe abnormalities in semantic processing by criminal psychopaths as revealed by functional magnetic resonance imaging,' *Psychiatry Research Neuroimaging, 130*:27–42.

Koenigs, M., Young, L., Adolphs, R., Tranel, D., Cushman, F., Hauser, M., and Damasio, A. (2007) 'Damage to the prefrontal cortex increases utilitarian moral judgements,' *Nature, 446*:908–911.

Laakso, M. P., Vaurio, O., Koivisto, E., Savolainen, L., Eronen, M., Aronen, H. J., . . ., and Tiihonen, J. (2001) 'Psychopathy and the posterior hippocampus,' *Behavioural Brain Research, 118*:187–193.

López, R., Poy, R., Patrick, C. J., and Moltó, J. (2013) 'Deficient fear conditioning and self-reported psychopathy: The role of fearless dominance,' *Psychophysiology, 50*:210–218.

Lozier, L. M., Cardinale, E. M., Vanmeter, J. W., and Marsh, A. A. (2014) 'Mediation of the relationship between callous–unemotional traits and proactive aggression by amygdala response to fear among children with conduct problems,' *JAMA Psychiatry, 71*:627–636.

Marsh, A. A., and Cardinale, E. M. (2012) 'When psychopathy impairs moral judgments: Neural responses during judgments about causing fear,' *Social Cognitive and Affective Neuroscience, 9*:3–11.

Marsh, A. A., Finger, E. C., Mitchell, D. G. V., Reid, M. E., Sims, C., Kosson, D. S., . . ., and Blair, R. J. R. (2008) 'Reduced amygdala response to fearful expressions in children and adolescents with callous–unemotional traits and disruptive behavior disorders,' *American Journal of Psychiatry, 165*:712–720.

Mendez, M. F., Anderson, E., and Shapira, J. S. (2005) 'An investigation of moral judgement in frontotemporal dementia,' *Cognitive and Behavioral Neurology*, *18*:193–197.

Motzkin, J. C., Newman, J. P., Kiehl, K. A., and Koenigs, M. (2011) 'Reduced prefrontal connectivity in psychopathy,' *Journal of Neuroscience*, *31*:17348–17357.

Müller, J. L., Gänßbauer, S., Sommer, M., Döhnel, K., Weber, T., Schmidt-Wilcke, T., and Hajak, G. (2008) 'Gray matter changes in right superior temporal gyrus in criminal psychopaths. Evidence from voxel-based morphometry,' *Psychiatry Research: Neuroimaging*, *163*:213–222.

Osumi, T., Nakao, T., Kasuya, Y., Shinoda, J., Yamada, J., and Ohira, H. (2012) 'Amygdala dysfunction attenuates frustration-induced aggression in psychopathic individuals in a non-criminal population,' *Journal of Affective Disorders*, *142*:331–338.

Pape, L. E., Cohn, M. D., Caan, M. W. A., Van Wingen, G., Van Den Brink, W., Veltman, D. J., and Popma, A. (2015) 'Psychopathic traits in adolescents are associated with higher structural connectivity,' *Psychiatry Research: Neuroimaging*, *233*:474–480.

Pujara, M. S., Motzkin, J. C., Newman, J. P., Kiehl, K. A., and Koenigs, M. (2014) 'Neural correlates of reward and loss sensitivity in psychopathy,' *Social Cognitive and Affective Neuroscience*, *9*:794–801.

Raine, A. (2018) 'Antisocial personality as a neurodevelopmental disorder,' *Annual Review of Clinical Psychology*.

Raine, A., Ishikawa, S. S., Arce, E., Lencz, T., Knuth, K. H., Bihrle, S., . . ., and Colletti, P. (2004) 'Hippocampal structural asymmetry in unsuccessful psychopaths,' *Biological Psychiatry*, *55*:185–191.

Raine, A., Lee, L., Yang, Y., and Colletti, P. (2010) 'Neurodevelopmental marker for limbic maldevelopment in antisocial personality disorder and psychopathy,' *British Journal of Psychiatry*, *197*:186–192.

Raine, A., Lencz, T., Bihrle, S., Lacasse, L., and Colletti, P. (2000) 'Reduced prefrontal gray matter volume and reduced autonomic activity in antisocial personality disorder,' *Archives of General Psychiatry*, *57*:119–127.

Raine, A., Lencz, T., Taylor, K., Hellige, H. B., Bihrle, S., Lacasse, L., Lee, M., . . ., and Colletti, P. (2003) 'Corpus callosum abnormalities in psychopathic antisocial individuals,' *Archives of General Psychiatry*, *60*:1134–1142.

Rijsdijk, F. V., Viding, E., De Brito, S., Forgiarini, M., Mechelli, A., Jones, A. P. & Mccrory, E. (2010) 'Heritable variations in gray matter concentration as a potential endophenotype for psychopathic traits,' *Archives of General Psychiatry*, *67*:406–413.

Sarkar, S., Craig, M. C., Catani, M., Dell'acqua, F., Fahy, T., Deeley, Q., and Murphy, D. G. M. (2013) 'Frontotemporal white-matter microstructural abnormalities in adolescents with conduct disorder: A diffusion tensor imaging study,' *Psychological Medicine*, *43*:401–411.

Sethi, A., Gregory, S., Dell'acqua, F., Thomas, E. P., Simmons, A., Murphy, D. G., . . ., and Craig, M. C. (2015) 'Emotional detachment in psychopathy: Involvement of dorsal default-mode connections,' *Cortex*, *62*:11–19.

Sobhani, M., Baker, L., Martins, B., Tuvblad, C., and Aziz-Zadeh, L. (2015) 'Psychopathic traits modulate microstructural integrity of right uncinate fasciculus in a community population,' *NeuroImage: Clinical*, *8*:32–38.

Soderstrom, H., Hultin, L., Tullberg, M., Wikkelso, C., Ekholm, S., and Forsman, A. (2002) 'Reduced frontotemporal perfusion in psychopathic personality,' *Psychiatry Research: Neuroimaging*, *114*:81–94.

Sundram, F., Deeley, Q., Sarkar, S., Daly, E., Latham, R., Craig, M., . . ., and Barker, G. J. (2012) 'White matter microstructural abnormalities in the frontal lobe of adults with antisocial personality disorder,' *Cortex*, *48*:216–229.

Tiihonen, J., Rossi, R., Laakso, M. P., Hodgins, S., Testa, C., Perez, J., . . ., and Aronen, H. J. (2008) 'Brain anatomy of persistent violent offenders: More rather than less,' *Psychiatry Research: Neuroimaging*, *163*:201–212.

Veit, R., Flor, H., Erb, M., Hermann, C., Lotze, M., Grodd, W., and Birbaumer, N. (2002) 'Brain circuits involved in emotional learning in antisocial behavior and social phobia in humans,' *Neuroscience Letters*, *328*:233–236.

Veit, R., Konicar, L., Klinzing, J. G., Barth, B., Yilmaz, Ö., and Birbaumer, N. (2013) 'Deficient fear conditioning in psychopathy as a function of interpersonal and affective disturbances,' *Frontiers in Human Neuroscience*, 7:706.

Viding, E., Sebastian, C. L., Dadds, M. R., Lockwood, P. L., Cecil, C. A. M., De Brito, S. A., and Mccrory, E. J. (2012) 'Amygdala response to preattentive masked fear in children with conduct problems: The role of callous–unemotional traits,' *American Journal of Psychiatry*, *169*:1109–1116.

Vieira, J. B., Almeida, P. R., Ferreira-Santos, F., Barbosa, F., Marques-Teixeira, J., and Marsh, A. A. (2013) 'Distinct neural activation patterns underlie economic decisions in high and low psychopathy scorers,' *Social Cognitive and Affective Neuroscience*, *9*:1099–1107.

Waller, R., Dotterer, H. L., Murray, L., Maxwell, A. M., and Hyde, L. W. (2017) 'White-matter tract abnormalities and antisocial behavior: A systematic review of diffusion tensor imaging studies across development,' *NeuroImage: Clinical*, *14*:201–215

White, S. F., Brislin, S., Sinclair, S., Fowler, K. A., Pope, K., and Blair, R. J. R. (2013) 'The relationship between large cavum septum pellucidum and antisocial behavior, callous-unemotional traits and psychopathy in adolescents,' *Journal of Child Psychology and Psychiatry*, *54*:575–581.

White, S. F., Marsh, A. A., Fowler, K. A., Schechter, J. C., Adalio, C., Pope, K., . . ., and Blair, R. J. R. (2012) 'Reduced amygdala response in youths with disruptive behavior disorders and psychopathic traits: Decreased emotional response versus increased top-down attention to nonemotional features,' *American Journal of Psychiatry*, *169*:750–758.

Wolf, R. C., Pujara, M. S., Motzkin, J. C., Newman, J. P., Kiehl, K. A., Decety, J., . . ., and Koenigs, M. (2015) 'Interpersonal traits of psychopathy linked to reduced integrity of the uncinate fasciculus,' *Human Brain Mapping*, *36*:4202–4209.

Yang, Y., Narr, K. L., Baker, L. A., Joshi, S. H., Jahanshad, N., Raine, A., and Thompson, P. M. (2015) 'Frontal and striatal alterations associated with psychopathic traits in adolescents,' *Psychiatry Research: Neuroimaging*, *231*:333–340.

Yang, Y., and Raine, A. (2009) 'Prefrontal structural and functional brain imaging findings in antisocial, violent, and psychopathic individuals: A meta-analysis,' *Psychiatry Research: Neuroimaging*, *174*:81–88.

Yang, Y., Raine, A., Colletti, P., Toga, A. W., and Narr, K. L. (2009) 'Abnormal temporal and prefrontal cortical gray matter thinning in psychopaths,' *Molecular Psychiatry*, *14*:561–563.

Yang, Y., Raine, A., Colletti, P., Toga, A. W., and Narr, K. L. (2010) 'Morphological alterations in the prefrontal cortex and the amygdala in unsuccessful psychopaths,' *Journal of Abnormal Psychology*, *119*:546–554.

Yang, Y., Raine, A., Joshi, A. A., Joshi, S. H., Chang, Y., Schug, R. A., . . ., and Narr, K. L. (2012) 'Frontal information flow and connectivity in psychopathy,' *The British Journal of Psychiatry*, *201*:408–409.

Yang, Y., Raine, A., Lencz, T., Bihrle, S., Lacasse, L., and Colletti, P. (2005) 'Volume reduction in prefrontal gray matter in unsuccessful criminal psychopaths,' *Biological Psychiatry*, *57*:1103–1108.

Yang, Y., Wang, P., Baker, L. A., Narr, K. L., Joshi, S. H., Hafzalla, G., . . ., and Thompson, P. M. (2015b) 'Thicker temporal cortex associates with a developmental trajectory for psychopathic traits in adolescents,' *PLoS One*, *10*:e0127025.

Zhang, J., Zhu, X., Wang, X., Gao, J., Shi, H., Huang, B., . . ., and Yao, S. (2014) 'Increased structural connectivity in corpus callosum in adolescent males with conduct disorder,' *Journal of the American Academy of Child & Adolescent Psychiatry*, *53*:466–475.e1.

11
Childhood and adolescent psychopathy

Olivier F. Colins and Henrik Andershed

Introduction

Personality disorders do not appear out of the blue in adulthood. Therefore, it should come as no surprise that antecedents of various personality disorders, including Borderline, Narcissistic, and Antisocial Personality Disorder, have been searched for in childhood and adolescence (Paris, 2003; Shiner & Tackett, 2014). This chapter will focus on a personality construct that is theorized to originate early in life, namely psychopathy or psychopathic personality; describe what is known and unknown about psychopathic personality in childhood and adolescence; and outline how future research endeavors can put theories about the origins and course of this personality construct to the test.

Although disputes among scholars fuel scientific progress, outsiders may have the impression that the area of psychopathy research is hallmarked more by disputes than by consensus. Various debates about which features should be included in the conceptualization and assessment of psychopathy personality are still ongoing. Therefore, this chapter starts with clarifying how we define child and adolescent psychopathy and why we do so.

The modern empirical study of child and adolescent psychopathic personality was instigated by the seminal work of Robert Hare, who standardized the study of adult psychopathy and developed what has become the best known expert-rater tool for research and applied forensic purposes, the Psychopathy Checklist–Revised (PCL–R; Hare, 2003). The development of the PCL: Youth Version (PCL: YV; Forth, Hart, & Hare, 1990; Forth & Kosson, 2003) was among the first attempts to extend PCL–R measured psychopathy to adolescence. The items of this youth version are almost identical to those of the PCL–R, though some items and their scoring criteria were excluded, changed, and/or modified to better reflect adolescents' life experiences (Forth & Kosson, 2003). Echoing PCL–R work (e.g., Hare & Neumann, 2008), research with the PCL: YV showed that its 20 items load on four facets or dimensions: interpersonal, affective, behavioral/lifestyle, and antisocial dimensions (e.g., Neumann, Kosson, Forth, & Hare, 2006; Salekin, Brannen, Zalot, Leistico, & Neumann, 2006). Paul Frick later developed a teacher- and parent-rating tool to assess psychopathic traits in 6- to 13-year-olds. This tool, the Antisocial Process Screening Device (APSD; Frick & Hare, 2001), was designed to assess as many of the PCL–R items as possible, though some items were excluded because they were not relevant for children (Frick, Bodin, & Barry, 2000; Frick, Obrien, Wootton, & Mcburnett, 1994). Even before Cooke and Michie (2001) favored a three-factor conceptualization of PCL–R measured psychopathy (which essentially excludes the antisocial dimension), Paul Frick favored a three-factor model in which the 18 of the 20 APSD items load on interpersonal (labeled narcissism), affective (labeled Callous–Unemotional), and behavioral/lifestyle (labeled impulsivity) dimensions (Frick et al., 2000). The sole APSD item that directly refers to criminal behavior ("Engages in illegal activities") is only included in the total score, which implies that the APSD does not involve a fourth, antisocial, dimension.

Based on the three-factor model of Cooke and Michie (2001), Henrik Andershed and colleagues developed the 50-item Youth Psychopathic Traits Inventory (YPI; Andershed, Kerr, Stattin, & Levander, 2002)(YPI) for adolescents, a self-report tool that also served as the base for the self-report YPI Short version (YPI–S; van Baardewijk et al., 2008) and self-report YPI Child version for use with 9–12-year-olds (YPI–C; van Baardewijk et al., 2010). The items of all YPI versions load on interpersonal (labeled grandiose/manipulation), affective (labeled Callous–Unemotional) and behavioral/lifestyle (labeled Impulsive–Irresponsible) dimensions. With the intent to enable a reliable assessment of psychopathic traits from early childhood onward, Henrik Andershed and colleagues more recently developed the Child Problematic Traits Inventory (CPTI; Colins, Andershed et al., 2014) for use in 3- to 12-year-olds. Though primarily intended to be a teacher-rating tool, evidence indicates that the CPTI also works well when using fathers and mothers as raters. In close resemblance with how psychopathy is often measured in adolescence and adulthood, the CPTI items load on interpersonal (labeled Grandiose–Deceitful), affective (labeled Callous–Unemotional), and behavioral/lifestyle (labeled Impulsivity–Need for Stimulation) dimensions.

Various other conceptualizations of psychopathy are available and came along with self-report tools (Lynam et al., 2011; Patrick, 2010; Lilienfeld & Andrews, 1996; Paulhus, Neumann, & Hare, 2012). Although these different conceptualizations and measures should receive a bit more attention than we can offer here, the crucial point we want to make is that these tools predominantly have been developed for use with and validated in (young) adults and fall outside the scope of this chapter.

Taken together, to reflect upon the status of childhood and adolescent psychopathy in a way that at least conceptually can be linked to adult psychopathy research, and to deal with the simple fact that merely one (i.e., the PCL: YV) of the aforementioned measures includes a dimension that primarily indexes criminality, the present chapter defines child and adolescent psychopathy as a construct incorporating three dimensions: interpersonal, callous–unemotional, and behavioral/lifestyle dimensions.

Psychopathic traits and psychopathic personality: a conceptual distinction

An important conceptual distinction we believe crucial is between psychopathic traits and psychopathic personality or psychopathy. We use the phrasing *psychopathic traits* to refer to one of the three psychopathy dimensions or to a total score comprising all of the dimensions. We use the phrasing *psychopathic personality or psychopathy* to refer to the co-occurring constellation of high levels of interpersonal, affective (from here on referred to as callous–unemotional), *and* behavioral/lifestyle traits. Put differently, an individual with a psychopathic personality is characterized by high scores on each of the three psychopathic traits dimensions. This implies that a study that only includes one psychopathic traits dimension, in our view, would not be considered highly informative for the study of psychopathic personality. Studies testing if correlations between one psychopathic traits dimension and an external construct of interest decrease substantially in strength when also controlling for the other two psychopathic traits dimension are, in our view, more informative for psychopathy research, as these studies may suggest that the relation between the psychopathic traits dimension and external constructs at least in part lies in the *combination* of all three psychopathic traits dimensions (e.g., Colins, Fanti, Larsson, & Andershed, 2017). Importantly, these latter studies are far from sufficient to further our understanding of psychopathic personality. Ideally, studies on youth psychopathic personality should include a three-way interaction term between the psychopathic traits dimensions or use person-oriented analyses to scrutinize if a group of individuals emerges who are high on all three psychopathic traits dimensions. Such person-oriented approaches can be explorative and thus data-driven (e.g., latent profile analyses), or a bit more theory-driven and confirmatory since one knows what one is looking for, namely youth high on all three psychopathic traits dimensions (e.g., using 1 *SD* above the mean as the cut-off).

Defining psychopathic personality in childhood and adolescence as being high on all three psychopathic traits dimensions converges with the view that adults with psychopathy are high on all psychopathic traits dimensions (e.g., Hare, 2016; Sprague, Javdani, Sadeh, Newman, & Verona, 2012; Gacono, 2015); conceptually makes sense since psychopathy is commonly defined as a multifaceted disorder (e.g., Frick et al., 2000; Hawes, Mulvey, Schubert, & Pardini, 2014; Colins, Fanti, Salekin, Mulder, & Andershed, 2017); and is tenable because mounting evidence shows that the three traits dimensions can be measured in a reliable and valid way in childhood and adolescence (Salekin & Lynam, 2010), and even early childhood.

The role we see for person-oriented analyses to identify children and adolescents with a putative psychopathic personality may need some additional reflection. The most likely counter-reaction when arguing that person-oriented analyses may foster what is known about child and adolescent psychopathy is that psychopathy "has been proven" to be dimensional and not a categorical construct or a taxon. Hence, this implies that there are no distinct qualitative differences between psychopathic and non-psychopathic individuals, and that individuals only differ in their *levels* of psychopathy. Yet, it has been argued that studies on the topic typically used statistical procedures that are fundamentally incapable of providing a test of taxonicity (Maraun & Hart, 2016), so it probably still remains an empirical question whether psychopathy is a taxon or not or contains both dimensional and categorical features (Ruscio, 2007). Notwithstanding that psychopathic personality eventually may appear not to be a taxon, it cannot be disregarded that a substantial number of PCL–R studies applied a PCL–R total score of 30 (e.g., Hicks, Markon, Patrick, Krueger, & Newman, 2004; Salekin, Rogers, & Sewell, 1997) or lower (e.g., Kiehl et al., 2001) as a cut-off to separate adults with psychopathy from those without psychopathy, and that a substantial number of studies use distribution-based cut-offs (e.g., top 5 percent or 30 percent; Drislane et al., 2014; Lee & Salekin, 2010) or model-based cluster analyses to enhance the study of psychopathy (e.g., Boduszek, Debowska, & Willmott, 2017; Colins, Fanti, Salekin, Mulder et al., 2017). Therefore, there are no strong arguments why the field cannot also value categorical approaches to identify a group of children and adolescents with a putative psychopathic personality. DeLisi (2016:84) takes it one step further and cogently argues that a categorical approach is even better than a dimensional approach, because

> it is a mistake to consider a person who is irresponsible, impulsive, and somewhat full of themselves as somewhat psychopathic because these traits would give them a non-zero score on a psychopathy scale. This approach is casting the net too wide.

Childhood and adolescent psychopathy: what is known?

Interest in child and adolescent psychopathy resulted in a proliferation of journal articles, culminating in the first handbook specific to the topic (Salekin & Lynam, 2010). Since the publication of this seminal handbook, the number of articles has continued to sharply increase. A Web of Science search (January 10, 2018) combining "psychopathy" or "psychopathic" with the following key terms (child* or adoles* or youth* or juven* or teenager or boy* or girl* or youngster* or toddl*) in the topic/title revealed 1,276 (topic)/470 (title) publications 2011–2017 as compared to 670 (topic)/294 (title) publications 2004–2010. Consequently, any attempt to be complete when reviewing this literature is doomed to fail when writing one brief chapter, so we do not even pretend that we strive for completeness. Instead, we briefly focus on what we think are the most robust and important conclusions that can be drawn when evaluating available child and adolescent psychopathy research. By doing so, we try to avoid duplicating information that was provided in recent, excellent reviews on callous–unemotional traits (e.g., Frick, Ray, Thornton, & Kahn, 2014a), as well as the interpersonal and behavioral/lifestyle traits (e.g., Salekin, 2016), and instead pay particular attention to important themes that, in our view, seems to be missed in contemporary research on child and adolescent psychopathy. So, what is, in our view, up-to-date, well-evidenced research within this particular field?

1 Factor-analytic work with the various non-expert rater tools mentioned earlier overall supports that youth psychopathic personality comprises a three-factor structure, capturing interpersonal, callous–unemotional, and behavior/lifestyle traits dimensions, though it must be noted that the APSD self-report version has trouble finding a stable factor structure (e.g., Colins, Bijttebier, Broekaert, & Andershed, 2014; Wang, Deng, Armour, Bi, & Zeng, 2015).
2 These measures most often generate dimension and total scores that are internally consistent to at least an acceptable degree. Of note, exceptions are not uncommon for the callous–unemotional traits dimension score of each tool, though poor internal consistency has most consistently been reported for the APSD self-report version (e.g., Poythress, Douglas, Falkenbach et al., 2006; Vanwoerden, Reuter, & Sharp, 2016).
3 A significant amount of research supports the criterion and convergent validity of the three psychopathic traits dimensions as measured by various of the aforementioned tools. A notable exception is the YPI–Child Version, which has received little empirical scrutiny, so future research is needed to confirm its convergent and criterion validity.
4 Studies in childhood, adolescence, or (emerging) adulthood (e.g., Cauffman, Skeem, Dmitrieva, & Cavanagh, 2016; Dadds, Fraser, Frost, & Hawes, 2005) support moderate temporal stability of psychopathic traits dimensions, that is, when using rank-order, mean-level, and individual-level stability (for reviews see, e.g., Andershed, 2010; Salekin, 2017). Studies also show that child and adolescent psychopathy scores correlate with adult psychopathy scores (e.g., Hemphälä, Kosson, Westerman, & Hodgins, 2015; Hawes, Byrd, Waller, Lynam, & Pardini, 2017), suggesting that the childhood psychopathy construct bears a relationship with the adult psychopathy construct.

We are well aware that it may seem as if we are unnecessarily harsh and over-critical for childhood and adolescent psychopathy research to draw only four major robust conclusions based on almost three decades of research in this area. We will explain this position in detail in the next section of this chapter.

Are callous–unemotional traits enough?

Notwithstanding that callous–unemotional (CU) traits only capture one of the psychopathic traits dimensions, there is a tendency to use CU traits interchangeably with psychopathic personality, especially when CU traits co-occur with conduct problems (e.g., Breeden, Cardinale, Lozier, Vanmeter, & Marsh, 2015; Jones, Laurens, Herba, Barker, & Viding, 2009). The main argument for this focus is that children and adolescents with CU traits often show the highest levels of other psychopathic traits, and that using only CU traits, therefore, often designates similar groups of youth with conduct problems as when using all psychopathic traits dimensions (e.g., Frick, 2009). Echoing findings among adults with a psychopathic personality, CU traits in youths with conduct problems indeed have been shown to be related to past and future conduct problems, aggression, and criminality (Frick et al., 2014a). From this point of view, the equation of CU traits and psychopathic personality seem justified. But is it? In our reading of the literature, and based on various strands of data, we think it clearly is not. For example:

1 Youth with conduct problems who are only high on CU traits can be differentiated from those who are high on all psychopathic traits dimensions, with the latter group displaying the highest levels of *concurrent* or *past* conduct problems, aggression, and antisocial behavior (e.g., Christian, Frick, Hill, Tyler, & Frazer, 1997; Colins, Noom, & Vanderplasschen, 2012).
2 A three-way interaction effect between the psychopathic traits dimensions exhibits a stronger relation with *concurrent* or *past* conduct problems (Colins, Andershed, Frogner et al., 2014), delinquency (Somma, Andershed, Borroni, & Fossati, in press) and proactive aggression (Orue & Andershed, 2015) than the CU traits dimension on its own.
3 Interpersonal and behavioral/lifestyle traits dimensions are uniquely positively related to *future* conduct problems, aggression, and criminality, whereas CU traits are not or are less strongly so (e.g., Colins, van Damme, Andershed, Fanti, & DeLisi, 2017; Colins, Andershed, & Pardini, 2015; Munoz & Frick, 2007), and the co-occurrence of conduct problems and CU traits as well as the co-occurrence of conduct problems with interpersonal and behavioral/lifestyle traits can lead to clinical levels of future conduct problems (Fanti, Kyranides, Lordos, Colins, & Andershed, in press).
4 A series of recent and novel studies were designed to empirically test if CU traits are enough to identify a subgroup of children and adolescents with conduct problems who show features associated with psychopathic personality, those of severe past and future antisocial behavior. All the studies reviewed next have in common that participants were assigned to mutually exclusive groups based on their conduct problem (CP) scores and scores on each of the three psychopathic traits dimensions, and that each study identified at least six groups of uttermost relevance given the topic under consideration (though in this chapter we focus on the two main groups of interest: groups 5 and 6). These six groups can be tentatively labeled as:

    1 Control: low CP, low on all three dimensions;
    2 CP only: high in CP, low on all three dimensions;
    3 Callous–Unemotional only: low in CP, only high on CU traits dimension;
    4 Psychopathic Personality only: low in CP; high on all three dimensions;
    5 Callous–Unemotional + CP: high in CP, only high on CU traits dimensions;
    6 Psychopathic Personality + CP: high in CP, high on all three dimensions.

Studies 1 (Frogner, Gibson, Andershed, & Andershed, 2018) and 2 (Frogner, Andershed, & Andershed, in press) were performed among 1,867 3- to 5-year-old Swedish boys and girls and relied on teacher ratings of the three CPTI-measured psychopathic traits dimensions at baseline and of conduct problems, fearlessness, and Attention-Deficit/Hyperactivity Disorder (ADHD) symptoms at baseline and 1- and 2-year follow-ups. Boys in the Psychopathic Personality + CP group displayed significantly higher levels of baseline conduct problems, similar levels of baseline CU traits, and were at a greater risk for future conduct problems at follow-up assessment and for stable conduct problems, stable fearlessness, and stable symptoms of ADHD. These main findings held among girls with the exception that the Psychopathic Personality + CP and the CU + CP groups did not significantly differ in their risk for future conduct problems.

Study 3 (Colins, Andershed, Salekin, & Fanti, 2018) was performed among 690 7- to 12-year-old Cypriot boys and girls and relied on parent-rated conduct problems and three psychopathic traits dimensions measured with the APSD (narcissism and impulsivity) and ICU (Callous–Unemotional). Conduct problems were reassessed 6 and 12 months later. At baseline, Psychopathic Personality + CP boys and girls were not significantly different in level of CU traits than their Callous–Unemotional + CP counterparts, whereas the first group displayed higher level of conduct problems in girls but not in boys. Across gender, Psychopathic Personality + CP children by far showed the most robust and highest risk for future and stable conduct problems, whereas CP only children were often equally and sometimes even at a higher risk than Callous–Unemotional + CP children.

In Study 4 (Andershed et al., in press), 996 Cypriot 12-year-old adolescents (56 percent girls) completed measures of conduct problems (CP) and the three psychopathic traits dimensions (as measured by the self-report versions of the APSD and ICU). The participants completed measures of conduct problems, aggression, and substance use at three annual follow-up assessments. Psychopathic Personality + CP and Callous–Unemotional + CP participants were not significantly different in terms of baseline conduct problems and CU traits. Psychopathic Personality + CP adolescents showed the most robust and highest risk for future *and* stable conduct problems, aggression, and substance use, whereas Callous–Unemotional + CP adolescents were only at risk for future conduct problems. Due to sample size issues, analyses could not be performed separately for boys and girls.

Taken together, these four studies together clearly suggest that merely using CU traits for subtyping children and adolescents with conduct problems is less sufficient than using the multidimensional psychopathy construct for predicting future and stable antisocial behaviors. Overall, this set of findings finding held when using various informants across various age groups and using different child and adolescent psychopathy tools and outcomes, suggesting that these results are not tool and sample specific. Admittedly, in some of these studies only a small number of adolescents with CP were assigned to the Callous–Unemotional + CP group relative to the number of adolescents with CP that could be assigned to the Psychopathic Personality + CP group, a finding supporting the view that being high on CU traits and being high on all three psychopathy dimensions identifies largely overlapping groups of children with CP (Frick, 2009). To illuminate how robust this overlap is, more work is needed.

Future studies robustly showing that only using CU traits is not sufficient enough to identify youth with putative psychopathic personalities would have important practical and theoretical information. First, these sets of findings suggest that researchers should use the entire psychopathy construct for identifying children and adolescents with conduct problems who are at risk for severe and stable antisocial behavior, as was the intention when the multidimensional adult psychopathy construct was downwardly extended to youth (e.g., Frick et al., 2000). Reconsidering the multidimensional features of the psychopathy construct may help to bridge youth psychopathy research with adult psychopathy research, where researchers rarely focus on CU traits alone to identify psychopathic adults, whether in community-based, clinic-referred, or forensic settings.

Next, being able to differentiate between Callous–Unemotional + CP and Psychopathic Personality + CP youth is relevant to avoid youth who merely display CU traits being misclassified as youth with "psychopathic personality." Some scholars may wonder what the fuzz is about and argue that youth with putative psychopathic personality would also have been identified when only using the CU traits dimension, since, for example, 17 of the 31 boys with conduct problems who were high in CU traits were also high on the interpersonal and behavioral/lifestyle traits dimensions (Colins et al., 2018). Our answer would be that if one can avoid "collateral damage" in 14 out of 31 boys (e.g., because children with the stigmatizing "psychopathy" label likely are not welcome in most treatment centers), it is worth the effort to scrutinize if and how we can improve our accuracy in identifying children and adolescents who display the entire constellation of co-occurring traits and those who do not. In addition, such efforts may also help clinicians identify youth who have the greatest need of intensive treatment; for example, some kids are not merely high in CU traits, but also present with a tendency to lie and manipulate and further jeopardize treatment programs through their impulsive, thrill-seeking, and irresponsible behavior. Finally, evidence that all three psychopathic traits dimensions are needed to improve the identification of youth with conduct problems who have putative psychopathic personality will also support the recent recommendation to incorporate interpersonal and behavioral/lifestyle traits as additional specifiers in DSM- or ICD-defined Conduct Disorder (e.g., Salekin, 2016).

Are callous–unemotional traits the core of psychopathic personality?

The CU traits dimension of the psychopathy construct has often been assumed to be the so-called core of psychopathy in child studies on this topic (e.g., Viding, Blair, Moffitt, & Plomin, 2005), but without a clear definition of the concept "core" (Salekin, 2016). A definition that captures its usage in the psychopathy literature is that the core comprises *the root of a problem, from which other traits and behaviors will develop, in interaction with the social environment* (Salekin & Andershed, in press). This implies that CU traits emerge first in life and that the interpersonal and behavior–lifestyle traits emerge later as downstream manifestations of these CU traits. Without doubt, the study of CU traits greatly contributed to our understanding of conduct problems. But is there enough evidence to be sure that CU traits constitute the core of psychopathic personality? We think it is not, for at least three reasons.

First, a tool that was specifically designed to assess the aforementioned three psychopathic traits dimensions in early childhood only recently became available: the CPTI. Various CPTI studies showed that these three dimensions can be measured in a reliable manner in 3–5-year-olds, are partially genetically undergirded (e.g., Tuvblad, Fanti, Andershed, Colins, & Larsson, 2017), and are associated with concurrent aggression, conduct problems, and fearlessness (e.g., Colins, Andershed, Frogner et al., 2014; Colins, Fanti, Larsson et al., 2017). There is also some evidence that the stability of early childhood CP that co-occurs with CU traits is associated with high levels of interpersonal and behavioral/lifestyle traits (Klingzell et al., 2016). Thus, this set of findings suggests that CU traits are not the only traits that must be considered when studying the early roots of psychopathic personality. Second, several pioneer studies that researched the developmental outcomes of CU in children used a CU measure that actually also tapped interpersonal traits (e.g., Waller et al., 2016; Rowe et al., 2010). This mix of traits raises the intriguing question to what extent the associations between CU traits and variables of interest are driven by interpersonal traits. Third, the widely accepted developmental psychopathology equifinality principle states that every developmental outcome could come about through multiple different pathways (Frick, Ray, Thornton, & Kahn, 2014b). As such, it is important to be open for the possibility that some children start their pathway towards psychopathic personality with CU traits, whereas others start with interpersonal or behavioral/lifestyle traits (Salekin, 2016), especially since a core deficit that gives rise to psychopathic personality is unlikely to be identified (e.g., Lilienfeld, Watts, Francis Smith, Berg, & Latzman, 2015; Miller & Lynam, 2015). To bolster what is known about the core, or more likely the cores, of psychopathic personality, longitudinal studies that consider all psychopathic traits dimensions from early childhood onwards are needed.

How stable is the constellation of co-occurring traits from early childhood onwards?

Studies that began to explore the viability of the psychopathy construct in early childhood are predominantly cross-sectional. Consequently, it remains largely unknown how stable these traits are from early childhood onwards. Specifically, we are aware of only one published study that assessed the stability of various psychopathic traits dimensions in children younger than 6 years of age. In one study, 4- to 9-year-old children (N = 900) were followed over 12 months, and a high rank-order stability (as indexed by Pearson correlation coefficients) of interpersonal (r = .55), affective (r = .63), and behavioral/lifestyle (r = .64) traits was revealed (Dadds et al., 2005). Yet, age-separate analyses of stability (for example in 4- and 5-year-olds) were not presented for these three psychopathic traits dimensions as measured by the parent version of the Antisocial Process Screening Device.

This knowledge gap is unfortunate since psychopathy has been described as a developmental disorder (like autism spectrum disorder) that is present by the age of 8 (Blair, 2010), with roots in early childhood (e.g., Raine, 2013), suggesting that adults with psychopathy already had fairly immutable levels of psychopathic traits early in life. Yet, adult psychopathic personality is thought to be a relatively rare disorder in the general population (estimated prevalence of 1–2 percent; Drislane & Patrick, 2013), and various traits that are part of the psychopathy construct can at some age be normative in children and adolescents (e.g., Seagrave & Grisso, 2002; Talwar & Lee, 2008). Therefore, studies that begin to explore the stability and change of psychopathic traits from early childhood onwards are highly warranted to scrutinize how many children and adolescents with elevated psychopathy scores will become tomorrow's adults with a psychopathic personality.

Given that psychopathic personality is commonly described as a constellation of co-occurring traits, future research should start to focus on ipsative change and stability, which as far as we know have not yet been used in the study of psychopathic personality. Ipsative change does not merely assess the change in each psychopathic traits dimension over time but also an individual's trait configuration or "profile" (e.g., Robins, Fraley, Roberts, & Trzesniewski, 2001). This is highly relevant for answering the intriguing question of how many children who are high on all three dimensions (which in our view is indicative of having a putative psychopathic personality) remain simultaneously high on all these dimensions over time. From this perspective, future studies that apply person-oriented analyses are needed to test if and how early this group of children can be identified (really at or even before the age of 8?), and how many of these children remain high on the various psychopathic traits dimensions later in life. Of course, psychopathic personality in (early) childhood does not necessarily manifest itself in the same way as adult psychopathy. However, child and adolescent psychopathy is commonly described as a constellation of co-occurring traits. Therefore, it makes sense to start looking for children who are high on all three psychopathic traits dimensions, which does not exclude the possibility that children with stable high scores on one or two psychopathic traits dimensions may also develop a psychopathic personality later in life.

How to differentiate between high and low levels of psychopathic traits?

Recommending the start of differentiating between children and adolescents with high and low levels of psychopathic traits in applied work is easier said than done. Clinicians with an interest in a standardized assessment of psychopathic personality traits may wonder which tool they should use to identify youth with elevated levels of psychopathic traits and likely have difficulties transferring research findings to their applied work.

Various tools that tap psychopathic traits dimensions have been developed and are currently available. Yet, mounting evidence shows that clinicians cannot assume that these tools can be used interchangeably. Indeed, notwithstanding that psychopathy measures enable the assessment of interpersonal, CU, and behavioral/lifestyle traits dimensions, the correlations between traits dimension scores as measured by various tools are sometimes poor to moderate at best. For example, in detained boys and girls, the CU dimension of the APSD self-report version is poorly to moderately correlated to the CU dimension of the YPI and YPI–S (e.g., Colins, Colins, Bijttebier et al., 2014; Poythress, Dembo, Wareham, & Greenbaum, 2006). In addition, whether or not a boy or a girl is considered to be high or low on psychopathy total or dimension scores greatly depends on the tool being used. For example, a study among detained girls used the ICU and the YPI to identify girls with Conduct Disorder who have high (versus low) levels of CU traits as categorically defined in DSM–5 (Colins & Andershed, 2015). This study showed that both tools identified 44 of 118 girls with Conduct Disorder to have CU traits, but that only 26 of these 44 girls were identified to have CU traits by both the ICU and the YPI. Another study among male youth offenders showed that only 0.5–1 percent of youths had a high total psychopathy score on all three tools that were used, compared with 13–15 percent on each individual tool (Cauffman, Kimonis, Dmetrieva, & Monahan, 2009).

Besides the poor overlap between measures designed to tap psychopathic personality traits, clinicians may wonder at what level a boy or girl can be considered to display high or normative levels of interpersonal, CU, and/or behavioral/lifestyle traits, respectively. Yet, for neither the APSD and ICU nor for the YPI, CPTI, or PCL: YV are there well-established, extensively tested, and validated cut-off scores that can aid in determining when scores on these measures are well outside a normative level. Echoing prior recommendations (e.g., Colins, Fanti, Salekin, Mulder et al., 2017; Ray, Frick, Thornton, Steinberg, & Cauffman, 2016), future research should fill this void, and we recommend editorial and review boards of scientific journals to consider such endeavors as scientifically and clinically relevant and important. Such research is also important to inform clinicians if assessing CU traits in a categorical manner (as for example is expected when using the Limited Prosocial Emotions specifier for Conduct Disorder) generates the same results as the body of research that used CU traits in a dimensional manner. Notwithstanding that such research is in its infancy, it seems that using different approaches yield different results (Colins, Damme et al., 2017; Hyde, Burt, Shaw, Donnellan, & Forbes, 2015). Admittedly, a lot of psychometric-related work is to be done to illuminate whether the same cut-off scores can be used across gender, age-groups, youth from various ethnic origins, settings, and countries.

To deal with the lack of such well-established cut-off scores, researchers often use distribution based cut-off scores (*SD*, median splits, and percentiles) to identify children with high levels of CU traits (e.g., Pasalich, Dadds, Hawes, & Brennan, 2012; Viding, Jones, Paul, Moffitt, & Plomin, 2008; Klapwijk et al., 2016) or high levels on all three psychopathy components (e.g., Colins et al., 2018) or total score (e.g., Van Baardewijk, Stegge, Bushman, & Vermeiren, 2009). Researchers also use model-based clustering techniques to identify groups of youth who differ in their permutations of psychopathic personality traits (e.g., Colins, Fanti, Salekin, Mulder et al., 2017; Fanti, Demetriou, & Kimonis, 2013; Kimonis, Frick, Cauffman, Goldweber, & Skeem, 2012). Findings from these studies may be easier to understand for clinicians than findings from variable-oriented studies using statistical techniques, such as structural equation modeling. Nevertheless, it is also important to keep in mind that these are group-based findings with large samples. Clinicians will need to make decisions when they work with one child and their families, long before data files are ready for in-depth analyses – if they ever are – within one's own institution, to estimate whether a child's score on psychopathy traits dimension is high relative to other children they see and work with (Colins, Fanti, Salekin, Mulder et al., 2017).

The road forward

The main aim of the present chapter was to critically review research, including our own work, on the child and adolescent psychopathy construct but also to constructively contribute in setting-up a research agenda for the upcoming decade. Basically, much more attention is needed to find the best way to identify children and adolescents who are high on the three psychopathic traits dimensions. Future work convincingly showing that it is indeed sufficient to use the CU traits dimension to identify antisocial and conduct disordered youth with putative psychopathic personality would be highly important, because this would increase confidence that the study of youth psychopathy does not drift away from adult psychopathy by using only one dimension of a multidimensional construct for identification purposes. Importantly, evidence that using CU traits alone does not identify the same group of youth as when using the three psychopathic traits dimensions would not at all imply that CU traits are not important for understanding heterogeneity among antisocial or conduct disordered youth. Such evidence, however, would imply that one cannot solely rely on CU traits to identify and study children and adolescents with psychopathic personalities.

Assessment development and evaluation may seem less attractive than, let's say, exploring the genetic and environmental bases of psychopathic personality traits or studying brain responses to emotional stimuli in youth with high psychopathy scores. Yet, assessment issues are very important and should remain a major focus in future work to ensure that researchers can include the most reliable and valid state-of-the-art measures in their future research projects. If it is uncertain whether the tool does a good job in assessing psychopathic traits dimensions, then the outcomes of the research endeavors may not really be informative for the study of psychopathic personality, regardless of the strengths and novelties of the design (e.g., large sample, repeated measures, brain imaging). Fortunately, a variety of well-tested measures are currently available, providing researchers with many more alternatives than was the case a decade ago, when researchers often depended on less reliable tools and/or (therefore) modified existing or created novel tools for a particular study that did not undergo in-depth psychometric scrutiny (e.g., Dadds et al., 2005; Viding et al., 2005; Rowe et al., 2010). As novel tools that have been developed for use among adults are more and more being tested with youth, such as the Triarchic Psychopathy Measure (Somma, Borroni, Drislane, & Fossati, 2016), the variety of potentially useful measures will soon become even greater. Also, a substantial body of knowledge is available to guide researchers in selecting the tool that will best serve their research questions when studying psychopathic personality. To highlight why it is so important to keep up with psychometric literature, an example is provided below. In this example, we focus on the APSD and the ICU because (1) these are among the two most widely used and tested measures in CU research; (2) these measures were used to develop the "Limited Prosocial Emotions" specifier for Conduct Disorder in DSM–5; and (3) various scholars argue that youth with Conduct Disorder who have CU traits (or

Limited Prosocial Emotions) are high on the other psychopathy components and thus have a personality that looks like adult psychopathy.

Evidence consistently showed that the APSD's Callous–Unemotional scale (six items) has trouble reliably assessing CU traits (e.g., Poythress, Douglas, Falkenbach et al., 2006). To more reliably and more comprehensively assess CU traits, the ICU was developed using the four items that have consistently loaded onto the Callous–Unemotional subscale of the APSD and by creating an additional six items for each of these four APSD items, leading to a total of 24 items. The APSD Callous–Unemotional scale has been used to propose the four criteria that are now part of the callous–unemotional specifier (labeled: "Limited Prosocial Emotions") for Conduct Disorder in DSM–5: (1) lack of remorse or guilt, (2) callous–lack of empathy, (3) shallow or deficient affect, and (4) unconcerned about performance. The APSD enables the assessment of each criterion by means of one item, whereas item response theory analyses with the ICU showed that nine (Kimonis et al., 2014) or eight (Kimonis et al., 2015) ICU items effectively assess the four criteria.[1] Thus, whereas the ICU was developed to enable a more comprehensible assessment of CU traits, it seems that researchers who use the original 24-item ICU will nevertheless have a limited number of items to assess the specifier (note that some items in the 8- and 9-item sets are items that were already in the APSD). Yet, it can even be questioned to what extent future research will be able to test the four criteria of the specifier by means of the ICU. In fact, to solve various psychometric problems that hallmarked the original ICU (e.g., Colins, Skeem, Dmitrieva, & Cavanagh, 2016; Wang et al., 2017), Hawes and colleagues developed a modified ICU version, including 12 items (ICU–12) of the original ICU (Hawes, Byrd, Henderson et al., 2014). Whereas the ICU–12 may resolve several psychometric problems that have been reported previously for the ICU, the ICU–12 includes zero and one item from the 8- or 9-item set selected to assess the DSM–5 specifier criteria "Concerned about performance" and "Shallow and Deficient Affect," respectively. This is worrisome since the APSD and the ICU are the only commonly used tools that enable the assessment of the criterion "Concerned about performance," which should not come as a surprise since only the APSD and the ICU were used to define the four Limited Prosocial Emotions (LPE) specifier criteria(Frick & Moffitt, 2010). We are currently in a situation in which researchers who plan to use psychometrically sound tools (e.g. YPI) or novel promising tools (e.g. ICU–12) are not able to assess CU traits as defined in DSM–5. It becomes even more complicated since an alternative, shorter version of the original ICU has been proposed that includes 10 items of the original 24-item ICU items (ICU–10; Ray, Frick, Thornton, Steinberg, & Cauffman, 2016). Specifically, the ICU–10 has only six items in common with the aforementioned ICU–12, and has three/two/zero and two ICU items that were selected to assess the LPE specifier criteria a, b, c, and d, respectively (Kimonis et al., 2014; Kimonis et al., 2015). Taken together, researchers who want to study CU traits in a way that closely resembles how these traits are defined in the DSM–5 will need to make careful decisions: use a tool that has been shown to have psychometric problems (in terms of factor structure and internal consistency) or use psychometrically sounder tools (ICU–12, YPI) that only enable the assessment of three of the four LPE specifier criteria.[2]

It is still unclear how many children and adolescents are expected to be identified (for research purposes) as having a psychopathic personality. Studies that used person-oriented analytical approaches may start to shed a light on this prevalence issue. Yet, in some studies this prevalence seems unrealistically high. For example, using model-based cluster analyses among criminal justice-involved youth, the rate of youth being high on all three psychopathic traits dimensions ranged from 46 percent (Kimonis et al., 2012) to 70 percent (Gill & Stickle, 2016) when relying on self-report tools and near 60 percent when relying on the PCL: YV (Kimonis, Skeem, Cauffman, & Dmitrieva, 2011). These rates vary substantially from the estimates of psychopathy among criminal justice-involved adults, for whom the estimated prevalence was 15–25 percent (Drislane & Patrick, 2013). Recall that the estimated prevalence of adult psychopathic personality in the general population is about 1–2 percent (Drislane & Patrick, 2013). Yet, some community-based studies that used various psychopathic traits dimensions reported that 12 to 16 percent of the sample is high on all used psychopathic traits dimensions (Colins et al., 2012; Frick et al., 2000; Colins, Fanti, Salekin, & Andershed, 2017).

Clearly, such high prevalence rates strongly suggest that current research attempts yield too many false positives, and that we should try to do better if we ever think that it is worth the effort and risk to start looking for children and adolescents with a psychopathic personality in real-world settings. Maybe in the future we will learn that we can definitely identify these kids very early in life, but with too much collateral damage it might be better that we not do so, at least not before a certain age. But this may be too pessimistic a view, and a lot of work must be done before such a tough conclusion can made. For example, more realistic prevalence rates may be revealed when using various sound tools and informants, when seeking for children and adolescents who remain high on the three psychopathic traits dimension over time, or when using more stringent cut-offs scores.

To ascertain that it is worth the effort to identify (young) children and adolescents with putative psychopathic personalities, future research is warranted to confirm that these kids differ from other youth in a theoretical and clinical meaningful way. For example, it has been theorized and showed that adults with psychopathy have anomalies in emotion processing, which involves emotion recognition, affective arousal, and expression of emotions. Adults with psychopathy have an impairment in the fundamental propensity to recognize fear and sadness, and these emotion recognition problems may extend across the full gamut of emotions (Dadds, Kimonis, Schollar-Root, Moul, & Hawes, 2017). Adults with psychopathy also seem to manifest significant abnormalities in their capacity to become affectively aroused by others' emotional states (fear and sadness), as indexed by physiological indices such as skin conductance (SC), heart rate (HR), and eye-blink startle reflex (Brook, Brieman, & Kosson, 2013). Research also strongly suggests that adults with psychopathy demonstrate reduced facial expressions when exposed to emotional stimuli (Fanti, Kyranides, & Panayiotou, 2015). In addition to emotion processing anomalies, adults with psychopathy also display planned (or cold-blooded) aggression (Cima & Raine, 2009), a preference for risk-taking behaviors (Weidacker, O'Farrell, Gray, Johnston, & Snowden, 2017), and an urge for immediate gratification (Hare, 1996).

From a theoretical perspective, it makes sense to expect that children and adolescents with putative psychopathic personalities will show these anomalies to a greater extent than youth with low levels on all three psychopathy components. But what about other youth? Future research may show quite consistently that children who are only high on the CU traits or the behavior–lifestyle traits dimension can and should be disentangled from youth with who display the entire constellation of traits (e.g., Christian et al., 1997; Colins et al., 2018; Frick et al., 2000; Colins, Fanti, Salekin et al., 2017). In this case, do we expect differences in emotion processing between children high in CU traits and children with a psychopathic personality? Among detained youth, substance use and misuse are highly prevalent (e.g., Colins et al., 2010), so if indices of substance use and misuse are relied upon as proxy for risk-taking behavior, do we really expect to show that youth with psychopathic personalities will display a higher level of substance use and misuse than youth who are only high in behavioral/lifestyle traits?

Finally, it has been argued that there is a need for ongoing research to test the field reliability and validity of psychological assessment instruments used in legal settings (Edens & Boccaccini, 2017). This is especially important when the instruments are being applied in a context where the information generated may have significant life consequences, such as clinical decision-making and judicial processing. Although studies on youth psychopathy or CU traits typically scrutinize the usefulness of assessment tools when guaranteeing confidentiality and anonymity of the participants, there is an urgent need to investigate how well these tools perform when being completed as part of a clinical protocol, where the information may have actual consequences for the child or adolescent. For example, youth detention settings often do not have the financial resources to rely on expert-based comprehensive evaluations for all youth entering the facility (e.g., Colins et al., 2012) and often experience difficulties in locating and finding parents and teachers able or willing to provide reliable diagnostic information (Colins, Vermeiren, Schuyten, Broekaert, & Soyez, 2008; Kroll et al., 2002). Therefore, self-reports represent an important tool for researchers and clinicians working with detained youth (e.g., Walters, 2015). Even though the development and validation of self-report instruments for psychopathy have been considered a recent advancement (e.g., Vitacco, Neumann, & Pardini, 2014), it remains to be seen if findings from studies that collected self-report data in the context of a research protocol can be generalized to studies that use self-report data collected in the context of a clinical protocol. Filling this void also bears great importance for the study of the LPE specifier, because self-report was an important source of information in developing the LPE specifier (Frick & Moffitt, 2010) and is still the most used source of information in LPE research with criminal justice-involved youth (e.g., Colins & Andershed, 2015; Kimonis et al., 2015; Colins, 2016).

Various well-described, large, and rich datasets are available that include multiple waves of assessments using a variety of methods, including measures that tap the three psychopathic traits dimensions. These datasets may be used to start testing how early children or adolescents who are high on all three psychopathic traits components over time can be found and how these juveniles differ from other youth (e.g., those only high in CU traits) in terms of indices of concurrent and future maladjustment. These studies may also test if, for example, adolescents with a putative psychopathic personality have already displayed notable features or anomalies in (early) childhood that put them at risk for being high on all three psychopathic traits dimensions in adolescence.

Researchers that plan to start new studies can rely on novel promising (e.g. CPTI) or potentially promising tools such as the Clinical Assessment of Prosocial Emotions (CAPE; Frick, 2013) to bolster what is known about child and adolescent psychopathic personality. For example, researchers can use the CAPE to measure the LPE specifier among conduct disordered adolescents exactly as described in DSM–5 and explore if Conduct Disorder youth with the LPE specifier can be further divided in a group that is high in interpersonal and behavioral/lifestyle traits and a group that is low on these two psychopathic traits dimensions. Hopefully, future research will support recent recommendations to include various psychopathy components as specifier for Conduct Disorder in future revisions of the DSM and ICD, for example, to identify youth with a psychopathic personality (Salekin, 2016).

Conclusion

Researchers should reconsider using the entire psychopathy construct for identifying and studying the etiology, stability, and prognosis of children and adolescents with a putative psychopathic personality. Our ideas and enthusiasm for furthering the study of psychopathic personality are greatly based upon earlier work, including the work that instigated the focus on CU traits. We want to emphasize that we will have no problem with learning that research will eventually show that it is indeed sufficient to solely rely on CU traits to identify children and adolescents with putative psychopathic personalities. Such evidence base increase confidence that studies that focus on CU traits and use fascinating and expensive techniques (e.g., MRI, epigenetics, and psychophysiology) are indeed highly informative for the study of the youth psychopathy personality, which is still defined as a constellation of co-occurring traits. Finally, great caution is needed when using the term "psychopathic personality," and for now we recommend only using this label for research purposes and not in applied work, especially when dealing with young children (Colins, Andershed, Frogner et al., 2014; Colins, Fanti, Larsson et al., 2017).

Notes

1 Nine item set: Items 1,3,5,8,13,15,16,17, and 24, of which three items (e.g., item 13) to assess criterion a; three items to assess criterion b, one item to assess criterion c, and two items to assess criterion d. The 8-item set does exclude item 13 from the 9-item set.

2 There are various reasons to wonder whether "unconcerned about poor performance" should be part of the Limited Prosocial Emotion specifier after all. First, this item was originally intended to tap a selfish/egocentric style (i.e., concern for one's own agenda and disregard for others) (Frick personal communication; cited in Salekin & Andershed, in press), which refers to the interpersonal traits dimensions rather than the CU dimension. Second, the relevance of "unconcerned about performance" in the definition of LPE can be questioned because this criterion is applicable to many other mental health problems, and, thus, may not be discriminating enough within youth with conduct disorder or the like (e.g. Salekin, 2016; Lahey, 2014).

References

Andershed, H. (2010) 'Stability and change of psychopathic-traits. What do we know?,' in R. T. Salekin & D. R. Lynam (Eds.), *Handbook of child and adolescent psychopathy*, New York, NY: The Guilford Press.

Andershed, H., Colins, O. F., Salekin, R. T., Lordos, A., Kyranides, M., and Fanti, K. A. (in press) 'Callous–Unemotional traits only versus the multidimensional psychopathy construct as predictors of various antisocial outcomes during early adolescence,' *Journal of Behavior Assessment and Psychopathology*.

Andershed, H., Kerr, M., Stattin, H., and Levander, S. (2002) 'Psychopathic traits in non-referred youths: Initial test of a new assessment tool,' in E. Blaauw & L. Sheridan (Eds.), *Psychopaths: Current international perspectives*, The Hague: Elsevier.

Blair, R. J. R. (2010) 'A cognitive neuroscience perspective on child and adolescent psychopathy,' *Handbook of Child and Adolescent Psychopathy*, 156–178.

Boduszek, D., Debowska, A., and Willmott, D. (2017) 'Latent profile analysis of psychopathic traits among homicide, general violent, property, and white-collar offenders,' *Journal of Criminal Justice*, *51*:17–23.

Breeden, A., Cardinale, E., Lozier, L., Vanmeter, J., and Marsh, A. (2015) 'Callous–unemotional traits drive reduced white-matter integrity in youths with conduct problems,' *Psychological Medicine*, *45*:3033–3046.

Brook, M., Brieman, C. L., and Kosson, D. S. (2013) 'Emotion processing in Psychopathy Checklist–assessed psychopathy: A review of the literature,' *Clinical Psychology Review*, *33*:979–995.

Cauffman, E., Kimonis, E. R., Dmetrieva, J., and Monahan, K. (2009) 'A multimethod assessment of Juvenile Psychopathy: Comparing the predictive utility of the PCL:YV, YPI, and NEO PRI,' *Psychological Assessment*, *21*:528–542.

Cauffman, E., Skeem, J., Dmitrieva, J., and Cavanagh, C. (2016) 'Comparing the stability of psychopathy scores in adolescents versus adults: How often is "fledgling psychopathy" misdiagnosed?,' *Psychology, Public Policy, and Law*, *22*:77.

Christian, R. E., Frick, P. J., Hill, N. L., Tyler, L., and Frazer, D. R. (1997) 'Psychopathy and conduct problems in children .2. Implications for subtyping children with conduct problems,' *Journal of Abnormal Psychology*, *36*:233–241.

Cima, M., and Raine, A. (2009) 'Distinct characteristics of psychopathy relate to different subtypes of aggression,' *Personality and Individual Differences*, *47*:835–840.

Colins, O., Andershed, H., and Pardini, D. A. (2015) 'Psychopathic traits as predictors of future criminality, intimate partner aggression, and substance use in young adult men,' *Law and Human Behavior*, *39*:547–558.

Colins, O., Andershed, H., Salekin, R. T., and Fanti, A. K. (2018) 'Comparing different approaches for subtyping children with conduct problems: Callous–unemotional traits only versus the multidimensional psychopathic personality construct,' *Journal of Behavior Assessment and Psychopathology, 40*:6–15.

Colins, O., Bijttebier, P., Broekaert, E., and Andershed, H. (2014) 'Psychopathic-like traits among detained female adolescents: Reliability and validity of the Antisocial Process Screening Device and the Youth Psychopathic Traits Inventory,' *Assessment, 21*:195–209.

Colins, O., Noom, M., and Vanderplasschen, W. (2012) 'Youth Psychopathic Traits Inventory–Short Version: A further test of the internal consistency and criterion validity,' *Journal of Behavior Assessment and Psychopathology, 34*:476–486.

Colins, O., van Damme, L., Andershed, H., Fanti, K., and DeLisi, M. (2017) 'Self-reported psychopathic traits and antisocial outcomes in detained girls: A prospective study,' *Youth Violence and Juvenile Justice, 15*:138–153

Colins, O., Vermeiren, R., Schuyten, G., Broekaert, E., and Soyez, V. (2008) 'Informant agreement in the assessment of disruptive behavior disorders in detained minors in Belgium: A diagnosis-level and symptom-level examination,' *The Journal of Clinical Psychiatry, 69*.

Colins, O., Vermeiren, R., Vreugdenhil, C., van Den Brink, W., Doreleijers, T., and Broekaert, E. (2010) 'Psychiatric disorders in detained male adolescents: A systematic literature review,' *Canadian Journal of Psychiatry–Revue Canadienne De Psychiatrie, 55*:255–263.

Colins, O. F. (2016) 'The clinical usefulness of the DSM–5 specifier for conduct disorder outside of a research context,' *Law and Human Behavior, 40*:310–318.

Colins, O. F., and Andershed, H. (2015) 'The DSM–5 with limited prosocial emotions specifier for conduct disorder among detained girls,' *Law and Human Behavior, 39*:198.

Colins, O. F., Andershed, H., Frogner, L., Lopez-Romero, L., Veen, V., and Andershed, A.-K. (2014) 'A new measure to assess psychopathic personality in children: The Child Problematic Traits Inventory,' *Journal of Psychopathology and Behavioral Assessment, 36*:4–21.

Colins, O. F., Andershed, H., Hawes, S. W., Bijttebier, P., and Pardini, D. A. (2016) 'Psychometric properties of the original and short form of the Inventory of Callous–Unemotional Traits in detained female adolescents,' *Child Psychiatry & Human Development, 47*:679–690.

Colins, O. F., Damme, L. V., Andershed, H., Fanti, K. A., and DeLisi, M. (2017) 'Self-reported psychopathic traits and antisocial outcomes in detained girls: A prospective study,' *Youth Violence and Juvenile Justice, 15*:138–153.

Colins, O. F., Fanti, K., Larsson, H., and Andershed, H. (2017) 'Psychopathic traits in early childhood: Further validation of the Child Problematic Traits Inventory,' *Assessment, 24*:602–614.

Colins, O. F., Fanti, K. A., Salekin, R. T., and Andershed, H. (2017) 'Psychopathic personality in the general population: Differences and similarities across gender,' *Journal of Personality Disorders, 31*:49–74.

Colins, O. F., Fanti, K. A., Salekin, R. T., Mulder, E., and Andershed, H. (2017) 'Psychopathy in detained boys: The search for primary and secondary variants in a clinical setting,' *Personality Disorders: Theory, Research, and Treatment*, in press.

Cooke, D. J., and Michie, C. (2001) 'Refining the construct of psychopathy: Towards a hierarchical model,' *Psychological Assessment, 13*:171–188.

Dadds, M. R., Fraser, J., Frost, A., and Hawes, D. J. (2005) 'Disentangling the underlying dimensions of psychopathy and conduct problems in childhood: A community study,' *Journal of Consulting and Clinical Psychology, 73*:400–410.

Dadds, M. R., Kimonis, E. R., Schollar-Root, O., Moul, C., and Hawes, D. J. (2017) 'Are impairments in emotion recognition a core feature of callous–unemotional traits? Testing the primary versus secondary variants model in children,' *Development and Psychopathology*, 1–11.

DeLisi, M. (2016) *Psychopathy as Unified Theory of Crime*, Basingstoke: Palgrave Macmillan.

Drislane, L. E., and Patrick, C. J. (2013) 'Psychopathy and antisocial personality disorder,' in M. Shally-Jensen (Ed.), *Mental health care issues in America: An encyclopedia*, Santa Barbara, CA: ABC-CLIO.

Drislane, L. E., Patrick, C. J., Sourander, A., Sillanmäki, L., Aggen, S. H., Elonheimo, H., . . ., and Kendler, K. S. (2014) 'Distinct variants of extreme psychopathic individuals in society at large: Evidence from a population-based sample,' *Personality Disorders: Theory, Research, and Treatment, 5*(2):154.

Edens, J. F., and Boccaccini, M. T. (2017) 'Taking forensic mental health assessment "out of the lab" and into "the real world": Introduction to the special issue on the field utility of forensic assessment instruments and procedures,' *Psychological Assessment*, 29:599.

Fanti, K. A., Demetriou, C. A., and Kimonis, E. R. (2013) 'Variants of callous–unemotional conduct problems in a community sample of adolescents,' *Journal of Youth and Adolescence, 42*:964–979.

Fanti, A. K., Kyranides, M. N., Lordos, A., Colins, O. F., and Andershed, H. (in press) 'Unique and interactive associations of callous–unemotional traits, impulsivity and narcissism with child and adolescent Conduct Disorder symptoms,' *Journal of Psychopathology & Behavioral Assessment.*

Fanti, K. A., Kyranides, M. N., and Panayiotou, G. (2015) 'Facial reactions to violent and comedy films: Association with callous–unemotional traits and impulsive aggression,' *Cognition and Emotion*, 1–16.

Forth, A., Hart, S. D., and Hare, R. D. (1990) 'Assessment of psychopathy in male young offenders,' *Psychological Assessment: A Journal of Consulting and Clinical Psychology*, *2*:342–344.

Forth, A., and Kosson, D. (2003) *The Hare PCL: YV*, Toronto, ON: Multi-Health Systems.

Frick, P. J. (2009) 'Extending the construct of psychopathy to youth: Implications for understanding, diagnosing, and treating antisocial children and adolescents,' *Canadian Journal of Psychiatry/Revue Canadienne de Psychiatrie*, *31*:803.

Frick, P. J. (2013) *Clinical Assessment of Prosocial Emotions: Version 1.1(CAPE 1.1)*, New Orleans, LA: University of New Orleans.

Frick, P. J., Bodin, S. D., and Barry, C. T. (2000) 'Psychopathic traits and conduct problems in community and clinic-referred samples of children: Further development of the psychopathy screening device,' *Psychological Assessment*, *12*:382–393.

Frick, P. J., and Hare, R. D. (2001) *Antisocial Process Screening Device technical manual*, Toronto, ON: Multi-Health Systems.

Frick, P. J., and Moffitt, T. E. (2010) *A proposal to the DSM–V childhood disorders and the ADHD and disruptive behavior disorders work groups to include a specifier to the diagnosis of conduct disorder based on the presence of callous–unemotional traits*, Washington, DC: American Psychiatric Association.

Frick, P. J., Obrien, B. S., Wootton, J. M., and Mcburnett, K. (1994) 'Psychopathy and conduct problems in children,' *Journal of Abnormal Psychology*, *103*:700–707.

Frick, P. J., Ray, J., Thornton, L., and Kahn, R. (2014a) 'Can callous–unemotional traits enhance the understanding, diagnosis, and treatment of serious conduct problems in children and adolescents? A Comprehensive Review,' *Psychological Bulletin*, *140*:1–57.

Frick, P. J., Ray, J. V., Thornton, L. C., and Kahn, R. E. (2014b) 'Annual research review: A developmental psychopathology approach to understanding callous-unemotional traits in children and adolescents with serious conduct problems,' *Journal of Child Psychology and Psychiatry*, *55*:532–548.

Frogner, L., Andershed, A. K., and Andershed, H. (in press) 'Psychopathic personality works better than CU traits for predicting fearlessness and ADHD symptoms among children with conduct problems,' *Journal of Psychopathology and Behavioral Assessment*.

Frogner, L., Gibson, C. L., Andershed, A.-K., and Andershed, H. (2018) 'Childhood psychopathic personality and callous–unemotional traits in the prediction of conduct problems,' *American Journal of Orthopsychiatry*, *88*:211–225.

Gacono, C. B. (2015) *The clinical and forensic assessment of psychopathy: A practitioner's guide*, Routledge: Taylor & Francis.

Gill, A. D., and Stickle, T. R. (2016) 'Affective differences between psychopathy variants and genders in adjudicated youth,' *Journal of Abnormal Child Psychology*, *44*:295–307.

Hare, R. D. (1996) 'Psychopathy: A clinical construct whose time has come,' *Criminal Justice and Behavior*, *23*:25–54.

Hare, R. D. (2003) *Hare Psychopathy Checklist–Revised (PCL–R): Second edition, technical manual*, Toronto, ON: Multi Health Systems.

Hare, R. D. (2016) 'Psychopathy, the PCL–R, and criminal justice: Some new findings and current issues,' *Canadian Psychology/Psychologie canadienne*, *57*:21.

Hare, R. D., and Neumann, C. S. (2008) 'Psychopathy as a clinical and empirical construct,' *Annual Review of Clinical Psychology*, *4*:217–246.

Hawes, S. W., Byrd, A. L., Henderson, C. E., Gazda, R. L., Burke, J. D., Loeber, R., and Pardini, D. A. (2014) 'Refining the parent-reported Inventory of Callous–Unemotional Traits in boys with conduct problems,' *Psychological Assessment*, *26*:256.

Hawes, S. W., Byrd, A. L., Waller, R., Lynam, D. R., and Pardini, D. A. (2017) Late childhood interpersonal callousness and conduct problem trajectories interact to predict adult psychopathy,' *Journal of Child Psychology and Psychiatry*, *58*:55–63.

Hawes, S. W., Mulvey, E. P., Schubert, C. A., Pardini, D. A. (2014) 'Structural coherence and temporal stability of psychopathic personality features during emerging adulthood,' *Journal of Abnormal Psychology*, *123*:623.

Hemphälä, M., Kosson, D., Westerman, J., and Hodgins, S. (2015) 'Stability and predictors of psychopathic traits from mid-adolescence through early adulthood,' *Scandinavian Journal of Psychology*, *56*:649–658.

Hicks, B. M., Markon, K. E., Patrick, C. J., Krueger, R. F., and Newman, J. P. (2004) 'Identifying psychopathy subtypes on the basis of personality structure,' *Psychological Assessment*, *16*:276.

Hyde, L. W., Burt, S. A., Shaw, D. S., Donnellan, M. B., and Forbes, E. E. (2015) 'Early starting, aggressive, and/or callous–unemotional? Examining the overlap and predictive utility of antisocial behavior subtypes,' *Journal of Abnormal Psychology, 124*:329.

Jones, A. P., Laurens, K. R., Herba, C. M., Barker, G. J., and Viding, E. (2009) 'Amygdala hypoactivity to fearful faces in boys with conduct problems and callous–unemotional traits,' *American Journal of Psychiatry, 166*:95–102.

Kiehl, K. A., Smith, A. M., Hare, R. D., Mendrek, A., Forster, B. B., Brink, J., and Liddle, P. F. (2001) 'Limbic abnormalities in affective processing by criminal psychopaths as revealed by functional magnetic resonance imaging,' *Biological Psychiatry, 50*:677–684.

Kimonis, E. R., Fanti, K., Goldweber, A., Marsee, M. A., Frick, P. J., and Cauffman, E. (2014) 'Callous–unemotional traits in incarcerated adolescents,' *Psychological Assessment, 26*:227.

Kimonis, E. R., Fanti, K. A., Frick, P. J., Moffitt, T. E., Essau, C., Bijttebier, P., and Marsee, M. A. (2015) Using self-reported callous-unemotional traits to cross-nationally assess the DSM-5 'with Limited Prosocial Emotions' specifier,' *Journal of Child Psychology and Psychiatry, 56*:1249–1261.

Kimonis, E. R., Frick, P. J., Cauffman, E., Goldweber, A., and Skeem, J. (2012) 'Primary and secondary variants of juvenile psychopathy differ in emotional processing,' *Development and Psychopathology, 24*:1091–1103.

Kimonis, E. R., Skeem, J., Cauffman, E., and Dmitrieva, J. (2011) 'Are secondary variants of juvenile psychopathy more reactively violent and less psychosocially mature than primary variants?,' *Law and Human Behavior, 35*:381.

Klapwijk, E. T., Aghajani, M., Colins, O. F., Marijnissen, G. M., Popma, A., Lang, N. D., Wee, N. J., and Vermeiren, R. R. (2016) 'Different brain responses during empathy in autism spectrum disorders versus conduct disorder and callous-unemotional traits,' *Journal of Child Psychology and Psychiatry, 57*:737–747.

Klingzell, I., Fanti, K. A., Colins, O. F., Frogner, L., Andershed, A.-K., and Andershed, H. (2016) 'Early childhood trajectories of conduct problems and callous–unemotional traits: The role of fearlessness and psychopathic personality dimensions,' *Child Psychiatry & Human Development, 47*:236–247.

Kroll, L., Rothwell, J., Bradley, D., Shah, P., Bailey, S., and Harrington, R. C. (2002) 'Mental health needs of boys in secure care for serious or persistent offending: A prospective, longitudinal study,' *Lancet, 359*:1975–1979.

Lahey, B. B. (2014) 'What we need to know about callous–unemotional traits: Comment on Frick, Ray, Thornton, and Kahn,' *Psychological Bulletin, 140*:58–63.

Lee, Z., and Salekin, R. T. (2010) 'Psychopathy in a noninstitutional sample: Differences in primary and secondary subtypes,' *Personality Disorders: Theory, Research, and Treatment, 1*:153.

Lilienfeld, S., and Andrews, B. (1996) 'Development and preliminary validation of a self-report measure of psychopathic personality traits in noncriminal population,' *Journal of Personality Assessment, 66*:488–524.

Lilienfeld, S. O., Watts, A. L., Francis Smith, S., Berg, J. M., and Latzman, R. D. (2015) 'Psychopathy deconstructed and reconstructed: Identifying and assembling the personality building blocks of Cleckley's chimera,' *Journal of Personality, 83*:593–610.

Lynam, D. R., Gaughan, E. T., Miller, J. D., Miller, D. J., Mullins-Sweatt, S., and Widiger, T. A. (2011) 'Assessing the basic traits associated with psychopathy: Development and validation of the Elemental Psychopathy Assessment,' *Psychological Assessment, 23*:108.

Maraun, M. D., and Hart, S. D. (2016) 'The taxonic latent structure and taxometrics in forensic mental health,' *Psychological Reports, 119*:450–486.

Miller, J. D., and Lynam, D. R. (2015) 'Understanding psychopathy using the basic elements of personality,' *Social and Personality Psychology Compass, 9*:223–237.

Munoz, L. C., and Frick, P. J. (2007) 'The reliability, stability, and predictive utility of the self-report version of the Antisocial Process Screening Device,' *Scandinavian Journal of Psychology, 48*:299–312.

Neumann, C. S., Kosson, D. S., Forth, A. E., and Hare, R. D. (2006) 'Factor structure of the Hare Psychopathy Checklist: Youth Version (PCL: YV) in incarcerated adolescents,' *Psychological Assessment, 18*:142.

Orue, I., and Andershed, H. (2015) 'The Youth Psychopathic Traits Inventory–Short Version in Spanish Adolescents–Factor structure, reliability, and relation with aggression, bullying, and cyber bullying,' *Journal of Psychopathology and Behavioral Assessment*, 1–13.

Paris, J. (2003) 'Personality disorders over time: Precursors, course and outcome,' *Journal of Personality disorders, 17*:479–488.

Pasalich, D. S., Dadds, M. R., Hawes, D. J., and Brennan, J. (2012) 'Attachment and callous–unemotional traits in children with early-onset conduct problems,' *Journal of Child Psychology and Psychiatry, 53*:838–845.

Patrick, C. (2010) 'Triarchic psychopathy measure (TriPM),' *PhenX Toolkit Online Assessment Catalog,' 813*:814.

Paulhus, D., Neumann, C. S., and Hare, R. D. (2012) *Manual for the self-report of psychopathy (SRP–III) scale*, Toronto, ON: Multi-Health Systems.

Poythress, N. G., Dembo, R., Wareham, J., and Greenbaum, P. E. (2006) 'Construct validity of the youth psychopathic traits inventory (YPI) and the antisocial process screening device (APSD) with justice-involved adolescents,' *Criminal Justice and Behavior, 33*:26–55.

Poythress, N. G., Douglas, K. S., Falkenbach, D., Cruise, K., Lee, Z., Murrie, D. C., and Vitacco, M. (2006) 'Internal consistency reliability of the self-report antisocial process screening device,' *Assessment, 13*:107–113.

Raine, A. (2013) *The anatomy of violence: The biological roots of crime*, London: Penguin Books Limited.

Ray, J. V., Frick, P. J., Thornton, L. C., Steinberg, L., and Cauffman, E. (2016) 'Positive and negative item wording and its influence on the assessment of callous–unemotional traits,' *Psychological Assessment, 28*:394.

Robins, R. W., Fraley, R. C., Roberts, B. W., and Trzesniewski, K. H. (2001) 'A longitudinal study of personality change in young adulthood,' *Journal of Personality, 69*:617–640.

Rowe, R., Maughan, B., Moran, P., Ford, T., Briskman, J., and Goodman, R. (2010) 'The role of callous and unemotional traits in the diagnosis of conduct disorder,' *Journal of Child Psychology and Psychiatry, 51*:688–695.

Ruscio, J. (2007) 'Taxometric analysis: An empirically grounded approach to implementing the method,' *Criminal Justice and Behavior, 34*:1588–1622.

Salekin, R. (2017) 'Research review: What do we know about psychopathic traits in children?,' *Journal of Child Psychology and Psychiatry, and Allied Disciplines.*

Salekin, R. T. (2016) 'Psychopathy in childhood: Toward better informing the DSM–5 and ICD–11 conduct disorder specifiers,' *Personality Disorders: Theory, Research, and Treatment*, 7:180.

Salekin, R. T., Brannen, D. N., Zalot, A. A., Leistico, A.-M., and Neumann, C. S. (2006) 'Factor structure of psychopathy in youth: Testing the applicability of the new four-factor model,' *Criminal Justice and Behavior, 33*:135–157.

Salekin, R. T., and Lynam, D. R. (2010) *Handbook of child and adolescent psychopathy*, New York, NY: The Guilford Press.

Salekin, R. T., Rogers, R., and Sewell, K. W. (1997) 'Construct validity of psychopathy in a female offender sample: A multitrait–multimethod evaluation' *Journal of Abnormal Psychology, 106*:576.

Seagrave, D., and Grisso, T. (2002) 'Adolescent development and the measurement of juvenile psychopathy,' *Law and Human Behavior, 26*:219–239.

Shiner, R. L., and Tackett, J. L. (2014) 'Personality disorders in children and adolescents,' *Child Psychopathology*, 848–896.

Somma, A., Andershed, H., Borroni, S., and Fossati, A. (in press) 'Psychopathic personality traits in relation to self-report delinquency in adolescence: Should we mind about interaction effects?,' *Journal of Psychopathology and Behavioral Assessment.*

Somma, A., Borroni, S., Drislane, L. E., and Fossati, A. (2016) 'Assessing the triarchic model of psychopathy in adolescence: Reliability and validity of the Triarchic Psychopathy Measure (TriPM) in three samples of Italian community-dwelling adolescents,' *Psychological Assessment, 28*:e36.

Sprague, J., Javdani, S., Sadeh, N., Newman, J. P., and Verona, E. (2012) 'Borderline personality disorder as a female phenotypic expression of psychopathy?,' *Personality Disorders: Theory, Research, and Treatment, 3*:127.

Talwar, V., and Lee, K. (2008) 'Social and cognitive correlates of children's lying behavior,' *Child Development, 79*:866–881.

Tuvblad, C., Fanti, K. A., Andershed, H., Colins, O. F., and Larsson, H. (2017) 'Psychopathic personality traits in 5 year old twins: The importance of genetic and shared environmental influences,' *European Child & Adolescent Psychiatry, 26*:469–479.

van Baardewijk, Y., Andershed, H., Stegge, H., Nilsson, K. W., Scholte, E., and Vermeiren, R. (2010) 'Development and Tests of Short Versions of the Youth Psychopathic Traits Inventory and the Youth Psychopathic Traits Inventory–Child Version,' *European Journal of Psychological Assessment, 26*:122–128.

van Baardewijk, Y., Stegge, H., Andershed, H., Thomaes, S., Scholte, E., and Vermeiren, R. (2008) 'Measuring psychopathic traits in children through self-report. The development of the Youth Psychopathic Traits Inventory–Child Version,' *International Journal of Law and Psychiatry, 31*:199–209.

van Baardewijk, Y., Stegge, H., Bushman, B. J., and Vermeiren, R. (2009) 'Psychopathic traits, victim distress and aggression in children,' *Journal of Child Psychology and Psychiatry*, *50*:718–725.
Vanwoerden, S., Reuter, T., and Sharp, C. (2016) 'Exploring the clinical utility of the DSM–5 conduct disorder specifier of 'with limited prosocial emotions' in an adolescent inpatient sample' *Comprehensive Psychiatry*, *69*:116–131.
Viding, E., Blair, R. J. R., Moffitt, T. E., and Plomin, R. (2005) 'Evidence for substantial genetic risk for psychopathy in 7-year-olds,' *Journal of Child Psychology and Psychiatry*, *46*:592–597.
Viding, E., Jones, A. P., Paul, J. F., Moffitt, T. E., and Plomin, R. (2008) 'Heritability of antisocial behaviour at 9: Do callous-unemotional traits matter?,' *Developmental Science*, *11*:17–22.
Vitacco, M. J., Neumann, C. S., and Pardini, D. A. (2014) 'Predicting future criminal offending in a community-based sample of males using self-reported psychopathy,' *Criminal Justice and Behavior*, *41*:345–363.
Waller, R., Dishion, T. J., Shaw, D. S., Gardner, F., Wilson, M. N., and Hyde, L. W. (2016) 'Does early childhood callous–unemotional behavior uniquely predict behavior problems or callous–unemotional behavior in late childhood?,' *Developmental Psychology*, *52*:1805.
Walters, G. D. (2015) 'A multi-wave cross-lagged regression analysis of the Youth Psychopathic Traits Inventory and Self-Reported Offending,' *Journal of Criminal Justice*, *43*:327–336.
Wang, M.-C., Deng, Q., Armour, C., Bi, X., and Zeng, H. (2015) 'The psychometric properties and factor structure of the Antisocial Process Screening Device self-report version in Chinese adolescents,' *Journal of Psychopathology and Behavioral Assessment*, *37*:553–562.
Wang, M.-C., Gao, Y., Deng, J., Lai, H., Deng, Q., and Armour, C. (2017) 'The factor structure and construct validity of the inventory of callous–unemotional traits in Chinese undergraduate students,' *PLoS One*, *12*:e0189003.
Weidacker, K., O'Farrell, K. R., Gray, N. S., Johnston, S. J., and Snowden, R. J. (2017) 'Psychopathy and impulsivity: The relationship of the triarchic model of psychopathy to different forms of impulsivity in offenders and community participants,' *Personality and Individual Differences*, *114*:134–139.

Part II

Measurement of psychopathy

12

The Elemental Psychopathy Assessment

Brandon Weiss, Donald R. Lynam, and Joshua D. Miller

Introduction

Psychopathy, which comprises traits such as egocentricity, manipulativeness, lack of remorse or concern for others, and impulsivity, has long been of interest to behavioral scientists given its relevance to the prediction of violent and nonviolent crime, substance use, and recidivism (Hare & Neumann, 2008). The Elemental Psychopathy Assessment (EPA; Lynam et al., 2011) is a 178-item self-report inventory based on the empirical work examining psychopathy from the Five-Factor Model (FFM) of general personality perspective. The EPA is distinguished from other assessments of psychopathy in being developed with the intent of representing basic elements of psychopathy, with clear links to the robust general structure of personality, rather than including compound factors based on clinical observation that embed multiple basic elements. The EPA yields a total psychopathy score, four empirically derived factors (i.e., Antagonism, disinhibition, Emotional Stability, narcissism), and 18 scales and exists in its original form as well as two shorter variants (EPA–Short Form: Lynam et al., 2013; EPA Super Short Form: Collison, Miller, Gaughan, Widiger, & Lynam, 2016). Traits from four of the five FFM domains were included in the EPA, including Neuroticism (e.g., EPA subscale Unconcern; Anger–Hostility), Extraversion (e.g., Coldness; Dominance), Agreeableness (e.g., Manipulation; callousness), and Conscientiousness (e.g., Impersistence; Rashness). Table 12.1 describes the factor structure of the 18 EPA scales, as well as the FFM domain that coincides with each scale, and example item content.

The present chapter reviews the psychometric and measurement issues that prompted the EPA's development and aims, presents the methodology by which the EPA was developed, examines the EPA's construct validity, and presents advantages and applications of the EPA in comparison to alternative measures of psychopathy.

The importance of an elemental structure

One of the main developments that prompted the expansion of research on psychopathy was the creation of a reliable and valid assessment tool, namely the Psychopathy Checklist (PCL) and its revision (PCL–R; Hare, 2003; Hare & Neumann, 2008), which typically involves an extensive

Table 12.1 Factor structure of the elemental psychopathy assessment

Higher-order factor	*EPA scale*	*FFM domain*	*Example item*
Antagonism	Coldness	Extraversion	"I don't feel a strong need to get close to people"
	Distrust	Agreeableness	"When someone does something nice for me, I wonder what they want from me"
	Manipulation	Agreeableness	"My tendency to be sneaky or deceptive has gotten me into trouble before"
	Self-Centeredness	Agreeableness	"I don't care if my actions have a negative impact on others"
	Callousness	Agreeableness	"The suffering of others is not my problem"
Disinhibition	Urgency	Neuroticism	"I often let my feelings get me into trouble"
	Thrill-seeking	Extraversion	"I've gotten in trouble because of some of the risks I've taken"
	Oppositional	Agreeableness	"I do what I want, not what others tell me to do"
	Disobliged	Conscientiousness	"I have gotten in trouble for failing to meet my obligations to others"
	Impersistence	Conscientiousness	"When something becomes boring or difficult, I move on to something else"
	Rashness	Conscientiousness	"I often find myself in trouble because I did not think far enough ahead"
Emotional Stability	Unconcern	Neuroticism	"I have fewer fears than most people I know"
	Self-Contentment	Neuroticism	"I have very few regrets about my past behavior"
	Invulnerability	Neuroticism	"I can remain calm in situations in which other people might panic"
Narcissism	Self-Assurance	Neuroticism	"I'm a pretty smooth talker"
	Anger	Neuroticism	"People who know me know not to make me angry"
	Dominance	Extraversion	"It is important to me to be the 'top dog' in a group"
	Arrogance	Agreeableness	"I do not believe it is bragging if you are telling the truth"

Note. FFM = Five-Factor Model.

file review and interview in order to score it. A considerable body of empirical literature surrounding the PCL/PCL–R has developed (Hare & Neumann, 2008; Patrick, 2006) and has led to the development of several self-report scales, including multiple iterations of the Self-Report Psychopathy Scale (SRP; Hare, 1985; Paulhus, Neumann, & Hare, in press) and the Levenson Self-Report Psychopathy Scale (LSRP; Levenson, Kiehl, & Fitzpatrick, 1995), which assess psychopathy in a manner associated with the PCL/PCL–R operationalization. Other models and assessments of psychopathy have been developed since then as well, with fewer direct links to the

PCL/PCL–R, including the Psychopathic Personality Inventory (PPI; Lilienfeld & Andrews, 1996) and its subsequent revision (PPI–R; Lilienfeld & Widows, 2005) and the triarchic model (Patrick, Krueger, & Fowles, 2009) and measure of psychopathy (TriPM; Patrick, 2010).

Much current work in psychopathy, by means of these measures, has endeavored to go beyond risk prediction and construct validation to uncover the basic structure of the psychopathy construct. These endeavors frequently rely on factor analyses of psychopathy scales (alone or in concert with other measures) and have led to much debate in the literature regarding psychopathy's underlying factor structure. For example, in the current version of the manual for the PCL–R (Hare, 2003), it is suggested that the PCL–R comprises four lower order facets and two higher order factors. However, Lynam and Widiger (2007) have argued that the repeated factor analyses of the PCL–R are unlikely to yield the basic dimensions of psychopathy itself (see also Skeem & Cooke, 2010). This argument also applies to self-report scales that were developed to assess the broad, multidimensional construct of psychopathy. The crux of the argument is that the items in the psychopathy assessments are themselves complex mixtures of different personality traits, or compounds, and that factor analyses of such compounds cannot yield basic elements. In the case of the PCL–R and self-report variants (e.g., SRP–III), many of the items refer to broad sets of behaviors or outcomes that could have occurred for a variety of reasons rather than distinct personality traits (e.g., poor probation or parole risk, early behavior problems, juvenile delinquency, promiscuous sexual behavior).

An alternative approach, utilized in the development of the EPA, is to use structural models of general personality to identify the basic elements of psychopathy (Lynam & Widiger, 2007). The main requirements for an elemental trait model are that its elements exist at the same level in the personality trait hierarchy and that the model be independent of any specific measure or theory of psychopathy. Although several such trait taxonomies were available, the Five-Factor Model (FFM) is arguably the predominant model of general and pathological personality available and was used in the development of the EPA. The model, and its primary associated measure, the Revised NEO Personality Inventory (NEO PI–R; Costa & McCrae, 1992), includes five broad domains. The domain of Neuroticism entails emotional adjustment and stability. Extraversion entails an individual's proneness to positive emotions and sociability. Openness to experience refers to an individual's interest in culture, and the preference and interest in experiencing and exploring new activities, ideas, and emotions. Agreeableness is concerned with an individual's interpersonal relationships and strategies; people high in Agreeableness tend to be trusting, straightforward, and empathic, whereas those who score low tend to be manipulative, arrogant, and unconcerned about others. Finally, Conscientiousness relates to the "control of impulses," as well as to the ability to plan, organize, and complete behavioral tasks. Within the NEO PI–R, each domain is made up of six lower-order facets. For example, the domain of Agreeableness (vs. Antagonism) consists of trust (vs. suspicion), straightforwardness (vs. deception), altruism (vs. exploitation), compliance (vs. aggression), modesty (vs. arrogance), and tendermindedness (vs. tough-mindedness).

The FFM was originally derived from the natural language, ensuring that important aspects of personality are represented (John & Srivastava, 1999). Although the specific facet selections of Costa and McCrae (1995) have been criticized for occurring outside the lexical tradition and for several notable secondary loadings (e.g., impulsiveness within Neuroticism is correlated with Conscientiousness; angry hostility within Neuroticism is correlated with Antagonism), most facets do not show large secondary loadings and are consistent with traits already recognized in the extant psychological literature. The FFM enjoys considerable empirical support in the form of convergent and discriminant validation across self, peer, and spouse ratings (Costa & McCrae, 1988); temporal stability across the life span (Roberts & DelVecchio,

2000); etic and emic cross-cultural support (Ashton & Lee, 2001; McCrae, Terracciano, & 78 members of the Personality Profiles of Cultures Project, 2005); behavioral genetic support for its structure (Yamagata et al., 2006); and relations to important outcomes (Ozer & Benet-Martinez, 2006), including academic achievement (Digman & Takemoto-Chock, 1981), antisocial behavior (Miller, Lynam, & Leukefeld, 2003), substance use and abuse (Flory, Lynam, Milich, Leukefeld, & Clayton, 2002), and risky sexual behavior (Miller et al., 2004). Perhaps most importantly, a number of articles examine psychopathy through the lens of the FFM (Lynam & Derefinko, 2006).

There is strong consensus about which FFM traits are most relevant to psychopathy across several different methods (Lynam & Widiger, 2007). Examinations of psychopathy through the lens of FFM have been conducted in a variety of ways, including translating the PCL–R items into the language of the FFM (i.e., PCL–R pathological lying: FFM low straightforwardness; Widiger & Lynam, 1998), generating expert ratings of the FFM traits considered most prototypical of psychopathic individuals (Miller, Lynam, Widiger, & Leukefeld, 2001), and examining correlations between the FFM and various psychopathy measures (Derefinko & Lynam, 2006; Gaughan, Miller, Pryor, & Lynam, 2009; Hicklin & Widiger, 2005; Lynam, Derefinko, Caspi, Loeber, & Stouthamer-Loeber, 2007; Skeem, Miller, Mulvey, Tiemann, & Monahan, 2005). Looking across these different approaches, Lynam and Widiger (2007) identified the following consensual FFM traits, rationally grouped into five clusters: interpersonal Antagonism (trust, straightforwardness, altruism, compliance, modesty, tendermindedness, warmth), impulsivity broadly construed (impulsiveness, excitement seeking, self-discipline, deliberation), interpersonal dominance (assertiveness), lack of self-directed negative affect (anxiety, depression, self-consciousness, vulnerability), and negative other directed affect (Anger).

Further, research has shown that the psychopathy-relevant traits within measures of the FFM (e.g., NEO PI–R) can be used to comprehensively assess psychopathy. Multiple studies show high convergence between FFM-assessed psychopathy and explicit measures of psychopathy, including the LSRP, SRP, and PPI/PPI–R (Derefinko & Lynam, 2006; Miller et al., 2001; Ross, Benning, Patrick, Thompson, & Thurston, 2009). For instance, across samples of undergraduates (Miller & Lynam, 2003; Miller et al., 2001) and drug abusers (Derefinko & Lynam, 2006), FFM psychopathy scores manifest relations with external criteria that mirror those found using explicit psychopathy assessments.

One concern often raised about using the NEO PI–R to assess psychopathy, and other personality disorders generally, is how capable a scale designed to assess the normal range of personality is of assessing the more pathological range of these traits (Haigler & Widiger, 2001). Walton, Roberts, Krueger, Blonigen, and Hicks (2008) demonstrated empirically that a general measure of personality, the Multidimensional Personality Questionnaire, captured the same portions of the latent psychopathy trait as the PPI (Lilienfeld & Andrews, 1996), one of the most widely used self-report psychopathy inventories. However, Walton et al. (2008) also noted that for both measures, "greater information was provided in the moderate regions of the trait with less information in the extreme regions" (p. 1642). One of the express aims in the development of the EPA was to represent the extreme regions (or pathological range) of traits thought relevant to psychopathy by modifying the item content of the NEO PI–R.

The development of the EPA scale was designed to overcome the problems found in both extant measures of psychopathy (involving compound traits) and extant measures of personality (involving normal range content). The specific traits included in the EPA have been identified across multiple methods and samples as characteristic of psychopathy (Lynam & Widiger, 2007). The EPA's development began with descriptions of the relevant facets and the construction of items that, though consistent with the initial facet, represented more maladaptive variants of these traits. The purpose of this was to develop an assessment of psychopathy that could be explicitly understood as a maladaptive variant of general personality structure.

Beginning with the 18 facets of the NEO PI–R identified as characteristic of psychopathy across multiple approaches, scales, and studies (Lynam & Widiger, 2007), the authors wrote items for the new scales, beginning with the original descriptions and items of the facets and describing more maladaptive manifestations. Specifically, they sought to represent each respective FFM facet using more maladaptive descriptions of the traits that would be apparent in pathological variants (e.g., "I have more important things to worry about than other people's feelings" for Self-Centeredness and "My stubbornness has frequently gotten me into trouble" for Opposition). The initial item writing yielded approximately 30 items per facet, which were edited, refined, and reduced to 14–18 items per facet. The ultimate set of EPA facets included distrust, manipulation, self-centeredness, opposition, arrogance, and callousness from FFM Agreeableness; impersistence, disobliged, and rashness from FFM Conscientiousness; coldness, dominance, and Thrill-seeking from FFM Extraversion; and Anger, urgency, unconcern, self-contentment, self-assurance, and invulnerability from FFM Neuroticism. Emphasizing the importance of working at the facet level, facets representing both pathologically low and high are included in the EPA for domains of Extraversion and Neuroticism.

When external criteria are included among the content of personality-based psychopathy scales (e.g., SRP–III antisocial), this can confound the scales' concurrent and predictive relations as they become tautological in nature (e.g., using explicitly antisocial items on a psychopathy scale to predict future antisocial behavior). In the development of the EPA, efforts were made to exclude explicitly antisocial content (e.g., "I have robbed someone") from the trait scales.

Enhancing practical utility

The EPA was designed with a number of practical measurement concerns in mind. These include the identification of invalid responders as well as the availability of shorter forms that may be better suited to long surveys in which psychopathy is but one of many important constructs being assessed.

Validity checks

There is a long-held notion that psychopathic individuals are either unwilling or unable to provide accurate information regarding the degree to which they manifest psychopathic traits. Although studies examining the self and informant reports of psychopathy demonstrate substantial convergence (Kelley, Edens, Donnellan, Mowle, & Sorman, 2017; Miller, Jones, & Lynam, 2011; Miller, Hyatt, Rauscher, Maples, & Zeichner, 2014), invalid responders still pose a serious threat to the validity of data. The EPA is distinguished among some measures of psychopathy in offering two validity scales for detecting individuals who may be providing invalid or distorted data. One set of validity items (i.e., Infrequency) was designed to identify individuals who were not paying attention to the items (e.g., "I never speak to anyone during the day"). The other set of items (i.e., Unlikely Virtue) was written to assess overly positive self-presentation; these items, the Too Good to Be True items, inquired about virtues or behaviors that few persons would possess (e.g., "I have never been envious of anyone else"). Practically, designating invalid responders involves identifying individuals who endorsed four or more Infrequency items and three or more Unlikely Virtue items using the two most extreme response categories (i.e., strongly agree/agree or strongly disagree/disagree), which equates to identifying individuals who are approximately 3 and 2.75 standard deviations above the Infrequency and Unlikely

Virtue scale score means, respectively, based on analysis of a large validation sample (Lynam et al., 2011).

Short-form development – 72-item EPA–SF

Although the self-reported nature of the EPA allows for its convenience in non-forensic settings and group-administered studies, its length (i.e., 178 items) may be prohibitive when assessment time is limited. A short form of the EPA (EPA–SF; Lynam et al., 2013) was developed using item response theory (IRT) to reduce administration time. Through this procedure, the 178-item EPA was reduced to 72 items (or 88 items if the two validity scales are used), which cuts the administration time by more than half. The short form was designed to provide a well-articulated description of psychopathic personality reflecting the 18 subscales of the original EPA. Research has shown that the short form compares very well to the full-length EPA in terms of internal structure and relations with psychopathy inventories, basic personality dimensions, and behavioral outcomes across undergraduate and incarcerated samples (Lynam et al., 2013). In general, validity coefficients are quite similar across the two forms. Total scores have shown virtually identical patterns of correlations with external criteria, and short-form subscales have shown a comparable set of correlations in relation to their long-form counterparts. Overall, Lynam et al. (2013) demonstrate that little is lost in terms of psychometric information or validity in moving from the long form to the short form, even at the level of the 18 subscales. Thus, the short form maintains the capacity to provide an articulated and fine-grained description of psychopathy. Subsequent studies have replicated the short form's validity in relation to correlates important to psychopathy, where criminologists, among others, have used it for its brevity to examine relations between psychopathy and modern forms of criminal behavior (Collison et al., 2016; Seigfried-Speller, Villacís-Vukadinović, & Lynam, 2017).

Super short form development – 18-item EPA–SSF

Developers of the EPA and EPA–SF have in recent years also developed a super short form (EPA–SSF; Collison et al., 2016) in order to serve researchers for whom even the 72-item EPA–SF form may be too time-consuming. Specifically, given the strong relations between psychopathy and criminal behaviors and recidivism, a well-validated and very brief psychopathy measure was thought to be of great value in criminology, wherein criminologists routinely develop large surveys in which psychopathy is but one of many important constructs being assessed. The EPA–SSF consists of 18 items, with each item corresponding to one of the 18 subscales from the long-form EPA. Items were chosen for the super-short form in a two-step process. First, EPA–SF's 72 items were factor analyzed in which the four EPA factors emerged. Next, two items from each subscale that loaded most highly on each of the four EPA factors were retained. Of these two items, items were retained that, according to previously reported IRT analyses, provide the most psychometric information at higher levels of their corresponding latent trait.

A factor analysis of the resultant 18 items suggested a three-factor solution that bore closest similarity to EPA factors of Antagonism, disinhibition, and Emotional Stability. Factor 1 (i.e., Antagonism) was marked by arrogance, Coldness, callousness, Distrust, Disobligation, Impersistence, Manipulativeness, and Self-Centeredness. Factor 2 (i.e., disinhibition) was marked by Anger, Opposition, Rashness, Thrill-seeking, and Urgency. Factor 3 (i.e., Emotional Stability) was marked by Unconcern, Self-Contentedness, Invulnerability, Dominance, and Self-Assuredness. Scales related to EPA narcissism (i.e., Anger, arrogance, Dominance, and Self-assuredness) were distributed across the resultant three factors with arrogance loading onto Factor 1 (i.e., Antagonism), Anger loading onto Factor 2 (i.e., disinhibition), and Dominance and Self-Assuredness loading onto Factor 3 (i.e., Emotional Stability). When compared to the EPA–SF factors, EPA–SSF Antagonism and disinhibition have evinced similar relations to multiple widely used measures of psychopathy (e.g., SRP–III, LSRP) and external criteria typically associated with psychopathy, including antisocial behavior, and substance use across student and incarcerated samples (Collison et al., 2016). EPA–SSF Emotional Stability has been most strongly related to the Fearless Dominance factor of the PPI and has shown a small relation to substance use. Overall, the EPA–SSF offers criminologists and other researchers an efficient way to measure psychopathy within larger surveys where psychopathy is one of many constructs being assessed, while retaining the EPA's strength in representing basic elements of psychopathic personality.

Convergent validity

General personality

Five-factor model

A unique feature of the EPA relative to other psychopathy assessment instruments is its explicit coordination with general personality structure (see Table 12.1). EPA subscales are strongly related to the respective NEO PI–R facet scales from which they were derived (Lynam et al., 2011; Miller et al., 2011a). EPA Antagonism, EPA disinhibition, and EPA Emotional Stability strongly map onto (low) Agreeableness, (low) Conscientiousness, and (low) Neuroticism, respectively, while EPA narcissism tends to show moderate relations with both FFM Extraversion and (low) Agreeableness (e.g., Crego & Widiger, 2014), consistent with the FFM structure of grandiose narcissism (e.g., Weiss & Miller, in press).

Although the EPA scales stayed true to their general trait origins, they out-predicted (i.e., demonstrated incremental validity) the original NEO PI–R facet scales in analyses involving three psychopathy measures consistent with the EPA's greater representation of maladaptive variants of FFM traits. Findings indicate that EPA scales also bear statistically stronger relations with other measures of psychopathy (i.e., SRP–III, LSRP, and PPI–R) than their general trait counterparts from the NEO PI–R in the majority of cases (Lynam et al., 2011).

HEXACO

EPA total and factor scores also demonstrate good convergent validity in relation to the Honesty-Humility, Emotionality, Extraversion, Agreeableness, Conscientiousness, and Openness to Experience (HEXACO) model of personality (Ashton & Lee, 2009), assessed using self- and informant-report formats (Miller et al., 2014). In general, the EPA factors were most strongly related to the general personality domains from which they were derived (e.g., EPA disinhibition uniquely related to Conscientiousness; EPA Antagonism uniquely related to Honesty–Humility and Agreeableness). The EPA total score manifested a trait profile generally consistent with previous research examining alternative measures of psychopathy (e.g., Decuyper, De Pauw, De Fruyt, De Bolle, & De Clerq, 2009), with the exception that the EPA total score is more strongly negatively correlated with HEXACO Emotionality than is typically found, most likely due to the substantial inclusion of the Emotional Stability content that accounts for a significant portion of the EPA. In addition, there is some evidence to suggest that EPA narcissism is not as closely related to HEXACO Extraversion as FFM Extraversion, though the reasons for this remain unclear.

Alternative psychopathy measures

Studies that have examined the EPA in relation to existing alternative psychopathy scales indicate excellent convergent (and discriminant) validity of the EPA's factor and individual scale scores across undergraduate (e.g., Miller et al., 2011), community (Miller et al., 2014), and incarcerated samples (Lynam et al., 2011) as well as when using self- or informant-reported EPA scores (Miller et al., 2014). EPA Antagonism has shown strong positive relations to almost all subscales from alternative psychopathy measures (Few, Miller, & Lynam, 2013), consistent with evidence from multiple frameworks – including meta-analyses of the empirical literature (Decuyper et al., 2009), expert ratings (Miller et al., 2001), and translations of the PCL–R into the language of the FFM (Widiger & Lynam, 1998) – that FFM Antagonism is central to most aspects of psychopathy (e.g., Lynam & Derefinko, 2006). Nevertheless, one exception to this pattern relates to subscales of PPI–R Fearless Dominance and Triarchic Psychopathy Measure Boldness (TriPM; Patrick et al., 2009), which do not bear strong relations to EPA Antagonism (e.g., see Miller & Lynam, 2012 meta-analysis; Crego & Widiger, 2014).

The strongest relations to EPA Antagonism have been found between conceptually similar scales. At the EPA scale level, SRP–III callous affect is most strongly related to EPA Coldness, Self-Centeredness, and callousness; SRP–III interpersonal manipulation has been most strongly related to EPA Manipulation and Self-Centeredness. Similarly, LSRP Factor 1 was most strongly related to EPA Coldness, Self-Centeredness, and callousness (Lynam et al., 2011). At the factor level, EPA Antagonism is most strongly related to PPI–R Factor 2 Self-centered Impulsivity, TriPM Meanness and disinhibition, and all subscales of the SRP–III (e.g., Crego & Widiger, 2014).

EPA disinhibition shows its largest correlations with subscales focused on behavioral dyscontrol (e.g., PPI–SCI; SRP–III Erratic Lifestyle; LSRP antisocial, TriPM disinhibition). At the EPA scale level, the strongest relations to EPA disinhibition have been found between conceptually similar subscales. SRP–III Erratic Lifestyle has been most strongly related to EPA Thrill-seeking, Opposition, and Rashness, while LSRP Factor 2 has been most strongly related to EPA Anger, Urgency, Impersistence, and Rashness (Lynam et al., 2011). At the factor level, EPA disinhibition seems almost interchangeable with PPI–R Self-centered Impulsivity and TriPM disinhibition and is strongly related to TriPM Meanness and all SRP–III subscales (e.g., Crego & Widiger, 2014).

The EPA Emotional Stability factor has shown strong relations to PPI–R Fearless Dominance/TriPM Boldness but weak correlations with the other subscales from the LSRP, PPI–R, SRP–III (Few et al., 2013), and TriPM (Crego & Widiger, 2014). This is consistent with evidence that suggests that PPI–R Fearless Dominance/TriPM Boldness includes content that is outside many psychopathy measures (Miller & Lynam, 2012) but is captured by the EPA.

Finally, EPA narcissism has been strongly associated with existing psychopathy scales that focus on the intrapersonal (e.g., LSRP egocentricity) and interpersonal (e.g., SRP–III interpersonal manipulation) styles and strategies psychopathic individuals use to manipulate their social environment (Few et al., 2013). Like EPA Emotional Stability, EPA narcissism bears strong relations with PPI–R Fearless Dominance/TriPM Boldness, which may owe to its common elevation on FFM Extraversion (e.g., Crego & Widiger, 2014), but captures more maladaptive content consistent with the grandiosity and entitlement associated with narcissism.

Providing further validation of the EPA as a standalone measure of the basic elements of psychopathy, the four EPA factors together account for a substantial amount of variance across the self-report psychopathy factors (Few et al., 2013; Lynam et al., 2011) and exhibits substantial incremental validity in accounting for variance in alternative psychopathy measures. Few, Miller, and Lynam (2013) found that, on average, EPA factors accounted for an additional 16 percent of the variance in psychopathy scores above and beyond the variance explained by other established measures of psychopathy (i.e., SRP–III, PPI–R, LSRP), whereas the factors from these alternative measures accounted for an additional 4 percent of the variance above and beyond the EPA factors.

In general, findings related to convergent validity have demonstrated the kind of differential relations one would expect. The interpersonal and affective aspects of psychopathy were most uniquely related to EPA Antagonism and EPA narcissism, whereas the erratic and antisocial components of psychopathy were most strongly uniquely related to the EPA disinhibition factor, and more controversial components of psychopathy concerning Fearless Dominance/Boldness are most uniquely related to EPA Emotional Stability and EPA narcissism.

Criterion validity

Externalizing behaviors

The EPA has demonstrated significant relations with a multitude of externalizing behaviors, including inmates' self-reported externalizing behavior, official reports of disciplinary infractions (Lynam et al., 2011), aggressive social cognitions (Miller et al., 2011) and reports of aggression (Wilson, Miller, Zeichner, Lynam, & Widiger, 2011; Wilson, Miller, Zeichner, Lynam, & Widiger, 2013), as well as substance use and antisocial behavior (e.g., Lynam et al., 2013). These finding have been shown in undergraduate (e.g., Wilson et al., 2011), community (Miller et al., 2014), and incarcerated samples (e.g., Lynam et al., 2011). Externalizing behaviors (e.g., antisocial behavior, proactive aggression) are most consistently and strongly related to EPA Antagonism and EPA disinhibition factors (e.g., Few et al., 2013), which is consistent with previous findings indicating relations between (low) Agreeableness/(low) disinhibition and externalizing (e.g., Miller, Lynam, & Jones, 2008).

Other EPA factor scores also show specific relations to certain outcomes. EPA narcissism may be most uniquely linked to reactive and proactive aggression (Miller et al., 2014) and, along with EPA Antagonism, direct, physical aggression assessed in laboratory settings (Miller, Wilson, Hyatt, & Zeichner, 2015; Hyatt, Weiss, Carter, Zeichner, & Miller, in press). These relations are consistent with the experimental literature documenting positive relations between narcissism and aggression (Reidy, Foster, & Zeichner, 2010), particularly behavior that follows some form of ego threat (e.g., Bushman & Baumeister, 1998; Twenge & Campbell, 2003).

EPA Emotional Stability, however, tends to bear null to weak relations with all externalizing behaviors when measured alone or in interaction with other EPA factors (e.g., Miller et al., 2014), challenging hypotheses that traits like Emotional Stability, Fearless Dominance, and Boldness may be related to problematic behaviors only when paired with elevated scores on other core aspects of psychopathy (e.g., Lilienfeld et al., 2012).

The EPA has also been examined in relation to computer crime, which includes attempting to gain unauthorized access to information systems and exploiting vulnerabilities in computer networks, writing and disseminating viruses, stealing and fraudulently using others' identities, monitoring network traffic, and defacing websites (Seigfried-Speller et al., 2017). EPA Antagonism and EPA disinhibition were moderately related to all forms of computer crime, while EPA narcissism was weakly related to all forms except for defacing websites. EPA Emotional Stability, on the other hand, was unrelated to computer crime.

DSM Personality Disorders

EPA scores also show associations with Personality Disorder (PD) constructs from the American Psychiatric Association's (APA) Diagnostic and Statistical Manual of Mental Disorders (DSM–5;

APA, 2013) that are indicative of an antagonistic interpersonal style. Consistent with the notion that psychopathic individuals manifest an interpersonal style characterized by aggression, manipulation, nonconformity with social mores, and callousness, EPA total scores are related to PDs characterized by these traits including DSM–IV (APA, 1994) Narcissistic PD, Antisocial PD, Paranoid PD, Histrionic PD, and Borderline PD (listed in order of magnitude), as well as trait narcissism, measured by the Narcissistic Personality Inventory (NPI; Raskin & Terry, 1988; Miller et al., 2011). Notably, this pattern of associations is highly similar to that manifested by PCL–R scores among male forensic patients (Hildebrand & de Ruiter, 2004).

Further, certain EPA factors overlap closely with pathological personality traits selected by the Personality and Personality Disorders Work Group to assess Antisocial Personality Disorder in Section III, Alternative Model of Personality Disorders included in DSM–5. Indeed, Antagonism and disinhibition traits from the Personality Inventory for DSM–5 (PID–5; Krueger, Derringer, Markon, Watson, & Skodol, 2012) exhibit strong relations to both EPA Antagonism and disinhibition and moderate to strong relations with EPA narcissism (Crego & Widiger, 2014). Both EPA Antagonism and disinhibition also bear strong relations to the Personality Diagnostic Questionnaire–4 Antisocial Personality Disorder (ASPD) scale (PDQ–4; Hyler, 1994), involving content related to criminal behavior, fighting, lying, and risk-taking.

Social cognition

Research examining EPA scores in relation to social cognition demonstrates that antagonistic and impulsive individuals as assessed by the EPA tend to manifest hostile and aggressive social cognition (Miller et al., 2011). Individuals with higher EPA scores may be more likely (1) to experience Anger in response to various interpersonal situations associated with a negative outcome, including situations in which the negative outcome is clearly accidental or ambiguous in nature – consistent with evidence of a hostile attribution bias; and (2) to report verbal and physical aggression to resolve the situation.

Important advantages and applications

There are several advantages offered by an elemental approach to assessing psychopathy, including the ability to granularly examine relations between psychopathic traits and external criteria, provide a bridge from psychopathy research to research on the FFM, examine the underlying structure of alternative psychopathy scales containing compound items and scales, and evaluate the centrality of certain psychopathy components versus others.

Fine-mapping relations between personality and external criteria

An elemental approach affords the ability to fine-map elements of psychopathy to the diversity of behavioral outcomes associated with psychopathy, including proactive and reactive aggression, nonviolent criminal behavior, and substance use and abuse. One may ask which elements are important for which particular outcomes (e.g., institutional aggression, recidivism, treatment resistance). Indeed, EPA's elemental structure operates in the service of delineating relations between narrow aspects of psychopathy and external criteria. For example, the EPA's granularity at the scale level has allowed researchers to identify important differences in the way negative emotionality relates to important criterion variables. Miller et al. (2011) demonstrated that EPA scales related to externalizing variants of negative emotionality (acting angrily or impulsively when upset) differed in important ways from EPA scales related to resiliency to negative emotionality such as shame, anxiety, depression, and embarrassment in their relations to criteria such as angry and aggressive social cognition and DSM–IV Cluster B PDs. In addition, one can use the EPA elemental structure to study the combinatorial effects, i.e., synergistic effects in which specific combinations of elements give rise to emergent properties. For example, although not yet examined in the empirical literature, facets reflecting poor constraint may moderate the influence of interpersonal Antagonism.

Linking psychopathy and criminal behavior to basic research on personality

The derivation of the EPA from a basic model of personality allows a bridge to be built between psychopathy and basic research on personality, which can help inform etiology, development, and treatment of disordered personality. Indeed, explicit links between the EPA and the FFM are an advantage of this model in that they allow the substantial literature on the FFM (e.g., heritability, cross-cultural consistency, temporal stability) to be brought to bear on the study of psychopathy. It may be possible to understand important issues surrounding psychopathy (e.g., gender or cultural differences, age-related changes, comorbidity) by examining it through the lens of general personality. For example, basic research on the FFM has been used to explain observed sex differences in psychopathy (Lynam & Derefinko, 2006) as well as the relation between psychopathy and age (Vachon et al., 2013). Additionally, several researchers are studying the basic processes underlying the various traits, including Antagonism (e.g., Graziano & Tobin, 2002; Meier, Robinson, & Wilkowski, 2006). Other researchers are examining general personality pathways to impulsive behavior, which appear as four facets from three different domains within the NEO PI–R (Whiteside & Lynam, 2001).

As a corollary, an elemental approach to psychopathy may facilitate the identification of endophenotypes related to psychopathy, with which researchers may be able to productively probe the biological and mechanistic underpinnings of externalizing behavior. For example, Bechara (2005) has recently placed the four traits related to impulsive behavior (i.e., EPA Urgency, Thrill-seeking, Impersistence, and Rashness) into a larger neurocognitive framework rooted in neurology. In addition, research in the emerging field of personality neuroscience may aid psychopathy researchers and criminologists in discovering the neurological underpinnings of antisocial behavior by demonstrating links between neurological features and FFM Agreeableness (e.g., DeYoung et al., 2010).

EPA scales and factors can be used as assays of other instruments to identify points of convergence and divergence, to clarify factor structures, and to explain relations among other instruments. For example, Lynam et al. (2013) used the EPA to show that the SRP–III, LSRP, and PPI–R all strongly represent particular traits related to interpersonal Antagonism (i.e., EPA Distrust, Manipulation, Self-Centeredness, Opposition, arrogance, and Coldness) and poor impulse control (i.e., EPA Urgency, Thrill-seeking, and Rashness). The SRP–III and PPI–R also appear to contain elements of low anxiety and interpersonal dominance (i.e., EPA Unconcern and Dominance). The LSRP diverges from other instruments in including higher, rather than lower, levels of negative affect (i.e., generally lower scores on EPA Self-Contentment, Self-Assurance, and Invulnerability), while the PPI–R stands alone in its focus on very low levels of negative affect (i.e., EPA Self-Contentment, Self-Assurance, and Invulnerability) and very high levels of positive affect, traits that are not included in the EPA with the exception of Dominance and Thrill-seeking (e.g., Benning, Patrick, Blonigen, Hicks, & Iacono, 2005; Gaughan et al., 2009**a**; Ross et al., 2009). Understanding the elemental structure underlying each of the most widely used psychopathy indices will benefit researchers by guiding an appropriate interpretation of the relations they bear with each other and external criteria.

Evaluating the centrality of psychopathic traits

One can identify which elements are most central, which are peripheral, and which are unnecessary to the construct of psychopathy (Lynam & Miller, 2012). Given recent writings by several of the present authors (Lynam & Miller, 2012; Miller & Lynam 2012) arguing against the centrality of traits related to Fearless Dominance/Boldness to psychopathy, it may surprise some that the EPA includes similar content. Their inclusion is due to the manner in which the EPA was developed, which prioritized the FFM traits identified via expert ratings, observed correlations between FFM inventories and psychopathy inventories, and a translation of the PCL–R. A strong motivation behind creating the EPA was to allow researchers to work at a more basic trait level so they could "examine which elements are most central, which are peripheral, and which are unnecessary to the construct of psychopathy" (p. 15). We suspect that some traits included within the EPA, particularly those most similar to Fearless Dominance/Boldness (e.g., Self-assurance, Self-contentment, and Invulnerability) will ultimately be shown to be relatively unimportant to psychopathy, at least in comparison to traits from Antagonism and disinhibition (i.e., Miller, Lamkin, Maples-Keller, & Lynam, 2016). The inclusion of this content in the EPA is important, however, as it enables psychopathy researchers to continue examining the importance of this content in a variety of ways (e.g., exploring additive and interactive effects of EPA Emotional Stability). As is the case with Fearless Dominance/Boldness (e.g., Lilienfeld et al., 2012; Marcus et al., 2013; Miller & Lynam, 2012), further research is needed to test whether the traits that compose the EPA Emotional Stability factor add important information necessary for the assessment and conceptualization of psychopathy.

Conclusion

The present chapter reviewed the literature on the Elemental Psychopathy Assessment (i.e., EPA), a measure of psychopathy built upon a view of the construct through the lens of a general personality framework. Through this lens, psychopathy is seen as a collection of maladaptive personality traits with clear links to general or "normal" personality. For the development of the EPA, core traits were identified across multiple approaches, and items were written to assess more extreme variants of the basic traits consistent with the understanding of psychopathy as disordered personality. As described in the chapter, short- and super-short forms of the EPA have also been developed. The EPA has been shown to be reliable across multiple studies using samples of undergraduates, samples from the community, and samples from forensic settings. The 18 subscales of the original and short-forms have been shown to be underlaid by four factors: Antagonism, disinhibition, Emotional Stability, and narcissism; only three subscales underlie the super-short version. The chapter reports on multiple studies attesting to the construct validity of the EPA, demonstrating that it relates to a variety of outcomes (e.g., other psychopathy scales, aggression, antisocial behavior, social cognition, and personality disorders) as predicted. Finally, the chapter discusses the advantages that come with thinking of psychopathy as a collection of traits from a general model of personality and of assessing it with the EPA.

References

American Psychiatric Association. (1994) *Diagnostic and statistical manual of mental disorders* (4th ed.), Washington, DC: American Psychiatric Association.

American Psychiatric Association. (2013) *Diagnostic and statistical manual of mental disorders* (5th ed.), Washington, DC: American Psychiatric Association.

Ashton, M. C., and Lee, K. (2001) 'A theoretical basis for the major dimensions of personality,' *European Journal of Personality*, *15*:327–353.

Ashton, M. C., and Lee, K. (2009) 'The HEXACO–60: A short measure of the major dimensions of personality,' *Journal of Personality Assessment*, *91*:340–345.

Bechara, A. (2005) 'Decision making, impulse control, and loss of willpower to resist drugs: A neurocognitive perspective,' *Nature Neuroscience*, *8*:1458–1463.

Benning, S. D., Patrick, C. J., Salekin, R. T., and Leistico, A.-M. R. (2005) 'Convergent and discriminant validity of psychopathy factors assessed via self-report: A comparison of three instruments,' *Assessment*, *12*:270–289.

Bushman, B. J., and Baumeister, R. F. (1998) 'Threatened egotism, narcissism, self-esteem, and direct and displaced aggression: Does self-love or self-hate lead to violence?,' *Journal of Personality and Social Psychology*, *75*:219–229.

Collison, K. L., Miller, J. D., Gaughan, E. T., Widiger, T. A., and Lynam, D. R. (2016) 'Development and validation of the super-short form of the Elemental Psychopathy Assessment,' *Journal of Criminal Justice*, *47*:143–150.

Costa, P. T., Jr., and McCrae, R. R. (1988) 'Personality in adulthood: A six-year longitudinal study of self-reports and spouse ratings on the NEO Personality Inventory,' *Journal of Personality and Social Psychology*, *54*:853–863.

Costa, P. T., Jr., and McCrae, R. R. (1992) *Revised NEO Personality Inventory (NEO–PI–R) and NEO Five-Factor Inventory (NEO–FFI) professional manual*, Odessa, FL: Psychological Assessment Resources.

Costa, P. T., Jr., and McCrae, R. R. (1995) 'Domains and facets: Hierarchical personality assessment using the Revised NEO Personality Inventory,' *Journal of Personality Assessment*, *64*:21–50.

Crego, C., and Widiger, T. A. (2014) 'Psychopathy, DSM–5, and a caution,' *Personality Disorders: Theory, Research, and Treatment*, *5*:335–347.

Decuyper, M., De Pauw, S., De Fruyt, F., De Bolle, M., and De Clercq, B. J. (2009) 'A meta-analysis of psychopathy-, antisocial PD- and FFM associations,' *European Journal of Personality*, *23*:531–565.

Derefinko, K. J., and Lynam, D. R. (2006) 'Convergence and divergence among self-report psychopathy measures: A personality-based approach,' *Journal of Personality Disorders*, *20*:261–280.

DeYoung, C. G., Hirsh, J. B., Shane, M. S., Papademetris, X., Rajeevan, N., and Gray, J. R. (2010) 'Testing predictions from personality neuroscience: Brain structure and the big five,' *Psychological Science*, *21*:820–828.

Digman, J. M., and Takemoto-Chock, N. K. (1981) 'Factors in the natural language of personality: Re-analysis, comparison, and interpretation of six major studies,' *Multivariate Behavioral Research*, *16*:149–170.

Few, L. R., Miller, J. D., and Lynam, D. R. (2013) 'An examination of the factor structure of the Elemental Psychopathy Assessment,' *Personality Disorders: Theory, Research, and Treatment*, *4*:247–253.

Flory, K., Lynam, D., Milich, R., Leukefeld, C., and Clayton, R. (2002) 'The relations among personality, symptoms of alcohol and marijuana abuse, and symptoms of comorbid psychopathology: Results from a community sample,' *Experimental and Clinical Psychopharmacology*, *10*:425–434.

Gaughan, E. T., Miller, J. D., Pryor, L. R., and Lynam, D. R. (2009) 'Comparing two alternative measures of general personality in the assessment of psychopathy: A test of the NEO PI–R and the MPQ,' *Journal of Personality*, *77*:965–996.

Gaughan, E. T., Miller, J. D., Pryor, L. R., and Lynam, D. R. (2009) 'Comparing two alternative measures of general personality in the assessment of psychopathy: A test of the NEO PI–R and the MPQ,' *Journal of Personality*, *77*:965–996.

Graziano, W. G., and Tobin, R. (2002) 'Agreeableness: Dimension of personality or social desirability artifact?,' *Journal of Personality*, *70*:695–727.

Haigler, E. D., and Widiger, T. A. (2001) 'Experimental manipulation of NEO–PI–R items,' *Journal of Personality Assessment*, *77*:39–358.

Hare, R. D. (1985) 'Comparison of procedures for the assessment of psychopathy,' *Journal of Consulting and Clinical Psychology*, *53*:7–16.

Hare, R. D. (2003) *Manual for the Psychopathy Checklist–Revised* (2nd ed.), Toronto, ON: Multi-Health Systems.

Hare, R. D., and Neumann, C. S. (2008) 'Psychopathy as a clinical and empirical construct,' *Annual Review of Clinical Psychology*, *4*:217–246.

Hicklin, J., and Widiger, T. A. (2005) 'Similarities and differences among antisocial and psychopathic self-report inventories from the perspective of general personality functioning,' *European Journal of Personality*, *19*:325–342.

Hildebrand, J., and de Ruiter, C. (2004) 'PCL–R psychopathy and its relation to DSM–IV Axis I and II disorders in a sample of male forensic psychiatric patients in the Netherlands,' *International Journal of Law and Psychiatry*, *27*:233–248.

Hyatt, C. S., Weiss, B., Carter, N. T., Zeichner, A., and Miller, J. D. (in press) 'The relation between narcissism and laboratory aggression is not contingent on environmental cues of competition,' *Personality Disorders: Theory, Research, and Treatment.*

Hyler, S. E. (1994) *PDQ-4+ personality questionnaire*, New York: Author.

John, O. P., and Srivastava, S. (1999) 'The Big Five trait taxonomy: History, measurement, and theoretical perspectives,' in L. A. Pervin & O. P. John (Eds.), *Handbook of personality: Theory and research* (2nd ed., pp. 102–138), New York, NY: Guilford Press.

Kelley, S. E., Edens, J. F., Donnellan, M. B., Mowle, E. N., and Sörman, K. (2017) 'Self-and informant perceptions of psychopathic traits in relation to the triarchic model,' *Journal of Personality*, in press.

Krueger, R. F., Derringer, J., Markon, K. F., Watson, D., and Skodol, A. E. (2012) 'Initial construction of a maladaptive personality trait model and inventory for DSM–5,' *Psychological Medicine*, *42*:1879–1890.

Levenson, M. R., Kiehl, K. A., and Fitzpatrick, C. M. (1995) 'Assessing psychopathic attributes in a noninstitutionalized population,' *Journal of Personality and Social Psychology*, *68*:151–158.

Lilienfeld, S. O., and Andrews, B. P. (1996) 'Development and preliminary validation of a self-report measure of psychopathic personality traits in noncriminal populations,' *Journal of Personality Assessment*, *66*:488–524.

Lilienfeld, S. O., Patrick, C. J., Benning, S. D., Berg, J., Sellbom, M., and Edens, J. F. (2012) 'The role of fearless dominance in psychopathy: Confusions, controversies, and clarifications,' *Personality Disorders: Theory, Research, and Treatment*, *3*:327–340.

Lilienfeld, S. O., and Widows, M. R. (2005) *PPI–R professional manual*, Lutz, FL: Psychological Assessment Resources.

Lynam, D. R., and Derefinko, K. J. (2006) 'Psychopathy and personality,' in C. J. Patrick (Ed.), *Handbook of the psychopathy* (pp. 133–155), New York, NY: Guilford Press.

Lynam, D. R., Derefinko, K. J., Caspi, A., Loeber, R., and Stouthamer-Loeber, M. (2007) 'The content validity of juvenile psychopathy: An empirical examination,' *Psychological Assessment*, *19*:363–367.

Lynam, D. R., Gaughan, E., Miller, J. D., Miller, D., Mullins-Sweat, S., and Widiger, T. A. (2011) 'Assessing the basic traits associated with psychopathy: Development and validation of the Elemental Psychopathy Assessment,' *Psychological Assessment*, *23*:108–124.

Lynam, D. R., and Miller, J. D. (2012) 'Fearless Dominance and psychopathy: Response to Lilienfeld et al.,' *Personality Disorders: Theory, Research, and Treatment*, *3*:341–353.

Lynam, D. R., Sherman, E., Samuel, D., Miller, J. D., Few, L. R., and Widiger, T. A. (2013) 'Development of a short form of the Elemental Psychopathy Assessment,' *Assessment*, *20*:659–669.

Lynam, D. R., and Widiger, T. A. (2007) 'Using a general model of personality to identify the basic elements of psychopathy,' *Journal of Personality Disorders*, *21*:160–178.

Marcus, D. K., Fulton, J. J., and Edens, J. F. (2013) 'The two-factor model of psychopathic personality: Evidence from the Psychopathic Personality Inventory,' *Personality Disorders: Theory, Research, and Treatment*, *4*:67–76.

McCrae, R. R., Terracciano, A., & 78 members of the Personality Profiles of Cultures Project. (2005) 'Universal features of personality traits from the observer's perspective: Data from 50 cultures,' *Journal of Personality and Social Psychology*, *88*:547–561.

Meier, B. P., Robinson, M. D., and Wilkowski, B. M. (2006) 'Turning the other cheek: Agreeableness and the regulation of aggression-related primes,' *Psychological Science*, *17*:136–142.

Miller, J. D., Lamkin, J., Maples-Keller, J. L., and Lynam, D. R. (2016) 'Viewing the triarchic model of psychopathy through general personality and expert-based lenses,' *Personality Disorders: Theory, Research, and Treatment*, 7:247–258.

Miller, J. D., and Lynam, D. R. (2003) 'Psychopathy and the five-factor model of personality: A replication and extension,' *Journal of Personality Assessment*, *81*:168–178.

Miller, J. D., and Lynam, D. R. (2012) 'An examination of the Psychopathic Personality Inventory's nomological network: A meta-analytic review,' *Personality Disorders: Theory, Research, and Treatment*, *3*:305–326.

Miller, J. D., Lynam, D., Zimmerman, R. S., Logan, T. K., Leukefeld, C., and Clayton, R. (2004) 'The utility of the Five Factor Model in understanding risky sexual behavior,' *Personality and Individual Differences*, *36*:1611–1626.

Miller, J. D., Gaughan, E. T., Maples, J., Gentile, B., Lynam, D. R., and Widiger, T. A. (2011a) 'Examining the Construct Validity of the Elemental Psychopathy Assessment,' *Assessment*, *18*:106–114.

Miller, J. D., Hyatt, C. S., Rausher, S., Maples, J. L., and Zeichner, A. (2014) 'A test of the construct validity of the Elemental Psychopathy Assessment scores in a community sample of adults,' *Psychological Assessment, 26*:555–562.

Miller, J. D., Jones, S. E., and Lynam, D. R. (2011b) 'Psychopathic traits from the perspective of self and informant reports: Is there evidence for a lack of insight?,' *Journal of Abnormal Psychology, 120*:758–764.

Miller, J. D., Lynam, D. R., and Jones, S. (2008) 'Externalizing behavior through the lens of the five-factor model: A focus on agreeableness and conscientiousness,' *Journal of Personality Assessment, 90*:158–164.

Miller, J. D., Lynam, D. R., Widiger, T. A., and Leukefeld, C. (2001) 'Personality disorders as extreme variants of common personality dimensions: Can the Five-Factor Model adequately represent psychopathy?,' *Journal of Personality, 69*:253–276.

Miller, J. D., Lynam, D., and Leukefeld, C. (2003) 'Examining antisocial behavior through the lens of the five factor model of personality,' *Aggressive Behavior, 29*:497–514.

Miller, J. D., Wilson, L. F., Hyatt, C. S., and Zeichner, A. (2015) 'Psychopathic traits and aggression: Which trait components predict aggressive responding in a laboratory task?,' *Personality and Individual Differences, 87*:180–184.

Ozer, D. J., and Benet-Martínez, V. (2006) 'Personality and the prediction of consequential outcomes,' *Annual Review of Psychology, 57*:401–421.

Patrick, C. J. (Ed.) (2006) *Handbook of psychopathy*, New York, NY: Guilford Press.

Patrick, C. J. (2010) *Operationalizing the triarchic conceptualization of psychopathy: Preliminary description of brief scales for assessment of boldness, meanness, and disinhibition.* Unpublished manual. Tallahassee, FL: Florida State University.

Patrick, C. J., Fowles, D. C., and Krueger, R. F. (2009) 'Triarchic conceptualization of psychopathy: Developmental origins of disinhibition, boldness, and meanness,' *Development and Psychopathology, 21*:913–938.

Paulhus, D. L., Robins, R. W., Trzesniewski, K. H., and Tracy, J. L. (2004) 'Two replicable suppressor situations in personality research,' *Multivariate Behavioral Research, 39*:303–328.

Raskin, R., and Terry, H. (1988) 'A principal–components analysis of the Narcissistic Personality Inventory and further evidence of its construct validity,' *Journal of Personality and Social Psychology, 54*:890–902.

Reidy, D. E., Foster, J. D., and Zeichner, A. (2010) 'Narcissism and unprovoked aggression,' *Aggressive Behavior, 36*:414–422.

Roberts, B. W., and DelVecchio, W. F. (2000) 'The rank-order consistency of personality traits from childhood to old age: A quantitative review of longitudinal studies,' *Psychological Bulletin, 126*:3–25.

Ross, S. R., Benning, S. D., Patrick, C. J., Thompson, A., and Thurston, A. (2009) 'Factor of the Psychopathic Personality Inventory: Criterion-related validity and relationship to the BIS/BAS and five-factor models of personality,' *Assessment, 16*:71–87.

Seigfried-Spellar, K. C., Villacís-Vukadinović, N., and Lynam, D. R. (2017) 'Computer criminal behavior is related to psychopathy and other antisocial behavior,' *Journal of Criminal Justice, 51*:67–73.

Skeem, J. L., and Cooke, D. J. (2010) 'One measure does not a construct make: Directions toward reinvigorating psychopathy research – reply to Hare and Neumann (2010),' *Psychological Assessment, 22*:455–459.

Skeem, J. L., Miller, J. D., Mulvey, E., Tiemann, J., and Monahan, J. (2005) 'Using a five-factor lens to explore the relation between personality traits and violence in psychiatric patients,' *Journal of Consulting and Clinical Psychology, 73*:454–465.

Twenge, J. M., and Campbell, W. K. (2003) 'Isn't it fun to get the respect that we're going to deserve? Narcissism, social rejection, and aggression,' *Personality and Social Psychology Bulletin, 29*:261–272.

Vachon, D. D, Lynam, D. R., Widiger, T. A., Miler, J. D., McCrae, R. R., and Costa, P. T. (2013) 'Basic traits predict the prevalence of personality disorder across the lifespan: The example of psychopathy,' *Psychological Science, 24*:698–705.

Walton, K. E., Roberts, B. W., Krueger, R. F., Blonigen, D. M., and Hicks, B. M. (2008) 'Capturing abnormal personality with normal personality inventories: An item response theory approach,' *Journal of Personality, 76*:1623–1648.

Weiss, B., and Miller, J. D. (in press) 'Distinguishing between grandiose narcissism, vulnerable narcissism, and narcissistic personality disorder,' in J. D. Foster, A. Brunell, & T. Hermann (Eds.), *The handbook of trait narcissism: Key advances, research methods, and controversies*, New York, NY: Springer.

Whiteside, S. P., and Lynam, D. R. (2001) 'The five factor model and impulsivity: Using a structural model of personality to understand impulsivity,' *Personality and Individual Differences, 30*:669–689.

Widiger, T. A., and Lynam, D. R. (1998) 'Psychopathy and the Five-Factor Model of personality,' in T. Millon, E. Simonson, M. Birket-Smith, & R. D. Davis (Eds.), *Psychopathy: Antisocial, criminal, and violent behavior* (pp. 171–187), New York, NY: Guilford Press.

Wilson, L., Miller, J. D., Zeichner, A., Lynam, D. R., and Widiger, T. A. (2011) 'An examination of the validity of the Elemental Psychopathy Assessment: Relations with other psychopathy measures, aggression, and externalizing behaviors,' *Journal of Psychopathology and Behavioral Assessment*, *33*:315–322.
Yamagata, S., Suzuki, A., Ando, J., Ono, Y., Kijima, N., Yoshimura, K., . . ., Jang, K. L. (2006) 'Is the genetic structure of human personality universal? A cross-cultural twin study from North America, Europe, and Asia,' *Journal of Personality and Social Psychology*, *90*:987–998.

13

Key findings and operational lessons in the measurement of psychopathy within the incarcerated serious and violent young offender study

Raymond R. Corrado and Evan McCuish

Introduction

The purpose of the current chapter is to review key findings from the Incarcerated Serious and Violent Young Offender Study (ISVYOS), with specific attention to what has been learned about the assessment of psychopathy within an adolescent offender population. The ISVYOS first received grant funding in 1998 from Canada's Social Sciences and Humanities Research Council (SSHRC). This initial grant was followed by four successive grants from SSHRC to continue the project, the most recent coming in spring 2016. Since most criminological studies primarily sampled from community populations of adolescents with relatively small subsamples of serious offenders, the research design of the ISVYOS involved a sample of primarily serious and/or violent incarcerated adolescent offenders. Essentially, the principal investigator (the lead author of this chapter) sought to forego the benefits of generalizability to explanations of delinquent behavior within high school populations in favor of a research design that facilitated a better understanding of the most serious and violent adolescent offenders. The objectives of this study thus focused on the role of key criminological constructs from a range of theories in explaining an array of serious and violent behaviors within custody centers as well as recidivism in the community. Another objective included examining the impact of intervention programs and other experiences that took place within the custody center.

Between 1998 and 2011, a series of interviews were conducted with approximately 1,400 adolescents incarcerated throughout different facilities in the province of British Columbia, Canada. In addition to the measurement of constructs core to classic criminological theories (e.g., family dynamics, school behavior, substance use, peer networks), a unique feature of this study was its role in helping to validate the Psychopathy Checklist: Youth Version (PCL: YV; Forth, 1995; Forth, Kosson, & Hare, 2003), one of the first standardized measures of adolescent psychopathic personality disturbance (PPD). The term PPD is used in place of psychopathy/psychopath given that personality is not fully formed in adolescence and symptoms are only moderately stable over this age (e.g., Hawes, Mulvey, Schubert, & Pardini, 2014). Since the implementation of this instrument, two other measures of PPD were also administered as part of the ISVYOS interview protocol[1]: the Antisocial Process Screening Device (APSD; Frick & Hare, 2001) and the Comprehensive Assessment of Psychopathic Personality–Institutional Rating Scale (CAPP–IRS; Cooke, Hart, Logan, & Michie, 2012).

The purpose of the present chapter is to review the key empirical findings from the ISVYOS as they relate to issues of reliability, structural validity, convergent validity, and predictive validity of this controversial theoretical construct in explaining serious and violent young offending patterns offenders. As well, inspired by Schubert et al. (2004), we discuss operational lessons that have emerged from the administration of measures of PPD over the course of the ISVYOS, including challenges with scoring these measures within an adolescent offender group. First, to provide a backdrop to key findings and operational lessons, the research design of the ISVYOS is described in greater detail.

The incarcerated serious and violent young offender study

The ISVYOS originated from theoretical and policy concerns related to the consistent identification in all the major cohort studies of the second half of the twentieth century of a small (i.e., single digit) percentage of delinquents that most frequently committed the most serious crimes (e.g., the Cambridge Study in Delinquent Development, the Philadelphia and Racine Birth Cohort Studies, the Denver Youth Survey, the Rochester Youth Development Study, the Pittsburgh Youth Study). It was this core group of serious and violent delinquents or young offenders that caused major political controversies throughout western industrialized nations concerning whether to transition towards more punitive, deterrence-based models of youth justice. The welfare model of juvenile justice laws originated in the first decade of the twentieth century in these countries but, by the end of the 1960s, initial research emerged that challenged the effectiveness of this approach to protect the public, especially regarding the above core group of violent delinquents. Laws in many U.S. states reduced the maximum age for juvenile justice jurisdiction and/or introduced mandatory waivers of violent older juvenile offenders to adult criminal courts.

Several theoretical issues associated with these serious and violent young offender (SVYO) trends were: (1) was there a specifiable set or pattern of beliefs that distinguished the motivations of SVYOs (e.g., rational choice, intense deviant peer pressures, moral disengagement), (2) what was the association of family structure and functioning with SVYOs, (3) were personality disorders evident, PPD in particular, among this group, (4) was there an association (harmful or beneficial) of government programs before, during, and post-incarceration, (5) was a pattern of neurological developmental disorders evident (e.g., fetal alcohol spectrum disorder [FASD]), and (6) what was the developmental course of criminal offending patterns that continued into adulthood? It was at this point that the lead author proposed a research project on several of these controversial themes regarding violent young offenders to the federal government of Canada's primary funding agency for research on crime, SSHRC.

Given that the classic cohort studies within criminology typically involved community studies with very small subsamples of serious and violent offenders (c.f., the Pathways to Desistance Study), the proposed ISVYOS research design focused on a sample of incarcerated youth to ensure that a sufficient range of SVYOs was captured to more fully address the types of theoretical questions described above. The focus of this chapter is on the contribution of the ISVYOS to explanations of SVYOs using PPD as the key theoretical construct of interest. Three related key theoretical PPD themes were: (1) whether PPD could be assessed validly in a sample of adolescents, (2) if evident, whether this personality disturbance was as powerfully predictive as it has been pertaining to serious and violent adult offenders, and (3) whether an assessment instrument utilizing a six-domain model of PPD could be validated in an adolescent sample. A more detailed breakdown of the study's methodology is described below.

Sample

The ISVYOS sample is separated into two cohorts based on the time of their recruitment to participate in the study. Cohort One includes approximately 500 participants, all of whom were recruited between 1998–2002, the time at which the *Young Offender's Act* (YOA) was the legislation that governed Canada's youth justice system. Cohort Two includes approximately 900 participants, all of whom were recruited between 2005–2011, the time at which the *Youth Criminal Justice Act* (YCJA) was the legislation that governed Canada's youth justice system. The YCJA was brought into law at least in part because adolescents were incarcerated at an inordinate rate under the YOA (Bala, Carrington, & Roberts, 2009). In both cohorts, females amount to approximately 15 percent of the sample, and approximately 25 percent of youth self-reported an Indigenous ethnic background. On average, youth were approximately age 16 at the time of their recruitment. For Cohort One, youth were recruited from a variety of different incarceration facilities within the Greater Vancouver Regional District (GVRD) in the province of British Columbia. A key principle of the YCJA involved a reduction in the use of custody for adolescent offenders. Consequently, at the time of data collection for Cohort Two, several of the custody facilities from Cohort One were no longer in existence. Instead, youth from Cohort Two were recruited from the lone youth custody center within the GVRD, located in Burnaby, as well as from the lone youth custody center on Vancouver Island, located in provincial capital city Victoria.

Procedure and interview schedule

The study received research ethics approval from the British Columbia Ministry of Child and Family Development (MCFD) as well as the Simon Fraser University research ethics board. MCFD is the legal guardian to all incarcerated youth in British Columbia, and this ministry gave consent to the research team to approach all incarcerated youth to participate in the ISVYOS. Following ethics approval, youth were approached in their unit in the custody center by research assistants (RAs). Approximately halfway through the study, refusal rates were recorded and revealed that approximately 5 percent of approached youth refused to participate. Informed assent was acquired from participating youth after an RA distributed and read aloud an information sheet describing the purpose of the study, how information would be collected (e.g., interview and file information), and that all information would be kept confidential apart from direct threats made against themselves or someone else. To help ensure confidentiality, participants were interviewed in an isolated room away from other youth and staff. Participants were told that their participation or non-participation would not affect the outcome of their trial/sentence, nor would it affect their treatment from staff while in custody.

For all participating youth, a structured intake interview was first performed. Over the course of the study, especially between Cohort One and Cohort Two, the intake interview varied slightly. However, all versions of the intake interview measured demographic characteristics, school behavior, family history, involvement with drugs and alcohol, involvement in aggressive behaviors, and perceptions of self-identity. For Cohort One, the completion of the intake interview was followed by the administration of the PCL: YV and the APSD. For Cohort Two, a wider range of interviews that followed the intake interview were completed to assess a broader range of domains (e.g., mental health issues, family functioning, foster care experiences, gang involvement, custody experiences, and treatment programming). For Cohort Two, also following the intake interview, the PCL: YV and CAPP–IRS were administered. The PCL: YV, APSD, and CAPP–IRS are discussed below.

Measures

The PCL family, which includes the PCL: YV, is often considered the gold standard with respect to the measurement of PPD. The manualized version of the PCL: YV was not available prior to 2003. As such, all PCL: YV assessments from Cohort One (*n* = 358) used the version developed by Forth (1995), and all assessments from Cohort Two (*n* = 184) used the version developed by Forth et al. (2003). Both versions of the PCL: YV included identical items with slightly different scoring rules for criminal behavior items (see Vincent, Odgers, McCormick, & Corrado, 2008). The PCL: YV is scored by a trained "expert" rater and was created to capture interpersonal, affective, and behavioral symptoms of PPD in adolescence. The 20 items of the PCL: YV are scored on a 0–2 scale (0 = item does not apply, 1 = item applies somewhat, 2 = item definitely applies) using information from a 60–90-minute semi-structured interview with the participant and a review of file information. Across the two cohorts, PCL: YV assessments were completed when the participant was approximately 17 years of age and the average score was approximately 20 out of 40, showing that participants from the ISVYOS averaged moderate symptoms of PPD. Approximately 25 percent of PCL: YV assessments involved Indigenous participants and 15 percent involved females, which resembled ethnic and gender breakdowns for the full sample.

The APSD was completed only for participants from Cohort One. A total of 100 youth completed this assessment, all of whom were male and were recruited three years after the start of the ISVYOS. The age and ethnicity of this subsample resembled the larger study. The APSD is like the PCL: YV in three ways: both were modeled after the PCL–R, both include items rated between 0–2, and both include a total of 20 items. Unlike the PCL: YV, the APSD is a self-report instrument. A PCL: YV assessment was administered for all participants with an APSD to allow for examinations of convergent validity. Participants averaged a score of 18.66 out of 40 on the APSD, which was also similar to participants' average score on the PCL: YV.

The CAPP–IRS was completed only for participants from Cohort Two. Thus far, ratings have been completed for a total of 272 youth, approximately 15 percent of whom are female. Indigenous youth represented approximately 30 percent of all participants that received a CAPP–IRS rating. The CAPP–IRS was based on the CAPP conceptual model developed by Cooke et al. (2004) in response to the observed need (e.g., Cooke & Michie, 2001; Skeem & Cooke, 2010) to make the assessment of PPD more inclusive of interpersonal and affective symptoms of the disorder and to avoid using criminal behavior as part of the measurement procedure. This conceptual model of PPD was developed using a lexical, "bottom-up" approach, in which the authors relied on clinical and research literature as well as surveys of clinicians to identify potential symptoms. Over-inclusiveness was favored as part of this approach based on the logic that statistical analysis could be used to cull irrelevant items. Thus, the CAPP–IRS is more likely to measure symptoms irrelevant to the disorder than it is to exclude symptoms relevant to the disorder. The CAPP conceptual model and its measurement tool, the CAPP–IRS, are defined by 33 symptoms that fall within six conceptual domains: attachment, Behavior, Cognitive, Dominance, Emotion, and Self. These 33 symptoms are rated on a 0–6 scale, and each symptom includes three adjectival descriptors thought to be related, but not identical, to the symptom being measured (see Cooke et al., 2004 for a detailed description). The symptoms can be scored using a fixed time-period (e.g., their strength over the last year) or based on lifetime severity. The latter strategy was used in the ISVYOS.

One of the principal aims in administering these different measures was to evaluate their predictive validity. To this end, offending outcomes were measured at each year of age between age 12 until the age at the end of the most recent data collection period (spring 2017). Offending outcomes were collected through CORNET, a software program that records, among other things, all criminal charges incurred within the province of British Columbia. In addition to the exact date, type of sentence, and crime-type, CORNET also includes the date of entry and date of exit from custody, which has allowed the study to control for exposure time. CORNET also included information on mortality and movements outside of British Columbia to control for instances of false desistance where an offender stops offending due to inopportunity (e.g., Eggleston, Laub, & Sampson, 2004). Using data collected from CORNET, the ISVYOS has examined the relationship between PPD and recidivism, PPD and types of offenders, and PPD and offending trajectories.

The reliability and validity of the PCL: YV, APSD, and CAPP–IRS

For each of the three instruments for which data are published, interrater reliability, internal reliability, structural validity (e.g., factor structure), convergent validity, discriminant validity, and predictive validity are discussed for Cohort One and Cohort Two (where applicable). Findings are also briefly summarized in Table 13.1.

Reliability and validity of the PCL: YV

In Cohort One, interrater reliability of the PCL: YV was evaluated based on 30 randomly selected cases coded by six raters who conducted interviews with these youth in pairs. Using intraclass correlation coefficients (ICC) for a two-way random effects model for absolute groups, the ICC was good for total scores (0.92) and adequate for Factor 1 (0.82) and Factor 2 (0.89). PCL: YV data for Cohort Two have not yet been published, but using the same method for calculating ICCs as used for Cohort One, based on paired ratings for nine youth, ICC was excellent for total scores (0.99). Different studies on the internal reliability of PCL: YV total scores and factor scores from Cohort One all report moderate to high internal consistency per Cronbach's alpha values. In a study that combined participants from Cohorts One and Two, McCuish, Mathesius, Lussier, and Corrado (2017) also showed that the internal consistency of PCL: YV was equally high across Indigenous and White youth. Using confirmatory factor analyses (CFA), this study found that both the three-factor and four-factor representations of the PCL: YV were a good fit to the full sample and that both factor structures were invariant across Indigenous and White youth. Several studies emerging from the ISVYOS examined convergent validity between the PCL: YV and other PPD instruments. As the PCL: YV is the gold standard to which the other instruments are compared, convergent validity is discussed in the sections that follow.

Given that a principal purpose of measuring PPD within the ISVYOS was to evaluate the construct's contribution to mainstream criminological theory, a substantial area of focus was on the predictive validity of the PCL: YV. Evaluations of predictive validity have measured offending outcomes based on recidivism, types of crime (e.g., sex offending, institutional misconduct), and offending trajectories. Beginning with recidivism outcomes, Corrado, Vincent, Hart, and Cohen (2004) studied the relationship between PCL: YV test scores and different types of recidivism outcomes among 182 males from the ISVYOS who were followed for an average of 14.5 months following release from custody. Controlling for age and ethnicity, PCL: YV

Table 13.1 Summary of key findings on three PPD instruments across both cohorts from the ISVYOS

	PCL: YV		*APSD*		*CAPP–IRS*	
	Cohort 1	*Cohort 2*	*Cohort 1*	*Cohort 2*	*Cohort 1*	*Cohort 2*
Interrater reliability	Total score ICC = .92	Total score ICC = .99	–	–	–	Total score ICC = .91
Internal reliability	Total score CA = .82 (boys); .70 (girls)	Total score CA = .81†	Total score CA = .77	–	–	Total score CA = .89
Structural validity	Support for three-factor model†† Four-cluster solution per *K*-means†††	Support for both a three- and four-factor model†	Weak support for three-factor model††††	–	–	Conceptual six-domain model a poor fit to the data; some support for a seven-domain model†††††
Convergent validity	Small to moderate *r* with APSD	High *r* with CAPP–IRS	Small to moderate *r* with PCL: YV	–	–	High *r* with PCL: YV; positive *r* with MACI–PCS
Discriminant validity	–	–	–	–	–	Negative *r* with anxiety
Predictive validity	Predicted recidivism for with males but not females; predicted offending trajectories	Predicted recidivism across White and Indigenous youth†	–	–	–	–

Note. ICC = intraclass correlation coefficient; CA = Cronbach's alpha; – = not applicable (either analysis not applicable, data unavailable, or not yet examined); PCL: YV = Psychopathy Checklist: Youth Version; APSD = Antisocial Process Screening Device; CAPP–IRS = Comprehensive Assessment of Psychopathic Personality–Institutional Rating Scale; MACI–PCS = Millon Adolescent Clinical Inventory Psychopathy Content Scale.

† Based on combined sample of both Cohort 1 and 2 (see McCuish et al., 2017); †† Vincent (unpublished doctoral dissertation); ††† Vincent et al. (2003); †††† Lee et al. (2003); ††††† McCormick (2015).

test scores, regardless of whether they were represented by a two-factor or three-factor model, significantly predicted both nonviolent and violent recidivism following release from custody. Using a cut-score of 28, high scores on the PCL: YV significantly reduced time until nonviolent and violent recidivism, and this was true for both the two-factor model and three-factor model.

Vincent, Vitacco, Grisso, and Corrado (2003) cluster-analyzed a group of males from Cohort One that received a PCL: YV rating. Using *K*-means cluster analysis of the three-factor model, four groups were specified and were named "Low traits cluster" (n = 74), "Callous–deceitful cluster" (n = 63), "Impulsive cluster" (n = 75), and "Psychopathic traits cluster" (n = 47). The latter cluster had the highest rates of general, nonviolent, and violent recidivism and had the shortest survival period for each outcome. The Impulsive cluster differed only from the Low traits cluster with respect to time until any recidivism. The findings supported the notion that PPD can contribute to explanations of offending beyond measures capturing elements of low self-control. Vincent et al. (2003) noted that the Impulsive cluster may be better suited to explanations of adolescent-limited offending, whereas the Psychopathic traits cluster was more suited to explanations of life course persistent offending.

Other studies using ISVYOS data examined the predictive validity of the PCL: YV across gender and ethnicity. With respect to gender, Vincent et al. (2008) compared the predictive validity of both the three-factor and four-factor models across males (n = 201) and females (n = 55) from Cohort One. Regardless of how test scores were represented, the PCL: YV was neither a significant predictor of general, nonviolent, nor violent recidivism for females. The opposite was observed for males, with all representations of test scores significantly increasing the odds of all recidivism outcomes. A series of Cox regression analyses separated by gender essentially replicated the above findings, showing that PCL: YV test scores were associated with significant decreases in time until recidivism for males but not for females. Vincent et al. (2008) questioned the applicability of the PCL: YV to females, noting that most instruments measuring PPD were developed and validated using male samples. The authors also questioned the utility of the PCL: YV with respect to making longer-term predictions about offending and with respect to the efficacy of the instrument's interpersonal and affective factors in predicting recidivism.

Looking at whether PCL: YV test scores functioned similarly across Indigenous and White youth, McCuish et al. (2017) examined whether PCL: YV test scores predicted general and violent recidivism in emerging adulthood (ages 18–23) and mature adulthood (ages 24–28). Overall, results tended to show that across both White and Indigenous participants, regardless of whether PCL: YV total scores, four-factor model scores, or three-factor model scores were examined, significant area under the curve (AUC) values were observed when predicting general and violent recidivism in emerging adulthood. For mature adulthood, the relationship between PCL: YV test scores and recidivism was less robust. For Indigenous youth, each representation of PCL: YV test scores (e.g., total, four-factor, and three-factor) predicted neither general nor violent recidivism in mature adulthood. For White youth, only PCL: YV total scores and four-factor scores predicted general recidivism, and none of the representations of PCL: YV test scores predicted violent recidivism. Nevertheless, overall, McCuish et al. (2017) suggested that the PCL: YV functioned equally well across Indigenous and White youth in terms of predicting recidivism outcomes in emerging adulthood. Other studies using ISVYOS data have examined more nuanced patterns of offending through emerging adulthood and mature adulthood.

In two separate studies, PCL: YV test scores from the ISVYOS were used to predict association with general offending trajectories (Corrado, McCuish, Hart, & DeLisi, 2015) and joint trajectories of violent and nonviolent offending (McCuish, Corrado, Hart, & DeLisi, 2015). Both analyses measured number of convictions incurred at each age between ages 12–28. Additional details about the two studies are discussed in another chapter in this book regarding the relationship between PPD and offending trajectories and thus we do not expand on the findings here. Importantly, however, both studies showed that controlling for demographic characteristics and other important risk and protective factors, the three-factor model of the PCL: YV, which excludes criminal behavior items, significantly predicted association with the highest rate general and violent offending trajectories identified for the sample. Such findings contrasted with previous research suggesting that the PCL: YV was uninformative of longer-term offending patterns. The difference between these and other studies may be related to the focus on recidivism versus offending trajectories, with the latter better capturing more serious patterns of offending. The study by McCuish et al. (2015) also showed that the relationship between PCL: YV test scores and chronic violent offending was principally related to the interpersonal and affective factors, which contrasted from prior recidivism-based studies, where items capturing criminal and behavioral problems were dominant (e.g., Corrado et al., 2004; Vincent et al., 2008). These two trajectory studies were in line with Vincent et al.'s (2003) conceptual description of PPD as a key explanatory variable for life course persistent offending and the need to look beyond hyperactive, impulsive, and attention-deficit traits.

Lastly, Cale, Lussier, McCuish and Corrado (2015) examined the relationship between PCL: YV test scores and sex offending outcomes, and Shaffer, McCuish, Corrado, Behnken, and DeLisi (2015) looked at involvement in institutional misconduct. Combining data from Cohort One and Two, Cale et al. (2015) showed that adolescents adjudicated for a sex offense had significantly higher scores on the PCL: YV's interpersonal and affective factors but not the lifestyle and antisocial factors. This latter finding was interesting given that a common finding both within the ISVYOS and across other PCL: YV studies was that the lifestyle and antisocial factors were most informative of general offending (e.g., Edens, Campbell, & Weir, 2007). With respect to examining institutional misbehavior, Shaffer et al. (2015) found that youth scoring high on the PCL: YV are at an increased likelihood of greater general misconduct as well as violent misconduct, though the effect sizes per AUC values were relatively small. Nevertheless, the studies by Cale et al. (2015) and Shaffer et al. (2015) helped illustrate that PPD may be helpful in explanations of more narrow forms of behavior in addition to general or violent offending.

The reliability and validity of the APSD

Lee, Vincent, Hart, and Corrado (2003) examined the reliability and validity of the APSD among a subsample of 100 males from the ISVYOS. The study was unique in that it allowed for an examination of one of the first self-report measures of adolescent PPD against the gold-standard, expert rating-based PCL: YV. The internal consistency of APSD total scores was adequate (Cronbach's α = .77) but the mean inter-item correlation was just 0.14. As well, the internal consistency of the three APSD subscales was lower than what is typically observed for the four factors of the PCL: YV (narcissism = .66; Callous–Unemotional = .48; impulsivity = .57). Lee et al. (2003) found just small to moderate correlations between the APSD and PCL: YV when examining correlations between total scores and correlations between factor scores. As well, convergent validity was affected by age, with correlations between the two measures decreasing when examining younger participants.

Given the similarities between the three-factor APSD model and the three-factor PCL: YV model, Lee et al. (2003) used CFA to examine whether method of assessment affected measurement of the latent trait. These authors observed that allowing the three factors scores of the APSD to load separately onto two method factors (i.e., clinical rating versus self-report) showed a significant improvement in model fit compared to a model where factor scores loaded onto two separate superordinate trait factors. Lee et al. (2003) suggested that this method effect, combined with the APSD's low correlations with the PCL: YV, implied that the APSD had low validity as a measure of adolescent PPD. To this point, the predictive validity of the APSD has not been examined among ISVYOS participants.

The reliability and validity of the CAPP–IRS

The CAPP–IRS is the newest of the three PPD measures and was only administered to a subsample of participants from Cohort Two. Studies were published while data collection remained ongoing, and thus there are differences in sample size across the reported studies. Interrater reliability was established by McCormick (2007). Using three pairs of raters to assess 30 participants, interrater reliability was excellent for total scores (ICC = 0.91) and adequate to excellent for domain scores (ICC 0.69–0.86). That ICC values were similar to the PCL: YV despite the CAPP–IRS using a wider 7-point scale is particularly important. Using this small subsample, McCormick (2007) also showed that apart from the Behavioral domain, domain scores were moderately to highly correlated with each other. The Dominance domain was most strongly correlated with CAPP–IRS total scores (r = .90).

Dawson, McCuish, Hart, and Corrado (2012) identified two youth from the ISVYOS expressed by clinical staff to be characterized by PPD. Consistent with the opinion of clinical staff, Dawson et al. (2012) observed that both youth scored high on the PCL: YV and the CAPP–IRS. The raters observed that between-case heterogeneity in symptom profiles was better captured by the CAPP–IRS because of its inclusion of a greater number of symptoms (33 versus 20) and broader rating scale (0–6 versus 0–2). In effect, ratings using the PCL: YV showed the two cases as showing relatively similar personality profiles, whereas ratings using the CAPP–IRS identified some relatively different personality profiles. Whereas the CAPP–IRS captured a more complex personality profile, the PCL: YV took less time to administer. The raters also noted that rating the Self domain of the CAPP–IRS was less challenging when the participant had stronger verbal skills and was older in age.

Building from the above studies, McCormick (2015) used classical test theory techniques to evaluate the internal structure of the CAPP–IRS among male and female youth (n = 185). Using domain scores, the internal consistency of the CAPP–IRS was excellent (Cronbach's α = .89) and corrected item–total correlation values between each domain, and CAPP–IRS total scores were all moderate to strong (r = .661–.761). Similar findings were observed when internal consistency and corrected item–total correlations were examined separately across gender. This finding was particularly important given the challenges with measuring PPD among female youth (Forouzan & Cooke, 2005). Looking within the six domains, Cronbach's α and corrected item–total correlations were lowest within the Behavior and Cognitive domains. Across the six domains, Attachment–Emotion, Dominance–Self, and Behavior–Cognitive pairings formed the strongest between-domain correlations, which was not surprising in that these three pairings resembled the interpersonal, affective, and lifestyle factors of the PCL: YV three-factor model.

The validity of the conceptually based six-domain representation of the CAPP was empirically tested using the CAPP–IRS. Using the male subsample, a CFA conducted by McCormick (2015) showed that this conceptual model was not an adequate fit to the data. This may be in part related to the purposeful over-inclusiveness of symptoms that characterize the CAPP model and in part related to inadequate sample size (n = 147). An exploratory factor analysis (EFA) showed that 28 symptoms loaded onto seven factors, with five symptoms failing to have a factor loading above .45. The seven factors were labeled Grandiose, Impulsive, Emotionless, Hostile, Callous, Superficial, and Fearless. The internal structure of the seven factors showed high corrected item–total correlations and Cronbach's α values were also high.

Looking specifically at the male subsample, McCormick (2015) also showed that the six domains of the CAPP–IRS had convergent validity with PCL: YV test scores and also showed convergent and divergent validity with other measures of psychological functioning. Unlike the relationship between the APSD and PCL: YV, the correlation between CAPP–IRS and PCL: YV total scores was high (r = .733). In line with expectation, the Dominance and Self domains had the strongest correlation with the interpersonal factor of the PCL: YV (r = .747 and .664, respectively) and the attachment and Emotion domains had the strongest correlation with the affective factor of the PCL: YV (r = .752 and .762, respectively). Regarding convergent validity with other measures of personality, CAPP–IRS scores were positively correlated with scales on the Millon Adolescent Clinical Inventory (MACI; Murrie & Cornell, 2000) that tapped into forceful and oppositional personality patterns. In terms of divergent validity, CAPP–IRS total scores were negatively correlated with anxiety. Although the CAPP–IRS includes a lack of anxiety as a symptom of the Emotion domain, there is some debate over whether this symptom should be included (e.g., Dawson et al., 2012). In line with expectation, CAPP–IRS total scores were also negatively correlated with submissiveness and conformist subscales from the MACI. Unexpectedly, introversion and inhibition subscales from the MACI were positively correlated with CAPP–IRS total scores.

To this point, the predictive validity of the CAPP–IRS has been considered solely at a conceptual level, and thus the relationship between the CAPP–IRS and offending outcomes is not reported here.

The ISVYOS and operational lessons in the measurement of PPD

Several theoretical and related conceptual challenges emerged concerning the attempts to measure PPD in this sample of SVYOs. Operational lessons are separated in this section according to (1) predictive validity versus measurement validity issues, (2) tailoring interviews to the appropriate developmental stage of the participant, and (3) nuances in the scoring of the CAPP–IRS that remain especially challenging in the absence of a manual specific to youth offenders.

First, as reported above, while the ISVYOS and others that used the PCL: YV found considerable support for utilizing the PPD construct for adolescents, the key challenge remains: the strongest predictor consistently has been the grouping of PCL: YV items from the lifestyle and antisocial factors rather than the items defining the affective and interpersonal factors that are more prototypical of PPD. The issue, therefore, has been whether the PCL: YV is validly assessing PPD and whether it is appropriate to use offending outcomes as the key basis of establishing predictive validity. In other words, as measures of PPD better predict offending outcomes, they also seem to move further away from the measurement of personality symptoms and instead rely heavily on behavioral indicators and thus raise tautological concerns.

To reiterate, our conclusion was that PPD necessarily required the specification of more domains, related symptoms, and indicators of the latter to enhance its construct validity. The fundamental assertion that the measurement of PPD should move away from behavioral indicators of the disorder is perhaps most important with respect to adolescents because several of these are, if not normative, at least not atypical traits of this developmental stage (e.g., impulsivity, lying, sensation seeking, and risk-taking behavior). In other words, a more elaborate set of symptoms and indicators for traditional domains likely increases the ability to more validly measure and distinguish the apparent wider variations in such traits among adolescents. The additional domains in the CAPP too provide a more theoretically complex attempt to explain the not atypical contradictions, emotional lability, identity confusion/rapid change, and spontaneous Anger of the adolescent stage. Of course, compared to the PCL: YV, a more complex PPD construct and related instrument such as the CAPP–IRS inevitably is more challenging for clinicians and researchers to utilize, especially for adolescents, because of its increased number and subtler symptom indicators, as well as the increased interview time and collateral data needed to complete it. The increased interview time required to complete the CAPP–IRS is a related challenge to weighing measurement and predictive validity, as appropriate tests of both require larger samples to appropriately identify the theoretically predicted wide range of profile types that likely would emerge from the six-domain CAPP–IRS.

Second, both the PCL: YV and the version of the CAPP–IRS used in the ISVYOS were adapted from instruments validated with adult samples. For the CAPP–IRS, in consultation with the developers of the instrument, we adapted several of the interview questions to be more tailored to youth living in Canada. RAs first noted that questions about political orientation and associated issues that were meant to capture intolerant/inflexible symptoms from the Cognitive domain resulted in minimal responses from participants. New questions were posed that aimed to address intolerant attitudes more typical for the developmental stage of adolescence (e.g., attitudes towards certain high school cliques, etc.).

Another important lesson was in the challenge of assessing PPD, especially when using the CAPP–IRS, with respect to the relatively limited verbal abilities of youth, especially those of younger ages. RA experiences were that older youth and youth with higher verbal abilities tended to provide more detailed responses to interview questions compared to younger youth and those with lower verbal IQ. It may be necessary to train RAs on different interview strategies and associated scoring procedures depending on the distinctive adolescent stage of the participant (e.g., questions specific to early versus late adolescence). Along with verbal IQ deficits was the broader issue of the generally lengthy and complex CAPP–IRS interview protocol that raised reliability issues concerning the ability of adolescents, those with FASD/ADD/ADHD specifically, to focus and respond truthfully throughout the entire time-period. Extensive RA training is necessary to mitigate against these internal reliability threats and recognize participant fatigue, as well as their routine debriefs with senior project staff and systematic review of potential interview bias. These issues were mitigated in part by activities with the youth between interview sections (e.g., ping pong) or to end the interview altogether and return later. Although inconvenient and possibly perceived as a limitation of the CAPP–IRS, we also think that the administration of the CAPP–IRS has provided valuable information about the potentially more serious limitations of lengthy self-report inventories. If participants are experiencing lapses in concentration and bouts of fatigue during interactions with RAs, the same is likely to occur during the completion of self-report questionnaires. The main difference between these questionnaires and the CAPP–IRS interview is that researchers can be aware of, and respond to, issues that may occur during the interview.

Third, with respect to lessons learned in scoring the CAPP–IRS, another important training component involved being careful not to be influenced by criminal charges/convictions when scoring PPD symptoms. RAs were trained to focus on whether the symptom was present across multiple domains of functioning (e.g., school, family, friends) rather than whether the youth, for example, lacked remorse for their criminal behavior against a rival gang member but showed remorse across other areas. A second scoring issue related to the importance of being aware of the chaotic and dysfunctional familial relationships often characterizing SVYOs. For example, although a youth may show severe lack of caring for their father, their father may also be abusive, unsupportive, and/or absent from this youth's life. In fact, being uncaring and uncommitted to a person with such a negative influence of the youth's development may be a sign of a positive, protective factor against potential future criminal behavior.

Future research directions for the incorporation of PPD within criminology

DeLisi (2016) has more fully articulated his assertion that the psychopathy construct is essential to criminological theories. His theoretical perspective reflects the inadequacies of traditional criminological theories in explaining SVYOs. Arguably, these theories have provided convincing understanding of delinquencies but, with few and more recent exceptions (e.g., Agnew's strain theory, Wikstrom and Treiber's situational action theory), these theories have not incorporated complex personality disorder constructs asserted to be necessary to predicting and explaining the variations in SVYOs patterns (Corrado, DeLisi, Hart, & McCuish, 2015). These constructs have evolved substantially across the five versions of the Diagnostic and Statistical

Manual (DSM–5) developed by psychiatrists and psychologists for clinical practice and research. Studies involving custody samples indicated that serious mental disorders were common for this group (e.g., Teplin et al., 2005; Cesaroni & Pederson-Badali, 2005), yet the criminological theoretical and empirical literature has been slower to integrate mental disorder perspectives into explanations of offending. The advances in explicating Axis II personality disorders as outlined in the DSM–5 are extremely important for criminological theories of SVYOs partly because of the insights provided by genetic, epigenetic, and brain scanning technologies (DeLisi & Vaughn, 2015).

For SVYOs, these insights focus on several themes. First, criminological theories that emphasize rational choice now should incorporate evidence that brain maturation essential to self-control and reasoned thought/choices typically occurs around the mid-20s age-range (Corrado & Mathesius, 2014). Second, neurological developmental disorders such as autistic spectral and fetal alcohol have several traits in common with PPD, which confounds valid diagnostic assessments necessary to explaining the multiple pathways hypothesized to lead to SVYO patterns/trajectories. Third, brain plasticity possibly explains the relative instability of personality traits across developmental stages (Roberts & DelVecchio, 2000), and this too confounds valid diagnostic assessments and especially longer-term predictive validity studies using PPD as a key explanatory variable.

Note

1 The Psychopathy Checklist: Screening Version (Hart, Hare, & Cox, 1995) and the Psychopathy Content Scale from the Millon Adolescent Clinical Inventory (Murrie & Cornell, 2000) were also administered, but these data have not yet been analyzed and thus are not discussed in this chapter.

References

Bala, N., Carrington, P., and Roberts, J. (2009) 'Evaluating the YCJA after five years: A qualified success,' *Canadian Journal of Criminology and Criminal Justice, 51*(2):131–167.

Cale, J., Lussier, P., McCuish, E. C., and Corrado, R. R. (2015) 'The prevalence of psychopathic personality disturbances among incarcerated youth: Comparing serious, chronic, violent and sex offenders,' *Journal of Criminal Justice, 43*(4):337–344.

Cesaroni, C., and Peterson-Badali, M. (2005) 'Young offenders in custody: Risk and adjustment,' *Criminal Justice and Behavior, 32*:251–277.Cooke, D. J., Hart, S. D., Logan, C., and Michie, C. (2012) 'Explicating the construct of psychopathy: Development and validation of a conceptual model, the Comprehensive Assessment of Psychopathic Personality (CAPP),' *International Journal of Forensic Mental Health, 11*:242–252.

Cooke, D. J., and Michie, C. (2001) 'Refining the construct of psychopathy: Towards a hierarchical model,' *Psychological Assessment, 13*(2):171–188.

Cooke, D. J., Michie, C., Hart, S. D., and Clark, D. A. (2004) 'Reconstructing psychopathy: Clarifying the significance of antisocial and socially deviant behavior in the diagnosis of psychopathic personality disorder,' *Journal of Personality Disorders, 18*:337–357.

Corrado, R. R., DeLisi, M., Hart, S. D., and McCuish, E. C. (2015) 'Can the causal mechanisms underlying chronic, serious, and violent offending trajectories be elucidated using the psychopathy construct?,' *Journal of Criminal Justice, 43*:251–261.

Corrado, R. R., and Mathesius, J. (2014) 'Developmental psycho-neurological research trends and their importance for reassessing key decision-making assumptions for children, adolescents, and young adults in juvenile/youth and adult criminal justice systems,' *Bergen Journal of Criminal Law & Criminal, 2*(2):141–163.

Corrado, R. R., Vincent, G. M., Hart, S. D., and Cohen, I. M. (2004) 'Predictive validity of the Psychopathy Checklist: Youth Version for general and violent recidivism. *Behavioral Sciences & the Law, 22*(1):5–22.

Corrado, R. R., McCuish, E. C., Hart, S. D., and DeLisi, M. (2015) 'The role of psychopathic traits and developmental risk factors on offending trajectories from early adolescence to adulthood: A prospective study of incarcerated youth,' *Journal of Criminal Justice, 43*(4):357–368.

Dawson, S. E., McCuish, E. C., Hart, S. D., and Corrado, R. R. (2012) 'Critical issues in the assessment of adolescent psychopathy: An illustration using two case studies,' *International Journal of Forensic Mental Health*, *11*(2):63–79.

DeLisi, M. (2016) *Psychopathy as unified theory of crime*, New York, NY: Palgrave Macmillan.

DeLisi, M., and Vaughn, M. G. (2015) 'Ingredients for criminality require genes, temperament, and psychopathic personality,' *Journal of Criminal Justice*, *43*(4):290–294.

Edens, J. F., Campbell, J. S., and Weir, J. M. (2007) 'Youth psychopathy and criminal recidivism: A meta-analysis of the psychopathy checklist measures,' *Law and Human Behavior*, *31*:53–75.

Eggleston, E. P., Laub, J. H., and Sampson, R. J. (2004) 'Methodological sensitivities to latent class analysis of long-term criminal trajectories,' *Journal of Quantitative Criminology*, *20*(1):1–25.

Forouzan, E., and Cooke, D. J. (2005) 'Figuring out la femme fatale: Conceptual and assessment issues concerning psychopathy in females,' *Behavioral Sciences & the Law*, *23*:765–778.

Forth, A. E. (1995) *Psychopathy and young offenders: Prevalence, family background, and violence*, Carleton University, Ottawa, Canada (Unpublished manuscript).

Forth, A. E., Kosson, D. S., and Hare, R. (2003) *The Hare Psychopathy Checklist: Youth Version*, New York, NY: Multi-Health Systems.

Frick, P. J., and Hare, R. D. (2001) *Antisocial Process Screening Device (APSD)*, Toronto, ON: Multi-Health Systems.

Hart, S. D., Hare, R. D., and Cox, D. N. (1995) *The Hare psychopathy checklist: Screening version (PCL: SV)*, Toronto, ON: Multi-Health Systems.

Hawes, S. W., Mulvey, E. P., Schubert, C. A., and Pardini, D. A. (2014) 'Structural coherence and temporal stability of psychopathic personality features during emerging adulthood,' *Journal of Abnormal Psychology*, *123*:623–633.

Lee, Z., Vincent, G. M., Hart, S. D., and Corrado, R. R. (2003) 'The validity of the Antisocial Process Screening Device as a self-report measure of psychopathy in adolescent offenders,' *Behavioral Sciences & the Law*, *21*(6):771–786.

McCormick, A. (2007) Interrater reliability of the comprehensive assessment of psychopathic personality disorder among a sample of incarcerated serious and violent young offenders (Doctoral dissertation, School of Criminology–Simon Fraser University).

McCormick, A. (2015) Validity of the comprehensive assessment of psychopathic personality disorder – Institutional rating scale in a Canadian sample of incarcerated serious and violent young offenders (Doctoral dissertation, Arts and Social Sciences: School of Criminology).

McCuish, E. C., Corrado, R. R., Hart, S. D., and DeLisi, M. (2015) 'The role of symptoms of psychopathy in persistent violence over the criminal career into full adulthood,' *Journal of Criminal Justice*, *43*:345–356.

McCuish, E. C., Mathesius, J. R., Lussier, P., and Corrado, R. R. (2017) 'The cross-cultural generalizability of the Psychopathy: Checklist Youth Version for adjudicated Indigenous youth,' *Psychological Assessment* (online first):1–12.

Murrie, D. C., and Cornell, D. G. (2000) 'The Millon Adolescent Clinical Inventory and psychopathy,' *Journal of Personality Assessment*, *75*(1):110–125.

Roberts, B. W., and DelVecchio, W. F. (2000) 'The rank-order consistency of personality traits from childhood to old age: A quantitative review of longitudinal studies,' *Psychological Bulletin*, *126*:3–25.

Schubert, C. A., Mulvey, E. P., Steinberg, L., Cauffman, E., Losoya, S. H., Hecker, T., . . ., and Knight, G. P. (2004) 'Operational lessons from the pathways to desistance project,' *Youth Violence and Juvenile Justice*, *2*(3):237–255.

Shaffer, C. S., McCuish, E. C., Corrado, R. R., Behnken, M. P., and DeLisi, M. (2015) 'Psychopathy and violent misconduct in a sample of violent young offenders,' *Journal of Criminal Justice*, *43*(4):321–326.

Skeem, J. L., and Cooke, D. J. (2010) 'Is criminal behavior a central component of psychopathy? Conceptual directions for resolving the debate,' *Psychological Assessment*, *22*(2):433–445.

Teplin, L. A., Elkington, K. S., McClelland, G. M., Abram, K. M., Mericle, A. A., and Washburn, J. J. (2005) 'Major mental disorders, substance use disorders, comorbidity, and HIV–AIDS risk behaviors in juvenile detainees,' *Psychiatric Services*, *56*:823–828.

Vincent, G. M., Odgers, C. L., McCormick, A. V., and Corrado, R. R. (2008) 'The PCL: YV and recidivism in male and female juveniles: A follow-up into young adulthood,' *International Journal of Law and Psychiatry*, *31*(3):287–296.

Vincent, G. M., Vitacco, M. J., Grisso, T., and Corrado, R. R. (2003) 'Subtypes of adolescent offenders: Affective traits and antisocial behavior patterns,' *Behavioral Sciences & the Law*, *21*(6):695–712.

14

Psychopathic Personality Traits Model (PPTM)

A new approach to defining psychopathy

Daniel Boduszek, Agata Debowska, and Dominic Willmott

Introduction

The concept of psychopathy, often conceptualized as the causal antecedent to violent offending, has long been of interest within the criminal justice system. Despite this, psychopathy has continued to be difficult to assess, with research in the area compromised by the absence of an established definition of the disorder (O'Kane, Fawcett, & Blackburn, 1996; Skeem, Polaschek, Patrick, & Lilienfeld, 2011). The first comprehensive conceptualization of psychopathy was proposed by Cleckley in 1941. Cleckley suggested the prototypical psychopath to be characterized by the following 16 traits: superficial charm, absence of delusions, absence of "nervousness," unreliability, untruthfulness, lack of remorse and shame, antisocial behavior, poor judgment and failure to learn by experience, pathological egocentricity, poverty in affective reactions, loss of insight, unresponsiveness in interpersonal relations, fantastic and uninviting behavior, rare suicidal behavior, impersonal sex life, and failure to follow any life plan.

This Cleckleyan representation of psychopathy served as the basis for designing some widely employed psychopathic assessment tools, such as the Psychopathy Checklist (PCL; Hare, 1980) and its updated version, the Psychopathy Checklist–Revised (PCL–R; Hare, 1991, 2003). The PCL–R is commonly presented as consisting of four correlated factors: (1) interpersonal manipulation, (2) callous affect, (3) Erratic Lifestyle, and (4) antisocial/criminal behavior. Psychopathy, as assessed using the PCL–R and associated measures, has been shown to be predictive of recidivism and aggression (see Dhingra & Boduszek, 2013 for a review). However, given that numerous items within the measure pertain directly to criminal and antisocial behavior alongside the suggestion that future behavior is best predicted by past behavior, such findings are not surprising. Indeed, the formulation of psychopathy as grasped by the PCL(–R) and its derivatives is weighted heavily towards indicators of behavioral expressions of the disorder, such as deviancy and maladjustment, which can have a profound influence on the scales' predictive utility for criminal behavior. For instance, the exclusion of factor 4 of the PCL–R (encompassing items that relate to antisocial behavior, including poor behavior controls, early behavior problems, juvenile delinquency, revocation of conditional release, and criminal versatility) reduces the predictive validity of the measure in regards to future reoffending (Polaschek, 2015; Yang, Wong, & Coid, 2010). Even though the affective and interpersonal manipulation components correspond with Cleckley's original conceptualization of a psychopathic personality, Erratic Lifestyle and antisocial behavior more closely resemble measures of criminal behavior and Antisocial Personality Disorder (Harpur, Hare, & Hakstian, 1989). Notably, prior research revealed that only the affective and interpersonal factors' items work equivalently well across race and gender (Bolt, Hare, Vitale, & Newman, 2004; Cooke, Kosson, & Michie, 2001), with poor generalizability of the remaining factors being reported (McDermott et al., 2000). Further still, antisocial traits were found to diminish over time, suggesting that the generalizability of this element of the construct may also be affected by the age of respondents. A recent empirical investigation by Debowska et al. (2018) demonstrated that Hare's model of psychopathy cannot be used in the same way in forensic and non-forensic populations due to inclusion of the antisocial factor. It appears, therefore, that items referring to criminal/antisocial tendencies should not be included in psychopathy measures.

The essence of psychopathy seems to be captured more successfully through assessments of affective deficits and interpersonal unresponsiveness. The proneness to contravene social and legal norms, on the other hand, appears to be *a possible behavioral outcome* of a psychopathic personality (Boduszek & Debowska, 2016; Skeem & Cooke, 2010a, 2010b). In line with such a notion, a growing body of evidence suggests that psychopathic personalities can thrive in both criminal and non-criminal contexts. For example, the prevalence of psychopathic traits was demonstrated to be higher in a corporate sample than that found in community samples (Babiak, Neumann, & Hare, 2010; Hassall, Boduszek, & Dhingra, 2015). Interestingly, heightened psychopathy scores in U.S. presidents were correlated with a better-rated presidential performance (Lilienfeld et al., 2012). As such, if criminal/antisocial tendencies are just one possible manifestation of psychopathy, other non-criminal/antisocial behaviors in which psychopaths may partake should also be accounted for. A simplified solution, therefore, would be to exclude antisocial/criminal items from psychopathy measures altogether (Boduszek & Debowska, 2016).

A new personality-based model of psychopathy: Psychopathic Personality Traits Model (PPTM)

Although Cleckley's conceptualization of psychopathy received the most widespread acceptance among researchers and clinicians, some of the traits listed in his clinical profile, such as pathological egocentricity, are largely missing from the existing psychopathy assessment tools. Further, we have recently suggested that criminal/antisocial tendencies are the consequence of psychopathic traits, rather than an integral part of the disorder, and individuals with increased psychopathic traits may be successful in both criminal and non-criminal endeavors (Boduszek & Debowska, 2016; Boduszek, Dhingra, Hyland, & Debowska, 2016). Thus, given the broad spectrum of activities in which psychopaths may engage, the inclusion of antisocial items in psychopathy construct appears counterproductive. Instead, there is a need for a clean personality model of psychopathy, which could be used among both forensic and non-forensic populations (Boduszek & Debowska, 2016; Johansson, Andershed, Kerr, & Levander, 2002). Accordingly, a new generation of research which distinguishes between personality deviation and social deviance is warranted (Skeem & Cooke, 2010b).

In an effort to address these issues, we sought to create and validate a new model of psychopathy – Psychopathic Personality Traits Model (PPTM) – with an associated brief self-report scale (the Psychopathic Personality Traits Scale – PPTS; Boduszek, Debowska, Dhingra, & DeLisi, 2016). The brief PPTS is used for research purposes only, but we are currently working on an extended version and a diagnostic tool. The PPTM grasps the essence of a psychopathic personality regardless of individuals' age, gender, cultural background, and criminal history. Central to our new model of psychopathy are four components: affective responsiveness, cognitive responsiveness, interpersonal manipulation, and egocentricity (see Figure 14.1).

The lack of *affective responsiveness* component reflects characteristics of low affective empathy and emotional shallowness. Individuals scoring high on this component are characterized by an inability to emotionally respond to another person's feelings. This dimension resembles the callous affect factor of the PCL–R, which has been constantly demonstrated to be the core feature of a psychopathic personality. The lack of *cognitive responsiveness* component, on the other hand, measures the inability to understand the emotional state of other, mentally represent another person's emotional processes, and emotionally engage with others at a cognitive level. The distinction between affective and cognitive responsiveness to others has been neglected in psychopathy research published to date. Nonetheless, a recent study demonstrated that prisoners with increased psychopathic traits were deficient in understanding affective states (emotions) but not cognitive states (beliefs) (Shamay-Tsoory, Harari, Aharon-Peretz, & Levkovitz, 2010). These findings indicate that reduced cognitive responsiveness to others' emotional states constitutes an important part of the psychopathy construct. Furthermore, although prior research has revealed the importance of intelligence (IQ) in psychopathy, past psychopathy models have failed to control for this aspect in psychopathy assessment. This is a serious limitation because individuals with high IQ are able to learn how to recognize certain emotions and respond in expected ways. For example, Bate, Boduszek, Dhingra and Bale (2014) demonstrated that intelligence is a moderator in the relationship between psychopathy and emotional responding, showing that individuals with increased psychopathic traits who score higher on intelligence (1 *SD* above the sample mean) are able to respond in a socially desirable manner to emotionally provoking stimuli. In order to verify whether deficiency in cognitive responsiveness to emotional states of others is a universal feature of psychopathy or is contingent on intelligence levels, future research using the PPTM should control for participants' IQ.

The third component of the PPTM, *interpersonal manipulation*, reflects characteristics such as superficial charm, grandiosity, and intentional deceitfulness. Manipulation is viewed as largely malicious and destructive of optimal human relationships. This aspect has been accounted for in past psychopathy models, including the PCL–R. Finally, *egocentricity* assesses an individual's tendency to focus on one's own interests, beliefs, and attitudes. In our opinion, egocentricity is one of the most important traits observed among individuals with increased psychopathic traits. According to Cleckley (1941), "the psychopath is always distinguished by egocentricity which is pathological and cannot be compared with the one witnessed is non-psychopathic individuals" (p. 346). This self-centeredness is closely linked with incapacity for love, other than self-love. Having said that, individuals with increased psychopathic traits are able to express positive feelings towards self and anyone whom they consider an "extension of self" (for example children or parents). However, this expression of feelings towards those who are regarded as an extension of self is only at the cognitive level. Items referring to egocentricity have been included in some established psychopathy measures (e.g., the PCL–R and the Psychopathic Traits Inventory–Revised [PPI–R; Lilienfeld & Widows, 2005]). However, since those items were not conceptualized as forming a separate psychopathy dimension, the predictive utility of self-centeredness over the remaining traits could not be investigated. Notably, Cooke, Hart, Logan, and Michie (2012) included "self domain," which resembles the PPTM egocentricity factor, as a separate dimension in their Comprehensive Assessment of Psychopathic Personality (CAPP) model. We also suggest that psychopaths' egocentricity and reduced affective responsiveness influence their ability to recognize other individuals' emotional states (cognitive responsiveness). Prominent conceptual models implicate structural and functional deficits in limbic brain systems, particularly the amygdala (see Debowska, Boduszek, Hyland, & Goodson, 2014), as the neurological

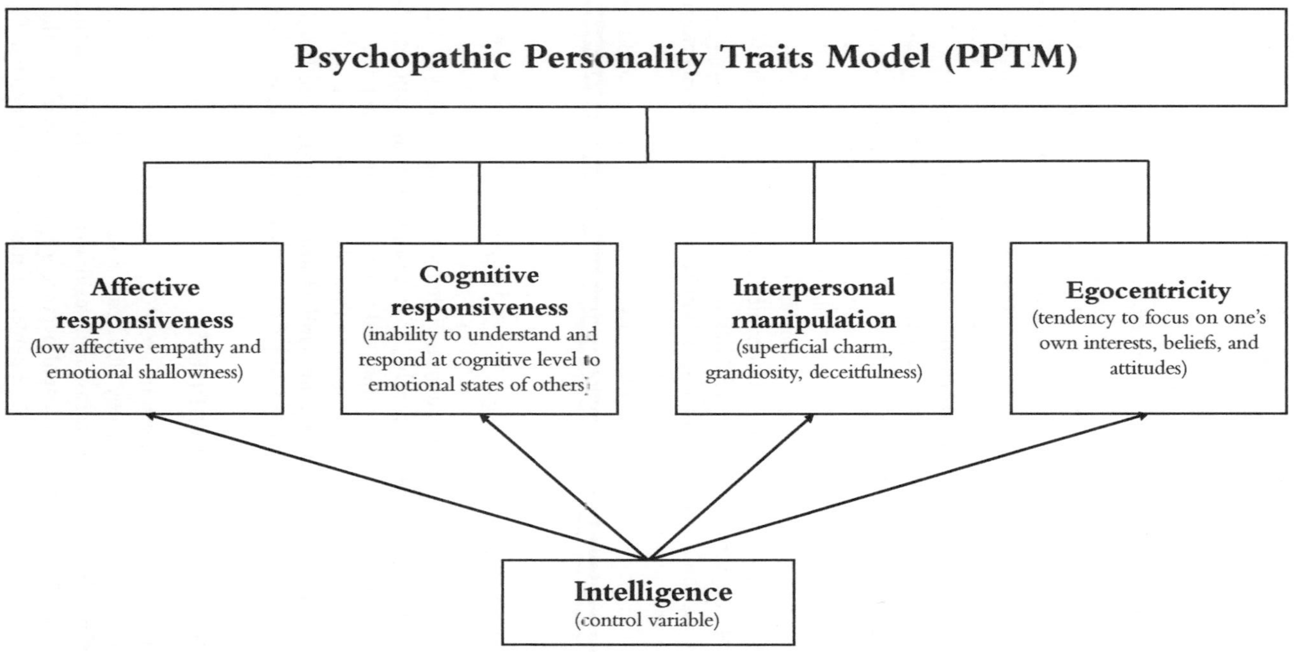

Figure 14.1 The Psychopathic Personality Traits Model (PPTM)

cause of the affective deficits in psychopathy. Prior research on empathic processing suggested that psychopathy is associated with overall recognition deficits (Dolan & Fullam, 2009; Hastings, Tangney, & Stuewig, 2008), as well as deficits in recognizing fear (Blair, Colledge, Murray, & Mitchell, 2001), sadness, and happiness (Dolan & Fullam, 2009; Hastings et al., 2008). In another study, incarcerated offenders with increased psychopathic traits showed deficiency in inferring emotional states (Shamay-Tsoory et al., 2010). Finally, Brook and Kosson (2013:162) reported impaired cognitive empathy and difficulty understanding "the full spectrum of emotions displayed by people" among psychopaths. This is congruent with Cleckley's (1941) suggestion that psychopathic individuals demonstrate general unresponsiveness and poverty in affect in interpersonal relations.

Our research explorations to date have displayed empirical evidence of this new conceptualization of psychopathy, validating the model's utility in a sample of 1,794 inmates from maximum and medium security prisons, and in excess of 3,000 participants from non-forensic settings, including community adults, university students, and children (age range 10–14 years). The appropriateness of the identified factorial solution was supported by the differential predictive validity of the four psychopathy facets in a large sample of prisoners (Boduszek et al., 2016). Inmates scoring higher on affective responsiveness, but not on cognitive responsiveness, were significantly more likely to commit violent offenses and have increased criminal social identity scores. Both affective responsiveness and cognitive responsiveness correlated significantly with self-esteem; however, those associations were in opposite directions. Specifically, affective responsiveness was associated with higher and cognitive responsiveness with lower levels of self-esteem. Additionally, cognitive responsiveness was significantly positively associated with child sexual abuse myths acceptance. In contrast, association between this external criterion and affective responsiveness was negative yet statistically non-significant.

Given the differing predictive utility of affective responsiveness and cognitive responsiveness, these two facets should be considered as unique and distinct from each other. As for the remaining psychopathy factors, interpersonal manipulation formed significant positive associations with child sexual abuse myths acceptance, criminal social identity, and a significant negative correlation with self-esteem. Egocentricity was found to predict increased scores on child sexual abuse myths scale, attitudes towards sexual dating violence, and criminal social identity. This psychopathy dimension was also associated with violent offending. In light of this evidence, the inclusion of egocentricity items within psychopathy measures is important, and failure to control for this aspect of the disorder as a separate and unique dimension appears misguided. Such research challenging the widely accepted notion of psychopathy and associated factors can also challenge the assumptions on which current criminal justice practices are based, subsequently leading to improved risk assessment, treatment provision, and prevention strategies.

Profiling psychopathy using the PPTM

Some psychopathy studies, mostly utilizing the PCL–R or its derivatives, have focused on establishing the prevalence of psychopathy. This past research revealed large discrepancies in the occurrence of psychopathic traits across samples drawn from different populations. More specifically, while the PCL–R-based estimated occurrence of psychopathy in the general population is between 0.3–2 percent (males: 1–2 percent, females: 0.3–0.7 percent; Patrick & Drislane, 2015), the prevalence of psychopathy in the offender population is suggested to oscillate between 15–25 percent (Lilienfeld & Arkowitz, 2007; Woodworth & Porter, 2002). Nonetheless, although the PCL–R scores were most often suggested to be best captured by a four-factor model, reflecting interpersonal, affective, lifestyle, and antisocial characteristics, studies into the prevalence of psychopathy tend to utilize total scale scores. Similarly, cut-off points used to diagnose the condition rely on the sum of scores rather than ratings obtained on these separate dimensions. Such an approach to measurement and diagnosis assumes variations in trait intensity (quantitative differences) but not in the constellation of psychopathic traits (qualitative differences) across individuals, which remains inconsistent with the literature (Colins, Fanti, Salekin, & Andershed, 2016). Relying on the PCL–R total scores could have led to exclusion of participants scoring high on core Interpersonal/Affective but low on lifestyle/antisocial traits of psychopathy, resulting in skewed findings. We suggest that psychopathy may be over-diagnosed in criminal populations due to (1) the widespread use of measures based upon behavioral conception of psychopathy (such as the PCL–R) and (2) the utilization of cut-off points derived from the sum of scores, which defies research suggesting that psychopathy is multidimensional in character (Boduszek & Debowska, 2016; Debowska, Boduszek, Kola, & Hyland, 2014; Kennealy, Skeem, Walters, & Camp, 2010).

In our recent study with the PPTM using a person- as opposed to variable-centered approach to data analysis (Boduszek, Debowska, & Willmott, 2017), we identify five meaningful classes (groups) of psychopathic traits among a systematically selected large representative sample of Polish prisoners. The results of latent profile analysis suggested that psychopathy should be interpreted as a continuum with varying levels of each dimension across individuals, rather than a dichotomous entity. Class 1, consisting of 44 percent of prisoners, was characterized by low mean scores on all four personality-based psychopathy dimensions and hence has been labeled the "low psychopathy group." Class 2, consisting of 16.8 percent of prisoners, was characterized by moderate mean scores on affective and cognitive responsiveness and relatively low ratings on interpersonal manipulation and egocentricity. This group was labeled the "moderate affective/cognitive responsiveness group." We also identified the "high interpersonal manipulation group" (class 3; 20.8 percent of prisoners), characterized by low mean scores on affective responsiveness, cognitive responsiveness, and egocentricity and high on interpersonal manipulation. Inmates in this class were significantly more likely to be convicted of property offenses than those in class 1. Consistent with earlier findings in regard to socioeconomic status of individuals with such traits, offenders in class 3, compared with class 1, were also more likely to engage in white-collar crime, which may be indicative of a higher social class background. Further, similar ratings on affective and cognitive responsiveness to those noted for class 2 in the present analysis were recorded for prisoners in class 4; yet this particular group (class 4) was also distinguished by moderate mean scores on egocentricity and high interpersonal manipulation (the "moderate psychopathy group"; 10.8 percent of inmates).

Finally, the "high psychopathy group" (class 5; with very high mean scores on affective responsiveness, moderate cognitive responsiveness, and high interpersonal manipulation and egocentricity) was identified. This group constituted 7.1 percent of prisoners, which indicates that most inmates (detained in maximum and medium security units) do not meet the diagnostic criteria for psychopathy. Using the same methodology, our most recent research revealed similar psychopathy profiles among various populations. Most interestingly, membership in high psychopathy group was comparable for all adult samples (772 U.S. prisoners = 7.6 percent; 1,201 U.K. community adults = 5.9 percent; 2,080 university students = 7.4 percent), but not for adolescents (n = 475), who were more likely than adults to have increased ratings on all PPTS dimensions (12.4 percent) (Boduszek, Debowska, Sherretts, Boulton & Willmott, 2017). High psychopathy groups were earlier extracted, among others, by Colins et al. (2016) and Dhingra, Boduszek, and Kola (2015); however, the class membership in the latter study amounted to 26.4 percent. Dhingra et al. profiled respondents using a behavioral measure of psychopathy (the Psychopathy Checklist: Screening Version [PCL: SV]; Hart, Cox, & Hare, 1995), and hence the current results are not directly comparable with this earlier research. Nonetheless, it appears that the high rates of psychopathy reported for some populations (those incarcerated and institutionalized in particular) may be accounted for by the inclusion of indicators of behavioral expressions of the condition (Boduszek & Debowska, 2016; Edens et al., 2001; Patrick, 2007; Patrick, Hicks, Nichol, & Krueger, 2007; Rogers, 1995).

Conclusion

As explicated in the current chapter, the PPTM offers an alternative psychopathy assessment based on personality traits. The PPTM consists of four dimensions, including affective responsiveness, cognitive responsiveness, interpersonal manipulation, and egocentricity. It is also conceptualized that intelligence levels moderate the relationship between the aforementioned psychopathic traits and behavioral outcomes. Importantly, while antisocial/criminal tendencies/behaviors may constitute one possible expression of psychopathy, they are not treated as integral to psychopathy construct within the newly developed framework. Using this personality approach to psychopathy assessment, we demonstrated that the prevalence of psychopathy among individuals incarcerated in medium and maximum security prisons amounts to approximately 7 percent of the total prison population and hence is *much lower* than previously speculated, comparable with the prevalence found among non-forensic adult samples (Boduszek, Debowska, Sherretts et al., 2017, Boduszek et al., 2017). Using a similar research methodology,[1] Colins et al. (2016) found that as much as 12 percent of adults in the general population belong in a psychopathic personality group. This may indicate that the difference in intensity of psychopathic traits between forensic and non-forensic populations is not as pronounced as reported to date. In light of this, it is recommended that both researchers and practitioners re-evaluate the previously utilized conceptualization of psychopathy and assessment methods. Additionally, psychopathy measures which index behavioral traits and rely on cut-off points for total scale ratings should be used with caution in clinical settings. We anticipate that the method of defining and measuring psychopathy upon which the PPTM is based, will (1) address the problems identified in past psychopathy research which treated antisocial/criminal behaviors as vital to psychopathy construct and (2) allow for reliable psychopathy assessment among forensic and non-forensic populations.

Note

1 With the exception of including some behavioral characteristics (i.e., impulsive–irresponsible traits) in the assessment of psychopathy, which could partly explain the high-class membership rates.

References

Babiak, P., Neumann, C. S., and Hare, R. (2010) 'Corporate psychopathy: Talking the walk,' *Behavioral Sciences & the Law*, *28*:174–193.

Bate, C., Boduszek, D., Dhingra, K., and Bale, C. (2014) 'Psychopathy, intelligence and emotional responding in a non-forensic sample: A physiological investigation,' *Journal of Forensic Psychiatry and Psychology*, *25*(5):600–612.

Blair, R. J. R., Colledge, E., Murray, L., and Mitchell, D. G. (2001) 'A selective impairment in the processing of sad and fearful expressions in children with psychopathic tendencies,' *Journal of Abnormal Child Psychology*, *29*(6):491–498.

Boduszek, D., Debowska, A., Dhingra, K., and DeLisi, M. (2016) 'Introduction and validation of Psychopathic Personality Traits Scale (PPTS) in a large prison sample,' *Journal of Criminal Justice*, *46*:9–17.

Boduszek, D., and Debowska, A. (2016) 'Critical evaluation of psychopathy measurement (PCL–R and SRP–III/SF) and recommendations for future research,' *Journal of Criminal Justice*, *44*:1–12.

Boduszek, D., Debowska., A., Sherretts, N., Boulton, M., and Willmott, D. (2017) 'Profiles of psychopathic personality traits among prisoners, community adults, university students, and adolescents' (Manuscript in preparation).

Boduszek, D., Debowska, A., and Willmott, D. (2017) 'Latent profile analysis of psychopathic traits among homicide, general violent, property, and white-collar offenders,' *Journal of Criminal Justice*, *51*:17–23.

Boduszek, D., Dhingra, K., Hyland, P., and Debowska, A. (2016) 'A bifactorial solution to the Psychopathy Checklist: Screening Version in a sample of civil psychiatric patients,' *Criminal Behaviour and Mental Health*, *26*(3):174–185.

Bolt, D. M., Hare, R. D., Vitale, J. E., and Newman, J. P. (2004) 'A multigroup item response theory analysis of the Psychopathy Checklist–Revised,' *Psychological Assessment*, *16*(2):155–168.

Brook, M., and Kosson, D. S. (2013) 'Impaired cognitive empathy in criminal psychopathy: Evidence from a laboratory measure of empathic accuracy,' *Journal of Abnormal Psychology*, *122*(1):156–166.

Cleckley, H. (1941) *The mask of sanity* (1st ed.), St. Louis, MO: C.V. Mosby.

Colins, O. F., Fanti, K. A., Salekin, R. T., and Andershed, H. (2016) 'Psychopathic personality in the general population: Differences and similarities across gender,' *Journal of Personality Disorders*, *30*:1–26.

Cooke, D. J., Hart, S. D., Logan, C., and Michie, C. (2012) 'Explicating the construct of psychopathy: Development and validation of a conceptual model, the Comprehensive Assessment of Psychopathic Personality (CAPP),' *International Journal of Forensic Mental Health*, *11*(4):242–252.

Cooke, D. J., Kosson, D. S., and Michie, C. (2001) 'Psychopathy and ethnicity: Structural, item, and test generalizability of the Psychopathy Checklist–Revised (PCL–R) in Caucasian and African American participants,' *Psychological Assessment*, *13*(4):531–542.

Debowska, A., Boduszek, D., Dhingra, K., Willmott, D., Sherretts, N., and DeLisi, M. (2018) 'Can we use Hare's psychopathy model within forensic and non-forensic populations? An empirical investigation,' *Deviant Behavior*, *39*(2):224–242.

Debowska, A., Boduszek, D., Hyland, P., and Goodson, S. (2014) 'Biological correlates of psychopathic traits,' *Mental Health Review Journal*, *19*(2):110–123.

Dhingra, K., and Boduszek, D. (2013) 'Psychopathy and criminal behaviour – A psychosocial research perspective,' *Journal of Criminal Psychology*, *3*(2):83–107.

Dhingra, K., Boduszek, D., and Kola, S. (2015) 'A latent class analysis of psychopathic traits in civil psychiatric patients,' *The Howard Journal of Criminal Justice*, *54*(3):237–249.

Dolan, M. C., and Fullam, R. S. (2009) 'Psychopathy and functional magnetic resonance imaging blood oxygenation level-dependent responses to emotional faces in violent patients with schizophrenia,' *Biological Psychiatry*, *66*(6):570–577.

Edens, J. F., Skeem, J. L., Cruise, K. R., and Cauffman, E. (2001) 'Assessment of "juvenile psychopathy" and its association with violence: A critical review,' *Behavioral Sciences and the Law*, *19*(1):53–80.

Hare, R. D. (1980) 'A research scale for the assessment of psychopathy in criminal populations,' *Personality and Individual Differences*, *1*(2):111–119.

Hare, R. D. (1991) *The Hare Psychopathy Checklist–Revised*, Toronto, ON: Multi-Health Systems.

Hare, R. D. (2003) *The Hare Psychopathy Checklist–Revised* (2nd ed.), Toronto, ON: Multi-Health Systems.

Harpur, T. J., Hare, R. D., and Hakstian, A. R. (1989) 'Two-factor conceptualization of psychopathy: Construct validity and assessment implications,' *Psychological Assessment: A Journal of Consulting and Clinical Psychology*, *1*(1):6–17.

Hart, S. D., Cox, D. N., and Hare, R. D. (1995) *Hare Psychopathy Checklist: Screening Version (PCL: SV)*, Toronto, ON: Multi-Heath Systems.

Hastings, M. E., Tangney, J. P., and Stuewig, J. (2008) 'Psychopathy and identification of facial expressions of emotion,' *Personality and Individual Differences*, *44*:1474–1483.

Hassall, J., Boduszek, D., and Dhingra, K. (2015) 'Psychopathic traits of business and psychology students and their relationship to academic success,' *Personality and Individual Differences*, *82*:227–231.

Johansson, P., Andershed, H., Kerr, M., and Levander, S. (2002) 'On the operationalization of psychopathy: Further support for a three-faceted personality oriented model,' *Acta Psychiatrica Scandinavica, 106*(s412):81–85.

Kennealy, P. J., Skeem, J. L., Walters, G. D., and Camp, J. (2010) 'Do core interpersonal and affective traits of PCL–R psychopathy interact with antisocial behavior and disinhibition to predict violence?,' *Psychological Assessment, 22*(3):569–580.

Lilienfeld, S. O., and Arkowitz, H. (2007) 'What "psychopath" means,' *Scientific American Mind, 18*(6):80–81.

Lilienfeld, S. O., Waldman, I. D., Landfield, K., Watts, A. L., Rubenzer, S., and Faschingbauer, T. R. (2012) 'Fearless dominance and the US presidency: Implications of psychopathic personality traits for successful and unsuccessful political leadership,' *Journal of Personality and Social Psychology, 103*:489–505.

Lilienfeld, S. O., and Widows, M. R. (2005) *PPI–R: Psychopathic Personality Inventory– Revised*, Lutz, FL: Psychological Assessment Resources, Incorporated.

McDermott, P. A., Alterman, A. I., Cacciola, J. S., Rutherford, M. J., Newman, J. P., and Mulholland, E. M. (2000) 'Generality of Psychopathy Checklist–Revised factors over prisoners and substance-dependent patients,' *Journal of Consulting and Clinical Psychology, 68*(1):181–186.

O'Kane, A., Fawcett, D., and Blackburn, R. (1996) 'Psychopathy and moral reasoning: A comparison of two classifications,' *Personality and Individual Differences, 20*(4):505–514.

Patrick, C. (2007) 'Back to the future: Cleckley as a guide to the next generation of psychopathy research,' in C. Patrick (Ed.), *Handbook of psychopathy* (pp. 605–617), New York, NY: Guilford Press.

Patrick, C. J., and Drislane, L. E. (2015) 'Antisocial personality disorder and psychopathy,' in P. H. Blaney, R. F. Krueger, & T. Millon (Eds.), *Oxford textbook of psychopathology* (pp. 681–706), New York, NY: Oxford University Press.

Patrick, C. J., Hicks, B. M., Nichol, P. E., and Krueger, R. F. (2007) 'A bifactor approach to modeling the structure of the Psychopathy Checklist–Revised,' *Journal of Personality Disorders, 21*(2):118–125.

Polaschek, D. L. (2015) '(Mis)understanding psychopathy: Consequences for policy and practice with offenders,' *Psychiatry, Psychology and Law, 22*(4):500–519.

Rogers R. (1995) *Diagnostic and structured interviewing: A handbook for psychologists*, Odessa, FL: PAR.

Shamay-Tsoory, S. G., Harari, H., Aharon-Peretz, J., and Levkovitz, Y. (2010) 'The role of the orbitofrontal cortex in affective theory of mind in criminal offenders with psychopathic tendencies,' *Cortex, 46*:668–677.

Skeem, J. L., and Cooke, D. J. (2010a) 'Is criminal behavior a central component of psychopathy? Conceptual directions for resolving the debate,' *Psychological Assessment, 22*(2):433–445.

Skeem, J. L., and Cooke, D. J. (2010b) 'One measure does not a construct make: Directions toward reinvigorating psychopathy research – reply to Hare and Neumann (2010),' *Psychological Assessment, 22*(2):455–459.

Skeem, J. L, Polaschek, D., Patrick, C. J., and Lilienfeld, S. O. (2011) 'Psychopathic personality: Bridging the gap between scientific evidence and public policy,' *Psychological Science in the Public Interest, 12*:95–162.

Woodworth, M., and Porter, S. (2002) 'In cold blood: Characteristics of criminal homicides as a function of psychopathy,' *Journal of Abnormal Psychology, 111*(3):436–445.

Yang, M., Wong, S. C., and Coid, J. (2010) 'The efficacy of violence prediction: A meta- analytic comparison of nine risk assessment tools,' *Psychological Bulletin, 136*(5):740–767.

15

The PCL–R family of psychopathy measures

Dimensionality and predictive utility of the PCL–R, PCL: SV, PCL: YV, SRP–III, and SRP–SF

Agata Debowska, Daniel Boduszek, and Russell Woodfield

Introduction

Although there is no consensus among researchers and clinicians as to what constitutes psychopathy, the description of the disorder which has received the most widespread acceptance is the one proposed by Cleckley (1941). In his publication entitled *The Mask of Sanity*, Cleckley suggested psychopathy to be composed of 16 traits, including egocentricity, lack of insight into the emotions of others, deficiency in emotional reactions, and no feelings of remorse or regret. In more recent publications, researchers have attempted to group Cleckleyan traits into latent factors, which resulted in the identification of four psychopathy dimensions representing interpersonal (e.g., deceitfulness, superficial charm, grandiosity), affective (e.g., lack of empathy, remorse, or guilt), lifestyle (e.g., impulsivity, irresponsibility), and behavioral (e.g., social deviance, criminality) features (Hare & Neumann, 2008). The characterization of psychopathy, reflecting these four latent domains, has served as the foundation for creating the Psychopathy Checklist (PCL; Hare, 1980), its updated version, the Psychopathy Checklist–Revised (PCL–R; Hare, 1991, 2003), as well as its progeny – the Psychopathy Checklist: Screening Version (PCL: SV; Hart, Cox, & Hare, 1995), the Psychopathy Checklist: Youth Version (PCL: YV; Forth, Kosson, & Hare, 2003), and the different versions of the Self-Report Psychopathy Scale – the SRP (Hare, 1985), SRP–II (Williams & Paulhus, 2004), and SRP–III (this version is also referred to as the SRP–IV and SRP: 4) (Paulhus, Neumann, & Hare, 2016).

The PCL–R and its derivatives are the dominant assessment of psychopathy in research and clinical practice, and studies examining the measures' construct validity, dimensionality, and predictive utility are abundant. However, as recently noted by Boduszek and Debowska (2016) in a critical evaluation of factor analytic research using the PCL–R and SRP–III, findings regarding the underlying factor structure of the scales are inconsistent, which has been explained by methodological and conceptual limitations of prior research. The purpose of this chapter is to summarize extant knowledge and critically evaluate research into construct validity, dimensionality, and predictive utility of the PCL–R, PCL: SV, PCL: YV, and SRP–III (including its abbreviated version, the Self-Report Psychopathy Scale–Short Form [SRP–SF]).

PCL–R

The PCL–R (Hare, 1991, 2003) is a 20-item scale completed by a trained clinician based on interviews and case history information. All items are rated on a 3-point scale (0 = does not apply, 1 = applies to a certain extent, 2 = definitely applies) and hence scores range from 0 to 40. The instrument was first developed and validated using data from North American samples of male offenders and forensic psychiatric patients, but its reliability and validity were later tested among more diverse samples, including offenders from different cultural backgrounds (e.g., Grann, Långström, Tengström, & Kullgren, 1999), adolescent offenders (e.g., Forth & Burke, 1998; Forth & Mailloux, 2000), female offenders (e.g., Salekin, Rogers, & Sewell, 1996), and substance abusers (e.g., Rutherford, Cacciola, Alterman, & McKay, 1996). Despite the scale's multidimensionality (see below for details), a cut-off point of 30, calculated based on the total PCL–R score, has been suggested for diagnosing psychopathy (Hare & Neumann, 2008).

Researchers generally agree that the scale is multidimensional in nature, but consensus has not been reached as to how many facets best represent the PCL–R ratings. Most frequently, the PCL–R scores were proposed to be captured by two-, three-, four-, or bi-factor models. The two-factor solution, proposed by Hare (1991), is composed of two distinct yet correlated dimensions – Factor 1 (Interpersonal/Affective) and Factor 2 (lifestyle/antisocial). Factor 1 incorporates eight scale items (charming, grandiose, lying, manipulate, no remorse, shallow, callous, and fail to accept responsibility), whereas Factor 2 consists of ten items (need for stimulation, parasitic, lack goals, impulsive, irresponsible, poor behavior controls, early behavior problems, juvenile delinquency, revocation of release, criminal versatility) (Harpur, Hakstian, & Hare, 1988; Harpur, Hare, & Hakstian, 1989; Krstic et al., 2017). The disproportion between the two factors in the number of items included has led to suggestions that the PCL–R is too heavily weighted towards behavioral expressions of psychopathy (Boduszek & Debowska, 2016; Patrick, 2007). In addition, two PCL–R items (promiscuous sexual behavior and many short-term marital relationships) do not load on any of the factors and are usually excluded from factorial analyses of the measure (Krstic et al., 2017).

The two-factor model presented above was found to be a statistically superior representation of the data in a number of studies. For example, in McDermott et al. (2000), research using exploratory factor analysis (EFA), this solution was reported as the best representation of the PCL–R scores obtained from a sample of 326 male offenders incarcerated in a prison in southern Wisconsin. However, within this same study, a one-factor model was found superior in grasping the PCL–R ratings among 620 (*n* = 442 men, *n* = 178 women) substance-dependent patients, suggesting that the scale may not work the same across samples drawn from different populations or the two sexes. In another study with offenders, Medina, Valdés-Sosa, García, Almeyda, and Couso (2013) suggested a two-factor model (Interpersonal/Affective and antisocial). As detailed earlier, promiscuous sexual behavior and many short-term marital relationships items did not load on any of the identified factors. These findings, however, should be tempered by the fact that a small sample size was used (124 Cuban violent offenders), only one possible factorial solution was tested, and fit statistics for the model were not reported. Further, Hildebrand, de Ruiter, de Vogel, and van der Wolf (2002) demonstrated the supremacy of a two-factor model in a sample of 107 Dutch psychiatric patients (*n* = 98 men, *n* = 9 women). Interestingly, the best-fitting model was not the two-factor model proposed by Hare (1991) but a modified two-factor model where item 14 (impulsivity) was allowed to load on both PCL–R facets. Although Hildebrand et al. (2002) tested seven alternative PCL–R solutions, most of them were not guided by theoretical considerations (e.g., two- and three-factor solutions with post hoc modifications, models with correlated errors of measurement), and it appears that the researchers were searching for a statistically rather than a conceptually superior representation of data. Of note, empirical research demonstrated that only Factor 1 items function equivalently well across race and gender (e.g., Bolt, Hare, Vitale, & Newman, 2004; Cooke, Kosson, & Michie, 2001). Poor generalizability of Factor 2 was reported for substance-dependent patients (McDermott et al., 2000) and antisocial traits were found to decline over time (Blonigen, Hicks, Krueger, Patrick, & Iacono, 2006; Gill & Crino, 2012).

The four-factor conceptualization of psychopathy is underpinned by the following correlated facets: interpersonal (including four items: charming, grandiose, lying, manipulate), affective (four items: no remorse, shallow, callous, fail to accept responsibility), lifestyle (five items: need for stimulation, parasitic, lack goals, impulsive, irresponsible), and antisocial (five items: poor behavior controls, early behavior problems, juvenile delinquency, revocation of release, criminal versatility) (Hare, 2003; Hare & Neumann, 2006). While this model is presented as the best model for the PCL–R scores in some of the most recent scholarship in the area, many of those studies do not test alternative factorial solutions (e.g., Krstic et al., 2017; León-Mayer, Folino, Neumann, & Hare, 2015; Mokros et al., 2011; Neumann, Hare, & Johansson, 2013; Neumann, Hare, & Pardini, 2014; Zwets, Hornsveld, Neumann, Muris, & van Marle, 2015), even if fit statistics for the four-factor model are not satisfactory or when correlations between the four factors are very high (e.g., Mokros et al., 2011; Zwets et al., 2015). Further, in Neumann, Hare, and Newman's (2007) study within three large samples drawn from prisons and forensic psychiatric hospitals, two models were assessed, including a correlated four-factor model and a hierarchical model with four first-order factors and one second-order factor. The researchers reported that the former model provided a better fit to the data, but comparisons between models were not made and fit statistics were reported only for the four-factor solution.

Based on 13 PCL–R items, Cooke and Michie (2001) argued for a three-factor hierarchical model, incorporating interpersonal (deceitful interpersonal style), affective (deficient affective experience), and behavioral (impulsive and irresponsible behavioral style) dimensions. This three-factor solution omits items referring to criminal/antisocial behavior, which, as the authors suggest, may be a correlate of psychopathy rather than its integral part (Skeem & Cooke, 2010a, 2010b). Cooke et al. (2001), Cooke, Michie, Hart, and Clark (2005b), and Johansson, Andershed, Kerr, and Levander (2002) found a three-factor or hierarchical three-factor model with 13 items to be the best model fit for the data, whereas the same models with testlets were reported as the best factorial solutions in six other studies (Cooke & Michie, 2001; Cooke, Michie, Hart, & Clark, 2005a; Cooke, Michie, & Skeem, 2007; Vitacco, Rogers, Neumann, Harrison, & Vincent, 2005; Weaver, Meyer, Van Nort, & Tristan, 2006; Weizmann-Henelius et al., 2010). However, this prior research is not free from limitations. In particular, the first problem pertains to repeated use of one data set for similar purposes. For example, Cooke and Michie (2001, study 4) and Cooke et al. (2005a, 2007) used the same sample of Scottish male prisoners, whereas Cooke et al. (2005a) and Cooke et al. (2005b) employed a sample of North American male adult and psychiatric offenders (N = 2,067). Second, the use of testlets with short scales, where there is no need to reduce the indicator-to-factor ratio, has been noted as questionable, and it has been advised that the technique should be avoided when examining the factor structure of the PCL–R (Boduszek & Debowska, 2016).

Some recent factor analytic work examined the utility of bi-factor models in grasping the PCL–R's dimensionality. Bi-factor modeling views covariation among observable indicators to be explained by both general factors and grouping/specific factors which, unlike in hierarchical models, exist at the same conceptual level. Flores-Mendoza, Alvarenga, Herrero, and Abad (2008), who assessed seven competing solutions, argued for the superiority of the bi-factor model with two specific factors and one general factor. However, in this particular study, the general and grouping factors had similar factor loadings and the researchers did not indicate what effect this might have on the subsequent use of the PCL–R in applied settings. Moreover, three of the scale items evidenced non-significant loadings and were removed from the model. In another study among 593 American male inmates, a bi-factor model with one general and three grouping (interpersonal, affective, and impulsivity) factors evidenced the best fit of the data. Although models with 13, 18, and 20 scale items were tested, the best-fitting model included the full set of 20 items (Patrick, Hicks, Nichol, & Krueger, 2007). This indicates that bi-factor modeling may be a viable alternative to traditional Confirmatory Factor Analysis (CFA) techniques, which allow for obtaining satisfactory results while modeling all PCL–R items. Thus, the inclusion of bi-factorial conceptualizations as comparison models has been recommended in all future PCL–R factor analytic research (Boduszek & Debowska, 2016).

Psychopathy, as indexed by the PCL/PCL–R, was noted to predict general and violent recidivism (Hart, Kropp, & Hare, 1988; Serin, 1996; Serin & Amos, 1995; Serin, Peters, & Barbaree, 1990) and sexual reoffending (Furr, 1993; Olver & Wong, 2015; Quinsey, Rice, & Harris, 1995; Rice, Harris, & Quinsey, 1990), which urged Rice and Harris (1995) to propose that the instrument should be used in clinical and legal decision-making. Using a sample of 81 Canadian offenders, Serin (1996) reported that the PCL–R Factor 1 (Interpersonal/Affective) was a better predictor of violent recidivism than Factor 2 (lifestyle/antisocial), but a growing body of evidence reveals that the PCL–R's predictive efficiency for crime is largely affected by Factor 2 rather than Factor 1 scores (Olver & Wong, 2015; Salekin et al., 1996; Skeem & Mulvey, 2001). In considering that Factor 2 embeds criminal behavior, this is unsurprising and indicates that the usefulness of the PCL–R in criminal justice settings may be attributable almost entirely to criminal history items (Polaschek, 2015). Yang, Wong, and Coid (2010), in a meta-analysis of predictive accuracy of the PCL–R, found that Factor 2 (effect size = 0.61) outperformed Factor 1 (effect size = 0.22) in predicting violent outcomes. While the total PCL–R score was a fairly good predictor of recidivism (effect size = 0.55), its predictive efficacy was comparable with violence prediction instruments. Based on these findings, the authors concluded that Factor 1, i.e., the core personality features of psychopathy, is not associated with violence. Walters (2012), in turn, found that three PCL–R factors (interpersonal, affective, and lifestyle) failed to predict general and violent recidivism beyond the contributions of age and past criminal history among 198 Canadian prisoners. In a study with 48 violent female offenders from Finland, Weizmann-Henelius, Virkkunen, Gammelgård, Eronen, and Putkonen (2015) established that the PCL–R does *not* predict the risk of violent reoffending in females, although violent recidivists tended to score higher on total PCL–R, as well as on antisocial behavior and lifestyle facets, than nonviolent recidivists. The PCL–R total and factor scores have also been correlated with non-criminal external criteria. For example, Factor 1 (interpersonal) and factor 4 (antisocial) facets were significantly positively associated with low anxiety and fearlessness (Neumann et al., 2013). Interestingly, Medina et al. (2013) found some theoretically unexpected correlations between the PCL–R facets and external measures. Specifically, the PCL–R total score as well as Factor 1 (Interpersonal/Affective) and Factor 2 (lifestyle/antisocial) scores formed significant negative correlations with physical aggression, verbal aggression, anger, and hostility.

PCL: SV

To enable quicker and less demanding psychopathy assessment in civil psychiatric populations, Hart et al. (1995) developed the PCL: SV, which can be used for screening for the presence of psychopathic traits. PCL: SV is a 12-item measure composed of two parts: part 1 consists of six items intended to reflect PCL–R Factor 1 (Interpersonal/Affective), whereas the remaining six items in part 2 correspond with PCL–R Factor 2 (lifestyle/antisocial). Most items are based on a subset of PCL–R items which were shortened and simplified. PCL: SV item 5 (lacks empathy) was derived by collapsing and simplifying two similar PCL–R items – 7 (shallow affect) and 8 (callous/lack of empathy). PCL: SV items tapping onto antisocial behavior dimension, in turn, were modified to enable administration without access to formal criminal record. All scale items are measured on a 3-point scale (0 = does not apply, 1 = applies to a certain extent, 2 = definitely applies) and so scores range from 0 to 24. A cut-off score of 18 was proposed for possible psychopathy, but a more comprehensive follow-up assessment is recommended for individuals scoring 18 or above. Even though not all PCL: SV items were found to be parallel to their PCL–R equivalent, the scale was dubbed an efficient abbreviated version of the PCL–R (Cooke, Michie, Hart, & Hare, 1999).

PCL: SV dimensionality research is guided by the same theoretical considerations as the one focusing on the PCL–R. In one of the earliest investigations, Forth, Brown, Hart, and Hare (1996) examined reliability and validity of the PCL: SV among 75 male and 75 female Canadian undergraduate students recruited for three independent studies. Sample 1 (25 males, 25 females) and 2 (25 males, 25 females) consisted of participants drawn from the general student population. Sample 3 (25 males, 25 females) were participants selected from a sample of 1,831 students with increased scores on Conduct Disorder (CD). Although participants who met the criteria for CD ($n = 38$) scored significantly higher than those who did not ($n = 112$) on total PCL: SV, the influence of part 2 items (i.e., those referring to antisocial behavior) on this difference was not investigated. Based on EFA, Forth et al. (1996:540) suggested a one-factor solution for both male and female participants, but the authors found the results difficult to interpret, especially for the female sample. Additionally, only nine items among men and five items among women had factor loadings above 0.4. In spite of these issues, it was concluded that the measure "can be used reliably with males and females in a nonforensic setting."

Latent structure of the PCL: SV was also investigated using CFA techniques. Hart et al. (1995) found a two-factor model to be acceptable (goodness-of-fit index [GFI] = 0.94) and superior to a unidimensional model. Rogers et al. (2000), in turn, argued for a higher-order factor solution for scores derived from a combined sample of female offenders and male forensic psychiatric patients. Although the robust Comparative Fit Index (CFI) was below the acceptable value of 0.90 (Bentler, 1995), the fit of the model was not compared with theoretically feasible competing solutions. Further, two-, three-, and four-factor models indicated acceptable fit to the scores from 149 inpatients within a maximum security psychiatric hospital, but the four-factor solution showed best overall fit (Hill, Neumann, & Rogers, 2004). Three- and four-factor models provided an acceptable fit to the data from 257 Lithuanian prisoners (Žukauskienė, Laurinavičius, & Čėsnienė, 2010).

Several studies assessed construct validity of the PCL: SV using data retrieved from 1,136 patients from the MacArthur Violence Risk Assessment Study. For example, Skeem and

Mulvey (2001) identified a two-factor solution as the best yet imperfect (corrected CFI = 0.89; Satorra & Bentler, 1988) representation of the data. In a subsequent study, Skeem, Mulvey, and Grisso (2003) assessed eight alternative models, including the traditional two-factor model and three-factor models based on all 12 items and, as suggested by Cooke and Michie (2001), after deleting three behavioral items (poor behavioral controls, adolescent antisocial behavior, and adult antisocial behavior). Offering an acceptable and the most parsimonious model fit was a 9-item non-hierarchical three-factor model composed of arrogant/deceitful style (superficial, grandiose, deceitful), deficient affective experience (lacks remorse, doesn't accept responsibility, lacks empathy), and impulsive–irresponsible lifestyle (impulsive, irresponsible, lacks goals) dimensions. The model was found factorially invariant across the two sexes and race (White vs. nonwhite). Finally, Vitacco, Neumann, and Jackson (2005) reported adequate fit statistics for three- and four-factor models, based on 9 and 12 items respectively.

In considering inconsistent results with respect to the PCL: SV dimensionality, it may be that traditional CFA techniques are insufficient to explain the complexity of psychopathy as captured by the measure. To address this important methodological issue, Boduszek, Dhingra, Hyland, and Debowska (2016) compared ten theory-informed models of the PCL: SV, including four alternative confirmatory bi-factor models, among the above-mentioned sample of civil psychiatric patients recruited as part of the MacArthur Violence Risk Assessment Study. Results indicated that a bi-factor model comprised of two general factors of psychopathy (Interpersonal/Affective, lifestyle/antisocial) and four subordinate factors (interpersonal, affective, lifestyle, antisocial) was a good and the most parsimonious fit to the data based on all fit indices. All items evidenced statistically significant factor loadings on the two general factors, and all factor loadings were above 0.4. Since factor loadings were poorer on the four subordinate factors compared with the general factors, it was suggested that the PCL: SV scoring scheme should be based on the latter. This solution, although not tested in previous PCL: SV scholarship, was consistent with Hare's (1991) two-factor representation of psychopathy. Correlated two-, three-, and four-factor models most frequently tested in prior research were rejected as poor approximations of the data. This further demonstrates the superiority of modeling multidimensional structures existing at the same conceptual level in this specific context. It is recommended that bi-factor solutions are further tested among more diverse populations and using other psychopathy measures derived from the PCL–R (see Hyland, 2015 for a guide to confirmatory bi-factor modeling).

As in PCL–R research, relationships between PCL: SV total and factor scores and external criteria were explored to gain an insight into the measure's predictive value. Forth et al. (1996) tested the association between PCL: SV total scores and Antisocial Personality Disorder. These correlations were statistically significant for both male and female participants, but the contribution of PCL: SV antisocial behavior items towards this result was not examined. Skeem and Mulvey (2001), in turn, suggested increased PCL: SV scores to be a relatively strong predictor of violence; however, the instrument's predictive efficiency, even though still statistically significant, was substantially reduced after controlling for additional criteria reflecting antisocial behavior and personality disorders. Additionally, when controlling for all PCL: SV dimensions in a four-factor model, only the antisocial behavior facet significantly correlated with criminal activity among Lithuanian offenders (Žukauskienė et al., 2010). Skeem et al. (2003) found total PCL: SV and antisocial behavior factor scores to be predictive of future violence, yet this predictive power was reduced when three items pertaining to criminality were deleted from the total measure score. Boduszek et al. (2016) demonstrated that Factor 2 (lifestyle/antisocial), but not Factor 1 (Interpersonal/Affective), formed significant positive correlations with Neuroticism, Barratt Impulsiveness Scale–Cognitive, and anxiety–depression; and negative correlations with openness and Conscientiousness. Both Factor 1 and 2 associated significantly positively with the number of violent acts and crime against property, but not with crime against people. All reported correlations were weak. Aggression among psychiatric patients with scores above the cut-off point for psychopathy, in turn, was predicted by interpersonal and antisocial psychopathy dimensions (Hill et al., 2004). These findings indicate that caution should be taken when using the PCL: SV as a violence risk assessment tool.

PCL: YV

Diagnosing personality disorders among youngsters is a controversial issue due to the malleability of personality prior to reaching adulthood and the stigmatizing effects such a diagnosis may entail (Freeman & Reinecke, 2007; Miller, Muehlenkamp, & Jacobson, 2008). On the other hand, some researchers have argued that assessing psychopathy in youths might be useful for risk assessment and case management of juveniles who offend (Corrado, Vincent, Hart, & Cohen, 2004). One of the concerns with respect to examining "fledgling" psychopathy (Lynam, 1996), however, is the applicability of assessment tools designed specifically for adults to adolescent samples. To exemplify, Rogers et al. (2000) applied the PCL: SV to a sample of 120 male adolescents, but three out of 12 items could not be rated. Two of these items inquired into adult behavior and relationships. The third item (relied excessively on family), in turn, could not be classed as pathological. To address these issues and enable reliable assessment of psychopathic traits among youths aged between 12 and 18 years, Forth et al. (2003) developed the PCL: YV. The measure is completed by a trained professional based on an interview with the youth and collateral information (such as court records, interview with parents). The measure consists of 20 items indexed on a 3-point scale (0 = does not apply to the youth, 1 = applies to a certain extent, 2 = applies to the youth). Scores vary from 0 to 40, with higher scores indicating increased levels of psychopathic characteristics. In contrast to the PCL–R, there is not a cut-off point for the PCL: YV to diagnose psychopathy. PCL: YV was designed to reflect two PCL–R factors: Factor 1 (Interpersonal/Affective) consists of eight items and Factor 2 (lifestyle/antisocial) consists of nine items. Three items (11, 17, and 20) do not appear in the factor scores but are used to calculate total score.

Although the PCL: YV was modeled after the PCL–R, researchers have sought to determine the factor structure of the instrument independently to enable its effective use. Jones, Cauffman, Miller, and Mulvey (2006) examined the structure of the PCL: YV among serious adolescent male (n = 1,170) and female (n = 184) offenders enrolled in the Pathways to Desistance study. Using CFA, four alternative models were tested, two of which provided a good model fit (three- and four-factor models). Both solutions, however, included additional parameters representing error covariation between item 1 (impression management) and 2 (grandiose sense of self-worth), as well as between item 18 (serious criminal behavior) and 20 (criminal versatility). Correlating errors of measurement is a serious methodological limitation which could have led to improved statistical performance of both solutions. In another study, Neumann, Kosson, Forth, and Hare (2006) reported that an 18-item four-factor model and a 13-item three-factor model provided satisfactory fit to the data retrieved from a sample of male adolescents incarcerated in North America and a sample of male adolescents from the U.K., but some of the fit indices were below the acceptable range (e.g., CFI = 0.83 and the root mean square error of approximation [RMSEA] = 0.09 for the four-factor model in the U.K. sample). The only model that evidenced good factor structure across the two groups was a four-factor parceled model. Acceptability of three- and four-factor models was also reported among mixed-gender (Salekin, Brannen, Zalot, Leistico, & Neumann, 2006) and male adolescent offenders (Vitacco, Neumann,

Caldwell, Leistico, & Van Rybroek, 2006), yet these findings should be tempered by the use of very small samples (N = 130 in Salekin et al., 2006 and N = 122 in Vitacco et al., 2006).

It has been demonstrated that some PCL: YV items function differently among male and female youths and hence generalizing psychopathy models identified with males to female samples appears problematic (Tsang et al., 2015). In spite of this, the focus in psychopathy research has been predominantly on men, and the PCL: YV factor analytic work with female populations is scarce. Of the rare studies, Kosson et al. (2013) assessed the suitability of one-, two-, three-, and four-factor models among a combined sample of 646 adolescent girls from Europe and North America who originally participated in 14 independent studies. The sample included incarcerated girls and those from less restrictive settings (short-term detention, community probation, clinic). Comparably to the above-cited research with boys, only three- and four-factor models evidenced adequate model fit in the full sample, the North American subsample (n = 285), and the subsample of girls from less restrictive settings (n = 277). Interestingly, only the three-factor model, i.e., the one excluding criminal items, yielded an acceptable fit in the European and incarcerated subsamples, suggesting that psychopathic characteristics may be expressed differently across cultures and settings. Sevecke, Pukrop, Kosson, and Krischer (2009), on the other hand, could not identify a single model which would adequately capture PCL: YV scores retrieved from girls.

Vitacco et al. (2006) tested an association between the three- and four-factor models of the PCL: YV and a single factor of instrumental aggression, using structural equation modeling (SEM). Results indicated that the four-factor model accounted for 20 percent of variance in the external criterion. The interpersonal psychopathy facet was positively associated with instrumental aggression, whereas antisocial behavior facet – negatively. Further, the three-factor model of the PCL: YV, i.e., the model without items referring to criminality, accounted for 8 percent of the variance for instrumental aggression, with the lifestyle psychopathy facet forming the only significant positive relationship with instrumental aggression. Since different psychopathy dimensions were associated with instrumental aggression in these two analyses, more studies among larger samples are warranted to corroborate the findings. With a similar focus on criminal and aggressive behaviors, Corrado, McCuish, Hart, and DeLisi (2015) demonstrated that chronic offending is *not* related to interpersonal and affective psychopathy symptoms as measured by the PCL: YV. In a three-year follow-up investigation, the PCL: YV was found to predict recidivism, but its predictive power was due primarily to the behavioral psychopathy characteristics. PCL: YV did not predict violent or nonviolent recidivism for girls. These findings ought to be considered by professionals who rely on the PCL: YV for violence risk assessment.

Apart from violence and recidivism, PCL: YV scores were associated with a range of external criteria. For example, in a small sample (N = 67) of Dutch female adolescents admitted to a secure treatment institution, increased PCL: YV Factor 1 (Interpersonal/Affective) scores were inversely associated with health concerns, low self-esteem, and anxiety. Factor 2 (lifestyle/antisocial) scores, in turn, were positively related to Anger, conduct problems, proneness to alcohol and drug problems, and psychological immaturity (Das, de Ruiter, & Doreleijers, 2008). In another empirical study with female adolescents recruited from an Illinois correctional facility for youth offenders (N = 80), total PCL: YV score was positively correlated with total number of charges and infractions, number of violent infractions, Conduct Disorder, Attention-Deficit/Hyperactivity Disorder (ADHD), and anxiety. Further, associations between four PCL: YV dimensions and behavioral and emotional functioning have been recently investigated among male (n = 40) and female (n = 40) adolescents incarcerated in Victoria, Australia. Two behavioral PCL: YV facets were related with delinquent and aggressive behaviors. ADHD was associated with affective deficits among girls. Item-level analyses revealed that seven of the 20 PCL: YV items, including "lack of remorse" and "callous/lack of empathy," significantly correlated with ADHD, suggesting that the PCL: YV may be identifying girls with ADHD as opposed to core psychopathic personality traits. Additionally, heightened scores on affective, lifestyle, and antisocial PCL: YV dimensions formed significant positive correlations with self-harming behaviors among girls but not among boys (Strand, Luebbers, & Shepherd, 2016).

SRP–III and SRP–SF

Clinician-administered psychopathy measures, despite requiring extensive resources, may be of value in applied settings, such as prisons and forensic hospitals, because they eliminate the problem of response bias. Such measures, however, are not practical for use with subclinical samples due to lack of clinical history data for participants from the general population (Lilienfeld & Fowler, 2007). To address this issue, Hare and colleagues created a self-report version of the PCL(–R), the SRP. The first edition of the SRP (Hare, 1985), consisting of 29 items, failed to adequately address the core features of a psychopathic personality, such as callousness and dishonesty (Lilienfeld & Fowler, 2007). The SRP–II included 60 items, 31 of which formed the core of the scale and aligned with the two factors of the PCL–R (Williams & Paulhus, 2004). In a validation study within a forensic sample, Hare (2003) reported a moderate correlation between the SRP–II and PCL–R (r = 0.54). The latest version of the measure, the SRP–III (Paulhus et al., 2016), consists of 64 items measured on a 5-point Likert scale. Paulhus et al. also developed a shortened, 29-item form of the scale (SRP–SF) to reduce administration time.

Factor analytic work tested one-, two-, three-, four-, and bi-factor models of the SRP–III and SRP–SF among student, community, and forensic populations. Mahmut, Menictas, Stevenson, and Homewood (2011) and Neal and Sellbom (2012) adopted an inquisitive approach to SRP–III factor structure assessment, testing four models in an Australian community sample (N = 500) and eight models in a North American college student sample (N = 602) respectively. Both studies found the four-factor model composed of interpersonal manipulation (IPM), callous affect (CA), erratic lifestyle (ELS), and antisocial behavior (AB) to be the best fit for the data. Mahmut et al. (2011), however, before proceeding to CFA, dropped 24 SRP–III items with loadings less than 0.30 in the EFA, rendering the results incomparable with other similar research. In five other studies, the SRP–III and SRP–SF scores demonstrated a good fit for the four-factor model; however, no competing model solutions were assessed (Declercq, Carter, & Neumann, 2015; Gordts, Uzieblo, Neumann, Van den Bussche, & Rossi, 2017; León-Mayer et al., 2015; Neumann et al., 2014; Neumann, Schmitt, Carter, Embley, & Hare, 2012). Debowska, Boduszek, Kola, and Hyland (2014), Gordts et al. (2017), and Neal and Sellbom (2012) failed to find an appropriate model fit when using all 64 SRP–III items as indicators. To reduce model complexity, the researchers employed the parceling technique/testlets,[1] which improved the overall model fit. Gordts et al. (2017) and Neal and Sellbom (2012) suggested the four-factor parceled model as the best fit for the data. Debowska et al. (2014), who used a Polish version of the SRP–III, included a bi-factor conceptualization of psychopathy with two general factors (Interpersonal/Affective and lifestyle/antisocial) and four grouping factors (IPM, CA, ELS, and ASB) and, after having examined eight competing solutions, found it to be a statistically superior representation of the data. Since standardized factor loadings were significantly stronger for the grouping factors than for the general factors, the Polish SRP–III was suggested to be measuring four primary factors of psychopathy and two hidden factors.

An important limitation identified in studies utilizing the SRP–SF pertains to the number of scale items used. While the original SRP–SF consists of 29 items, some researchers have reduced the number of indicators. For example, Gordts et al. (2017) used a 28-item scale. Neumann et al. (2014) utilized a 19- and 26-item (but the figure provided suggests the inclusion of 18 items only) SRP–SF, without explaining which scale items were excluded. Neumann et al. (2012) analyzed the factor structure of an experimental 19-item version of the SRP. This lack of consistency significantly undermines the generalizability of research findings and the reliability of the measure. More recently, Debowska et al. (2018) tested the construct validity, factor structure, and factorial invariance of the 29-item SRP–SF, using data from 730 U.K. and U.S. inmates (sample 1) and 2,506 U.K. students (sample 2). From among seven models, the one with two factors (Interpersonal/Affective and lifestyle/antisocial) while controlling for four grouping factors (CA, IPM, ELS, and ASB) best represented the underlying structure of the scale in both samples. Nonetheless, the solution was factorially *variant* for the two groups, indicating that the measure cannot be used in the same way with student and offender populations. This was suggested to be due to inclusion of the criminal/antisocial items. Dotterer et al. (2016) found a bi-factor solution with one general and four grouping factors to provide the best approximation to the 29-item SRP–SF scores within a sample of 2,554 young adults (a model with two general factors was not tested). This model was factorially invariant across gender, but some scale items worked differently among men and women. Unexpectedly and in opposition to unacceptably low fit indices (the Tucker–Lewis Index [TLI] = 0.88, CFI = 0.89 for the total sample), the authors also stated that a correlated four-factor model "showed good fit to the data" (p. 1).

Research has assessed correlations between SRP–III/SF factors and external criteria. SRP–III–IPM factor was found to be positively associated with aggression, drinking, bullying, blame externalizing, alienation, relational and physical aggression, fraud, and narcissism; and negatively correlated with impression management, deception, honesty, and Agreeableness. SRP–III–CA facet formed significant positive correlations with drinking, anxiety, avoidance, verbal and physical bullying, and callousness/unemotional traits; and negative correlations with impression management, deception, empathy, and Agreeableness. SRP–III–ELS was positively related with aggression, three bullying dimensions (verbal, social, physical), boredom proneness, excitement seeking, disconstraint, general externalizing behavioral style, alcohol and drug problems, Extraversion, and openness; and negatively with impression management, deception, planful control, Agreeableness, and Conscientiousness. Lastly, SRP–III–ASB associated positively with physical bullying, destructive aggression, theft, and alcohol and drug problems; and negatively with impression management and deception (Debowska et al., 2014; Gordts et al., 2017; Freeman & Samson, 2012; Neal & Sellbom, 2012). While most of these associations were in the expected direction, some were atheoretical, such as the negative correlation between IMP and impression management, or the positive relationship between CA and anxiety. Further, despite some very high correlations between the SRP–III factors (up to 0.88 between IPM and CA; Debowska et al., 2014), the differential predictive validity of the different dimensions was mostly weak to moderate in the above-cited studies (see Boduszek & Debowska, 2016).

IPM as indexed using SRP–SF correlated positively with social bullying, criminal offenses, internalizing, externalizing, maternal mortality rate (MMR), infant mortality rate (IMR), fertility rate, and pathogen levels; and negatively with gross domestic product per capita (GDPpc), progressive sex-role ideology, and body mass index (BMI). SRP–SF–CA factor associated positively with avoidance, verbal and physical bullying, criminal offenses, externalizing, and internalizing. SRP–SF–ELS formed significant positive correlations with bullying (verbal, social, physical), criminal offenses, internalizing, externalizing, and cultural masculinity. SRP–SF–ASB created positive links with physical bullying, MMR, IMR, and fertility rate; and negative with progressive sex-role ideology and BMI (Gordts et al., 2017; Neumann et al., 2012; Neumann, Hare, & Pardini, 2014). The choice of some of those correlates, however, is unclear from the theoretical perspective (e.g., MMR, IMR, fertility rate, GDPpc). Of importance, in Gordts et al.'s (2017) study corresponding SRP–III and SRP–SF facets formed some differing associations with external variables. For example, SRP–III–IPM, but not SRP–SF–IPM, correlated significantly with the Adolescent Peer Relations Instrument–Social Target subscale (Parada, 2000). The SRP–III–CA associated positively and SRP–SF–CA associated negatively with the Adolescent Peer Relations Instrument–Verbal Target subscale, but these correlations were statistically non-significant.

Conclusion

Although the PCL–R and its derivatives are the most frequently used psychopathy assessment tools in both research and practice, the instruments' construct and predictive validity have been challenged (Boduszek & Debowska, 2016; Cooke & Michie, 2001; Skeem & Cooke, 2010a, 2010b). In considering that the PCL–R is often equated with the concept that it contends to measure and the significant role it plays in criminal justice settings, such methodological limitations may distort our understanding of psychopathy and subsequently lead to ill-informed decisions affecting the lives of people being assessed. In light of the above, it is of paramount importance that *critical* reviews of research into the PCL–R family of psychopathy measures with suggestions for surmounting all identified limitations are regularly conducted and published.

Based on the review of studies presented herein, all PCL–R-based measures are characterized by multidimensionality. However, there is a lack of consensus among researchers as to the model structure that best represents the instruments' scores. Studies conducted among student, community, offending, adult, youth, and mixed-gender or exclusively male/female populations from a number of different cultural settings suggest that the scales' scores can be captured by two-, three-, four-, bi-factor, and hierarchical models. While the correlated four-factorial model seems to be identified as the best solution most frequently, especially in research using the PCL–R and SRP–III, it was oftentimes the case that only this particular model was tested, rendering comparisons between competing, theoretically sound models impossible (e.g., Declercq et al., 2015; Gordts et al., 2017; Krstic et al., 2017; León-Mayer et al., 2015; Mokros et al., 2011; Neumann et al., 2013, 2014; Zwets et al., 2015). One interesting recent innovation in factor analytic literature looking at the PCL–R and its derivatives is the inclusion of bi-factor models, which have been demonstrated to be superior in capturing the instruments' scores (e.g., Boduszek et al., 2016; Debowska et al., 2014; Dotterer et al., 2016; Flores-Mendoza et al., 2008), even when all PCL–R scale items are modeled, including those traditionally regarded as not belonging to any latent factor (e.g., Patrick et al., 2007). Of importance, despite the multifaceted nature of the PCL–R, the cut-off point used to diagnose psychopathy relies on the total instrument score, hence assuming variations in trait intensity (quantitative differences) but not in the constellation of psychopathic traits (qualitative differences) across individuals. A recent statistical study into the validity of this approach revealed in excess of 8.5 million different response combinations that amounted to the score of 30, and over 14.2 million that amounted to 30 or more. This suggests that "applying cut scores on this measure results in imprecise quantifications of psychopathy" (Balsis, Busch, Wilfong, Newman, & Edens, 2017:1). Additionally, the inclusion of criminality items in total score calculations could have led to an overestimation of psychopathy in offending samples. Therefore, it is recommended that future research seeks to address this issue, possibly by excluding all behavioral items, which may be an outcome of psychopathic personality traits. Offering a promising alternative to traditional cut-off points are person-centered statistical techniques (such as latent profile/class analysis), which have the power to reveal patterns of co-occurrence between different psychopathic traits and establish how the resultant psychopathy profiles predict external criteria, such as aggression or reoffending (Boduszek, Debowska, & Willmott, 2017).

Other limitations identified in the extant research include the use of parceling procedure with short scales (e.g., Cooke & Michie, 2001; Cooke et al., 2005a, 2007; Vitacco, Rogers, Neumann et al., 2005; Weizmann-Henelius et al., 2010), correlating errors of measurement (e.g., Hildebrand et al., 2002; Jones et al., 2006), dropping scale items based on statistics rather than theoretical considerations (e.g., Mahmut et al., 2011), use of small samples (e.g., Das et al., 2008; Medina et al., 2013; Salekin et al., 2006; Vitacco et al., 2006), repeated use of the same sample for similar purposes (e.g., Cooke et al., 2005a, 2005b, 2007; Cooke & Michie, 2001), and descriptions/recommendations which do not follow on from/match study results (e.g., Dotterer et al., 2016; Forth et al., 1996). All future research should aim to surpass these problems, in an effort to challenge the status quo of psychopathy research and promote knowledge development.

Note

1 The terms "parcels" and "testlets" are normally used interchangeably (Reeve & Lam, 2005).

References

Balsis, S., Busch, A. J., Wilfong, K. M., Newman, J. W., and Edens, J. F. (2017) 'A statistical consideration regarding the threshold of the Psychopathy Checklist–Revised,' *Journal of Personality Assessment, 1*:1–9.

Bentler, P. M. (1995) *EQS structural equations program manual*, Encino, CA: Multivariate Software.

Blonigen, D. M., Hicks, B. M., Krueger, R. F., Patrick, C. J., and Iacono, W. G. (2006) 'Continuity and change in psychopathic traits as measured via normal-range personality: A longitudinal-biometric study,' *Journal of Abnormal Psychology, 115*(1):85–95.

Boduszek, D., and Debowska, A. (2016) 'Critical evaluation of psychopathy measurement (PCL–R and SRP–III/SF) and recommendations for future research,' *Journal of Criminal Justice, 44*:1–12.

Boduszek, D., Debowska, A., and Willmott, D. (2017) 'Latent profile analysis of psychopathic traits among homicide, general violence, property, and white-collar offenders,' *Journal of Criminal Justice, 51*:17–23.

Boduszek, D., Dhingra, K., Hyland, P., and Debowska, A. (2016) 'A bifactorial solution to the Psychopathy Checklist: Screening Version in a sample of civil psychiatric patients,' *Criminal Behaviour and Mental Health, 26*(3):174–185.

Bolt, D. M., Hare, R. D., Vitale, J. E., and Newman, J. P. (2004) 'A multigroup item response theory analysis of the Psychopathy Checklist–Revised,' *Psychological Assessment, 16*(2):155–168.

Cleckley, H. (1941) *The mask of sanity* (1st ed.), St. Louis, MO: C.V. Mosby.

Cooke, D. J., Kosson, D. S., and Michie, C. (2001) 'Psychopathy and ethnicity: Structural, item, and test generalizability of the Psychopathy Checklist–Revised (PCL–R) in Caucasian and African American participants,' *Psychological Assessment, 13*(4):531–542.

Cooke, D. J., and Michie, C. (2001) 'Refining the construct of psychopathy: Towards a hierarchical model,' *Psychological Assessment, 13*(2):171–188.

Cooke, D. J., Michie, C., Hart, S. D., and Clark, D. (2005a) 'Assessing psychopathy in the UK: Concerns about cross-cultural generalisability,' *The British Journal of Psychiatry, 186*(4):335–341.

Cooke, D. J., Michie, C., Hart, S. D., and Clark, D. (2005b) 'Searching for the pan-cultural core of psychopathic personality disorder,' *Personality and Individual Differences, 39*(2):283–295.

Cooke, D. J., Michie, C., Hart, S. D., and Hare, R. D. (1999) 'Evaluating the Screening Version of the Hare Psychopathy Checklist–Revised (PCL: SV): An item response theory analysis,' *Psychological Assessment, 11*(1):3–13.

Cooke, D. J., Michie, C., and Skeem, J. (2007) 'Understanding the structure of the Psychopathy Checklist–Revised: An exploration of methodological confusion,' *The British Journal of Psychiatry, 190*(49):s39–s50.

Corrado, R. R., McCuish, E. C., Hart, S. D., and DeLisi, M. (2015) 'The role of psychopathic traits and developmental risk factors on offending trajectories from early adolescence to adulthood: A prospective study of incarcerated youth,' *Journal of Criminal Justice*, *43*(4):357–368.

Corrado, R. R., Vincent, G. M., Hart, S. D., and Cohen, I. M. (2004) 'Predictive validity of the Psychopathy Checklist: Youth Version for general and violent recidivism,' *Behavioral Sciences & the Law*, *22*(1):5–22.

Das, J., de Ruiter, C., and Doreleijers, T. (2008) 'Reliability and validity of the Psychopathy Checklist: Youth Version in Dutch female adolescents,' *International Journal of Law and Psychiatry*, *31*(3):219–228.

Debowska, A., Boduszek, D., Dhingra, K., Sherretts, N., Willmott, D., and DeLisi, M. (2018) 'Can we use Hare's psychopathy model within forensic and non-forensic populations? An empirical investigation,' *Deviant Behavior*, *39*(2):224–242.

Debowska, A., Boduszek, D., Kola, S., and Hyland, P. (2014) 'A bifactor model of the Polish version of the Hare Self-Report Psychopathy Scale,' *Personality and Individual Differences*, *69*:231–237.

Declercq, F., Carter, R., and Neumann, C. S. (2015) 'Assessing psychopathic traits and criminal behavior in a young adult female community sample using the Self-Report Psychopathy Scale,' *Journal of Forensic Sciences*, *60*(4):928–935.

Dotterer, H. L., Waller, R., Neumann, C. S., Shaw, D. S., Forbes, E. E., Hariri, A. R., and Hyde, L. W. (2016) 'Examining the factor structure of the Self-Report of Psychopathy Short-Form across four young adult samples,' *Assessment*, 23:1–18.

Flores-Mendoza, C. E., Alvarenga, M. A. S., Herrero, Ó., and Abad, F. J. (2008) 'Factor structure and behavioural correlates of the Psychopathy Checklist–Revised [PCL–R] in a Brazilian prisoner sample,' *Personality and Individual Differences*, *45*(7):584–590.

Forth, A. E., Brown, S. L., Hart, S. D., and Hare, R. D. (1996) 'The assessment of psychopathy in male and female noncriminals: Reliability and validity,' *Personality and Individual Differences*, *20*(5):531–543.

Forth, A. E., and Burke, H. C. (1998) 'Psychopathy in adolescence: Assessment, violence, and developmental precursors,' in D. J. Cooke, A. E. Forth, & R. D. Hare (Eds.), *Psychopathy: Theory, research and implications for society* (pp. 205–229), Dordrecht: Springer Netherlands.

Forth, A. E., Kosson, D., and Hare, R. (2003) *The Hare Psychopathy Checklist: Youth Version*, New York, NY: Multi-Health Systems.

Forth, A. E., and Mailloux, D. L. (2000) 'Psychopathy in youth: What do we know,' in C. B. Gacono (Ed.), *The clinical and forensic assessment of psychopathy: A practitioner's guide* (pp. 25–54), Mahwah, NJ: Erlbaum.

Freeman, A., and Reinecke, M. A. (2007) *Personality disorders in childhood and adolescence*, Hoboken: John Wiley & Sons.

Freeman, J. E., and Samson, F. (2012) 'Are you telling the truth? Psychopathy assessment and impression management in a community sample,' *The Open Criminology Journal*, *5*:16–23.

Furr, K. D. (1993) 'Prediction of sexual or violent recidivism among sexual offenders: A comparison of prediction instruments,' *Annals of Sex Research*, *6*(4):271–286.

Gill, D. J., and Crino, R. D. (2012) 'The relationship between psychopathy and age in a non- clinical community convenience sample,' *Psychiatry, Psychology and Law*, *19*(4):547–557.

Gordts, S., Uzieblo, K., Neumann, C., Van den Bussche, E., and Rossi, G. (2017) 'Validity of the Self-Report Psychopathy Scales (SRP–III full and short versions) in a community sample,' *Assessment*, *24*(3):308–325.

Grann, M., Långström, N., Tengström, A., and Kullgren, G. (1999) 'Psychopathy (PCL–R) predicts violent recidivism among criminal offenders with personality disorders in Sweden,' *Law and Human Behavior*, *23*(2):205–217.

Hare, R. D. (1980) 'A research scale for the assessment of psychopathy in criminal populations,' *Personality and Individual Differences*, *1*(2):111–119.

Hare, R. D. (1985) 'Comparison of procedures for the assessment of psychopathy,' *Journal of Consulting and Clinical Psychology*, *53*(1):7–16.

Hare, R. D. (1991) *The Hare Psychopathy Checklist–Revised*, Toronto, ON: Multi-Health Systems.

Hare, R. D. (2003) *The Hare Psychopathy Checklist–Revised* (2nd ed.), Toronto, ON: Multi-Health Systems.

Hare, R. D., and Neumann, C. S. (2006) 'The PCL–R assessment of psychopathy: Development, structural properties, and new directions,' in C. Patrick (Ed.), *Handbook of Psychopathy* (pp. 58–90), New York, NY: The Guilford Press.

Hare, R. D., and Neumann, C. S. (2008) 'Psychopathy as a clinical and empirical construct,' *Annual Review of Clinical Psychology*, *4*:217–246.

Harpur, T. J., Hakstian, A. R., and Hare, R. D. (1988) 'Factor structure of the Psychopathy Checklist,' *Journal of Consulting and Clinical Psychology*, *56*(5):741–747.
Harpur, T. J., Hare, R. D., and Hakstian, A. R. (1989) 'Two-factor conceptualization of psychopathy: Construct validity and assessment implications,' *Psychological Assessment: A Journal of Consulting and Clinical Psychology*, *1*(1):6–17.
Hart, S. D., Cox, D. N., and Hare, R. D. (1995) *Hare Psychopathy Checklist: Screening Version (PCL: SV)*, Toronto, ON: Multi-Heath Systems.
Hart, S. D., Kropp, P. R., and Hare, R. D. (1988) 'Performance of male psychopaths following conditional release from prison,' *Journal of Consulting and Clinical Psychology*, *56*(2):227–232.
Hildebrand, M., de Ruiter, C., de Vogel, V., and van der Wolf, P. (2002) 'Reliability and factor structure of the Dutch language version of Hare's Psychopathy Checklist–Revised,' *International Journal of Forensic Mental Health*, *1*(2):139–154.
Hill, C. D., Neumann, C. S., and Rogers, R. (2004) 'Confirmatory factor analysis of the Psychopathy Checklist: Screening Version in offenders with axis I disorders,' *Psychological Assessment*, *16*(1):90–95.
Hyland, P. (2015) 'Application of bifactor models in criminal psychology research: A guide to researchers,' *Journal of Criminal Psychology*, *5*(2):65–74.
Johansson, P., Andershed, H., Kerr, M., and Levander, S. (2002) 'On the operationalization of psychopathy: Further support for a three-faceted personality oriented model,' *Acta Psychiatrica Scandinavica*, *106*(s412):81–85.
Jones, S., Cauffman, E., Miller, J. D., and Mulvey, E. (2006) 'Investigating different factor structures of the psychopathy checklist: Youth version: Confirmatory factor analytic findings,' *Psychological Assessment*, *18*(1):33–48.
Kosson, D. S., Neumann, C. S., Forth, A. E., Salekin, R. T., Hare, R. D., Krischer, M. K., and Sevecke, K. (2013) 'Factor structure of the Hare Psychopathy Checklist: Youth Version (PCL: YV) in adolescent females,' *Psychological Assessment*, *25*(1):71–83.
Krstic, S., Neumann, C. S., Roy, S., Robertson, C., Knight, R. A., and Hare, R. D. (2017) 'Using latent variables- and person-centered approaches to examine the role of psychopathic traits in sex offenders,' *Personality Disorders: Theory, Research, and Treatment*, in press.
León-Mayer, E., Folino, J. O., Neumann, C., and Hare, R. D. (2015) 'The construct of psychopathy in a Chilean prison population,' *Revista Brasileira de Psiquiatria*, *37*(3):191–196.
Lilienfeld, S. O., and Fowler, K. A. (2007) 'The self-report assessment of psychopathy: Problems, pitfalls, and promises,' in C. J. Patrick (Ed.), *Handbook of psychopathy* (pp. 107–132), New York, NY: The Guilford Press.
Lynam, D. R. (1996) 'Early identification of chronic offenders: Who is the fledgling psychopath?,' *Psychological Bulletin*, *120*(2):209–234.
Mahmut, M. K., Menictas, C., Stevenson, R. J., and Homewood, J. (2011) 'Validating the factor structure of the Self-Report Psychopathy Scale in a community sample,' *Psychological Assessment*, *23*(3):670–678.
McDermott, P. A., Alterman, A. I., Cacciola, J. S., Rutherford, M. J., Newman, J. P., and Mulholland, E. M. (2000) 'Generality of Psychopathy Checklist–Revised factors over prisoners and substance-dependent patients,' *Journal of Consulting and Clinical Psychology*, *68*(1):181–186.
Medina, P., Valdés-Sosa, M., García, L. G., Almeyda, S. V., and Couso, O. (2013) 'Reliability and validity of the Psychopathy Checklist–Revised (PCL–R) in a Cuban prison sample,' *Salud Mental*, *36*:439–444.
Miller, A. L., Muehlenkamp, J. J., and Jacobson, C. M. (2008) 'Fact or fiction: Diagnosing borderline personality disorder in adolescents,' *Clinical Psychology Review*, *28*(6):969–981.
Mokros, A., Neumann, C. S., Stadtland, C., Osterheider, M., Nedopil, N., and Hare, R. D. (2011) 'Assessing measurement invariance of PCL–R assessments from file reviews of North American and German offenders,' *International Journal of Law and Psychiatry*, *34*(1):56–63.
Neal, T. M., and Sellbom, M. (2012) 'Examining the factor structure of the Hare self-report psychopathy scale,' *Journal of Personality Assessment*, *94*(3):244–253.
Neumann, C. S., Hare, R. D., and Johansson, P. T. (2013) 'The Psychopathy Checklist–Revised (PCL–R), low anxiety, and fearlessness: A structural equation modeling analysis,' *Personality Disorders: Theory, Research, and Treatment*, *4*(2):129–137.
Neumann, C. S., Hare, R. D., and Newman, J. P. (2007) 'The super-ordinate nature of the Psychopathy Checklist–Revised,' *Journal of Personality Disorders*, *21*(2):102–117.
Neumann, C. S., Hare, R. D., and Pardini, D. A. (2014) 'Antisociality and the construct of psychopathy: Data from across the globe,' *Journal of Personality*, *83*(6):678–692.

Neumann, C. S., Kosson, D. S., Forth, A. E., and Hare, R. D. (2006) 'Factor structure of the Hare Psychopathy Checklist: Youth Version (PCL: YV) in incarcerated adolescents,' *Psychological Assessment*, *18*(2):142–154.

Neumann, C. S., Schmitt, D. S., Carter, R., Embley, I., and Hare, R. D. (2012) 'Psychopathic traits in females and males across the globe,' *Behavioral Sciences & the Law*, *30*:557–574.

Olver, M. E., and Wong, S. C. (2015) 'Short- and long-term recidivism prediction of the PCL–R and the effects of age: A 24-year follow-up,' *Personality Disorders: Theory, Research, and Treatment*, *6*(1):97–105.

Parada, R. (2000) Adolescent Peer Relations Instrument: A theoretical and empirical basis for the measurement of participant roles in bullying and victimization of adolescence: An interim test manual and a research monograph: A test manual. Publication Unit, Self-concept Enhancement and Learning Facilitation (SELF) Research Centre, University of Western Sydney.

Patrick, C. (2007) 'Back to the future: Cleckley as a guide to the next generation of psychopathy research,' in C. Patrick (Ed.), *Handbook of psychopathy* (pp. 605–617), New York, NY: Guilford Press.

Patrick, C. J., Hicks, B. M., Nichol, P. E., and Krueger, R. F. (2007) 'A bifactor approach to modeling the structure of the Psychopathy Checklist–Revised,' *Journal of Personality Disorders*, *21*(2):118–141.

Paulhus, D. L., Neumann, C. S., and Hare, R. D. (2016) *Manual for the Self-Report Psychopathy Scale*, Toronto, ON: Multi-Health Systems.

Polaschek, D. L. (2015) '(Mis)understanding psychopathy: Consequences for policy and practice with offenders,' *Psychiatry, Psychology and Law*, *22*(4):500–519.

Quinsey, V. L., Rice, M. E., and Harris, G. T. (1995) 'Actuarial prediction of sexual recidivism,' *Journal of Interpersonal Violence*, *10*(1):85–105.

Reeve, C. L., and Lam, H. (2005) 'The psychometric paradox of practice effects due to retesting: Measurement invariance and stable ability estimates in the face of observed score changes,' *Intelligence*, *33*(5):535–549.

Rice, M. E., and Harris, G. T. (1995) 'Violent recidivism: Assessing predictive validity,' *Journal of Consulting and Clinical Psychology*, *63*(5):737–748.

Rice, M. E., Harris, G. T., and Quinsey, V. L. (1990) 'A follow-up of rapists assessed in a maximum security psychiatric facility,' *Journal of Interpersonal Violence*, *5*(4):435–448.

Rogers, R., Salekin, R. T., Hill, C., Sewell, K. W., Murdock, M. E., and Neumann, C. S. (2000) 'The Psychopathy Checklist–Screening Version: An examination of criteria and subcriteria in three forensic samples,' *Assessment*, 7(1):1–15.

Rutherford, M. J., Cacciola, J. S., Alterman, A. I., and McKay, J. R. (1996) 'Reliability and validity of the Revised Psychopathy Checklist in women methadone patients,' *Assessment*, *3*(2):145–156.

Salekin, R. T., Brannen, D. N., Zalot, A. A., Leistico, A. M., and Neumann, C. S. (2006) 'Factor structure of psychopathy in youth: Testing the applicability of the new four-factor model,' *Criminal Justice and Behavior*, *33*(2):135–157.

Salekin, R. T., Rogers, R., and Sewell, K. W. (1996) 'A review and meta-analysis of the psychopathy checklist and psychopathy checklist-revised: Predictive validity of dangerousness,' *Clinical Psychology: Science and Practice*, *3*(3):203–215.

Satorra, A., and Bentler, P. M. (1988, August) 'Scaling corrections for chi-square statistics in covariance structure analysis,' *Proceedings of the American Statistical Association*, *1*:308–313.

Serin, R. C. (1996) 'Violent recidivism in criminal psychopaths,' *Law and Human Behavior*, *20*(2):207–217.

Serin, R. C., and Amos, N. L. (1995) 'The role of psychopathy in the assessment of dangerousness,' *International Journal of Law and Psychiatry*, *18*(2):231–238.

Serin, R. C., Peters, R. D., and Barbaree, H. E. (1990) 'Predictors of psychopathy and release outcome in a criminal population,' *Psychological Assessment: A Journal of Consulting and Clinical Psychology*, *2*(4):419–422.

Sevecke, K., Pukrop, R., Kosson, D. S., and Krischer, M. K. (2009) 'Factor structure of the Hare Psychopathy Checklist: Youth version in German female and male detainees and community adolescents,' *Psychological Assessment*, *21*(1):45–56.

Skeem, J. L., and Cooke, D. J. (2010a) 'Is criminal behavior a central component of psychopathy? Conceptual directions for resolving the debate,' *Psychological Assessment*, *22*(2):433–445.

Skeem, J. L., and Cooke, D. J. (2010b) 'One measure does not a construct make: Directions toward reinvigorating psychopathy research – reply to Hare and Neumann (2010),' *Psychological Assessment*, *22*(2):455–459.

Skeem, J. L., and Mulvey, E. P. (2001) 'Psychopathy and community violence among civil psychiatric patients: Results from the MacArthur Violence Risk Assessment Study,' *Journal of Consulting and Clinical Psychology*, *69*(3):358–374.

Skeem, J. L., Mulvey, E. P., and Grisso, T. (2003) 'Applicability of traditional and revised models of psychopathy to the Psychopathy Checklist: Screening Version,' *Psychological Assessment, 15*(1):41–55.
Strand, S., Luebbers, S., and Shepherd, S. M. (2016) 'Psychopathic features in young incarcerated females,' *Journal of Criminal Psychology, 6*(2):63–75.
Tsang, S., Schmidt, K. M., Vincent, G. M., Salekin, R. T., Moretti, M. M., and Odgers, C. L. (2015) 'Assessing psychopathy among justice involved adolescents with the PCL: YV: An item response theory examination across gender,' *Personality Disorders: Theory, Research, and Treatment, 6*(1):22–31.
Vitacco, M. J., Neumann, C. S., Caldwell, M. F., Leistico, A. M., and Van Rybroek, G. J. (2006) 'Testing factor models of the Psychopathy Checklist: Youth Version and their association with instrumental aggression,' *Journal of Personality Assessment, 87*(1):74–83.
Vitacco, M. J., Neumann, C. S., and Jackson, R. L. (2005) 'Testing a four-factor model of psychopathy and its association with ethnicity, gender, intelligence, and violence,' *Journal of Consulting and Clinical Psychology, 73*(3):466–476.
Vitacco, M. J., Rogers, R., Neumann, C. S., Harrison, K. S., and Vincent, G. (2005) 'A comparison of factor models on the PCL–R with mentally disordered offenders the development of a four-factor model,' *Criminal Justice and Behavior, 32*(5):526–545.
Walters, G. D. (2012) 'Psychopathy and crime: Testing the incremental validity of PCL–R- measured psychopathy as a predictor of general and violent recidivism,' *Law and Human Behavior, 36*(5):404–412.
Weaver, C. M., Meyer, R. G., Van Nort, J. J., and Tristan, L. (2006) 'Two-, three-, and four- factor PCL–R models in applied sex offender risk assessments,' *Assessment, 13*(2):208–216.
Weizmann-Henelius, G., Putkonen, H., Grönroos, M., Lindberg, N., Eronen, M., and Häkkänen-Nyholm, H. (2010) 'Examination of psychopathy in female homicide offenders – Confirmatory factor analysis of the PCL–R,' *International Journal of Law and Psychiatry, 33*(3):177–183.
Weizmann-Henelius, G., Virkkunen, M., Gammelgård, M., Eronen, M., and Putkonen, H. (2015) 'The PCL–R and violent recidivism in a prospective follow-up of a nationwide sample of female offenders,' *The Journal of Forensic Psychiatry & Psychology, 26*(5):667–685.
Williams, K. M., and Paulhus, D. L. (2004) 'Factor structure of the Self-Report Psychopathy scale (SRP–II) in non-forensic samples,' *Personality and Individual Differences, 37*(4):765–778.
Yang, M., Wong, S. C., and Coid, J. (2010) 'The efficacy of violence prediction: A meta-analytic comparison of nine risk assessment tools,' *Psychological Bulletin, 136*(5):740–767.
Žukauskienė, R., Laurinavičius, A., and Česnienė, I. (2010) 'Testing factorial structure and validity of the PCL: SV in Lithuanian prison population,' *Journal of Psychopathology and Behavioral Assessment, 32*(3):363–372.
Zwets, A. J., Hornsveld, R. H., Neumann, C., Muris, P., and van Marle, H. J. (2015) 'The four-factor model of the Psychopathy Checklist–Revised: Validation in a Dutch forensic inpatient sample. *International Journal of Law and Psychiatry, 39*:13–22.

16

The triarchic psychopathy model

Theory and measurement

Martin Sellbom

Introduction

Individuals high on psychopathy can be identified in every culture and society. In one way or another, most people have met someone high on psychopathy – many have been deceived and manipulated by them and forced to live with the harm they have caused (Hare, 2007). As evident from the many chapters in this book, psychopathy has become a very important construct in the criminal justice system (e.g., risk classifications in sentencing cases). Although some estimates based on the Psychopathy Checklist–Revised (PCL–R; Hare, 2003) indicate that psychopathy comprises 0.5–1 percent of the population, individuals with psychopathy are estimated to account for 15–20 percent of prison inmates (Hare, Hart, & Harpur, 1991) and can have a tremendous effect on society as a whole. These individuals are responsible for a disproportionate amount of criminal conduct, have long-lasting and varied criminal careers, and are at substantial risk for violence and sexual aggression, as well as future offending (Skeem, Polaschek, Patrick, & Lilienfeld, 2011). The most obvious manifestations of psychopathy involve blatant violation of societal rules and laws (Hare, 1994); however, many psychopathic individuals manage to avoid incarceration, using interpersonal manipulation to exploit and otherwise cause distress in others (Hare, 2007; see e.g., http://aftermath-surviving-psychopathy.org for a website for psychopathy survivors). In the business world, psychopaths can be responsible for creating hostile work environments, corruption, malfeasance, and other egregious violations of the public trust that cause financial hardship (Babiak, Neumann, & Hare, 2010). Yet, others have argued that some aspects of psychopathy might even be adaptive, with Lykken (1982:22) classically suggesting that the hero and the psychopath are "twigs from the same branch." Some recent research has indeed confirmed that psychopathy can be associated with heroism and situational altruism, but these findings are not consistent or particularly robust (Smith, Lilienfeld, Coffey, & Dabbs, 2013).

The scientific psychopathy field has been engaged in major and important debates over the past few decades with respect to the conceptual formulation of this construct. Throughout history, there have been many theories and formulations of the psychopathic personality, with a considerable number of divergences and differential emphases on what traits are considered most important. Such disagreements have persisted to the present time, with debates concerning the ultimate factor structure of psychopathy (e.g., Cooke & Michie, 2001; Hare & Neumann,

2006), which have had significant conceptual implications; the role of criminal behavior in defining and operationalizing psychopathy (e.g., Hare & Neumann, 2010; Skeem & Cooke, 2010); whether the domain of Boldness/Fearless Dominance is a central psychopathy domain (e.g., Lilienfeld et al., 2012; Miller & Lynam, 2012); and even whether a classic trait such as impulsivity should be considered a core characteristic (Poythress & Hall, 2011). The triarchic psychopathy model (Patrick, Fowles, & Krueger, 2009; Patrick, 2010a) represents an attempt to integrate these various perspectives into a unified model for this important personality disorder.

Historical and contemporary antecedents for the triarchic psychopathy model

Psychopathy has been discussed in the literature for centuries, with descriptions such as *moral insanity* (Pinel, 1806/1962), *morally depraved and sadistic* (Krafft-Ebing, 1904), and *swindlers* (Kraeplin, 1915), to mention a few. The contemporary formulations of psychopathy originated with Hervey Cleckley's (1941) classic monograph *The Mask of Sanity*, which described a series of cases he observed in a psychiatric hospital that he deemed representative of psychopathy. Cleckley contended that the psychopath often presented outwardly as relatively free of psychological maladjustment and, rather, would present (at least superficially) with good intelligence and lacking in serious neurosis, anxiety, or debilitating mental health problems, giving rise to the "mask." On the other hand, Cleckley (1941 | 1988) also indicated that the psychopath exhibited gross behavioral maladjustment, including impulsivity and irresponsibility, and seemed incapable of forming close emotional attachments to others or learning from punishing experiences. These characteristics led Cleckley (1941:355) to famously summarize that the psychopath superficially charming and gregarious, yet "carries disaster lightly in each hand." In the fifth edition of his book, Cleckley organized the psychopathy descriptions into 16 behavioral criteria, which influenced various formal operationalizations of the disorder. More recently, Patrick (2006) organized Cleckley's criteria into three broad domains reflecting positive *psychological adjustment* (i.e., good intelligence and social adeptness, absence of delusions or irrationality, absence of nervousness, and low incidence of suicide), *emotional unresponsiveness and social detachment*, and *behavioral deviancy*, which map onto several contemporary psychopathy models and measurements. It is noteworthy that only three of Cleckley's 15 cases were described as violent, cruel, or antagonistic (Patrick et al., 2009).

It is important to note that the conceptual formulations of psychopathy seem to be at least in part dependent on the context in which it has been examined. In a now classic monograph titled *The Psychopath: An Essay on the Criminal Mind*, William and Joan McCord described a far more vicious phenotype (McCord & McCord, 1964). More specifically, they described the psychopath as emotionally cold, guiltless, loveless, highly aggressive, and motivated by Anger or rage more than by anxiety or fear. This perspective was to an extent also championed by Lee Robins (1966), who focused on developmental antecedents to psychopathy and its aggressive and disinhibited manifestations; this perspective was eventually highly influential in the DSM–III (and beyond) operationalization of Antisocial Personality Disorder.

David Lykken (1957) theorized and empirically demonstrated that psychopathic offenders showed an attenuated affective response and, in particular, a deficit in fear processing. The findings from this seminal study were initially replicated in a series of experiments by Robert Hare and colleagues (see, e.g., Hare, 1978, for a review) and, much later, Patrick and colleagues (Patrick, Bradley, & Lang, 1993; Patrick, 1994) using a startle reflex paradigm, leading Lykken (1995) to conclude that psychopathy was the result of a low fear quotient. Although research has generally been in support of the role of fearlessness and with several neurobiological theories rooted in amygdala dysfunction (e.g., Blair, 2006), others have argued for a broader range of deficits (e.g., Kiehl, 2006; Patrick & Bernat, 2009), or even that other cognitive functions like attention can completely account for the association between fearlessness and psychopathy (e.g., Newman, Curtin, Bertsch, & Baskin-Sommers, 2010).

Arguably the single most influential development in psychopathy theory and research was the construction of the Psychopathy Checklist (PCL; Hare, 1980) and its revised version, the Psychopathy Checklist–Revised (PCL–R; Hare, 1991, 2003). The PCL–R consists of 20 trait and behavioral criteria that are rated by a trained clinician on the basis of a semi-structured interview and records. Factor analyses of the PCL items initially yielded two factors (Harpur, Hakstian, & Hare, 1988) that reflected affective–interpersonal and social deviance deficits (Harpur, Hare, & Hakstian, 1989), and this two-factor conceptualization quickly came to dominate the field. Later, Cooke and Michie (2001) conducted a series of confirmatory factor analyses in several large offender samples and proposed that a subset of 13 PCL–R items would provide for an optimal three-factor model (interpersonal, affective, and lifestyle factors) while reducing the saturation of criminal behavior within the psychopathy structure. Hare (2003) and Hare and Neumann (2006) later offered a four-factor structure that augmented Cooke and Michie's model with a fourth factor (labeled antisocial) comprised of the remaining PCL–R items. The role of criminality/antisociality as a structural component of psychopathy has become a source of significant debate (e.g., Hare & Neumann, 2010; Skeem & Cooke, 2010), with proponents arguing that such behavior is an integral part of the disorder and the opponents contending that this perspective confuses cause (personality) with consequence (manifest behavior). Nevertheless, the PCL–R has been a (if not *the*) major operationalization of psychopathy since its publication, with at times the unfortunate consequence of many equating the measure with the construct (Skeem & Cooke, 2010). Undoubtedly, a major source of knowledge regarding psychopathy has been generated through research with the PCL–R, which has served to further move psychopathy theory in the direction of its constituent underlying domains. Many recent self-report inventories were indeed influenced by the PCL–R (e.g., Levenson's Self-Report Psychopathy Scale [Levenson, Kiehl, & Fitzpatrick, 1995]; Hare Self-Report Psychopathy Scale [SRP–III; Paulhus, Neumann, & Hare, in press]).

Despite the influence and utility of the PCL–R, it is not practical or suitable for research in community samples. This limitation led Scott Lilienfeld to develop the Psychopathic Personality Inventory (PPI; Lilienfeld, 1990; Lilienfeld & Andrews, 1996; later revised into PPI–R; Lilienfeld & Widows, 2005), which is a 187-item self-report inventory. The PPI item generations were heavily influenced by a range of psychopathy theories, with a significant emphasis on Cleckley's and Lykken's conceptualizations of psychopathic personality, from which Lilienfeld believed the PCL–R had drifted away (Lilienfeld & Andrews, 1996). The effort resulted in eight individual subscales (Machiavellian egocentricity, Social Potency, Coldheartedness, fearlessness, Carefree Nonplanfulness, Blame Externalization, Impulsive Nonconformity, and Stress Immunity). Benning, Patrick, Hicks, Blonigen, and Krueger (2003) subjected these PPI subscales to a factor analysis, which yielded a two-factor structure (or three-factors, where Coldheartedness loaded singularly on a third factor) labeled Fearless Dominance and impulsive/antisocial.[1] These two factors have been the subject of a disproportionate amount of PPI research, culminating in two meta-analyses (Miller & Lynam, 2012; Marcus, Fulton, & Edens, 2013). Although impulsive/antisocial is quite similar in terms of its nomological network to PCL–R Factor 2, it is clear that Fearless Dominance differs more substantially from other measures reflecting PCL–R Factor 1. Some (e.g., Miller & Lynam, 2012) have gone as far as to suggest that Fearless Dominance is peripheral to psychopathy and should not be viewed as a central component, whereas others (e.g., Lilienfeld et al., 2012) have replied that the Fearless Dominance traits encompass important psychopathy features identified by Cleckley but subsequently ignored in other psychopathy measures that model the PCL–R. (This issue is discussed further in a later section).

The youth psychopathy literature has largely, albeit not exclusively, been modeled after the adult PCL–R tradition. The Psychopathy Checklist–Youth Version (PCL: YV; Forth, Kosson, & Hare, 2003) is a direct translation of the PCL–R constructs into adolescence. Andershed and colleagues (2002) developed the Youth Psychopathic Traits Inventory (YPI), which is a self-report questionnaire modeled after Cooke and Michie's (2001) three-factor PCL–R model. This factor structure reflects grandiose/manipulation, callous–unemotional, and impulsive/irresponsible psychopathy traits. Frick and Hare (2001) developed the Antisocial Process Screening Device – a parent and teacher rating form for children – to assess childhood psychopathy, and its factor structure focuses on callous–unemotional, narcissistic (grandiosity/manipulation), and impulsivity traits. An explosion of research within the past decade has focused the child and adolescent literature specifically on callous–unemotional traits as a specifier for children with conduct problems, and was eventually incorporated into DSM–5 (re-labeled Limited Prosocial Emotions; American Psychiatric Association [APA], 2013).

Triarchic psychopathy model

Patrick et al. (2009) argued that three broad phenotypic themes could be distilled from the similarities and differences of these varying perspectives on psychopathy. The first broad domain was referred to as *disinhibition*. Virtually all theories and measurements include a domain that reflects impulsivity, irresponsibility, inability to delay gratification, nonplanfulness, and poor frustration tolerance, which would render a significant proneness to externalizing behavior.

The second domain was labeled *meanness*. It reflects a dispositional proclivity towards deficient empathy, callousness, attenuated capacity to and outright dislike for forming close attachments with other people, exploitativeness and deceitfulness, and relational aggression (Patrick et al., 2009). This phenotypic domain is emphasized in numerous psychopathy theories and measures, albeit to varying degrees. For instance, McCord and McCord (1964) viewed these traits as the cornerstone on psychopathy and it is clearly heavily emphasized in the first factor (affective–interpersonal) of the PCL–R. Meanness is also highly similar to callous–unemotional traits that are often viewed as the core of psychopathy in the youth literature (e.g., White & Frick, 2010). However, Cleckley focused on a limited range of meanness traits whereby he emphasized the lack of attachment, unemotionality, manipulativeness, and egocentricity, but did not otherwise characterize those with psychopathy as instrumentally aggressive, cruel, sadistic, or vicious.

The third domain, Boldness, represents the nexus of social dominance, thrill seeking/fearlessness, and low stress-reactivity (Patrick et al., 2009) and can be traced back to Cleckley's and Lykken's (1995) descriptions of psychopathy. More specifically, Cleckley's "mask" reflects positive psychological adjustment (i.e., good intelligence and social adeptness, absence of delusions or irrationality, absence of nervousness, and low incidence of suicide) and immunity to internalizing psychopathology and fear, in that it entails the presence of severe underlying pathology masked by an outward appearance of robust mental health. Similarly, Lykken (1995) proposed that fearlessness could explain many of the characteristics associated with psychopathy. At the measurement level, this position has primarily been emphasized in the PPI/PPI–R through the Fearless Dominance domain and the interpersonal facet of the PCL–R (Venables, Hall, & Patrick, 2014; Wall, Wygant, & Sellbom, 2015).

Research on the triarchic psychopathy model

Subsequent research on the triarchic psychopathy model initially focused on validating various hypotheses set forth based on the degree to which it should associated with other models and measures (e.g., Sellbom & Phillips, 2013; Drislane, Patrick, & Arsal, 2014). The literature on this model has grown substantially over the past eight years and covers a range of psychopathy-relevant areas, including links to cognitive and affective mechanisms, environmental influences, overlap with normal and abnormal personality traits, and associations with various outcomes.

Explaining variance in other psychopathy models

Much of the validity work to date has centered on the degree to which the triarchic domains can explain variance in other psychopathy models and measures per hypotheses derived from triarchic theory. Patrick (2010a) presented initial data on associations between the PCL–R and the Triarchic Psychopathy Measure (TriPM). All three of the latter domains were meaningfully associated with total PCL–R scores (*r*s = .20 [boldness], .29 [meanness], and .32 [disinhibition]; βs = .22–.27, all *p*s < .05) in a male prison sample (*n* = 148). In terms of specific PCL–R facet scores, boldness was preferentially associated with the interpersonal facet; meanness with the affective facet; and disinhibition with the lifestyle facet; all three triarchic domains contributed uniquely to the prediction of the antisocial facet, which indicates that all three domains are relevant to criminal and antisocial conduct throughout the lifespan. Venables et al. (2014) and Wall et al. (2015) have replicated these general associations. Thus, although the PCL–R contains more meanness and disinhibition variance than boldness variance, as predicted from triarchic theory, all three domains are represented within this measure.

Similar evidence has emerged when various self-report measures of psychopathy have served as the main criteria in both offender and undergraduate samples (Drislane et al., 2014a; Sellbom & Phillips, 2013; Stanley, Wygant, & Sellbom, 2013). From the perspective of the PPI/PPI–R, boldness is preferentially associated with PPI/PPI–R Fearless Dominance, as expected; meanness with PPI/PPI–R Coldheartedness; and both meanness and disinhibition with PPI/PPI–R Self-Centered Impulsivity (Drislane et al., 2014b; Sellbom & Phillips, 2013; Stanley et al., 2013). For the latter PPI domain, meanness is primarily the best predictor of the Machiavellian egocentricity subscale, whereas disinhibition is the best predictor of Carefree Nonplanfulness (Drislane et al., 2014a; Sellbom & Phillips, 2013). Furthermore, Drislane et al. (2014b) and Sellbom and Phillips (2013) have also shown that Levenson Self-Report Psychopathy Scale (LSRP) scores are primarily accounted for by meanness and disinhibition, but not boldness, as described in the LSRP section earlier. Drislane et al. further showed that meanness and disinhibition primarily accounted for variance in the Hare Self-Report Psychopathy Scale–III, with meanness being preferentially associated with interpersonal manipulation and callous affect, whereas disinhibition being primarily related to Erratic Lifestyle; both uniquely predicted Criminal Tendencies. Boldness was also significantly and uniquely associated with the former two subscales, but to a considerably smaller degree than meanness.

In terms of associations with a range of youth psychopathy measures, Drislane et al. (2014a) showed that the Youth Psychopathic Traits Inventory (YPI), Inventory of Callous Unemotional Traits (ICU), Antisocial Process Screening Device (APSD), and Child Psychopathy Scale (CPS) were primarily associated with meanness and disinhibition, with only YPI scores also being associated with boldness (primarily subscales reflecting grandiosity and manipulation; see Sellbom & Phillips [2013] for similar results for APSD and ICU). Thus, for the most part, the youth psychopathy measures that have primarily been influenced by the PCL–R tend to favor meanness and disinhibition with respect to content coverage.

Multivariate associations among various psychopathy subscales have been articulated by means of exploratory factor analysis in two samples from the same university population (Marion et al., 2013; Sellbom & Phillips, 2013). The TriPM domain scales, along with subscales from the PPI, LSRP, APSD, and the ICU, were subjected to a maximum likelihood estimated EFA. In both studies, EFA results revealed three latent factors reflecting *boldness* (TriPM Boldness and PPI Fearless Dominance subscales), *meanness* (TriPM Meanness, PPI Machiavellian egocentricity and Coldheartedness subscales, LSRP egocentricity and Callous scales, APSD Callous–Unemotional and narcissism subscales, and the ICU), and *disinhibition* (PPI Carefree Nonplanfulness, rebellious nonconformity, and Blame Externalization subscales; LSRP antisocial subscale; and the APSD impulsivity–conduct problems subscale). In both samples, the TriPM displayed the highest loading scale for two of the factors and the second highest loading on a third.

In sum, the above referenced research clearly indicates that the triarchic psychopathy domains map onto other psychopathy models and measures as hypothesized by Patrick et al. (2009). These findings provide evidence for situating this model as comprehensive framework that captures most elements emphasized in various psychopathy theories and measures. Of course, it is important that a nomological network is elaborated upon with respect to the triarchic domains themselves, which is described in the next sections.

Neurobehavioral links

An important theme in psychopathy has been linking its underlying dimensions to various neurobiological referents. Patrick and Drislane (2015) noted that the triarchic domains have bio-behavioral referents that map onto neurobiological markers. More specifically, drawing from the broader psychopathy research using measures that generally represent these domains (e.g., general externalizing propensity for disinhibition; Fearless Dominance for boldness; callous–unemotional traits in youth for meanness), they proposed a pattern of robust findings. More specifically, they viewed disinhibition as rooted in the neurobehavioral dimension of *inhibitory control*, which is linked to a variety of mostly prefrontal cortical processes (Patrick, Durbin, & Moser, 2012), including executive cognitive control (Young et al., 2009) and reduction in P3 brain potential response (e.g., Yancey, Venables, Hicks, & Patrick, 2013). Boldness is purported to reflect the neurobehavioral dimension of threat sensitivity in light of research that has been conducted with the PPI Fearless Dominance scale (which measures the boldness construct). Such research has shown evidence for an attenuated startle response in the context of aversive stimuli (e.g., Benning, Patrick, & Iacono, 2005), which is also the case for PCL–R Factor 1, which is mostly a measure of meanness, but to a smaller degree boldness (e.g., Venables et al., 2014; Wall et al., 2015). Meanness is less clear with respect to these neurobehavioral dimensions, but Patrick and Drislane (2015) tentatively linked this domain to *disaffiliated agency* defined as "aggressive resource seeking without concern for others" (p. 630) in light of the literature on callous–unemotional traits in childhood and adolescence. It is noteworthy, however, that Patrick et al. (2009) hypothesized that fearless temperament could potentially explain what boldness and meanness have in common owing to the robust findings of attenuated startle response for both PCL–R Factor 1 and PPI Fearless Dominance.

The emerging research conducted directly on the triarchic psychopathy constructs has generally been consistent with these general findings and conclusions, particularly for boldness and meanness. Esteller, Poy, and Molto (2016) examined the triarchic model with respect to startle reflex potentiation in light of both erotic and threatening stimuli in a mixed gender Spanish university sample. They found that boldness, but not meanness, was associated with an attenuated startle response to threatening stimuli. These findings support the notion of an underlying threat (in)sensitivity for boldness, but not the initial hypothesis set forth by Patrick et al. (2009) that this effect would be related to the overlap in boldness and meanness. Kyranides et al. (2017) examined associations between the triarchic domains and various physiological measures of autonomic activity and startle reflex in relation to both violence and erotic stimuli in a Greek Cypriot community sample. All three triarchic domains were associated with lower autonomic arousal at baseline, but only boldness was negatively associated with arousal while watching violent video content. Boldness was also associated with lower ratings of fear relative to violent videos. Meanness, but not boldness, was associated with an attenuated startle response during violent videos. Thus, it appears as if the nature of the stimuli (violence/aggression vs. threat/fear) dictates which domain is linked to these affective deficits.

Environmental influences

A considerable amount of psychopathy research has been focused on biologically based mechanisms for understanding psychopathy development. Far fewer studies have examined environmentally related mechanisms in a systematic fashion. A recent line of research in the triarchic psychopathy literature has specifically focused on the role of attachment in these psychopathy domains.

Craig, Gray, and Snowden (2013) examined associations between triarchic psychopathy domains and attachment models and parental care in an online undergraduate sample from the U.K. They found that parental care and over-protection were negatively associated with disinhibition, via the mediation of anxious and avoidant attachment styles, whereas maternal care was positively associated with boldness as mediated via (low) anxious attachment. In other words, the model was consistent with the possibility that maternal care contributed to a reduction of anxious attachment, which in turn associated with increases in boldness. Christian, Wilkinson, and Sellbom (2016) replicated and extended these findings in two Australian and U.S. online community samples using multiple well-established measures of attachment theory. Boldness was consistently negatively associated with insecure attachment styles, whereas meanness was reliably associated with avoidant attachment. disinhibition was consistently associated with insecure attachment styles, particularly anxious attachment.

Overall, these studies provide preliminary support for considering attachment theory in psychopathy research, particularly for understanding the interpersonal relations of triarchic psychopathy domains. These studies also provide tentative support for further consideration of relational and environmental experience in the development of psychopathy which could compliment current neurobiological explanations of the construct. Although interesting, these studies were associated with significant limitations in design (cross-sectional study, non-clinical participants, and retrospective reporting), and future research needs to elucidate these associations using longitudinal designs in more pathological samples.

Associations with externalizing and other maladaptive behaviors

Several studies have examined the association between triarchic psychopathy domains and various forms of externalizing and other socially deviant behaviors, which further elucidate how the three domains manifest behaviorally. Coffee, Cox, and Koplin (2017) recently examined associations between what they referred to as "normative" deviance and the triarchic domains in a large online U.S. community sample. They found that boldness and disinhibition, in particular, were associated with various forms of deviant behavior, whereas meanness did not evince meaningful associations with these variables. Although disinhibition was correlated with most forms of deviance, boldness was specifically related to school misconduct, substance use, general deviance, assault, and overall lifetime involvement in deviant behavior. The two domains displayed additive (but not non-additive) effects in a regression model for each of these forms of deviance.

Neo, Sellbom, Smith, and Lilienfeld (2016) examined a latent structural regression model in a large U.S. community sample of employed individuals and found that disinhibition was primarily associated with counterproductive workplace behavior and a passive leadership style. Meanness was associated with unethical decision-making in a workplace context, engagement of hardline approach to influencing others, and refusal to engage in teamwork. Boldness was primarily associated with more covert tactics of influence, but also an assertive, team-oriented leadership approach.

Furthermore, Snowden, Gray, and Smith (2017) recently showed, in a sample of 81 U.K. prison inmates, that boldness, but not Meanness or disinhibition, was uniquely associated with an experimental task (Balloon Analogue Risk Task) indexing risk taking behavior. This finding is consistent with fearlessness and thrill and adventure seeking as part of the broader boldness construct. Rogers, Viding, and Chamorro-Premuzic (2013) considered financial risk taking in particular and examined the association between triarchic domains and instrumental vs disinhibited financial risk-taking in a very large online community sample. They found that both boldness and meanness were associated with instrumental but not disinhibited financial risk-taking, whereas disinhibition yielded the opposite pattern.

Weidacker, O'Farrell, Gray, Johnston, and Snowden (2017) used both offender and community participants in an examination of associations between triarchic psychopathy domains and various forms of impulsivity. Regression results showed a clear picture in that boldness was preferentially associated with sensation seeking but low levels of positive and negative urgency. disinhibition evinced moderate to large correlations with all forms of impulsivity, but in a regression model was primarily associated with urgency, whereas meanness was preferentially associated with lack of premeditation and lack of perseverance. Along similar lines, Gatner, Douglas, and Hart (2016) showed in a university sample that meanness and disinhibition were both associated with impulsive behavior, whereas boldness was preferentially associated with risk-taking behaviors. Thus, different constellations of triarchic psychopathy domains will likely manifest in different patterns of impulsive behavior.

A smaller literature has focused specifically on aggression and antisocial behavior. Van Dongen, Drislane, Nijman, Soe-Agnie, and van Marle (2017) recently examined the triarchic domains in a Dutch forensic psychiatric sample. They showed that meanness and disinhibition were meaningfully associated with both self-reported proactive and reactive aggression; Donnellan and Burt (2016) showed similar findings in a university sample. Other studies have found that these two psychopathy domains (and disinhibition in particular) are associated with self-reported delinquency and antisocial behavior in Portuguese, U.S., Chinese, and Italian community samples (Almeida et al., 2015; Coffee et al., 2017; Shou, Sellbom, Xu, Chen, & Sui, in press; Somma, Borroni, Drislane, & Fossati, 2016). Fanti, Kyranides, Drislane, Colins, and Andershed (2016) and Kyranides et al. (2017) showed that all three domains were associated with various forms of aggression in a Cypriot university sample, whereas Gatner et al. (2016) found that meanness was the best predictor of self-reported physical violence and disinhibition of non-physical violence in a Canadian student sample.

In sum, all three triarchic domains have been linked to various forms of externalizing and maladaptive behaviors across contexts. Boldness is associated with maladaptive risk taking and fearlessness, which in some cases lead to problematic and maladaptive outcomes (e.g., school misconduct, substance abuse), but those high on this domain will not necessarily engage in a highly nonplanful or emotionally mediated impulsive behavior. disinhibition, on the other hand, is broadly associated with externalizing, impulsivity, and especially reactive aggression, with little thought to the consequences. Meanness seems to be specifically associated with aggression, hardline approaches to handling others, and egocentric decision-making with little concern for others.

Rooting the triarchic domains in broader personality and psychopathology

It is important to keep in mind that the triarchic psychopathy domains, more broadly, reflect dispositions that are anchored in broader personality and psychopathology structure. There is nothing distinctly unique about these domains beyond the specific trait aggregates they represent (Patrick & Drislane, 2015; see also e.g., Lynam & Miller, 2015, for situating psychopathy within the Five Factor Model of personality [FFM]). Several studies have linked the triarchic psychopathy domains to various models of both normative and abnormal personality traits. From the FFM perspective, several studies have indicated that boldness is primarily associated with Extraversion and Neuroticism, and inconsistent negative associations with Agreeableness (Blagov, Patrick, Oost, Goodman, & Pugh, 2015; Donnellan & Burt, 2016; Drislane et al., 2014; Miller, Lamkin, Lynam, & Maples-Keller, 2016; Poy, Segarra, Esteller, Lopez, & Molto, 2014; Shou, Sellbom, & Han, 2016; Sica et al., 2015; Stanley et al., 2013). The latter association is primarily due to Boldness being moderately associated with low modesty and low straightforwardness (Donnellan & Burt, 2016; Drislane et al., 2014; Poy et al., 2014). Meanness tends to consistently display large negative correlations with Agreeableness and weak to moderate negative correlations with Conscientiousness, whereas disinhibition has shown the opposite pattern with the same two FFM domains (Blagov et al., 2015; Donnellan & Burt, 2016; Drislane et al., 2014; Miller et al., 2016; Poy et al., 2014; Shou et al., 2016; Sica et al., 2015; Stanley et al., 2013). Disinhibition is also weakly to moderately associated with Neuroticism (Blagov et al., 2015; Donnellan & Burt, 2016; Miller et al., 2016; Poy et al., 2014; Stanley et al., 2013), with Anger/hostility and impulsivity driving these associations (Donnellan & Burt, 2016; Poy et al., 2014).

Drislane et al. (2014) also reported associations between the triarchic domains and an abbreviated version of the Multidimensional Personality Questionnaire (MPQ; Tellegen, 1982) in a large sample of undergraduate students. Boldness was primarily associated with Social Potency, well-being, and achievement orientation (i.e., agentic positive emotionality), and low levels of stress reactivity and harm avoidance. Meanness, on the other hand, was most strongly associated with aggression and, to a much lesser degree, alienation, low behavioral control, low social closeness, and low harm avoidance. Finally, disinhibition was negatively associated with behavioral control and positively associated with aggression, alienation, and stress reactivity.

Research on the alternative model of personality disorder (AMPD) listed in Section III of the DSM–5 has also yielded robust links between its maladaptive personality trait model and triarchic psychopathy constructs in a range of correctional, community, and university settings (Anderson, Sellbom, Wygant, Salekin, & Krueger, 2014; Strickland, Drislane, Lucy, Krueger, & Patrick, 2013; Wygant et al., 2016). These studies typically used the Personality Inventory for DSM–5 (PID–5; Krueger et al., 2012), but Wygant et al. (2016) also used clinician-ratings for these personality traits. These studies indicate that meanness is preferentially associated with PID–5 Antagonism and its facets; disinhibition with PID–5 disinhibition and its facets; and Boldness with low PID–5 Negative Affectivity and low Detachment. Boldness is also specifically associated with PID–5 Risk Taking, Grandiosity, Attention Seeking, and Manipulativeness – indicating stronger associations with aspects of Antagonism than its FFM counterpart, (low) Agreeableness. Moreover, these three studies confirmed that the DSM–5 AMPD Antisocial Personality Disorder trait constellation is primarily reflective of meanness and disinhibition, whereas a new psychopathy specifier includes traits that are akin to boldness (Anderson et al., 2014; Strickland et al., 2013; Wygant et al., 2016), thereby moving the operationalization towards "primary" psychopathy (see Venables et al., 2014; Wall et al., 2015).

Overall, these studies point to a clear constellation of personality traits across theoretical models which comprise these conceptual triarchic domains. The results indicate that this model can easily be conceptualized from dimensional trait perspectives beyond psychopathy specific measurements. As suggested by Lynam, Miller, Widiger and their colleagues (see e.g., Lynam & Miller, 2015), psychopathy is little more than a personality trait constellation that is rooted in dimensional personality traits. Regardless of theoretical perspective on either psychopathy or personality trait models, the former can be successfully mapped onto the latter. The triarchic domains represent three such higher-order constellations, with demonstrated meaningful empirical correlates, but it will behoove researchers to determine if these constellations are inherently meaningful beyond any other similar trait constellation that does not map perfectly onto these.

Overall, research on the triarchic psychopathy model has exploded over the past several years and has generally been supportive of this perspective. The triarchic psychopathy domains do account for variance in other psychopathy models to the degree that is theoretically indicated. These domains have also begun to map onto neurobehavioral domains in the ways anticipated and theorized based on extant psychopathy and broader psychopathology research (Patrick & Drislane, 2015), with promising links to more putative environmental influences (i.e., interpersonal attachment) as well. Indeed, the triarchic psychopathy domains link with other personality trait models in expected ways and support contentions that psychopathy (or domains of psychopathy) reflects a particular maladaptive personality constellation(s). Finally, psychopathy is also associated with a host of negative outcomes, as would be expected based on psychopathy theory, though the boldness domain is less predictive of maladaptivity than the other two domains.

The role of boldness in psychopathy

The boldness domain has proven quite controversial with respect to its relevance to the psychopathic personality. As stated earlier, this domain was conceived as a phenotypic manifestation of the characteristics discussed by Cleckley, Lykken, and measured primarily by the PPI/PPI–R (Patrick et al., 2009) and has become the foundation for the Antisocial Personality Disorder psychopathy specifier in the DSM–5 AMPD (APA, 2013). Some scholars have been quite critical of boldness as a psychopathy domain and suggest it is peripheral or even irrelevant to psychopathy (e.g., Gatner et al., 2016; Miller & Lynam, 2012). Given that boldness is obviously viewed as highly relevant to psychopathy from the triarchic psychopathy model perspective, this debate will be briefly summarized here.

Summary of criticisms

Miller and Lynam (2012) published a meta-analysis on the PPI, and based on these findings, they argued that PPI/PPI–R Fearless Dominance (i.e., an operational cognate of boldness) measures something that is largely irrelevant or at best peripheral to the psychopathy construct. They based this conclusion on small associations between Fearless Dominance with other measures of psychopathy (in particular PCL–R) as well as the lack of robust associations between this scale and maladaptive externalizing outcomes (see also Marcus et al., 2013, meta-analysis for similar findings, albeit less strong conclusions).

Subsequently, scholars have continued to question this construct of boldness in light of a series of studies that have generally failed to provide support for boldness as a pathological construct. Gatner et al. (2016) examined the associations between the triarchic domains and various measures of aggression, rule breaking, impulsivity, substance abuse, and risk-taking in a Canadian undergraduate sample. Although boldness was the best predictor of risk-taking behaviors (as consistent with the literature reviewed earlier), it was not associated with the other constructs, did not increment the other triarchic domains in the prediction of those constructs, and was not associated with non-additive effects in conjunction with other domains in any predictions. Moreover, Vize, Lynam, Lamkin, Miller, and Pardini (2016) examined the predictive validity of a childhood index of Fearless Dominance psychopathy, based on mapping items from the common language Q-set (Caspi et al., 1992) onto the PPI–R scales and factors. This index was measured in the Pittsburgh Youth Study at age 13 and a range of concurrent and predictive (at age 24) correlates were examined. Surprisingly, the associations between FD and FFM domains were negligible at age 24, whereas the typical pattern of observations was observed concurrently.

Miller et al. (2016) examined associations between the FFM and triarchic psychopathy domains from multiple perspectives. As documented in the earlier review, boldness was primarily associated with low Neuroticism and high Extraversion. It was also strongly associated with experts' FFM-rated profile for primary psychopathy (.50), similar to meanness (.64) and higher than disinhibition (.24). On the other hand, boldness failed to meaningfully associate with a meta-analytical FFM profile, unlike the other two domains. Furthermore, in a second study, Miller et al. summarized the ratings of triarchic FFM profiles by 48 academic clinical psychologists in terms of symptoms of various forms of psychopathology, including psychopathy and other personality disorders. They found that the description associated with the meanness FFM profile corresponded with a very high mean rating of psychopathy, whereas the mean ratings for boldness and disinhibition were smaller (but not significantly different from one another). The boldness FFM profile was associated with narcissism to a similar degree as the other domains but was otherwise rated low on psychopathology symptoms. Miller et al. concluded that meanness is the core of psychopathy and Boldness is more peripheral. Finally, Gatner, Douglas, and Hart (in press) asked university students to read descriptions of the three triarchic psychopathy domains and rate the degree of similarity to natural language traits in the FFM and the CAPP. They found that meanness and disinhibition both were associated with high FFM and CAPP ratings to the degree they deemed theoretically expected, but boldness descriptions evinced far lower ratings on typical FFM psychopathy traits and CAPP symptoms, and was more highly associated with CAPP "foil" items. Thus, from the perspective of the FFM and CAPP perspectives of psychopathy, Gatner et al. concluded that boldness is highly dissimilar and generally irrelevant. Gatner et al. failed to mention that the FFM and CAPP perspectives of psychopathy are based on the work of authors highly critical of the boldness construct (e.g., Miller, Lynam, Hart).

Summary of proponents' perspectives

Other scholars have strongly disagreed with many of these criticisms and offered evidence to counter some of these negative findings. Lilienfeld et al. (2012) argued, among other things, that proponents and opponents appear to associate with dissimilar nomological networks of psychopathy, with the latter scholars' views leaving little room for adaptivity of the psychopathy construct. Indeed, Cleckley's (1941 | 1988) writings clearly include descriptions of characteristics that are reflective of Boldness, which comprise the putative "mask" of sanity. Indeed, Crego and Widiger (2016) asked community participants to rate each of Cleckley's 15 original cases on a variety of characteristics, including triarchic psychopathy and FFM traits. Their findings showed that Cleckley's psychopaths were rated as high on Boldness. Moreover, as acknowledged by Miller et al. (2016), when experts are asked to rate the prototypical Cleckley psychopath on FFM traits (Miller, Lynam, Widiger, & Leukefeld, 2001), the mean profile converges strongly with Boldness.

Lilienfeld et al. (2016a) conducted a meta-analysis that excluded the PCL–R and its self-report derivatives. They found considerably stronger links between Boldness (based on TriPM, PPI, or other direct estimates) and other psychopathy measures (weighted r = .39; and r = .44 when limited to well-validated psychopathy measures) compared to meta-analyses including such measures (Miller & Lynam, 2012; Marcus et al., 2013). In particular, the correlations between Boldness and two factors from Lynam and Miller's own Elemental Psychopathy Assessment (EPA; Lynam et al., 2011) were .73 (Emotional Stability) and .58 (narcissism). Lilienfeld et al. contended that if Boldness is irrelevant to psychopathy, then over 40 percent of the item content of the EPA is construct-irrelevant, which indeed seems like an improbable assertion in light of Lynam and colleagues' careful approach to test construction. Moreover, Lilienfeld et al. (2012; Lilienfeld, Smith, & Watts, 2016; Lilienfeld, Smith, Sauvigné et al. 2016b) also reported that Boldness is moderately to strongly correlated with scores on the Hare Self-Report Psychopathy scale (Paulhus et al., in press; see also Marcus et al., 2013). Finally, it is also noteworthy that a factor analysis of CAPP self-ratings revealed a Boldness factor with promising concurrent validity (Sellbom, Cooke, & Hart, 2015). Thus, Boldness is associated with other psychopathy measures despite evincing smaller associations with PCL–based measures, which theoretically are less anchored in Boldness.

Lilienfeld et al. (2012; Lilienfeld, Smith, Sauvigné et al., 2016) also argued that Boldness traits might differentiate primary psychopathy from secondary psychopathy and cited research that indicates that emotional stability and other relevant traits indeed separate the two manifestations (e.g., Drislane, Patrick, Sourander et al., 2014; Hicks, Markon, Patrick, Krueger, & Newman, 2004). Indeed, as discussed earlier, two studies have also demonstrated that boldness, but not Meanness or disinhibition, differentiate PCL–R psychopathy from traditional diagnosis of Antisocial Personality Disorder (Venables et al., 2014; Wall et al., 2015). Such research supports the inclusion of boldness traits as the psychopathy specifier to Antisocial Personality Disorder diagnosis in the DSM–5.

Research has also suggested that mental health professionals as well as forensic practitioners also deem boldness relevant to psychopathy, which is in contrast to Miller et al.'s (2016) and Gatner et al.'s (in press) findings. Sörman et al. (2016) surveyed three samples of forensic mental health practitioners, probation officers, and community participants being considered for jury duty. Each of the samples rated boldness descriptors as moderately to highly prototypical of psychopathy and similar to average ratings of CAPP items. Most recently, Berg, Lilienfeld, and Sellbom (in press) asked both academic and clinical mental health professionals (including graduate students) to rate seven different vignettes of the same person with boldness, meanness, or disinhibition descriptions as well as all possible combinations of the three with respect to classic psychopathy and various psychopathy and personality disorder traits. Overall, the findings revealed that descriptions that included boldness were more likely to be perceived as high on classical psychopathy than if not present, albeit not in isolation. Thus, in the presence of other psychopathy traits, and in particular meanness, boldness traits seem necessary with respect to perceived resemblance to the classic psychopathic personality.

Finally, Gatner et al. (2016) and Vize et al. (2016) failed to find evidence for interaction effects for boldness with other psychopathy factors in the prediction of externalizing criteria.

However, readers should be aware that there are other studies that have indeed found such support. For instance, Kastner and Sellbom (2012) found that estimated PPI Fearless Dominance traits exponentiated the association between estimated PPI impulsive/antisocial and sexual risk-taking (but see Fulton, Marcus, & Ziegler-Hill, 2014). Rock, Sellbom, Ben-Porath, and Salekin (2013) found that estimated PPI Fearless Dominance traits moderated the association between estimated PPI impulsive/antisocial and failure to complete a court-ordered domestic violence treatment program, in that those high on both domains were associated with greater levels of non-completion. Similarly, Smith, Edens, and McDermott (2013) found that PPI–R Fearless Dominance and PPI Self-Centered Impulsivity were both associated with predatory aggression in a sample of 200 forensic psychiatric patients, with evidence for a statistically significant interaction effect whereby being high on both domains was associated with even greater levels of predatory aggression.

Overall, both sides of this debate have produced arguments and data that are supportive of their respective perspectives. As noted in the beginning of this section, it is important to first fully delineate the nomological network associated with psychopathy to fully resolve these issues. It is certainly not in dispute (at least by this author) that meanness represents a (if not *the*) core of psychopathy, but the question is the degree of relevance of boldness (and disinhibition, but this is less widely disputed; cf. Poythress & Hall, 2011). Boldness seem to be associated with the interpersonal and resilience traits that have been observed in what others view as primary or classic psychopathy (e.g., Cleckley's mask); these traits differentiate primary and secondary psychopathy (including PCL–R from ASPD), and when comprehensive models of psychopathic personality are articulated (triarchic psychopathy model, CAPP, and Lynam and Millers' EPA/FFM), boldness traits do emerge. However, unlike meanness, boldness does not seem directly relevant to all manifestations of psychopathy and might be particularly pertinent to the more "successful" community variants or primary (as opposed to secondary) offender psychopaths. More research is clearly needed to better understand what Boldness traits do manifest in the context of psychopathy.

Assessment of the Triarchic Psychopathy Model

There are several ways to operationalize the triarchic constructs that have emerged in the literature. Although the Triarchic Psychopathy Measure (TriPM; Patrick, 2010b) has been viewed as synonymous with the model as its original operationalization, it is important to consider that these domains are theoretical and "open" constructs (Meehl, 1986) that should not necessarily be tied to one measurement modality. As such, the various methods of operationalizing the Triarchic Psychopathy Model will be discussed in this section, starting of course with the original and most commonly used measure, the TriPM.

Triarchic Psychopathy Measure

The TriPM is a 58-item self-report inventory on which individuals respond "true," "mostly true," "mostly false," or "false" to each statement as it applies to them. The TriPM evolved through research on two separate inventories designed to measure conceptual models of externalizing psychopathology (Krueger, Markon, Patrick, Benning, & Kramer, 2007) and fear and threat sensitivity (Kramer et al., 2012; see also Patrick & Drislane, 2015). The disinhibition and Meanness scales are composed of items from the Externalizing Spectrum Inventory (ESI; Krueger et al., 2007) and, more specifically, those that best represent (1) a broad dimension of general externalizing propensity (disinhibition), entailing impulsive–irresponsible, rule-breaking tendencies, and (2) a residual dimension of callous–aggression (meanness), reflecting uncaring/ exploitative tendencies. The boldness items were derived from a separate inventory that was designed to index differing thematic expressions of fearless–dominant tendencies that relate in turn to a broad bio-behavioral dimension of fear vs. fearlessness (Kramer et al., 2012) or threat sensitivity (Yancey et al., 2013). The TriPM places primary emphasis on assessment of psychopathy in terms of these distinguishable facets, as opposed to psychopathy as a unitary global construct (Patrick & Drislane, 2015; Skeem et al., 2011).

The TriPM has been formally translated into Dutch (Soe-Agnie et al., 2011), Spanish (Poy et al., 2014), Portuguese (Almeida et al., 2015), Italian (Sica et al., 2015; Somma et al., 2016), Cypriot Greek (Fanti et al., 2016), and Chinese (Shou et al., 2016). These various validation studies have documented a pattern of findings that is remarkably consistent with those of the English version.

Internal psychometrics

The TriPM scales have generally evinced good internal consistency reliability coefficients across various studies. Cronbach's alpha for these scales range from .77 to .89 for boldness; .83–.91 for meanness; and .79–.89 for disinhibition (see Sellbom, Lilienfeld, Fowler, & McCrary, in press, for a review). Moreover, the scales are typically correlated at different levels; boldness and disinhibition are generally uncorrelated (e.g., $r = -.05$ in Poy et al., 2014; $r = .03$ in Strickland, Drislane, Lucy, Krueger, & Patrick, 2013). Boldness and meanness are reported to have weak positive correlations ($r = .17$ in Poy et al., 2014; $r = .20$ in Strickland et al., 2013). In contrast, disinhibition and meanness were found to be highly correlated ($r = .54$ in Poy et al., 2014; $r = .62$ in Strickland et al., 2013).

Shou, Sellbom, and Xu (in press) conducted an item response theory (IRT) analysis with the Chinese TriPM in a large Chinese university sample. They also examined differential item functioning (DIF) relative to American university students. Shou et al. (in press) found that meanness and disinhibition represented robust unidimensional scales with most (albeit not all) items providing meaningful information to their respective total scores; indeed, Shou et al. recommended that 16-item and 13-item scales of disinhibition and meanness respectively would work equally well as their full-length counterparts, at least in Chinese student samples. Furthermore, Shou, Sellbom, and Xu (in press) failed to find unidimensional support for boldness and instead recommended a two-facet structure of emotional stability (nine items) and social dominance (eight items), which performed well in the IRT analyses. Furthermore, a substantial number of items were associated with significant DIF values and thus evinced lack of measurement invariance across Chinese and American students' TriPM item responses. Shou and her colleagues offered a number of culturally oriented explanations for these differences, but their overarching conclusions was that the TriPM scale scores were associated with different levels of measurement precision as well as severity levels with respect to psychopathy. Therefore, actual TriPM scores cannot be directly compared across these cultures even in light of sharing similar positions in the domains' nomological networks (Shou et al., 2016; Shou, Sellbom, Xu et al., in press). Further research along these lines with other translated measures is important.

Construct validity

The TriPM has considerable support for its construct validity. Much of the research reported earlier on the triarchic psychopathy model generally has been conducted using the TriPM and will therefore not be repeated here. Sellbom et al. (in press) reviewed the psychometric properties of the TriPM. They reported that the TriPM domains account for variance in other psychopathy measures to a degree that is theoretically expected from triarchic theory. The TriPM domain scales also converge with dimensional personality traits from established models in ways that would be conceptually expected.

The TriPM is a promising self-report questionnaire, as demonstrated by its encouraging convergent and discriminant validity. Of course, given the relative recency of the TriPM, additional research is necessary to elaborate on its construct validity and clinical utility. For instance, these domain scores need to be further empirically linked to the neuroscience constructs that are theoretically associated with them. In addition, given the relevance of psychopathy to forensic decision-making in the criminal justice system, the TriPM will need to be incorporated into risk assessment paradigms as well to document its predictive validity.

Other self-report inventories

The triarchic psychopathy domains can also be operationalized through other self-report inventories for which triarchic scales have been developed. These efforts include using items from different psychopathy measures (e.g., PPI/PPI–R, YPI) and omnibus personality inventories (e.g., MPQ, MMPI-2-RF) to measure the three triarchic constructs based on a three-step procedure. First, experts familiar with the triarchic model independently rate items from the source inventory for their conceptual relevance to each of the triarchic constructs. Next, the provisional scales are refined through internal psychometric analyses to optimize item specificity (i.e., selective convergence with targeted scale) and maximizing internal consistency. In the final validation step, the final triarchic scales are evaluated for convergent and discriminant relations with other psychopathy inventories and personality measures.

Psychopathic personality inventory

Hall et al. (2014) were the first to explore this method by using items from the PPI in large undergraduate and offender samples. The PPI–boldness scale was associated selectively with TriPM boldness, with MPQ personality traits of Social Potency, Stress Immunity, and fearlessness, and with scores on the PCL–R interpersonal facet. PPI–meanness was associated most strongly with the TriPM meanness scale, and with scales of the LSRP and SRP–III indexing callousness, egocentricity, affective detachment, and antisocial behavior; PPI–meanness also showed robust associations with personality traits reflecting detachment, Antagonism, and aggression, and with symptoms of Antisocial Personality Disorder. Finally, scores on PPI–disinhibition were preferentially associated with psychopathy scales indexing impulsivity, sensation seeking, and antisocial tendencies. PPI–disinhibition also showed associations with MPQ traits of aggression, alienation, and stress reactivity, and child and adult symptoms of Antisocial Personality Disorder.

Sellbom, Wygant, and Drislane (2015) examined the PPI/PPI–R triarchic scales in male prison inmate and mixed-gender community samples. They found that these scales were associated with PCL–R, TriPM, and LSRP scales as conceptually indicated, replicating Hall et al.'s findings. Sellbom et al. also showed a pattern of convergent and discriminant validity for the PPI/PPI–R triarchic scales with various measures of maladaptive personality traits (PID–5) and antisocial behavior and substance abuse, with PPI–disinhibition being preferentially associated with the latter two, though PPI–Boldness contributed uniquely to these predictions in a regression model.

Youth Psychopathic Traits Inventory

Drislane and colleagues (2015) developed triarchic scales for the YPI using data from a large university sample. They reported that the YPI–Triarchic scores showed good internal consistency and promised convergent and discriminant validity in relation to factor scores on other psychopathy inventories. YPI–boldness showed strong associations with counterpart boldness scales of the TriPM and PPI as well as with scores on the PPI's Fearless Dominance factor. YPI–meanness showed expected robust associations with TriPM and PPI meanness scales, the PPI Coldheartedness scale, SRP–III callous affect and interpersonal manipulation scales, other measures of callous–unemotional traits, and subscales of the Child Psychopathy Measure (Lynam, 1997) reflecting lack of guilt and poverty of affect. Also, as hypothesized, YPI–disinhibition showed robust convergence with TriPM and PPI disinhibition scales, the PPI impulsive/antisocial scale, the SRP–III Erratic Lifestyle and LSRP secondary scales, and subscales of the CPS reflecting impulsive–antisocial tendencies. However, some lack of discriminant validity was evident for the YPI–boldness scale in particular, as it correlated more strongly with both the YPI–disinhibition and meanness scales than observed for other operationalizations (e.g., TriPM, PPI, MMPI-2-RF), and showed larger-than-expected associations with impulsive–antisocial subscales of the SRP–III and CPS. These findings for the YPI–boldness scale, which likely reflect the generally correlated nature of the YPI's items, indicate that the item content of certain inventories may constrain the effectiveness of triarchic facet measures derivable from them (Drislane & Patrick, 2017; Patrick & Drislane, 2015).

Minnesota Multiphasic Personality Inventory–2–restructured form (MMPI-2–RF)

Sellbom et al. (2016) recently developed triarchic scales for the MMPI-2–RF (Ben-Porath & Tellegen, 2008/2011), which is a broadband inventory for clinical and maladaptive personality symptoms and traits. The authors used the same methodology in very large prison inmate and university samples to develop the MMPI-2-RF–Tri scales and validated them in independent female correctional and mixed gender university samples. In terms of associations with TriPM and PPI triarchic scales, the same patterns as observed for the other efforts were found for the MMPI-2–RF–Tri scales. In addition, MMPI-2–RF meanness was associated with Machiavellianism and various measures of callous–unemotional traits (though at times at equivalent levels as MMPI-2–RF disinhibition), whereas Boldness was associated with narcissism. Sellbom et al. also demonstrated incremental validity above and beyond standard MMPI-2–RF scales in predicting scores on the TriPM in each of these samples. Overall, the findings from these studies are quite similar to those reported for the PPI/PPI–R and YPI, though the MMPI-2–RF meanness scale was somewhat questionable with respect to how well the instrument's items can capture the Coldheartedness/callousness variance germane to this construct.

Kutchen et al. (2017) examined the MMPI-2–RF Triarchic scales in a male correctional sample and two university samples. Many of the findings with other psychopathy measures (PCL–R, PPI–R) were replicated and the scales showed a good pattern of convergent and discriminant validity with scales from the PID–5 and Personality Assessment Inventory (PAI; Morey, 1991). The most notable finding was that the MMPI-2–RF Meanness scale continued to be less supported than the other two triarchic scales. Although many hypotheses with respect to convergent validity were borne out (e.g., PPI–R Self-Centered Impulsivity, measures of aggression, Antagonism, alienation), correlations with key measures such as the PCL–R affective facet and Antisocial Personality Disorder symptoms were weak or non-significant. Thus, the utility of the MMPI-2–RF Meanness scale might be somewhat compromised in that it does not sufficiently cover the full range of the construct (in particular, callousness and Coldheartedness items), but further research will be necessary to fully elucidate the utility of this scale.

Multidimensional personality questionnaire

More recently, triarchic scales have also been developed for the MPQ (Brislin, Drislane, Smith, Edens, & Patrick, 2015). These scales were validated in both community samples and with federal prison inmates. The pattern of results was virtually identical for those reported for the PPI–Tri, YPI–Tri, and MMPI-2–RF–Tri scales in terms of associations with PCL–R scores and a range of other personality constructs. Brislin and colleagues (2017) most recently replicated these MPQ–Tri scales in a range of university and male and female offender samples.

Primate behavior ratings

In a highly innovative effort, Latzman and colleagues (2016) used a 41-item personality rating questionnaire developed for chimpanzees to construct triarchic scales using the same method as described earlier. These scales yielded good internal consistency estimates and inter-correlations in a sample of socially housed chimpanzees similar to what are reported for other studies. Validation efforts indicated that the CHMP–Tri boldness scale was negatively associated with ratings of depression in the chimpanzees, whereas CHMP–Tri disinhibition, and meanness to a lesser degree, were positively correlated with ratings of physical aggression. Moreover, Latzman and colleagues also collected data from an online community sample with the CHMP–Tri scales (in self-report format) and the TriPM and found a pattern of convergent and discriminant validity similar to those of other triarchic measures. Finally, in a separate sample of chimpanzees, Latzman et al. (2016) showed that the CHMP–Tri boldness scale was associated with approach behavior, whereas CHMP–Tri disinhibition showed a trend towards being related to inability to delay gratification.

In a subsequent study, Latzman and colleagues (2017) examined the heritability of the triarchic psychopathy domains operationalized by the CHMP–Tri ratings in two samples of chimpanzees with different social learning experiences. They found that all three triarchic domains were associated with significant heritability estimates (.36 [disinhibition], .65 [meanness], and .66 [boldness]) in the mother-reared sample, but not the nursery-reared sample. Thus, early social learning has an impact on ultimate genetic contributions, which makes conceptual sense, as the nursery-reared apes were removed from their mothers due to inadequate care and thus experience highly atypical childhood development (Latzman et al., 2017). Furthermore, Latzman et al.'s analyses revealed that a genetic higher-order domain for the triarchic scales could be estimated, with meanness being the clear central marker, suggesting some etiological centrality for this domain with respect to psychopathy (consistent with Lynam and Miller's [2015] contention that Antagonism is the central psychopathy domain).

Other developments

At the time of this writing, there are a number of other triarchic psychopathy measurement projects ongoing that readers might want to consider, especially since they will very likely be published soon. Patrick and colleagues have developed a Triarchic Psychopathy Interview, which shows good convergent and discriminant validity in relation to the PCL–R, but also provides incremental validity above and beyond the latter in the prediction of various forms of internalizing psychopathology (C. Patrick, personal communication, August 2017). These findings indicate that the boldness component in particular can be very useful in complementing the PCL–R in psychopathy assessment. Furthermore, Drislane, Jones, Brislin, and Patrick (2017) have developed NEO PI–R triarchic scales, which also demonstrate a pattern of promising convergent and discriminant validity in relation to the TriPM and a host of other personality inventories – much in the same vein as the scales for the PPI, YPI, MMPI-2–RF, and MPQ.

The assessment of triarchic psychopathy domains can be operationalized with very promising construct validity across a number of self-report inventories in addition to the TriPM. More recent efforts have shown utility with respect to interview-based ratings of humans (C. Patrick, personal communication, August 2017) and behavior ratings of chimpanzees. As noted earlier, any measure (e.g., self-report, other-report, clinician-rating) constitutes merely one operationalization of a construct. It therefore stands to reason that any item pool with sufficient content coverage of a construct from a particular theoretical perspective could be used to index the construct, although (as highlighted by the potential weaknesses of the YPI–boldness scale and MMPI-2–RF meanness scale; Drislane et al., 2015; Sellbom et al., 2016) caution is warranted, and demonstrations of convergent and discriminant validity essential, before assuming that a derived measure effectively indexes the intended construct. Latent variables from confirmatory-structural models of target constructs, specified using existing validated scale indicators, can serve as useful referents for evaluating the equivalency of new scale measures (Drislane & Patrick, 2017). Future research should continue to evaluate these strategies, especially given the potential benefits they hold for advancing psychopathy research in valuable ways through use of unique existing samples and datasets.

Conclusion

The triarchic model represents a promising and integrative perspective of the psychopathic personality. This model can certainly serve as an important framework for further elucidating the key ingredients of this seemingly elusive concept. Research does appear to indicate that meanness is indeed a core trait (see e.g., Lynam & Miller, 2015; Miller et al., 2016) that is critical for all manifestations of psychopathy, but boldness and disinhibition moderate the expression (see also Drislane, Patrick, Sourander et al., 2014). It will be very important for future research to further clarify just how these different combinations are manifested (including elevations on all three) and the degree to which they are important for clinical and forensic practice.

Research has been promising in terms of linking triarchic psychopathy domains to various putative etiological mechanisms, including neurophysiological correlates of these domains as they relate to processing of various types of information and decision-making. However, considerably more work is needed in this regard to more fully understand the distinct mechanisms that underlie these domains. Patrick and Drislane (2015), for instance, have persuasively linked boldness to threat insensitivity and disinhibition to lack of (frontally mediated) inhibitory control, but more research with actual triarchic model measures is needed. It will also be essential to more broadly examine how these mechanisms overlap with general (maladaptive) personality for a broader framework. For instance, do meanness and Antagonism share the same mechanisms? In addition, systematic consideration of environmental factors, including how they interact with neurobehavioral domains, in the development and manifestation of psychopathy is critical to further our understanding of this important clinical disorder.

Another area that is very under-developed with respect to the triarchic model of psychopathy is how well it translates into criminal justice-related practice. There has been very little research using forensic and correctional populations and even fewer studies that has explicitly considered criminal or offender risk outcomes. Indeed, psychopathic personality disorder is viewed as an important clinical construct at least in part owing to its high relevance in risk formulation and prediction in such settings. It will therefore behoove psychopathy scholars from the triarchic framework to more fully elaborate on the role of these triarchic constructs in offender management and risk assessment.

Note

1 On the PPI–R, a three higher-order scale is used, with Coldheartedness serving as the third factor and impulsive/antisocial renamed Self-Centered Impulsivity.

References

Almeida, P. R., Seixas, M. J., Ferreira-Santos, F., Vieira, J. B., Paiva, T. O., Moreira, P. S., and Costa, P. (2015) 'Empathic, moral and antisocial outcomes associated with distinct components of psychopathy in healthy individuals: A Triarchic model approach,' *Personality and Individual Differences*, *85*:205–211.

American Psychiatric Association. (2013) *Diagnostic and statistical manual of mental disorders* (5th ed.), Washington, DC: American Psychiatric Press.

Andershed, H., Kerr, M., Stattin, H., and Levander, S. (2002) 'Psychopathic traits in non-referred youths: Initial test of a new assessment tool,' in E. Blaauw, J. M. Philippa, K. C. M. P. Ferenschild, & B. van Lodensteijn (Eds.), *Psychopaths: Current international perspectives* (pp. 131–158), The Hague: Elsevier.

Anderson, J. L., Sellbom, M., Wygant, D. B., Salekin, R. T., and Krueger, R. F. (2014) 'Examining the associations between DSM–5 section III antisocial personality disorder traits and psychopathy in community and university samples,' *Journal of Personality Disorders*, *28*(5):675–697.

Babiak, P., Neumann, C. S., and Hare, R. D. (2010) 'Corporate psychopathy: Talking the walk,' *Behavioral Sciences & the Law*, *28*(2):174–193.

Benning, S. D., Patrick, C. J., Hicks, B. M., Blonigen, D. M., and Krueger, R. F. (2003) 'Factor structure of the psychopathic personality inventory: Validity and implications for clinical assessment,' *Psychological Assessment*, *15*(3):340–350.

Benning, S. D., Patrick, C. J., and Iacono, W. G. (2005) 'Psychopathy, startle blink modulation, and electrodermal reactivity in twin men,' *Psychophysiology*, *42*(6):753–762.

Ben-Porath, Y. S., and Tellegen, A. (2008/2011) *MMPI-2-RF: Manual for Administration, Scoring, and Interpretation*, Minneapolis, MN: University of Minnesota Press.

Berg, J. M., Lilienfeld, S. O., and Sellbom, M. (in press) 'The role of boldness in psychopathy: A study of academic and clinical perceptions,' *Personality Disorders: Theory, Research, and Treatment*.

Blagov, P. S., Patrick, C. J., Oost, K. M., Goodman, J. A., and Pugh, A. T. (2015) 'Triarchic psychopathy measure: Validity in relation to normal-range traits, personality pathology, and psychological adjustment,' *Journal of Personality Disorders*, Advance online publication.

Blair, R. J. R. (2006) 'The emergence of psychopathy: Implications for the neuropsychological approach to developmental disorders,' *Cognition*, *101*(2):414–442.

Brislin, S. J., Drislane, L. E., Smith, S. T., Edens, J. F., and Patrick, C. J. (2015) 'Development and validation of triarchic psychopathy scales from the Multidimensional Personality Questionnaire,' *Psychological Assessment*, *27*(3):838–851.

Brislin, S. J., Venables, N. C., Drislane, L. E., Blonigen, D. M., Iacono, W. G., Tellegen, A., . . ., and Patrick, C. J. (2017) 'Further validation of triarchic psychopathy scales from the Multidimensional Personality Questionnaire: Setting the stage for large-sample etiological studies,' *Assessment*, Advance online publication.

Caspi, A., Block, J., Block, J. H., Kloop, B., Lynam, D., Moffitt, T. E., and Stouthamer-Loeber, M. (1992) 'A "common language" version of the California Child Q-set for personality assessment,' *Psychological Assessment*, *4*:512–523.

Christian, E., Sellbom, M., and Wilkinson, R. B. (2016) 'Clarifying the associations between individual differences in general attachment styles and psychopathy,' *Personality Disorders: Theory, Research, and Treatment*, Advance online publication.

Cleckley, H. (1941 | 1988) *The mask of sanity* (7th ed.), St. Louis, MO: Mosby.

Coffee, C. A., Cox, J., and Koplin, M. (2017) 'Examining the relationships between the triarchic psychopathy constructs and behavioral deviance in a community sample,' *Journal of Personality Disorders*, Advance online publication.

Cooke, D. J., Hart, S. D., Logan, C., and Michie, C. (2012) 'Explicating the construct of psychopathy: Development and validation of a conceptual model, the Comprehensive Assessment of Psychopathic Personality (CAPP),' *International Journal of Forensic Mental Health, 11*(4):242–252.

Cooke, D. J., and Michie, C. (2001) 'Refining the construct of psychopathy: Towards a hierarchical model,' *Psychological Assessment, 13*(2):171–188.

Craig, R. L., Gray, N. S., and Snowden, R. J. (2013) 'Recalled parental bonding, current attachment, and the triarchic conceptualisation of psychopathy,' *Personality and Individual Differences, 55*(4):345–350.

Crego, C., and Widiger, T. A. (2016) 'Cleckley's psychopaths: Revisited,' *Journal of Abnormal Psychology, 125*(1):75–87.

Donnellan, M. B., and Burt, S. A. (2016) 'A further evaluation of the triarchic conceptualization of psychopathy in college students,' *Journal of Psychopathology and Behavioral Assessment, 38*(2):172–182.

Drislane, L. E., Brislin, S. J., Kendler, K. S., Andershed, H., Larsson, H., and Patrick, C. J. (2015) 'A triarchic model analysis of the Youth Psychopathic Traits Inventory,' *Journal of Personality Disorders, 29*(1):15–41.

Drislane, L. E., Jones, S., Brislin, S. J., and Patrick, C. J. (2017) *Interfacing five-factor model and triarchic conceptualizations of psychopathy*, Manuscript submitted for publication.

Drislane, L. E., and Patrick, C. J. (2017) 'Integrating alternative conceptions of psychopathic personality: A latent variable model of triarchic psychopathy constructs,' *Journal of Personality Disorders, 31*(1):110–132.

Drislane, L. E., Patrick, C. J., and Arsal, G. (2014a) 'Clarifying the content coverage of differing psychopathy inventories through reference to the triarchic psychopathy measure,' *Psychological Assessment, 26*(2):350–362.

Drislane, L. E., Patrick, C. J., Sourander, A., Sillanmäki, L., Aggen, S. H., Elonheimo, H., . . ., and Kendler, K. S. (2014b) 'Distinct variants of extreme psychopathic individuals in society at large: Evidence from a population-based sample,' *Personality Disorders: Theory, Research, and Treatment, 5*(2):154–163.

Esteller, À., Poy, R., and Moltó, J. (2016) 'Deficient aversive-potentiated startle and the Triarchic model of psychopathy: The role of boldness,' *Biological Psychology, 117*:131–140.

Fanti, K. A., Kyranides, M. N., Drislane, L. E., Colins, O. F., and Andershed, H. (2016) 'Validation of the Greek Cypriot translation of the triarchic psychopathy measure,' *Journal of Personality Assessment, 98*(2):146–154.

Forth, A. E., Kosson, D. S., and Hare, R. D. (2003) *Hare Psychopathy Checklist: Youth Version*, Toronto, ON: Multi-Health Systems.

Frick, P. J., and Hare, R. D. (2001). *Antisocial process screening device*, Toronto, ON: Multi- Health Systems.

Fulton, J. J., Marcus, D. K., and Zeigler-Hill, V. (2014) 'Psychopathic personality traits, risky sexual behavior, and psychological adjustment among college-age women,' *Journal of Social and Clinical Psychology, 33*(2):143–168.

Gatner, D. T., Douglas, K. S., and Hart, S. D. (2016) 'Examining the incremental and interactive effects of boldness with meanness and disinhibition within the triarchic model of psychopathy,' *Personality Disorders: Theory, Research, and Treatment*, 7(3):259–268.

Gatner, D. T., Douglas, K. S., and Hart, S. D. (in press) 'Comparing the lexical similarity of the triarchic model of psychopathy to contemporary models of psychopathy,' *Journal of Personality*.

Hall, J. R., Drislane, L. E., Patrick, C. J., Morano, M., Lilienfeld, S. O., and Poythress, N. G. (2014) 'Development and validation of Triarchic construct scales from the psychopathic personality inventory,' *Psychological Assessment, 26*(2):447–461.

Hare, R. D. (1978) 'Electrodermal and cardiovascular correlates of psychopathy,' in R. D. Hare & D. Schalling (Eds.), *Psychopathic behavior: Approaches to research* (pp. 107–143), Chichester: Wiley.

Hare, R. D. (1980) 'A research scale for the assessment of psychopathy in criminal populations,' *Personality and Individual Differences, 1*(2):111–119.

Hare, R. D. (1991/2003) *Hare Psychopathy Checklist–Revised*, Toronto, ON: Mental Health Systems.

Hare, R. D. (1994) *Predators: The disturbing world of the psychopaths among us*. Psychology Today, Jan/Feb, 1994.

Hare, R. D. (2007) 'Forty years are not enough: Recollections, random musings, and prognostications,' in H. Hervé & J. Yuille (Eds.), *The psychopath: Theory, research, and practice* (pp. 3–29), Mahwah, NJ: Lawrence Erlbaum and Associates.

Hare, R. D., Hart, S. D., and Harpur, T. J. (1991) 'Psychopathy and the DSM–IV criteria for antisocial personality disorder,' *Journal of Abnormal Psychology, 100*(3):391–398.

Hare, R. D., and Neumann, C. S. (2006) 'The PCL–R assessment of psychopathy,' in C. J. Patrick (Ed.), *Handbook of psychopathy* (pp. 58–88), New York, NY: Guilford Press.

Hare, R. D., and Neumann, C. S. (2010) 'The role of antisociality in the psychopathy construct: Comment on Skeem and Cooke (2010),' *Psychological Assessment, 22*:446–454.
Harpur, T. J., Hakstian, A. R., and Hare, R. D. (1988) 'Factor structure of the Psychopathy Checklist,' *Journal of Consulting and Clinical Psychology, 56*:741–747.
Harpur, T. J., Hare, R. D., and Hakstian, A. R. (1989) 'Two-factor conceptualization of psychopathy: Construct validity and assessment implications,' *Psychological Assessment: A Journal of Consulting and Clinical Psychology, 1*(1):6–17.
Hicks, B. M., Markon, K. E., Patrick, C. J., Krueger, R. F., and Newman, J. P. (2004) 'Identifying psychopathy subtypes on the basis of personality structure,' *Psychological Assessment, 16*(3):276–288.
Kastner, R. M., and Sellbom, M. (2012) 'Hypersexuality in college students: The role of psychopathy,' *Personality and Individual Differences, 53*(5):644–649.
Kiehl, K. A. (2006) 'A cognitive neuroscience perspective on psychopathy: Evidence for paralimbic system dysfunction,' *Psychiatry Research, 142*(2):107–128.
Kraepelin, E. (1915) *Psychiatrie: Ein lehrbuch* (8th ed.), Leipzig: Barth.
Krafft-Ebing, R. V. (1904) *Text book of insanity* (Translated by Chaddock CG), Philadelphia, PA: FA Davies.
Kramer, M. D., Patrick, C. J., Krueger, R. F., and Gasperi, M. (2012) 'Delineating physiologic defensive reactivity in the domain of self-report: Phenotypic and etiologic structure of dispositional fear,' *Psychological Medicine, 42*(6):1305–1320.
Krueger, R. F., Markon, K. E., Patrick, C. J., Benning, S. D., and Kramer, M. D. (2007) 'Linking antisocial behavior, substance use, and personality: An integrative quantitative model of the adult externalizing spectrum,' *Journal of Abnormal Psychology, 116*(4):645–666.
Krueger, R. F., Derringer, J., Markon, K. E., Watson, D., and Skodol, A. E. (2012) 'Initial construction of a maladaptive personality trait model and inventory for DSM–5,' *Psychological Medicine, 42*(9):1879–1890.
Kutchen, T. J., Wygant, D. B., Tylicki, J. L., Dieter, A. M., Veltri, C. O., and Sellbom, M. (2017) 'Construct validity of the MMPI–2–RF Triarchic Psychopathy scales in correctional and collegiate samples,' *Journal of Personality Assessment, 99*(4):408–415.
Kyranides, M. N., Fanti, K. A., Sikki, M., and Patrick, C. J. (2017) 'Triarchic dimensions of psychopathy in young adulthood: Associations with clinical and physiological measures after accounting for adolescent psychopathic traits,' *Personality Disorders: Theory, Research, and Treatment, 8*(2):140–149.
Latzman, R. D., Drislane, L. E., Hecht, L. K., Brislin, S. J., Patrick, C. J., Lilienfeld, S. O., . . ., and Hopkins, W. D. (2016) 'A chimpanzee (pan troglodytes) model of triarchic psychopathy constructs: Development and initial validation,' *Clinical Psychological Science, 4*(1):50–66.
Latzman, R. D., Patrick, C. J., Freeman, H. D., Schapiro, S. J., and Hopkins, W. D. (2017) 'Etiology of triarchic psychopathy dimensions in Chimpanzees (Pan troglodytes),' *Clinical Psychological Science, 5*(2):341–354.
Levenson, M. R., Kiehl, K. A., and Fitzpatrick, C. M. (1995) 'Assessing psychopathic attributes in a noninstitutionalized population,' *Journal of Personality and Social Psychology, 68*(1):151–158.
Lilienfeld, S. O. (1990) *Development and preliminary validation of a self-report measure of psychopathic personality*, University of Minnesota, Minneapolis, Unpublished doctoral dissertation.
Lilienfeld, S. O., and Andrews, B. P. (1996) 'Development and preliminary validation of a self-report measure of psychopathic personality traits in noncriminal population,' *Journal of Personality Assessment, 66*(3):488–524.
Lilienfeld, S. O., Patrick, C. J., Benning, S. D., Berg, J., Sellbom, M., and Edens, J. F. (2012) 'The role of fearless dominance in psychopathy: Confusions, controversies, and clarifications,' *Personality Disorders: Theory, Research, and Treatment*, 3:327–340.
Lilienfeld, S. O., Smith, S. F., Sauvigné, K. C., Patrick, C. J., Drislane, L. E., Latzman, R. D., and Krueger, R. F. (2016a) 'Is boldness relevant to psychopathic personality? Meta-analytic relations with non-Psychopathy Checklist-based measures of psychopathy,' *Psychological Assessment, 28*(10):1172–1185.
Lilienfeld, S. O., Smith, S. F., and Watts, A. L. (2016b) 'Fearless dominance and its implications for psychopathy: Are the right stuff and the wrong stuff flip sides of the same coin?,' in V. Zeigler-Hill & D. K. Marcus (Eds.), *The dark side of personality: Science and practice in social, personality, and clinical psychology* (pp. 65–86), Washington, DC: American Psychological Association.
Lilienfeld, S. O., and Widows, M. R. (2005) *Psychological assessment inventory-revised (PPI–R)*, Lutz, FL: Psychological Assessment Resources.
Lykken, D. T. (1957) 'A study of anxiety in the sociopathic personality,' *The Journal of Abnormal and Social Psychology, 55*(1):6–10.
Lykken, D. T. (1982) 'Fearlessness – its carefree charm and deadly risks,' *Psychology Today, 16*(9):20–28.
Lykken, D. T. (1995) *The antisocial personalities*, Hillsdale, NJ: Erlbaum.

Lynam, D. R. (1997) 'Pursuing the psychopath: Capturing the fledgling psychopath in a nomological net,' *Journal of Abnormal Psychology, 106*:425–438.

Lynam, D. R., and Miller, J. D. (2015) 'Psychopathy from a basic trait perspective: The utility of a five-factor model approach,' *Journal of Personality, 83*(6):611–626.

Lynam, D. R., Gaughan, E. T., Miller, J. D., Miller, D. J., Mullins-Sweatt, S., and Widiger, T. A. (2011) 'Assessing the basic traits associated with psychopathy: Development and validation of the Elemental Psychopathy Assessment,' *Psychological Assessment, 23*:108–124.

Marcus, D. K., Fulton, J. J., and Edens, J. F. (2013) 'The two-factor model of psychopathic personality: Evidence from the Psychopathic Personality Inventory,' *Personality Disorders: Theory, Research, and Treatment, 4*(1):67–76.

Marion, B. E., Sellbom, M., Salekin, R. T., Toomey, J. A., Kucharski, L. T., and Duncan, S. (2013) 'An examination of the association between psychopathy and dissimulation using the MMPI-2–RF validity scales,' *Law and Human Behavior, 37*(4):219–230.

McCord, W., and McCord, J. (1964) *The psychopath: An essay on the criminal mind*, Princeton, NJ: Van Nostrand.

Meehl, P. (1986) 'Diagnostic taxa as open concepts: Metatheoretical and statistical questions about reliability and construct validity in the grand strategy of nosological revision,' in T. Millon & G. L. Klerman (Eds.), *Contemporary directions in psychopathology: Toward the DSM–IV* (pp. 215–232), New York, NY: Guilford Press.

Miller, J. D., Lamkin, J., Maples-Keller, J. L., and Lynam, D. R. (2016) 'Viewing the triarchic model of psychopathy through general personality and expert-based lenses,' *Personality Disorders: Theory, Research, and Treatment,* 7(3):247–258.

Miller, J. D., and Lynam, D. R. (2012) 'An examination of the Psychopathic Personality Inventory's nomological network: A meta-analytic review,' *Personality Disorders: Theory, Research, and Treatment, 3*(3):305–326.

Miller, J. D., Lyman, D. R., Widiger, T. A., and Leukefeld, C. (2001) 'Personality disorders as extreme variants of common personality dimensions: Can the five factor model adequately represent psychopathy?,' *Journal of Personality, 69*(2):253–276.

Morey, L. C. (1991) *Personality Assessment Inventory*, Lutz, FL: Psychological Assessment Resources.

Neo, B., Sellbom, M., Smith, S. F., and Lilienfeld, S. O. (2016) 'Of boldness and badness: Insights into workplace malfeasance from a Triarchic psychopathy model perspective,' *Journal of Business Ethics*, Advance online publication.

Newman, J. P., Curtin, J. J., Bertsch, J. D., and Baskin-Sommers, A. R. (2010) 'Attention moderates the fearlessness of psychopathic offenders,' *Biological Psychiatry, 67*(1):66–70.

Patrick, C. J. (1994) 'Emotion and psychopathy: Startling new insights,' *Psychophysiology, 31*:319–330.

Patrick, C. J. (2006) 'Back to the Future: Cleckley as a Guide to the Next Generation of Psychopathy Research,' in C. J. Patrick (Ed.), *Handbook of psychopathy*, New York, NY: Guilford Press.

Patrick, C. J. (2010a) 'Conceptualizing the psychopathic personality: Disinhibited, bold, . . . Or just plain mean?,' in R. T. Salekin & D. R. Lynam (Eds.), *Handbook of Child and Adolescent Psychopathy* (pp. 15–48), New York, NY: Guilford Press.

Patrick, C. J. (2010b) Operationalizing the triarchic conceptualization of psychopathy: Preliminary description of brief scales for assessment of boldness, meanness, and disinhibition, Department of Psychology, Florida State University, Tallahassee, FL (Unpublished manual). Retrieved April 25, 2018, from www.phenxtoolkit.org.

Patrick, C. J., and Bernat, E. M. (2009) 'Neurobiology of psychopathy: A two-process theory,' in G. G. Berntson & J. T. Cacioppo (Eds.), *Handbook of neuroscience for the behavioral sciences* (pp. 1110–1131), New York, NY: John Wiley & Sons.

Patrick, C. J., Bradley, M. M., and Lang, P. J. (1993) 'Emotion in the criminal psychopath: Startle reflex modulation,' *Journal of Abnormal Psychology, 102*(1):82–92.

Patrick, C. J., and Drislane, L. E. (2015) 'Triarchic model of psychopathy: Origins, operationalizations, and observed linkages with personality and general psychopathology,' *Journal of Personality, 83*(6):627–643.

Patrick, C. J., Durbin, C. E., and Moser, J. S. (2012) 'Reconceptualizing antisocial deviance in neurobehavioral terms,' *Development and Psychopathology, 24*(3):1047–1071.

Patrick, C. J., Fowles, D. C., and Krueger, R. F. (2009) 'Triarchic conceptualization of psychopathy: Developmental origins of disinhibition, boldness, and meanness,' *Development and Psychopathology, 21*(3):913–938.

Paulhus, D. L., Neumann, C. S., and Hare, R. D. (in press) *Manual for the Hare Self-Report Psychopathy scale*, Toronto, ON: Multi-Health Systems.

Pinel, P. (1962) *A treatise on insanity* (D. Davis, Trans.), New York, NY: Hafner. (Original work published 1806)
Poy, R., Segarra, P., Esteller, À., López, R., and Moltó, J. (2014) 'FFM description of the triarchic conceptualization of psychopathy in men and women,' *Psychological Assessment, 26*(1):69–76.
Poythress, N. G., and Hall, J. R. (2011) 'Psychopathy and impulsivity reconsidered,' *Aggression and Violent Behavior, 16*(2):120–134.
Robins, L. N. (1966) *Deviant children grown up: A sociological and psychiatric study of sociopathic personality*, Baltimore, MD: Williams & Wilkins.
Rock, R. C., Sellbom, M., Ben-Porath, Y. S., and Salekin, R. T. (2013) 'Concurrent and predictive validity of psychopathy in a batterers' intervention sample,' *Law and Human Behavior, 37*(3):145–154.
Rogers, J., Viding, E., and Chamorro-Premuzic, T. (2013) 'Instrumental and disinhibited financial risk taking: Personality and behavioural correlates,' *Personality and Individual Differences, 55*(6):645–649.
Sellbom, M., Cooke, D. J., and Hart, S. D. (2015) 'Construct validity of the Comprehensive Assessment of Psychopathic Personality (CAPP) concept map: Getting closer to the core of psychopathy,' *International Journal of Forensic Mental Health, 14*(3):172–180.
Sellbom, M., Drislane, L. E., Johnson, A. K., Goodwin, B. E., Phillips, T. R., and Patrick, C. J. (2016) 'Development and validation of MMPI-2-RF Scales for indexing triarchic psychopathy constructs,' *Assessment, 23*(5):527–543.
Sellbom, M., Lilienfeld, S. O., Fowler, K., and McCrary, K. L. (in press) 'The self-report assessment of psychopathy: Challenges, pitfalls, and promises,' in C. J. Patrick (Ed.), *Handbook of psychopathy* (2nd ed.), New York, NY: Guilford.
Sellbom, M., and Phillips, T. R. (2013) 'An examination of the triarchic conceptualization of psychopathy in incarcerated and nonincarcerated samples,' *Journal of Abnormal Psychology, 122*(1):208–214.
Sellbom, M., Wygant, D. B., and Drislane, L. E. (2015) 'Elucidating the construct validity of the psychopathic personality inventory triarchic scales,' *Journal of Personality Assessment, 97*(4):374–381.
Shou, Y., Sellbom, M., and Han, J. (2016) 'Development and validation of the Chinese triarchic psychopathy measure,' *Journal of Personality Disorders, 30*(4):436–450.
Shou, Y., Sellbom, M., and Xu, J. (in press) 'Psychometric properties of the triarchic psychopathy measure: An item response theory approach,' *Personality Disorders: Theory, Research, and Treatment.*
Shou, Y., Sellbom, M., Xu, J., Chen, T., and Sui, A. (in press) 'Elaborating on the construct validity of triarchic psychopathy measure in Chinese clinical and nonclinical samples,' *Psychological Assessment.*
Sica, C., Drislane, L., Caudek, C., Angrilli, A., Bottesi, G., Cerea, S., and Ghisi, M. (2015) 'A test of the construct validity of the Triarchic Psychopathy Measure in an Italian community sample,' *Personality and Individual Differences, 82*:163–168.
Skeem, J. L., and Cooke, D. J. (2010) 'Is criminal behavior a central component of psychopathy? Conceptual directions for resolving the debate,' *Psychological Assessment, 22*(2):433–445.
Skeem, J. L., Polaschek, D. L., Patrick, C. J., and Lilienfeld, S. O. (2011) 'Psychopathic personality: Bridging the gap between scientific evidence and public policy,' *Psychological Science in the Public Interest, 12*(3):95–162.
Smith, S. F., Lilienfeld, S. O., Coffey, K., and Dabbs, J. M. (2013) 'Are psychopaths and heroes twigs off the same branch? Evidence from college, community, and presidential samples' *Journal of Research in Personality, 47*(5):634–646.
Smith, S. T., Edens, J. F., and McDermott, B. E. (2013) 'Fearless dominance and self-centered impulsivity interact to predict predatory aggression among forensic psychiatric inpatients,' *International Journal of Forensic Mental Health, 12*(1):33–41.
Snowden, R. J., Smith, C., and Gray, N. S. (2017) 'Risk taking and the triarchic model of psychopathy,' *Journal of Clinical and Experimental Neuropsychology*, Advance online publication.
Soe-Agnie, S. E., Van Dongen, J. D. M., Loomans, M. M., Patrick, C. J., Nijman, H. L. I., De Jong, C. A. J., and Van Marle, H. J. C. (2011) *Dutch version of the Triarchic Psychopathy Measure* (Unpublished manuscript).
Somma, A., Borroni, S., Drislane, L. E., and Fossati, A. (2016) 'Assessing the triarchic model of psychopathy in adolescence: Reliability and validity of the Triarchic Psychopathy Measure (TriPM) in three samples of Italian community-dwelling adolescents,' *Psychological Assessment, 28*(4):e36–e48.
Sörman, K., Edens, J. F., Smith, S. T., Clark, J. W., Kristiansson, M., and Svensson, O. (2016) 'Boldness and its relation to psychopathic personality: Prototypicality analyses among forensic mental health, criminal justice, and layperson raters,' *Law and Human Behavior, 40*(3):337–349.

Stanley, J. H., Wygant, D. B., and Sellbom, M. (2013) 'Elaborating on the construct validity of the Triarchic Psychopathy Measure in a criminal offender sample,' *Journal of Personality Assessment, 95*(4):343–350.
Strickland, C. M., Drislane, L. E., Lucy, M., Krueger, R. F., and Patrick, C. J. (2013) 'Characterizing psychopathy using DSM–5 personality traits,' *Assessment, 20*(3):327–338.
Tellegen, A. (1982) Brief manual for the multidimensional personality questionnaire, University of Minnesota (Unpublished manuscript).
van Dongen, J. D., Drislane, L. E., Nijman, H., Soe-Agnie, S. E., and van Marle, H. J. (2017) 'Further evidence for reliability and validity of the Triarchic Psychopathy Measure in a forensic sample and a community sample,' *Journal of Psychopathology and Behavioral Assessment, 39*(1):58–66.
Venables, N. C., Hall, J. R., and Patrick, C. J. (2014) 'Differentiating psychopathy from antisocial personality disorder: A triarchic model perspective,' *Psychological Medicine, 44*(5):1005–1013.
Vize, C. E., Lynam, D. R., Lamkin, J., Miller, J. D., and Pardini, D. (2016) 'Identifying essential features of juvenile psychopathy in the prediction of later antisocial behavior: Is there an additive, synergistic, or curvilinear role for fearless dominance?,' *Clinical Psychological Science, 4*(3):572–590.
Wall, T. D., Wygant, D. B., and Sellbom, M. (2015) 'Boldness explains a key difference between psychopathy and antisocial personality disorder,' *Psychiatry, Psychology and Law, 22*(1):94–105.
Weidacker, K., O'Farrell, K. R., Gray, N. S., Johnston, S. J., and Snowden, R. J. (2017) 'Psychopathy and impulsivity: The relationship of the triarchic model of psychopathy to different forms of impulsivity in offenders and community participants,' *Personality and Individual Differences, 114*:134–139.
White, S. F., and Frick, P. J. (2010) 'Callous–unemotional traits and their importance to causal models of severe antisocial behavior in youth,' in R. T. Salekin & D. R. Lynam (Eds.), *Handbook of child and adolescent psychopathy* (pp. 135–155), New York, NY: Guilford Press.
Wygant, D. B., Sellbom, M., Sleep, C. E., Wall, T. D., Applegate, K. C., Krueger, R. F., and Patrick, C. J. (2016) 'Examining the DSM–5 alternative personality disorder model operationalization of antisocial personality disorder and psychopathy in a male correctional sample,' *Personality Disorders: Theory, Research, and Treatment*, 7(3):229–239.
Yancey, J. R., Venables, N. C., Hicks, B. M., and Patrick, C. J. (2013) 'Evidence for a heritable brain basis to deviance-promoting deficits in self-control,' *Journal of Criminal Justice, 41*(5):309–317.
Young, S. E., Friedman, N. P., Miyake, A., Willcutt, E. G., Corley, R. P., Haberstick, B. C. et al. (2009) 'Behavioral disinhibition: Liability for externalizing spectrum disorders and its genetic and environmental relation to response inhibition across adolescence,' *Journal of Abnormal Psychology, 118*:117–130.

17

The triarchic model of psychopathy among incarcerated male youths

A psychometric study

Pedro Pechorro, Matt DeLisi, Isabel Alberto, James V. Ray, and Mário R. Simões

We wish to thank the following Portuguese juvenile detention centers: Bela Vista, Mondego, Navarro de Paiva, Olivais, Padre António Oliveira, Santo António, Santa Clara, and Prisão-Escola de Leiria.

In memory of George Palermo, esteemed editor of the *International Journal of Offender Therapy and Comparative Criminology*.

Introduction

Patrick, Fowles, and Krueger's (2009) triarchic model is one of the newest conceptual models of psychopathy, one that highlights boldness, meanness, and disinhibition as being noteworthy features to the disorder. According to their historical review of the psychopathy construct, boldness, meanness, and disinhibition have been recurrent, central themes of the disorder. In their conceptualization, boldness relates to an assertive, socially dominant interpersonal style and venturesomeness. It is the ability to recover quickly from stressful situations, having high self-assurance, and having a tolerance for unfamiliarity and danger. Boldness encompasses social functioning and is clearly not intended to be limited to antisocial or criminal individuals but is instead a general population feature.

In contrast, meanness captures the callous, cold, cruel, aggressive features of psychopathy and draws on the tradition of criminal psychopathy seen in works from decades earlier (for a review, see DeLisi, 2016). Meanness captures the angry, hostile, aggressive, and violent aspects of the disorder. According to Patrick (2010), meanness is seen in many behavioral manifestations displayed in psychopaths' life histories. These include arrogance and verbal derisiveness, defiance of authority, physical cruelty to animals (especially during childhood), and humans (during adolescence and adulthood), various forms of aggression, destructiveness, and the targeted exploitation of others for gain.

Disinhibition relates to impulsivity, irresponsibility, impatience, and a general tendency to fail to inhibit one's conduct. It broadly captures the notion that psychopaths have severe self-regulation deficits and are unable to control themselves in a variety of contexts. Whereas non-psychopathic individuals are frequently able to inhibit their conduct in part by using self-sanctioning emotions such as shame, embarrassment, and guilt, psychopaths lack these emotions and by extension lack the emotional inhibitions to negative behavior.

In a study using samples of female prison inmates and university students, Sellbom and Phillips (2013) found that among college students, meanness correlated positively with measures of Coldheartedness, callous and unemotional traits, egocentricity, and narcissism. Disinhibition correlated positively with measures of antisocial behavior, impulsivity, Blame Externalization, rebellious nonconformity, and Carefree Nonplanfulness. Boldness was correlated positively with Social Potency, Stress Immunity, and fearlessness. Among female prisoners, boldness was associated positively with narcissism, sensation seeking, thrill and adventure seeking, and negatively associated with the behavioral inhibition system (BIS). Meanness was negatively correlated with empathy and BIS and positively associated with Machiavellianism and sensation seeking. Disinhibition associated positively with sensation seeking, boredom susceptibility, behavioral activation system (BAS) drive, BAS fun seeking, and BAS reward responsiveness.

Less is known about the psychometric properties of the Triarchic Psychopathy Model based on the Youth Psychopathic Traits Inventory, namely the YPI–Triarchic (YPI–Tri). In a study of university students, Drislane and colleagues (2015) found the measure had good internal consistency and convergent validity with other psychopathy measures, including the Inventory of Callous Unemotional Traits, Antisocial Process Screening Device, Child Psychopathy Scale, Youth Psychopathic Inventory, Self-Report Psychopathy Scale, and Levenson Self-Report Psychopathy Scale. There were also significant associations with negative traits associated with general personality functioning, including Social Potency, well-being, achievement, social closeness, stress reaction, alienation, aggression, control, harm avoidance, and traditionalism from the Multidimensional Personality Questionnaire and Antagonism (low scores on trust, straightforwardness, altruism, compliance, modesty, and tendermindedness) from the NEO Personality Inventory–Revised. While these are important findings, it is not clear how well the measure translates to a correctional/clinical sample of youth.

To our knowledge, no previous study has examined the psychometric properties of the YPI–Tri among incarcerated male youths, which may limit generalizability of this measure to forensic or correctional populations with a higher base rate of psychopathy (Drislane et al., 2014). Thus, the main goal of the present study was to fill that research gap. It was predicted that the YPI–Tri would: (1) present a three-factor structure; (2) show adequate internal consistency values as measured by Cronbach's alpha; (3) show convergent validity with other measures of psychopathy and discriminant validity with a measure of basic empathy; and (4) show criterion-related validity (e.g., with Conduct Disorder, crime seriousness).

Method

Participants

A sample of 221 male participants (M = 16.75 years; SD = 1.41 years; age range = 13–20 years) from the nation-wide juvenile detention centers managed by the Ministry of Justice of Portugal agreed to voluntarily participate in the study. Most of them were white Europeans (54.3 percent), but the sample also included black Africans (20.5 percent), mixed race South Americans (18.6 percent), and other ethnic minorities (6.8 percent). Most of them (87.6 percent) were convicted of having committed serious and/or violent crimes (e.g., robbery, assault, rape). The participants were incarcerated by the court's decision, the harshest disposition a court in Portugal can decide. Seven of the detention centers are considered low to medium security, and one is considered maximum security and is exclusively used for youths tried as adults.

Measures

The Youth Psychopathic Traits Inventory–Triarchic (YPI–Tri; Drislane et al., 2015) is a 33-item self-report measure derived from items of the YPI with distinct relevance to constructs of the Triarchic Psychopathy Model. The YPI–Tri was designed using a three-step procedure. First, in a development phase, candidate items of the original item set of the YPI (Andershed, Kerr, Stattin, & Levander, 2002) were selected through a consensus-based construct rating approach used in prior work (Hall et al., 2014). Second, the YPI–Tri scales underwent a refinement phase and finally a psychometric evaluation phase. Each item is scored on an ordinal 4-point Likert scale (ranging from 0 = does not apply at all to 3 = applies very well). The YPI–Tri consists of three scales, namely: boldness (10 items), disinhibition (14 items), and meanness (10 items). Higher scores reflect an increased presence of psychopathic traits.

The Youth Psychopathic Traits Inventory (YPI; Andershed et al., 2002) is a 50-item self-report measure designed to assess the core personality traits of the psychopathic personality constellation in youth aged 12 years old and up. Each item is scored on an ordinal 4-point Likert scale (ranging from 0 = does not apply at all to 3 = applies very well). The YPI consists of ten subscales (with five items each) designed in line with Cooke and Michie's (2001) three-dimensional conceptualization of the psychopathy construct, namely: the grandiose/manipulation dimension (Dishonest charm, Grandiosity, Lying, and Manipulation subscales), the Callous–Unemotional dimension (Callousness, Unemotionality, and Remorselessness subscales), and the Impulsive–Irresponsible dimension (Impulsivity, Thrill-seeking, and Irresponsibility subscales). Higher scores reflect an increased presence of the characteristics associated, namely psychopathic traits. The Portuguese version of the YPI was used (Pechorro, Andershed, Ray, Maroco, & Gonçalves, 2015; Pechorro, Ribeiro da Silva, Andershed, Rijo, & Gonçalves, 2016). The internal consistency for the current study, estimated by Cronbach's alpha, was .87.

The Antisocial Process Screening Device (APSD; Frick & Hare, 2001) is a multidimensional 20-item measure designed to assess psychopathic traits in adolescents, modeled after the Hare Psychopathy Checklist (Hare, 2003). Each item is anchored on a 3-point ordinal scale (0 = never, 1 = sometimes, 2 = often). The APSD–SR (Caputo, Frick, & Brodsky, 1999) has been used with pre-adolescents and adolescents ages 11–18 years old. Scores are calculated by reverse-scoring the reversible items and then summing the items to obtain the total score and the factors scores. This scale possesses three main factors: Callous–Unemotional, narcissism, and impulsivity. Higher scores indicate an increased presence of psychopathic traits. The Portuguese version of the APSD–SR was used (Pechorro, Maroco, Poiares, & Vieira, 2013; Pechorro, Hidalgo, Nunes, & Jiménez, 2016). The internal consistency for the current study, estimated by Cronbach's alpha, was .81.

The Basic Empathy Scale (BES; Jolliffe, & Farrington, 2006) is a 20-item self-report measure designed to assess empathy in youths. The BES was developed as a concise and coherent scale with the aim of measuring two distinct factors: affective empathy and cognitive empathy. Each item is scored on a 5-point ordinal scale (from 1 = strongly disagree to 5 = strongly agree). The BES has been used with pre-adolescents and adolescents aged 9–18 years old. Scores are calculated by reverse-scoring the positively worded items and then summing the items to obtain the total score and the factors scores. Higher scores indicate an increased presence of empathic characteristics. The Portuguese version of the BES was used (Pechorro, Ray, Salas-Wright, Maroco, & Gonçalves, 2015). The internal consistency for the current study, estimated by Cronbach's alpha, was .91.

The Sellin–Wolfgang Index of Crime Seriousness (ICS)guided the delinquency seriousness classification of the official court reports. Level 0 consists of no delinquency. Level 1 consists of minor delinquency committed at home, such as stealing minor amounts of money from mother's purse. Level 2 consists of minor delinquency outside the home, including shoplifting something worth less than 5 euros, vandalism, and minor fraud (e.g., not paying bus fare). Level 3 consists of moderately serious delinquency, such as any theft over 5 euros, gang fighting, carrying weapons, and joyriding. Level 4 consists of serious delinquency such as car theft and breaking and entering. Level 5 consists of having performed at least two of each of the behaviors in level 4.

A questionnaire was also constructed to describe the socio-demographic characteristics of the participants. This questionnaire included variables such as participants' age, nationality, ethnic group, and highest level of schooling completed. Some questions regarding alcohol abuse and drug use during the last year were also included (coded as 5-point ordinal variables from 0 = almost never/never to 4 = almost always/always).

Procedures

The original translation of the YPI into the European Portuguese language was used in the present study. The translation and retroversion followed appropriate procedures (e.g., avoiding item bias or differential item functioning). The questionnaire was then independently back-translated into English. The original and the back-translated items were compared for non-equivalence of meaning and items were revised when any discrepancies in meaning were detected until no semantic differences were identified between the English version and the Portuguese version (for more details, see Pechorro, Andershed, Ray, Maroco, & Gonçalves, 2015).

Authorization to assess youths from the eight existing Juvenile Detention Centers in Portugal that admit male youths was obtained from the Ministry of Justice. The detainees were informed about the nature of the study and asked to voluntarily participate. The participation rate was approximately 92 percent. Reasons for not participating in the present study included refusal to participate (5 percent), inability to participate due to not understanding the Portuguese language (2 percent), and inability to participate due to security issues (1 percent). The measures were administered by means of individual face-to-face interviews. Some of the information (e.g., socio-demographic variables) was obtained from self-reports. Institutional files were also used to complement the information obtained (e.g., prior criminal activity and detentions, psychiatric diagnosis). The first author and a colleague made the diagnosis of Conduct Disorder (American Psychiatric Association, 2013) after interviewing each youth and taking into consideration the institutional files (which also included the official psychiatric and psychological assessments of each youth).

Analytic plan

The data were analyzed using SPSS v24 (IBM SPSS, 2016) and EQS 6.3 (Bentler & Wu, 2015). Principal Components Analysis (PCA) with Varimax rotation was done using SPSS and Confirmatory Factor Analysis (CFA) with the robust estimation methods was done using EQS. Goodness-of-fit indices included Satorra–Bentler chi-square/degrees of freedom, comparative fit index (CFI), incremental fit index (IFI), and root mean square error of approximation

(RMSEA). A chi-square/degrees of freedom value < 5 is considered acceptable, a value ≤ 2 is considered good, and a value of 1 is considered very good (Blunch, 2016; Maroco, 2014; West, Taylor, & Wu, 2012). A CFI ≥ .90 and RMSEA ≤ .08 indicate adequate fit, whereas a CFI ≥ .95 and RMSEA ≤ .06 indicate good model fit. The incremental fit index, also known as Bollen's IFI, is relatively insensitive to sample size where values ≥ .90 are considered acceptable. The CFA was performed on the ordinal items and standardized loadings above .30 were considered. No modification indices were used. Polychoric correlations were used together with robust methodologies to perform the CFA because they provide a more accurate estimate (Byrne, 1996).

Cronbach's alpha (α) (considered satisfactory if above .70), mean inter-item correlations (MIIC; considered good if within the .15–.50 range), and corrected item–total correlation ranges (CITCR; considered adequate if above .20) were used to assess reliability (Clark & Watson, 1995; Nunnally & Bernstein, 1994). Pearson correlations were used to analyze associations between scale variables, Spearman correlations were used to analyze associations between ordinal and scale variables, and point-bisserial correlations were used to analyze associations between scale and nominal dichotomous variables (Leech, Barrett, & Morgan, 2015). Correlations were considered low if below .20, moderate if between .20 and .50, and high if above .50.

Results

The first step in examining the psychometric properties of the YPI–Tri was to explore its factor structure using PCA with Varimax rotation. The Kaiser–Myer–Olkin measure of sampling adequacy (.82) and Bartlett Test of Sphericity (χ^2 = 1405.21, $p \leq .001$) indicated the suitability of the data for exploratory factor analysis. Preliminary PCA was undertaken using a criterion of greater than or equal to .30 as the level of loading significance (Nunnally & Bernstein, 1994), with the results compatible with the presumed three-factor solution. A three-component solution was subsequently forced with the components accounting for 43 percent of the common variance in scale items. However, several items obtained low loadings, below the recommend level of .30, and/or high cross-loadings, especially regarding the boldness factor (items 2 and 41) and the meanness factor (items 23, 35, and 49). Corrected item–total correlations revealed these items obtained low associations (i.e., below .20), and they were excluded from subsequent analysis. Each factor retained seven items. Regarding the disinhibition factor, item 50 was excluded and no substantial additional problems in terms of low item loadings or item–total correlations were found. However, in order to create a more parsimonious short version of the YPI–Tri while attempting to preserve the content coverage, redundant items were deleted (i.e., items 4, 9, 13, 26, 34, and 43) until only seven items remained on each factor. This strategy also took into account the guidelines established by Smith, McCarthy, and Anderson (2000) for developing valid and reliable alternative short-form measures. The reduced measure was hereafter referred to as Youth Psychopathic Traits Inventory Triarchic Short version (YPI–Tri-S).

The next step was to test the three-factor first-order structure proposed for this instrument by means of CFA. The following goodness of fit indices were obtained: one-factor model S-Bχ^2 / df = 2.97, IFI = .83, CFI = .83, RMSEA = .09 (.08–.10); three-factor first-order model S-Bχ^2 / df = 1.84, IFI = .92, CFI = .92, RMSEA = .06 (.05–.07); and three-factor second-order model S-Bχ^2 / df = 1.91, IFI = .81, CFI = .81, RMSEA = .06 (.05–.07). Based on these appropriate goodness-of-fit indices, we found support for the three-factor first-order model (Maroco, 2014; West et al., 2012). Presented in Table 17.1 are the loadings for the three-factor first-order inter-correlated model. All loadings were above .30.

Table 17.2 presents Pearson correlations between the YPI–Tri-S total and its dimensions. As expected, mostly positive moderate to high correlations were obtained.

Table 17.1 Loadings for the confirmatory three-factor structure of the YPI–Tri-S

	Factor 1	*Factor 2*	*Factor 3*
Boldness			
1 I like to be where exciting things happen.	.40		
11 I can make people believe almost anything.	.78		
15 I am good at getting people to believe in me when [. . .].	.77		
19 I have talents that go far beyond other people's.	.44		
20 It's easy for me to manipulate people.	.81		
22 I like to do things just for the thrill of it.	.66		
36 What scares others usually doesn't scare me.	.43		
Disinhibition			
3 I prefer to spend my money right away rather than save it.		.46	
5 I have probably skipped school or work more than most [. . .].		.63	
16 I have often been late to work or classes in school.		.72	
18 It often happens that I talk first and think later.		.50	
29 I get bored quickly by doing the same thing over and over.		.43	
32 It often happens that I do things without thinking ahead.		.45	
40 I often don't/didn't have my school or work assignments [. . .].		.67	
Meanness			
8 I have the ability not to feel guilt and regret about things [. . .].			.71
12 I think that crying is a sign of weakness, even if no one [. . .].			.38
17 When other people have problems, it is often their own [. . .].			.47
21 I seldom regret things I do, even if other people feel that [. . .].			.67
39 I don't understand how people can be touched enough [. . .].			.49
44 To feel guilty and remorseful about things you have done [. . .].			.45
48 To feel guilt and regret when you have done something [. . .].			.64

Note. YPI–Tri-S = Youth Psychopathic Traits Inventory Triarchic short version.

Table 17.2 Pearson correlation matrix for the YPI–Tri-S

	YPI–Tri-S total	*Boldness*	*Disinhibition*	*Meanness*
YPI–Tri-S total	1			
Boldness	.85***	1		
Disinhibition	.73***	.44***	1	
Meanness	.81***	.56***	.33***	1

Note. YPI–Tri-S = Youth Psychopathic Traits Inventory Triarchic short version.

***$p \leq .001$ level.

Table 17.3 displays the alphas, mean inter-item correlations, and corrected item-total correlation ranges for the YPI–Tri-S. The YPI–Tri-S showed good internal consistency (alpha above the recommended cut-off value of .70), mean inter-item correlations (within the recommended value range of .15–.50), and corrected item–total correlations (above .20).

Table 17.4 presents the correlations of the YPI–Tri-S with other psychometric measures. The convergent validity with the original YPI and the APSD–SR revealed mostly moderate to high statistically significant correlations. Discriminant validity with the BES total revealed non-significant correlations. The meanness scale showed a significant negative correlation with the

Table 17.3 Cronbach's alphas, mean inter-item correlations, and corrected item–total correlation ranges for the YPI–Tri-S

	Alpha	*MIIC*	*CITCR*
YPI–Tri-S total	.84	.20	.23–.57
Boldness	.77	.32	.35–.62
Disinhibition	.72	.27	.34–.51
Meanness	.71	.26	.32–.52

Note. YPI–Tri-S = Youth Psychopathic Traits Inventory Triarchic short version; Alpha = Cronbach's Alpha; Omega = Omega coefficient; MIIC = mean inter-item correlation; CITCR = corrected item–total correlation range.

Table 17.4 Convergent and discriminant validity of the YPI–Tri-S

	YPI–Tri-S total	*Boldness*	*Disinhibition*	*Meanness*
YPI total	.95***	.85***	.66***	.76***
YPI G–M	.79***	.81***	.44***	.62***
YPI I–I	.76***	.60***	.84***	.39***
YPI C–U	.81***	.64***	.36***	.91***
APSD total	.58***	.56***	.41***	.41***
APSD narcissism	.50***	.53***	.31***	.36***
APSD impulsivity	.45***	.38***	.45***	.25***
APSD CU	.26***	.24***	.14*	.24***
BES total	–.00	.03	.08	–.11
BES affective	–.09	–.07	.01	–.15*
BES Cognitive	.11	.13*	.14*	–.00

Note. YPI–Tri-S = Youth Psychopathic Traits Inventory Triarchic short version; YPI = Youth Psychopathic Traits Inventory; YPI G–M grandiose/manipulation dimension; YPI I–I Impulsive–Irresponsible dimension; YPI C–U Callous–Unemotional dimension; APSD = Antisocial Process Screening Device – Self-Report; APSD CU = Callous–Unemotional dimension; BES = Basic Empathy Scale.

***$p \leq .001$ level, * $p \leq .05$ level.

BES affective scale, and the Boldness and disinhibition scales showed significant positive correlations with the BES cognitive scale.

Table 17.5 shows the criterion-related validity. Results showed mostly statistically significant correlations varying from low to moderate in magnitude.

Discussion

The main aim of the present study was to test the psychometric properties of the YPI–Tri among incarcerated male juvenile delinquents. Our study mostly confirms the applicability of the triarchic model of psychopathy to incarcerated male youths, adding support for the psychometric properties previously obtained among undergraduate students (Drislane et al., 2014). However, the YPI–Tri measure underwent a refining process that excluded items, leading to the creation of a shortened version with only seven items per scale – the YPI–Tri-S.

The PCA results were compatible with the presumed three-factor solution and the CFA results strongly supported the three-factor inter-correlated model, while the one-factor model

Table 17.5 Criterion-related validity of the YPI–Tri-S

	YPI–Tri-S total	*Boldness*	*Disinhibition*	*Meanness*
ACO	–.25***	–.29***	–.11	–.18**
AFPL	–.15*	–.15*	–.09	–.10
ICS	.25***	.21***	.23***	.16*
VC	.11	.16*	.00	.08
CD diagnostic	.22***	.20**	.18**	.11
Alcohol	.24***	.23***	.21***	.16*
Cannabis	.33***	.27***	.26***	.26***
Coca/Hero	.31***	.30***	.29***	.15*

Note. YPI–Tri-S = Youth Psychopathic Traits Inventory Triarchic short version; ACO = age of crime onset; AFPL = age of first problem with the law; ICS = index of crime seriousness; VC = violent crime; CD diagnostic = DSM-5 Conduct Disorder diagnostic; Coca/Hero = Cocaine/Heroin.

***p ≤ .001 level, ** p ≤ .01 level, * p ≤ .05 level.

and the three-factor second-order model did not fit the data well. All factor loadings were above the .30 level, with the lowest one obtained for item 12 ("I think that crying is a sign of weakness, even if no one sees you") of the meanness scale and the highest one obtained for item 20 ("It's easy for me to manipulate people") of the boldness scale. The Pearson correlations matrix between the YPI–Tri-S total and its dimensions showed mostly positive moderate to high statistically significant associations. The strongest association among the YPI–Tri-S scales was between meanness and boldness and the lowest between meanness and disinhibition. These values were similar to the ones found for the YPI–Tri by Drislane et al. (2014).

The YPI–Tri-S total and its three scales presented satisfactory Cronbach's alpha values above the .70 recommended level (Nunnally & Bernstein, 1994). However, these values were somewhat lower than the ones obtained by Drislane et al. (2014), which might be explained by reduced number of items of the YPI–Tri-S. In terms of the mean inter-item correlations, good values were found because the YPI–Tri-S total and the scales were within the .15–.50 range (Clark & Watson, 1995), showing appropriate homogeneity. The corrected item–total correlation ranges were all above the minimum recommended value of .20 (Kaplan & Saccuzzo, 2013), demonstrating appropriate associations between the items.

The convergent validity of the YPI–Tri-S with the original YPI and the APSD–SR revealed mostly positive moderate to high statistically significant correlations demonstrating the expected overlap in line with Drislane et al.'s (2014) study. The discriminant validity with the BES total revealed the expected null or negative low correlations due to non-overlapping constructs (American Educational Research Association [AERA], 2014; Kaplan & Saccuzzo, 2013). The exceptions were the significant positive correlations of the boldness and disinhibition scales with the BES cognitive scale, which can be explained by the fact that some males with high psychopathic traits appear to overcome deficits in cognitive empathy as they move through the pubertal years (Dadds et al., 2009).

The criterion-related validity of the YPI–Tri-S and its scales with the criminal variables revealed mostly the existence of moderate–low negative associations with age of crime onset, age of first problem with the law. Negative associations between psychopathy scores and the age of crime onset have been consistently reported in the literature (e.g., Forth et al., 2003; Pechorro, Maroco, Gonçalves, Nunes, & Jesus, 2014). Moderate–low positive associations were found with crime seriousness, but in terms of the violent crime variable only the boldness scale obtained a statistically significant correlation. Such positive associations between psychopathy scores and antisocial and criminal behavior variables have been consistently reported in the literature (e.g., Forth et al., 2003; Poythress, Dembo, Wareham, & Greenbaum, 2006).

The criterion-related validity of the YPI–Tri-S and its scales with DSM's Conduct Disorder (American Psychiatric Association, 2013) showed mostly the positive moderate statistically significant associations typically provided by youth psychopathy instruments (e.g., Forth et al., 2003; Pechorro et al., 2013); the exception was the meanness scale, with a lower correlation. The correlations of the YPI–Tri-S with alcohol use, cannabis use, and cocaine/heroin were positive and low to moderate, to as expected from other short self-report measures of psychopathic traits (e.g., Colins, Noom, & Vanderplasschen, 2012). Overall, the YPI–Tri-S presented satisfactory relations to external correlates.

The findings of our study provide some additional support for the extension of the triarchic model of psychopathy to adolescents and its potential generalization across different cultures and ethnic groups. We were able to demonstrate some appropriate psychometric properties that justify the future use of the YPI–Tri-S. However, some caution is advised. Further psychometric procedures are needed and should be done in the near future (e.g., cross-validation using other samples, test–retest reliability, known-groups validity). Additionally, our study relied mostly on self-report measures, which may artificially inflate the associations found due to shared method variance. Another serious limitation was the relatively small sample size, which is an important issue given that CFA was used (both Type I and II errors are much more likely with smaller samples, and this concern is elevated when the data are skewed).

Conclusion

To our knowledge, this is the first study attempting to investigate the psychometric properties of a measure of the triarchic model of psychopathy especially designed with youths in mind among incarcerated male juvenile delinquents. We hope that our study may promote future research/ use of these instruments with different samples (e.g., clinical, community) and contribute to the study of the psychopathy construct among youths. In conclusion, the present study generally lends support to the structural, criterion, external, and divergent validity and reliability of the YPI–Tri-S among incarcerated male youths.

References

American Educational Research Association (AERA), American Psychological Association (APA), and National Council for Measurement in Education (NCME). (2014) *Standards for educational and psychological testing*, Washington, DC: AERA.

American Psychiatric Association. (2013) *Diagnostic and statistical manual of mental disorders* (5th ed.), Washington, DC: Author.

Andershed, H., Kerr, M., Stattin, H., and Levander, S. (2002) 'Psychopathic traits in non-referred youths: Initial test of a new assessment tool,' in E. Blaauw & L. Sheridan (Eds.), *Psychopaths: Current international perspectives* (pp. 131–158), The Hague: Elsevier.

Bentler, P., and Wu, E. (2015) *Supplement to EQS 6.3 for Windows user's guide*, Temple City, CA: Multivariate Software, Inc.

Blunch, N. (2016) *Introduction to structural equation modeling using IBM SPSS statistics and EQS*, Thousand Oaks, CA: Sage Publications.

Byrne, B. M. (1996) *Measuring self-concept across the life span: Issues and instrumentation*, Washington, DC: American Psychological Association.

Caputo, A., Frick, P., and Brodsky, S. (1999) 'Family violence and juvenile sex offending,' *Criminal Justice and Behavior*, *26*:338–356.

Clark, L., and Watson, D. (1995) 'Constructing validity: Basic issues in objective scale development,' *Psychological Assessment*, 7:309–319.
Colins, O. F., Noom, M., and Vanderplasschen, W. (2012) 'Youth Psychopathic Traits Inventory–Short Version: A further test of the internal consistency and criterion validity,' *Journal of Psychopathology and Behavioral Assessment*, *34*:476–486.
Cooke, D., and Michie, C. (2001) 'Refining the construct of psychopathy: Towards a hierarchical model,' *Psychological Assessment*, *13*:171–188.
Dadds, M. R., Hawes, D. J., Frost, A., Vassallo, S., Bunn, P., Hunter, K., and Merz, S. (2009) 'Learning to "talk the talk": The relationship of psychopathic traits to deficits in empathy across childhood,' *Journal of Child Psychology and Psychiatry*, *50*:599–606.
DeLisi, M. (2016) *Psychopathy as unified theory of crime*, New York, NY: Palgrave Macmillan.
Drislane, L. E., Brislin, S. J., Kendler, K. S., Andershed, H., Larsson, H., and Patrick, C. J. (2015) 'A triarchic model analysis of the Youth Psychopathic Traits Inventory,' *Journal of Personality Disorders*, *29*(1):15–41.
Drislane, L. E., Patrick, C. J., and Arsal, G. (2014) 'Clarifying the content coverage of differing psychopathy inventories through reference to the Triarchic Psychopathy Measure,' *Psychological Assessment*, *26*:350–361.
Forth, A. E., Kosson, D. S., and Hare, R. D. (2003) *Hare Psychopathy Checklist: Youth Version*, Toronto, ON: Multi-Health Systems.
Frick, P., and Hare, R. (2001) *The Antisocial Process Screening Device (APSD): Technical manual*, Toronto, ON: Multi-Health Systems.
Hall, J. R., Drislane, L. E., Patrick, C. J., Morano, M., Lilienfeld, S. O., and Poythress, N. G. (2014) 'Development and validation of triarchic construct scales from the Psychopathic Personality Inventory,' *Psychological Assessment*, *26*:447–461.
Hare, R. (1991/2003) *The Hare Psychopathy Checklist–Revised: Manual*, Toronto, ON: Multi-Health Systems.
IBM Corp. (2016) *IBM SPSS statistics for Windows (version 24)*, Armonk, NY: Author.
Jolliffe, D., and Farrington, D. (2006) 'Development and validation of the Basic Empathy Scale,' *Journal of Adolescence*, *29*:589–611.
Kaplan, R., and Saccuzzo, D. (2013) *Psychological testing: Principles, applications, and issues* (8th ed.), Belmont, CA: Cengage.
Leech, N., Barrett, K., and Morgan, G. (2015) *IBM SPSS for intermediate statistics: Use and interpretation* (5th ed.), New York, NY: LEA.
Maroco, J. (2014) *Análise de Equações Estruturais: Fundamentos teóricos, software & aplicações* [Structural equations analysis: Theoretical foundations, software and applications], Pero Pinheiro: ReportNumber, Ltd.
Nunnally, J., and Bernstein, I. (1994) *Psychometric theory* (3rd ed.), New York, NY: McGraw-Hill.
Patrick, C. J. (2010) 'Conceptualizing the psychopathic personality: Disinhibited, bold, . . . or just plain mean?,' in R. T. Salekin & D. R. Lynam (Eds.), *Handbook of child & adolescent psychiatry* (pp. 15–48), New York, NY: The Guilford Press.
Patrick, C. J., Fowles, D. C., and Krueger, R. F. (2009) 'Triarchic conceptualization of psychopathy: Developmental origins of disinhibition, boldness, and meanness,' *Development and Psychopathology*, *21*:913–938.
Pechorro, P., Andershed, H., Ray, J., Maroco, J., and Gonçalves, R. (2015) 'Validation of the Youth Psychopathic Traits Inventory and Youth Psychopathic Traits Inventory–Short among incarcerated juvenile delinquents,' *Journal of Psychopathology and Behavioral Assessment*, *37*:576–586.
Pechorro, P., Hidalgo, V., Nunes, C., and Jiménez, L. (2016) 'Confirmatory factor analysis of the Antisocial Process Screening Device: Self-Report among incarcerated male juvenile offenders,' *International Journal of Offender Therapy and Comparative Criminology*, *60*:1856–1872.
Pechorro, P., Maroco, J., Poiares, C., and Vieira, R. (2013) 'Validation of the Portuguese version of the Antisocial Process Screening Device–Self-report (APSD–SR) with a focus on delinquent behavior and behavior problems,' *International Journal of Offender Therapy and Comparative Criminology*, *57*:112–126.
Pechorro, P., Ray, J. V., Salas-Wright, C., Maroco, J., and Gonçalves, R. A. (2015) 'Adaptation of the Basic Empathy Scale among a Portuguese sample of incarcerated juvenile offenders,' *Psychology, Crime and Law*, *21*:699–714.
Pechorro, P., Maroco, J., Gonçalves, R., Nunes, C., and Jesus, S. (2014) 'Psychopathic traits and age of crime onset in male juvenile delinquents,' *European Journal of Criminology*, *11*:288–302.
Pechorro, P., Ribeiro da Silva, D., Andershed, H., Rijo, D., and Gonçalves, R. A. (2016) 'The Youth Psychopathic Traits Inventory: Measurement invariance and psychometric properties among Portuguese youths,' *International Journal of Environmental Research and Public Health*, *13*:852–857.

Poythress, N., Dembo, R., Wareham, J., and Greenbaum, P. (2006) 'Construct validity of the Youth Psychopathic Features Inventory (YPI) and the Antisocial Process Screening Device (APSD) with justice-involved adolescents,' *Criminal Justice and Behavior, 33*(1):26–55.
Sellbom, M., and Phillips, T. R. (2013) 'An examination of the triarchic conceptualization of psychopathy in incarcerated and nonincarcerated samples,' *Journal of Abnormal Psychology, 122*:208–214.
Smith, G. T., McCarthy, D. M., and Anderson, K. G. (2000) 'On the sins of short-form development,' *Psychological Assessment, 12*:102–111.
West, S., Taylor, A., and Wu, W. (2012) 'Model fit and model selection in structural equation modeling,' in R. Hoyle (Ed.), *Handbook of structural equation modeling* (pp. 209–231), New York, NY: The Guilford Press.

Part III

Homicide, sexual offending, and psychopathy

18
Psychopathy and homicide

Bryanna Fox

Introduction

The idea that homicide and psychopathy are strongly linked been part of pop culture for decades, largely starting with Alfred Hitchcock's portrayal of Norman Bates in the classic film *Psycho* in 1960. Other films, such as *The Texas Chainsaw Massacre* (1974), *Halloween* (1978), and *A Nightmare on Elm Street* (1984), found great success by propelling the psychopathic serial killer character into the mainstream. However, the genre hit a fever pitch after Anthony Hopkins' portrayal of Hannibal Lecter in *The Silence of the Lambs* in 1991. Indeed, the number of films featuring a cold, calculating, manipulative, and ruthless murderer increased sharply thereafter, with films such as *Se7en* (1995), *Scream* (1996), *Kiss the Girls* (1997), *The Bone Collector* (1999), and the undeniably relevant *American Psycho* (2000) to follow. However, during this time, no empirical research had been conducted to determine the true base rate of murderers who qualify as psychopaths, or the features of psychopaths who commit homicide.

It is clear, however, that there is a strong link between psychopathy and violent behavior. For instance, while psychopaths are estimated to make up just 1 percent of the population, they are responsible for upwards of 50 percent of all violent crime (Patrick, 2007; Porter & Woodworth, 2006; Salekin, Rogers, Ustad, & Sewell, 1998). Psychopathy has also been able to predict an individual's future violent behavior with 78 percent accuracy (Harris, Rice, & Cormier, 1991), and psychopathy scores have been more successful at predicting future violence than actuarial instruments designed specifically to predict violent recidivism (Hemphill, Templeman, Wong, & Hare, 1998:393). As murder is the most severe form of violence, it seems like that psychopathy would be a key trait of many offenders. Or, as Woodworth and Porter (2002:436–437) stated, "a relationship between psychopathy and some forms of homicide seems likely."

Indeed, many researchers from fields including psychology, psychiatry, criminology, neuroscience, and law enforcement have all investigated the relationship between homicide offenders and psychopathy. However, a formal systematic review of the research on psychopathy and homicide has not yet been conducted. Therefore, this chapter aims to identify and summarize the state of the field on psychopaths who commit homicide and address key questions such as: "How many murderers are psychopaths?" and "What are the most common features of the victim, offense, and psychopaths that commit murder?" The chapter concludes with suggestions for future theoretical and empirical research on psychopathy and homicide.

Psychopathy

As readers of this chapter are likely familiar with the construct of psychopathy, only a brief description of the traits, assessments, and research on psychopaths will be discussed. In short, a psychopath is typically defined as an individual who shows an overall lack of remorse and empathy for others, feels little emotion, has low behavioral control, engages in risky and sensation seeking behaviors, is self-centered, manipulative, a pathological liar, and does not consider the consequences of his or her actions (Cleckley, 1941; Hare, 2003).

There are several available instruments used to measure levels of psychopathy and identify those considered to be "psychopathic." The original and most common assessment is Hare's suite of Psychopathy Checklists (PCL), which include the PCL–R (revised), PCL: SV (screening version), and PCL: YV (youth version) (Hare, 2003). Each of these utilizes an itemized list of 20 traits and behaviors that represent psychopathic tendencies, which include affective/interpersonal issues such as low affect and empathy, manipulative personality, egocentricity, impulsiveness, and antisocial lifestyle factors such as sexual promiscuity, juvenile delinquency, and criminal versatility (Hare, 1991).

Based largely on research using the PCL–R, psychopathy has been shown to be one of the strongest predictors of violence (Hare, 1991; Harris et al., 1991; Salekin, Rogers, & Sewell, 1996; Salekin, 2008; Serin & Amos, 1995; Vaughn, Howard, & DeLisi, 2008; Weizmann-Henelius, Virkkunen, Gammelgård, Eronen, & Putkonen, 2015) and violent recidivism (Douglas, Vincent, & Edens, 2006; Hare, Clark, Grann, & Thornton, 2000). Additionally, the core traits of psychopathy, such as low self-control, callous and unemotional traits, behavioral problems, negative emotionality, and low empathy are highly similar to the key predictors of violent behavior (Fox, Jennings, & Farrington, 2015; Lynam, 1998; Lynam, Miller, Vachon, Loeber, & Stouthamer-Loeber, 2009; Raine, 1993). This similarity between psychopathic traits and risk factors for violence has led some to assert that "there is a synergy between the violent criminals' personality traits, lifestyle, and observed behavior that dovetails so exquisitely that it is as if their criminality is wrapped up in a box. That box is psychopathy" (Vaughn & DeLisi, 2008:164).

Homicide

In the United States alone, over 15,000 murders are committed each year (Murphy, Xu, & Kochanek, 2013). While the loss of each of those lives is devastating, the impact on those directly affected by homicide, as well as the criminal justice system and society at large, is substantial. Upwards of 9 percent of all American adults have been directly affected by a homicide experience, and the total costs associated with homicide in terms of policing, prosecution, incarceration, and lost productivity was estimated at $250 billion nationwide, a figure which exceeds $17 million per offense (DeLisi et al., 2010).

While there is considerable motivation to prevent homicide, this has proven a difficult task for variety of reasons. One of the foremost issues is that homicide is largely a heterogenous offense in terms of the characteristics of the offenders and/or why and how the crime takes place (Porter & Woodworth, 2006). For instance, some homicides are highly planned "instrumental" acts, while others are more reactive in nature and typically occur in response to a situational provocation or emotional dispute (i.e., "crimes of passion") (Porter & Woodworth, 2006). As instrumental violence is motivated by objectives such as monetary gain or elevated social status, and is typically premeditated and not emotionally driven (Berkowitz, 1993; Glenn & Raine, 2009), offenders who commit instrumental offenses are believed to be calculating, manipulative, callous–unemotional, and goal-directed (Cornell et al., 1996; Flight & Forth, 2007). Conversely, reactive homicides are unplanned and generally preceded by an emotionally provoking or threatening situation in which the offender, who is believed to be more explosive and impulsive, lashes out violently to address the situation (Woodworth & Porter, 2002). This dichotomy makes any single homicide prevention strategy largely ineffective, as at best, the approach will address one of the offender types or underlying causes for the crime.

While several studies have been conducted to examine the specific relationship between psychopathic traits and homicide, no systematic analysis has yet been conducted to determine the state of the literature, and what conclusions on the link between homicide and psychopathy can currently be drawn. Therefore, this chapter aims to address this gap by achieving two specific goals: (1) identify all literature conducted on the relationship between psychopathy and homicide, and (2) determine the average level and proportion of psychopaths who commit homicide, and all relevant additional information to help understand, identify, and potentially develop policy to address this group of ruthless killers.

Methodology

This study aimed to identify and review all peer-reviewed empirical studies on the relationship between psychopathy and homicide to determine the rate and level of psychopathy among homicide offenders. To do this, an exhaustive electronic search of major psychological, criminological, and medical journal databases and Google Scholar was conducted. Each database was searched using the terms "homicide" and "psychopathy" and all variants, including psychopath, psychopathic, PCL, homicidal, murder, murderer, and killer, in order to identify all suitable scientific publications to be included in this study. The search period was January 1, 1941[1] through June 30, 2017. As sexual homicide (a subtype of murder) is categorically unique from non-sexual homicide, only studies on general homicide were retained for this analysis.

Initially, 24 studies on psychopathy and all forms of homicide were identified. However, after conducting checks to ensure each study met the inclusion criteria, several articles were eliminated from the sample. In total, 13 articles met the criteria and were included in this review. Each article was analyzed for results relating to the prevalence of psychopathy and key findings on homicide offenders. Results of these studies will be discussed in order of year of publication.

Results

Woodworth and Porter (2002)

The first empirical study to examine the level of psychopathy among homicide offenders was conducted by Woodworth and Porter (2002). While the primary goal was to examine differences in the motivation for homicide among psychopathic and non-psychopathic offenders, this study was also the first to provide statistical data on the proportion of homicides committed by psychopaths and details on the motivation for their crimes.

Based upon a sample of 125 offenders incarcerated for homicide in Canada in 2000, Woodworth and Porter (2002) administered the PCL–R to the sample and coded each of their offenses on a Likert-type scale from purely reactive (i.e., impulsive, spontaneous, crime of passion) to purely instrumental (i.e., to achieve a premeditated goal such as revenge, material gain, or inflicting pain) in nature. Results of the study showed that the mean total PCL–R score for the offenders was 22.3 (SD = 8.8, range = 1–37), and 27.2 percent (n = 34) of the sample scored above 30, which is the psychopathic cut-off in Western nations (Hare, 1991).

Additional analyses by Woodworth and Porter (2002) indicate that homicides committed by the psychopathic offenders showed a higher degree of instrumentality, or "cold-bloodedness," in the offense compared to non-psychopaths, as 93.3 percent of psychopaths committed a primarily instrumental homicide. Higher PCL–R scores were significantly correlated with higher levels of instrumental violence (r = .45, p < .001). Comparatively, the majority (51.6 percent) of non-psychopaths committed predominantly reactive homicides. This variation in the type of homicide committed by psychopathic status was statistically significant (p < .001).

An analysis of the two sub-factors in the PCL–R, affective/interpersonal traits (Factor 1) and antisocial lifestyle (Factor 2) indicated that only Factor 1 scores play a role in predicting the level of instrumentality of the homicide. This suggests that the personality traits assessed in Factor 1 may have more to do with the planning and self-interest related to instrumental homicides, while the antisocial and aggressive behaviors evaluated in Factor 2 may be more related to reactive emotional crimes and counter-active to instrumental offending. Finally, Woodworth and Porter (2002) also found a significant relationship between victim gender and offender psychopathic status. Specifically, non-psychopathic offenders murdered men and women in near equal proportions, while 73.5 percent of psychopaths' homicides were against females and just 23.5 percent were against males.

Although some have suggested that psychopaths may be more likely to commit spontaneous and reactive murders based upon their high level of impulsivity and poor behavioral controls (e.g., Hare, 1998), Woodworth and Porter's (2002) landmark study supported the hypothesis that psychopaths are "more likely to engage in instrumental or cold-blooded homicides compared with non-psychopathic individuals" (p. 442).

Nestor, Kimble, Berman, and Haycock (2002)

The second study on homicide and psychopathy was conducted by Nestor, Kimble, Berman, and Haycock (2002) using a sample of 26 murderers with mental disorders that were committed to a maximum security forensic hospital in the United States between 1987 and 1995. The all-male sample included individuals who varied on levels of psychosis and psychopathy, as well as intellectual abilities, learning disabilities, and social intelligence. Nestor and colleagues (2002) used diagnostic records to determine the presence or absence of a psychotic disorder, including schizophrenia, schizoaffective disorder, schizophreniform disorder, bipolar disorder with psychotic features, depressive disorder with psychotic features, delusional disorder, or psychotic disorder not otherwise specified. They also administered the PCL–R to determine levels of psychopathy for each offender in the sample.

A cluster analysis was utilized to identify subgroups within the murderers based upon their level of psychosis and psychopathy. Results showed there are two underlying groups: one with a high incidence of psychosis and low level of psychopathy called the "psychotic" murderers (n = 13), and another with a high level of psychopathy and low rate of psychosis called the "psychopathic" murderers (n = 13). While the psychopathy scores and rate of psychosis for the entire sample were not reported, Nestor and colleagues (2002) stated that those in the "psychopathic" group had an average PCL–R score of 21.3 (SD = 7.2), while those in the "psychotic" group had an average PCL–R score of 9.3 (SD = 6.1).

Sizable differences in affective/interpersonal traits (Factor 1) and antisocial lifestyle (Factor 2) were also found between the psychotic and psychopathic murderer groups. The psychopathic offenders scored higher than the psychotic offenders on both Factors, but both groups scored slightly higher on Factor 2 than on Factor 1. This finding contrasts with Woodworth and Porter's (2002) results and may indicate that among homicide offenders with mental disorders, antisocial and aggressive behaviors in Factor 2 may be slightly more common than the low affect and interpersonal traits included in Factor 1.

Other key findings from Nestor et al. (2002) stand contrary to pop culture portrayals of psychotic versus psychopathic killers. For instance, offenders in the psychotic group, on average, had more years of education than the psychopathic offenders; psychotic killers scored significantly higher on verbal intelligence, and no significant difference in overall intelligence was found between the psychopathic and psychotic homicide offenders.

Laurell and Dåderman (2005) and (2007)

In a pair of studies conducted by Laurell and Dåderman (2005, 2007), a sample of 35 men convicted of homicide in Sweden that were referred for a forensic psychiatric assessment between 1979 and 1986 were analyzed for their level of psychopathy using the PCL–R, as well as other characteristics of their crime, criminal history, and background. Unlike Nestor et al. (2002), all killers diagnosed with a psychotic disorder were eliminated from the study.

Laurell and Dåderman (2007) reported that the mean PCL–R score for the sample of murderers was 20.2 (SD = 11.1, range = 1.6–34.8), and that 40 percent of the sample qualified as psychopathic using the Scandinavian cut-off of 27 on the PCL–R. When using the Western cut-off of 30 on the PCL–R, 31.4 percent of the sample qualified as psychopaths. After dividing the offenders into two groups corresponding to whether they qualified as psychopathic or not, Laurell and Dåderman (2005) examined how psychopathy relates to other features of the murderers and their past and future crimes.

Of the 14 offenders in the psychopathic group, 78.5 percent (n = 11) committed a crime after their homicide conviction, while just one-third (n = 6) of the 17 non-psychopathic offenders recidivated (p = .008). The difference in mean PCL–R scores for those who recidivated or did not recidivate resulted in an effect size of d = .7. These results support the hypothesis that psychopaths show a persistent disregard for social norms and laws, and often show a high rate of recidivism throughout their life (Hare, 1999b; Serin & Amos, 1995).

While Laurell and Dåderman (2005) found that only two of the 35 murderers (5.7 percent) had at least one criminal parent, both offenders were psychopathic, with PCL–R scores of 31.0 and 31.8. A t-test of mean PCL–R scores for murderers with or without any criminal parents resulted in a statistically significant difference across groups (p < .0001). Specifically, killers with a criminal parent had a mean PCL–R score of 31.4 (SD = 0.5), while killers without any criminal parent had a mean PCL–R score of 19.5 (SD = 11.1). This difference in mean PCL–R scores produced an effect size of d = .5.

With respect to relationship of the offenders to their victims, Laurell and Dåderman found that the median PCL–R score was nearly identical for the offenders who had a social relationship with their murder victims and those who did not. No significant association was found between psychopathy and relationship with the homicide victim. In other words, psychopaths were not more likely to target victims that they knew or strangers as compared to the non-psychopathic killers.

Overall, these studies both support and refute findings from past research. First, Laurell and Dåderman (2005) found a significant positive association between psychopathy scores and recidivism, which supports the literature indicating that psychopaths are more likely to recidivate than non-psychopaths. Laurell and Dåderman (2005) also found that those with a criminal parent tend to have a higher PCL–R score than those with no criminal parents. However, the proportion of those in the high psychopathy group with a criminal parent (14 percent) was much lower than the proportion in past studies (see e.g., Farrington, 2000; Marshall & Cooke, 1999). This finding supports Hare's (1999a) proposition that there is no causal relationship between having criminal parents and incidence of psychopathy, as psychopaths with unstable family backgrounds simply commit more violent crimes than psychopaths with stable backgrounds. Finally, while Laurell and Dåderman (2005) found no difference in psychopathy between those with known versus stranger murder victims, this does not support Hare's (1999a) hypothesis that it is more common for psychopaths to murder strangers than for non-psychopaths.

Porter and Woodworth (2007)

In the follow-up to their original study on psychopathy and homicide in 2002, Porter and Woodworth (2007) examined the psychopathy scores of 50 men incarcerated for homicide across three federal prisons in Canada. Using the PCL–R, the mean total psychopathy score for the sample was 20.6 ($SD = 7.9$, range = 3–33), and just 18 percent ($n = 9$) of the offenders scored a 30 or above, the diagnostic cut-off for psychopathy. While the psychopaths had higher Factor 1 and 2 scores in general, the mean Factor 2 scores were highest for both the psychopathic and non-psychopathic killers.

Porter and Woodworth (2007) also examined the characteristics of the homicide victims, their relationship to the offenders, and aspects of the offense such as sexual violence and level of instrumentality or reactivity in the offense. In contrast to Woodworth and Porter (2002), in this study non-psychopaths killed nearly three times more men than women (73.2 percent vs. 26.8 percent, respectively), while psychopathic killers had slightly more female (56.6 percent) versus male (44.4 percent) victims. Additionally, psychopaths predominantly killed known victims (77.8 percent), as did the non-psychopaths (70.7 percent). These findings support Laurell and Dåderman (2005), which found no significant relationship between psychopathy and relationship of offender to victim. However, as just 22 percent of psychopaths and 29 percent of non-psychopaths murdered strangers, the findings do not support Hare's (1999a) hypothesis that psychopaths are more likely to kill strangers compared to non-psychopaths.

Overall, 10 percent of the offenders engaged in some form of sexual activity with the victim during the homicide. While this activity was slightly more prevalent among non-psychopaths than psychopaths, the proportion of psychopaths who engaged in sexual violence (22.2 percent) was considerably larger than the proportion of non-psychopaths (7.3 percent). Additionally, the murders committed by the psychopaths were more instrumental (88.9 percent) than those committed by the non-psychopaths (42.1 percent). Like Woodworth and Porter's (2002) findings, total PCL–R scores were positively correlated with instrumental violence ($r = .33, p < .05$). Additionally, Factor 1 scores were positively correlated with instrumental violence ($r = .41, p < .001$), while Factor 2 scores were not. This again suggests that low affect/empathy may have more to do with the "cold-blooded" instrumentality of certain murders versus antisocial lifestyle.

Finally, Porter and Woodworth (2007) found that psychopaths and non-psychopaths did not significantly differ on the quality of their memories about the offense. However, when the level of instrumentality and reactivity of each crime was rated using official and self-reported accounts of the offense, scores were significantly lower for the official reports than self-reports for all offenders ($p < .05$). In other words, murderers described their crimes as more reactive in nature than the official reports suggested. There was no significant difference found in the misrepresentation of the offense between psychopaths and non-psychopaths, which surprisingly indicates that both groups of offenders were equally likely to lie (or mislead) the researchers about their crimes in the self-reports. However, psychopaths were significantly more likely than non-psychopaths to leave out a critically important detail of the murder in their self-reported description of the crime (66.7 percent vs. 30.6 percent, respectively). This suggests that psychopaths may be more likely to deceive on issues of greater importance regarding their crime.

Serafim, de Barros, Valim, and Gorenstein (2009)

Serafim, de Barros, Valim, and Gorenstein (2009) conducted a unique study, as it was the first to include a control group in which to compare the murderers' levels of psychopathy and emotional responses. In addition to the 35 university students and staff in the control group (deemed non-psychopathic and non-criminal), another 75 male homicide offenders serving a prison sentence and undergoing sanity evaluations in Brazil were included in the study and separated into psychopathic and non-psychopathic murderers based upon PCL–R score. Serafim et al. (2009) examined variations in each group's level of state- and trait-anxiety and emotional response to various types of images.

While an average psychopathy score for all murderers was not reported, the psychopathic murderers had a mean PCL–R score of 31.5 (SD = 1.3), non-psychopathic murderers had a mean score of 20.9 (SD = 1.4), and those in the control group had a mean PCL–R score of 4.9 (SD = 1.0). This variation in psychopathy across groups was statistically significant ($p <$ .001); however, the sample groups were based upon level of psychopathy, so this variation is to be expected. As seen in past studies (Woodworth & Porter, 2002; Porter & Woodworth, 2007), Factor 2 scores were higher for all homicide offenders compared to Factor 1 scores; however, those considered psychopathic scored higher overall on both Factors. Notably, while scoring low in general, the participants in the control group had higher scores for Factor 1 compared to Factor 2.

When emotional response and anxiety of the various groups were examined, Serafim et al.'s (2009) findings largely support past research and theory on the affective component of psychopathy. Specifically, no significant difference in heart rate among the psychopathic murderers was found regardless of whether they observed a neutral, pleasant, or unpleasant image. Conversely, non-psychopathic murderers showed a significant increase in heart rate when observing a pleasant image as compared to a neutral or unpleasant image ($p <$ .001). With respect to trait- and state-anxiety among the groups, psychopathic murderers showed the lowest levels overall on the inventories (mean = 26.7 and 29.5, respectively), followed by the non-psychopathic murderers (mean = 36.6 and 40.4, respectively) and then the, control group (43.9 and 41.8, respectively). Together, these findings suggest that psychopathic murderers may have a deficit in their autonomic response to positive or negative emotional stimuli, supporting the idea that these offenders have very low empathy and affectivity (Raine, Lencz, Bihrle, LaCasse, & Colletti, 2000).

Häkkänen-Nyholm and Hare (2009)

In Finland, Häkkänen-Nyholm and Hare (2009) collected data on 546 homicide offenders prosecuted for homicide between 1995 and 2004. The goal of this study was to compare psychopathy scores, as well as motivation for offending, post-offense behavior, and sentencing decisions for solo and multiple offender killers. Of the full sample, 471 (86 percent) were solo offenders while 75 (14 percent) had accomplices involved in the homicide. Additionally, while most of the sample was male (n = 414), over a quarter of the subjects were female (n = 151).

To determine levels of psychopathy, the authors identified elements of the PCL–R retrospectively using information available in the case files and forensic reports on each offender.

Results indicated that multi-perpetrator killers had higher average levels of psychopathy than solo offenders, with the multiple offenders' average PCL–R score at 23.1 (*SD* = 8.3) and solo offenders' average score at 18.4 (*SD* = 10.0). This difference in level of psychopathy was statistically significant ($p < .001$). No data on the average PCL–R score for the full sample or the proportion of offenders meeting the cut-off for psychopathy was provided.

With respect to the crime and sentencing measures, there were many interesting findings that both support and contradict prior research on psychopathy and homicide offenders. Specifically, high PCL–R scores were associated with (falsely) claiming a reactive justification for the killing (i.e., "self-defense"), denying responsibility for the murder, and shifting blame to external forces or even the victim (see e.g., Porter & Woodworth, 2007). Häkkänen-Nyholm and Hare (2009) also found that higher psychopathy scores were significantly related to having a male victim, a stranger victim, and leaving the scene of the killing. However, some of these findings contradict prior research. For instance, Woodworth and Porter (2002) and Porter and Woodworth (2007) both found that psychopaths tend to kill female victims (as much as three times more than male victims), and that psychopaths tend to murder fewer stranger victims, or at least the same proportion of stranger and known victims (Laurell & Dåderman, 2005).

Other novel findings from the study are that PCL–R scores are associated with receiving a final sentence from a higher-level court (indicating higher likelihood of appeals by psychopaths) and psychopathy is associated with being convicted for a less serious crime. Häkkänen-Nyholm and Hare (2009) hypothesize that these outcomes are likely the result of the psychopaths being more successful in covering up the crime and preventing law enforcement from considering them as suspects, influencing court proceedings, and finding other ways to successfully manipulate aspects of the criminal justice system. Or, as the authors put it, "a good show often trumps common sense (Babiak & Hare, 2006), even when the audience consists of those whose job it is to detect deception and dissimulation" (Häkkänen-Nyholm & Hare, 2009:773).

Juodis, Woodworth, Porter, and Brinke (2009)

Similar to the study by Häkkänen-Nyholm and Hare (2009) conducted a few months earlier, Juodis, Woodworth, Porter, and Brinke (2009) examined the crime, victim, and offender characteristics for those who commit homicides individually and with multiple offenders. Using a sample of 124 male homicide offenders serving sentence in two federal prisons in Canada, a total of 84 (68 percent) single offender and 40 (32 percent) multiple offender murderers were analyzed. The average age of the solo offenders was 31.4 (*SD* = 9.8), while the multi-offenders were several years younger, with a mean age of 26.8 (*SD* = 8.2).

The PCL–R is routinely administered to inmates in Canada using interviews and file reviews. Based upon data from solo homicide offenders, the mean total PCL–R score was 21.8 (*SD* = 9.4). The mean PCL–R score for the multi-perpetrator murderers was 23.6 (*SD* = 7.4), but the difference in scores between the offender groups was not statistically significant. No average PCL–R score for the full sample was provided. Using the Western cut-off for psychopathy, 29.8 percent of solo and 22.5 percent of multi-perpetrator murderers qualify as psychopaths, but there was also not a statistically significant difference.

While Häkkänen-Nyholm and Hare (2009) focused on criminal justice outcomes, Juodis and colleagues (2009) focused on the murder, victim, and motivation for the offense and their association with individual versus multiple offender homicide. Among these, few significant differences in the crime scene behaviors were found. For instance, nearly equal proportions of individual and multiple offenders used stabbing/cutting, shooting, or "other" methods as the cause of death. Nearly 12 times as many solo murderers used strangulation/smothering (25.6 percent vs. 2.8 percent), while twice as many multiple offenders killed via beating or assault (22.2 percent vs. 12.8 percent). Of these, just shooting and strangulation among the solo offenders were significantly correlated with PCL–R scores ($r = -.30, p < .01$ and $r = .29, p < .05$, respectively). This indicates that solo offenders with higher psychopathy scores were less likely to shoot their victims but more likely to strangle their victims.

Among victim traits, there were very similar proportions of victims who were strangers, friends, and family members to the murderer in both offender types. The killers with accomplices were most likely to murder an acquaintance (37.5 percent), which is almost double the proportion of solo murderers (19.5 percent). The solo murderers were most likely to kill a stranger (36.6 percent), with the second most common victims being current or former intimate partners (20.7 percent). Only 7.5 percent of multi-offender killers murdered a current or former intimate partner. Psychopathy scores and killing a stranger victim were significantly and positively correlated ($r = .28, p < .05$).

A significant difference was found between offender type and gender of the victim. Solo killers most often murdered female victims (65.0 percent), compared to just 38.5 percent of murderers with accomplices. Multi-offender murderers were more likely to kill men (61.5 percent), compared to just 35 percent of solo killers. The victim's gender and offender's PCL–R score were significantly associated for both individual ($r = .24, p < .05$) and multi-perpetrator ($r = .31, p < .05$) murderers, indicating higher psychopathy scores for both groups were associated with female victims.

Finally, when examining the level of instrumentality and reactivity in each offense, there are several considerable differences reported. First, the individual murderers were much more reactive in their motivation than multi-perpetrator murderers (48.1 percent vs. 21.1 percent, respectively), while the killers with accomplices were more likely to have more instrumental motivations (78.9 percent vs. 51.9 percent, respectively). Interestingly, only high psychopathy scores and instrumental motivations among the multi-perpetrator murderers were significantly correlated ($r = .35, p < .05$).

Due to the similarity between the Juodis et al. (2009) and Häkkänen-Nyholm and Hare (2009) studies, many direct comparisons on the supporting and contrasting findings between the studies can be made. For instance, Juodis and colleagues' Canadian sample had over twice as many multi-perpetrator murderers compared to Häkkänen-Nyholm and Hare's sample (32.0 percent vs. 14.0 percent, respectively). This may the result of Juodis and colleagues' all-male sample, while Häkkänen-Nyholm and Hare included female homicide offenders (who may be more likely to offend alone). Also, no significant difference in PCL–R scores was found between the solo- and multi-offender killers in Juodis et al.'s Canadian sample, but there was a significant difference in Häkkänen-Nyholm and Hare's Finnish sample (the multi-perpetrator killers scored higher). When examining associations between psychopathy scores and features of the offense, Häkkänen-Nyholm and Hare found that high psychopathy scores were significantly related to male victims. However, Juodis and colleagues found that offenders with higher psychopathy scores tend to kill female victims, which is in line with results from Porter and Woodworth (2007) and Woodworth and Porter (2002). Finally, both Häkkänen-Nyholm and Hare and Juodis et al. found a significant positive relationship between psychopathy scores and stranger victims (for Juodis and colleagues, it was only among solo murderers). These findings are in contrast to prior research which suggests that psychopaths tend to murder fewer stranger victims than known victims (Laurell & Dåderman, 2005; Porter & Woodworth, 2007). In short, more work in this area needs to be done.

Häkkänen-Nyholm, Repo-Tiihonen, Lindberg, Salenius, and Weizmann-Henelius (2009)

Based upon a sample of 633 Finnish offenders who committed a homicide between 1995 and 2004, this study examined differences in the level of psychopathy among sexual and non-sexual murderers. As the goal of this review is to examine psychopathy among general homicide offenders, and the fact that there are so few (n = 18) sexual murderers in the sample, the focus of this review will be on the non-sexual (n = 615) homicide offenders. However, results from Häkkänen-Nyholm, Repo-Tiihonen, Lindberg, Salenius, and Weizmann-Henelius (2009) suggest that there are few significant differences in the sexual and non-sexual murderers in terms of demographics, background, and offense characteristics.

Based upon PCL–R scores collected from offender interviews, the mean psychopathy score for non-sexual homicide offenders was 18.9 (*SD* = 9.8), while the mean score for sexual homicide offenders was 25.3 (*SD* = 8.9). This gap in psychopathy was one of the few statistically significant differences to appear between the sexual and non-sexual homicide offenders (p = .008). Using the Scandinavian cut-off of 26 or above on the PCL–R, 29.2 percent of non-sexual and 55.6 percent of sexual homicide offenders fall into the psychopath classification. This difference was also found to be statistically significant (p = .017). Using the standard cut-off of 30, the proportion of psychopaths decreased to 33.3 percent among sexual murderers, and 17.3 percent of non-sexual homicide offenders. This difference was not statistically significant.

An analysis of psychopathy sub-factors indicated that the sexual murderers had higher Factor 1 and Factor 2 scores compared to the non-sexual homicide offenders. The difference in Factor 1 scores was statistically significant (p < .001), but the difference in Factor 2 scores was not. Häkkänen-Nyholm et al. (2009) also examined a considerable number of offense and offender characteristics to evaluate differences between the sexual and non-sexual murderers. The vast majority of characteristics were not significantly different between the offender types. In fact, just six of the 32 characteristics showed a significant difference between the killer groups. These include leaving the body at the crime scene, using ligature or manual strangulation or suffocation, having a co-offender/accomplice, experiencing sexual abuse as a child, receiving mental health treatment before age 18, and having a history of committing sexual crimes. For each of these characteristics, except leaving the body at the scene, the sexual murderers were at least twice but up to eight times as likely to have the characteristic compared to the non-sexual offenders. Non-sexual murderers were more likely than the sexual offenders to leave the body at the crime scene.

Other notable findings include that sexual and non-sexual murderers were both far more likely to have an acquaintance, current/former intimate partner, or relative as a victim (83.3 percent and 92.8 percent, respectively) compared to strangers (16.7 percent and 7.2 percent, respectively). Also, while not statistically different among the offender types, the vast majority in both groups have a criminal history (sexual murderers: 88.9 percent, non-sexual murderers: 69.3 percent), and most have a known history of violence (sexual murderers: 55.6 percent, non-sexual murderers: 51.0 percent). Unfortunately, both groups had very high rates of physical abuse committed by family members (each around 41 percent), while nearly 19 percent of sexual murderers and 5 percent of non-sexual murderers experienced sexual abuse in childhood. These findings support research which suggests that adverse childhood experiences such as physical and sexual abuse significantly increase the risk of serious, violent, and chronic criminal behavior (Fox, Jennings, & Farrington, 2015) and sexual offending (Fox, 2017; Fox & DeLisi, 2017). As Häkkänen-Nyholm et al. (2009) noted, it appears that there is a link between childhood abuse and both forms of homicide (particularly the sexual offenses), and that early intervention and follow-up of cases where trauma and abuse are reported in childhood may help prevent some of these crimes from occurring in the future.

Weizmann-Henelius, Putkonen, Grönroos, Lindberg, Eronen and Häkkänen-Nyholm (2010)

In the first study to examine the level of psychopathy solely among female homicide offenders, Weizmann-Henelius and colleagues (2010) used a sample of 97 women convicted for homicide between 1993 and 2005 in Finland. The PCL–R was administered to the entire sample, and the mean total score was 16.8 ($SD = 9.7$, range = 0–34). Just 9.3 percent ($n = 9$) of the female murderers qualified for psychopathy using the Western cut-off of 30, but using a lower cut-off of 25 (in line with research from other Scandinavian nations), 21.6 percent of the sample ($n = 21$) met the designation for psychopathy. The mean score and proportion of psychopaths in Weizmann-Henelius and colleagues' (2010) sample were both considerably lower than findings from each of the studies previously noted. It is possible that this reflects the Finnish sample, or the fact that the homicide offenders were all female. However, the sample also showed a low base rate of criminal history and prior violence (42.3 percent and 30.9 percent, respectively) and 11 of the 97 women (11.5 percent) were not considered legally responsible for their murder due to a psychosis diagnosis. Consequently, more research on female homicide offenders is needed to disentangle these issues and better evaluate the level of psychopathy in this population.

Putkonen, Weizmann-Henelius, Repo-Tiihonen, Lindberg, Saarela, Eronen, and Häkkänen-Nyholm (2010)

Using another unique sample, Putkonen et al. (2010) evaluated psychopathy among 50 offenders incarcerated for homicide in Finland between 1995 and 2004. Within the sample, 25 murderers were aged 60 or over, while a random sample of 25 homicide offenders under age 60 served as the comparison group. The average age of the older offenders was 66.8 ($SD = 5.7$, range = 60–82), while the mean age for the younger offenders was 34.8 ($SD = 10.8$, range = 19–59). Based upon the PCL–R assessment, level of psychopathy was calculated for each offender. No data was provided for the average PCL–R score for the entire sample. The average PCL–R score for the older offenders was 9.2 ($SD = 8.7$, range = 0–35), while the younger murderers showed a higher mean PCL–R score of 17.6 ($SD = 9.4$, range = 2.0–37.8). The difference in PCL–R scores between these groups was statistically significant ($p < .002$) and resulted in an effect size of $d = .93$.

When comparing the proportion of murderers who scored in the psychopathic range, there was a substantial variation between the two groups. When assessing the level of psychopaths in the murder sample according to a Scandinavian cut-off at 25, only 8 percent ($n = 2$) of older offenders versus 24 percent ($n = 6$) of the younger homicide offenders qualified as psychopaths. Using the Western cut-off of PCL–R of 30 or above, just 4 percent ($n = 1$) of the older offenders and 24 percent ($n = 6$) of the younger killers qualified as psychopaths. Among the sub-factors, younger murderers scored higher overall, but a significant difference between the older and younger offenders was only found for Factor 2 scores ($p < .001$).

In sum, while the younger murderers showed psychopathy scores that were lower than most others seen in the previously mentioned studies, the older offenders scores were considerably lower. This indicates that the mechanisms (and explanation) for the association between psychopathy and homicide requires more examination to be better understood.

Laajasalo, Salenius, Lindberg, Repo-Tiihonen and Häkkänen-Nyholm (2011)

While pop culture often associates psychopathic murderers with psychotic disorders such as schizophrenia, research suggests this is a rare occurrence, with comorbidity under 5 percent (Hart & Hare, 1997; Rice & Harris, 1995). However, as there is limited research on these atypical psychotic murderers, Laajasalo and colleagues (2011) aimed to examine the prevalence of psychopathic traits among these offenders. Using a sample of 72 offenders prosecuted for murder in Finland between 1995 and 2004 and diagnosed with schizophrenia, and a matched sample of 72 offenders convicted of homicide during the same time frame, an analysis of psychopathy and characteristics of the offenders was conducted. The sample of schizophrenic murderers represents 9.6 percent of all homicide offenders in Finland during the sampled time frame. The mean age of the schizophrenic offenders was 34.8 years old ($SD = 11.3$), and the majority ($n = 64$) were men while eight of the offenders were female.

Based upon the PCL–R administered during standard psychiatric evaluations, the average PCL–R score for the total sample of 144 murderers was 17.7 ($SD = 9.8$). Using the Scandinavian cut-off of 26, 23.6 percent of the sample qualified as psychopaths, while 13.2 percent fit the definition using the Western standard of 30 or above on the PCL–R. Among the schizophrenic and general homicide offenders, a significant difference in mean PCL–R scores was found ($p = .005$). Specifically, the schizophrenic murderers showed a mean PCL–R score of 15.4 ($SD = 9.8$), while the average score for the general homicide offenders was nearly five points higher at 20.0 ($SD = 9.0$). The difference in PCL–R scores between these groups resulted in an effect size of $Z = -2.81$.

With respect to the background characteristics of the offenders, Laajasalo and colleagues (2011) found that the general homicide offenders had significantly higher rates of alcohol dependence ($n = 31$) compared to the schizophrenic murderers ($n = 16$; $p < .001$). Also, while the general homicide offenders were not diagnosed with schizophrenia, all but four (94.4 percent) were diagnosed with another psychiatric disorder. The two groups had no significant differences in IQ, which was unexpected; however, there was considerable missing data for this measure among the schizophrenic murderers, which may correspond to offenders too ill to complete the IQ testing.

Finally, analysis of correlations between crime behavior characteristics and PCL–R scores were also conducted, but surprisingly, no variables reflecting the method or location of the murder were significantly correlated with either group's PCL–R scores. With respect to homicide behaviors, excessive violence was more common among the schizophrenic murderers than general homicide offenders (26.0 percent vs. 16.4 percent, respectively), but this difference also did not reach statistical significance.

In sum, this study shows that contrary to popular belief, schizophrenic murderers tend to score significantly lower on psychopathy compare to general homicide offenders. However, contrary to prior academic findings (e.g., Hare, 2003), the comorbidity of schizophrenia and psychopathy among homicide offenders occurs more often than previously believed.

Cope, Ermer, Gaudet, Steele, Eckhardt, Arbabshirani, Caldwell, Calhoun, and Kiehl (2014)

In the most recent study conducted on this topic, Cope and colleagues (2014) were the first to examine the relationship between psychopathy and homicide among juvenile offenders. Using data collected on 20 adolescent males who committed homicide between 2007 and 2011 and were incarcerated at a maximum security youth detention facility in the United States, an analysis of psychopathy and other neurological and psychological issues such as abnormality in brain structure, traumatic brain injuries, and callous–unemotional traits was conducted. Due to the age of the sample (mean = 17.5, *SD* = 1.2), the youth version of the PCL assessment (PCL: YV) was utilized. Additionally, a comparison group of 135 non-homicide juvenile offenders who committed lesser crimes such as burglary, assault, rape, drug possession, theft, and fraud and 21 "healthy" adolescents with no criminal history were drawn upon to compare the adolescent murderer group scores.

Using the PCL: YV, the mean total score for the juvenile homicide offenders (JHOs) was 29.1 (*SD* = 5.2). This is the highest average psychopathy score for any of the general homicide offender groups reviewed, except the Serafim et al. (2009) sample which consisted entirely of psychopaths. Even so, these JHOs scored just 2.4 points lower than the Serafim et al. (2009) psychopathic murderer group, and they scored 6.8 points higher than the second highest average scoring group, which was reported in Woodworth and Porter's (2002) original study. In short, while the exact proportion of the JHOs that qualify as psychopaths was not reported, given the extremely high scores of these offenders it seems likely that it is a sizable proportion. The non-homicide offenders had an average total score of 23.1 (*SD* = 6.0). No PCL: YV scores were reported for the "healthy" youth.

In line with prior research, both sub-factor scores for the JHOs were high, with Factor 2 much higher than the Factor 1 scores. A statistically significant difference was found between the JHOs and non-homicide juvenile offender on the total and individual factor scores in the PCL: YV. However, when other demographic and psychological features were compared between JHOs and healthy youth, several significant differences were found. For instance, the median household income for each participant's home zip code (socioeconomic status [SES]) of the healthy youth was over $16,000 more per year than the JHOs ($p < .001$), and the average IQ of the JHOs (mean = 93.0) was 17.6 points lower than the healthy youth (mean = 110.6, $p < .001$). The JHO group also had significantly higher levels of regular substance use than the healthy ($p < .001$) and non-homicide juvenile offenders ($p = .006$), and significantly higher levels of substance dependence than both the healthy ($p < .001$) and non-homicide juvenile offenders ($p = .001$). However, when examining personality features such as impulsivity and callous–unemotional traits, the JHOs scored higher on both than non-homicide offenders, but this difference was not statistically significant. Personality data was not collected for the healthy youth.

With respect to brain abnormalities, two major areas were assessed: number of traumatic brain injuries with loss of consciousness (TBI) and various deficits in brain matter volume. TBIs were self-reported by the youth, while deficits in brain volume were evaluated using high-resolution T1-weighted structural magnetic resonance imaging (MRI) scans. Results showed that JHOs had more neurological abnormalities compared to the healthy youth and non-homicide juvenile offenders. Specifically, JHOs were more than five times as likely to have a TBI than healthy youth, with an average of 1.1 TBI for each JHO, but only 0.2 average TBI for the healthy adolescents ($p < .001$). Head injuries have been shown to relate to higher rates of serious criminal and violent behavior, with studies suggesting that up to 87 percent of prison inmates experience at least one severe TBI (Farrer & Hedges, 2011; León-Carrión & Ramos, 2003; Slaughter, Fann & Ehde, 2003), compared to just 8 percent of all Americans (Silver, Kramer, Greenwald, & Weissman, 2001), but 100 percent of sampled death-row inmates in the United States (Lewis, Pincus, Feldman, Jackson, & Bard, 1986).

Based upon the MRI results, Cope and colleagues (2014) reported that there were significantly lower total brain volumes in the JHOs compared to healthy youth ($p < .001$) and their offender counterparts ($p = .007$). The JHOs also had reduced gray matter volumes compared to both the healthy youth ($p < .001$) and the non-homicide offenders ($p = .006$). In total, it was estimated that the JHOs had nearly 5 percent less brain volume for all measures, as compared to the non-homicide offenders. Finally, in addition to the many global differences in brain volume and gray matter volume, there were also several regional differences in gray matter volume in the hippocampus, posterior insula, and other areas of the medial and lateral temporal cortex between the JHOs and non-homicide offenders. Specifically, most regional gray matter reduction was found in the temporal lobes of the JHOs, which supports prior findings on specific brain volume deficits among violent males with Antisocial Personality Disorder (ASPD) (Barkataki, Kumari, Das, Taylor, & Sharma, 2006). Additional research suggests that individuals with ASPD, a disorder analogous to (but less severe than) psychopathy, showed an 11 percent reduction in prefrontal gray matter volume compared to healthy subjects (Raine et al., 2000). Finally, Cope et al. (2014) identified that the JHO sample also showed reduced gray matter volumes in the temporal poles of the brain, which has previously been associated with higher psychopathic traits (Ermer, Cope, Nyalakanti, Calhoun, & Kiehl, 2013).

While this study was one of the first to examine neuropsychological deficits in adolescent homicide offenders, it should be noted that these youths are largely those who were so extreme and violent that their age of criminal onset, particularly for homicide, was extremely young, and that these offenders were the ones who were caught. As Yang and colleagues (2005) found, unsuccessful psychopaths, but not "successful" psychopaths (i.e., those who were not caught for their offenses) had a 22.3 percent reduction in prefrontal gray matter volume as compared to healthy subjects. In other words, more research on both incarcerated and self-reported JHOs should take place to better understand the relationship between psychopathy, homicide, and neuropsychological deficits such as reduced gray matter volume in the brain.

Discussion

This chapter presents the results of a systematic review on the state of the literature on psychopathy and homicide offenders. Specifically, this review identified and summarized all original empirical studies published on this topic from January 1941 to June 2017 and addressed key questions regarding the prevalence and characteristics of psychopaths who commit homicide. This review indicates that a considerable amount of knowledge has been gained from the 13 empirical studies conducted on psychopathic murderers, but there are also several gaps in our understanding of these dangerous offenders that have not been addressed in the literature. A summary of the results of the 13 studies included in this systematic review are presented in Table 18.1. Answers to the key questions posed at the onset of this chapter, as well as suggestions for future research, are to follow.

How many murderers are psychopaths?

The prevalence of psychopathy among homicide offenders was surprisingly variant in the eight studies. Specifically, rates ranged from a low of 5.6 percent to 55.6 percent, depending largely upon the location, subsample, and type of homicide committed. For instance, Laajasalo et al. (2011) reported that 5.6 percent of a subsample of murderers qualified as psychopaths; however, the offenders in this sample were diagnosed schizophrenics, which has been shown to be inversely correlated with psychopathy (Hart & Hare, 1997; Rice & Harris, 1995). Additionally, the sample used in Laajasalo et al. (2011) was Finnish, and Scandinavians are believed to have lower rates of psychopathy compared to other regions (Hare, 1991). Another subsample with a

Table 18.1 Summary of research and findings on psychopathy and homicide offenders

Study	*n*	*Sample*	*Country*	*Mean PCL score*	*Psychopathy prevalence**	*Other notable findings*
Woodworth and Porter (2002)	125	Homicide offenders	Canada	22.3	27.2%	• 73.5% of psychopaths killed women • 93.3% of psychopaths commit primarily instrumental murder • PCL–R scores correlated with instrumental violence ($r = .45$) • Factor 1 scores highest, predict level of instrumentality
Nestor, Kimble, Berman, and Haycock (2002)	26	Male homicide offenders with a mental disorder	USA	21.3 (psychopath) 9.3 (psychotic)	–	• Factor 2 scores highest for both groups • Psychotic killers had higher education and verbal IQ • Psychopathic killers had higher performance IQ
Laurell and Dåderman (2005), (2007)	35	Homicide offenders	Sweden	20.2	40.0%	• 78.5% of psychopathic killers recidivated • 14% of psychopathic killers had criminal parent • 78.5% of psychopathic killers knew the victim
Porter and Woodworth (2007)	50	Homicide offenders	Canada	20.6	18.0%	• 56.6% of psychopaths killed women • 77.8% of psychopathic killers knew the victim • 22.2% of psychopaths engaged in sexual violence • 88.9% of psychopaths commit primarily instrumental murder • PCL–R scores correlated with instrumental violence ($r = .33$) • Factor 2 scores highest, Factor 1 scores correlated with instrumentality ($r = .41$)
Serafim, de Barros, Valim, and Gorenstein (2009)	75	Male homicide offenders	Brazil	31.5 (psychopath) 20.9 (non-psychopath)	–	• No significant difference in heart rate among psychopathic killers when shown neutral, pleasant, or unpleasant images • Psychopathic killers scored lowest on trait- and state-anxiety • Factor 2 scores highest among both murderer groups
Häkkänen-Nyholm and Hare (2009)	546	Solo and multi-perp homicide offenders	Finland	23.1 (multi-offender) 18.4 (solo offender)	–	• High PCL–R scores correlated with male victims, stranger victims, and being convicted of a less serious crime • Psychopathic killers more likely to falsely claim a reactive justification, deny responsibility, and shift blame for murder

(*Continued*)

Table 18.1 (Continued)

Study	*n*	*Sample*	*Country*	*Mean PCL score*	*Psychopathy prevalence**	*Other notable findings*
Judis, Woodworth, Porter, and Brinke (2009)	124	Male solo and multi-perp homicide offenders	Canada	23.6 (multi-offender) 21.8 (solo offender)	22.5% (multi-offender) 29.8% (solo offender)	• Psychopathic killers more likely to kill women • PCL–R scores correlated with stranger victims ($r = .28$), strangulation ($r = .29$), and shooting victims ($r = -.30$). • 48.1% of solo murderers reactive, while 78.9% of multi-offender killers had instrumental motivations to kill
Häkkänen-Nyholm et al. (2009)	633	Sexual & non-sexual homicide offenders	Finland	25.3 (sexual homicide) 18.9 (non-sexual homicide)	55.6% (sexual homicide) 29.2% (non-sexual homicide)	• 83.3% of sexual, 92.8% of non-sexual killers knew victim • Sexual killers more likely to strangle/suffocate victim, have co-offender, history of sex crimes, abused sexually as a child, received mental health treatment in childhood • All murderers had low average IQs, long criminal history, and high rates of abuse in childhood • Factor 2 scores highest for both groups
Weizmann-Henelius et al. (2010)	97	Female homicide offenders	Finland	16.8	21.6%	• 42.3% had criminal history, 30.9% commit violence in past • 11.5% not considered legally responsible due to psychosis
Putkonen et al. (2010)	50	Homicide offenders	Finland	17.6 (under age 60) 9.2 (age 60 or over)	24.0% (under age 60) 8.0% (age 60 or over)	• Factor 2 scores higher for younger killers, Factor 1 scores higher for older killers
Laajasalo et al. (2011)	144	Homicide offenders with psychotic disorders	Finland	15.4 (schizophrenic) 20.0 (non-psychotic)	5.60% (schizophrenic) 20.8% (non-psychotic)	• 94.4% of non-psychotic killers had a psychiatric disorder • Schizophrenic killers showed more excessive violence
Cope et al. (2014)	20	Juvenile homicide offenders	USA	29.1	–	• JHOs 5x more likely to have a traumatic head injury, had lower total brain volume, reduced gray matter volume, and lower gray matter in temporal poles versus healthy youth • JHOs had nearly 5% less brain volume compared to non-homicide offenders • Factor 2 higher than Factor 1

* Psychopathy prevalence reported with regional customary cut-offs (PCL = 30+ in Western nations, 25–27+ in Scandinavian nations.)

particularly low prevalence of psychopathy was seen in Putkonen et al. (2010), where 8 percent of the older murderers were psychopathic. But, like Laajasalo et al. (2011), this subsample of homicide offenders are unique in that they were aged 60 and over, and from Finland. Due to these demographics the risk of psychopathy is lower, and a low base rate of psychopathy for this offender subsample is therefore not surprising.

On the other hand, the highest rate of psychopathy was reported in Häkkänen-Nyholm et al. (2009)'s subsample of sexual homicide offenders. While this study was also conducted in Finland, the prevalence of psychopathy among sexual homicide offenders has consistently been shown to be higher than non-sexual offenders, as sexual killers are believed to be more prone to particularly callous and manipulative behavior, lack of empathy, pathological lying, and disregard for social norms, even when compared to other murderers (DeLisi & Vaughn, 2007).

Excluding these outlier samples, the base rate of psychopathy among homicide offenders was found to be between 18 percent (Porter & Woodworth, 2007) and 40 percent (Laurell & Dåderman, 2007). Most studies reported prevalence in the 20 to 29 percent range. These findings are more in line with previous, albeit limited, reports on the base rate of psychopathy among murderers. For instance, using four empirical studies on the topic, Dhingra and Boduszek (2013) reported a prevalence between 11 percent and 32 percent. In short, it appears that while the prevalence of psychopathic killers may vary greatly depending on the type of murder, location of the offense, age, gender, and mental health status of the offender, in general, *about one in four murderers is a psychopath.*

What are the most common features of the victims of psychopaths that commit murder?

As shown in Table 18.1, there are a plethora of findings regarding the crime and victim features, and the background, traits, and criminal history associated with psychopaths and the crimes they commit. To begin, the results of research on the victims that psychopaths tend to target will be discussed.

Most studies examining the gender of victims found that the majority of psychopaths target females, with estimates of the *proportion of female victims among psychopathic killers between 57 percent and 73 percent* (Juodis et al., 2009; Porter & Woodworth, 2007; Woodworth & Porter, 2002). One study, Häkkänen-Nyholm and Hare (2009), found that higher PCL–R scores were significantly correlated with killing male victims, but Juodis and colleagues (2009) found the opposite, as higher PCL–R scores in their sample were significantly correlated with murdering female victims.

With respect to Hare's (1999a) hypothesis that psychopaths are more likely to kill strangers compared to non-psychopaths, three of the five studies which examined the issue found that most psychopaths murdered victims that they knew (Häkkänen-Nyholm et al., 2009; Laurell & Dåderman, 2005, 2007; Porter & Woodworth, 2007). Specifically, results of the three studies show that *78 percent to 93 percent of psychopathic murderers targeted a victim that was known to them* as an acquaintance, former or current intimate partner, or relative. Conversely, two studies (Häkkänen-Nyholm & Hare 2009; Juodis et al., 2009) found that high PCL–R scores were correlated with killing stranger victims. From the lack of consistency in the available research on common features of victims murdered by psychopaths, it is clear that more research on this topic is needed.

What are the most common offense features of psychopathic murders?

One of the ongoing debates is regarding the level of instrumentality and reactivity involved in homicides committed by psychopaths (Porter & Woodworth, 2006). While Cleckley (1941) originally predicted that psychopaths would be highly reactive due to their impulsivity and low behavioral controls, and studies suggested that psychopaths often engage in reactive violence (Cornell et al., 1996; Williamson, Hare & Wong, 1987), other studies show that psychopaths are more callous and cold-blooded in their criminal activity and tend to commit more instrumental violent offenses (Hart & Dempster, 1997; Porter, Birt & Boer, 2001).

Results from this review support the "cold-blooded" hypothesis for psychopaths' motivation for offending, as each of the studies on the topic found considerable support for high levels of instrumentality in the murders committed by psychopaths (Porter & Woodworth, 2007; Woodworth & Porter, 2002; Juodis et al., 2009). Specifically, *89 percent to 93 percent of the general homicides committed by psychopaths were primarily instrumental* (Porter & Woodworth, 2007; Woodworth & Porter, 2002). Among multi-perpetrator psychopathic killers, the proportion of instrumental offenses was 79 percent, and it was 52 percent among solo psychopathic murderers (Juodis et al., 2009).

A secondary debate has also arisen regarding the traits of psychopaths which primarily contribute to the commission of cold-blooded instrumental offenses. Prior research suggests that higher Factor 1 scores are related to higher levels of instrumentality, as the offenders who are "particularly ruthless" would be more likely to commit cold-blooded violence (Porter, Birt & Boer, 2001; Porter & Woodworth, 2006:484). This review supports these findings, as *higher Factor 1 scores were shown to relate to higher levels of instrumentality* in both studies which examined the issue (Porter & Woodworth, 2007; Woodworth & Porter, 2002). However, it should be noted that six of the seven studies to report sub-factor scores on the PCL–R show that, overall, Factor 2 scores were higher than Factor 1 scores for offenders in their sample (Cope et al., 2014; Häkkänen-Nyholm et al., 2009; Nestor et al., 2002; Porter & Woodworth, 2007; Putkonen et al., 2010; Serafim et al., 2009). Only Woodworth and Porter (2002) found that Factor 1 scores were highest among the killers in their sample, while Putkonen et al. (2010) found that Factor 1 scores were highest only for the murderers over age 60.

Other notable findings on the characteristics of murders committed by psychopaths include that PCL–R scores were positively correlated with strangulation, but negatively correlated with shooting their victims (Juodis et al., 2009). Nearly a quarter of psychopaths engaged in sexual violence during their murders (Porter & Woodworth, 2007), but surprisingly, few offense characteristics were significantly different for sexual versus non-sexual killers (Häkkänen-Nyholm et al., 2009).

What are the most common features of the psychopaths that commit murder?

Finally, with respect to features of psychopaths who commit murder, a wide variety of findings can also be found. While research already suggests that the majority of risk factors for violent behavior are also defining characteristics of psychopaths (Porter, Campbell, Woodworth & Birt, 2001), this review tended to focus on new information that is not typically reviewed in the literature on psychopathy, violence, and homicide offenders.

For instance, Serafim and colleagues (2009) found that there was no significant difference in heart rate among psychopathic killers when shown neutral, pleasant, or unpleasant images, and that psychopathic killers scored lowest on trait- and state-anxiety compared to non-psychopathic offenders and a control group. This provides empirical support for the fact that psychopathic murderers tend to commit more instrumental violence, and that high Factor 1 scores are more likely to be associated with extreme violence as compared to Factor 2 scores.

On a related note, Cope and colleagues (2014) found that juvenile homicide offenders were five times as likely to have a traumatic head injury, and had five percent less brain volume compared to non-homicide offenders. While this study did not isolate psychopathic offenders, the findings by Cope et al. support studies which found highly similar neurological and psychological deficits among violent offenders with Antisocial Personality Disorder (Barkataki et al., 2006) and higher psychopathic traits (Ermer et al., 2013). Interestingly, psychopathic killers were also found to have lower education and verbal IQ compared to psychotic murderers (Nestor et al., 2002), and both sexual and non-sexual killers were found to have low average IQs, high rates of abuse in childhood, and a long criminal record (Häkkänen-Nyholm et al., 2009).

With respect to the criminal history of the psychopathic murderers, 42.3 percent commit a crime and 30.9 percent commit violence in the past (Weizmann-Henelius et al., 2010). Additionally, 78.5 percent of psychopathic killers reoffended after their murder, and 14 percent had at least one criminal parent (Laurell & Dåderman, 2005, 2007). High PCL–R scores were also correlated with manipulation of the criminal justice system, including shifting blame, falsely claiming self-defense, and denying responsibility for the murder, as well as being convicted of a less serious crime than non-psychopathic murderers (Häkkänen-Nyholm & Hare, 2009).

Conclusion

Future research should aim to collect more data on the development of psychopathy and the overlap between other risk factors for criminal behavior, ideally using prospective longitudinal studies. This will allow for more causal inferences to be developed, as well as evaluation of within-individual changes that may lead to psychopathy or homicide, for instance after a severe head injury or trauma and abuse occurs. The more advanced study designs would help researchers to better address the complexity found in psychopathic offenders, and better test the many hypotheses surrounding psychopathic killers which are currently still being debated.

Additionally, given the considerable overlap in risk factors for psychopathy and violence, as well as the high base rate of psychopathy among homicide offenders, the construct of psychopathy should be specifically incorporated into mainstream criminological theories. To this end, Fox, Jennings, and Farrington (2015) outlined the direct integration of psychopathy into the ten leading developmental and life-course theories in criminology, while DeLisi (2009, 2016) detailed specifics on how psychopathy can be utilized as the unified theory of crime. In short, it is only after psychopathy is incorporated as a mainstream construct in criminological theory and research that significant leaps in the understanding and prediction of criminal behavior, and empirical tests of the relationship between psychopathy and homicide, can be conducted.

While this review indicates that the quantity, and quality, of empirical research on psychopathy and homicide has risen substantially over the past 15 years, it is also clear that much more work needs to be done. Although little to no evidence has suggested that psychopathy is a treatable condition (DeLisi, 2016), we should instead focus our efforts on early risk assessment and prevention. Given that this review of all empirical research on psychopathy and homicide suggests that an average of one in four murderers qualifies as a psychopath, there should be a renewed effort to identify risk factors for psychopathy, and develop intervention programs for those at greatest risk, when possible. For instance, more research should be conducted on issues identified in studies in this review, such as head trauma and abuse or trauma in childhood, to determine if these are risk factors for developing psychopathic tendencies. If so, far more research and prevention efforts on these topics should be pursued. If even one homicide can be prevented through our continued research on the nature and origins of psychopathy, it is certainly an effort that is well worth our while.

Note

1 This is the year that Hervey Cleckley's pioneering book on psychopathy, *The Mask of Sanity*, was released.

References

Babiak, P., and Hare, R. D. (2006) *Snakes in suits: When psychopaths go to work*, New York, NY: Regan Books.

Barkataki, I., Kumari, V., Das, M., Taylor, P., and Sharma, T. (2006) 'Volumetric structural brain abnormalities in men with schizophrenia or antisocial personality disorder,' *Behavioural Brain Research*, *169*(2):239–247.

Berkowitz, L. (1993) *Aggression: Its causes, consequences, and control*, New York, NY: McGraw-Hill.

Cleckley, H. (1941) *The mask of sanity*, St. Louis, MO: Mosby.

Cope, L. M., Ermer, E., Gaudet, L. M., Steele, V. R., Eckhardt, A. L., Arbabshirani, M. R., . . ., and Kiehl, K. A. (2014) 'Abnormal brain structure in youth who commit homicide,' *Neuroimage: Clinical*, *4*:800–807.

Cornell, D. G., Warren, J., Hawk, G., Stafford, E., Oram, G., and Pine, D. (1996) 'Psychopathy in instrumental and reactive violent offenders,' *Journal of Consulting and Clinical Psychology*, *64*(4):783–790.

DeLisi, M. (2009) 'Psychopathy is the unified theory of crime,' *Youth Violence and Juvenile Justice*, 7:256–273.

DeLisi, M. (2016) *Psychopathy as unified theory of crime*, New York, NY: Palgrave Macmillan.

DeLisi, M., Kosloski, A., Sween, M., Hachmeister, E., Moore, M., and Drury, A. (2010) 'Murder by numbers: Monetary costs imposed by a sample of homicide offenders,' *The Journal of Forensic Psychiatry & Psychology*, *21*(4):501–513.

DeLisi, M., and Vaughn, M. G. (2007) 'Still psychopathic after all these years,' in M. DeLisi & P. J. Conis (Eds.), *Violent offenders: Theory, research, public policy, and practice*. (pp. 171–184), Sudbury, MA: Jones and Bartlett.

Dhingra, K., and Boduszek, D. (2013) 'Psychopathy and criminal behaviour: A psychosocial research perspective,' *Journal of Criminal Psychology*, *3*(2):83–107.

Douglas, K. S., Vincent, G M., and Edens, J. F. (2006) 'Risk for criminal recidivism: The role of psychopathy,' in C. J. Patrick (Ed.), *The handbook of psychopathy* (pp. 533–554), New York, NY: Guilford Press.

Ermer, E., Cope, L. M., Nyalakanti, P. K., Calhoun, V. D., and Kiehl, K. A. (2013) 'Aberrant paralimbic gray matter in incarcerated male adolescents with psychopathic traits,' *Journal of the American Academy of Child & Adolescent Psychiatry*, *52*(1):94–103.

Farrer, T. J., and Hedges, D. W. (2011) 'Prevalence of traumatic brain injury in incarcerated groups compared to the general population: A meta-analysis,' *Progress in Neuro-Psychopharmacology and Biological Psychiatry*, *35*(2):390–394.

Farrington, D. P. (2000) 'Psychosocial predictors of adult antisocial personality and adult convictions,' *Behavioral Sciences and the Law*, *18*:605–622.

Flight, J. I., and Forth, A. E. (2007) 'Instrumentally violent youths: The roles of psychopathic traits, empathy, and attachment,' *Criminal Justice and Behavior*, *34*(6):739–751.Fox, B. (2017) 'What makes a difference? Evaluating the key distinctions and predictors of sexual and non-sexual offending among male and female juvenile offenders,' *Journal of Criminal Psychology*, 7(2):134–150.

Fox, B., and DeLisi, M. (2017) 'From criminological heterogeneity to coherent classes: Developing a typology of juvenile sex offenders,' *Youth Violence and Juvenile Justice*, doi:10.1177/1541204017699257.

Fox, B. H., Jennings, W. G., and Farrington, D. P. (2015) 'Bringing psychopathy into developmental and life-course criminology theories and research,' *Journal of Criminal Justice*, *43*(4):274–289.

Fox, B. H., Perez, N., Cass, E., Baglivio, M. T., and Epps, N. (2015) 'Trauma changes everything: Examining the relationship between adverse childhood experiences and serious, violent and chronic juvenile offenders,' *Child Abuse & Neglect*, *46*:163–173.

Glenn, A. L., and Raine, A. (2009) 'Psychopathy and instrumental aggression: Evolutionary, neurobiological, and legal perspectives,' *International Journal of Law and Psychiatry*, *32*(4):253–258.

Häkkänen-Nyholm, H., and Hare, R. D. (2009) 'Psychopathy, homicide, and the courts: Working the system,' *Criminal Justice and Behavior*, *36*(8):761–777.

Häkkänen-Nyholm, H., Repo-Tiihonen, E., Lindberg, N., Salenius, S., and Weizmann-Henelius, G. (2009) 'Finnish sexual homicides: Offence and offender characteristics,' *Forensic Science International*, *188*(1):125–130.

Hare, R. D. (1991) *The Hare Psychopathy Checklist–Revised*, Toronto, ON: Multi-Health Systems.

Hare, R. D. (1998) 'Psychopaths and their nature: Implications for the mental health and criminal justice systems,' in T. Millon, E. Simonsen, M. Birket-Smith, & R. D. Davis (Eds.), *Psychopathy: Antisocial, criminal, and violent behavior* (pp. 188–214), New York, NY: Guilford.

Hare, R. D. (1999a) *Without conscience: The disturbing world of the psychopaths among us*, New York, NY: Guilford Press.

Hare, R. D. (1999b) 'Psychopathy as a risk factor for violence,' *Psychiatric Quarterly*, *70*(3):181–197.

Hare, R. D. (2003) *The Hare Psychopathy Checklist–Revised* (2nd ed.), Toronto, ON: Multi-Health Systems.

Hare, R. D., Clark, D., Grann, M., and Thornton, D. (2000) 'Psychopathy and the predictive validity of the PCL–R: An international perspective,' *Behavioral Science and the Law, 18*:623–645.

Harris, G. T., Rice, M. E., and Cormier, C. A. (1991) 'Psychopathy and violent recidivism,' *Law and Human Behavior, 15*:625–637.

Hart, S. D., and Dempster, R. (1997) 'Impulsivity and psychopathy,' In C. Webster & M. Jackson (Eds.), *Impulsivity: Theory, assessment and treatment* (pp. 212–232), New York, NY: Guilford Press.

Hart, S. D., and Hare, R. D. (1997) 'Psychopathy: Assessment and association with criminal conduct,' in D. M. Stoff & J. Breiling (Eds.), *Handbook of antisocial behaviour* (pp. 22–35), Hoboken, NJ: Wiley & Sons.

Hemphill, J. F., Templeman, R., Wong, S., and Hare, R. D. (1998) 'Psychopathy and crime: Recidivism and criminal careers,' in D. J. Cooke, A. E. Forth, & R. D. Hare (Eds.), *Psychopathy: Theory, research and implications for society* (pp. 375–399), Dordrecht: Kluwer Academic.

Juodis, M., Woodworth, M., Porter, S., and Ten Brinke, L. (2009) 'Partners in crime: A comparison of individual and multi-perpetrator homicides,' *Criminal Justice and Behavior, 36*(8):824–839.

Laajasalo, T., Salenius, S., Lindberg, N., Repo-Tiihonen, E., and Häkkänen-Nyholm, H. (2011) 'Psychopathic traits in Finnish homicide offenders with schizophrenia,' *International Journal of Law and Psychiatry, 34*(5):324–330.

Laurell, J., and Dåderman, A. M. (2005) 'Recidivism is related to psychopathy (PCL–R) in a group of men convicted of homicide,' *International Journal of Law and Psychiatry, 28*(3):255–268.

Laurell, J., and Dåderman, A. M. (2007) 'Psychopathy (PCL–R) in a forensic psychiatric sample of homicide offenders: Some reliability issues,' *International Journal of Law and Psychiatry, 30*(2):127–135.

Leon-Carrion, J., and Ramos, F. J. C. (2003) 'Blows to the head during development can predispose to violent criminal behaviour: Rehabilitation of consequences of head injury is a measure for crime prevention,' *Brain Injury, 17*(3):207–216.

Lewis, D. O., Pincus, J. H., Feldman, M., Jackson, L., and Bard, B. (1986) 'Psychiatric, neurological, and psychoeducational characteristics of 15 death row inmates in the United States,' *American Journal of Psychiatry, 143*(7):838–845.

Lynam, D. R. (1998) 'Early identification of the fledgling psychopath: Locating the psychopathic child in the current nomenclature,' *Journal of Abnormal Psychology, 120*:209–234.

Lynam, D. R., Miller, D. J., Vachon, D., Loeber, R., and Stouthamer-Loeber, M. (2009) 'Psychopathy in adolescence predicts official reports of offending in adulthood,' *Youth Violence and Juvenile Justice*, 7:189–207.

Marshall, L. A., and Cooke, D. J. (1999) 'The childhood experiences of psychopaths: A retrospective study of familial and societal factors,' *Journal of Personality Disorders, 13*(3):211–225.

Murphy, S. L., Xu, J., and Kochanek, D. (2013) 'Deaths: Final data for 2010,' *National Vital Statistics Reports, 61*(4):1–118.

Nestor, P. G., Kimble, M., Berman, I., and Haycock, J. (2002) 'Psychosis, psychopathy, and homicide: A preliminary neuropsychological inquiry,' *American Journal of Psychiatry, 159*(1):138–140.

Patrick, C. J. (2007) 'Getting to the heart of psychopathy,' in H. Herve & J. C. Yuille (Eds.), *Psychopathy: Theory, research, and social implications* (pp. 207–252), Hillsdale, NJ: Erlbaum.

Porter, S., Birt, A. R., and Boer, D. P. (2001) 'Investigation of the criminal and conditional release histories of Canadian federal offenders as a function of psychopathy and age,' *Law and Human Behavior, 25*:647–661.

Porter, S., Campbell, M. A., Woodworth, M., and Birt, A. R. (2001) 'A new psychological conceptualization of the sexual psychopath,' in F. Columbus (Ed.), *Advances in psychology research* (Vol. 7, pp. 21–36), New York, NY: Nova Science.

Porter, S., and Woodworth, M. (2006) 'Psychopathy and aggression,' in C. J. Patrick (Ed.), *Handbook of psychopathy* (pp. 481–494), New York, NY: Guilford Press.

Porter, S., and Woodworth, M. (2007) '"I'm sorry I did it . . . but he started it": A comparison of the official and self-reported homicide descriptions of psychopaths and non-psychopaths,' *Law and Human Behavior, 31*(1):91–107.

Putkonen, H., Weizmann-Henelius, G., Repo-Tiihonen, E., Lindberg, N., Saarela, T., Eronen, M., and Häkkänen-Nyholm, H. (2010) 'Homicide, psychopathy, and aging – A nationwide register-based case-comparison study ofhomicide offenders aged 60 years or older,' *Journal of Forensic Sciences, 55*(6):1552–1556.

Raine, A. (1993) *The psychopathology of crime: Criminal behavior as a clinical disorder*, San Diego, CA: Academic Press.

Raine, A., Lencz, T., Bihrle, S., LaCasse, L., and Colletti, P. (2000) 'Reduced prefrontal gray matter volume and reduced autonomic activity in antisocial personality disorder,' *Archives of General Psychiatry, 57*(2):119–127.

Rice, M. E., and Harris, G. T. (1995) 'Violent recidivism: Assessing predictive validity,' *Journal of Consulting and Clinical Psychology, 63*(5):737–748.

Salekin, R. T. (2008) 'Psychopathy and recidivism from mid-adolescence to young adulthood: Cumulating legal problems and limiting life opportunities,' *Journal of Abnormal Psychology, 117*:386–395.

Salekin, R. T., Rogers, R., and Sewell, K. W. (1996) 'A review and meta-analysis of the Psychopathy Checklist and Psychopathy Checklist-Revised: Predictive validity of dangerousness,' *Clinical Psychology: Science and Practice, 3*(3):203–215.

Salekin, R. T., Rogers, R., Ustad, K. L., and Sewell, K. W. (1998) 'Psychopathy and recidivism among female inmates,' *Law and Human Behavior, 22*:109–128.

Serafim, A. D. P., Barros, D. M. D., Valim, A., and Gorenstein, C. (2009) 'Cardiac response and anxiety levels in psychopathic murderers,' *Revista Brasileira de Psiquiatria, 31*(3):214–218.

Serin, R. C., and Amos, N. L. (1995) 'The role of psychopathy in the assessment of dangerousness,' *International Journal of Law and Psychiatry, 18*:231–238.

Silver, J. M., Kramer, R., Greenwald, S., and Weissman, M. (2001) 'The association between head injuries and psychiatric disorders: Findings from the New Haven NIMH Epidemiologic Catchment Area Study,' *Brain Injury, 15*(11):935–945.

Slaughter, B., Fann, J. R., and Ehde, D. (2003) 'Traumatic brain injury in a county jail population: Prevalence, neuropsychological functioning and psychiatric disorders,' *Brain Injury, 17*(9):731–741.

Vaughn, M. G., and DeLisi, M. (2008) 'Were Wolfgang's chronic offenders psychopaths? On the convergent validity of psychopathy and career criminality,' *Journal of Criminal Justice, 36*:33–42.

Vaughn, M. G., Howard, M. O., and DeLisi, M. (2008) 'Psychopathic personality traits and delinquent careers: An empirical examination,' *International Journal of Law and Psychiatry, 31*:407–416.

Weizmann-Henelius, G., Putkonen, H., Grönroos, M., Lindberg, N., Eronen, M., and Häkkänen-Nyholm, H. (2010) 'Examination of psychopathy in female homicide offenders – Confirmatory factor analysis of the PCL-R,' *International Journal of Law and Psychiatry, 33*(3):177–183.

Weizmann-Henelius, G., Virkkunen, M., Gammelgård, M., Eronen, M., and Putkonen, H. (2015) 'The PCL-R and violent recidivism in a prospective follow-up of a nationwide sample of female offenders,' *The Journal of Forensic Psychiatry & Psychology, 26*(5):667–685.

Williamson, S. E., Hare, R. D., and Wong, S. (1987) 'Violence: Criminal psychopaths and their victims,' *Canadian Journal of Behavioral Science, 19*:454–462.

Woodworth, M., and Porter, S. (2002) 'In cold blood: Characteristics of criminal homicides as a function of psychopathy,' *Journal of Abnormal Psychology, 111*:436–445.

Porter, S., and Woodworth, M. (2006) 'Psychopathy and aggression,' in C. J. Patrick (Ed.), *Handbook of psychopathy* (pp. 481–494). New York, NY: Guilford Press.

Yang, Y., Raine, A., Lencz, T., Bihrle, S., LaCasse, L., and Colletti, P. (2005) 'Volume reduction in prefrontal gray matter in unsuccessful criminal psychopaths,' *Biological Psychiatry, 57*(10):1103–1108.

19

The perpetual influence of dark traits on alienists

Enzo Yaksic

Introduction

The aggressiveness exhibited toward future colleagues by probationers from what Christin (2017) calls the expert fields – comprised here of law enforcement, journalistic, and academic domains – typifies the character of those surviving rigors heaped upon them. Rites of passage perform as selection mechanisms that allow experts withstanding such rituals access to the sanctity derived from possession of credentials. The propensity to direct lingering animosity at associates after the passage of these trials, coupled with the inclination to lure others into the oppressive fray, compels trainees of the expert fields to behave in defective ways. Because the best are inevitably led astray by systems that gradually reward the wrong behaviors (Apple, 2017), such transgressions became tautologically linked to their professions. These transformations are now inextricably infused to the initiate's temperament and serve as the harbinger of the malevolent side of human nature to these sectors. The antisocial nature required to participate, flourish, and thrive in these institutions may, as Muris, Merckelbach, Otgaar, and Meijer (2017) postulate, foster dark features in those encountering what Christin (2017:2) calls "strict barriers to entry." This chapter will explore the heterogeneous and multidimensional (Kowalski, Vernon, & Schermer, 2017) dark characteristics that influence six dark personality-derived profiles (referred to hereinafter as profiles) specific to the expert fields: Phony Charlatans, Mystic Defenders, Harboring Imposters, False Mentors, Foraging Collaborators, and Disreputable Profiteers.

Beacons in the dark?

Criminals receive undue attention from the expert fields while non-offenders – whose traits, attitudes, and circumstances aid in a renouncement of unlawful behavior – are ignored (DeLisi, 2017). Society relies on the law enforcement officer (LEO), journalist, and academic to function as beacons of order and knowledge in dark times, those marked by Kajonius, Persson, and Jonason (2015) as decreasing in empathy for others and contemporary culture. Although they continue to swear to abide by oaths of honor and integrity in their service to the public, the unmitigated power assumed by these disciplines has attracted some with nefarious intent (Barker, 2014). Given the centrality afforded to expert knowledge in modern society (Christin, 2017), when autonomy, relatedness, and competence (Furnham, Hyde, & Trickey, 2014) come into dissonance with context, a transmogrification occurs that facilitates the utilization of behaviors such as wanton hostility, threats of excommunication, and fear of rebuke to aid in obtaining stature and control. Future prosocial efforts to be truthful, honest, fair, sincere, and faithful (Muris et al., 2017) are enveloped once the dark traits are understood to carry minimal threat of negative psychosocial consequences (Furnham et al., 2014; Jonason, Webster, Schmitt, Li, & Crysel, 2012) and be beneficial to the possessor.

The dark tetrad of Machiavellianism, narcissism, psychopathy, and "everyday sadism" (Black, Woodworth, & Porter, 2014; Paulhus & Williams, 2002) are evolved and adaptive strategies (Jones & Figueredo, 2013) consisting of inter-correlated personality traits (Paulhus, Curtis, & Jones, 2018) and exist in the framework of transgressive behavior (Muris et al., 2017). These enduring styles of thinking, acting, and feeling are measured on a continuum of individual differences (Paulhus et al., 2018), often tied together with Social Dominance Orientation (Sidanius, Liu, Shaw & Pratto, 1994), and are abundant among those that study and capture serial homicide offenders. No research addresses the commonalities across the investigative and social professions of the expert fields, as Hare (2017) believes viewing clinical descriptions and empirical findings through a prism of dysfunction regarding these traditionally respected roles is difficult.

Hare (1980) undertook study of psychopaths around the time interest in serial murder compelled researchers and practitioners to invest in that construct. The terms became conflated (Sherretts, Boduszek, Debowska, & Willmott, 2017) due to the nature in which offenders treat their victims (Hickey, Walters, Drislane, & Patrick, 2014). The quest to understand how serial murder and psychopathy interface (Hickey et al., 2014) and questions regarding why individuals with characteristics and experiences similar to those of the multiple murderer do not commit serial killings (Schlesinger, 1998) required experts to begin studying this phenomenon from the perspective of the serial homicide offender (Culhane, Hilstad, Freng, & Gray, 2011). It has since been discovered that most perpetrators of homicide (Boduszek, Debowska, & Willmott, 2017; Sherretts et al., 2017) and serial homicide (Beasley, 2004; Hickey et al., 2014; Culhane et al., 2011; Reid, 2017) fail to rank adequately high enough on the revised Psychopathy Checklist (Venables, Hall, & Patrick, 2014) to be considered psychopathic. This suggests that the difference in intensity of traits between forensic and non-forensic populations is not as pronounced as once thought (Boduszek et al., 2017). Although some argue that the core characteristics of psychopathic personality disorder are incompatible with successful functioning (Brooks & Fritzon, 2016), mediating violent drives with everyday sadism may allow the profiles to operate efficiently while venting Anger and demeaning others for pleasure (Jones, 2017). These findings place the pursuers in closer proximity to the pursued, as use of the dark tetrad has been identified as aiding in professional endeavors (Furnham et al., 2014; Jonason et al., 2012).

Valuing the principled use of dark traits

Because dark traits – characterized by Kajonius et al. (2015) as entitlement, superiority, and dominance (i.e., narcissism), glib social charm and manipulativeness (i.e., Machiavellianism), callous social attitudes, impulsivity, and interpersonal Antagonism (i.e., psychopathy) and enjoyed cruelty (i.e., sadism) – are understood to be practical responses to everyday life, they must be thought of as learned values. The exclusion of others is encouraged by leaders of the three domains viewing them as businesses. Individuals high on dark tetrad traits, craving stimulation, achievement, and power (Kajonius, Persson, & Jonason, 2015), are often heralded while supervisors mistake meretricious dominance for being effective and persuasive. The value systems maintained by employees of the expert fields are inconsistent with most simply due to the type of specialized focus and subject matter with which each contends. While repeated exposure desensitizes homicide investigators to death, some in the expert fields display empathy strategically to further goals and resort to surface and deep acting to depersonalize and distance themselves. Therefore, the darkness of the tetrad does not necessarily originate from some latent evilness but rather a difference in principles (Kajonius et al., 2015).

The rigid rule structure imposed upon staff at each of the three institutions has existed for hundreds of years, standing as a challenge to the most dark and imaginative to invent ways of circumventing such regulations and directives. The normalization of corruption in law enforcement organizations (Ashforth & Anand, 2003), entitlement in academic environments (Turnipseed & Cohen, 2015), elitism (Christin, 2017), and sensationalism in the news media (Parmley, 1995; Pauli, 2017) are byproducts of dark personalities learning boundaries and breaking rules. Muris et al. (2017:183) might categorize those in the expert fields as "living in circumstances under which they no longer observe rules." While most occupations may not sponsor the use of transgressive behaviors to advance society (Muris et al., 2017), members of the expert fields that engage in violations of social norms and moral values are often seen as just, curious, creative, and influential in retrospect, where narcissism is confused with self-confidence and Antisocial Personality Disorder is a marker of decisiveness and courage (Furnham et al., 2014). Perhaps dark personalities intentionally activate facets of their character when advantageous to accomplishing goals or when course correcting after forced by hindrances to stray from their true providence. In response to hazards experienced during daily work routines of the expert fields, Paulhus et al. (2018) note that Machiavellians utilize relational aggression to establish social hierarchies or to assert power, sadists perform boring tasks for the opportunity to harm others, and narcissists show aggressive reactions to insults to their intellectual ability.

Fortunately, most activities begun by dark personalities progress no further than providing opportunities for the profiles to showcase themselves, as these endeavors are often founded in myth (Beauge, 2013). For this reason, the dark personalities' inclination to destroy others may appear trite or even conventional by modern standards (Paulhus & Williams, 2002). The tendencies common to dark personalities – self-promotion, emotional–interpersonal coldness and aggressiveness (Paulhus & Williams, 2002) – manifest through a common core of disagreeableness and inevitably result in overlap throughout current measures of the dark tetrad (Paulhus et al., 2018) and across career sectors (Kijak, 2016). While significant relationships exist between narcissism and leadership, Machiavellianism and competitive roles, psychopathy and positions of authority and power, Machiavellians in particular are suited to investigative (policing, journalism) and social (education) careers (Kijak, 2016). This review demonstrates that the profiles contain less of the psychopath's erratic lifestyle and deficiencies in impulse control and more of their disinhibited, coercively parasitic orientation and bold but superficially conning natures; less of the Machiavellianist's cynical disregard for morality and more of their long-term deliberate calculation and goal-directed strategic planning; less of the narcissist's pursuit of gratification from vanity and more of their arrogance, egotism, and exaggeration of attributes to appear superior.

Illuminating the path forward

Research is needed to discern if the dark tetrad concept is redundant with the variance in the dark personality traits contained in the Big Five factors of openness to experience, Conscientiousness, Extraversion, Agreeableness, and Neuroticism (Rantanen, Metsäpelto, Feldt, Pulkkinen, Kokko, 2007). This review followed the roadmap laid forth by Muris et al. (2017), which suggested future research focus on populations other than student samples, approaches beyond the cross-sectional, and results produced from consideration paid to the dimensionality of personality and the proximal examination of the dark traits. Because individuals in community samples with dark traits tend to underreport negative behaviors (Paulhus & John, 1998), the paucity of factor analytic work using measurement instruments such as the Self-Report Psychopathy Scale–Short Form (SRP–SF) precludes any firm conclusions from being made regarding its dimensionality (Debowska et al., 2017).

The use of alternative observational methods was required in this review to gauge the existence and impact of dark traits among those that study and capture serial homicide offenders. Since self-report questionnaires may aid narcissists, Machiavellians, psychopaths, and sadists in presenting themselves in a disguised way (Muris et al., 2017), ethnographers, as Christin (2017) notes, should be keenly sensitive to discrepancies between outward statements and private sentiments. Those under the employ of these three vocations are hyperaware of dark traits and would be less forthcoming about potentially latent characteristics lingering within themselves. The author, whose presence and work among the expert fields has spanned nearly two decades, acts as the primary informant and utilizes an ethnographic strategy as a means to bypass the observer effect, attribution errors, and fake-good reporting biases. Because the traits and characteristics of these disorders are a product of complex interactions between biological and temperamental predispositions and social forces (Babiak et al., 2012), it is important to frame this review as concentrating on those whose efforts to make inroads to become well-established experts in their careers cause distress to others through use of transgressive behavior and antagonistic schemes.

Consequences of transgressive behavior and antagonistic schemes

Complaints regarding etiquette can appear unfounded given the seemingly positive impact dark traits have had on these sectors. Research demonstrates that serial homicide is declining as a result of alienists magnifying qualities shared with the pursued (Yaksic, DeSpirito, & Reid, 2017). But the psychopathic personality condition, which results in substantial destruction to the self and others (Colins, Fanti, Salekin, & Andershed, 2017), alongside the mercurial nature of many industry standouts, has caused derailment (Furnham et al., 2014) to occur. Because older scientists champion the regnant paradigm out of emotional connection and prestige (Gobry, 2016), timeworn tropes and outmoded perspectives dictate much of what is known regarding serial murder. The use of structured and systematically collected data was explored to combat the deleterious proliferation of myths overtaking the study and pursuit of serial homicide offenders due to the reliance on anecdata and obsession with archaic crimes (Evans, 2017; Haigney, 2017; Killelea, 2017; Notes, 2017) over the past half century. The abandonment and collapse of this initiative, which intended to freely offer information on serial murderers, is attributable to a multitude of factors – misplaced political affiliations, deep personal biases, open disdain for credit sharing, and a commodification of the work of others for personal gain (Yaksic, 2017a). Such characteristics, indigenous to the realms of law enforcement, journalism, and academia (Babiak et al., 2012), lead those composed of dark personality traits to unceremoniously obtain influence, collude with like minds to maintain power, and prevent open and transparent discussion.

Skepticism about the quality and quantity of information held in datasets is a healthy exercise (Long, 2017) in the era of big data but one often viewed as setting the stage for adversarial relationships. Few support open science or the confrontation of errors (Oransky & Marcus, 2017) in order to keep data hidden and protect against the discovery of its limitations and flaws. The nonrational psychological mechanisms of psychic numbing, pseudoinefficacy and the prominence effect (Slovic & Slovic, 2015) impact efforts to provide meaning to data as the profiles ensure that the good of the few outweigh the needs of the many. Consortiums among the expert fields serve as feedback chambers rather than true exchanges of ideas because public sector employees are less likely to involve others in work activities and have a weaker social presence than those in the private sector (Furnham et al., 2014). The depth and length of teamwork determines the speed with which alliances deteriorate and fail, leading to what Black et al. (2014) call short-term exploitative relationships as the realness of colleagues is divulged after the need to feign empathy wanes. Results of the present author's collaborative experiment demonstrate that the cognitive importance, perception of resemblance, and positive emotional valence associated with belonging to the in-group is central to the self-concept (Sherretts et al., 2017) of the expert fields. Resultantly, faction forming, segregation, and disavowal of others' work are the chosen methods of dealing with viewpoints counter to the mainstream. For example, the theory regarding the decline in serial homicide (Yaksic et al., 2017), which would taper the wild exaggerations behind the estimations of serial homicide victimization (Fridg, 2017; Gellatly, 2017; Whiffen, 2017; Montgomery, Rice, & Cummings, 2017; Dumcius, 2017) and effectively curtail the agendas of profit seekers, is at the mercy of such obstacles and may culminate in negative backlash directed towards the authors.

Refracting light upon the dark archetypes

Behavior enabling ruthless subjugation has become commonplace in the twenty-first century as those in power exercise their will over others regardless of consequence. Power, domination, and control play a large part in the lives of serial homicide offenders because serial murder is about the practiced masking of true intentions through use of duality and presentation of self to exert masculinity. Although "prosocial" dark personalities behave similarly, they remain unchecked and insulated by status and rationalizations while spouting support for the victims and their families. The emergence of the profiles coincides with the witting utilization of strategies and reliance on fiendish tactics to accomplish nefarious goals to forward reputations, increase stature, garner awards, and collect payment.

Members of the profiles attempt to halt the process of impermanence by carving out niches, altering origin stories, rewriting histories, and protecting legacies. The battle to stave off irrelevancy parallels the journey embarked upon by serial homicide offenders to avoid capture, the associated pitfall of obscurity, and the forced consideration of the scope of their wake. The continuous distribution of some aspects of the profiles ensures their dimensional, as opposed to categorical, classification. The idea that psychopathic personality traits in adults are best viewed on a continuum was posited by DeLisi (2009), even in the context of the popular opinion that psychopaths are inhuman and qualitatively different from other individuals. Babiak et al. (2012) concur, asserting that there is a range between highly psychopathic persons to those with the same number or fewer traits in a milder form. Because the expert fields exercise immense control over their turf and care fanatically about structure of positions within these spaces (Christin, 2017), navigating antagonistic personalities within these subclinical worlds involves being aware of the components of which each is comprised.

The Phony Charlatan (PC) plies inspirational platitudes and peddles false hope to a victim's surviving family (Ferak, 2017) to manufacture celebrity by proxy. Forming symbiotic relationships with successful individuals and attaching themselves to high profile cases grants these professional connections access to aggrandizing quotations later used as promotional material for merchandising opportunities such as tomes detailing the life experiences (Mains, 2017) of these dissemblers. Experts at self-promotion, PCs deceive themselves with unrealistic perceptions of their "superhero" quality (Paulhus, 1998). Lacking requisite talent, PCs cast aside contrary judgments and garishly thrust their way into the mainstream. PCs prioritize the practice of appearing on media forums willing to host their unrelenting yet empty pitch messages of redemption in the face of adversity ahead of generating actual meaningful contributions as they yearn for virality ("TV show," 2015). PCs exist as a packaged set of goods and services as their wares must be presented to migrating audiences in a readily consumable format. PCs are masters at advancing their commercial stature but sacrifice integrity on a quest to attain the wealth to which they feel entitled. Cultivating a besotted, sycophantic fanbase and pandering to those spectators aids PCs in alchemizing their once obscure status to that of "living legend" but sometimes requires harnessing misfortune and any semblance of personal connection to tragedy.

The Mystic Defender (MD) calls attention to an ongoing war of good against evil proclaimed to be waged throughout society. MDs scoring high on dark traits are seen more as "warriors" (Muris et al., 2017) with an unchallenged messianic complex and assure themselves of an eventual triumph over sinister forces. These fabulists are the embodiment of fantastical thinking and invent elaborate stories that serve as mechanisms to inject themselves into the chronology of others' lives (Beauge, 2015). MDs are supremely capable of persuading others to believe a deluded version of reality where intervention requires insight only they possess as few can comprehend the actions of criminals as they are able. MDs wish to be trumpeted as visionaries and demand that others bask in the glory of their creations. Their trajectories remain aimed towards favorable outcomes regardless of the preponderance of voices clamoring for evidence of such masterful deeds. For example, MD's frame unresolved homicides as stories without finite endings in an ingenious ploy that absolves them from any expectations of providing a conclusion. To MDs, bringing attention to cases is enough of a contribution as blame is placed on LEOs for any stall in momentum. Inactivity is interpreted to be the byproduct of a territorial workforce (Ferak, 2015) whose burdens can be alleviated by taking advantage of the consultation services offered by the MD and their cadre of "super friends" (Brandolph, 2014). Imagery is broadcast as propaganda to indoctrinate, instill a sense of valor and Boldness, and be emulated by underlings, because MDs desire to subvert pre-existing cultures and transition herds to higher plains of existence (Hiller, 2013). Without acknowledging the often-complex network of circumstances that affect outcomes in the criminal justice system, MDs erroneously assume that the dedication of will and attention can conquer all problems.

The Harboring Imposter (HI) capitalizes on their target's benevolence and requests assistance traversing the landscape of the expert fields only to jettison their guides once they establish their own foothold. HIs can be classified as prototypical "users" intent on fulfilling personal agendas under the guise of acting on the instruction of larger entities such as media conglomerates, newspapers, or television companies. HIs are characterized by a compulsive need for limelight by generating "look-at-me" reportage (Nazaryan, 2017) and attempting to bring literary aspirations to true crime (Miller, 2017). An unwavering belief in their superiority causes HIs to wield others as pawns to attain the endless litany of awards reserved for those whose offerings outmatch their peers (Clarion-Ledger, 2017). These individuals precipitate narratives and nurture timelines that serve to place the storyteller at the forefront (Quinn, 2017; Smith, 2017) using modern techniques such as doublespeak or the humblebrag.

The False Mentor (FM) molds conscripted lieges into loyal subjects while using this oftentimes uncredited talent to sustain their own interests. Youthful energy is syphoned by FMs as the student's naivety and willingness to contribute is misused. Because mentor relationships are parasitic and transactionary alliances conducted under the equivocal façade of loyal friendship, the eventual realization that such manipulation occurred leads to a deterioration of the relationship. Future career prospects are hampered when the relationship becomes irreparable because the student's network is comprised of individuals recommended by FMs. Wary of heirs to claim their kingdom, valid suggestions are often unheeded due to the FM's fragile sense of self. Although FMs have poor follow-through, the mistakes of their henchmen are seldom overlooked. Refusal to allow others to validate the work of FMs inspires siloed teams, resulting in unbalanced projects loaded with errors and missing data (Anonymous, 2017). Some lives are defined by achievements and the inflated stature garnered from work done by others, perhaps encouraging the intellectual theft, blatant plagiarism, and ethics violations in the expert fields.

The Foraging Collaborator (FC) feigns loyalty and respect when offering their services, only to disappear after periods of dormancy. The intelligence amassed by FCs is traded to competitors to increase their stake in the next in-group. FCs are acutely aware that titles equate to worth and build reputations intended to be enamored by those outside of their expert field. FCs pledge allegiance to themselves, alienating those that helped them acquire reverence. Oftentimes trained by FMs, FCs come to view relationships as transient, ephemeral, and disposable. Inhuman metrics meant to judge individual competency fuel the FC's search for partnership, but the process of leveraging connections sanitizes all meaningful interactions and trumps any measure of authenticity. The FC's miniscule contributions, transformed by politics, can surpass those of the primary investigators in the eyes of outsiders.

The Disreputable Profiteer (DP) gains from the suffering and pain of victims and their surviving family, being careful to avoid any missteps that affect the marketability of their products and complete their mission no matter the cost. DPs develop a meritorious attitude where both adulation and compensation are deserved with no mode of monetization beyond their grasp. The golden age of true crime (Stewart, 2017) relieves the DP from concerns that the denigration of victims should be regarded as anything more than a wayward interest (Beck, 2014; Flynn, 2017) but closer inspection demonstrates how exploitative this pastime of murder tourism can be (Miller, 2017; Nicholson, 2017). DPs flout limits and expand their reach into taboo areas (i.e., necrophilia) as a means to channel the fleeting attention of true crime connoisseurs. DPs are without serious credentials and instead deploy methods devised to cloak those deficits by means of misdirection (e.g., artificial padding of H-Indexes, outright plagiarism, focus on niche markets, or use of anecdotes instead of data). These techniques often lead to struggles over a subject's purview while DPs uphold the status quo by answering serious inquiries with carbon copy, assembly line responses (Gross, 2017; Montgomery et al., 2017). DPs maintain a predisposition to embellish facts, a defect directly attributable to the same weak core tenets and underpinnings responsible for the formulaic mainstay of befriending serial killers solely to profit from the demise of others (Bonn, 2014; Phelps, 2017).

An unspoken kinship between the pursuers and the pursued

Many professions are populated with those nurturing some proportion of the dark traits – discourteous physicians, rude bus drivers, impolite waitresses, ill-mannered executives, disrespectful bartenders, uncivil engineers, ungracious insurers, unscrupulous attorneys, lurid personal trainers, egotistical models, antisocial social workers, and vile truckers – but dark personalities emerge only when callousness and manipulation function as one. To be considered intentionally harmful, one must be simultaneously dishonest and lack concern for others (Jones & Figueredo, 2013; Paulhus et al., 2018). The duties of LEO, journalist, and professor are given to those with high levels of cognitive abilities, Extraversion, and Agreeableness – characterized by Muris et al. (2017) as trustworthiness, straightforwardness, altruism, compliance, modesty, and tender mindedness – but the profiles often deceive to ensure that their subjects (e.g., informants, sources, or research assistants) cooperate while remaining apathetic to considerations for their long-term well-being. Here, the absence of honesty and empathy converge across the profiles and constitute the malevolent personality representing a "dark core" of covariance (Jones & Figueredo, 2013). These three industries also employ creative and narcissistic individuals (Muris et al., 2017), each with high levels of verbal fluency, originality, and speed of processing which concurrently enable them to produce more credible lies and contribute to feelings of entitlement and engagement in unethical behaviors as the benefits of deceptive behaviors (Sarzyńskam et al., 2017) are recognized.

There is an invariable parallel between the mechanisms directing the behavior of the serial murderer and those of the profiles. Each enacts plans after a series of past successes while accommodating a level of social disengagement alongside feelings of "otherness" (Hickey et al., 2014). Stalwarts of these vocations cannot insert bias as they keep the general public at arm's length while protecting, quoting, and studying them. But those from the profiles fostering sentiments of discontent and their doppelgängers (i.e., serial murderers) rely on callous–unemotional features to readily bend the narrative to fit their worldview. The anticipation and attainment of reward motivates both while each operates at the behest of the antisocial dimensions of psychopathy (Hare, 2017) and commit their offenses in a secretive, highly compartmentalized manner (Hickey et al., 2014). Levin and Fox (2008) argue that sadistic serial killers do not differ from other people in terms of their ability to exercise empathy, manage the impression they make on others, compartmentalize, and dehumanize. Instead, killers merely lack a position of dominance in the legitimate system. The same proneness to deviancy that serial murderers express during their progression towards enactment (Hickey et al., 2014) conversely aids some in the expert fields to make strides after attaining appointments laden with esteem. The expert fields demand excellent memory retention, as does a serial homicide offender's ability to recall facets of crimes decades afterwards. Novel ideas often arise in the expert fields as intrusive thoughts, along the same wavelengths that inspire offenders to act at the insistence of knowledge gleaned during periods of introspection and imaginative thinking. Investment in reputation is as crucial to the expert fields as the serial murderer's need to control how they are portrayed. LEOs, journalists, professors, and offenders are consumingly self-aware and share mental processes beyond the detestable outcome of violent phases and acts.

Whatever spawns the initial attraction to investigate serial murderers, the expert fields come to find qualities intrinsic to serial killers commingled with their own personalities. Curiosity regarding the amount of tethering and overlap between the pursuers and the pursued often reveals the path towards self-revelation but concomitantly undoes most internal progress. The absence of morality and reliance on excuses, rampant in the expert fields, makes connections to others counterfeit in soulless and bankrupt self-serving ventures. Methods used by the expert fields – such as crafting clever origin stories meant to assist in preying on targets – are unabashedly disingenuous and matched only by fraudulently questionable motives. The collateral damage caused by the profiles is often outright ignored, belatedly celebrated, or quickly justified, in turn preventing them from comprehending that such a myopic pursuit of grandiosity diverged from the orthodox. Like serial murderers, the profiles institute ruses and concoct façades to avoid criticism and are often confused by those in opposition to their messages. The profiles experience anxiety regarding the desperation to advance and are acutely aware that judgment may arrive from those peering under the surface to penetrate their veneer. Each in the expert fields is described as working towards missions believed to be accomplishable by them alone due to their cunning and devious ways. The influence of others' goodwill is insignificant to the profiles, as each remains convinced that their success materialized solely due to their own knowhow.

Displays of high Antagonism and low Conscientiousness are hallmarks of the disorder of psychopathy but may be extreme levels of normally distributed personality traits (DeLisi, 2009) similar to those sustained by serial murderers. To persist in the expert fields requires a falsification of entire features of one's persona. In presenting a forward-facing image, the profiles cajole others to believe that they are adept at meeting the demands of participating in teams, meanwhile securing their individual vested interests. Implementing moral disengagement (Egan, Hughes, & Palmer, 2015) allows the profiles to capitalize on their standing to ardently protect territory, destroy the prospects of others, falsely claim credit and authorship over the ideas of others, injudiciously refuse to collaborate, exploit the good will of colleagues, emanate false confidence, demean the contributions of others and control the narrative. As social media amplifies the ability to share branded messages beyond unhealthy levels (Clemente, 2017), members of the profiles shun mutualistic social strategies in favor of antagonistic ones where others are regarded as objects to be abused or rivals to be defeated (Jones & Figueredo, 2013). Those with dark personalities thrive when presented with opposing goals, relying on dubious practices and evoking gamesmanship rules to steal the advantage from their nemeses.

A dark playground entrenched in lore

According to Branson (2013), to secure funding for the mission of the Federal Bureau of Investigation (FBI), agents of the Behavior Science Unit invented the existence of super predators to be uniquely dangerous villains (Jenkins, 2002) stoppable only by a law enforcement agency equipped with the prognostication method of criminal profiling.[1] FBI agents, acting as advisors to the works of author Thomas Harris, romanticize the idea that a damaging interplay occurs in interactions between interviewers and their subjects. Interviewers are pulled from the brink of insignificance and receive meaning from killers filled with implications for cases and, by extension, their own lives. This *folie à deux* arises as retired agents are coaxed to form symbiotic relationships with offenders via unorthodox methods that eventually decimate their life. Because of the congenital appeal the presumed infectious madness has on those in extended close proximity to serial homicide offenders, such iconography continues to spawn fictional works (Gardiner, 2017) which have precipitated a legion of dogmatic references to the necessity of becoming a monster to catch one. Exaggerations in Kevin Williamson's *The Following*, Neil Cross' *Luther*, Eric Overmyer's *Bosch*, Nic Pizzolatto's *True Detective*, Stieg Larsson's *Men Who Hate Women*, and Joe Penhall's *Mindhunter* pale in comparison to Jo Nesbo's *The Snowman*, which adheres to all of the fabled trappings designed to placate fans: a completely insane killer that is never going to stop taunting or playing games with the damaged detectives.

Due to these depictions, the uninitiated perceive the process of meeting a serial murderer as involving great sacrifice, since interviewers allow offenders to occupy their headspace. It should be noted that examiners do not become disgruntled or disfigured by their respondents and even form friendships with these killers (Bonn, 2014; Phelps, 2017). Some interrogators are gleeful at the importance their work provides them and the effect such dealings have on their friends and family (Williams, 2017). Society must determine if it owes a debt to those claiming to possess unique insight – garnered not from a systematic analysis of data (Northeastern University Atypical Homicide Research Group, 2017a) – often based on speculation (Byrne, 2017) or classified as erroneous (Gerber, 2017). Such covenants have become profitable dalliances to promoters with fictitious titles such as "criminal profiler" (Gerber, 2017; Mains, 2015; Snierson, 2017; X-G Productions, 2017), experts that command respect and expect adulation for shouldering the supposed burden of exposure to serial offenders. By securing access to multiple murderers, members of the profiles have transformed this arena into an exclusive province and safeguarded their positions as experts. DeLisi (2009) praises criminologists for their ability to study antisocial behavior without expressing contempt or making value judgments about offenders, but, because those that study and pursue offenders are so intertwined with killers, such condemnations would stand as an indictment of the shared attitudes maintained by the latter and echoed by the former.

Turning perception inward

Few are employed to understand the abject suffering of others like LEOs, journalists, and professors. These groups may have initially gravitated towards dark personalities to discern the meaning behind some undeveloped yet detectable qualities within themselves, but the observance of such a dichotomous phenomenon as serial murder may have inadvertently imprinted parts of the pursued upon the pursuers. Fallon (2014) pioneered the idea of turning perception inward to unveil the commonalities shared between researchers and psychopathic criminals. The belief that some might become murderers without the proper structures in place has been further explored by others that claim all have a latent capacity to kill under the right circumstances (Phelps, 2017). Some in the expert fields may indeed rival serial murderers in feeling attracted to death (Malizia, 2017) and experiencing excitement garnered from the discovery of illicit images or stories of murder, but symptoms of Post-Traumatic Stress Disorder (Chopko, Palmieri, & Adams, 2015; Kopel & Friedman, 1997), burnout, and compassion fatigue (Sollie, Kop, & Euwema, 2017) may be induced in investigators not equipped with a dark personality. Psychometric testing might uncover an immunity held by those harboring aspects of the profiles by deciphering how they became hardened to human suffering (Sollie et al., 2017), unresponsive to the intrusive memories, avoidance, negative changes in thinking and mood, alterations in physical and emotional reactions (Center for Substance Abuse Treatment, 2014), and ignorance to the instinct of being repulsed by death (Malizia, 2017) experienced by the general population.

But not all involved in the study and apprehension of serial murderers stay the course. Some criminal justice students yearn to find themselves on the hunt for the whereabouts of such offenders, but most researchers move on to other topics after publishing one or two articles on the subject (Dowden, 2005). Although leadership roles on serial murder taskforces are avoided by LEOs,[2] even tangential exposure to this environment could engender a subsummation of dark qualities (e.g., lack of empathy, assertion and egocentrism, use of manipulation, and being unconcerned by the negative consequences of actions). More research is needed to coax out which triggers and stressors urge dark personalities to cope with trauma by responding with hostility. It is doubtful that other professional fields of inquiry stimulate such inharmonious dispositions, duplicity, and discordant functions within operatives like in the expert fields. Professors must collaborate with others while also generating enough unique ideas to be considered independent investigators, LEOs are paid to actively deceive others to meet their objectives, and journalists are to remain secretive of their sources while expecting others to trust them implicitly. Perhaps those that have retired from the expert fields were cognizant that transformations can produce anxiety such as loss of structure and isolation (Turnage, 2017). Those dedicating their time to understanding serial offenders may have self-actualized and come to accept that present in them are traits shared with killers. Reveling in the gore and most gruesome aspects of death suits the expert fields, folks rarely committing to projects for altruistic purposes, the love of science, or the advancement of self-discovery. Such processes were the last vestiges before the expert fields surrendered to the burgeoning entertainment complex.

No fear of the dark

Several fixtures of popular culture – *Harry Potter*, Iron Maiden, The Legend of Zelda, *Twin Peaks*, and *Stranger Things* – have juxtaposed light and dark, each remarking on those dual influences on the inhabitants of those universes. Society has slowly awoken to the existence of what lies in wait through these mediums. The expert fields of this world have been trying for decades to engineer an interest in crime as recreation and cultivate a desire to connect to its storytellers.

In necessitating an attraction to serial offenders, the expert fields fleshed out their careers long before movie stars attached themselves to serial murderers when reclassifying their roles from novice newbies to serious actors (Ford & Kit, 2017; Lovitt, 2016; Stack, 2017). Fascination with the devastation wrought by violent offenders may be explained by a need to satiate the call from within to locate likeminded people and capitulate to an equal sense of belonging. The urge to form a fanbase dedicated to the exploits of murderers and rapists (Bond, 2016) suggests that the origins of psychopathy extend beyond biology and heritable genes: the disorder may be a learned response to contagious external stimuli. The communicable spread of dark characteristics does run counter to the established myth of the solitary disposition attributed to the offenders at the center of such fawning.

Some measure of dissonance enables fans to label offenders as otherworldly beings, celebrate the actions of dark personalities, and avoid direct comparison with their own commensurate behavior. As originators of monetizing the expedition for higher status, many in the expert fields openly embrace the creation of games (Britto, 2017; Sykes, 2017), true crime summer camps (Pettler, 2017), "profiling" classes (Mellor, 2017), escape rooms (Moss, 2017), tangible merchandise (Hafford, 2017), conventions (Fitzpatrick, 2017), podcasts (Palmer, 2017), and homicide hunk type personalities (DiscoveryID, 2017) – exploitative services purposely catering to an ever widening collective eager to ingest anything related to the criminal justice system, even if most products merely repackage criminal cases from past eras for new audiences. The ubiquity of podcasters and cold case "analysts" endowing true crime aficionados with titillating tales on the pitfalls suffered by prior homicide victims under the guise of providing actionable advice arises from our need to have complex topics reduced to consumable constructs (Colin-Thome, 2017). Only the darkest personalities can mine the experiences of those whose lives were taken to highlight potential mistakes. The worst and most desperate attempts to placate fans, though, result in feigned existential crises meant to enhance the author's account of near consumption by the abyss (Kaplan, 2017; Mallie, Aguiar, Mendez, & Clark, 2017; McNamara, 2018; Williamson, 2017; Quinn, 2017). If authors were scarred by such proximal distance to depravity, why traumatize the public by subjecting them to these accounts if not to appear heroic for emerging unscathed?

Conclusion

Nowhere are there more confrontational encounters and conflict than among stakeholders in making murder profitable. Several members of the expert fields have lent their voice to efforts that reinforce the tropes related to how serial murderers function and operate, dutiful servants reflexively progressing archaic theories with the expectation that such stagnant ramblings are owed renown. But these actions allow the ethos surrounding serial killers to endure beyond the current age of myth busting and stereotype dismantling. Those that mold and shape how offenders are scrutinized fortify their standpoints with the fierceness and solemnity reserved for those answering to a self-imposed higher calling. Within such an insular world, Edwards and Roy (2017) wonder what kind of profession is being creating for the next generation as perverse incentives and hypercompetition have given rise to misconduct and a reduction of scientific progress. Those without what are deemed proper qualifications are segregated and forced to prove their worth through meritorious service frequently benefiting the arbiters.

Up to this point, retention of talented and spirited members of the expert fields has depended upon the interplay between their willingness to continue traditions rooted in legend and their own resilience when treated improperly. The Northeastern University Atypical Homicide Research Group (NUAHRG) was created to correct decades of misinformation and construct deep collaborations to supersede those begun by the profiles (Northeastern University Atypical Homicide Research Group, 2017b). Adventurous investigators should be given opportunities to explore novel techniques (Yaksic, 2017b) and avenues (Keatley, Marono, Reid, Yaksic, & Clarke, 2017) in interstitial science (Greenleaf, 2017) without the threat of reprisal from colleagues. Instead of struggling to reincorporate emotional intelligence into callous brains (Hagerty, 2017), the NUAHRG forum comforts those with vulnerabilities that were initially drawn to and subsequently exploited by dark personalities (Black et al., 2014). The application of dispositional empathy is critical when enticing prospective contributors to overlook a history of mistreatment. Gobry (2016) calls for the career track for science to be delivered back to mavericks from the elder careerists so often rewarded for forcing the youngest scientists to kowtow to their theories to avoid professional risk. Without the injection of new and righteous energy, the expert fields will be in dire straits for decades to come.

Society is banding together to hold industries accountable for their erroneous ways and salacious behaviors (Reader, 2017). It is time for the expert fields to celebrate those challenging regnant paradigms and embodying the spirit of science (Gobry, 2016), to do away with the bias of hostile attribution (Paulhus et al., 2018), to admonish those writing exhibitionistic and superfluous memoirs (Miller, 2017), and abolish the profiles, scrubbing the historical record of their abuses. Psychopathy is more prevalent in community samples than once hypothesized (Sest & March, 2017; Paulhus et al., 2018), meaning that it may be the dominant trait of the dark tetrad and hold a superordinate position over the malicious yet subordinate features of narcissism and Machiavellianism (Muris et al., 2017). Since almost two-thirds of the publications on the dark tetrad appeared in recent years (Muris et al., 2017), this area of inquiry remains fertile ground for new discoveries. To properly address the identity crisis discussed in this review, the expert fields must disentangle from the pull of the dark traits and ironically give into the period of darkness called "via negativa," a silence and fasting of the soul allowing for new growth and maturation of the human spirit (Seaward, 2014). A former agent of the FBI stated that arrogance and narcissism were fatal traits held by many killers that led to their demise (Gerber, 2017). The expert fields may be doomed to suffer the same fate by repeating patterns from the past and being unwilling to reform.

Notes

1 The fabled abilities of this organization are so ingrained into societal fabric that it has been intimated that the Long Island Serial Killer case languishes unresolved because the FBI was initially shut out (Killoran, 2016).

2 Andreu, N. (5 May 2017). Research assistance. Message posted to NUAHRG electronic mailing list. Archived at yaksic.e@alumni.neu.edu

References

Anonymous. (2017) 'Of monsters and mentors: PhD disasters, and how to avoid them,' *Times Higher Education*. Retrieved April 25, 2018 from www.timeshighereducation.com/features/monsters-and-mentors-phd-disasters-and-how-to-avoid-them#survey-answer

Apple, S. (2017) 'John Arnold made a fortune at Enron. Now he's declared war on bad science,' *Wired*. Retrieved April 25, 2018 from www.wired.com/2017/01/john-arnold-waging-war-on-bad-science/

Ashforth, B. E., and Anand, V. (2003) 'The normalization of corruption in organizations,' *Research in Organizational Behavior, 25*:1–52.

Babiak, P., Folino, J., Hancock, J., Hare, R. D., Logan, M., Mayer, E. L., . . ., and Woodworth, M. (2012) 'Psychopathy: An important forensic concept for the 21st century,' *FBI Law Enforcement Bulletin, 81*:28–34.

Barker, E. (2014) 'Which professions have the most psychopaths? The fewest?' *Time*. Retrieved April 25, 2018 from http://time.com/32647/which-professions-have-the-most-psychopaths-the-fewest/

Beasley, J. O. (2004) 'Serial murder in America: Case studies of seven offenders,' *Behavioral Sciences & the Law*, *22*:395–414.

Beauge, J. (2013) 'Fascination with unsolved mysteries prompts detective to form cold case group,' *PennLive*. Retrieved April 25, 2018 from www.pennlive.com/midstate/index.ssf/2013/10/cold_cases_intrigue_lycoming_c.html

Beauge, J. (2015) 'Wrong person may have been identified as killer of 10-year-old girl, investigator says,' *PennLive*. Retrieved April 25, 2018 from www.pennlive.com/midstate/index.ssf/2015/02/investigator_says_wrong_person.html

Beck, J. (2014) 'The grisly, all-American appeal of serial killers,' *The Atlantic*. Retrieved April 25, 2018 from www.theatlantic.com/national/archive/2014/10/the-grisly-all-american-appeal-of-serial-killers/381690/

Black, P. J., Woodworth, M., and Porter, S. (2014) 'The Big Bad Wolf? The relation between the Dark Triad and the interpersonal assessment of vulnerability,' *Personality and Individual Differences*, *67*:52–56.

Boduszek, D., Debowska, A., and Willmott, D. (2017) 'Latent profile analysis of psychopathic traits among homicide, general violent, property, and white-collar offenders,' *Journal of Criminal Justice*, *51*:17–23.

Bond, M. (2016) 'Why are we eternally fascinated by serial killers?' *BBC – Future*. Retrieved April 25, 2018 from www.bbc.com/future/story/20160331-why-are-we-eternally-fascinated-by-serial-killers

Bonn, S. (2014) *Why we love serial killers: The curious appeal of the world's most savage murderers*, New York, NY: Skyhorse Publishing.

Brandolph, A. (2014) 'Wecht gets role on cold case unit,' *TribLive.com*. Retrieved April 25, 2018 from http://triblive.com/news/allegheny/5316976-74/wecht-cases-cold

Branson, A. L. (2013) 'African American serial killers: Over-represented yet underacknowledged,' *Howard Journal of Crime and Justice*, *52*(1):1–18.

Britto, B. (2017) 'Murder mystery subscription box challenges players to "Hunt a Killer",' *The Washington Post*. Retrieved April 25, 2018 from www.washingtonpost.com/local/murder-mystery-subscription-box-challenges-players-to-hunt-a-killer/2017/04/15/03b2c736-212e-11e7-a0a7–8b2a45e3dc84_story.html

Brooks, N., and Fritzon, K. (2016) 'Psychopathic personality characteristics amongst high functioning populations,' *Crime Psychology Review*, *2*:22–44.

Byrne, M. (2017) 'Two crime profilers for Anthony Sanborn Jr. say clues suggest a serial killer,' *Portland Press Herald*. Retrieved April 25, 2018 from www.pressherald.com/2017/06/21/two-crime-profilers-for-anthony-sanborn-jr-clues-suggest-a-serial-killer/

Center for Substance Abuse Treatment. (2014) *Trauma-informed care in behavioral health services*. Rockville, MD: Substance Abuse and Mental Health Services Administration (US). (Treatment Improvement Protocol (TIP) Series, No. 57.) Chapter 3, Understanding the Impact of Trauma. Retrieved April 25, 2018 from www.ncbi.nlm.nih.gov/books/NBK207191/

Chopko, B. A., Palmieri, P. A., and Adams, R. E. (2015) 'Critical incident history questionnaire replication: Frequency and severity of trauma exposure among officers from small and midsize police agencies,' *Journal of Trauma Stress*, *28*(2):157–161.

Christin, A. (2017) 'Algorithms in practice: Comparing web journalism and criminal justice,' *Big Data & Society*, *4*(2):1–14.

Clarion-Ledger. (2017) 'Clarion-Ledger, journalists win big at press awards,' *Clarion Ledger*. Retrieved April 25, 2018 from www.clarionledger.com/story/news/2017/07/08/clarion-ledger-journalists-win-big-press-awards/462380001/

Clemente, J. #Oxygen #CrimeCon #XGProductions @realcrimeprofil realcrimeprofile @CM_Set Report 9:01 AM – 9 Jun 2017 Tweet. Retrieved April 25, 2018 from https://twitter.com/JimClemente/status/873178358208749571/photo/1

Colins, O. F., Fanti, K. A., Salekin, R. T., and Andershed, H. (2017) 'Psychopathic personality in the general population: Differences and similarities across gender,' *Journal of Personality Disorders*, *31*(1):49–74.

Colin-Thome, D. (2017) 'This is why we're all obsessed with true crime stories, according to "Up and Vanished" Creator Payne Lindsey,' *Bustle*. Retrieved April 25, 2018 from www.bustle.com/p/this-is-why-were-all-obsessed-with-true-crime-stories-according-to-up-vanished-creator-payne-lindsey-63415

Culhane, S. E., Hilstad, S. M., Freng, A., and Gray, M. J. (2011) 'Self-reported psychopathology in a convicted serial killer,' *Journal of Investigative Psychology and Offender Profiling*, *8*(1):1–21.

Debowska, A., Boduszek, D., Dhingra, K., Sherretts, N., Willmott, D., and DeLisi, M. (2017). 'Can we use Hare's psychopathy model within forensic and non-forensic populations? An empirical investigation,' *Deviant Behavior*, 1–19.

DeLisi, M. (2009) 'Psychopathy is the unified theory of crime,' *Youth Violence and Juvenile Justice*, 7(3):256–273.

DeLisi, M. (2017) 'Elucidating both the non-existent and extensive violent criminal career,' *The Lancet Psychiatry*, *4*(6):429–430.

DiscoveryID. Happy #ManCrushMonday, #IDAddicts! You're welcome. #MurderChoseMe 2:04 PM – 24 Jul 2017 Tweet. Retrieved April 25, 2018 from https://twitter.com/DiscoveryID/status/889561893924417536

Dowden, C. (2005) 'Research on multiple murder: Where are we in the state of the art?,' *Journal of Police and Criminal Psychology*, *20*(2):8–18.

Dumcius, G. (2017) 'There's no one out there killing these kids' found in the water, Boston's top cop says,' *MassLive.com*. Retrieved April 25, 2018 from www.masslive.com/news/index.ssf/2017/05/theres_no_one_out_there_killin.html

Edwards, M. A., and Roy, S. (2017) 'Academic research in the 21st century: Maintaining scientific integrity in a climate of perverse incentives and hypercompetition,' *Environmental Engineering Science*, *34*(1):51–61.

Egan, V., Hughes, N., and Palmer, E. J. (2015) 'Moral disengagement, the dark triad, and unethical consumer attitudes,' *Personality and Individual Differences*, *76*:123–128.

Evans, M. (2017) 'Has the true identity of Jack the Ripper been revealed? Victorian diary proven genuine contains huge clue,' *The Telegraph*. Retrieved April 25, 2018 from www.telegraph.co.uk/news/2017/08/06/true-identity-jack-ripper-revealed-diary-confirmed-genuine/

Fallon, J. H. (2014) *The psychopath inside: A neuroscientist's personal journey into the dark side of the brain*, New York, NY: Current.

Ferak, J. (2015) 'Murder victim's family has few options,' *Appleton Post-Crescent*. Retrieved April 25, 2018 from www.postcrescent.com/story/news/investigations/2015/11/06/murder-victims-family-has-few-options/74676838/

Ferak, J. (2017) 'FBI: Bones from suspect's yard not Bobby Joe Fritz,' *Appleton Post-Crescent*. Retrieved April 25, 2018 from www.postcrescent.com/story/news/investigations/2017/06/27/fbi-bones-suspects-yard-not-bobby-joe-fritz/417234001/

Fitzpatrick, M. (2017) 'DNA or it didn't happen,' *The Ringer*. Retrieved April 25, 2018 from https://theringer.com/crimecon-true-crime-nancy-grace-making-a-murderer-67136cc7ac3a

Flynn, E. (2017) 'Fatal attraction: Inside the dark world of true crime fans who obsess over sick murders and idolize killers,' *The Sun*. Retrieved April 25, 2018 from www.thesun.co.uk/news/3487694/inside-the-dark-world-of-true-crime-fans-who-obsess-over-sick-murders-and-idolise-killers/

Ford, R., and Kit, B. (2017) 'Cannes: Zac Efron to play Ted Bundy in "Extremely Wicked, Shockingly Evil and Vile",' *The Hollywood Reporter*. Retrieved April 25, 2018 from www.hollywoodreporter.com/news/cannes-zac-efron-play-ted-bundy-extremely-wicked-shockingly-evil-vile-1003797

Fridg, M. (2017) 'The Dewey Decimal System of death,' *Freethink*. Retrieved April 25, 2018 from www.youtube.com/watch?v=5jSQ9v60rUY

Furnham, A., Hyde, G., and Trickey, G. (2014) 'Do your dark side traits fit? Dysfunctional personalities in different work sectors,' *Applied Psychology: An International Review*, *63*(4):589–606.

Gardiner, M. (2017) *UNSUB: A novel*, New York, NY: Dutton.

Gellatly, M. (2017) 'Probe into 3 deaths complicated by lack of cause,' *The Robesonian*. Retrieved April 25, 2018 from www.robesonian.com/news/99949/probe-into-3-deaths-complicated-by-lack-of-cause

Gerber, M. (2017) 'How an ex-FBI profiler helped put an innocent man behind bars,' *Los Angeles Times*. Retrieved April 25, 2018 from www.latimes.com/local/california/la-me-profiler-wrongful-conviction-20170720-htmlstory.html

Gobry, P.-E. (2016) 'Big science is broken,' *The Week*. Retrieved April 25, 2018 from http://theweek.com/articles/618141/big-sciencebroken

Greenleaf, C. (2017) 'Adventurous scientist fellows program,' *Massachusetts Institute of Technology Media Lab*. Retrieved April 25, 2018 from www.media.mit.edu/posts/adventurous-science-faq/

Gross, D. J. (2017) 'Families, experts believe Kohlhepp may have more victims,' *GoUpstate.com*. Retrieved April 25, 2018 from www.goupstate.com/news/20170527/families-experts-believe-kohlhepp-may-have-more-victims

Hafford, M. (2017) 'The gang's all here! Serial killer shot glasses thanks to @swordandscale The gang's all here! Serial killer shot glasses thanks to @swordandscale,' 8:45 PM 30 May 2017 Tweet. Retrieved April 25, 2018 from https://twitter.com/mirandahafford/status/869731575704977412

Hagerty, B. B. (2017) 'When your child is a psychopath,' *The Atlantic*. Retrieved April 25, 2018 from www.theatlantic.com/magazine/archive/2017/06/when-your-child-is-a-psychopath/524502/

Haigney, S. (2017) 'Quentin Tarantino exploring new movie on Manson family,' *The New York Times.* Retrieved April 25, 2018 from www.nytimes.com/2017/07/12/movies/quentin-tarantino-charles-manson-film.html

Hare, R. D. (1980) 'A research scale for the assessment of psychopathy in criminal populations,' *Personality and Individual Differences, 1*(2):111–119.

Hare, R. D. (2017) 'A person-centered approach to research on the nature and meaning of psychopathy–brain relations,' *Biological Psychiatry: Cognitive Neuroscience and Neuroimaging, 2*:111–112.

Hickey, E., Walters, B. K., Drislane, L. E., and Patrick, C. J. (2014) 'Deviance at its darkest: Psychopathy and serial murder,' in C. J. Patrick (Ed.), *Handbook of psychopathy* (2nd ed.), New York, NY: Guilford Press.

Hiller, H. (2013) 88 Dragon Design Studio. Retrieved April 25, 2018 from www.88dragon.com/images/stock_images/KMains_2723A.jpg

Jenkins, P. (2002) 'Catch me before I kill more: Seriality as modern monstrosity,' *Cultural Analysis*, 3:1–17.

Jonason, P. K., Webster, G. D., Schmitt, D. P., Li, N. P., and Crysel, L. (2012) 'The antihero in popular culture: Life history theory and the dark triad personality traits,' *Review of General Psychology, 16*(2):192–199.

Jones, D. N., and Figueredo, A. J. (2013) 'The core of darkness: Uncovering the heart of the dark triad,' *European Journal of Personality, 27*:521–531.

Jones, M. (2017) 'Are we angrier or is it simply easier to be?' *Tulsa World.* Retrieved April 25, 2018 from www.tulsaworld.com/opinion/mikejones/mike-jones-are-we-angrier-or-is-it-simply-easier/article_04f3ce82-fb08-5fb0–8d4b-8aba34880d67.html

Kajonius, P. J., Persson, B. N., and Jonason, P. K. (2015) 'Hedonism, achievement, and power: Universal values that characterize the Dark Triad,' *Personality and Individual Differences*, 77:173–178.

Kaplan, M. (2017) 'This is what it's like to be friends with a serial killer,' *NY Post.* Retrieved April 25, 2018 from http://nypost.com/2017/07/23/this-is-what-its-like-to-be-friends-with-a-serial-killer/

Keatley, D., Marono, A., Reid, S., Yaksic, E., and Clarke, D. (2017) 'A behavior sequence analysis of serial killers' lives: From childhood abuse to methods of murder,' *Journal of Interpersonal Violence*, in press.

Kijak, M. (2016) 'Investigating the Dark Triad in relation to career choices, job satisfaction and career suitability' (Unpublished manuscript).

Killelea, E. (2017) '"American Ripper": Inside new investigation into serial killer H.H. Holmes,' *Rolling Stone.* Retrieved April 25, 2018 from www.rollingstone.com/culture/news/inside-investigation-into-serial-killer-hh-holmes-w491708

Killoran, E. (2016) 'Why hasn't the Long Island serial killer case been solved?' *Rolling Stone.* Retrieved April 25, 2018 from www.rollingstone.com/culture/features/why-hasnt-the-long-island-serial-killer-case-been-solved-w453872

Kopel, H., and Friedman, M. (1997) 'Posttraumatic symptoms in South African police exposed to violence,' *Journal of Trauma Stress, 10*(2):307–317.

Kowalski, C. M., Vernon, P. A., and Schermer, J. A. (2017) 'Vocational interests and dark personality: Are there dark career choices?,' *Personality and Individual Differences*, 104:43–47.

Levin, J., and Fox, J. (2008) 'Normalcy in behavioral characteristics of the sadistic serial killer.' Retrieved April 25, 2018 from http://jacklevinonviolence.com/articles/Normalcyofserialmurder.pdf

Long, K. (2017) 'We crashed UW's class on calling BS. Here's what we learned about sleuthing "big data",' *The Seattle Times.* Retrieved April 25, 2018 from www.seattletimes.com/seattle-news/education/popular-uw-class-teaches-students-when-to-call-bs-on-big-data-claims/

Lovitt, B. (2016) '"My Friend Dahmer": Inside movie adaptation of serial killer's teen life,' *Rolling Stone.* Retrieved April 25, 2018 from www.rollingstone.com/culture/features/my-friend-dahmer-inside-movie-adaptation-of-serial-killers-teen-life-w431165

Malizia, N. (2017) 'Serial killer: The mechanism from imagination to the murder phases,' *Sociology Mind*, 7:44–59.

Mains, K. (2015) 'Back by popular demand "Ken's Corner",' 3:26 PM 4 Feb 2015 Tweet. Retrieved April 25, 2018 from https://twitter.com/detectivemains/status/563071204215783425

Mains, K. L. (2017) *Unsolved no more: A cold case detective's fight for justice*, Denver, CO: WildBlue Press.

Mallie, S., Aguiar, L., Mendez, G. K., and Clark, L. (2017) 'The Golden State Killer,' *48 Hours.* Retrieved April 25, 2018 from www.cbsnews.com/news/michelle-mcnamara-patton-oswalt-true-crime-writers-relentless-search-for-the-golden-state-killer/

McNamara, M. (2018) *I'll be gone in the dark: One woman's obsessive search for the Golden State Killer*, New York, NY: HarperCollins.

Mellor, L. (2017) 'Criminal profiling classes taught by professional,' *Kijiji*. Retrieved April 25, 2018 from www.kijiji.ca/v-classes-lessons/city-of-toronto/criminal-profiling-classes-taught-by-professional/1271842384

Miller, L. (2017) 'True crime gets pretty,' *Slate*. Retrieved April 25, 2018 from www.slate.com/articles/arts/books/2017/08/the_true_crime_memoir_when_mfa_grads_and_literary_aspirants_write_true_crime.html

Montgomery, R., Rice, G. E., and Cummings, I. (2017) 'After four slayings, anxiety stalks trails in south Kansas City,' *The Kansas City Star*. Retrieved April 25, 2018 from www.kansascity.com/news/local/crime/article154240664.html

Moss, T. (2017) 'Ever wonder what it'd be like to escape a serial killer's lair? New Bluffton business can help you with that,' *The Island Packet*. Retrieved April 25, 2018 from www.islandpacket.com/news/business/article157200379.html

Muris, P., Merckelbach, H., Otgaar, H., and Meijer, E. (2017) 'The malevolent side of human nature: A meta-analysis and critical review of the literature on the dark triad (Narcissism, Machiavellianism, and Psychopathy),' *Perspectives on Psychological Science*, *12*(2):183–204.

Nazaryan, A. (2017) 'The Grim Sleeper' is the story of the South L.A. serial killer and the women who were his victims,' *Los Angeles Times*. Retrieved April 25, 2018 from www.latimes.com/books/jacketcopy/la-ca-jc-grim-sleeper-20170706-story.html

Nicholson, R. (2017) 'True crime makes great TV. But must it linger on women's corpses?' *The Guardian*. Retrieved April 25, 2018 from www.theguardian.com/commentisfree/2017/aug/07/true-crime-tv-linger-womens-corpses-disturbing

Northeastern University Atypical Homicide Research Group. (2017a) 'Behavioral analysis unit 5.' Retrieved April 25, 2018 from www.northeastern.edu/homicide/behavioral-analysis-unit-5/

Northeastern University Atypical Homicide Research Group. (2017b) 'Conference 2017.' Retrieved April 25, 2018 from www.northeastern.edu/homicide/conference/

Notes, G. (2017) 'How a Son of Sam detective realized "This Has Got to Be the Guy",' *The New York Times*. Retrieved April 25, 2018 from www.nytimes.com/2017/08/06/nyregion/son-of-sam-killings-david-berkowitz.html

Oransky, I., and Marcus, A. (2017) 'A shrimp study's jumbo error – and what other researchers can learn,' *STAT News*. Retrieved April 25, 2018 from www.statnews.com/2017/06/01/shrimp-study-error/

Palmer, L. (2017) 'Hunt a killer launches first podcast series, "Behind True Crime",' *prweb*. Retrieved April 25, 2018 from www.prweb.com/releases/2017/08/prweb14601177.htm

Parmley, W. W. (1995) 'Sensationalism and the news media,' *Journal of the American College of Cardiology*, *26*(3):836–837.

Paulhus, D. L., Curtis, S. R., and Jones, D. N. (2018) 'Aggression as a trait: The dark tetrad alternative,' *Current Opinion in Psychology*, *19*:88–92.

Paulhus, D. L., and John, O. P. (1998) 'Egoistic and moralistic biases in self-perception: The interplay of self-deceptive styles with basic traits and motives,' *Journal of Personality*, *66*(6):1025–1060.

Paulhus, D. L., and Williams, K. M. (2002) 'The Dark Triad of personality: Narcissism, Machiavellianism, and psychopathy,' *Journal of Research in Personality*, *36*:556–563.

Pauli, H. (2017) 'Why I quit: Local newspapers can needlessly ruin lives for empty clicks,' *The Guardian*. Retrieved April 25, 2018 from www.theguardian.com/media/2017/aug/08/local-news-crime-reporting-quitting-journalism

Pettler, L. (2017) 'You love True Crime & we love True Crime so join LPA's True Crime Summer Fun! Online camps for kids . . . AND YOU ASKED FOR IT . . . CAMP 4 ADULTS!You love True Crime & we love True Crime so join LPA's True Crime Summer Fun! Online camps for kids . . . AND YOU ASKED FOR IT . . . CAMP 4 ADULTS!,' 5:17 PM 19 May 2017 Tweet. Retrieved April 25, 2018 from https://twitter.com/DrLauraPettler/status/865692864038264832

Phelps, M. W. (2017) *Dangerous ground: My friendship with a serial killer*, New York, NY: Kensington.

Quinn, A. (2017) '"The Spider and the Fly" gets stuck in a web of self-regard,' *NPR Book Reviews*. Retrieved April 25, 2018 from www.npr.org/2017/01/26/510816523/the-spider-and-the-fly-gets-stuck-in-a-web-of-self-regard

Rantanen, J., Metsäpelto, R. L., Feldt, T., Pulkkinen, L., and Kokko, K. (2007) 'Long-term stability in the Big Five personality traits in adulthood,' *Scandinavian Journal of Psychology*, *48*(6):511–518.

Reader, R. (2017) 'Uber's implosion marks a tipping point for overt workplace sexism,' *Fast Company*. Retrieved April 25, 2018 from www.fastcompany.com/40431116/ubers-implosion-marks-a-tipping-point-for-overt-workplace-sexism

Reid, S. (2017) 'Developmental pathways to serial homicide: A critical review of the biological Literature,' *Aggression and Violent Behavior, 35*:52–61.
Sarzyńskam J., Falkiewicz, M., Riegel, M., Babula, J., Margulies, D. S., Nęcka, E., . . ., and Szatkowska, I. (2017) 'More intelligent extraverts are more likely to deceive,' *PLoS One, 12*(4):1–17.
Schlesinger, L. B. (1998) 'Pathological narcissism and serial homicide: Review and case study,' *Current Psychology, 17*:212–221.
Seaward, B. L. (2014) *Managing stress: Principles and strategies for health and well-being*, Sudbury, MA: Jones & Bartlett Learning.
Sest, N., and March, E. (2017) 'Constructing the cyber-troll: Psychopathy, sadism, and empathy,' *Personality and Individual Differences, 119*:69–72.
Shao, R., and Lee, T. M. C. (2017) 'Are individuals with higher psychopathic traits better learners at lying? Behavioural and neural evidence,' *Translational Psychiatry*, 7:e1175.
Sherretts, N., Boduszek, D., Debowska, A., and Willmott, D. (2017) 'Comparison of murderers with recidivists and first time incarcerated offenders from U.S. prisons on psychopathy and identity as a criminal: An exploratory analysis,' *Journal of Criminal Justice, 51*:89–92.
Sidanius, J., Liu, J. H., Shaw, J. S., and Pratto, F. (1994) 'Social dominance orientation, hierarchy attenuators and hierarchy enhancers: Social dominance theory and the criminal justice system,' *Journal of Applied Social Psychology, 24*(4):338–366.
Slovic, S., and Slovic, P. (2015) *Numbers and nerves: Information, emotion, and meaning in a world of data*, Corvallis, OR: Oregon State University Press.
Smith, E. E. (2017) The two kinds of stories we tell about ourselves. *Ideas.Ted.Com*. Retrieved April 25, 2018 from http://ideas.ted.com/the-two-kinds-of-stories-we-tell-about-ourselves/
Snierson, D. (2017) See Paul Bettany as the Unabomber in new Discovery series. *Entertainment Weekly*. Retrieved April 25, 2018 from http://ew.com/tv/2017/05/19/paul-bettany-unabomber-discovery-manhunt/
Sollie, H., Kop, N., and Euwema, M. C. (2017) 'Mental resilience of crime scene investigators: How police officers perceive and cope with the impact of demanding work situations,' *Criminal Justice and Behavior*, in press.
Stack, T. (2017) Darren Criss on going from a warbler on *Glee* to a killer in *The Assassination of Gianni Versace. Entertainment Weekly*. Retrieved April 25, 2018 from http://ew.com/tv/2017/06/23/darren-criss-assassination-of-gianni-versace/
Stewart, A. (2017) 'My Favorite Murder' and the growing acceptance of true-crime entertainment. *The Washington Post*. Retrieved April 25, 2018 from www.washingtonpost.com/lifestyle/my-favorite-murder-and-the-growing-acceptance-of-true-crime-entertainment/2017/05/07/7c9b53d8–2f71–11e7–9dec-764dc781686f_story.html
Sykes, T. (2017) Bloody stealth-'em-up Serial Cleaner is out now. *PC Gamer*. Retrieved April 25, 2018 from www.pcgamer.com/bloody-stealth-em-up-serial-cleaner-is-out-now/
Turnage, C. (2017) More than a 'summer slump': How the loss of structure affects academics. *The Chronicle of Higher Education*. Retrieved April 25, 2018 from www.chronicle.com/article/More-Than-a-Summer/240357
Turnipseed, D. L., and Cohen, S. R. (2015) 'Academic entitlement and socially aversive personalities: Does the Dark Triad predict academic entitlement?,' *Personality and Individual Differences, 82*:72–75.
Venables, N. C., Hall, J. R., and Patrick, C. J. (2014) 'Differentiating psychopathy from antisocial personality disorder: A triarchic model perspective,' *Psychological Medicine, 44*(5):1005–13.
Whiffen, G. (2017) No indication St. Anthony missing-person cases linked: Expert. *The Telegram*. Retrieved April 25, 2018 from www.thetelegram.com/news/local/2017/6/15/no-indication-st–anthony-missing-person-cases-linked–expert.html
Williams, J. (2017) 075: Mary Ellen O'Toole – serial killers, sexual sadists. *FBI Retired Case File Review*. Retrieved April 25, 2018 from https://overcast.fm/+GAzzrHcrw
Williamson, B. (2017) 'Serial killer whisperer' Amanda Howard gets inside notorious criminal minds. *ABC Radio Adelaide*. Retrieved April 25, 2018 from www.abc.net.au/news/2017-06-29/serial-killer-whisperer-true-crime-author-amanda-howard-talks/8658896
X-G Productions. (2017) Our work. Retrieved April 25, 2018 from www.xgproductions.com/portfolio/
Yaksic, E. (2015) 'Addressing the challenges and limitations of utilizing data to study serial Homicide,' *Crime Psychology Review, 1*(1):108–134.
Yaksic, E., DeSpirito, L., and Reid, S. (2017) 'Detecting an observable decline in serial homicide: Have we banished the devil from the details?,' *Homicide Studies*, in press.

Yaksic, E. (2017a) Open letter to the atypical homicide research community. *Serial Homicide Expertise and Information Sharing Collaborative*. Retrieved April 25, 2018 from http://serialhomicidecollaborative.blogspot.com/2017/01/open-letter-to-atypical-homicide.html

Yaksic, E. (2017b) 'Novel techniques to detect the multiple–event murderer: An exploration of a researcher's field notes,' in M. DeLisi & P. J. Conis (Eds.), *Violent offenders: Theory, research, public policy and practice* (3rd ed.), Burlington, MA: Jones & Bartlett Learning.

20

Psychopathy among juvenile homicide offenders

Jonathan W. Caudill and Henriikka Weir

Acknowledgment: The authors would like to thank Erika Weliever for collecting news media content used within this chapter.

Introduction

> Sometime around 10 p.m., Paris convinced the babysitter she could go home. It was after that, according to detectives, that Paris grabbed a kitchen knife and walked into the bedroom where Ella was sleeping. He then proceeded to beat, choke, and stab his 4-year-old sister 17 times – an autopsy report noted a cluster of deep stab wounds on Ella's chest, along with numerous cuts to her fingers, wrists, and forearms, indicating she fought back.
>
> (Barajas, 2013:1)

After contemplating how to handle the gruesome scene he created in 2007, Paris Lee Bennett – 13 years old at the time and currently serving a 40-year sentence in the Texas Department of Criminal Justice for Capital Murder – called 911 and reported that he had stabbed his sister to death "while in the throes of a vivid hallucination . . . [that included] . . . a demonic version of his sister, engulfed in flames . . . [and] . . . laughing maniacally at him" (Barajas, 2013:1). The investigation, however, found evidence suggesting Mr. Bennett's description of the situation misrepresented what really occurred that fateful evening. Evidence suggested that Mr. Bennett did not provide resuscitation efforts to his sister even though he told the 911 dispatcher that he was doing so while he counted alleged chest compressions. Detectives recounted that Mr. Bennett attempted unsuccessfully to cry while being interviewed shortly after the crime. While only circumstantial to Mr. Bennett's motivations, the investigation revealed the discovery of semen on the inside of Mr. Bennett's shorts from that evening and on the bed where his sister died. If this was not twisted enough, Mr. Bennett's mother reported from her visit with him in the detention facility, "Paris got quiet, then there was this whole shift in his demeanor . . . it was like this whole other person took over [and] he just started laughing at me [and said,] 'well it took you fucking long enough'" (Barajas, 2013:1). After his mother confronted him about the discovered semen, Mr. Bennett's anger devolved and he again became violent (Barajas).

Homicides committed by juvenile offenders shock the conscience and lead the public and social scientists to search for answers – answers to inquiries about why they would take such drastic action and what drove them to commit the ultimate act of aggression against another person. It is a common human behavior to want to understand and be able to explain in simple terms the motivations of people that exact lethal violence against another human, especially when the perpetrator is young and, presumably, less culpable. While homicides committed by juveniles are rare (Rodway et al., 2011), homicide in itself is extreme and costly enough to garner substantial attention (DeLisi et al., 2010). Understanding the individual-level correlates, such as personality deficits and pathological behaviors, of juvenile homicide offending are of particular interest here and the focus of this chapter.

A common perspective in explaining severely violent behaviors of juvenile offenders is one that demonstrates a lack of empathy and disregard for the consequences of behavior. Psychopathy is a term often used to describe clusters of characteristics that persist over a period of time in individuals such as a lack of empathy, impulsivity, callousness, narcissism, manipulation, and deceitfulness (DeLisi & Vaughn, 2012; Hare & Neumann, 2008; Porter & Woodworth, 2006). However, psychopathy is not a clinically recognized diagnosis in DSM–5 (Diagnostic and Statistical Manual of Mental Disorders 5th Edition – the most prevalent guide used by healthcare professionals in the U.S. to diagnose mental health disorders; APA, 2013). Instead, the DSM–5's Antisocial Personality Disorder diagnosis most closely resembles that of psychopathy (Salekin, 2016). This diagnosis includes significant impairments in personality functioning (i.e., narcissism/grandiosity or disregard for laws and norms and lack of empathy or incompetence with intimacy) and pathological personality traits (i.e., Antagonism and disinhibition).[1] A limitation relevant here, though, is that diagnosis of psychopathy requires that the subject be at least 18 years old to be diagnosed with Antisocial Personality Disorder (APA, 2013). While this age requirement may assist practitioners in recognizing the developing personality and brain structure of juveniles, it is also worth noting that the DSM is an ever-evolving diagnostic manual and, thus, its applicability in understanding psychopathic traits among juveniles that commit homicide may also be limited.

To be clear, the prevalence of personality disorders among the general population is rare. For example, it is estimated that approximately 4 to 6 percent of the male population and 1.5 to 2 percent of the female population suffer from Antisocial Personality Disorder. However, these estimates are dramatically higher for the incarcerated population. Black and colleagues (Black, Gunter, Loveless, Allen, & Sieleni, 2010) found that greater than one-third (35 percent) of their sample of newly incarcerated offenders at Iowa Department of Corrections' Medical and Classification Center met the criteria for Antisocial Personality Disorder.[2] Despite the rare occurrence of personality disorders among the general population and the reluctance of the mental health community to diagnose juveniles with Antisocial Personality Disorder, there is evidence that some adolescents exhibit psychopathic traits (Andershed, 2010); it has been posited that perceiving psychopathic traits on a continuum is superior to the traditional categorical classifications (DeLisi, 2016).

Speaking to this point, a study focused on Finnish youths convicted of homicides revealed through the PCL–R (Hare's (2003) Psychopathy Checklist–Revised) that 21 percent of the juvenile homicide offenders (JHOs) would have been classified as psychopaths if using a cut-off criterion of 26 points or more. Twelve percent would have been classified as psychopaths if using a cut-off criterion of 30 points or more (Lindberg et al., 2009). Studies on mixed aged (i.e., adolescent and adult) samples have drawn similar conclusions. For example, Woodworth and Porter (2002) discovered among a sample of incarcerated Canadian homicide offenders – ranging in age from 14 to 55 years old at the time of the homicide – that 27 percent scored within the psychopathic range on PCL–R. Interestingly, this estimate aligns with estimates of Antisocial Personality Disorder found among the broader inmate population (as opposed to only homicide offenders) (DeLisi & Vaughn, 2012).

Exploring situational and social characteristics of the most consequential violence perpetrated by youth may help to shed light on the relationship between psychopathy and juvenile homicide offending. When looking at specialized JHOs, the incidence of psychopathy or psychopathic tendencies vary depending on the type of JHO. For example, it has been estimated that about 10 percent of youth who kill their caregivers are dangerously antisocial (Heide, 1995, 2013). On the other hand, a study of juvenile sexual murders discovered that 20 out of 22 (91 percent) offenders examined were diagnosed with Conduct Disorder (Myers, Chan, Vo, & Lazarou, 2010). This was by far the most common diagnosis among this group of JHOs. Additionally, the majority of studies focused on adolescent mass murderers report a history of violent behavior and/or antisocial and narcissistic characteristics among these offenders (see McGee & DeBernardo, 1999; Meloyv et al., 2004; Meloy, Hempel, Mohandie, Shiva, & Gray, 2001). The prevalence of these psychopathic traits estimated among youthful offenders in the scholarly literature provides the antithesis to the DSM–5's requirement that Antisocial Personality Disorder, which closely resembles the classification for psychopathy, can only occur in adulthood. This discrepancy calls for further exploration of the relationship between juvenile homicide offending and psychopathy.

State of the knowledge

Not all adolescents engaging in crime and delinquency score high on the scales intended to measure psychopathy. Frankly, many scholars consider delinquency to be a normative developmental phase during adolescence (Moffitt, 1993; Patterson, Reid, & Dishion, 1992; Sampson & Laub, 1995), and some scholars have presented empirically based limitations (such as reliability and factor structure, as well as criterion-related construct and predictive validity) of scales typically used to diagnose psychopathy among juvenile offenders (Cauffman, Kimonis, Dmitrieva, & Monahan, 2009; Sharp & Kine, 2008). Coupled with these concerns is the ethical dilemma that such a diagnosis may have far-reaching impacts for the diagnosed youth (Sharp & Kine, 2008). Indeed, even the youth who commit homicides more often than not do not meet the clinical cut-off for psychopathy or develop into having an Antisocial Personality Disorder (Lindberg et al., 2009). Nonetheless, a body of literature has clearly recognized several main characteristics of psychopathy present in a small but identifiable group of young offenders (Andershed, 2010). Furthermore, studies have shown that youth with significant psychopathic/antisocial traits impose disproportionate consequences on society in terms of the severity, frequency, and longevity of their offending trajectories (Vaughn & Howard, 2005). Understanding the individual-level characteristics of JHOs may help to shed light on underlying personality deficits among this population of serious and violent offenders.

Situational factors: for whom the bell tolls

Juveniles that commit homicide are more likely to kill known victims as opposed to family members or strangers (Rodway et al. 2011; Rowley, Ewing, & Singer, 1987), and the majority of the murders involving known suspects are typically the result of interpersonal conflict (Cornell, Benedek, & Benedek, 1987). Rowley and associates discovered in their review of 787 JHOs that approximately one-half (49 percent) of the sample murdered an acquaintance, approximately one-third murdered a stranger, and approximately 17 percent murdered a family member (including eight present that murdered a parental figure). When juveniles murder family members, their parental figures are most commonly the victims (Rowley et al).

The distinction of whether the JHO knows the victim is relevant to how JHOs approach their crimes. While most JHOs report being under the influence of substances (including alcohol) during the crime (DiCataldo & Everett, 2008), JHOs that kill a known victim are less likely to report being intoxicated during their crime than those JHOs that kill strangers (Cornell et al. 1987). Furthermore, mass murdering juvenile offenders typically refer back to an affront from known victims prior to their acts. Meloy and associates (Meloy et al.,2001) discovered that approximately two-thirds of their sample of mass murdering juvenile offenders experienced a triggering event, such as dismissal from someone the offender held in high regard. It is important, however, to not confuse being triggered with reactive, uncontrollable behavior, as over 60 percent of Meloy and associates' mass murdering JHOs classified as family annihilators and classroom avengers discussed lethal violence prior to their offenses. This suggests some level of premeditation, planning, and callousness instead of their offense being the product of an uncontrollable emotional outburst, especially when it involved known victims.

The making of juvenile homicide offenders: all in the family

The family is one of the most common threads explored when studying JHOs. Although some research suggests JHOs recall positive memories of their family (DiCataldo & Everett, 2008), most studies report that they regularly recall problematic familial environments (Busch, Zagar, Hughes, Arbit, & Bussell, 1990; DeLisi, Piquero, & Cardwell, 2016; Rodway et al. 2011). In comparing 33 JHOs to 28 mainstream violent juvenile offenders, DiCataldo and Everett suggested that JHOs and non-homicide violent juvenile offenders reported similar levels of parental criminality, and JHOs were less likely than their less violent counterparts to report sibling criminality. However, many other studies focusing on familial influences of JHOs suggest more deleterious relationships. For example, Rodway and colleagues (2011) discovered that more than one-quarter of their sample of JHOs reported familial histories of alcohol/drug abuse and/or criminality and approximately 40 percent of them reported mental health disabilities within their families.

Beyond the narrow focus of parental criminality and violence, research has observed the influence of adverse childhood experiences on violent offending. Counter to expectations, however, research suggests that exposure to adverse childhood experiences is a poor indicator of the propensity to commit homicide among juvenile offenders (DeLisi et al., 2017). The exception to these findings is among Hispanic JHOs, where the culminating effects of adverse childhood experiences was predictive of being incarcerated for a homicide. Interesting in this context is that JHOs are more likely to result from disorganized communities (DeLisi et al., 2016), suggesting a potential confounding effect of neighborhood and culture.

A common familial theme among JHOs is the substantial exposure to violence. Research has revealed that JHOs are more likely than comparison groups of offenders to report being exposed to violence (DeLisi et al., 2016) and exposed to it through the family (Busch et al., 1990; Darby, Allan, Kashani, Hartke, & Reid, 1998; Hill-Smith, Hugo, Hughes, Fonagy, & Hartman, 2002). Busch and colleagues observed the distinctions between 71 juveniles convicted of homicide and 71 low-level juvenile delinquents. They found that 58 percent of the JHOs had criminally violent family members, while only 20 percent of the comparison group reported similar influences. Darby et al. discovered that JHOs reporting previously abuse at the hands of a family member were also more likely to report previous suicide attempts. These findings provide support for the "lockage phenomenon" (see Mohr & McKnight, 1971), where juveniles resort to lethal violence either against themselves or others as a last-ditch effort to escape abuse and the chaotic home environment. Indeed, for those youth who kill their caregivers, serious childhood maltreatment is a persistent correlate of homicidal violence. It has been estimated that over 90 percent of children who kill their parents have been seriously abused, while the remaining (fewer than 10 percent) could be classified either as severely mentally ill or seriously antisocial (Heide, 1995). Hill-Smith and associates' results coincide with these findings, as their sample of JHOs were more likely to report harsh parenting from both parents than a comparison group of juvenile property crime (burglary) offenders (32 percent compared to 5 percent, respectively).

Whether the abuse was at the hands of a family member or someone else, evidence suggests that JHOs are more likely to have experienced abuse prior to their crime. In a study of 221 JHOs, Caudill and Trulson (2016) found that approximately 15 percent of their sample reported being abused physically and Busch et al. (1990) found that 25 percent of their JHOs (compared to 20 percent of the low-level juvenile delinquents, $p < 0.01$) experienced physical abuse. The consequence of physical abuse run deep, as JHOs with a history of being abused physically are more likely to recidivate after release from incarceration (Trulson & Caudill, 2017).

A lack of conformity

The challenges of chaotic home environments and abuses may be further complicated by developmental and school problems. Although Heide (1995; 2013) suggested that mental retardation is relatively rare among JHOs, Busch and colleagues revealed that 21 percent of their sample of JHOs suffered mental retardation (compared to 10 percent of the comparison group) and Rodway et al. (2011) reported that approximately one-half of their 363 JHOs in England and Wales were considered developmentally delayed. Myers and colleagues (2010), in a study of juvenile sexual murderers, discovered that 91 percent (20 out of 22) of offenders were diagnosed with some form of Conduct Disorder – the most common diagnosis among this group of JHOs.

In addition to lower IQ scores (DeLisi et al. 2016), juvenile homicide offenders tend to present other psychological challenges as well. Subclasses of JHOs – juvenile sexual homicide offenders and juvenile mass murderers – present more troubling psychological abnormalities, including a tendency to have emotional and personality disturbances (McGee & DeBernardo, 1999; Meloy et al., 2004; Myers & Blashfield, 1997) and "a pathologically narcissistic sense of entitlement" (Meloy et al. 2001:726). These psychological complications seem to permeate offenders' social situations. Rodway et al. found that JHOs fared poorly in school, with almost three-quarters (73 percent) of them reporting disciplinary problems. Hill-Smith et al. (2002) reported similar scholastic problems for JHOs compared to other offenders, in that JHOs reported significantly greater frequencies of being excluded from school activities.

Given the familial adversities and inability to conform in regular activities (such as school), it is of little surprise that JHOs report elevated levels of substance abuse. Research suggests that alcohol abuse among JHOs ranges from 40 percent to 63 percent (Busch et al., 1990; Darby et al., 1998; Rodway et al., 2011). To put it in context, Busch and colleagues found that 38 percent of their sample of JHOs reported alcohol abuse compared to only 24 percent of their comparison group. Illicit drug abuse is also a common finding among JHOs, with estimates ranging from 58 percent to 80 percent (Busch et al., 1990; Caudill & Trulson, 2016; Darby et al., 1998).

The combination of psychological abnormalities, substance abuse issues, and school problems may develop into a sense of non-belonging for these violent offenders. Studies have shown that JHOs report higher rates of gang affiliation (Busch et al., 1990; Caudill & Trulson, 2016), which may lend support to a hedonistic perspective. Caudill and Trulson discovered that approximately 30 percent of their sample of JHOs were gang affiliated, and Busch et al. revealed that 41 percent of the JHOs were gang affiliated compared to only 14 percent of the comparison group of nonviolent delinquents. The complications of gang affiliated JHOs is highlighted by research suggesting that gang-related homicides or gang-affiliated JHOs are significantly more likely to continue their criminality after being released from incarceration (Trulson, Caudill, Haerle, & DeLisi, 2012).

Behavioral continuity

Psychopathic tendencies during adolescence, especially callousness, have been closely "associated with a pattern of serious aggressive behavior . . . and can signal a pattern of persistent and violent behavior" (Porter & Woodworth, 2006:482). In their book chapter on psychopathy and aggression, Porter and Woodworth discuss multiple studies that have shown that psychopathic traits in adolescence increase violent offense convictions, aggression while incarcerated, and violent reoffending (see also Brandt, Kennedy, Patrick, & Curtain, 1997; Campbell, Porter, & Santor, 2004; Forth & Mailloux, 2000; Frick, 1998; Lynam, 2002). However, when discussing behavioral continuity regarding psychopathy in JHOs and other violent juvenile offenders, several issues must be considered. These include diagnostic issues, criminal histories, and viability of rehabilitation among JHOs.

Pathological considerations

Due to their still developing brains and personalities, clinicians and practitioners have been careful not to consider personality disorders among juveniles (Meyers, 2014). However, the DSM–5 recognizes two potential precursors for Antisocial Personality Disorder in juveniles: Oppositional Defiant Disorder and Conduct Disorder (APA, 2013). Oppositional Defiant Disorder includes symptoms such as angry and irritable mood, argumentative and defiant behavior, and vindictiveness and can be identified in even very young children (APA, 2013). This disorder can be characterized as mild, moderate, or severe, depending on pervasiveness across different settings, and must be independent of culturally accepted and age-based norms and/or other mental health diagnosis (APA, 2013). A Conduct Disorder can be diagnosed in individuals who show "a repetitive and persistent pattern of behavior in which the basic rights of others or major age-appropriate societal norms or rules are violated" (i.e., aggression, vandalism, theft, deceitfulness, and serious rule violations) and "the disturbance in behavior causes clinically significant impairment in social, academic, or occupational functioning" (APA, 2013, 312.8x (F91.x)). Conduct Disorder can have a childhood (i.e., younger than 10) or adolescent onset. It can also be diagnosed in those who are 18 or older if the criteria for Antisocial Personality Disorder are not met (APA, 2013). There is often a progression from Oppositional Defiant Disorder to Conduct Disorder to Antisocial Personality Disorder; however, not all children with Oppositional Defiant Disorder develop Conduct Disorder and not all conduct-disordered youth will progress to having an Antisocial Personality Disorder (Holmes, Slaughter, & Kashani, 2001). It is estimated that approximately 25 to 40 percent of youth with Conduct Disorder will later meet the diagnostic criteria for Antisocial Personality Disorder (Meyers, 2014). Among JHOs, scholarship has demonstrated a continuity of criminal behaviors through their criminal histories.

Criminal histories

A one-time offense most definitely causes detrimental consequences for those involved, but the serious and violent offender that continues their criminality after being detected and punished presents an even greater threat to the community. Observing the criminal histories of JHOs has produced mixed findings. While DiCataldo and Everett's (2008) comparison of 33 JHOs to 38 non-homicide violent juvenile offenders revealed that JHOs had fewer previous delinquent referrals, fewer referrals for violent crimes, and experienced fewer out-of-home placements than the non-homicide violent offenders, other studies have suggested a more serious, and potentially pathological, criminal history associated with JHOs (Caudill & Trulson, 2016; Darby et al., 1998; Rodway et al., 2011).

Darby et al. (1998) found that the majority of juveniles convicted for a homicide-related offense had backgrounds that included a history of aggressive behaviors. Rodway et al. (2011) found that approximately one-half of their sample of JHOs had a previous conviction (52 percent) or previous reprimand (47 percent), with approximately 20 percent of the sample of juvenile homicide offenders having been previously convicted for a violent offense and 10 percent convicted previously for a weapons offense. Caudill and Trulson (2016) discovered among their sample of incarcerated JHOs that, on average, these offenders had over two previous felony offense referrals and, from a behavioral continuity perspective, approximately one-half (47 percent) of them continued their violent behavior by engaging in peer assaults while incarcerated.

Criminally involved homicides

The discrepancy found in the criminal histories of JHOs may be partially explained by the involvement of JHOs in other crimes. Cornell et al. (1987:390) suggested that criminally involved JHOs "tended to murder strangers and some familiar persons (e.g., neighbors, acquaintances), but rarely family members." Khachatryan, Heide, Rad, and Hummel (2016) furthered this line of thought by observing the unique characteristics of lone versus group JHOs and discovered that 60 percent of the offenders committed their crime against strangers, but those acting as lone offenders were statistically more likely to have murdered a known victim than a stranger (69 percent compared to 28 percent, respectively, $p < 0.01$). Furthermore, lone offenders were significantly more likely to have committed their violence as a result of interpersonal conflict than as part of a criminal activity (63 percent compared to 14 percent, respectively, $p < 0.001$). These findings suggest that there is a distinction in motivation and execution of crimes carried out by JHOs that are involved in other criminal activities and, thus, may present differing psychological traits.

Beyond the victim characteristics and group behavior of JHOs, other scholars have addressed the type of crimes in which the criminally involved JHOs engage. Rowley and associates (1987) found that approximately 58 percent of the stranger murders were associated with a theft motivation, and Mencken, Nolan, and Berhanu (2004) revealed mixed support for the hypothesis that involvement in the illicit drug market increased the likelihood that juveniles were involved in a capital crime (the murder of a law enforcement officer). Trulson and Caudill (2017) revealed further support for behavioral continuity and use of instrumental violence among a subsample of JHOs. They suggested that homicide offenders that participated in assaults on other inmates while incarcerated were significantly more likely to be rearrested post-incarceration.

Viability of rehabilitation among juvenile homicide offenders

Inherent in the correctional supervision and treatment of juvenile offenders is the idea of limited cognitive abilities and the opportunity to rehabilitate, or change, the offender's criminal trajectory. This is evinced through state legislative efforts to handle juvenile homicide offenders differently than adult homicide offenders and court rulings requiring such differential treatment (see, for example, *Graham v. Florida*, 2010; *Roper v. Simmons*, 2005). While sentencing JHOs to less severe punishments than adult homicide offenders may appear to be the morally correct action, it may not account for the impact these JHOs have on the community after being released from incarceration.

Estimates of JHO recidivism range depending on the follow-up time and diversity of samples, but all demonstrate recidivism rates over 50 percent. Heide and colleagues (Heide, Spencer, Thompson, & Solomon, 2001) revealed that 58 percent of their sample of offenders were returned to the Florida Department of Corrections within 16 years after being released for their offense, and the majority (80 percent) of those recidivists recidivated within three years post-release. Although Trulson et al. (2016) found that homicide offenders were no more likely to recidivate within five years post-incarceration than other non-sexual/non-robbery violent offenders, Trulson et al. (2012) revealed that JHOs were significantly more likely to be rearrested than non-homicide related offenders when considering only felony recidivism. Specific to felony recidivism, Caudill and Trulson (2016) discovered that approximately 60 percent (58 percent) of the released juvenile homicide offenders were rearrested within ten years of release.

Given that over one-half of JHOs studied recidivated after being released from incarceration and many of them recidivated for felony-level criminality, it is important to understand the factors associated with recidivism among these serious and violent offenders. Khachatryan et al. (2016) found that JHOs committing their violence as part of group were more likely to be rearrested following their release than were the lone offenders. Trulson and Caudill (2017) found no statistical distinction in recidivism rates between those JHOs convicted of non-capital and capital homicides (48 percent compared to 54 percent, respectively) during their three-year follow-up period. However, they did discover that those JHOs that continued their use of violence while incarcerated (assault on staff) and presented other behavioral problems (i.e., program disruption) while incarcerated were at a significantly greater risk of recidivism post-release (Caudill & Trulson, 2016). This persistent criminality among these serious and violent offenders, while not diagnosed as psychopathic, may well represent the behavioral outcomes of personality traits – such as callousness, apathy, narcissism, hostility, disregard for laws, impulsivity, irresponsibility, and risk-taking – that naturally result in a threat to public safety. How society deals with JHOs, especially those that demonstrate antisocial abnormalities, is of paramount interest.

Social consequences

Juvenile homicide offending is clearly of concern and is shocking to the conscience of society. Evidence suggests that JHOs have distinctly different social histories than their non-homicide juvenile offender counterparts, with many of them experiencing exposure to violence through abuse and familial criminality. While there is evidence to suggest JHOs use instrumental violence to achieve some end, these ends appear to differ depending on the circumstances of the crime, the victim, and the offender's background. The findings of behavioral continuity among JHOs translate to a continued threat to the community once these offenders are released from incarceration and, thus, understanding to greater degree the underlying mechanism that perpetuate serious violent offending patterns among youthful offenders deserves attention. As discussed, the psychological abnormalities, use of illicit substances and alcohol, and troubles integrating into social institutions – such as school – present unique challenges among those juveniles that kill. Toward this end, examining the incidence of psychopathy among the JHOs has started to receive considerable attention, with a desire to be able to separate the most dangerous (i.e., those most likely to reoffend in terms of serious violent crimes) from the JHOs who could potentially be rehabilitated.

Because of the DSM–5's limited ability to recognize psychopathy among juveniles, the three-factor model of child and adolescent psychopathy has been recommended in the literature examining psychopathy among those under the age of 18 (Salekin, 2016). Indeed, during the past few decades, research on child and adolescent psychopathy has demonstrated that this is a multifaceted disorder, underlined by grandiose/manipulation, callous–unemotional, and daring–impulsive traits (Dong, Wu, & Waldman, 2014; Salekin & Lynam, 2010). This body of research is especially important in distinguishing psychopathy from Conduct Disorder, a DSM–5 diagnosis that has been criticized by some experts for not including all three facets of child psychopathy in its criteria (Salekin, 2016).

While many of the individual items as well as the factors themselves may be highly correlated with each other depending on the scale used, a mounting body of evidence shows that both child and adolescent psychopathy can be best described with three-factor models (Dong et al., 2014). These factors can be roughly divided as explained below, and not all children/adolescents who score high on one dimension will automatically score high on another (Salekin, 2016). Grandiose/manipulation facet, depending on the scale, measures mostly interpersonal traits, which may include items attempting to gauge an individual's thoughts about him/herself as more important than others, excessive bragging, using others as means, exhibitions of superficial charm, bullying, sensitivity to perceived criticism, pathological lying, parasitic orientation, and shallow emotions (Dong et al., 2014; Salekin, 2016). Callous–unemotional component, again, depending on the scale, measures mostly affective characteristics, which may include items attempting to evaluate the individual's lack of concern for others, lack of guilt and remorse, lack of concern about school work or other responsibilities, undependability, irresponsibility, inability to show/feel emotions, and lack of stable friendships. Finally, daring–impulsive measures mostly behavioral dimensions of personality, which may include items involving the individual's tendency to act without thinking, short sightedness, engagement in risky activities, boredom, blaming others for his/her mistakes, early problem behavior, criminal versatility, and poor Anger control (Dong et al., 2014;Salekin, 2016).

Implications

The safety of citizens and the humane treatment of adolescent offenders must be weighed against one other when attempting to determine which JHOs would be most suitable candidates for rehabilitation and early release. Since a vast body of empirical literature has consistently shown the connection between psychopathy and an elevated risk of future violence among adolescents (Brandt et al., 1997; Campbell et al., 2004; Forth & Mailloux, 2000; Frick, 1998; Lynam, 2002) and adults (Douglas, Vincent, & Edens, 2006; Hare, 1999), it is unsurprising that instruments such as PCL: YV (Psychopathy Checklist: Youth Version) have been increasingly utilized in assessing serious juvenile offenders, including JHOs, in criminal justice settings. Results from these assessments could potentially influence decisions, ranging from whether the juvenile will be tried as an adult (OJJDP, n.d.) to a jury's sentencing decision (Boccaccini, Murrie, Clark, & Cornell, 2008). Due to far-reaching and in many cases life-altering consequences that these assessments can potentially have on the JHOs and other serious juvenile delinquents, it is important to understand the validity and reliability of these instruments.

Literature on the predictive validity of various juvenile psychopathy assessment instruments regarding violent recidivism has been mixed. Several studies find support for one type of instrument but not others (Hilterman, Nicholls, & Chjis van Nieuwenhuizen, 2014; Marczyk,

Heilbrun, Lander, & DeMatteo, 2003), while others (see Catchpole & Gretton, 2003) assert that most commonly used youth psychopathy scales are accurate in predicting violent reoffending. To gain a more comprehensive picture of the discrepancies, Sharp and Kine (2008) conducted a meta-review on the strengths and weaknesses of current assessments used to measure psychopathy in juveniles. In their review, the authors included aspects such as reliability and factor structure, as well as criterion-related construct and predictive validity. While Sharp and Kine pointed out some issues relating to criterion-related validity and internal consistency, they also appeared optimistic that future research will provide more confidence in these constructs, likely evaporating some fears and confusion.

Perhaps the most frequently evaluated youth psychopathy assessment tool is the PCL: YV.[3] The Hare Psychopathy Checklist: Youth Version (PCL: YV, Forth, Kosson, & Hare, 2003) is a 20-item checklist (each item having a potential score varying from 0 to 2), measuring clusters of affective, interpersonal, and behavioral characteristics similar to the DSM–5 diagnosis criteria for Antisocial Personality Disorder (i.e., grandiosity/narcissism, deceitfulness, manipulativeness, lack of empathy, callousness, hostility, disregard for laws, impulsivity, irresponsibility, and risk-taking) (OJJDP, n.d.). As with the adult scale, a score of 30 (out of a maximum of 40 points) is considered the cut-off criterion for psychopathy (Fort et al.; MacArthur Foundation, 2006). However, there is some evidence that a lower threshold (those with scores of 20 or higher) exhibit significant personality impairment and may be at increased risk of criminal behavior and violence (Meyers, 2014). A study by Cauffman and colleagues (2009) compared the accuracy of predicting recidivism across several assessment measures of juvenile psychopathy, including the PCL: YV. Consistent with previous comparisons, they concluded that there were substantial discrepancies between the different scales. More specifically, they cautioned that while the scores obtained from the different psychopathy assessment instruments might be useful in affording short-term increases in monitoring juveniles with elevated scores, practitioners should be careful in making long-term predictions regarding adolescent recidivism based on the scores obtained from these instruments. "Moreover, the lack of long-term predictive power for the PCL: YV and the inconsistent psychopathy designations obtained with different measures raise serious questions about the use of such measures as the basis for legal or clinical treatment decisions" (Cauffman et al. p. 528). Odgers, Reppucci, and Moretti (2005) reached similar conclusions in a sample of 125 female juvenile offenders. Using advanced statistical modeling, the authors found that PCL: YV scores failed to significantly predict recidivism.

That said, there is a vein of literature countering this perspective and suggesting that the PCL: YV is predictive of recidivism. Catchpole and Gretton (2003) conducted a one-year evaluation of criminal outcomes in 74 violent juvenile offenders and found PCL: YV scores to be significantly predictive of both general and violent reoffending. Gretton, Hare and Catchpole (2004) conducted a ten-year follow-up study of adolescent boys ranging from ages 12 to 18 and demonstrated that the total PCL: YV score was significantly and positively correlated with violent recidivism. Similarly, Corrado, Vincent, Hart, and Cohen (2004) discovered among a sample of 182 adolescent male offenders that the PCL: YV significantly predicted both general and violent reoffending. They estimated that the predictive accuracy of PCL: YV for violent recidivism was 65 percent (as compared to 63 percent for nonviolent and 68 percent for overall recidivism). However, Corrado and his colleagues suggested that the predictive validity of PCL: YV was explained mostly through the behavioral dimensions of psychopathy rather than affective or interpersonal dimensions. In the three-factor model of child and adolescent psychopathy, discussed earlier in this chapter, this would correspond to the daring–impulsive facet.

Being able to accurately measure psychopathy in serious and violent juvenile offenders, especially among those juveniles who have committed homicides, could be vital in individualizing sentences. With two recent U.S. Supreme Court cases, *Jackson v. Hobbs* (2011) and *Miller v. Alabama* (2012), ruling that "life without parole" sentences for juveniles was unconstitutional for even the most serious of offenses (see *Graham v. Florida*, 2010), it is expected that states may need to resentence numerous offenders sentenced to life without parole as juveniles. Consequently, state parole boards will take on the important but difficult task of making the risk–benefit assessment regarding which individuals to release from state custody and when. On one end of the spectrum is the reality that the longer we keep the young offenders in the criminal justice system, the more institutionalized they become and more money they will cost to society (MacArthur Foundation, 2006). On the other end of the spectrum is the inherent risk presented by releasing juvenile homicide offenders and research suggesting that longer incarcerations may reduce recidivism risks (Caudill & Trulson, 2016; MacArthur Foundation, 2006).

Conclusion

This chapter explored the potential relationship between psychopathy and juvenile homicide offending. The current literature supports the notion that juvenile homicide offenders have unique and, in many cases, deleterious experiences, such as exposure to violence, through their families and at the hands of those they hold in high regard. While the origins of psychopathy are less clear (see DeLisi 2016) and there is concern that branding a youthful offender with a personality disorder may have negative effects over the individual's life course, what is clear is that psychopathic traits do present themselves in juvenile offenders (Salihovic, Özdemir, Kerr, 2014). More specifically, the literature on juvenile offenders has identified the three-factor model of child and adolescent psychopathy, which recognizes that there are three distinct but often overlapping and correlated facets to child and adolescent psychopathy: grandiose/manipulation, callous–unemotional, and daring–impulsive traits (Dong et al. 2014; Salekin & Lynam, 2010).

Although juvenile homicide offending is a rare event, those juveniles that commit murder evince some troubling psychological characteristics. Of these most violent juvenile offenders, a subclass of them exhibit traits aligned with the three-factor model of psychopathy, such as callousness, grandiosity, manipulativeness, impulsivity, disregard for law and the welfare of others, and risk taking. Further complicating matters is the continuity of behavior among JHOs. Research suggests that more than one-half of the juveniles that commit homicide recidivate for another felony offense after being punished for their crimes. While the scholarly evidence suggests a prevalence of psychopathic traits among the most serious, violent, and habitual juvenile offenders; the social conscience has limited the criminal justice system's abilities to deal effectively with the threat they pose. Thus, being able to accurately diagnose those who may possess the most serious risk of future harm to society (i.e., severe psychopathic traits) would seem beneficial. Yet, as can be seen from the discussion presented in this chapter, the diagnostic tools available (i.e., DSM–5 and different youth psychopathy scales) have documented weaknesses in this regard. While the DSM–5's revised diagnostic criteria for Antisocial Personality Disorder has considerable overlap with the empirically and clinically recognized construct of "psychopathy," Antisocial Personality Disorder cannot be diagnosed in individuals younger than 18 (APA, 2013). Alternatively, several clinical instruments developed to measure psychopathy in youth, such as PCL: YV, have been criticized for their potential lack of predictive validity regarding recidivism and other issues (Cauffman et al., 2009; Odgers et al., 2005; Sharp & Kine, 2008).

Indeed, while most clinicians report using psychopathy instruments as tools when making risk assessments with juveniles, most also express extreme concern about labeling juveniles as psychopaths (Viljoen, McLachlan, & Vincent, 2010). Rather, "juvenile risk reports were more likely than adult reports to routinely discuss treatment and protective factors, and provide recommendations to reevaluate risk" (Viljoen et al. 2010:377). Further, labeling juveniles as "psychopaths" has also shown to influence jury's decisions regarding sentence severities for the same offenses (Boccaccini et al., 2008). A couple studies have suggested that violent delinquents may be worth treating as they showed benefits of intensive treatment programs over the traditional criminal justice system responses (see Caldwell, Vitacco, & Van Rybroek, 2006). Similar results have been achieved among those youth scoring high on the PCL: YV: "Treatment is associated with relatively slower and lower rates of serious recidivism, even after controlling for the effects of nonrandom assignment to treatment groups and release status" (Caldwell, Skeem, Salekin, & Van Rybroek, 2006:571).

Ultimately, the goal here is to recognize the individual nature of criminality and, thus, the need for more individualized sentences of those juvenile offenders that commit the most heinous of crimes. The juvenile justice system was designed under the auspices of the *parens patriae* doctrine – the government acts in the best interest of the juvenile – and this allows for agents and organizations to move beyond the legal aspects of the crime. In many respects, the juvenile court attempts to balance the best interests of the offender and the public safety needs of the community, and there may be further opportunity here to be more refined in this process. While there may be value in treatment for JHOs that express psychopathic traits (Caldwell, Vitacco, & Van Rybroek, 2006), the ability of the court to recognize these individual characteristics in invaluable. Collectively, "broad-brush approaches . . . hinder the utility of the criminal justice system by overlooking the individualized and situational nature of behavior" (Caudill & Ptacek, 2017:32–33). As demonstrated in this chapter, the only absolute characteristics of juvenile homicide offending is the statutory nature of the offenders and the serious and violent nature of their crimes. Some, indeed, also express psychopathic traits and, for them, more serious and deliberate mechanisms of formal social control should be available.

Notes

1 The antagonist pathological personality traits involve manipulativeness, deceitfulness, callousness, and hostility. The disinhibitionist pathological personality traits include irresponsibility, impulsivity, and risk taking. In addition, these traits must be free of cultural context, expressed persistently over a period of time, occur in different life settings, and not be solely a result of a medical condition or substance use (APA, 2013).

2 Black et al. (2010) found no statistical difference in the prevalence of Antisocial Personality Disorder for males and females among their incarcerated sample of offenders.

3 Multiple questionnaire measures of juvenile psychopathy have been developed over the past 30 years, including the Antisocial Process Screening Devise (APSD; Frick & Hare, 2001; Frick, O'Brien, Wootton, & McBurnett, 1994), the Child Psychopathy Scale (CPS; Lynam, 1997), the Psychopathy Content Scale (PCS; Murrie & Cornell, 2000); and the Youth Psychopathic Traits Inventory (YPI; Andershed, Kerr, Sattin, & Levander, 2002). However, perhaps one of the most widely used instruments to measure psychopathy in psychiatric, correctional, and research settings, the Hare's (2003) Revised Psychopathy Checklist (PCL-R), has also been modified to measure psychopathic tendencies in youth from 12 to 18 (Sharp & Kine, 2008).

References

American Psychiatric Association. (2013) *Diagnostic and statistical manual of mental disorders* (5th ed.), Arlington, VA: American Psychiatric Publishing.

Andershed, H. (2010) 'Stability and change of psychopathic traits: What do we know?,' in R. Salekin & D. R. Lynam (Eds.), *Handbook of child and adolescent psychopathy* (pp. 233–250), New York, NY: Guilford Press.

Andershed, H., Kerr, M., Sattin, H., and Levander, S. (2002) 'Psychopathic traits in non-referred youths: A new assessment tool,' in E. Blauuw & L. Sheridan (Eds.), *Psychopaths: Current International Perspectives* (pp. 131–158), The Hague: Elsevier.

Barajas, M. (2013) Murder destroyed Charity Lee's family, forever altered her concept of justice. *San Antonio Current*, June 11, 2013. Retrieved August 18, 2017 from www.sacurrent.com/sanantonio/murder-destroyed-charity-lees-family-forever-altered-her-concept-of-justice/Content?oid=2246452

Black, D. W., Gunter, T., Loveless, P., Allen, J., and Sieleni, B. (2010) 'Antisocial personality disorder in incarcerated offenders: Psychiatric comorbidity and quality of life,' *Annals of Clinical Psychiatry*, *22*(2):113–120.

Boccaccini, M. T., Murrie, D. C., Clark, J. W., and Cornell, D. G. (2008) 'Describing, diagnosing, and naming psychopathy: How do youth psychopathy labels influence jurors?,' *Behavioral Sciences and the Law*, *26*:487–510.

Brandt, J. R., Kennedy, W. A., Patrick, C. J., and Curtain, J. J. (1997) 'Assessment of psychopathy in a population of incarcerated adolescent offenders,' *Psychological Assessment*, *9*:429–435.

Busch, K. G., Zagar, R., Hughes, J. R., Arbit, J., and Bussell, R. E. (1990) 'Adolescents who kill,' *Journal of Clinical Psychology*, *46*(4):472–485.

Caldwell, M. F., Skeem, J., Salekin, R., and Van Rybroek, G. J. (2006) 'Treatment response of adolescent offenders with psychopathy features: A 2-year follow-up?,' *Criminal Justice and Behavior*, *33*(5):571–596.

Caldwell, M. F., Vitacco, M., and Van Rybroek, G. J. (2006) 'Are violent delinquents worth treating?,' *Journal of Research in Crime and Delinquency*, *43*(2):148–168.

Campbell, M. A., Porter, S., and Santor, D. (2004) 'Psychopathic traits in adolescent offenders: An evaluation of criminal history, clinical, and psychosocial correlates,' *Behavioral Science and the Law*, *22*:22–47.

Catchpole, R. E. H., and Gretton, H. M. (2003) 'The predictive validity of risk assessment with violent young offenders: 1-year examination of criminal outcome,' *Criminal Justice and Behavior*, *30*(6):688–708.

Caudill, J. W., and Ptacek, P. (2017) 'Sentencing: Individualized considerations of broad-brush reforms,' *ACJS Today*, *42*(3):29–35.

Caudill, J. W., and Trulson, C. R. (2016) 'The hazards of premature release: Recidivism outcomes of blended-sentenced juvenile homicide offenders,' *Journal of Criminal Justice*, *46*:219–227.

Cauffman, E., Kimonis, E. R., Dmitrieva, J., and Monahan, K. (2009) 'A multimethod assessment of juvenile psychopathy: Comparing the predictive utility of the PCL:YV, YPI, and NEO PRI,' *Psychological Assessment*, *21*(4):528–542.

Cornell, D. G., Benedek, E. P., and Benedek, D. M. (1987) 'Juvenile homicide: Prior adjustment and a proposed typology,' *American Journal of Orthopsychiatry*, *57*(3):383–393.

Corrado, R. R., Vincent, G. M., Hart, S. D., and Cohen, I. M. (2004) 'Predictive validity of the Psychopathy Checklist: Youth Version for general and violent recidivism,' *Behavioral Science and the Law*, *22*:5–22.

Darby, P. J., Allan, W. D., Kashani, J. H., Hartke, K. L., and Reid, J. C. (1998) 'Analysis of 112 juveniles who committed homicide: Characteristics and a closer look at family abuse,' *Journal of Family Violence*, *13*(4):365–375.

DeLisi, M. (2016) *Psychopathy as unified theory of crime*, New York, NY: Palgrave Macmillan.

DeLisi, M., Alcala, J., Kusow, A., Hochstetler, A., Heirigs, M. H., Caudill, J. W., . . ., and Baglivio, M. T. (2017) 'Adverse childhood experiences, commitment offense, and race/ethnicity: Are the effects crime-, race-, and ethnicity-specific?,' *International Journal of Environmental Research and Public Health*, *14*:331–342.

DeLisi, M., Kosloski, A., Sween, M., Hachmeister, E., Moore, M., and Drury, A. (2010) 'Murder by the numbers: Monetary costs imposed by a sample of homicide offenders,' *The Journal of Forensic Psychiatry & Psychology*, *21*(4):501–513.

DeLisi, M., Piquero, A. R., and Cardwell, S. M. (2016) 'The unpredictability of murder: Juvenile homicide in the Pathways to Desistance Study,' *Youth Violence & Juvenile Justice*, *14*(1):26–42.

DeLisi, M. & Vaughn, M. G. (2012) 'Still psychopathic after all these years?,' in M. DeLisi & P. J. Conis (Eds.), *Violent offenders: Theory, research, policy, and practice* (2nd ed., pp. 67–76), Burlington, MA: Jones & Bartlett Learning.

DiCataldo, F., and Everett, M. (2008) 'Distinguishing juvenile homicide from violent juvenile offending,' *International Journal of Offender Therapy and Comparative Criminology*, *52*(2):158–174.

Dong, L., Wu, H., and Waldman, I. D. (2014) 'Measurement and structural invariance of the Antisocial Process Screening Device,' *Psychological Assessment*, *26*:598–608.

Douglas, K. S., Vincent, G. M., and Edens, J. F. (2006) 'Risk for criminal recidivism: The role of psychopathy,' in C. J. Patrick (Ed.), *Handbook of psychopathy* (pp. 533–554), New York, NY: Guilford Press.

Forth, A. E., Kosson, D. S., and Hare, R. D. (2003) *The Psychopathy Checklist: Youth Version*, Toronto, ON: Multi-Health Systems.
Forth, A. E., and Mailloux, D. L. (2000) 'Psychopathy in youth: What do we know?,' in C. B. Gacono (Ed.), *The Clinical and Forensic Assessment of Psychopathy: A Practitioner's Guide* (pp. 25–54), Mahwah, NJ: Erlbaum.
Frick, P. J. (1998) *Conduct disorders and severe antisocial behavior*, New York, NY: Plenum Press.
Frick, P. J., and Hare, R. D. (2001) *The Antisocial Process Screening Device*, Toronto, ON: Multi-Health Systems.
Frick, P. J., O'Brien, B. S., Wootton, J. M., and McBurnett, K. (1994) 'Psychopathy and conduct problems in children,' *Journal of Abnormal Psychology*, *103*:700–707.
Graham v. Florida, 560 U.S. 48 (2010).
Gretton, H. M., Hare, R. D., and Catchpole, R. E. H. (2004) 'Psychopathy and offending from adolescence to adulthood: A 10-year follow-up,' *Journal of Consulting and Clinical Psychology*, *72*(4):636–645.
Hare, R. D. (1999) 'Psychopathy as a risk factor for violence,' *Psychiatric Quarterly*, *70*(3):181–197.
Hare, R. D. (2003) *The Hare Psychopathy Checklist–Revised*, Toronto, ON: Multi-Health Systems.
Hare, R. D., and Neumann, C. S. (2008) 'Psychopathy as a clinical and empirical construct,' *Annual Review of Clinical Psychology*, *4*:217–246.
Heide, K. M. (1995) *Why kids kill parents*, London: Sage Publications.
Heide, K. M. (2013) Understanding parricide: When sons and daughters kill parents, New York, NY: Oxford University Press.
Heide, K. M., Spencer, E., Thompson, A., and Solomon, E. (2001) 'Who's in, who's out, and who's back: Follow-up data on 59 juveniles incarcerated in adult prison for murder or attempted murder in the early 1980s,' *Behavioral Sciences and the Law*, *19*:97–108.
Hill-Smith, A. J., Hugo, P., Hughes, P., Fonagy, P., and Hartman, D. (2002) 'Adolescents murderers: Abuse and adversity in childhood,' *Journal of Adolescence*, *25*:221–230.
Hilterman, L. B., Nicholls, T. L., and van Nieuwenhuizen, C. (2014) 'Predictive validity of risk assessments in juvenile offenders: Comparing the SAVRY, PCL:YV, and YLS/CMI with unstructured clinical assessments,' *Assessment*, *21*(3):324–339.
Holmes, S. E., Slaughter, J. R., and Kashani, J. (2001) 'Risk factors in childhood that lead to the development of conduct disorder and antisocial personality disorder,' *Child Psychiatry and Human Development*, *31*(3):183–193.
Jackson v. Hobbs, 132 S. CT. 548 (2011).
Khachatryan, N., Heide, K. M., Rad, J., and Hummel, E. V. (2016) 'Post-incarceration recidivism of lone versus group juvenile homicide offenders,' *Behavioral Sciences and the Law*, *34*:709–725.
Lindberg, N., Laajasalo, T., Holi, M., Putkonen, H., Weizmann-Henelius, G., and Häkkänen-Nyholm, H. (2009) 'Psychopathic traits and offender characteristics – a nationwide consecutive sample of homicidal male adolescents,' *BMC Psychiatry*, *9*:18–29.
Lynam, D. R. (1997) 'Pursuing the psychopath: Capturing the fledgling psychopath in a nomological net,' *Journal of Abnormal Psychology*, *106*:425–438.
Lynam, D. R. (2002) 'Fledgling psychopathy: A view from personality theory,' *Law and Human Behavior*, *26*:255–259.
MacArthur Foundation: Research Network on Adolescent Development and Juvenile Justice. (2006, September) *Issue brief 4: Assessing juvenile psychopathy: Developmental and legal implications*. Retrieved March 29, 2018 from https://ncfy.acf.hhs.gov/library/2006/assessing-juvenile-psychopathy-developmental-and-legal-implications
Marczyk, G. R., Heilbrun, K., Lander, T., and DeMatteo, D. (2003) 'Predicting juvenile recidivism with the PCL:YV, MAYSI, and YLS/CMI,' *International Journal of Forensic Mental Health*, *2*(1):7–18.
McGee, J., and DeBernardo, C. (1999) 'The classroom avenger,' *Forensic Examiner*, *8*:16–18.
Meloy, J. R., Hempel, A., Gray, T., Mohandie, K., Shiva, A, and Richards, T. C. (2004) 'Comparative analysis of North American adolescent and adult mass murderers,' *Behavioral Sciences and the Law*, *22*:291–309.
Meloy, J. R., Hempel, A., Mohandie, K., Shiva, A, and Gray, T. (2001) 'Offender and offense characteristics of a nonrandom sample of adolescent mass murderers,' *Journal of the American Academy of Child Adolescent Psychiatry*, *40*:719–728.
Mencken, F. C., Nolan, J., and Berhanu, S. (2004) 'Juveniles, illicit drug activity, and homicides against law enforcement officers,' *Homicide Studies*, *8*(4):327–349.
Meyers, S. (2014, February 3) The sociopathic child: Myths, parenting tips, what to do. *Psychology Today*. Retrieved March 29, 2018 from www.psychologytoday.com/blog/insight-is-2020/201402/the-sociopathic-child-myths-parenting-tips-what-do

Miller v. Alabama, 132 S. Ct. 2455 (2012).

Moffitt, T. E. (1993) 'Adolescence-limited and life-course-persistent antisocial behavior: a developmental taxonomy,' *Psychological Review*, *100*:674–701.

Mohr, J. W., and McKnight, C. K. (1971) 'Violence as a function of age and relationship with special reference to matricide,' *Canadian Psychiatric Association Journal*, *16*(1):29–32.

Murrie, D. C., and Cornell, D. G. (2000) 'The Millon adolescent clinical inventory and psychopathy,' *Journal of Personality Assessment*, *75*:110–125.

Myers, W. C., and Blashfield, R. (1997) 'Psychopathology and personality in juvenile sexual homicide offenders,' *Journal of the American Academy of Psychiatry and the Law*, *25*(4):497–508.Myers, W. C., Chan, H. C., Vo, E. J., and Lazarou, E. (2010) 'Sexual sadism, psychopathy, and recidivism in juvenile sexual murderers,' *Journal of Investigative Psychology and Offender Profiling*, 7:49–58.

Odgers, C. L., Reppucci, N. D., and Moretti, M. M. (2005) 'Nipping psychopathy in the bud: An examination of the convergent, predictive, and theoretical utility of the PCL–YV among adolescent girls,' *Behavioral Sciences and the Law*, *23*(6):743–763.

Office of Juvenile Justice and Delinquency Prevention (OJJDP) (n.d.). *Instrument profile: Psychopathy Checklist: Youth Version (PCL–YV)*. Retrieved March 29, 2018 from www.nttac.org/index.cfm?event=gsg.WebtoolSearchResultsInstrumentDetails&id=65

Patterson, G. R., Reid, J. R., and Dishion, T. J. (1992) *Antisocial boys*, Eugene, OR: Castalia.

Porter, S., and Woodworth, M. (2006) 'Psychopathy and aggression,' in C. J. Patrick (Ed.), *Handbook of psychopathy* (pp. 481–494), New York, NY: Guilford Press.

Rodway, C., Norrington-Moore, V., While, D., Hunt, I. M., Flynn, S., Swinson, N., Roscoe, A., Appleby, L., and Shaw, J. (2011) 'A population-based study of juvenile perpetrators of homicide in England and Wales,' *Journal of Adolescence*, *34*:19–28.

Roper v. Simmons, 543 U.S. 551 (2005).

Rowley, J. C., Ewing, C. P., and Singer, S. I. (1987) 'Juvenile homicide: The need for an interdisciplinary approach,' *Behavioral Sciences & the Law*, *5*(1):1–10.

Salekin, R. T. (2016) 'Psychopathy in childhood: Why should we care about grandiose–manipulative and daring–impulsive traits?,' *British Journal of Psychiatry*, *209*:189–191.

Salekin, R. T., and Lynam, D. R. (2010) *Handbook of child and adolescent psychopathy*, New York, NY: Guilford Press.

Salihovic, S., Özdemir, M., and Kerr, M. (2014) 'Trajectories of adolescent psychopathic traits,' *Journal of Psychopathology and Behavioral Assessment*, *36*(1):47–59.

Sampson, R. J., and Laub, J. H. (1995) 'Understanding variability in lives through time: Contributions of life-course criminology,' *Studies on Crime & Crime Prevention*, *4*(2):143–158.

Sharp, C., and Kine, S. (2008) 'The assessment of juvenile psychopathy: Strengths and weaknesses of currently used questionnaire measures,' *Child and Adolescent Mental Health*, *13*(2):5–95.

Trulson, C. R., and Caudill, J. W. (2017) 'Juvenile homicide offender recidivism,' *Journal of Criminal Psychology*, 7(2):93–104.

Trulson, C. R., Caudill, J. W., Haerle, D. R., and DeLisi, M. (2012) 'Cliqued up: The postincarceration recidivism of young gang-related homicide offenders,' *Criminal Justice Review*, *37*(2):174–190.

Trulson, C. R., Caudill, J. W., Haerle, D. R., and DeLisi, M. (2016) *Lost causes: Blended sentencing, second chances, and the Texas Youth Commission*, Austin, TX: University of Texas Press.

Vaughn, M. G., and Howard, M. O. (2005) 'The construct of psychopathy and its potential contribution to the study of serious, violent, and chronic youth offending,' *Youth Violence and Juvenile Justice*, *3*:235–252.

Viljoen, J. L., McLachlan, K., and Vincent, G. M. (2010) 'Assessing violence risk and psychopathy in juvenile and adult offenders: A survey of clinical practices,' *Assessment*, *17*(3):377–395.

Woodworth, M., and Porter, S. (2002) 'In cold blood: Characteristics of criminal homicides as a function of psychopathy,' *Journal of Abnormal Psychology*, *111*(3):436–445.

21

Psychopathy and sexual aggression

A review of empirical research

Jesse Cale and Melanie Burton

Introduction

The interpersonal, affective, and behavioral characteristics of psychopathy have direct relevance for understanding sexual aggression. However, the link between psychopathy and sexual aggression is multifaceted and varies across different dimensions of sexual aggression. Several theoretical models of sexual aggression incorporate psychopathy as a key explanatory construct (e.g., Knight & Sims-Knight 2003; Malamuth 2003; Seto & Barbaree 1997; Lalumière, Harris, Quinsey, & Rice, 2005). Furthermore, some researchers have argued that psychopathy and psychopathic traits are an integral component of sexual aggression. For example, Knight and Sims-Knight (2003) suggested there are at least two developmental pathways to sexual aggression associated with the presence of psychopathic personality characteristics. The first is the "antisocial pathway," characterized by a general versatile pattern of criminal behavior. In this pathway, sex offenses are opportunistic and reflect a combination of precocious sexuality and a general tendency to act in an aggressive and antisocial manner. The second is the "callous–unemotional pathway," characterized by a lack of emotional responsivity/emotional inhibitions to causing pain, suffering, and distress in others. As a result of the absence of internal emotional inhibitions, certain individuals characterized by callousness and unemotional traits who also experience deviant sexual fantasies that disinhibit their sexual behaviors may be particularly at risk of committing acts of sexual aggression (see also Malamuth, 1998, 2003).

Finally, these pathways are not necessarily mutually exclusive; a third pathway characterized by the combination of the callous–unemotional and antisocial pathways represents a more complete picture of psychopathy and possibly the most serious sexual aggressors. These pathways have been hypothesized to characterize both juvenile and adult sexual aggression (e.g., Knight & Sims-Knight 2004).

In order to investigate characteristics of these pathways more closely, below we examine the empirical evidence on the link between psychopathy and sexual aggression in studies of incarcerated sexual aggressors with an aim to scrutinize: (1) the prevalence of psychopathy across types of sexual aggressors; (2) empirical evidence on the link between psychopathy and sexual deviance; (3) empirical evidence on the relationship between psychopathy and recidivism; and (4) empirical evidence on the relationship between psychopathy and juvenile sexual aggression.

The measurement of psychopathy among sexual aggressors

Since the early 1990s, the number of studies examining the link between psychopathy and sexual aggression has increased substantially, and the majority of studies use the Psychopathy Checklist–Revised version (PCL–R; Hare, 1991, 2003). The PCL–R consists of 20 items rated on a 3-point scale (0 = item does not apply to the individual, 1 = item applies in some circumstances, 2 = item definitely applies to the individual) measuring the personality, interpersonal, and behavioral aspects of the psychopathy construct. The two main factors that constitute the disorder involve: (1) interpersonal/affective traits (i.e., Factor 1); and (2) lifestyle/antisocial behavior (i.e., Factor 2). The interpersonal facet of factor one involves traits including glibness/superficial charm, a grandiose sense of self-worth, pathological lying, and a conning/manipulative interpersonal style. The affective facet of Factor 1 includes traits reflecting lack of remorse, shallow affect, lack of empathy, and not accepting responsibility. The lifestyle facet of Factor 2 involves the need for stimulation, a parasitic lifestyle, lack of goals, impulsivity, and irresponsibility. Finally, the antisocial facet of Factor 2 includes poor behavioral controls, early behavioral problems, juvenile delinquency, revocation of conditional release, and criminal versatility. While a total score of 40 on the PCL–R is possible, Hare (1991) and others suggest that a score of 30 represents the clinical cut-off that distinguishes psychopathic individuals. Most studies using the PCL–R with samples of sexual aggressors report overall scores, with fewer reporting facet level findings.

The PCL–R is intended for the assessment of psychopathic personality characteristics by clinicians who have received specialized training, drawing information on individuals from multiple sources (e.g., interviews, case files, etc.). For several studies with incarcerated sexual aggressors, researchers have accessed institutional case files (e.g., in forensic psychiatric facilities, prisons) where clinicians have previously assessed and recorded PCL–R assessments. In others, researchers have received specialized training and conducted PCL–R assessments through interviews with research participants in addition to using corroborating file-based information/evidence. Finally, some studies rely specifically on file-based information on individuals; researchers may receive training to conduct PCL–R assessments and score them solely according to file-based information on participants and then conduct interrater reliability analysis for specific cases. It is important to note these differences in procedures in studies of psychopathy and sexual aggression because there is evidence of discrepancies in scoring between trained clinicians, trained researchers, and researchers using solely file-based information (e.g., see Murrie, Boccaccini, Caperton, & Rufino, 2012).

Although the PCL–R is intended for use with adults, some studies have applied it in the context of assessing psychopathic personality characteristics among sexually aggressive youth (e.g., Långström & Grann 2000; Långström & Lindblad 2000; Myers & Blashfield, 1997), modifying certain questions so they are more age appropriate. More commonly in studies with sexually aggressive youth, the Psychopathy Checklist–Youth Version (PCL: YV; Forth, Kosson, & Hare, 2003) is utilized. The PCL: YV is derived from the PCL–R and intended for use with adolescents based on interviews and corroborating information. Similar to the PCL–R, it is based on 20 items across four factors (interpersonal, affective, behavioral, and antisocial) with items that have been modified for use with adolescents. The interpersonal factor consists of items including: impression management; grandiose sense of self-worth; pathological lying; and manipulation for personal gain. The affective factor includes: lack of remorse; shallow affect; callousness/lack of empathy; and failure to accept responsibility. The behavioral factor involves: need for stimulation; parasitic orientation; lack of goals; impulsivity; and irresponsibility. Finally, the antisocial factor of the PCL: YV includes: poor anger control; early behavioral problems;

serious criminal behavior; serious violations of release; and criminal versatility. While there is no cut-off score for a diagnosis of psychopathy among youth (i.e., compared to a cut-off score of 30 for the PCL–R with adults), several studies with sexually aggressive youth nonetheless delineate specific cut-off scores, usually between 25 to 30.

The PCL–R and PCL: YV are the most common instruments used to assess psychopathic personality characteristics in studies of sexually aggressive youth and adults. The current review focuses primarily on studies based on these instruments with incarcerated sexual aggressor populations. We also make note of studies that have utilized other instruments assessing psychopathic personality characteristics among sexual aggressors, including: the Psychopathic Personality Inventory (PPI; Lilienfeld & Andrews, 1996; e.g., Strassberg, Eastvold, Kenney, & Suchy, 2012); the Antisocial Process Screening Device (APSD) (Frick & Hare, 2001; e.g., Caputo, Frick, & Brodsky, 1999); the Youth Psychopathic Traits Inventory (YPI; Andershed, Kerr, Stattin, & Levander, 2002; e.g., Boonmann et al., 2015). and specific scales related to psychopathic personality traits based on the Multidimensional Inventory of Development, Sex, and Aggression (MIDSA; Augur Enterprises Inc, 2007; Netland & Miner 2012).

The prevalence of psychopathy among adult sexual aggressors

The prevalence of psychopathy varies substantially between types of sexual aggressors. It also varies within certain types, where certain facets of psychopathy are associated with different aspects of sexual aggression (e.g., the presence of sexual deviance, the level of violence in sex offenses, and recidivism). In custodial and forensic settings, sexual aggressors of women display similar or elevated levels of psychopathy compared to non-sex offenders (Book, Clark, Forth, & Hare, 2006:153). Furthermore, ample empirical evidence shows that the prevalence of psychopathy varies substantially between sexual aggressors of women, sexual aggressors of children, and polymorphic sexual aggressors (i.e., those who offend against multiple victim types) across different samples.

In a sample of 2,514 incarcerated adult males in the United States, Brown, Dargis, Mattern, Tsonis, and Newman (2015) reported that prevalence rates of psychopathy using a cut-off score of 30 and above on the PCL–R ranged from 32.5 percent for polymorphic sexual aggressors, 25.5 percent for sexual aggressors of women, 22.0 percent for non-sex offenders, and 13.7 percent for sexual aggressors of children. Here, the corresponding average PCL–R scores for the groups were: 26.7 (standard deviation = 6.2) for polymorphic sexual aggressors; 24.3 (standard deviation = 7.0) for sexual aggressors of women; 23.7 (standard deviation = 6.9) for non-sex offenders; and 21.3 (standard deviation = 7.5) for sexual aggressors of children. Furthermore, polymorphic sexual aggressors displayed significantly higher Factor 1 scores compared to the other groups, and significantly higher Factor 2 scores compared to sexual aggressors of children but not sexual aggressors of women or non-sex offenders. In other words, polymorphic sexual aggressors displayed the highest level of callous and unemotional traits compared to other types, but their antisocial behavior was in line with that of sexual aggressors of women and non-sex offenders.

Porter et al. (2000) investigated the prevalence of psychopathy in a sample of 329 incarcerated sexual aggressors and non-sex offenders in Canada. They used a cut-off score of 30 or higher on the PCL–R and found the prevalence of psychopathy between groups from highest to lowest was: 64.0 percent for polymorphic sexual aggressors, 35.9 percent for sexual aggressors of women; 34.0 percent for non-sex offenders; 10.8 percent for intrafamilial sexual aggressors of children; and 6.3 percent for extrafamilial sexual aggressors of children. The corresponding average PCL–R scores for the groups were: 29.0 (standard deviation = 6.5) for polymorphic sexual aggressors; 25.9 (5.9) for sexual aggressors of women; 25.8 (standard deviation = 7.0) for non-sex offenders; 21.2 (standard deviation = 6.4) for intrafamilial sexual aggressors of children; and, 20.9 (standard deviation = 6.1) for extrafamilial sexual aggressors of children. Porter et al. (2000:227) noted that polymorphic sexual aggressors were between two and ten times more likely than other groups to be characterized by psychopathy. They also reported that many sexual aggressors of children scored highly on Factor 1 of the PCL–R, where Factor 2 scores largely differentiated the degree of antisocial behavior displayed between sexual aggressors of women and sexual aggressors of children (Porter et al., 2000:227).

Olver and Wong (2006) reported a similar pattern in the prevalence of psychopathy measured by the PCL–R in a sample of 156 incarcerated adult sexual aggressors in Canada, using cut-off scores of 25 and above and 30 and above. For the total sample, the respective prevalence rates were 29 percent and 13 percent. For polymorphic sexual aggressors, the respective prevalence rates were 42 percent and 19 percent, followed by sexual aggressors of women at 37 percent and 17 percent, incestuous sexual aggressors of children at 17 percent and 3 percent, and extrafamilial sexual aggressors of children at 4 percent and 4 percent. The corresponding average PCL–R scores were: 20.2 (standard deviation = 7.4) for the total sample; 22.7 (standard deviation = 7.3) for polymorphic sexual aggressors; 21.9 (standard deviation = 7.3) for sexual aggressors of women; 17.7 (standard deviation = 6.8) for incestuous sexual aggressors of children; and 15.9 (standard deviation = 5.8) for extrafamilial sexual aggressors of children.

In short, the pattern is fairly consistent; the prevalence of psychopathy is highest among polymorphic sexual aggressors, followed by sexual aggressors of women, and then sexual aggressors of children. Indeed, this general pattern has also been observed in several other studies to varying extents, depending on the nature and size of samples (e.g., Firestone, Bradford, Greenberg, & Serran, 2000; Harris et al., 2003; Harris, Rice, Hilton, Lalumiere, & Quinsey, 2007; Jackson & Richards, 2007; Serin, Malcolm, Khanna, & Barb, 1994; Quinsey, Rice, & Harris, 1995; Rice & Harris 1997; Seto & Barbaree 1999; Skovran, Huss, & Scalora, 2010). Part of the basis for these differences is the fact that polymorphic sexual aggressors and sexual aggressors of women are more criminally active than sexual aggressors of children. At the same time, callousness and unemotional traits are differentially related to certain aspects of sexual offending, such as the motivation for sexual aggression.

Sexual aggressors of women

One of the most prominent typologies of sexual aggressors of women is based on the motivation for acts of sexual aggression (Knight & Prentky, 1990). Knight and Prentky (1990) identified five key motivation types that include: opportunistic; pervasively angry; sexual sadistic; sexual non-sadistic; or vindictive types. The opportunistic type are individuals characterized by an impulsive and antisocial lifestyle where sexual offenses are typically unplanned and do not involve high levels of violence (i.e., the violence is instrumental). Here the primary goal here reflects sexual gratification, and aggression is a tactic employed: (1) to create an opportunity for a sexual encounter; or (2) if conventional opportunities for a sexual encounter are blocked. The pervasively angry type are individuals characterized by undifferentiated anger (i.e., not specifically directed towards women). Furthermore, they generally also have extensive violent and criminal histories where high levels of expressive violence characterize the sex offenses they commit. In contrast, the sadistic type reflects individuals whose motivation is to act out sadistic sexual fantasies. These are individuals sexually aroused by sadism and violence, who plan sex offenses that are particularly violent and ritualistic, and severely harm and, in some cases, kill their victims. The non-sadistic sexual type, on the other hand, are individuals who are characterized by deviant sexual fantasies, such as rape fantasies, who plan their offenses and use physical aggression to the extent that it secures the compliance of their victims. These individuals are motivated by dominance and power over the victim, but not necessarily sexual sadism. Finally, the vindictive type reflects individuals characterized by rage exclusively focused toward women. They are not typically characterized by extensive and violent criminal histories (i.e., compared to the pervasively anger type); however, their offenses are characterized by a high degree of expressive violence.

The link between psychopathy and motivation types of sexual aggressors of women has been directly examined in two studies. Barbaree, Seto, Serin, Amos, and Preston (1994) compared PCL–R scores of vindictive, opportunistic, non-sadistic, and sadistic sexual aggressors of women. The sample was based on 60 adult sexual aggressors of women involved in treatment at a sexual behavior clinic in Canada. The average PCL–R scores across the types were: opportunistic (mean = 20.5, standard deviation = 6.1); sadistic (mean = 20.0, standard deviation = 9.5); vindictive (mean = 17.5, standard deviation = 1.4); and non-sadistic (mean = 13.7, standard deviation = 6.5). The "sadistic" type had significantly higher Factor 2 scores than the "non-sadistic" type; the former were more likely to have a criminal history/antisocial lifestyle (see also DeLisi et al., 2017). However, there were no statistically significant differences in overall PCL–R or Factor 1 scores across the sample (Barbaree et al., 1994).

Using the same typology in another study of 60 sexual aggressors of women drawn from one medium and one maximum security institution in Canada, Brown and Forth (1997) reported the prevalence of psychopathy in the combined sample was 35 percent, using a PCL–R cut-off score of 30 and above. The highest prevalence of psychopathy was reported for the opportunistic type (52.4 percent) (854) and, congruent with findings from the study of Barbaree et al. (1994), psychopathy was also associated with the number of prior non-sexual offenses (852).

In a larger study of 958 sexual aggressors from several different treatment settings in the United States, Krstic et al. (2017) found that the four facets of the PCL–R were differentially associated with specific elements of sex offenses. While they did not directly test the motivation-based typology of Knight and Prentky (1990) described above, they did find that the affective and antisocial facets of the PCL–R were associated with increased violence (i.e., expressive aggression, victim injury, sadistic violence, stabbing) in sexual offenses, consistent with certain dimensions of sexual sadism. The antisocial facet was also positively associated with physical control (i.e., blindfolding, gagging, tying up the victim), consistent with the instrumental dimension of opportunistic offenses. Taken together, the findings from these studies provide evidence that psychopathy is associated with opportunistic and sadistic motivations for sexual aggression against women, possibly over and above other types.

Sexual aggressors of children

As discussed earlier, across studies, the prevalence of psychopathy is lowest among sexual aggressors of children.[1] However, there is mixed empirical evidence as to whether psychopathy varies between subtypes of sexual aggressors of children. On the one hand, some studies have reported prevalence differences between different types of sexual aggressors of children. Strassberg et al. (2012) used the PPI to compare pedophilic and non-pedophilic sexual aggressors of children from three different residential treatment sites in the United States. In their study, non-pedophilic sexual aggressors of children scored significantly higher on psychopathy measured by the PPI compared to pedophilic sexual aggressors of children.

Other studies that have examined psychopathy between types of sexual aggressors of children have compared extrafamilial (i.e., where the child victim is unrelated to the perpetrator) and intrafamilial (i.e., the child is biologically or legally related to the perpetrator) aggressors. In the study by Olver and Wong (2006) discussed earlier, using a cut-off score of 25 and above, the prevalence of psychopathy among intrafamilial sexual aggressors of children was 17 percent, compared to only 4 percent among extrafamilial sexual aggressors of children. However, using a cut-off score of 30 and above on the PCL–R, the prevalence rates were much lower and virtually identical (4 percent for extrafamilial aggressors and 3 percent for intrafamilial aggressors).

Other studies have produced directly contrary results. In a study by Beggs and Grace (2008) that was based on 216 treated sexual aggressors of children in New Zealand, they reported that extrafamilial sexual aggressors of children had significantly higher scores on the PCL–R (mean = 9.5, standard deviation = 8.1) compared to intrafamilial sexual aggressors of children (mean = 7.2, standard deviation = 6.4), averages far below clinical cut-offs. Furthermore, at a cut-off score of 25 the overall prevalence of psychopathy in their sample was low (4.6 percent) compared to other studies discussed above. These differences between intra- and extrafamilial sexual aggressors of children compared to other studies may be explained at least in part by the sample composition and context (i.e., sexual aggressors of children/treatment completers).

In contrast, several studies have failed to uncover any differences in the prevalence of psychopathy between types of sexual aggressors of children. In a study by Kingston, Firestone, Moulden, and Bradford (2007) there were no differences in PCL–R scores between pedophilic and non-pedophilic extrafamilial sexual aggressors of children sampled from a sexual behavior clinic in Canada. Seto and Barbaree (1999) and Porter et al. (2000) did not uncover any differences between intrafamilial and extrafamilial sexual aggressors of children on PCL–R scores in their samples of incarcerated sexual aggressors in Canada. Similarly, Firestone, Bradford, Greenberg, and Serran (2000) did not uncover any significant differences in overall PCL–R scores, Factor 1, or Factor 2 scores between intrafamilial and extrafamilial sexual aggressors of children referred for assessment to a sexual behavior clinic in Canada. Finally, in a more recent study, Walters, Knight, Looman, and Abracen (2016) also did not observe differences in the PCL–R scores between extrafamilial and incestuous sexual aggressors of children, in a sample of sexual aggressors admitted to a federal corrections assessment unit in Canada.

Evidence pertaining to the prevalence of psychopathy across types of sexual aggressors sheds some light on the characteristics of individuals on different developmental pathways leading to sexual aggression. First, the prevalence of psychopathy is highest among polymorphic sexual aggressors, followed by sexual aggressors of women, and then sexual aggressors of children. Second, psychopathy is differentially associated with motivations for sexual aggression against women, specifically opportunistic and sadistic motivations. Third, the link between psychopathy and sexual aggression against children is complex; the balance of evidence suggests that psychopathy functions equivalently across types of sexual aggressors of children. Finally, the role of psychopathy in sexual aggression is likely most evident among serious and violent repeat sexual aggressors characterized by antisocial and callous–unemotional traits. Krstic et al. (2017) showed that sexual aggressors rated highly on all four facets of the PCL–R display the highest levels of sexual violence. Furthermore, Kaseweter, Woodworth, Logan, and Freimuth (2016) compared PCL–R scores in a sample of 92 "high risk sex offenders" drawn from the Integrated Sexual Predator Information Network (ISPIN) in Canada. The ISPIN is a database of some of the highest risk sexual aggressors in Canada. The average PCL–R score for the entire sample was 28.4 (standard deviation = 7.1), and they reported no differences in average PCL–R scores between "coercive child molesters" (mean = 27.0, standard deviation = 6.7), "sadistic rapists" (mean = 29.7, standard deviation = 3.8), and "stranger focused child molesters" (mean = 30.7, standard deviation = 6.9). In effect, the most serious and violent repeat sexual aggressors are those likely characterized by high levels of psychopathy in addition to deviant sexual preferences (e.g., deviant sexual fantasies, sadistic paraphilia, or pedophilia). Therefore, below we investigate the empirical evidence on the relationship between psychopathy and sexual deviance.

Psychopathy and sexual deviance

Clinical psychologists have emphasized the role of sexual deviance in sexual aggression, with a specific emphasis deviant sexual arousal and the presence of paraphilia. Deviant sexual arousal typically refers to the presence of deviant sexual fantasies such as those involving violence and sexualized violence, children, or both. On the other hand, paraphilias are atypical sexual urges and arousal patterns beyond what is considered "normal" and, at the extreme, cause significant distress and/or dysfunction. The Diagnostic and Statistical Manual of Mental Disorders fifth edition (DSM–5) identifies eight paraphilias: voyeuristic; exhibitionistic; frotteuristic; sexual masochism; fetishistic; transvestic; pedophilic; and sexual sadism disorders.

Serin et al. (1994) examined the relationship between psychopathy and deviant sexual arousal measured by phallometric assessment (which refers to the measurement of penile tumescence upon exposure to deviant sexual stimuli such as sexual violence and/or sexual depictions of children) in a sample of 65 incarcerated adult sexual aggressors in Canada, between 33 sexual aggressors of women and 32 sexual aggressors of children. In the total sample, the prevalence of psychopathy was low; using a cut-off score of 29 and above on the PCL–R, the prevalence of psychopathy was 9.9 percent (12.2 percent for sexual aggressors of women and 7.5 percent for sexual aggressors of children). In terms of PCL–R scores, sexual aggressors of women scored slightly higher on average (mean = 17.1, standard deviation = 8.6) compared to sexual aggressors of children (mean = 13.2, standard deviation = 7.8). They found a low-to-approaching moderate significant correlation between phallometrically assessed deviant sexual arousal and psychopathy scores. This relationship held specifically for sexual aggressors of children and, and to a lesser extent, sexual aggressors of women (here the correlation was marginally significant). Furthermore, differentiating between incestuous and extrafamilial sexual aggressors of children, they found some evidence that the association between psychopathy and deviant sexual arousal better characterized extrafamilial sexual aggressors of children (Serin et al., 1994).

This is also consistent with findings presented by Firestone et al. (2000) based on a sample of 539 adult sexual aggressors referred for sexual behavior assessment to a clinic in Canada. They utilized three sets of deviant sexual stimuli involving: (1) sexual depictions of children; (2) sexual depictions of violence involving children; and (3) sexual depictions of violence against women. First, sexual aggressors of women had significantly higher PCL–R scores compared to extrafamilial sexual aggressors of children and incestuous sexual aggressors of children. Second, in the entire sample, total PCL–R scores were positively associated with arousal to sexual depictions of violence against women. More specifically, Factor 2 scores on the PCL–R were significantly correlated with arousal to sexual depictions of violence against women, as well as sexual depictions of violence involving children. However, when they controlled for sexual aggressor type, the relationship between psychopathy and deviant sexual arousal was only evident among extrafamilial sexual aggressors of children. More specifically, overall PCL–R scores were associated with arousal to sexual depictions of children among extrafamilial sexual aggressors of children. In addition, Factor 1 and Factor 2 PCL–R scores were correlated with deviant sexual arousal to violence involving children as well as violence against women among extrafamilial sexual aggressors of children.

In terms of paraphilia, a key focus concerns the link between psychopathy and sexual sadism. Sexual sadism refers to sexual arousal to causing pain, humiliation, fear, or physical and/or mental harm to another person. For example, some sexual aggressors of women are motivated by a sexual preference for rape/non-consensual sex involving violence (i.e., the sadistic type; Knight & Prentky, 1990). Indeed, psychopathy and sadism share several common features, such as the preparedness to inflict pain or injuries and emotional detachment from the suffering of others (Cooke, 2001; Meloy, 2002; Mokros, Osterheider, Hucker, & Nitschke, 2011).

There is ample empirical evidence supporting the association between psychopathy and sadism among serious sexual aggressors. As discussed earlier, Barbaree et al. (1994) found that PCL–R scores were positively associated with sadism among sexual aggressors of women. In a sample of 41 adult inmates from a maximum security prison in the USA, Holt, Meloy, and Strack (1999) found that those with a PCL–R score of 30 or greater scored significantly higher on measures of sexual sadism. Woodworth et al. (2013) investigated the association between psychopathy and nonviolent, sadistic, and "other" paraphilia in a sample of 139 "high risk sex offenders" from across a Canadian province. They found that aggressors characterized by sadistic paraphilia were more likely to score in the 30–40 range on the PCL–R (Woodworth et al., 2013).

In another study of 100 male forensic patients convicted of sex offenses in Germany, Mokros et al. (2011) found that sexual aggressors classified as "sexual sadists" had higher PCL–R scores (mean = 21.5, standard deviation = 7.8) compared to "non-sadistic sex offenders" (mean = 17.1, standard deviation = 7.0). More specifically, affective deficits and behavioral disinhibition were associated with sexual sadism over and above interpersonal and lifestyle factors. This suggests that affective deficits and behavioral disinhibition are critical precursors to sexually sadistic behavior in sex offenses (Mokros et al., 2011). Robertson and Knight (2014) similarly showed that sadism was correlated with overall PCL–R scores in two samples of incarcerated and civilly committed sexual aggressors. They uncovered positive associations between measures of sadism and the affective, interpersonal, and antisocial facets of the PCL–R. In terms of antisociality, DeLisi et al. (2016) similarly showed that sexual sadism was associated with non-sexual criminal versatility in a sample of federally incarcerated sexual aggressors in the United States.

The evidence is quite clear that psychopathy and sexual deviance characterize the most serious and violent sexual aggressors. As such, studies of sexual homicide provide a unique context for investigating this relationship. Porter, Woodworth, Earle, Drugge, and Boer (2003) measured psychopathy in a sample of 125 incarcerated adult homicide offenders in Canada, 38 of whom committed a sexual homicide. In the overall sample, the prevalence of psychopathy using a cut-off score of 30 and above was 27.2 percent. For those who committed a sexual homicide, the prevalence of psychopathy was 47.4 percent. In terms of homicide characteristics, psychopathic sexual homicide offenders committed more gratuitous and sadistic violence compared to non-psychopathic offenders, and callous–unemotional traits were associated with the presence of sadistic violence (Porter, Woodworth, Earle, Drugge, & Boer, 2003).

A similar pattern characterizes extrafamilial sexual aggressors of children who kill their victims. Firestone, Bradford, Greenberg, Larose, and Curry (1998) compared 17 homicidal extrafamilial sexual aggressors of children with 35 non-homicidal extrafamilial sexual aggressors of children in terms of their PCL–R scores. First, homicidal sexual aggressors of children had significantly higher total PCL–R scores (mean = 28.7, standard deviation = 5.8) on average compared to non-homicidal sexual aggressors of children (mean = 16.6, standard deviation = 6.6). Second, higher Factor 1 PCL–R scores differentiated homicidal from non-homicidal sexual aggressors of children. In a similar study, Firestone, Bradford, Greenberg, and Larose (1998) compared 48 sexual aggressors (not differentiating between types) who killed their victims to 50 incestuous sexual aggressors of children in terms of their PCL–R scores. Again, homicidal sexual aggressors scored significantly higher in terms of their overall PCL–R score (mean = 26.6, standard deviation = 7.6) compared to incestuous sexual aggressors of children (mean = 18.7, standard deviation = 7.0), and here this pattern held across both factors of the PCL–R.

In short, the evidence on the link between psychopathy and sexual deviance among sexual aggressors is substantial. Sexual aggressors characterized by psychopathy are more likely to act on their sexual urges, whether they represent deviant sexual fantasies and paraphilia or not. Furthermore, there are several shared features between psychopathy and certain deviant sexual fantasies and paraphilia, particularly those involving violence. Centrally, the common thread involves the ability to inflict harm, pain, and/or suffering on a repeated basis without any sort of empathetic response. Importantly, while psychopathy and sexual deviance are associated with the characteristics of sexual crimes, there is also strong evidence on their link to the repetition of them.

Psychopathy and recidivism among sexual aggressors

Antisociality and sexual deviance are the key predictors of sexual recidivism (Hanson & Morton-Bourgon, 2005). Furthermore, psychopathy can be conceptualized as an extreme manifestation of antisociality (e.g., DeLisi, 2009, 2016). However, the link between psychopathy and recidivism among sexual aggressors is not straightforward. First, while the base-rate of sexual recidivism among sexual aggressors increases with the length of follow-up period, it is comparably lower than the base rate of violent and nonviolent recidivism among sexual aggressors (Hanson & Bussière, 1998). Therefore, it is important to understand how psychopathy is associated with different recidivism outcomes among sexual aggressors. Second, recidivism rates, as with psychopathy, vary across different sexual aggressor types. Third, as discussed above, sexual deviance manifests in different ways among sexual aggressors, and there is evidence that sexual deviance, as with recidivism, is differentially associated with certain facets of psychopathy over others.

In terms of direct associations between psychopathy and sexual recidivism, the empirical literature is characterized by mixed results. In a study of 409 adult sexual aggressors convicted of a contact sexual offense under community supervision in Canada, Hanson and Harris (2000) compared PCL–R scores of sexual recidivists and non-recidivists. Using a cut-off score of 29, the prevalence of psychopathy among sex offense recidivists was 20.5 percent compared to 8.0 percent among non-recidivists. The corresponding average PCL–R scores were 23.4 (standard deviation = 6.8) and 16.7 (standard deviation = 8.0). Looman, Abracen, Serin, and Marquis (2005) uncovered a similar pattern in sample of 102 adult sexual aggressors in an institutional treatment program in Canada. Using a cut-off score of 25 on the PCL–R, they observed that those in the high psychopathy group were more likely to be characterized by recidivism. In this study, the recidivism outcome was a combination of sexual or violent recidivism. In contrast, Murrie et al. (2012) found PCL–R scores were not predictive of sexual recidivism in a mixed sample (i.e., sexual aggressors of children, sexual aggressors of women, and polymorphic sexual aggressors) of 398 adult sexual aggressors evaluated for civil commitment in the United states. Here, the antisocial facet of the PCL–R approached statistical significance in predicting combined violent/sexual recidivism.

In a study of 216 incarcerated adult sexual aggressors who participated in an institutional treatment program in Canada, Barbaree, Seto, Langton, and Peacock (2001) found that the PCL–R alone predicted general and serious recidivism but not sexual recidivism. Similarly, Rettenberger, Matthes, Boer, and Eher (2010) also found that PCL–R scores alone did not predict sexual recidivism but did predict violent and nonviolent recidivism among 394 sexual aggressors assessed at a regional intake facility in Austria. Importantly, they also showed that the PCL–R was differentially associated with recidivism across different sexual aggressor types; PCL–R scores predicted sexual, violent, and nonviolent recidivism among extrafamilial sexual aggressors of children and general recidivism among incestuous sexual aggressors of children (Rettenberger et al., 2010).

In effect, there are unique associations between psychopathy and different recidivism outcomes for specific sexual aggressor types. Furthermore, sexual deviance also factors into these patterns. Quinsey et al. (1995) examined the relationship between psychopathy and recidivism among sexual aggressors of women, sexual aggressors of children, and polymorphic sexual aggressors in a sample of 178 adult sexual aggressors at a maximum security psychiatric facility in Canada. Sexual aggressors of children displayed the lowest PCL–R scores (mean = 12.9, standard deviation = 6.3) compared to sexual aggressors of women (mean = 18.4, standard deviation = 9.2) and polymorphic sexual aggressors (mean = 16.7, standard deviation = 7.9). Sexual aggressors of women and polymorphic sexual aggressors were characterized by the poorest survival rates to sexual reconvictions and violent reconvictions compared to sexual aggressors of children. Furthermore, psychopathy and sexual deviance each independently predicted sexual recidivism among the entire sample (Quinsey et al., 1995).

In another study of 288 adult sexual aggressors at a maximum security psychiatric facility (partially comprised of the sample from the study of Quinsey et al., 1995), Rice and Harris (1997) found a large effect of psychopathy on violent recidivism. At the same time, the interaction between psychopathy and sexual deviance was primarily associated with sexual recidivism (see also Olver & Wong, 2006). Sexual aggressors of women and polymorphic sexual aggressors were at a higher risk of violent recidivism compared to sexual aggressors of children, and the latter were at a higher risk for subsequent sexual offenses. Serin, Mailloux, and Malcolm (2001) conducted a follow-up study of 65 incarcerated sexual aggressors of children and sexual aggressors of women from their previous study (Serin et al., 1994) and found that those who displayed psychopathic characteristics in addition to deviant sexual arousal reoffended faster and at higher rates compared to those individuals characterized by sexual deviance but not psychopathy.

Taken together, these findings demonstrate that psychopathy and sexual deviance, independently and combined, contribute to different recidivism outcomes among sexual aggressors. First, psychopathy is associated with recidivism generally; prior convictions and criminal versatility, two of the antisocial facet items of the PCL–R, feature heavily in many risk assessment instruments and are key predictors of future offending. However, the wide variation in criminal careers across sexual aggressor types likely explains, at least in part, discrepant findings on the direct link between psychopathy and sexual recidivism among sexual aggressors. In effect, the antisocial facet of psychopathy is associated with higher rates of non-sexual recidivism. Second, sexual deviance manifests in different forms across sexual aggressors (e.g., sexual sadism vs. pedophilia, in some cases both). It has a differential impact on the offending process for certain sexual aggressors over others; the evidence suggests sexual deviance is independently associated with sexual recidivism among certain sexual aggressors of children. Third, where psychopathy and sexual deviance overlap, regardless of sexual aggressor type, the outcomes in terms of recidivism generally, and sexual recidivism specifically, are more pronounced. The combination of psychopathy and sexual deviance is associated with general and sexual recidivism across different types of sexual aggressors.

Psychopathy and juvenile sexual aggression

Compared to studies of adult sexual aggressors, there is comparably less empirical research on the link between psychopathy and juvenile sexual aggression. Similar to studies with adults, the prevalence of psychopathic personality characteristics among juvenile sexual aggressors varies substantially, and much of this variation has to do with differences in the assessment instruments used in studies, study contexts (e.g., incarcerated versus treatment settings), and composition of samples. For example, in a sample of 46 juvenile sexual aggressors who were incarcerated in

Sweden, Långström and Grann (2000) reported the prevalence rate of psychopathy was 20 percent, using a cut-off score of 26 on the PCL–R. Using the PCL: YV, Cale, Lussier, McCuish, and Corrado (2015) examined the prevalence of psychopathy in a sample of 263 incarcerated juvenile males (40 juvenile sexual aggressors; 223 juvenile non-sex offenders). Using cut-off scores of 25 and above and 30 and above, the prevalence of psychopathic personality characteristics, respectively, were: 32.7 percent and 12.9 percent for the total sample; 27.4 percent and 9.4 percent for non-sex offenders; and, 62.5 percent and 32.5 percent for juvenile sexual aggressors. In another Canadian study consisting exclusively of 220 juvenile sexual aggressors in an outpatient treatment program, Gretton, McBride, Hare, O'Shaughnessy, and Kumka (2001) reported that only approximately 13 percent of the sample scored higher than 30 on the PCL: YV.

Other studies with juvenile sexual aggressors have focused more specifically on the presence of callous and unemotional characteristics. For example, in a sample of 69 incarcerated juvenile males in the United States, using the PSD, Caputo et al. (1999) reported that the prevalence of callous and unemotional characteristics was significantly higher among juvenile sexual aggressors (34.8 percent) compared to violent offenders (5.9 percent) and nonviolent offenders (6.9 percent). Lawing, Frick, and Cruise (2010) found a slightly higher prevalence rate of callous and unemotional characteristics (54 percent) in another sample of 150 juvenile sexual aggressors incarcerated in the United States. Furthermore, they showed that callous–unemotional characteristics were associated with specific characteristics of sex crimes, including a higher frequency of sex offenses and higher levels of violence against victims.

Importantly, several studies have produced contrary results to the general patterns described above, failing to note any differences between juvenile sexual aggressors and non-sex offenders in terms of psychopathy and/or callous–unemotional characteristics (e.g., Boonmann et al., 2015; Fanniff, Schubert, Mulvey, Iselin, & Piquero, 2017; Freeman, Dexter-Mazza, & Hoffman, 2005; Caldwell, Ziemke, & Vitacco, 2008; Zakireh, Ronis, & Knight, 2008), or associations between psychopathic personality characteristics and specific aspects of sexual crimes (e.g., Morrell & Burton 2014). In addition, very few studies have examined the presence of psychopathic personality characteristics in subtypes of juvenile sexual aggressors. In a recent study of juvenile sexual aggressors in the Netherlands, Boonmann et al. (2015) did not observe any differences in YPI scores of incarcerated juvenile sexual aggressors classified as "child molesters," "peer/adult solo offenders," or "peer/adult group offenders." Using scales reflecting psychopathic characteristics from the MIDSA, Netland and Miner (2012) did not uncover any differences in psychopathic personality characteristics between juveniles classified as sexual aggressors of children, those who offended against peer or adult victims, or polymorphic juvenile sexual aggressors. However, Parks and Bard (2006) made similar comparisons using the PCL: YV in a sample of 156 incarcerated juvenile sexual aggressors and found that polymorphic juvenile sexual aggressors displayed the highest scores on the PCL: YV compared to juvenile sexual aggressors with child or peer/adult victims. More specifically, the polymorphic juvenile sexual aggressor group rated higher on affective and behavioral facets of the PCL: YV compared to juvenile sexual aggressors with child victims.

There is also evidence of complex associations between psychopathy, sexual deviance, and recidivism among juvenile sexual aggressors, some of which parallel those found in studies with adult sexual aggressors. Gretton et al. (2001) found that psychopathy and sexual deviance were not associated in their sample of juvenile sexual aggressors. However, psychopathy alone was associated with recidivism, and psychopathy and sexual deviance together predicted violent and nonviolent reoffending. Långström and Grann (2000) similarly reported that psychopathy was associated with general recidivism in a sample of juvenile sexual aggressors in Sweden. Furthermore, they provided some evidence linking sexual deviance and sexual recidivism using early onset sexually abusive behavior, any male victims, and multiple victims as proxy measures for sexual deviance. Parks and Bard (2006) showed that polymorphic juvenile sexual aggressors were characterized by the highest levels of sexual drive and preoccupation (measured by the Juvenile Sex Offender Assessment Protocol–II (JSOAP–II; Prentky & Righthand, 2003) compared to those with child and peer/adult victims. In addition, juvenile sexual aggressors with child victims also scored significantly higher than those with peer/adult victims on sexual drive and preoccupation. However, these measures for sexual deviance were not predictive of sexual or non-sexual recidivism; rather, the interpersonal and antisocial facets of the PCL: YV predicted sexual recidivism, whereas the behavioral and antisocial facets of the PCL: YV predicted non-sexual recidivism. Finally, as with adults, there is some evidence for the role of sexual sadism and psychopathy among juveniles who commit sexual homicide, particularly in terms of reoffending in this context (Myers & Blashfield, 1997; Myers, Chan, Vo, & Lazarou, 2010).

Conclusion

The link between psychopathy and sexual aggression is complex; certain facets of psychopathy are differentially associated with specific dimensions of sex crimes, and these relationships vary between types of sexual aggressors. One way to make sense of these differences is to consider the role of psychopathy on different pathways to sexual aggression. First, an antisocial pathway to sexual aggression characterizes certain sexual aggressors of women. These are individuals whose sexual aggression occurs against the backdrop of generally versatile antisocial/criminal behavior and precocious sexual behavior. Indeed, the evidence shows that psychopathic traits are associated with non-sexual recidivism over and above sexual recidivism for sexual aggressors of women. In the sexual context, psychopathic personality characteristics may reflect sensation seeking characterized by high-risk sexual behaviors (Meloy 2002; Skovran et al., 2010). In effect, this pathway is characterized by individuals for whom achieving sexual encounters may not be problematic, but in the face of blocked opportunities they will resort to antisocial tactics, be it deception, coercion, or aggression, for example, to facilitate their goals. For others on this pathway who have problematic sexual lives, resorting to sexual aggression may simply be more expedient. Either way, the motivation for sexual aggression in this context is opportunistic in nature. Cale and Lussier (2011) described this overall pattern of behavior in the sexual context as antisocial sexuality. Furthermore, the antisocial pathway may characterize a substantial proportion of juvenile sexual aggressors (e.g., Butler & Seto 2002; Cale et al., 2016). Indeed, adolescent males are at several disadvantages when it comes to achieving sexual encounters in this developmental period (e.g., lack of employment/money, status, etc.). In this context, psychopathic personality characteristics facilitate overcoming such disadvantages.

Another way to overcome such disadvantages, be it among adolescent or adult males, is to select victims more likely to comply with sexual advances, or in other words, who are vulnerable. In this context, the antisocial pathway characterizes certain sexual aggressors of children, and one possibility is that this pathway cuts across pedophilic, non-pedophilic, extrafamilial, and intrafamilial types. Psychopathic personality traits likely play a key role in differentiating those who act on their urges from those who do not. Furthermore, opportunity structures also play an important role in sexual aggression (Smallbone & Cale 2015). In the intrafamilial context, the average age of sexual abuse perpetration coincides with the average age of emerging adolescence in families with children (e.g., around the mid-thirties). In the extrafamilial context, there is substantial evidence for the role of opportunistic motivations for sexual aggression against children in youth-oriented institutions, all consistent with an antisocial pathway to sexual aggression.

The callous–unemotional pathway is also central to sexual aggression, but possibly in very different contexts than those described above. Indeed, as Knight and Guay (2006) point out, the callous–unemotional aspect of psychopathy is central to the quality of violence in sexual crimes. Therefore, the callous–unemotional pathway may best characterize the interaction of psychopathic personality traits and different sadistic and non-sadistic sexual motivations for sexual aggression. In addition, this relationship is especially pertinent when sexual preferences involving paraphilia are involved; the empirical evidence suggests the relationship between callous–unemotional traits and sexual deviance is evident across sex aggressor types and, possibly, even certain juvenile sexual aggressors. The intersection of callous–unemotional traits and sexual deviance is reflected in characteristics of sexual crimes, such as sexualized violence, and, to some extent, the repetition of these acts. The affective deficits of psychopathy facilitate sexualized violence, be it against children or adults; essentially, the lack of inhibition to cause severe pain, humiliation, fear, or physical, sexual, and/or mental harm to another individual. Furthermore, it is well known that possibly the vast majority of sex crimes go unreported, and that incarcerated sexual aggressors represent only a small portion of men who commit acts of sexual aggression (i.e., specifically those who are caught) (DeLisi et al., 2016). Therefore, another possibility is that this pathway may characterize "non-criminal" or undetected sexual aggressors (i.e., those with minimal-to-no contact with the criminal justice system). This may characterize individuals who perpetrate serious sexual violence in the intimate partner context, where the motivation may not necessarily be sadistic, but reflect power and dominance motives.

Finally, the mixed callous–unemotional antisocial pathway presents the complete picture of psychopathy as it relates to the quality and quantity of sexual violence among the most serious and violent sexual aggressors. First, this pathway is characterized by criminal and sexual versatility. Criminal versatility is reflected in the extensive and diverse antisocial backgrounds, nonviolent, violent, and sexual reoffending of sexual aggressors on this pathway reflecting the antisocial facet of psychopathy (e.g., Cale & Lussier, 2014). Sexual versatility is evident in patterns of victim switching: those who indiscriminately target children, adolescents, adults, males, and/or females. On the one hand, some have argued this reflects sensation seeking in the sexual context, congruent with the thrill-seeking dimension of psychopathy (e.g., Skovran et al., 2010). However, others have argued it reflects multiple paraphilia where callous and unemotional traits facilitate sexualized violence and disinhibition to pain and suffering in different contexts (e.g., Woodworth et al., 2013). Either way, when the affective, interpersonal, and antisocial dimensions of psychopathy coincide with persistent and harmful deviant sexual fantasies and/or paraphilia, the outcome tends to be the most serious and violent sexual crimes.

Note

1 In a study by Schimmenti, Passanisi, and Caretti (2014) that compared sexual aggressors of children to non-sex offenders in a sample of incarcerated inmates in Italy, they showed that sexual aggressors of children had significantly higher Factor 1 scores (i.e., interpersonal and affective facets) on the PCL-R. Unfortunately, it was not possible to determine differences between subtypes of sexual aggressors of children.

References

Andershed, H. A., Kerr, M., Stattin, H., and Levander, S. (2002) 'Psychopathic traits in non-referred youths: A new assessment tool,' in E. Blaauw & L. Sheridan (Eds.), *Psychopaths: Current International Perspectives* (pp. 131–158), Den Haag: Elsevier.

Augur Enterprises Inc. (2007) *MIDSA clinical manual*, Bend, OR: Augur Enterprises Inc.

Barbaree, H. E., Seto, M. C., Langton, C. M., and Peacock, E. J. (2001) 'Evaluating the predictive accuracy of six risk assessment instruments for adult sex offenders,' *Criminal Justice and Behavior*, *28*(4):490–521.

Barbaree, H. E., Seto, M. C., Serin, R. C., Amos, N. L., and Preston, D. L. (1994) 'Comparisons between sexual and nonsexual rapist subtypes,' *Criminal Justice and Behavior*, *21*(1):95–114.

Beggs, S. M., and Grace, R. C. (2008) 'Psychopathy, intelligence, and recidivism in child molesters,' *Criminal Justice and Behavior*, *35*(6):683–695.

Book, A. S., Clark, H. J., Forth, A. E., and Hare, R. D. (2006) 'The PCL-R and PCL: YV: Forensic applications and limitations,' in R. P. Archer (Ed.), *Forensic uses of clinical assessment instruments* (pp. 147–179), Mahwah, NJ: Erlbaum.

Boonmann, C., Jansen, L. M., 't Hart-Kerkhoffs, L. A., Vahl, P., Hillege, S. L., Doreleijers, T. A., and Vermeiren, R. R. (2015) 'Self-reported psychopathic traits in sexually offending juveniles compared with generally offending juveniles and general population youth,' *International Journal of Offender Therapy and Comparative Criminology*, *59*(1):85–95.

Brown, A. R., Dargis, M. A., Mattern, A. C., Tsonis, M. A., and Newman, J. P. (2015) 'Elevated psychopathy scores among mixed sexual offenders,' *Criminal Justice and Behavior*, *42*(10):1032–1044.

Brown, S. L., and Forth, A. E. (1997) 'Psychopathy and sexual assault: Static risk factors, emotional precursors, and rapist subtypes,' *Journal of Consulting and Clinical Psychology*, *65*(5):848–857.

Butler, S. M., and Seto, M. C. (2002) 'Distinguishing two types of adolescent sex offenders,' *Journal of the American Academy of Child & Adolescent Psychiatry*, *41*(1):83–90.

Caldwell, M. F., Ziemke, M. H., and Vitacco, M. J. (2008) 'An examination of the Sex Offender Registration and Notification Act as applied to juveniles: Evaluating the ability to predict sexual recidivism,' *Psychology, Public Policy, and Law*, *14*(2):89–114.

Cale, J., and Lussier, P. (2011) 'Toward a developmental taxonomy of adult sexual aggressors of women: Antisocial trajectories in youth, mating effort, and sexual criminal activity in adulthood,' *Violence and Victims*, *26*(1):16–32.

Cale, J., and Lussier, P. (2014) 'A criminal career approach to sex offender subtypes: Is there a relationship between pathways in the offending process and the criminal career of extrafamilial sex offenders?,' in J. Proulx et al. (Eds.), *Pathways to sexual aggression* (pp. 229–258), New York, NY: Routledge.

Cale, J., Lussier, P., McCuish, E., and Corrado, R. (2015) 'The prevalence of psychopathic personality disturbances among incarcerated youth: Comparing serious, chronic, violent and sex offenders,' *Journal of Criminal Justice*, *43*(4):337–344.

Cale, J., Smallbone, S., Rayment-McHugh, S., and Dowling, C. (2016) 'Offense trajectories, the unfolding of sexual and non-sexual criminal activity, and sex offense characteristics of adolescent sex offenders,' *Sexual Abuse*, *28*(8):791–812.

Caputo, A. A., Frick, P. J., and Brodsky, S. L. (1999) 'Family violence and juvenile sex offending: The potential mediating role of psychopathic traits and negative attitudes toward women,' *Criminal Justice and Behavior*, *26*(3):338–356.

Cooke, D. J. (2001) 'Psychopathy, sadism and serial killing,' in A. Raine & J. Sanmartin (Eds.), *Violence and psychopathy* (pp. 123–137), New York, NY: Kluwer Academic/Plenum Publishers.

DeLisi, M. (2009) 'Psychopathy is the unified theory of crime,' *Youth Violence and Juvenile Justice*, 7(3):256–273.

DeLisi, M. (2016) *Psychopathy as unified theory of crime*, New York, NY: Palgrave MacMillan.

DeLisi, M., Caropreso, D. E., Drury, A. J., Elbert, M. J., Evans, J. L., Heinrichs, T., and Tahja, K. M. (2016) 'The dark figure of sexual offending: New evidence from federal sex offenders,' *Journal of Criminal Psychology*, *6*(1):3–15.

DeLisi, M., Drury, A., Elbert, M., Tahja, K., Caropreso, D., and Heinrichs, T. (2017) 'Sexual sadism and criminal versatility: Does sexual sadism spillover into nonsexual crimes?,' *Journal of Aggression, Conflict and Peace Research*, *9*(1):2–12.

Fanniff, A. M., Schubert, C. A., Mulvey, E. P., Iselin, A. M. R., and Piquero, A. R. (2017) 'Risk and outcomes: Are adolescents charged with sex offenses different from other adolescent offenders?,' *Journal of Youth and Adolescence*, *46*(7):1394–1423.

Firestone, P., Bradford, J. M., Greenberg, D. M., and Larose, M. R. (1998) 'Homicidal sex offenders: Psychological, phallometric, and diagnostic features,' *Journal of the American Academy of Psychiatry and the Law*, *26*(4):537–552.

Firestone, P., Bradford, J. M., Greenberg, D. M., Larose, M. R., and Curry, S. (1998) 'Homicidal and nonhomicidal child molesters: Psychological, phallometric, and criminal features,' *Sexual Abuse*, *10*(4):305–323.

Firestone, P., Bradford, J. M., Greenberg, D. M., and Serran, G. A. (2000) 'The relationship of deviant sexual arousal and psychopathy in incest offenders, extrafamilial child molesters, and rapists,' *Journal of the American Academy of Psychiatry and the Law*, *28*(3):303–308.

Forth, A. E., Kosson, D. S., and Hare, R. D. (2003) *Hare psychopathy checklist: Youth version*. Toronto, ON: Multi-Health Systems.

Freeman, K. A., Dexter-Mazza, E. T., and Hoffman, K. C. (2005) 'Comparing personality characteristics of juvenile sex offenders and non-sex offending delinquent peers: A preliminary investigation,' *Sexual Abuse*, *17*(1):3–12.

Frick, P. J., and Hare, R. D. (2001) *The Psychopathy Screening Device*, Toronto, ON: Multi-Health Systems.

Gretton, H. M., McBride, M., Hare, R. D., O'Shaughnessy, R., and Kumka, G. (2001) 'Psychopathy and recidivism in adolescent sex offenders,' *Criminal Justice and Behavior*, *28*(4):427–449.

Hanson, R. K., and Bussière, M. T. (1998) 'Predicting relapse: A meta-analysis of sexual offender recidivism studies,' *Journal of Consulting and Clinical Psychology*, *66*(2):348–362.

Hanson, R. K., and Harris, A. J. R. (2000) 'Where should we intervene? Dynamic predictors of sexual offense recidivism,' *Criminal Justice and Behavior*, *27*(1):6–35.

Hanson, R. K., and Morton-Bourgon, K. E. (2005) 'The characteristics of persistent sexual offenders: A meta-analysis of recidivism studies,' *Journal of Consulting and Clinical Psychology*, *73*(6):1154.

Hare, R. D. (1991) *The Hare Psychopathy Checklist–Revised*, Toronto, ON: Multi-Health Systems.

Hare, R. D. (2003) *The Psychopathy Checklist–Revised* (2nd ed.), Toronto, ON: Multi Health Symptoms.

Harris, G. T., Rice, M. E., Hilton, N. Z., Lalumiere, M. L., and Quinsey, V. L. (2007) 'Coercive and precocious sexuality as a fundamental aspect of psychopathy,' *Journal of Personality Disorders*, *21*(1):1–27.

Harris, G. T., Rice, M. E., Quinsey, V. L., Lalumière, M. L., Boer, D., and Lang, C. (2003) 'A multisite comparison of actuarial risk instruments for sex offenders,' *Psychological Assessment*, *15*(3):413–425.

Holt, S. E., Meloy, J. R., and Strack, S. (1999) 'Sadism and psychopathy in violent and sexually violent offenders,' *Journal of the American Academy of Psychiatry and Law*, *27*(1):23–32.

Jackson, R. L., and Richards, H. J. (2007) 'Diagnostic and risk profiles among civilly committed sex offenders in Washington State,' *International Journal of Offender Therapy and Comparative Criminology*, *51*(3):313–323.

Kaseweter, K., Woodworth, M., Logan, M., and Freimuth, T. (2016) 'High-risk sexual offenders: Towards a new typology,' *Journal of Criminal Justice*, *47*(Supplement C):123–132.

Kingston, D. A., Firestone, P., Moulden, H. M., and Bradford, J. M. (2007) 'The utility of the diagnosis of pedophilia: A comparison of various classification procedures,' *Archives of Sexual Behavior*, *36*(3):423–436.

Knight, R. A., and Guay, J.-P. (2006) 'The role of psychopathy in sexual coercion against women,' in C. J. Patrick (Ed.), *Handbook of psychopathy* (pp. 512–532), New York, NY: Guilford Press.

Knight, R. A., and Prentky, R. A. (1990) 'Classifying sexual offenders,' in W. L. Marshall, D. R. Laws, & H. E. Barbaree (Eds.), *Handbook of sexual assault: Issues, theories, and treatment of the offender* (pp. 23–52), Boston, MA: Springer US.

Knight, R. A., and Sims-Knight, J. E. (2003) 'The developmental antecedents of sexual coercion against women: Testing alternative hypotheses with structural equation modeling,' *Annals of the New York Academy of Sciences*, *989*(1):72–85.

Knight, R. A., and Sims-Knight, J. E. (2004) 'Testing an etiological model for male juvenile sexual offending against females,' *Journal of Child Sexual Abuse*, *13*(3–4):33–55.

Krstic, S., Neumann, C. S., Roy, S., Robertson, C. A., Knight, R. A., and Hare, R. D. (2017) 'Using latent variable- and person-centered approaches to examine the role of psychopathic traits in sex offenders,' *Personality Disorders: Theory, Research, and Treatment*, in press.

Lalumière, M. L., Harris, G. T., Quinsey, V. L., and Rice, M. E. (2005) 'The causes of rape,' *Canadian Psychology*, *46*(4):254–256.

Långström, N., and Grann, M. (2000) 'Risk for criminal recidivism among young sex offenders,' *Journal of Interpersonal Violence*, *15*(8):855–871.

Långström, N., and Lindblad, F. (2000) 'Young sex offenders: Background, personality, and crime characteristics in a Swedish forensic psychiatric sample,' *Nordic Journal of Psychiatry*, *54*(2):113–120.

Lawing, K., Frick, P. J., and Cruise, K. R. (2010) 'Differences in offending patterns between adolescent sex offenders high or low in callous–unemotional traits,' *Psychological Assessment*, *22*(2):298–305.

Lilienfeld, S. O., and Andrews, B. P. (1996) 'Development and preliminary validation of a self-report measure of psychopathic personality traits in noncriminal population,' *Journal of Personality Assessment*, *66*(3):488–524.

Looman, J., Abracen, J., Serin, R., and Marquis, P. (2005) 'Psychopathy, treatment change, and recidivism in high-risk, high-need sexual offenders,' *Journal of Interpersonal Violence, 20*(5):549–568.
Malamuth, N. M. (1998) 'An evolutionary-based model integrating research on the characteristics of sexually coercive men,' *Advances in Psychological Science, 1*:151–184.
Malamuth, N. M. (2003) 'Criminal and noncriminal sexual aggressors,' *Annals of the New York Academy of Sciences, 989*(1):33–58.
Meloy, J. R. (2002) 'The "polymorphously perverse" psychopath: Understanding a strong empirical relationship,' *Bulletin of the Menninger Clinic, 66*(3):273–289.
Mokros, A., Osterheider, M., Hucker, S. J., and Nitschke, J. (2011) 'Psychopathy and sexual sadism,' *Law and Human Behavior, 35*(3):188–199.
Morrell, L. M., and Burton, D. L. (2014) 'An exploration of psychopathy in self-report measures among juvenile sex offenders,' *International Journal of Offender Therapy and Comparative Criminology, 58*(5):550–566.
Murrie, D. C., Boccaccini, M. T., Caperton, J., and Rufino, K. (2012) 'Field validity of the Psychopathy Checklist–Revised in sex offender risk assessment,' *Psychological Assessment, 24*(2):524–529.
Myers, W. C., and Blashfield, R. (1997) 'Psychopathology and personality in juvenile sexual homicide offenders,' *Journal of the American Academy of Psychiatry and the Law Online, 25*(4):497–508.
Myers, W. C., Chan, H. C. O., Vo, E. J., and Lazarou, E. (2010) 'Sexual sadism, psychopathy, and recidivism in juvenile sexual murderers,' *Journal of Investigative Psychology and Offender Profiling*, 7(1):49–58.
Netland, J. D., and Miner, M. H. (2012) 'Psychopathy traits and parental dysfunction in sexual offending and general delinquent adolescent males,' *Journal of Sexual Aggression, 18*(1):4–22.
Olver, M. E., and Wong, S. C. P. (2006) 'Psychopathy, sexual deviance, and recidivism among sex offenders,' *Sexual Abuse: A Journal of Research and Treatment, 18*(1):65.
Parks, G. A., and Bard, D. E. (2006) 'Risk factors for adolescent sex offender recidivism: Evaluation of predictive factors and comparison of three groups based upon victim type,' *Sexual Abuse: A Journal of Research and Treatment, 18*(4):319–342.
Porter, S., Fairweather, D., Drugge, J., Herve, H., Birt, A., and Boer, D. P. (2000) 'Profiles of psychopathy in incarcerated sexual offenders,' *Criminal Justice and Behavior, 27*(2):216–233.
Porter, S., Woodworth, M., Earle, J., Drugge, J., and Boer, D. (2003) 'Characteristics of sexual homicides committed by psychopathic and nonpsychopathic offenders,' *Law and Human Behavior, 27*(5):459–470.
Prentky, R., and Righthand, S. (2003) *Juvenile sex offender assessment protocol–II (J-SOAP–II) manual,* Washington, DC. U.S. Department of Justice Office of Juvenile Justice and Delinquency Prevention.
Quinsey, V. L., Rice, M. E., and Harris, G. T. (1995) 'Actuarial prediction of sexual recidivism,' *Journal of Interpersonal Violence, 10*(1):85–105.
Rettenberger, M., Matthes, A., Boer, D. P., and Eher, R. (2010) 'Prospective actuarial risk assessment,' *International Journal of Offender Therapy and Comparative Criminology, 54*(2):169–186.
Rice, M. E., and Harris, G. T. (1997) 'Cross-validation and extension of the Violence Risk Appraisal Guide for child molesters and rapists,' *Law and Human Behavior, 21*(2):231–241.
Robertson, C. A., and Knight, R. A. (2014) 'Relating sexual sadism and psychopathy to one another, non-sexual violence, and sexual crime behaviors,' *Aggressive Behavior, 40*(1):12–23.
Schimmenti, A., Passanisi, A., and Caretti, V. (2014) 'Interpersonal and affective traits of psychopathy in child sexual abusers: Evidence from a pilot study sample of Italian offenders,' *Journal of Child Sexual Abuse, 23*(7):853–860.
Serin, R. C., Mailloux, D. L., and Malcolm, P. B. (2001) 'Psychopathy, deviant sexual arousal, and recidivism among sexual offenders,' *Journal of Interpersonal Violence, 16*(3):234–246.
Serin, R. C., Malcolm, P. B., Khanna, A., and Barbaree, H. E. (1994) 'Psychopathy and deviant sexual arousal in incarcerated sexual offenders,' *Journal of Interpersonal Violence, 9*(1):3–11.
Seto, M. C., and Barbaree, H. E. (1997) 'Sexual aggression as antisocial behavior: A developmental model,' in D. M. Stoff, J. Brieling, & J. Maser (Eds.), *Handbook of antisocial behavior* (pp. 524–533), Hoboken, NJ: John Wiley & Sons Inc.
Seto, M. C., and Barbaree, H. E. (1999) 'Psychopathy, treatment behavior, and sex offender recidivism,' *Journal of Interpersonal Violence, 14*(12):1235–1248.
Skovran, L. C., Huss, M. T., and Scalora, M. J. (2010) 'Sexual fantasies and sensation seeking among psychopathic sexual offenders,' *Psychology, Crime & Law, 16*(7):617–629.
Smallbone, S., and Cale, J. (2015) 'Situational theories,' in T. Ward & A. Beech (Eds.), *Theories of sexual offending*, New York, NY: Wiley.

Strassberg, D. S. Eastvold, A., Kenney, J. W., and Suchy, Y. (2012) 'Psychopathy among pedophilic and nonpedophilic child molesters,' *Child Abuse & Neglect*, *36*(4):379–382.
Walters, G. D., Knight, R. A., Looman, J., and Abracen, J. (2016) 'Child molestation and psychopathy: A taxometric analysis,' *Journal of Sexual Aggression*, *22*(3):379–393.
Woodworth, M., Freimuth, T., Hutton, E. L., Carpenter, T., Agar, A. D., and Logan, M. (2013) 'High-risk sexual offenders: An examination of sexual fantasy, sexual paraphilia, psychopathy, and offence characteristics,' *International Journal of Law and Psychiatry*, *36*(2):144–156.
Zakireh, B., Ronis, S. T., and Knight, R. A. (2008) 'Individual beliefs, attitudes, and victimization histories of male juvenile sexual offenders' *Sexual Abuse*, *20*(3):323–351.

22

Sadism, psychopathy, and sexual offending

Sonja Krstic, Nicholas Longpré, Raymond Knight, and Carrie Robertson

Introduction

The concept of sadism originated in the writings of Marquis de Sade (1740–1814). The diagnosis bears his name because of his literary works, which are imbued with eroticism of violence and cruelty. The term sadism appeared in the medical literature in the work of the Richard von Krafft-Ebing (1886), who in his book *Psychopathia Sexualis* defined sadism as the experience of pleasure caused by acts of cruelty and corporal punishment inflicted on humans or animals. This can also involve the desire to humiliate, hurt, hit, or even destroy others to experience sexual pleasure.

Sexual sadism has been included in the Diagnostic and Statistical Manual of Mental Disorders (DSM; American Psychiatric Association, 1951, 2013) since the mid-twentieth century. The DSM paraphilias subgroup has defined sadism as sexual pleasure and arousal that are rooted in fantasized or actual infliction of psychological or physical suffering on a victim and has required for its diagnosis that the fantasies or behaviors must be severe, recurrent, and last for at least six months. In addition, the behaviors must be directed towards non-consenting partners, or the sexual urges or fantasies must cause marked distress or interpersonal difficulty.

The actual diagnosis of sadism is fraught with problems, such as low validity and poor consistency across assessments (Levenson, 2004; Marshall, Kennedy, & Yates, 2002). The absence of pathognomonic symptoms has been cited as an explanation for several of these problems (Marshall et al., 2002). Symptoms that are supposedly characteristic of those diagnosed sadistic are regularly found among non-pathological samples (Crépault & Couture, 1980; Malamuth & Check; 1983). Moreover, a large number of behaviors purportedly related to sexual sadism are found among non-sadistic sexual offenders (Groth & Birnbaum, 1979; Marshall & Hucker, 2006). It appears that many behaviors attributed to sadistic offenders (e.g., violence), many underlying motivations (e.g., aggressive fantasies), and many of the consequences on victims (e.g., humiliation) are not exclusive to those diagnosed as sadistic (Marshall & Kennedy, 2003).

The absence of pathognomonic symptoms weakens the assumption of a categorical diagnosis and leads to the conclusion that sadism may be represented better as a dimension. In recent years, taxometric studies have shown that sadism is distributed dimensionally (Knight, Sims-Knight, & Guay, 2013; Longpré, Guay, Knight, & Benbouriche, 2017; Longpré, Sims-Knight,

Guay, Thornton, & Knight, manuscript in preparation; Mokros, Schilling, Weiss, Nitschke, & Eher, 2014). According to Knight (2014), there is no empirical evidence to support the hypothesis of the taxonic structure of sadism in self-report data, archivally derived crime-scene data, or non-offense behaviors. The sum of the empirical evidence clearly warrants a dimensional interpretation of sadism. Moreover, in this dimensional interpretation extreme sadistic violence represents only a small part of the coercion spectrum (Knight, 2014; Longpré, Proulx, & Brouillette-Alarie, 2016). Knight and colleagues (Knight, 2010, 2014; Knight et al., 2013; Longpré et al., manuscript in preparation; Sims-Knight & Guay, 2011) found ample evidence to support the existence of an agonistic continuum ranging from non-sadistic sexual coercion to severe sadism. Knight et al. (2013) concluded that there is a single sexual aggression construct, in which non-sadistic coercive fantasies and behaviors are present at the lower end of the continuum, and sadistic fantasies and behaviors are present at the upper end of the continuum.

Psychopathy

Psychopathy is a serious personality disorder, notorious for its hallmark features, such as lack of guilt and conscience, callous disregard of others, marked impulsivity, and chronic antisocial behavior (Hare, 1991, 2003). The phenomenon of psychopathy, and the "mask of sanity" (Cleckley, 1941) that psychopaths present to the world, obscuring their stark emotional dysfunction, have long been the subject of fascination among scientists and laymen alike. Psychopathy is of particular interest because of its strong association with criminal and violent behavior (Coid, Yang, Ullrich, Roberts, & Hare, 2009; Hare, 2003; Hare & Neumann, 2008; Porter & Woodworth, 2006), coupled with the pronounced resistance to treatment (Harris & Rice, 2006; Kiehl & Hoffman, 2011). Psychopathic individuals are overrepresented among felons (Hare, 2003); they tend to be more violent during crime commission (Robertson & Knight, 2014) and to recidivate more frequently than non-psychopathic offenders (Douglas, Vincent, & Edens, 2006; Kennealy, Skeem, Walters, & Camp, 2010). Moreover, the core components of psychopathy seem to be strongly related to sexually coercive behaviors (Knight & Guay, 2006:in press).

Even though psychopathy seems so inextricably linked with forensic settings, with the estimated prevalence of 15–25 percent among convicted male felons (Hare, 2003), psychopaths are not at all uncommon in general population. It is estimated that about 1–2 percent of individuals may be psychopathic, some of whom even seem to greatly benefit from the specific set of personality traits they possess, rising to the top of corporate ladders, all the while wreaking havoc with the lives of those in their power (Babiak, Neumann, & Hare, 2010; Hall & Benning, 2006). There is, however, substantially less empirical research devoted to the phenomenon of "successful" psychopathy (Babiak et al., 2010; Hall & Benning, 2006). What psychopaths in all walks of life seem to have in common is their frightening capability to commit even the most socially devastating, ruthless acts and violent crimes with no sense of guilt, concomitant with the ability to deceptively mask true intentions and eagerly manipulate and exploit others.

Psychopathy is a complex disorder, characterized by a constellation of interpersonal, affective, and lifestyle/behavioral features, such as superficial charm, callousness and lack of empathy, impulsivity, and chronic antisocial behavior (Hare, 1991, 2003). The number of studies dedicated to the exploration of various aspects of this syndrome has dramatically increased over the past two decades, and there is a growing body of literature addressing the underlying structure of psychopathic traits, the associations of these traits with various forms of criminal behavior, the covariation of components of psychopathy with neural mechanisms and cognitive performance, and implications of the syndrome for intervention and treatment. Psychopathic traits appear to be the result of a complex interplay of genetic (Viding & McCrory, 2012) and environmental factors (Krstic, Knight, & Robertson, 2016). These traits and their cognitive and neural correlates (Herpers, Scheepers, Bons, Buitelaar, & Rommelse, 2014) emerge in childhood and show considerable stability over the course of the lifetime (Lynam, Caspi, Moffitt, Loeber, & Stouthamer-Loeber, 2007). The treatment of the disorder in adults has been shown to be difficult and unreliable (Harris & Rice, 2006; Salekin, Worley, & Grimes, 2010), and psychopathic individuals are considered to be high-risk and high-need offenders (Olver, Lewis, & Wong, 2013). Early interventions may be more successful, however (Caldwell, Skeem, Salekin, & Van Rybroek, 2006; Somech & Elizur, 2012).

Even though the conceptualization of psychopathy has varied throughout the history, Cleckley's (1976) definition of the disorder has been essential to the way we now think about it. His description of psychopathy comprised 16 personality and behavioral traits that provided the basis for the 20 items of Psychopathy Checklist (PCL; Hare, 1991) and its successor, Psychopathy Checklist Revised (PCL–R; Hare, 2003), arguably the most extensively used and best-validated measure in the evaluation of psychopathy. Four underlying factors, or facets, are now considered to best represent the components of psychopathy, as measured with PCL–R (Hare & Neumann, 2005; Vitacco, Neumann, & Jackson, 2006; Vitacco, Rogers, Neumann, Harrison, & Vincent, 2005). Thus, the traits reflected in the superficial, dishonest, and manipulative interactions with others are subsumed under the interpersonal facet, whereas the affective facet captures affective dysfunction. The lifestyle and the antisocial facets capture impulsivity, and chronic and pervasive antisocial behavior, respectively (Hare, 2003). Applying the earlier two-factor model to PCL–R, the interpersonal and affective facets can be incorporated in the original Factor 1, and the lifestyle and antisocial facets in Factor 2.

Despite the success of the PCL–R, its wide acceptance as a diagnostic indicator of psychopathy, and its contribution to advancing empirical research, disagreements about what constitutes the core components of psychopathy have been abundant (Hare & Neumann, 2005; Skeem & Cooke, 2010). Two competing conceptualizations of the disorder were proposed in the past, one based on personality and the other based on its behavioral features (Lilienfeld, 1994; Lilienfeld, 1998). The proponents of the personality-based approach to psychopathy, originating with Cleckley (1976), viewed psychopathy in the light of personality features associated with the disorder and considered the antisocial aspect to be secondary. In contrast, the behavior-oriented approach focused on the behavioral, antisocial outcomes of psychopathy (Lilienfeld, 1998). The triarchic model of psychopathy (Patrick, Fowles, & Krueger, 2009) provided an integrated conceptualization, incorporating the personality structuring of the personality-focused approach and the consideration of the disinhibitory psychopathology into the three components: Boldness, Meanness, and disinhibition. Although the components of the Triarchic Psychopathy Model have been found to correlate significantly and differentially with the interpersonal, lifestyle, and antisocial facets of PCL–R, their association with the affective facet has been found modest at best (Baskin-Sommers et al., 2015; Venables, Hall, & Patrick, 2014).

The association between psychopathy and sexual aggression is of particular interest and significance. Psychopathic traits among incarcerated offenders have been associated with the commission of sexually coercive crimes (Coid, 1992; DeGue, DiLillo, & Scalora 2010; Knight & Guay, 2006; Krupp, Sewall, Lalumière, Sheriff, & Harris, 2013); such traits have also been both empirically and theoretically linked to major elements of sexually aggressive behavior, such as inability to respond to victim's distress cues (Blair, Mitchell, & Blair, 2005), failure to inhibit sexual arousal when faced with victim resistance (Firestone, Bradford, Greenberg, & Serran, 2000; Lalumière, Quinsey, Harris, Rice, & Trautrimas, 2003), hypersexuality, sexual compulsivity, and preoccupation (Graham & Knight, 2017; Knight & Guay, 2006:in press). These associations are seen both among offenders and in the general population, and these findings have emerged consistently across studies and diverse samples. Thus, it is reasonable to hypothesize that psychopathy and sexual aggression have some etiological pathways in common (Knight & Guay, 2006:in press; Knight & Sims-Knight, 2013).

Empirical similarities between sadism and psychopathy

Sadism and psychopathy have both been theoretically, clinically, and empirically related to violence (Robertson & Knight, 2014) and to sexually coercive behaviors (Knight & Guay, 2006). Several studies have found that the two constructs covary (Knight & Guay, 2006; Mokros, Osterheider, Hucker, & Nitschke, 2011; Robertson & Knight, 2014). These two phenomena share several common features, such as emotional detachment from the suffering of others and a proclivity to inflict severe injuries (Mokros et al., 2011). These significant similarities have led some authors to speculate that there should be a sadistic psychopath (Murphy & Vess, 2003), for whom sadism may be a symptom of psychopathy and not a comorbid phenomenon. In the last few years, however, several studies have shown that these two phenomena may be distinct from a phenomenological point of view, despite their clear overlap (Kirsch & Becker, 2007; Mokros et al., 2011; Robertson & Knight, 2014).

Psychopathy is highly prevalent among sexual offenders and among sexual murderers (Langevin, 2003; Porter, Woodworth, Earle, Drugge, & Boer, 2003). Base rates of psychopathy can be quite elevated among sexual offenders (as high as 64 percent), especially among individuals who tend to have mixed victims (both children and adults), suggesting a more opportunistic approach among psychopathic offenders (Hare, 2003; Porter, ten Brinke, & Wilson, 2009; Rice & Knight, in press). In addition, it has been estimated that nearly 85 percent of sexual murderers have moderate to high psychopathy scores, with nearly 48 percent of them scoring above the clinical cut-off PCL–R score of 30 (Porter et al., 2003). This same study also found that, unsurprisingly, psychopathic offenders were more likely to perpetrate sadistic and gratuitous violence compared to non-psychopathic counterparts. A higher incidence of psychopathy has also been found among sadistic sexual offenders when compared to non-sadistic sexual offenders (Kirsch, Becker, Fanniff, & Martens, 2006). Kirsch et al. (2006) reported that 90 percent of their sadistic offenders had scores greater than 25 on the PCL–R. Psychopathy has also been related to sexually deviant penile plethysmography indices and violent and sexual recidivism (Firestone, Bradford, Greenberg, & Serran, 2000). Although some sexual murderers exhibit an extreme form of sexual sadism, it not certain whether all would be diagnosed as sadists (James & Proulx, 2014).

Mokros et al. (2011) recently explored the empirical relation between the severe sexual sadism scale (SeSaS; Nitschke, Osterheider, & Mokros, 2009) and the PCL–R in a sample of 100 male forensic patients from Germany. They reported that sadistic offenders scored significantly higher than non-sadistic offenders on the PCL–R. They also reported a significant correlation between both measures. Only PCL–R's affective and antisocial facets, however, showed significant correlations with the SeSaS. Finally, an exploratory factor analysis yielded a clear two-factor solution, in which sexual sadism and psychopathy loaded on separate factors. Their results indicated that although sadism and psychopathy are significantly correlated, they remain two distinct constructs.

Robertson and Knight (2014) also investigated the relation between sexual sadism and psychopathy. They found that self-reported sadism correlated with PCL–R total score, as well as with interpersonal, lifestyle and antisocial facets. They also reported a relation between sadism based on archival-classification and PCL–R total score as well as interpersonal, affective, and antisocial facets. Whereas the affective facet was found to be a good predictor of violence and abnormal sexual behavior, the antisocial facet was found to be a good predictor of sexual violence and physical control in the offense. These results indicated that PCL–R and sexual sadism were related. Furthermore, these results indicated that PCL–R affective and antisocial facets were good predictors of violence in the sexual offense. Similar results were reported in a recent study that employed both variable and trait-centered approaches to examining psychopathic traits in sex offenders. Affective and antisocial facets showed the greatest power in predicting violent sexual behaviors, and the subtype of offenders characterized by highest affective and antisocial facet scores were also most likely to engage in expressive aggression and sadistic assault before, during, and after the commission of sexual crimes (Krstic et al., 2017). Although the association between antisocial scores and violence has been consistently reported across a number of studies (e.g., Kennealy et al., 2010; Olver, Neumann, et al., 2013), the apparently important relation of the affective psychopathic traits with violent sexual crimes has not received enough attention.

Conclusion

In summary, these results indicated that sadism, whether measured by self-report or rated from archival files, whether assessed as dimensional or as categorical, is correlated with psychopathy and PCL–R scores. Furthermore, both constructs appear to be distinguishable from a phenomenological point of view, as Mokros et al.'s (2011) two-factor solution suggested. Finally, PCL–R Factor 1 and 2 are implicated in both the severity of the offense and recidivism. Importantly, it is reasonable to hypothesize that some core components of psychopathy may be inextricably linked to sexual violence and sadistic behaviors.

References

American Psychiatric Association. (1951) *Diagnostic and statistical manual of mental disorders* (1st ed.), Washington, DC: Author.

American Psychiatric Association. (2013) *Diagnostic and statistical manual of mental disorders* (5th ed.), Washington, DC: Author.

Babiak, P., Neumann, C. S., and Hare, R. D. (2010) 'Corporate psychopathy: Talking the walk,' *Behavioral Sciences and the Law, 28*(2):174–193.

Baskin-Sommers, A. R., Curtin, K. J., and Newman, J. P. (2015) 'Altering the cognitive–affective dysfunctions of psychopathic and externalizing offender subtypes with cognitive remediation,' *Clinical Psychology Science, 1*(3):45–57.

Blair, J., Mitchell, D., and Blair, K. (2005) *The psychopath: Emotion and the brain*, Malden, MA: Blackwell.

Caldwell, M., Skeem, J., Salekin, R., and Van Rybroek, G. (2006) 'Treatment response of adolescent offenders with psychopathy features: A 2-year follow-up,' *Criminal Justice and Behavior, 33*(5):571–596.

Cleckley, H. (1976) *The mask of sanity* (6th ed.), St. Louis, MO: Mosby.

Coid, J. W. (1992) 'DSM–III diagnosis in criminal psychopaths: A way forward,' *Criminal Behaviour & Mental Health, 2*:78–94.

Coid, J., Yang, M., Ullrich, S., Roberts, A., and Hare, R. D. (2009) 'Prevalence and correlates of psychopathic traits in the household population of Great Britain,' *International Journal of Law and Psychiatry, 32*(2):65–73.

Crépault, E., and Couture, M. (1980) 'Men's erotic fantasies,' *Archives of Sexual Behavior, 9*:565–581.

DeGue, S., DiLillo, D., and Scalora, M. (2010) 'Are all perpetrators alike? Comparing risk factors for sexual coercion and aggression,' *Sexual Abuse: A Journal of Research and Treatment, 22*:402–426.

Douglas, K. S., Vincent, G. M., and Edens, J. F. (2006) 'Risk for criminal recidivism: The role of psychopathy,' in C. J. Patrick (Ed.), *Handbook of psychopathy* (pp. 533–554), New York, NY: Guilford Press.

Firestone, P., Bradford, J. M., Greenberg, D. M., and Serran, G. A. (2000) 'The relationship of deviant sexual arousal and psychopathy in incest offenders, extrafamilial child Molesters, and rapists,' *Journal of the American Academy of Psychiatry and Law, 28*:303–308.

Knight, R. A., and Graham, F. J. (2017) 'Hypersexuality: Equifinal, cohesive, clinical presentation or symptom cluster with multiple underlying mechanisms?,' *Archives of Sexual Behavior, 46*:2261–2264.

Groth, A. N., and Birnbaum, H. J. (1979) *Men who rape: The psychology of the offender*, New York, NY: Plenum.

Hall, J. R., and Benning, S. D. (2006) 'The "successful" psychopath: Adaptive and subclinical manifestations of psychopathy in the general population,' in C. J. Patrick (Ed.), *Handbook of psychopathy* (pp. 459–478), New York, NY: Guilford Press.

Hare, R. D. (1991) *The Hare Psychopathy Checklist–Revised*, Toronto, ON: Multi-Health Systems.

Hare, R. D. (2003) *The Hare Psychopathy Checklist–Revised* (2nd ed.), Toronto, ON: Multi-Health Systems.

Hare, R. D., and Neumann, C. S. (2005) 'Structural models of psychopathy,' *Current Psychiatry Reports*, 7(1):57–64.

Hare, R. D., and Neumann, C. S. (2008) 'Psychopathy as a clinical and empirical construct,' *Annual Review of Clinical Psychology*, *4*(2):217–246.

Harris, G. T., and Rice, M. (2006) 'Treatment of psychopathy: A review of empirical findings,' in C. J. Patrick (Ed.), *Handbook of psychopathy* (pp. 555–572), New York, NY: Guilford Press.

Herpers, P., Scheepers, F. E., Bons, D., Buitelaar, J. K., and Rommelse, N. N. (2014) 'The cognitive and neural correlates of psychopathy and especially callous–unemotional traits in youths: A systematic review of the evidence,' *Development and Psychopathology*, *26*(1):245–273.

James, J., and Proulx, J. (2014) 'A psychological and developmental profile of sexual murderers: A systematic review,' *Aggression and Violent Behavior*, *19*:592–607.

Kennealy, P. K., Skeem, J. L., Walters, G. D., and Camp, J. (2010) 'Do core interpersonal and affective traits of PCL–R psychopathy interact with antisocial behavior and disinhibition to predict violence?,' *Psychological Assessment*, *22*:569–580.

Kiehl, K. A., and Hoffman, M. B. (2011) 'The criminal psychopath: History, neuroscience, treatment, and economics,' *Jurimetrics*, *51*:355–397.

Kirsch, L. G., and Becker, J. V. (2007) 'Emotional deficits in psychopathy and sexual sadism: Implications for violent and sadistic behavior,' *Clinical Psychology Review*, *27*:904–922.

Kirsch, L. G., Becker, J. V., Fanniff, A. M., and Martens, A. (2006) *Childhood sexual abuse by a female and the development of sexual sadism*. Poster presented at the annual meeting of the Association for the Treatment of Sexual Abusers, Chicago, IL.

Krafft-Ebing, R. (1998) *Psychopathia sexualis*, Philadelphia, PA: F.A. Davis. (Original work published in 1886).

Knight, R. A. (2010) 'Is a diagnostic category for paraphilic coercive disorder defensible?,' *Archive of Sexual Behavior*, *39*(2):419–426.

Knight, R. A. (2014) *Sadism: End of an agonistic continuum*, Paper presented at the 33rd conference of the Association for the Treatment of Sexual Abusers (ATSA), San Diego, California.

Knight, R. A., and Guay, J.-P. (2006) 'The role of psychopathy in sexual coercion against women,' in C. J. Patrick (Ed.), *Handbook of psychopathy* (pp. 512–532), New York, NY: Gilford Press.

Knight, R. A., and Guay, J.-P. (in press) 'The role of psychopathy in sexual coercion against women: An update and expansion,' in C. J. Patrick (Ed.), *Handbook of psychopathy* (Vol II), New York, NY: The Guilford Press.

Knight, R. A., and Sims-Knight, J. E. (2013) 'Risk factors for sexual violence,' in J. White, M. P. Koss, & A. Kazdin (Eds.), *Violence against women and girls* (Vol. I, pp. 125–172), Washington, DC: American Psychological Association.

Knight, R. A., Sims-Knight, J., and Guay, J.-P. (2013) 'Is a separate diagnostic category defensible for paraphilic coercion?,' *Journal of Criminal Justice*, *41*:90–99.

Krstic, S., Knight, R. A., and Robertson, C. A. (2016) 'Developmental antecedents of the facets of psychopathy: The role of multiple abuse experiences,' *Journal of Personality Disorders*, *30*(5):677–693.

Krstic, S., Neumann, C. S., Roy, S., Robertson, C. A., Knight, R. A., and Hare, R. D. (2017) 'Using latent variable- and person-centered approaches to examine the role of psychopathic traits in sex offenders,' *Personality Disorders: Theory, Research, And Treatment*, doi:10.1037/per0000249

Krupp, D. B., Sewall, L. A., Lalumière, M. L., Sheriff, C., and Harris, G. T. (2013) 'Psychopathy, adaptation and disorder,' *Frontiers in Psychology*, *27*(4):139–148.

Lalumière, M., Quinsey, V., Harris, G., Rice, M., and Trautrimas, C. (2003) 'Are rapists differentially aroused by coercive sex in phallometric assessments?,' *Annals of the New York Academy of Sciences*, *989*:211–24.

Langevin, R. (2003) 'A study of the psychosexual characteristics of sex killers: Can we identify them before it is too late?,' *International Journal of Offender Therapy and Comparative Criminology*, *47*:366–382.

Levenson, J. S. (2004) 'Reliability of sexually violent predator civil commitment criteria in Florida,' *Law and Human Behavior*, *28*(3):57–68.

Lilienfeld, S. O. (1994) 'Conceptual problems in the assessment of psychopathy,' *Clinical Psychology Review*, *14*(1):17–38.

Lilienfeld, S. O. (1998) 'Recent methodological advances and developments in the assessment of psychopathy,' *Behavior Research and Therapy*, *36*:99–125.

Longpré, N., Proulx, J., and Brouillette-Alarie, S. (2016) 'Convergent validity of three measures of sexual sadism: Value of a dimensional measure,' *Sexual Abuse: A Journal of Research and Treatment*, in press.

Longpré, N., Guay, J. P., Knight, R. A., and Benbouriche, M. (2017) 'Sadistic offender or sexual sadism? Taxometric evidence for a dimensional structure of sexual sadism,' *Archives of Sexual Behavior*, in press.

Longpré, N., Sims-Knight, J. E., Guay, J. P., Thornton, D., and Knight, R. A. (2018) Is Paraphilic coercion a different construct from sadism or simply the lower end of a continuum anchored at the high end by sadism? Manuscript in preparation.

Lynam, D. R., Caspi, A., Moffitt, T. E., Loeber, R., and Stouthamer-Loeber, M. (2007) 'Longitudinal evidence that psychopathy scores in early adolescence predict adult psychopathy,' *Journal of Abnormal Psychology*, *116*(1):155–176.

Marshall, W. L., Kennedy, P., and Yates, P. (2002) 'Issues concerning the reliability and validity of the diagnosis of sexual sadism applied in prison settings,' *Sexual Abuse: A Journal of Research and Treatment*, *14*(4):301–311.

Malamuth, N. M., and Check, J. V. C. (1983) 'Sexual arousal to rape depictions: Individuals differences,' *Journal of Abnormal Psychology*, *92*:55–67.

Marshall, W. L., and Hucker, S. J. (2006) 'Issues in the diagnosis of sexual sadism,' *Sexual Offender Treatment*, *1*(2):1–4.

Marshall, W. L., and Kennedy, P. (2003) 'Sexual sadism in sexual offenders: An elusive diagnosis,' *Aggression and Violent Behavior*, *8*(1):1–22.

Mokros, A., Osterheider, M., Hucker, S. J., and Nitschke, J. (2011) 'Psychopathy and sexual sadism,' *Law and Human Behavior*, *35*(3):188–199.

Mokros, A., Schilling, F., Weiss, K., Nitschke, J., and Eher, R. (2014) 'Sadism in sexual offenders: Evidence for dimensionality,' *Psychological Assessment*, *26*(1):138–147.

Murphy, C., and Vess, J. (2003) 'Subtypes of psychopathy: Proposed differences between narcissistic, borderline, sadistic, and antisocial psychopaths,' *Psychiatric Quarterly*, *74*:11–29.

Nitschke, J., Osterheider, M., and Mokros, A. (2009) 'A cumulative scale of severe sexual sadism,' *Sexual Abuse: A Journal of Research and Treatment*, *21*:262–278.

Olver, M. E., Lewis K., and Wong, S. C. (2013) 'Risk reduction treatment of high-risk psychopathic offenders: The relationship of psychopathy and treatment change to violent recidivism,' *Personality Disorders*, *4*:160–167.

Olver, M. E., Neumann, C. S., Wong, S. C. P., and Hare, R. D. (2013) 'The structural and predictive properties of the Psychopathy Checklist–Revised in Canadian Aboriginal and non-Aboriginal offenders,' *Psychological Assessment*, *25*:167–179.

Patrick, C. J., Fowles, D. C., and Krueger, R. F. (2009) 'Triarchic conceptualization of psychopathy: Developmental origins of disinhibition, boldness, and meanness,' *Development and Psychopathology*, *21*(3):913–938.

Porter, S., ten Brinke, L., and Wilson, K. (2009) 'Crime profiles and conditional release performance of psychopathic and non-psychopathic sexual offenders,' *Legal and Criminological Psychology*, *14*:109–118.

Porter, S., and Woodworth, M. (2006) 'Psychopathy and aggression,' in C. J. Patrick (Ed.), *Handbook of psychopathy* (pp. 481–494), New York, NY: Guilford Press.

Porter, S., Woodworth, M., Earle, J., Drugge, J., and Boer, D. (2003) 'Characteristics of sexual homicides committed by psychopathic and nonpsychopathic offenders,' *Law and Human Behavior*, *27*:459–470.

Robertson, C., and Knight, R. A. (2014) 'Relating sexual sadism and psychopathy to one another, non-sexual violence, and sexual crime behaviours,' *Aggressive Behavior*, *40*(1):12–23.

Rice, J., and Knight, R. A. (in press) 'Differentiating adults with mixed age victims from those who exclusively sexually assault children or adults,' *Sexual Abuse: A Journal of Research and Treatment*, in press.

Salekin, R. T., Worley, C., and Grimes, R. D. (2010) 'Treatment of psychopathy: A review and brief introduction to the mental model approach for psychopathy,' *Behavioral Sciences and the Law*, *28*(2):235–266.

Skeem, J. L., and Cooke, D. J. (2010) 'Is criminal behavior a central component of psychopathy? Conceptual directions for resolving the debate,' *Psychological Assessment*, *22*(2):433–445.

Sims-Knight, J. E., and Guay, J. P. (2011) *Is PCD a construct distinct from sadism?* Paper presented at the 30th Annual Conference of the Association for the Treatment of Sexual Abusers (ATSA), Toronto, ON.

Somech, L. Y., and Elizur, Y. (2012) 'Promoting self-regulation and cooperation in pre-kindergarten children with conduct problems: A randomized controlled trial,' *Journal of the American Academy of Child and Adolescent Psychiatry*, *51*(4):412–422.

Venables, N. C., Hall, J. R., and Patrick, C. J. (2014) 'Differentiating psychopathy from antisocial personality disorder: A triarchic model perspective,' *Psychological Medicine, 44*(5):1005–1013.

Viding, E., and McCrory, E. J. (2012) 'Genetic and neurocognitive to the development of psychopathy,' *Developmental Psychopathology, 24*(3):969–983.

Vitacco, M. J., Neumann, C. S., and Jackson, R. L. (2006) 'Testing a four-factor model of psychopathy and its association with ethnicity, gender, intelligence, and violence,' *Journal of Consulting Clinical Psychology, 73*(3):466–476.

Vitacco, M. J., Rogers, R., Neumann, C. S., Harrison, K. S., and Vincent, G. M. (2005) 'A comparison of factor models on the PCL–R with mentally disordered offenders: The development of a four-factor model,' *Criminal Justice and Behavior, 32*(5):526–545.

23

Psychopathy and sexual offending

Vincent Egan and Simon Duff

Introduction

The current chapter explores the relationship between psychopathy and sexual offending and can be seen as complementary to Seto, Harris, and Lalumière's (2015) chapter on the same topic. We conclude that although there is an association, it is because of the broader association between psychopathy and offending of all types, and that this in turn often reflects general Antagonism. Disproportionately attributing sexual offending to psychopathy belies the many pathways into sexual offending, which is itself a very broad criminological classification, ranging from hands-off, remote offenses (for example, viewing indecent material online or stealing items for fetishistic purposes) to hands-on/contact offenses (rape and sexual assault). Moreover, some aspects of psychopathy are more associated with sexual offending than others; the core traits (affective and interpersonal) are less strongly associated than behavioral and criminal lifestyle facets. Also, concurrent sexual deviation is a key risk-increasing factor, as are emotional–neurotic elements emerging from secondary psychopathy, such as obsessionality and compulsivity. Given the nature of this volume, we do not intend to review the background literature on the psychopathy construct, which is well covered elsewhere in this book.

While not everybody holds that psychopathy and sexual offending are isomorphically associated, psychopathy may help differentiate offender profiles. For example, Porter et al. (2000) examined a large sample (N = 329) of offenders categorized by their crimes, finding that although all sex offender groups showed more of the interpersonal and affective characteristics of psychopathy, mixed rapist/abusers and rapists were more psychopathic than child abusers. Significantly, they found that of the crossover sexual offenders (sexual offenders who victimize persons across boundaries of age and/or gender; Heil, Ahlmeyer, & Simons, 2003), 64 percent were psychopathic. At the same time, the significance of psychopathy as a general explanatory concept for sexual offending may be exaggerated; Langevin (2003) compared a group of sexual murderers to a large cohort of other sexual offenders regarding their sexual, criminological, and psychological histories. The sex killers started their criminal careers earlier, had been more commonly in young offenders' institutions, had been gang members, and were arsonists, sadistic, fetishist, and voyeuristic, but were also more likely to be diagnosed with Antisocial Personality Disorder than psychopathy. A large German study also found that Antisocial, Borderline,

Sadistic, and Schizoid Personality Disorders were more common in sexual murderers, with multiple sexual murderers also characterized by expressing more sexual sadism, voyeurism, and a lower incidence of mood disorder than single sexual murderers (Hill, Habermann, Berner, & Briken, 2007). Intelligent psychopaths may be able to find ways of expressing deviant desires without obviously breaking laws, meaning that psychopaths with lower IQ are four times more likely to be sexually reconvicted (Beggs & Grace, 2008).

Broadly speaking, there appear two clear strands to the literature on psychopathy and sexual offending; psychopathy as a predictor of sexual recidivism; and psychopathy as a marker for sexual deviance. There is also likely to be a population of people who have high levels of psychopathy and high levels of deviance but do not offend, or at least not in a way that draws attention; a psychopathic individual with money may well find that it is more strategically expedient to pay for a sex worker than to commit a sexual assault. We suspect it likely that there are hidden cohorts of such persons. The lifestyles of these persons would be an interesting cohort to examine.

Methodological and conceptual issues

The methods by which psychopathy is assessed vary, but in criminal and forensic mental health settings, many have settled on the revised Psychopathy Checklist (PCL–R, Hare, 2003) as a useful broad-spectrum tool to assess the construct. This is a widely used assessment tool with one factor that is a recognized structure of core psychopathic features (none of which are inherently criminal; F1) and a second factor comprising antisocial lifestyle features (F2). Some controversy arose when Cooke, Michie, and Skeem (2007) presented a rigorous analysis of PCL–R data from over 1,200 British prisoners and found the best model to describe the instrument required the addition of a specific criminal behavior element over these two factors. Subsequent work revealed a hierarchical model in which the two factors further divided themselves into four facets, so F1 comprised facets of arrogant and deceitful interpersonal style (f1) and deficient affective experience (f2), while F2 comprised facets of impulsive and irresponsible behavioral style (f3) and criminal lifestyle (f4), a good-fitting model which has been observed in a large cohort of adult sex offenders (Weaver, Meyer, Van Nort, & Tristan, 2006).

The concern with the structure of the PCL–R has been because it has sometimes seemed that psychopathy is nothing but the PCL–R, with the criminal behavior the central element of the construct, whereas evidence suggests that this is not the case (Skeem & Cooke, 2010). One is left in the unusual position of observing that the core traits of psychopathy in a person will undoubtedly make them difficult and unpleasant, but it is the antisocial behavioral facets of F2 captured by the PCL–R that predict many antisocial outcomes, not psychopathy's underlying interpersonal and affective facets.

Another aspect of psychopathy that is conceptually difficult but germane to the consideration of sexual offenders is the clinical distinction between primary and secondary psychopathy. Primary psychopathy is regarded as a condition in which persons have an inability to recognize or perceive emotions, so may lack anxiety; it is this lack of physiological response that may mean psychopathic individuals may literally not feel fear or empathy for others (the "somatic marker" model of psychopathy). Secondary psychopathy is seen in persons who present with psychopathic behaviors, but who are emotionally disturbed and so may have comorbid neurotic disorders such as anxiety or obsessive–compulsive difficulties (Yildirim & Derksen, 2015). It is in the latter population one will see the not uncommon comorbidity of antisocial and Borderline Personality Disorder; it has been suggested they have similar genetic etiology, but primary psychopathy is protective of secondary psychopathic expression (Hunt, Bornovalova, & Patrick,

2015). From this, one might predict that primary psychopaths will have opportunistic or impersonal appetitive sex if they desire so, but it will not have any emotional or relational meaning, nor be associated with neurotic difficulties, whereas secondary psychopathic sexual offenders may have many sexual complexes and disorders and prior courtship difficulties.

Finally, an important consideration for this chapter that the reader must bear in mind, as with many other reviews that investigate the possible relationship between psychopathy and other behavior, is the inconsistent application of cut-offs for the identification of psychopathy. A variety of scores are used, commonly 25 (e.g., Olver & Wong, 2006) and 30 (e.g., Brown & Forth, 1997), and this will impact on the populations that are identified as offending and recidivating psychopaths and non-psychopaths.

Evidence for psychopathy as a risk factor for sexual recidivism

The evidence for psychopathy as a risk-increasing factor for recidivism is unambiguous, and we will examine some of that evidence below. Before doing so, there is an important finding that should be kept in mind when considering the link between psychopathy and recidivism. Recidivism can only be measured within incarcerated populations when individuals are released, and if psychopathic individuals were denied release, psychopathy would not be a risk-increasing factor for sexual recidivism. However, research by Porter, ten Brinke, and Wilson (2009) found that in their sample of 310 Canadian males in a medium secure prison, psychopathic individuals were 2.5 times more likely to be granted release than non-psychopathic individuals (based on PCL–R scores with a clinical cut-off of 30) and that psychopathic sex offenders were 2.4 times more likely to be released than non-psychopathic sexual offenders. This is important, as it may suggest psychopathic individuals are no more likely to reoffend than their non-psychopathic counterparts due to psychopathy *per se*, but spending less time in institutions may expose them to fewer treatment opportunities, place them back into antisocial environments, and allow them more time to offend.

Over 20 years ago, Salekin, Rogers, and Sewell (1996) performed a meta-analysis of the 18 studies that up to that point had investigated the relationship between the PCL/PCL–R and violent and nonviolent recidivism, finding moderate to strong effect sizes and an ability to predict violence and general recidivism. Around this time, Hanson and Bussière (1998) examined sexual offense recidivism, finding that although the general reconviction rate for this kind of offense was low (13.4 percent; n = 23,393), some subgroups of offenders were much more likely to commit another offense of this kind. Hanson et al. found sexual offense recidivism best predicted by measures of sexual deviancy (e.g., deviant sexual preferences, prior sexual offenses) and generic criminological factors (e.g., age, total prior offenses). Those who failed to complete treatment were at higher risk for reoffending than those who completed treatment.

A more extensive study by Hanson and Morton-Bourgon (2005) comprising 82 recidivism studies (1,620 findings, 29,450 sexual offenders) reaffirmed this earlier finding. Deviant sexual preferences and antisocial orientation were the major predictors of sexual recidivism for adult and adolescent sexual offender populations. Antisocial orientation was the major predictor of violent recidivism and general (any) recidivism. The review also identified some dynamic risk factors that have the potential of being useful treatment targets (e.g., sexual preoccupations, general self-regulation problems). Predicting current belated recognitions, many constructs included in sex offender treatment programs (e.g., psychological distress, denial of sex crime, victim empathy, stated motivation for treatment) were found to have little or no relationship with sexual or violent recidivism. Within this study was a meta-analysis of the association between total PCL–R scores and sexual recidivism, which found an effect size of 0.29.

Using the two-factor, four-facet hierarchical structure model of the PCL–R, Hawes, Boccaccini, and Murrie (2013) broke down the measure into these constituent factors and facets for a meta-analysis, examining their specific value predicting sexual recidivism across 20 studies (n = 5,239). The effect size for the total PCL–R predicting sexual recidivism was d = 0.40. F2 – antisocial lifestyle and behavior – had the highest effect (d = 0.44), and facet 4 (criminal lifestyle) the strongest association (d = 0.40) relative to the other factor or facet scores (d = 0.01 to 0.17). Echoing a theme of this chapter, offenders who scored high on both the PCL–R and a measure of sexual deviance were more likely to reoffend sexually than other offenders (odds ratio = 2.80 to 3.21, k = 6).

These results reiterate that it is the combination of particular high PCL–R scores and sexual deviance that are most relevant to estimating risk of future sexual offending (see also Olver & Wong, 2006). Nevertheless, the observation that psychopathy and sexual deviance are a "deadly combination" (Hare, 1999:189) is perhaps best moderated to antisocial behavioral habits and sexual deviance as "the deadly combination." Olver and Wong (2006) observed that PCL–R scores, however fractionated, were a weak predictor of sexual recidivism (but, primarily via Factor 2, a predictor of violent non-sexual and general recidivism), and that sexual deviance is negatively correlated with psychopathy (which was also found in Gretton et al.'s 2001 study looking at adolescents assessed with the PCL: YV, where a score of 30 or above was categorized as "high"). This is because not all psychopaths are sexual offenders, and sexual offending is a far more complex and diverse area of offending, among whom are many persons with neurotic–emotional disorders who have courtship, attachment, and emotional congruence issues rather than being driven by the callous and remorseless use of others. What, then, of psychopathy when expressed sexually?

Are psychopaths more inclined to sexual deviance?

Sexual behavior is inherently risky, and therefore humans are typically cautious about who they have sex with; interpersonal anxieties, impregnation and the responsibilities and commitments associated, sexually transmitted diseases, and performance anxiety may all contribute to sexual inhibition unless one is very confident of their partner's accepting them or genuine commitment. Such concerns are less cardinal to persons who lack anxiety and are emotionally detached. It is therefore to be expected that psychopaths may have a different pattern of sexual behavior relative to the general population.

If so, one might expect inconsiderate unprotected sex or the transmission of sexually transmitted diseases (STDs) to be more common in psychopathic individuals. Evidence upholds this prediction: risky sexual behavior is higher in subclinically psychopathic individuals, with the impulsive antisociality facet of psychopathy a significant predictor for both genders, but especially so for males, who also tend to have the raised Fearless Dominance needed for the exploratory behavior in the first place (Fulton, Marcus, & Payne, 2010). Unprotected sex and HIV-related sexual risk behavior is also elevated in more psychopathic adolescent drug misusers (Malow et al., 2007). However, thoughtless and inconsiderate or irresponsible sexual activity is not itself sexually deviant. One possible explanation for elements of deviant sex is the fact that psychopathic individuals have been shown, in some circumstances, to be poorer at delay gratification (identified as an important component of socialization; Wilson & Herrnstein, 1985); rather than waiting until, for example, a partner clearly consents, being unable to delay gratification may lead individuals to be sexually impulsive. These studies tend to be carried out where the rewards are monetary (e.g., Newman, Kosson, & Patterson, 1992), and it is important to find ways to examine delay gratification in response to potential sexual rewards.

"Sexual deviance" is a very emotive and loaded term, which provokes the Anger of sexual radicals keen to embrace marginal sexual practices as much as social conservatives seeking to legislate or pathologize people's private sexual lives (De Block & Adriaens, 2013). DSM has progressively improved from the times when homosexuality appeared in the index as a mental disorder (Drescher, 2015), and introduced the term paraphilia ("deviant attraction") to replace the term "sexual deviation." A paraphilia is a persistent, intense, atypical sexual arousal pattern that exists independent of whether it causes an individual distress or impairment; this means "furries" (persons who dress up for sexual purposes as large cartoon animals) can be seen as having a paraphilia, even if nobody is hurt (Soh & Cantor, 2015). A disordered paraphilia involves persistent and intense atypical sexual arousal patterns accompanied by clinically significant distress or impairment to the individual, or the focus of this desire (First, 2014). In practice, DSM–5 specifies the most common of these disorders as voyeurism (watching), exhibitionism, frotteurism (rubbing), pedophilia, sexual sadism, sexual masochism, non-specific fetishism, and transvestism (American Psychiatric Association, 2013).

Five of these eight categories are commonly seen in the context of sexual offending; sexual masochism can be likewise criminalized if the person(s) delivering the pain to the sexual masochists are believed to have committed a criminal offense, as in the case of the men in the U.K. who were prosecuted under "Operation Spanner" for committing assault involving actual bodily harm during consensual sadomasochism (White, 2006): the operation was called "Spanner" as the police officers involved said that "the acts involved made their nuts tighten." Fetishism may also be identified as a more serious forensic concern if a person, for example, steals fetishistic items (e.g., underwear, nappies) associated with their kink (Schlesinger & Revitch, 1999).

Psychopathy and sexual sadism

While psychopathy and sexual sadism are serious risk factors for criminal offending (Woodworth et al., 2013; Meere & Egan, 2017), it is less certain if psychopaths are necessarily sexually deviant. Mokros, Osterheider, Hucker, and Nitschke (2011) assessed psychopathy and sexual sadism in 100 mentally disordered offenders and found their data best explained by two separate latent variables reflecting these constructs, in which f2/f3 (affective–behavioral) psychopathic facets preceded sexually sadistic conduct. Elsewhere, Robertson and Knight (2014) also examined sexual sadism and the PCL–R in two large samples of sexual offenders; they found sadism and psychopathy correlated, but were not synonymous, and sexual sadism was primarily underpinned by f1 and f4 (interpersonal–criminal lifestyle) and total PCL–R scores. PCL–R facets collectively predicted the violence and paraphilic factors. It is easy to see how the how emotion recognition and emotional experience deficits in psychopaths may lead some to be unempathic and so behave in a sexually sadistic way (Kirsch & Becker, 2007; Marsh & Blair, 2008).

However, the question remains: are psychopaths actually deriving pleasure and arousal from sexual sadism, or do they simply have a deficit in perceiving that they are causing suffering? We know, for example, that persons high in F1 (primary, interpersonal–emotional psychopathy) show diminished galvanic skin responses to both pleasant and unpleasant noises (Verona, Patrick, Curtin, Bradley, & Lang, 2004). Psychopaths are less likely to react spontaneously to aversive and upsetting images (Levenston, Patrick, Bradley, & Lang, 2000). Moreover, reflecting the idea that primary and secondary psychopaths differ emotionally, and thus their emotional needs will likewise vary, evidence that psychopathic males have higher high basal urinary oxytocin, and so could be said to feel like they are in love – with themselves – is intriguing (Mitchell et al., 2013).

That psychopaths are less sensitive to, or more easily able to ignore, contextual information that might moderate deviant behavior appears to be a shared view across much research.

Newman (1997) has suggested an additional factor that may work to make such information even less available, and that is specific forms of Central Nervous System (CNS) arousal. He suggests that some aspects of psychopathy may be explained by increased arousal in systems that are sensitive to reward cues and reduced arousal in behavioral inhibitory systems that are responsible for directing attending to significant stimuli that may lead to ongoing behavior being interrupted. This may include ongoing antisocial behavior. It is thought that without the broad range of influences that CNS arousal and personality has on physical and cognitive systems, sexual behavior may be generally less frequent in humans (Derefinko et al., 2014; Hald & Malamuth, 2015), so we know that CNS arousal plays a facilitative role in nondeviant sex even in the non-psychopathic individual.

There is some evidence that psychopathic individuals derive inverted social reward, in that they derive pleasure from another person's discomfort and the callous treatment of others; they also less enjoy positive social interactions (Foulkes, McCrory, Neumann, & Viding, 2014). Foulkes et al. believe that the self-serving and cruel social behavior seen in psychopathy may in part be explained by what these individuals find rewarding. Elsewhere, Međedović (2017) observed that elevated positive emotions experienced when observing violent stimuli and negative emotions as a reaction to peaceful stimuli predicted sadism, even when psychopathy variance was controlled. An implicit association study examining violence-dependent stimuli and terms describing positive and negative emotions also found that the combination of callous affect and lower negative associations to violent stimuli predicted sadism. Phallometric studies of rapists have found that a sexual interest in (or indifference to) non-consent is as important for predicting tumescent response arousal to violence and injury (Harris, Lalumiere, Seto, Rice, & Chaplin, 2012). Thus, the distress of others may be inherently arousing to more psychopathic individuals.

Psychopathy and pedophilia

Pedophilia is one of the more common sexual offenses. If psychopathy was linked either through sexual deviance or a lack of concern for the law's views of the appropriateness of a sexual partner, one would expect high levels of psychopathy in people convicted for sexual offenses against children. Studies have shown that not only are rates of psychopathy low in child molesters (8 percent, Serin, Malcolm, Khanna, & Barbaree, 1994; 9.4 percent Porter et al., 2000), but rates differ between different forms of sexual offense. For example, in Porter's study 35.9 percent of rapists exceeded the PCL–R cut-off of 30.

Like many other sexual offenses, pedophilia can involve direct or indirect contact. Persons committing hands-on contact offenses may be different to persons looking at indecent images of children on line (and so non-contact), but even then there is nuance and idiosyncrasy; the person paying to view another person commit a sexual offense with a child over the Internet is probably more committed to their deviation, as what they see will be explicitly sexual in nature. Babchishin, Hanson, and VanZuylen (2015) conducted an analysis of over 5,000 sexual offenders, comparing persons convicted for possession of child pornography, contact sexual offenses, and those who committed both kinds of offense. The crossover from remote to active offending occurred in those persons who expressed a sexual interest in children, had practical access to victims, a significant previous criminal history, and a lack of internal controls to inhibit acting on sexually deviant interests. Sexual offenses against children can be clustered into aggressive, intimate, or criminal-opportunist types (Canter, Hughes, & Kirby, 1998). Non-pedophiles who engage in offenses driven by criminal opportunism or aggression are significantly more psychopathic than purely pedophilic intimate-type offenders (Strassberg, Eastvold, Kenney, & Suchya,

2012), who are driven by more emotional needs. Again, crossover-type offenders (trisexuals – they will try anything) present as being of the most concern.

Crossover offenders are presumably more polymorphously perverse, and this reflects the importance of sexual preoccupation and sexual obsessive–compulsivity when assessing sexual offenders, whether they are psychopathic or not. Examining a large corpus of data on British sexual offenders, Tully, Browne, and Craig (2015) found the sexual interests/ preoccupation subscale of the Structured Assessment of Risk and Need–Treatment Needs Analysis (SARN–TNA, Thornton, 2002) most effective for predicting future risk of reconviction for a sexual offense, while the SARN's other subscales (offense-supportive attitudes, troubled relationships, poor self-management) showed no significant predictive effects on reconviction and risk outcomes. A raised sexual preoccupation subscale meant an individual was five times more likely to be reconvicted, whereas the next strongest effect was for offense supportive attitudes, which was not statistically significant. Egan, Kavanagh and Blair (2005) found the most sexually deviant offenders to be the most obsessional, and that this relationship maintained even when corrected for Neuroticism.

Compulsive use of Internet pornography can be explained by a general addictive model that integrates Neuroticism, low Agreeableness, and obsessive–compulsive difficulties, and these constructs also predict clinical problems such as negative urgency and behavioral dyscontrol (Egan & Parmar, 2013). Compulsive sexual behavior tends to be associated with neurotic difficulties; for instance, Odlaug et al. (2013) found such persons also reported more depressive and anxiety symptoms, higher levels of stress, poorer self-esteem, and higher rates of social anxiety disorder, Attention-Deficit/Hyperactivity Disorder, compulsive buying, pathological gambling, and kleptomania. These concurrent disorders are in the neurotic/ impulse-control domains. Likewise, exhibitionism and voyeurism is characterized by a generalized sexual compulsivity and a variety of neurotic indicators (Långström & Seto, 2006). The active move from non-contact to contact sexual offending is modest; a review of 12 studies of exhibitionists and voyeurs followed up for five years more found 5–10 percent of such offenders escalating to contact sexual offenses, as compared to 25 percent who committed a further exhibitionistic offense. They found the most supported risk factor for escalation was a generic antisocial behavior, including a history of sexual and non-sexual convictions (McNally & Fremouw, 2014). These findings strongly point towards secondary, emotionally associated psychopathy being more common for sexual offenders. There is no strong evidence that primary psychopathy is disproportionately associated with pedophilia in whatever form, even though psychopaths are higher on sexual sensation seeking generally (Skovran, Huss, & Scalora, 2010); however, should psychopathy be present in the offender, it is likely the offenses will be more common, serious and incorrigible (Porter, ten Brinke, & Wilson, 2009).

Mechanisms underlying psychopathy and sexual offending

While inferring sexual deviation or paraphilias can be identified using self-report, this requires a context in which the interviewee is open to discussing private and intimate aspects of their life, with no problematic consequences for their frankness. This openness may be compromised when there are legal or criminal-justice implications to what is disclosed (Boer, 2016). As a result, research has sought what David Glasgow (personal communication) describes as "the holy grail" of sex offender research; objective methodologies to identify arousal in relation to sexual stimuli in an individual. One difficulty with such approaches is that emotive physiological responses from a primarily psychopathic individual may be weaker, as they are inherently low in anxiety or excitability. Results in the field are mixed. A meta-analysis of 95 studies by Lorber (2004) examined heart rate (HR) and electrodermal activity (EDA) with aggression, psychopathy, and conduct problems, finding autonomic patterns did not always generalize across antisocial spectrum behavior constructs. Low resting EDA and low task EDA (indicative of less stress, less sweating, and less activity by the subject's sympathetic nervous system) are associated with psychopathy/sociopathy and conduct problems. However, EDA reactivity is *positively* associated with aggression, and negatively associated with psychopathy/sociopathy. Likewise, low resting HR and high HR reactivity were associated with aggression and conduct problems. Similar findings have been found with community cohorts assessed for psychopathy with startle blink tasks (Benning, Patrick, & Iacono, 2005). Does this mean that psychopathic individuals are lower in arousal generally, but quicker to show change in response to a suitable stimulus?

Irrespective of the cognitive state of a psychopath, and notwithstanding that many sexual offenses are committed by impotent or aging males whose spirit remains willing despite their flesh being weak, penile plethysmography (PPG) remains a face-valid methodology to assess sexual, and thus potentially deviant, arousal. The PPG measures increased blood flow to the penis relative to baseline when a person shown an image that may or may not be arousing. Labial plethysmography for women shows similar effects (Huberman, Dawson, & Chivers, 2017). Integrating 37 studies (a combined sample of 6,785) examining PPG in relation to pedohebephilic interests, and the significance of this to reconviction found the paradigm worked better with stronger visual and audio-visual stimuli, and also worked relatively; relative PPG increase over baseline led to more valid phallic measurement. This measurement was able to significantly predict reconviction, and supports the view that PPG can be an objective measure of sexual interest, at least for children (McPhail et al., 2017). However, this study reviewed sexual offenders generally; psychopathy, specifically measured by the PCL–R, and phallometric indexes of deviant sexual arousal were only modestly significantly correlated, in a sample of 63 convicted sexual offenders (r = 0.28, p < .02; Serin, Malcolm, Khanna, & Barbaree, 1994); Firestone, Bradford, Greenberg, and Serran (2000) found that sexual deviance (as measured by PPG) and psychopathy only correlated significantly in their sample of non-incestuous child molesters. Similarly, psychopathy scores (as measured by the PCL: YV) and deviant sexual arousal measured by PPG were not significantly correlated in an adolescent sample (Gretton, McBride, Hare, O'Shaughnessy, & Kumka, 2001).

The limitations of directly physiological tasks have led to a drift back to more experimental cognitive measures such as implicit association and viewing time paradigms. Implicit association tasks appear to accurately identify pedophilic associations of children and sexual activity, and the paradigm can be adapted to similar atypical associations with violence in psychopathic murderers (Gray, Brown, MacCulloch, Smith, & Snowden, 2005; Gray, MacCulloch, Smith, Morris, & Snowden, 2003).

Ongoing questions about psychopathy and sexual offending

Psychopathic individuals are commonly involved in incestuous offenses (Firestone et al., 2000). It might be that the emotional factors involved in such an offense, such as emotional congruence, courtship misallocation, and neediness are unlikely to be raised in persons with primary psychopathy due to their lack of emotional needs. Though this does not preclude a primary psychopath committing an incestuous offense and, if they do, the chance of a reconviction is higher (Kingston, Firestone, Wexler, & Bradford, 2008), a psychopath may be less likely to be so inclined in the first place. However, it may be for more prosaic reasons that antisocial psychopaths are far less likely to be able to maintain a successful relationship, and as such their access to their own children is less likely. Perhaps in this situation the presence of psychopathy may be considered almost a protective factor against incest. For example, Ellis (1987) identifies a substantial association between psychopathy and unstable pair bonding (e.g., marital desertion, extramarital sex), and this relationship instability may undermine the social environment that might otherwise enable incest.

One concern is that if psychopaths are good at manipulating others, this could include manipulation through controlling their responses to sexual deviance measures. Objective or experimental cognitive indices of deviant arousal might be subject to performance strategies that could hinder their objectivity. Vitacco and Rogers (2009) suggest denial and defensiveness are more common than antisocial and psychopathic motivations when evaluating and treating offenders, and the present authors have no reason to disagree with this view. For instance, Babchishin, Curry, Fedoroff, Bradford, and Seto (2017) tested the degree to which men could inhibit their sexual arousal during phallometric assessment when instructed to do and found small to moderate effects, this change being no more than would be predicted by measurement error for the methodology. The ability to suppress sexual arousal was not associated with sexual offense recidivism. Some researchers have tested whether eye-movement paradigms may indicate if competing covert processes seek to inhibit erectile inhibition during a PPG task. Trottier, Rouleau, Renaud, and Goyette (2014) found attempts to control erectile responses involved specific eye-movement variations that were characterized by a general deceleration of the exploration process and limited exploration of the erogenous zone(s) in the image. If psychopathic individuals are more polymorphously perverse, one might expect them to be more undiscriminating in their arousal to a wider variety of stimuli, nor to care about this arousal, even in custodial settings. This is precisely what is found in relation to social desirability, where psychopathic respondents are typically less likely attempt to fake good, indicative of their lesser concern for social convention (Verschuere et al., 2014).

Conclusion

This chapter has explored the association of psychopathy and sexual offending. There is an assumption that psychopathy moderates all forms of antisocial behavior, which is possibly exaggerated; though psychopathy can be expressed in many ways, it is by no means the only influence on offending, and particularly not in the area of sexual offending, where neurotic, interpersonal, and emotional factors are also highly implicated. Different constellations of psychopathic behavior in different people may be, paradoxically, protective, if, for example, the guilt and shame associated with an unmet sexual desire in a more neurotic individual is irrelevant to the psychopathic individual who simply chooses to use a sex worker or casual sex with a like-minded person met on social media; they may not find themselves frustrated, and then, when over-aroused, may take sex from a non-consenting or vulnerable other. This model would fit with the idea of non-offending psychopaths and that offending psychopaths are not 'globally' deviant but tend to 'focus' on specific areas. When assessing the psychopathic sexual offender, many of their other qualities – substance misuse, intelligence, sexual preoccupation, rational and adaptive expression of sexual needs – are also critical to understanding the individual pathways that may lead to their offending.

References

American Psychiatric Association. (2013) 'Paraphilic disorders,' in *Diagnostic and statistical manual of mental disorders* (5th ed., pp. 685–686), Arlington, VA: American Psychiatric Publishing.

Babchishin, K. M., Hanson, R. K., and VanZuylen, H. (2015) 'Online child pornography offenders are different: A meta-analysis of the characteristics of online and offline sex offenders against children,' *Archives of Sexual Behavior*, *44*(1):45–66.

Babchishin, K. M., Curry, S. D., Fedoroff, J. P., Bradford, J., and Seto, M. C. (2017) 'Inhibiting sexual arousal to children: Correlates and its influence on the validity of penile plethysmography,' *Archives of Sexual Behavior*, *46*(3):671–684.

Beggs, S. M., and Grace, R. C. (2008) 'Psychopathy, intelligence, and recidivism in child molesters: Evidence of an interaction effect,' *Criminal Justice and Behavior*, *35*(6):683–695.

Benning, S. D., Patrick, C. J., and Iacono, W. G. (2005) 'Psychopathy, startle blink modulation, and electrodermal reactivity in twin men,' *Psychophysiology*, *42*(6):753–762.

Boer, D. P. (Ed.) (2016) *The Wiley handbook on the theories, assessment and treatment of sexual offending*, London: Wiley-Blackwell.

Brown, S. L., and Forth, A. E. (1997) 'Psychopathy and sexual assault: Static risk factors, emotional precursors, and rapist subtypes,' *Journal of Consulting and Clinical Psychology*, *65*(5):848–857.

Canter, D., Hughes, D., and Kirby, S. (1998) 'Paedophilia: Pathology, criminality, or both? The development of a multivariate model of offence behaviour in child sexual abuse,' *The Journal of Forensic Psychiatry*, *9*(3):532–555.

Cooke, D. J., Michie, C., and Skeem, J. (2007) 'Understanding the structure of the Psychopathy Checklist–Revised,' *The British Journal of Psychiatry*, *190*(49):s39–s50.

De Block, A., and Adriaens, P. R. (2013) 'Pathologizing sexual deviance: A history,' *The Journal of Sex Research*, *50*(3–4):276–298.

Derefinko, K. J., Peters, J. R., Eisenlohr-Moul, T. A., Walsh, E. C., Adams, Z. W., and Lynam, D. R. (2014) 'Relations between trait impulsivity, behavioral impulsivity, physiological arousal, and risky sexual behavior among young men,' *Archives of Sexual Behavior*, *43*(6):1149–1158.

Drescher, J. (2015) 'Out of DSM: Depathologizing homosexuality,' *Behavioral Sciences*, *5*(4):565–575.

Egan, V., Kavanagh, B., and Blair, M. (2005) 'Sexual offenders, personality and obsessionality,' *Sexual Abuse*, *17*(2):223–240.

Egan, V., and Parmar, R. (2013) 'Dirty habits? On-line pornography use as a function of personality, obsessionality, and compulsivity,' *Journal of Sexual and Marital Therapy*, *39*(5):394–409.

Ellis, L. (1987) 'Relationships of criminality and psychopathy with eight other apparent behavioral manifestations of sub-optimal arousal,' *Personality and Individual Differences*, *8*(6):905–925.

Firestone, P., Bradford, J. M., Greenberg, D. M., and Serran, G. A. (2000) 'The relationship of deviant sexual arousal and psychopathy in incest offenders, extrafamilial child molesters, and rapists,' *Journal of the American Academy of Psychiatry and Law*, *28*:303–308.

First, M. B. (2014) 'DSM-5 and paraphilic disorders,' *Journal of the American Academy of Psychiatry and the Law*, *42*(2):191–201.

Foulkes, L., McCrory, E. J., Neumann, C. S., and Viding, E. (2014) 'Inverted social reward: Associations between psychopathic traits and self-report and experimental measures of social reward,' *PLoS One*, *9*(8):e106000.

Fulton, J. J., Marcus, D. K., and Payne, K. T. (2010) 'Psychopathic personality traits and risky sexual behavior in college students,' *Personality and Individual Differences*, *49*(1):29–33.

Gray, N. S., MacCulloch, M. J., Smith, J., Morris, M., and Snowden, R. J. (2003) 'Forensic psychology: Violence viewed by psychopathic murderers,' *Nature*, *423*:497–498.

Gray, N. S., Brown, A. S., MacCulloch, M. J., Smith, J., and Snowden, R. J. (2005) 'An implicit test of the associations between children and sex in pedophiles,' *Journal of Abnormal Psychology*, *114*(2):304–308.

Gretton, H. M., McBride, M., Hare, R. D., O'Shaughnessy, R., and Kumka, G. (2001) 'Psychopathy and recidivism in adolescent sex offenders,' *Criminal Justice and Behavior*, *28*(4):427–449.

Hald, G. M., and Malamuth, N. N. (2015) 'Experimental effects of exposure to pornography: The moderating effect of personality and mediating effect of sexual arousal,' *Archives of Sexual Behavior*, *44*(1):99–109.

Hanson, R. K., and Bussiere, M. T. (1998) 'Predicting relapse: A meta-analysis of sexual offender recidivism studies,' *Journal of Consulting and Clinical Psychology*, *66*(2):348–362.

Hanson, R. K., and Morton-Bourgon, K. E. (2005) 'The characteristics of persistent sexual offenders: A meta-analysis of recidivism studies,' *Journal of Consulting and Clinical Psychology*, *73*(6):1154–1163.

Hare, R. D. (1999) 'Psychopathy as a risk factor for violence,' *Psychiatric Quarterly*, *70*:181–197.

Hare, R. D. (2003) *The Psychopathy Checklist–Revised* (2nd ed.), Toronto, ON: Multi-Health Systems.

Harris, G. T., Lalumière, M. L., Seto, M. C., Rice, M. E., and Chaplin, T. C. (2012) 'Explaining the erectile responses of rapists to rape stories: The contributions of sexual activity, non-consent, and violence with injury,' *Archives of Sexual Behavior*, *41*(1):221–229.

Hawes, S. W., Boccaccini, M. T., and Murrie, D. C. (2013) 'Psychopathy and the combination of psychopathy and sexual deviance as predictors of sexual recidivism: Meta-analytic findings using the Psychopathy Checklist–Revised,' *Psychological Assessment*, *25*(1):233–243.

Heil, P., Ahlmeyer, S., and Simons, D. (2003) 'Crossover sexual offenses,' *Sexual Abuse*, *15*(4):221–236.

Hill, A., Habermann, N., Berner, W., and Briken P. (2007) 'Psychiatric disorders in single and multiple sexual murderers,' *Psychopathology*, *40*(1):22–28.

Huberman, J. S., Dawson, S. J., and Chivers, M. L. (2017) 'Examining the time course of genital and subjective sexual responses in women and men with concurrent plethysmography and thermography,' *Biological Psychology*, *129*:359–369.

Hunt, E., Bornovalova, M. A., and Patrick, C. J. (2015) 'Genetic and environmental overlap between borderline personality disorder traits and psychopathy: Evidence for promotive effects of factor 2 and protective effects of factor 1,' *Psychological Medicine*, *45*(7):1471–1481.

Kingston, D. A., Firestone, P., Wexler, A., and Bradford, J. M. (2008) 'Factors associated with recidivism among intrafamilial child molesters,' *Journal of Sexual Aggression*, *14*(1):3–18.

Kirsch, L. G., and Becker, J. V. (2007) 'Emotional deficits in psychopathy and sexual sadism: Implications for violent and sadistic behavior,' *Clinical Psychology Review*, *27*(8):904–922.

Langevin, R. (2003) 'A study of the psychosexual characteristics of sex killers: Can we identify them before it is too late?,' *International Journal of Offender Therapy and Comparative Criminology*, *47*(4):366–382.

Långström, N., and Seto, M. C. (2006) 'Exhibitionistic and voyeuristic behavior in a Swedish national population survey,' *Archives of Sexual Behavior*, *35*(4):427–435.

Levenston, G. K., Patrick, C. J., Bradley, M. M., and Lang, P. J. (2000) 'The psychopath as observer: Emotion and attention in picture processing,' *Journal of Abnormal Psychology*, *109*(3):373–385.

Lorber, M. F. (2004) 'Psychophysiology of aggression, psychopathy, and conduct problems: A meta-analysis,' *Psychological Bulletin*, *130*(4):531–552.

Malow, R. M., Dévieux, J., Rosenberg, R., Nair, M., McMahon, R., Brown, E. J., and Kalichman, S. C. (2007) 'Antisocial psychopathy and HIV risk among alcohol and other drug (AOD) abusing adolescent offenders,' *American Journal of Infectious Diseases*, *3*(4):230–239.

Marsh, A. A., and Blair, R. J. R. (2008) 'Deficits in facial affect recognition among antisocial populations: A meta-analysis,' *Neuroscience & Biobehavioral Reviews*. *32*(3):454–465.

McNally, M. R., and Fremouw, W. J. (2014) 'Examining risk of escalation: A critical review of the exhibitionistic behavior literature,' *Aggression and Violent Behavior*, *19*(5):474–485.

McPhail, I. V., Hermann, C. A., Fernane, S., Fernandez, Y. M., Nunes, K. L., and Cantor, J. M. (2017) 'Validity in phallometric testing for sexual interests in children: A meta-analytic review,' *Assessment* (in press).

Međedović, J. (2017) 'Aberrations in emotional processing of violence-dependent stimuli are the core features of sadism,' *Motivation and Emotion*, *41*(2):273–283.

Meere, M., and Egan, V. (2017) 'Everyday sadism, the Dark Triad, personality, and disgust sensitivity,' *Personality and Individual Differences*, *112*(1):157–161.

Mitchell, I. J., Smid, W., Troelstra, J., Wever, E., Ziegler, T. E., and Beech, A. R. (2013) 'Psychopathic characteristics are related to high basal urinary oxytocin levels in male forensic patients,' *The Journal of Forensic Psychiatry & Psychology*, *24*(3):309–318.

Mokros, A., Osterheider, M., Hucker, S. J., and Nitschke, J. (2011) 'Psychopathy and sexual sadism,' *Law and Human Behavior*, *35*(3):188–199.

Newman, J. P. (1997) 'Conceptual models of the nervous system: Implications for antisocial behavior,' in D. M. Stoff, J. Brieling, & J. Maser (Eds.), *Handbook of Antisocial Behavior* (pp. 324–335), Toronto, ON: Wiley.

Newman, J. P., Kosson, D. S., and Patterson, M. C. (1992) 'Delay of gratification in psychopathic and nonpsychopathic offenders,' *Journal of Abnormal Psychology*, *101*(4):630–636.

Odlaug, B. L., Lust, K., Schreiber, L. R., Christenson, G., Derbyshire, K., Harvanko, A., Golden, D, and Grant, J. E. (2013) 'Compulsive sexual behavior in young adults,' *Annals of Clinical Psychiatry*, *25*:193–200.

Olver, M., and Wong, S. (2006) 'Psychopathy, sexual deviance, and recidivism among sex offenders,' *Sexual Abuse: A Journal of Research and Treatment*, *18*(1):65–82.

Porter, S., Fairweather, D., Drugge, J., Hervé, H., Birt, A., and Boer, D. P. (2000) 'Profiles of psychopathy in incarcerated sexual offenders,' *Criminal Justice and Behavior*, *27*(2):216–233.

Porter, S., ten Brinke, L., and Wilson, K. (2009) 'Crime profiles and conditional release performance of psychopathic and non-psychopathic sexual offenders,' *Legal and Criminological Psychology*, *14*(1):109–118.

Robertson, C. A., and Knight, R. A. (2014) 'Relating sexual sadism and psychopathy to one another, non-sexual violence, and sexual crime behaviors,' *Aggressive Behavior, 40*(1):12–23.
Salekin, R. T., Rogers, R., and Sewell, K. W. (1996) 'A review and meta-analysis of the Psychopathy Checklist and Psychopathy Checklist–Revised: Predictive validity of dangerousness,' *Clinical Psychology: Science and Practice, 3*(3):203–215.
Schlesinger, L. B., and Revitch, E. (1999) 'Sexual burglaries and sexual homicide: Clinical, forensic, and investigative considerations,' *Journal of the American Academy of Psychiatry and the Law, 27*(2):227–238.
Serin, R. C., Malcolm, P. B., Khanna, A., and Barbaree, H. E. (1994) 'Psychopathy and deviant sexual arousal in incarcerated sexual offenders,' *Journal of Interpersonal Violence, 9*(1):3–11.
Seto, M. C., Harris, G. T., and Lalumière, M. L. (2015) *Psychopathy and sexual offending. The clinical and forensic assessment of psychopathy: A practitioner's guide* (pp. 403–418), New York, NY: Routledge.
Skeem, J. L., and Cooke, D. J. (2010) 'Is criminal behavior a central component of psychopathy? Conceptual directions for resolving the debate,' *Psychological Assessment, 22*(2):433–445.
Skovran, L. C., Huss, M. T., and Scalora, M. J. (2010) 'Sexual fantasies and sensation seeking among psychopathic sexual offenders,' *Psychology, Crime & Law, 16*(7):617–629.
Soh, D. W., and Cantor, J. M. (2015) 'A peek inside a furry convention,' *Archives of Sexual Behavior, 44*(1):1–2.
Strassberg, D. S., Eastvold, A., Kenney, J. W., and Suchya, Y. (2012) 'Psychopathy among pedophilic and nonpedophilic child molesters,' *Child Abuse & Neglect, 36*(4):379–382.
Trottier, D., Rouleau, J. L., Renaud, P., and Goyette, M. (2014) 'Using eye tracking to identify faking attempts during penile plethysmography assessment,' *The Journal of Sex Research, 51*(8):946–955.
Tully, R. J., Browne, K. D., and Craig, L. A. (2015) 'An examination of the predictive validity of the Structured Assessment of Risk and Need Treatment Needs Analysis (SARN–TNA) in England and Wales,' *Criminal Justice and Behavior, 42*(5):509–528.
Verona, E., Patrick, C. J., Curtin, J. J., Bradley, M. M., and Lang, P. J. (2004) 'Psychopathy and physiological response to emotionally evocative sounds,' *Journal of Abnormal Psychology, 113*(1):99–108.
Verschuere, B., Uzieblo, K., De Schryver, M., Douma, H., Onraedt, T., and Crombez, G. (2014) 'The inverse relation between psychopathy and faking good: Not response bias, but true variance in psychopathic personality,' *The Journal of Forensic Psychiatry & Psychology, 25*(6):705–713.
Vitacco, M. J., and Rogers, R. (2009) 'The assessment of psychopathy and response styles in sex offenders,' *Sex Offenders: Identification, Risk Assessment, Treatment, and Legal Issues*, 130–143.
Weaver, C. M., Meyer, R. G., Van Nort, J. J., and Tristan, L. (2006) 'Two-, three-, and four-factor PCL–R models in applied sex offender risk assessments,' *Assessment, 13*(2):208–216.
Wilson, J. Q., and Herrnstein, R. J. (1985) *Crime and human nature: The definitive study of the causes of crime*, New York, NY: Simon & Schuster.
White, C. (2006) 'The Spanner trials and the changing law on sadomasochism in the UK,' *Journal of Homosexuality, 50*(2–3):167–187.
Woodworth, M., Freimuth, T., Hutton, E. L., Carpenter, T., Agar, A. D., and Logan, M. (2013) 'High-risk sexual offenders: An examination of sexual fantasy, sexual paraphilia, psychopathy, and offence characteristics,' *International Journal of Law and Psychiatry, 36*(2):144–156.
Yildirim, B. O., and Derksen, J. J. (2015) 'Clarifying the heterogeneity in psychopathic samples: Towards a new continuum of primary and secondary psychopathy,' *Aggression and Violent Behavior, 24*(1):9–41.

24

Psychopathy and sexuality

Impersonal and exploitive

Beth A. Visser

Introduction

In both fiction and non-fiction, the psychopath tends to be portrayed as a serial killer (television's Dexter Morgan, or Hannibal Lecter from the movie *Silence of the Lambs*) who might or might not also be a sexual predator (e.g., convicted killers/rapists Ted Bundy and Clifford Olson). The popular stereotype of the psychopath might lead people to be concerned about sadistic sexual homicide as opposed to being wary of the smooth-talker who uses deception and aggression for financial, social, and sexual gain. The psychopathy literature clearly demonstrates that psychopaths and individuals with elevated levels of psychopathic traits exploit others for their own purposes, and that these tactics generalize to the realm of sexual behavior.

Core features of psychopathy include callousness, manipulativeness, an irresponsible, parasitic lifestyle, and social deviance (Hare, 2003). These personal characteristics would seem to make the psychopath a threat in terms of sexuality, particularly since the glibness and superficial charm may, at least initially, serve to conceal underlying social malevolence. The coldness and lack of empathy associated with psychopathy could mean a lack of concern for the distress of a sexual partner or victim. The impulsivity and disregard for consequences could mean acting inappropriate and/or illegally on sexual impulses, particularly since psychopathy is characterized by reward-driven behavior and a lack of sensitivity to punishment (Visser, Ashton, & Pozzebon, 2012; Wallace, Malterer, & Newman, 2009). All of these characteristics would seem to make the psychopathic sexual offender a challenging candidate for treatment, risking treatment dropout or subsequent reoffending despite program completion.

Sexuality in psychopathy definitions

In psychiatrist Herve Cleckley's (1941/1988:360) seminal book on psychopathy, *The Mask of Sanity*, he identified "sex life impersonal, trivial, and poorly integrated" as a definitional characteristic of psychopathy. Cleckley suggested that when psychopaths engaged in what he called "abnormal relations," it was typically not a function of a strong sexual orientation or paraphilia but often for "just the hell of it." In 15 case studies, Cleckley described the promiscuous and risky sexual activity of psychopaths (13 of them male) as being impulsive, with little consideration of legal or social consequences. The profiled psychopaths tended to marry on whims, then abandon the partner or take on additional sexual partners almost immediately. Although the psychopaths often managed to elicit devotion from others, they seemed to experience no such deep feelings themselves.

Cleckley (1941/1988) emphasized the lack of emotional connection and commitment that was core to psychopathic sexuality. Cleckley suggested that although the sex life of the psychopath was "abnormal" there was no reason to believe that it was related to sexual disorders, including paraphilias. Cleckley did not propose that psychopaths were more inclined than others to use coercion or aggression to obtain sexual gratification. He described a psychopathic physician who bit a prostitute's nipple off, but Cleckley attributed this incident to "injudicious blunderings" (p. 206) as opposed to aggression. Cleckley also noted that the psychopath who is also a sexual sadist would be a particularly dangerous individual (p. 291).

Like Cleckley, Hare (2003) considered sexuality sufficiently core to psychopathy to identify "promiscuous sexual behavior" as a defining feature and included it as an item on the 20-item Psychopathy Checklist Revised (PCL–R; Hare, 2003:41), a tool widely used in the forensic assessment of psychopathy. Hare also noted the impersonal nature of the psychopath's sexual relationships, as well as the "willingness to participate in a wide variety of sexual activities." Unlike Cleckley, Hare also noted the possibility that the psychopath might utilize coercion to obtain sex and may even have a history of sexual assault charges. To some extent, Hare's focus on illegal sexual behavior may be a function of his greater interest in offender samples as opposed to Cleckley's hospital samples. Alternatively, Hare's inclusion of coercion may reflect a shift in the psychopathy construct from a psychiatric issue to a criminal justice issue since Cleckley's writings.

Overall, the defining characteristics of the psychopath suggest an under-controlled, manipulative, and possibly coercive individual who engages in sexual relations for the temporary pleasure they offer, as opposed to furthering any lasting personal or emotional connection. The lack of empathy for others and willingness to exploit that are also psychopathy features seem to pave the way for coercive tactics around sexual behavior. Indeed, Harris, Rice, Hilton, Lalumière, and Quinsey (2007) concluded that early, promiscuous, and coercive sexual activity was a core feature of psychopathy.

Evolutionary basis

Although psychopathy is frequently described using the terminology of "disorder," several authors have suggested that psychopathy is better conceptualized as an evolved strategy (e.g., Book & Quinsey, 2004; Book et al., 2016; Glenn, Kurzban, & Raine, 2009; Harris et al., 2007; Harris, Rice, & Quinsey, 1994; Mealey, 1995). Behavioral genetics studies show substantial heritability (about 50 percent) to psychopathy (e.g., Blonigen, Carlson, Krueger, & Patrick, 2003). Consistent with the view that psychopathy might be a successful adaptation as opposed to a disorder is the fact that offenders with high scores on the PCL–R do not have the facial asymmetry seen in other offenders and in individuals with neurodevelopmental disorders (Lalumière, Harris, & Rice, 2001).

Mealey (1995) proposed that psychopaths are cheaters who are apt to exploit the cooperation of others. Further, Mealey suggested that psychopathy was a frequency-dependent strategy in that it could only be successful in populations where the majority of individuals were cooperative and adhered to group rules. Book and Quinsey (2004) likewise proposed that psychopathy was characterized by not only a cheater versus cooperator strategy, but also a hawk versus dove strategy. That is, not only are psychopaths cheaters who exploit the cooperation of others, but they also tend to be "warrior-hawks," characterized by impulsive aggression even in situations where others would not find aggression appropriate. In terms of sexual behavior, this "cheater-hawk" strategy would seem to suggest tactics such as lying to potential sexual partners (e.g., feigning love and/or commitment) as well as using other coercive tactics to attain sex (e.g., threats, force, assaulting an incapacitated individual).

In terms of "life history strategy" (LHS; Figueredo et al., 2006), psychopathy has been associated with a "fast" LHS. That is, reproductive success is attained by having many short-term sexual partners and not investing in those partners or in subsequent offspring. A "slow" LHS would involve a stable relationship and a small number of highly nurtured children. Consistent with theory around psychopathy as a fast life strategy, Harris et al. (2007) reported that male psychopathic offenders had more offspring than their male non-psychopathic offender counterparts. These authors suggested that such a strategy of having many children but failing to care for them could only be successful if one parent (the mother, in Harris et al.'s theory) nurtured the subsequent children. Harris et al. proposed that this psychopathic strategy relied on early and coercive sexuality.

Research has generally supported these evolutionary theories. For example, Harris et al. (2007) reported that in a sample of adult male sex offenders, psychopathy could be well described as consisting of the traditional Factor 1 (interpersonal and affective aspects), Factor 2 (lifestyle and social deviance features), and a third, moderately correlated factor of precocious and coercive sexuality (having many partners before the age of 15 years, forced sex on someone before the age of 15, etc.). Jonason, Koenig, and Tost (2010) reported that psychopathy scores were correlated with scores on a measure of fast life history and reported having had more sexual partners.

Subclinical psychopathy

There has been a great deal of recent research interest in subclinical psychopathy, both in its own right and as part of the "dark triad" of personality (Paulhus & Williams, 2002), which also includes narcissism and Machiavellianism. There is much evidence that psychopathy is continuous in nature and little to suggest a qualitative difference between psychopaths and those with psychopathic traits who would not meet criteria for a psychopath diagnosis (Edens, Marcus, Lilienfeld, & Poythress, 2006; Miller, Lynam, Widiger, & Leukefeld, 2001).

In student and community samples, there are consistent findings around psychopathy and sexual behavior that are in keeping with Cleckley's (1941/1988) and Hare's (2003) descriptions of psychopaths. Kosson, Kelly, and White (1997), for example, found that in an undergraduate student sample, psychopathy was associated with sexual aggression (e.g., threats, taking advantage of an intoxicated person). Visser, Pozzebon, Bogaert, and Ashton (2010) reported that in a sample of 198 students and community members, both men's and women's psychopathic traits were associated with a pattern of early onset sexual activity, more sexual partners, and more sexual affairs while already in a relationship.

Evidence for evolutionary hypotheses of psychopathy have been found in subclinical, non-offender samples. Jonason et al. (2010) reported evidence consistent with psychopathy as a fast life strategy in two undergraduate student samples. Such findings provide support for the notions that findings in non-offender samples may inform the forensic research, and also that subclinical psychopathy or "psychopathic traits" are important constructs in non-clinical populations and are predictive of important life outcomes.

In a small sample of community men, Seto, Khattar, Lalumiere, and Quinsey (1997) found that psychopathy was associated with sexual deception. However, these authors reported that psychopathy was not related to sexual deception to a greater extent than with non-sexual deception, suggesting that deception could be a broadly utilized psychopathic tactic. In this sample, psychopathy was also highly negatively correlated ($r = -.45$) with checking with a sexual partner about contraception, a finding that seems consistent with the impulsivity and disregard for consequences described by both Cleckley (1941/1988) and Hare (2003).

Sexual violence

Psychopathy is a well-established predictor of both reactive and proactive aggression (see Blais, Solodukhin, & Forth, 2014 for a meta-analysis) as well as violent and nonviolent recidivism. Further, psychopaths are more diverse in their criminal behavior than non-psychopaths, suggesting that they are opportunists rather than specialists. A particular concern, then, is around sexual violence. For this reason, PCL–R scores tend to be weighted heavily on risk assessment tools such as the Violent Risk Assessment Guide (VRAG; Quinsey, Harris, Rice, & Cormier, 2006), which has been found to be a useful tool in the prediction of recidivism in sex offenders (see Hanson, Morton-Bourgon, Hanson, & Morton-Bourgon, 2009 for a meta-analysis).

Kiehl and Hoffman (2011:355) described the criminal justice resources consumed by psychopaths as "astonishing," noting that although about 1 percent of the adult male non-institutionalized general population is estimated to meet criteria for psychopathy, about 16 percent of offender populations meet criteria. In the PCL–R manual, Hare (2003) reported that from pooling samples available at the time, about 34 percent of rapists met criteria for a psychopath diagnosis, 66 percent of mixed rapists/child molesters did, and only 6 percent of child molesters did, suggesting that there is good reason to be concerned about psychopathic sex offenders. In looking more closely at the characteristics of psychopathic rapists versus non-psychopathic rapists, Brown and Forth (1997) found that psychopaths were, contrary to hypothesis, no more likely to target strangers than non-psychopaths, nor did they inflict greater injury on their victims. The psychopaths in this study started their criminal careers at a younger age but did not start sexually offending any younger than the non-psychopaths. The psychopaths were more likely, however, to be opportunistic or pervasively angry, leading Brown and Forth to speculate that treatment strategies might target the psychopathic impulsive and erratic lifestyle.

Quinsey, Rice, and Harris (1995) reported that in a sample of 178 male sex offenders, psychopathy predicted sexual and violent recidivism. Further, these authors reported that psychopathy could be clearly differentiated from sexual deviance (i.e., a preference for children or for coercion) and that both were risk factors for future recidivism. In keeping with these findings, Serin, Mailloux, and Malcolm (2001) reported that in a sample of 68 sex offenders, those with the highest levels of psychopathy and deviant sexual arousal recidivated earlier and at higher rates. In Hawes et al.'s (2013) meta-analysis of 20 PCL–R studies, the authors found that PCL–R psychopathy was a strong predictor of sexual recidivism, but Factor 2 was a stronger predictor than Factor 1 or total scores. This finding suggests that the erratic, impulsive, antisocial lifestyle aspects of psychopathy are more central to sexual recidivism than the cold and manipulative personality aspects.

Also, Hawes et al. (2013) concluded that with the exception of one of the constituent studies, the evidence indicated that offenders who were high scorers on both the PCL–R and a measure of sexual deviance were twice as likely to reoffend sexually as other offenders. Thus, in keeping with Cleckley's (1941/1988) hypothesis, those individuals who are psychopaths and also have deviant sexual attractions are dangerous people. Paul Bernardo, for example, a Canadian psychopath with sexually sadistic interests, was convicted of kidnapping, killing, and sexually assaulting two young women with the assistance of his then-wife, Karla Homolka (Williams,

1998). Williams noted that the two video-recorded the sexual assaults of the two women and many others (including Karla's own sister) for their later enjoyment. Bernardo also admitted to being the notorious "Scarborough Rapist" who sexually assaulted numerous women, typically as they walked along from bus stops (Williams, 1998). Bernardo would seem to represent the dangerous combination of a callous, manipulative, exploitive psychopath who also enjoyed sexually humiliating women.

In Porter et al.'s (2000) sample of 329 Canadian offenders, they found the highest rate of psychopaths (64.0 percent) in offenders categorized as mixed rapist/child molester. This group included offenders with convictions for sexual crimes against individuals of 14 years or less as well as over the age of 14 years. Similarly, Olver and Wong (2006) reported that the highest PCL–R scores were found in the group of sex offenders that had victimized both children and adults. In *Without Conscience*, Hare (1999) quoted a psychopath who was convicted of sexually assaulting the 8-year-old daughter of his girlfriend as saying, "I just take what's available," (p. 110), suggesting no particular pedophilic interest but also no moral sanctions again sexually violating a child. This consistent finding that psychopaths are most prevalent in the mixed adult/child victim group (see also Skovran, Huss, & Scalora, 2010) emphasizes the point that psychopaths are opportunistic thrill-seekers who are diverse in their crimes and their victims.

Porter et al. (2000) reported that for the group of offenders who victimized only children aged 14 years and less, rates of psychopaths were comparatively low (6.3 percent to 10.8 percent) as compared to rapists (35.9 percent), whose sexual assault victims were all older than 14 years. The authors noted that the psychopathy rate of the group of offenders who sexually victimized children was lower than in the general prison population, suggesting that the high recidivism rate of this group may be due to a strong pedophilic orientation as opposed to psychopathy, and that psychopathy may add less to the prediction of risk in this group.

Porter, Campbell, Woodworth, and Birt (2001) proposed a subgroup of sexual offenders that they called "sexual psychopaths." The authors suggested that this group of perpetrators was more diverse and more violent in their sexual offenses because they are driven by Thrill-seeking as opposed to sexual deviancy. Porter et al. noted that psychopathic American serial killer Ted Bundy would meet criteria for the sexual psychopath, as evidenced by his many victims of very different ages and appearances. Likewise, Canadian serial killer Clifford Olson sexually victimized children and young adults of both genders. Meloy (2002) likewise suggested that the high levels of sensation seeking in psychopaths was related to sexual offending in diverse ways and with diverse victim groups. Meloy suggested that the psychopath's need for excitement led to rapid habituation and boredom with sexual partners and activities.

Sexual fantasy

One strategy for learning more about the link between psychopathy and sexuality is to study people's sexual fantasies. Fantasies should reflect individual preferences and be less contaminated by social norms and by practical limitations than sexual behavior. Additionally, if truthful reports of fantasies could be obtained, they might shed light on whether psychopaths differ from non-psychopaths in the deviant content of their fantasies, or whether psychopaths are simply more inclined than other people to act on their deviant fantasies. This question is an important one in that there is evidence that sexual offenders are influenced, at least to some extent, by their sexual fantasies (Baumgartner, Scalora, & Huss, 2002).

Skovran et al. (2010) found that in a sample of 199 men in a maximum security forensic hospital, psychopaths reported more sexual fantasies than did non-psychopaths. Psychopathy was associated with all fantasy categories except those relating to incest/molesting. The fact that psychopaths reported higher levels of fantasizing about what the authors described as "exploratory" fantasies (e.g., group sex, mate-swapping) is in keeping with explanations that psychopaths are sensation seekers with a preference for novelty in their sexual behavior. However, in the 36 sex offenders in the sample, Skovran et al. reported no relation between psychopathy and sadomasochistic fantasies.

In a large undergraduate student sample ($N = 643$), Baughman, Jonason, Veselka, and Vernon (2014) reported that of the dark triad personality traits (i.e., narcissism, Machiavellianism, and subclinical psychopathy), psychopathy was associated with a wider range of sexual fantasies than the other dark triad variables. The authors reported that psychopathy was particularly related to exploratory (sexual variety), impersonal, and sadomasochistic fantasies.

In a sample of male undergraduate students, Williams, Cooper, Howell, Yuille, and Paulhus (2009) reported that the overwhelming majority (95 percent) had reported at least one deviant fantasy, which the authors defined as incorporating object fetishism, transvestitism, sadism, bondage, voyeurism, exhibitionism, frotteurism, pedophilia, or sexual assault. The authors reported that psychopathy mediated the relation between deviant fantasies and behavior, such that only at higher levels of psychopathic traits were men also engaging in the fantasized sexual behaviors.

Visser, DeBow, Pozzebon, Bogaert, and Book (2015) examined fantasy content and psychopathic traits in two student/community samples. In study 1, participants provided an open-ended fantasy narrative and two raters rated the narratives for predetermined themes. For both men and women, individuals who reported higher levels of psychopathic traits wrote fantasies that were less romantic and referred to more numerous partners who tended to be uncommitted.

In study 2, participants rated various sexual fantasy items as well as indicating how frequently they had engaged in that activity in real life. Visser et al. (2015) reported that psychopathy was related to greater pornography use and, for women only, with greater frequency of engaging in sexual fantasizing. The authors reported that in regression analyses, psychopathy predicted fantasizing about many uncommitted partners, adventurous/risky sex, dominance, submission, and deviance (e.g., exhibitionism, voyeurism). That is, psychopathy was associated with fantasizing about every sexual theme except for romance, suggesting again that psychopathy seems to be related to variety and novelty in sexual interests. Similarly, when asked about the frequency of engaging in fantasized behaviors, psychopathy was a significant predictor of every behavior except romance, even after controlling for the level of fantasizing about that behavior. Further, psychopathy moderated the relation between fantasizing about both deviant and uncommitted sexual activity and engaging in both deviant and uncommitted sexual behavior. The nature of this interaction was such that only at high levels of psychopathy was fantasizing about uncommitted and deviant sexual activities a significant predictor of the corresponding real-life behaviors.

Thus, it seems that people with psychopathic traits are more apt to be engaging in fantasized behaviors that other individuals might limit to the realm of fantasy. Visser et al. (2015) noted that another explanation for their results could lie in the fact that people with higher levels of psychopathic traits have a broader range of sexual experiences. Leitenberg and Henning (1995) noted that many people fantasize about previous sexual activities and partners. Thus, individuals who are more psychopathic may use their more varied sexual experiences as fodder for subsequent fantasies. This study highlights the consistency between fantasies and behavior, as well as the degree to which psychopathy is associated with diverse sexual interests even in these non-forensic samples.

The findings of these reviewed studies around the role of psychopathy in linking fantasy to real-life behavior support the previous findings that the combination of psychopathy and deviant interests is a dangerous one. Whereas people with low psychopathy might inhibit such interests or find ways to negotiate consent with a partner, more psychopathic individuals might resort to manipulation, deceit, and/or coercion to satisfy their sexual desires.

Gender differences

Women are less psychopathic than men in general (Hare, 2003; Miller, Watts, & Jones, 2011; Visser et al., 2010), and the base rate of psychopaths is lower in female offender populations (Hare, 2003) than in male offender populations. Mealey (1995) suggested that men and women would have different thresholds for expressing psychopathy, in that men would require less environmental contribution to become psychopathic. Likewise, women would require a greater genetic diathesis to express psychopathic tendencies.

The structure, personality, and behavioral correlates of psychopathy seem to be quite similar for men and women (e.g., Visser et al., 2010; Warren et al., 2003). although there is some evidence that the role of sexuality may be different. In validating the Psychopathy Checklist Revised (PCL–R; Hare, 2003), Hare found that the promiscuous sexual behavior item failed to load on either PCL–R factor in men, but loaded onto Factor 2 (lifestyle and behavioral aspects of psychopathy) in female samples. Thus, sexual promiscuity might relate to parasitic lifestyle and social deviance to a greater extent for women than for men. Indeed, Forouzan and Cooke (2005) suggested that whereas promiscuous sexual activity might reflect sensation seeking in men, it might be a tool for exploitation and manipulation when used by women.

Mealey (1995) noted that for women, psychopathy does not seem to be a risk factor for sexual offending. Even in the case of serial killer Aileen Wuornos, perhaps the most famous female psychopath, Myers, Gooch, and Meloy (2005) suggested that there it was unclear whether there was any sexual motivation or gratification involved in her crimes, which were typically carried out when Wuornos was engaging in prostitution.

In Cleckley's (1941/1988:53) 15 case studies, only two are female. Cleckley described 20-year-old Roberta as having sexual intercourse with numerous men and experiencing "a moderate, half-warmed pleasure, but nothing like intense passion." He noted that she was never particularly motivated or tempted by sex, nor did she experience any passion for or emotional connection to her many partners. In the second case, 40-year-old Anna had a history of engaging in impersonal sexual activity with a group of teenage boys when she was in high school. This pattern of varied and impersonal sexual activity continued over the years, with Anna seemingly unable to form loving attachments, although her charm and intelligence attracted men who seemed to feel great love for her. Of Anna, Cleckley wrote:

> It seems likely that she has frequently experienced the physiologic reactions of orgasm but that these reactions have been a minor factor in her behavior pattern. Sometimes, while having technically satisfactory relations with a husband, she would continue intercourse with other men who, it seems, failed entirely to arouse or to gratify her in the usual sense. As a matter of fact, while living with the husband who, more regularly than any other man she can recall, made her "respond," she initiated and continued relations with several other men. From some of these she neither particularly wanted nor ever received pleasure that could be called sensual or romantic.
>
> *(Cleckley, 1941/1988:115)*

The impersonal sexual behavior of the two female patients seems highly consistent with those of Cleckley's male patients who similarly charmed then discarded numerous sexual partners. Cleckley's male and female patients were generally described as engaging in varied casual sexual relations with inappropriate partners, but unlike Hare's psychopathic offenders, they do not seem particularly coercive in their sexuality.

In student samples, psychopathy seems to relate to women, like men, having an earlier onset of sexual activity, more sexual partners, more sexual "affairs" (Visser et al., 2010), and more "poaching" of other people's partners (Sunderani, Arnocky, & Vaillancourt, 2013). Muñoz, Khan, and Cordwell (2011) reported that in an undergraduate student sample, although men reported greater use of all kinds of sexual coercion (e.g., touching/arousing the other person, emotional manipulation, exploiting by intoxication, and physical force), primary psychopathy predicted sexual coercion by women as well. Despite reporting less sexually coercive behavior on average, women with higher levels of psychopathic traits reported using coercive tactics in a similar fashion as their male counterparts (the exception was exploiting by intoxication, which was used more extensively by men with psychopathic traits than by women with psychopathic traits). Such evidence suggests that psychopathy is associated with a willingness to use coercive tactics to achieve a goal. It seems possible, though, that women's tactics are less likely to reach levels where partners call for police assistance and thus go unreported.

Treatment

For many years, it was thought that treatment was ineffective or even counterproductive for psychopathic offenders (Rice, Harris, & Cormier, 1992). A particular concern emerged when some early studies suggested that psychopaths not only failed to benefit from treatment but were able to persuade therapeutic staff that they have made progress (e.g., Rice et al., 1992; Seto & Barbaree, 1999). As with treatment of psychopathic offenders in general, it seems that treatment with psychopathic sex offenders can have some effectiveness (Olver & Wong, 2009). Despite their increased risk of reoffending compared to non-psychopathic counterparts, psychopathic sex offenders who completed treatment recidivated violently at lower rates than those who did not complete treatment (Olver & Wong, 2009).

A concern about the studies on the effectiveness of treatment for psychopathic sex offenders is that they are quite limited in number. Doren and Yates (2008) reviewed the research, which included data on psychopath versus non-psychopath treatment response to cognitive behavioral therapies for sex offenders. They found only ten studies, all coming from only four different treatment programs. The authors concluded that sex offender treatment is as successful for some psychopaths as non-psychopaths, whereas other psychopaths do not seem to benefit to the same extent. Doren and Yates also concluded that treatment did not lower serious recidivism by psychopaths to the same levels as for treated non-psychopaths. Because the characteristics that distinguished the psychopaths who benefited from treatment from those who did not varied across the studies, the authors recommended more research to better understand and replicate these features.

Another issue is that psychopathic sex offenders seem to be at particular risk of dropout from treatment. Olver and Wong (2011) reported that in a Canadian sample of 154 male incarcerated sex offenders receiving intensive treatment, psychopathy in general, and callous affect (a PCL–R facet) in particular, was a risk factor for treatment dropout. The authors suggested that shallow emotionality/coldness could impair therapeutic alliance and perhaps indicate to treatment staff that such individuals are not engaged in the process. Also, therapeutic attempts to induce empathy in the offender would fail, perhaps causing frustration in staff and offender. The authors noted that guidelines for treating psychopathic sex offenders (e.g., resisting manipulation tactics) could be helpful in working with this group of offenders and minimizing dropout.

Conclusion

Overall, this chapter has pointed to the dangerousness posed by the male sex offender who is also a psychopath. To find very high rates of psychopathy, one can look to the group of incarcerated men who are perpetrators of sexual assaults against both adults and children. Furthermore, these individuals are likely to drop out of treatment, and even when they do complete treatment, they may or may not be as successful as their non-psychopathic counterparts. Thus, the stereotypical psychopath seems to have a real-life, equally frightening counterpart.

Although the evidence reviewed has emphasized that psychopathy combined with deviant sexuality is a dangerous combination, most psychopaths will not have strong, deviant sexual interests. However, psychopaths are very likely to bring their pervasive manipulation, deception, and exploitation to the realm of sexual behavior. Thus, the individual who is susceptible to the charms of the psychopath may find himself or herself abandoned, cheated on, lied to, and financially exploited. Psychopaths may use threats, force, or other forms of coercion to obtain sex from a non-consenting partner. The varied antisociality of the psychopath is likely to manifest itself in both sexual and non-sexual ways in the context of interpersonal relationships.

Although psychopathic men are far more likely than psychopathic women to be the perpetrators of sexual violence, there is evidence that female psychopaths use their sexuality as a tool of manipulation and exploitation. Evolutionary theories suggest that a cheating, aggressive, "fast" life strategy is core to psychopathy, and the research generally supports such theories. Even at the subclinical level, both men and women with higher levels of psychopathy report earlier sexual activity, more sexual partners, cheating on partners, and greater use of coercion. Even in their sexual fantasies, people with higher levels of psychopathic traits report a greater variety of sexual fantasies, and a stronger fantasy/real life behavior link for fantasies around both impersonal and deviant sexual activities.

Overall, the impersonal, deceptive, and exploitive sensation seeking of the psychopath is reflected in his or her sexuality. To the extent that a psychopathic individual has sexual interests around non-consensual activities, there appears to be a greater likelihood that the individual will fail to inhibit the corresponding behavior. Although the forensic literature tends to emphasize the lifestyle and behavioral correlates of these activities, it seems likely that the emotional coldness and lack of empathy play an important role as well. There is a need for greater research into sex offender treatment for psychopaths, including how to reduce dropout rates of psychopathic participants.

References

Baughman, H. M., Jonason, P. K., Veselka, L., and Vernon, P. A. (2014) 'Four shades of sexual fantasies linked to the Dark Triad,' *Personality and Individual Differences*, *67*:47–51

Baumgartner, J., Scalora, M., and Huss, M. (2002) 'Assessment of the Wilson Sex Fantasy Questionnaire among child molesters and nonsexual forensic offenders,' *Sexual Abuse: A Journal of Research and Treatment*, *14*:19–30.

Blais, J., Solodukhin, E., and Forth, A. (2014) 'A meta-analysis exploring the relationship between psychopathy and instrumental versus reactive violence,' *Criminal Justice and Behavior*, *41*:797–821.

Blonigen, D. M., Carlson, S. R., Krueger, R. F., and Patrick, C. J. (2003) 'A twin study of self-reported psychopathic personality traits,' *Personality and Individual Differences*, *35*(1):79–197.

Brown, S., and Forth, A. (1997) 'Psychopathy and sexual assault: Static risk factors, emotional precursors, and rapist subtypes,' *Journal of Consulting and Clinical Psychology*, *64*:848–847.

Book, A., Methot-Jones, T., Blais, J., Hosker-Field, A., Volk, A., Visser, B., . . ., and D'Agata, M. (2016) 'Psychopathic traits and the cheater-hawk hypothesis,' *Journal of Interpersonal Violence*, in press.

Book, A. S., and Quinsey, V. L. (2004) 'Psychopaths: Cheaters or warrior-hawks?,' *Personality and Individual Differences*, *36*:33–45.
Cleckley, H. (1988) *The mask of sanity* (5th ed.), St. Louis, MO: Mosby. (Original work published in 1941).
Doren, D., and Yates, P. (2008) 'Effectiveness of sex offender treatment for psychopathic sexual offenders,' *International Journal of Offender Therapy and Comparative Criminology*, *52*:234–245.
Edens, J. F., Marcus, D. K., Lilienfeld, S. O., and Poythress Jr., N. G. (2006) 'Psychopathic, not psychopath: Taxometric evidence for the dimensional structure of psychopathy,' *Journal of Abnormal Psychology*, *115*:131–144.
Figueredo, A. J., Vasquez, G., Brumbach, B. H., Schneider, S. M. R., Sefcek, J. A., Tal, I. R., . . ., and Jacobs, W. J. (2006) 'Consilience and life history theory: From genes to brain to reproductive strategy,' *Developmental Review*, *26*(2):243–275.
Forouzan, E., and Cooke, D. J. (2005) 'Figuring out la femme fatale: Conceptual and assessment issues concerning psychopathy in females,' *Behavioral Sciences & the Law*, *23*:765–778.
Glenn, A. L., Kurzban, R., and Raine, A. (2009) 'Evolutionary theory and psychopathy,' *Aggression and Violent Behavior*, *16*:371–380.
Hanson, R. K., Morton-Bourgon, K. E., Hanson, R. K., and Morton-Bourgon, K. E. (2009) 'The accuracy of recidivism risk assessments for sexual offenders: A meta-analysis of 118 prediction studies,' *Psychological Assessment*, *21*:1–21.
Hare, R. D. (1999) *Without conscience: The disturbing world of the psychopaths among us*, New York, NY: Guilford Press.
Hare, R. D. (2003) *The Psychopathy Checklist–Revised* (2nd ed.), Toronto, ON: Multi-Health Systems.
Harris, G. T., Rice, M. E., Hilton, N. Z., Lalumière, M. L., and Quinsey, V. L. (2007) 'Coercive and precocious sexuality as a fundamental aspect of psychopathy,' *Journal of Personality Disorders*, *21*(1):1–27.
Harris, G. T., Rice, M. E., and Quinsey, V. L. (1994) 'Psychopathy as a taxon: Evidence that psychopaths are a discrete class,' *Journal of Consulting and Clinical Psychology*, *62*:387–397.
Hawes, S. W., Boccaccini, M. T., Murrie, D. C., Hawes, S. W., Boccaccini, M. T., and Murrie, D. C. (2013) 'Psychopathy and the combination of psychopathy and sexual deviance as predictors of sexual recidivism: Meta-analytic findings using the psychopathy Checklist–Revised,' *Psychological Assessment*, *25*:233–243.
Jonason, P. K., Koenig, B. L., and Tost, J. (2010) 'Living a fast life: The dark triad and life history theory,' *Human Nature*, *21*:428–442.
Kiehl, K. A., and Hoffman, M. B. (2011) 'The criminal psychopath: History, neuroscience, treatment, and economics,' *Jurimetrics*, *51*(4):355–398.
Kosson, D. S., Kelly, J. C., and White, J. W. (1997) 'Psychopathy-related traits predict self-reported sexual aggression among college men,' *Journal of Interpersonal Violence*, *12*:241–254.
Lalumière, M. L, Harris, G. T., and Rice, M. E. (2001) 'Psychopathy and developmental instability,' *Evolution and Human Behavior*, *22*:75–92.
Leitenberg, H., and Henning, K. (1995) 'Sexual fantasy,' *Psychological Bulletin*, *3*:469–496.
Mealey, L. (1995) 'The sociobiology of sociopathy: An integrated evolutionary model,' *Behavioral and Brain Sciences*, *18*:523–541.
Meloy, J. (2002) 'The "polymorphously perverse" psychopath: Understanding a strong empirical relationship,' *Bulletin of the Menninger Clinic*, *66*:273–289.
Miller, J. D., Lynam, D. R., Widiger, T. A., and Leukefeld, C. (2001) 'Personality disorders as extreme variants of common personality dimensions: Can the five-factor model adequately represent psychopathy?,' *Journal of Personality*, *69*:253–276.
Miller, J. D., Watts, A., and Jones, S. E. (2011) 'Does psychopathy manifest divergent relations with components of its nomological network depending on gender?,' *Personality and Individual Differences*, *50*(5):564–569.
Muñoz, L. C., Khan, R., and Cordwell, L. (2011) 'Sexually coercive tactics used by university students: A clear role for primary psychopathy,' *Journal of Personality Disorders*, *25*(1):28–40.
Myers, W. C., Gooch, E., and Meloy, J. R. (2005) 'The role of psychopathy and sexuality in a female serial killer,' *Journal of Forensic Science*, *50*:1–6.
Olver, M., and Wong, S. C. P. (2006) 'Psychopathy, sexual deviance, and recidivism among sex offenders,' *Sexual Abuse: A Journal of Research and Treatment*, *18*(1):65–82.
Olver, M. E., and Wong, S. C. P. (2009) 'Therapeutic responses of psychopathic sexual offenders: Treatment attrition, therapeutic change, and long-term recidivism,' *Journal of Consulting and Clinical Psychology*, 77:328–336.
Olver, M. E., and Wong, S. (2011) 'Predictors of sex offender treatment dropout: Psychopathy, sex offender risk, and responsivity implications,' *Psychology, Crime & Law*, *17*:457–471.

Paulhus, D. L., and Williams, K. M. (2002) 'The dark triad of personality: Narcissism, Machiavellianism, and psychopathy,' *Journal of Research in Personality, 36*:556–563.

Porter, S., Campbell, M. A., Woodworth, M., and Birt, A. R. (2001) 'A new psychological conceptualization of the sexual psychopath,' in F. Columbus (Ed.), *Advances in psychological research* (Vol. 7, pp. 21–36), New York, NY: Nova Science.

Porter, S., Fairweather, D., Drugge, J., Herve, H., Birt, A., and Boer, D. P. (2000) 'Profiles of psychopathy in incarcerated sexual offenders,' *Criminal Justice and Behavior, 27*:216–233.

Quinsey, V. L., Harris, G. T., Rice, M. E., and Cormier, C. A. (2006) *Violent offenders: Appraising and managing risk* (2nd ed.). *The law and public policy*, Washington, DC: American Psychological Association.

Quinsey, V. L., Rice, M. E., and Harris, G. T. (1995) 'Actuarial prediction of sexual recidivism,' *Journal of Interpersonal Violence, 10*:85–105.

Rice, M. E., Harris, G. T., and Cormier, C. A. (1992) 'An evaluation of a maximum security therapeutic community for psychopaths and other mentally disordered offenders,' *Law and Human Behavior, 16*(4):399–412.

Serin, R., Mailloux, D., and Malcolm, P. (2001) 'Psychopathy, deviant sexual arousal, and recidivism among sexual offenders,' *Journal of Interpersonal Violence, 16*(3):234–246.

Seto, M. C., and Barbaree, H. (1999) 'Psychopathy, treatment behavior, and sex offender recidivism,' *Journal of Interpersonal Violence, 14*:1235–1248.

Seto, M. C., Khattar, N. A., Lalumière, M. L., and Quinsey, V. L. (1997) 'Deception and sexual strategy in psychopathy,' *Personality and Individual Differences, 22*:301–307.

Skovran, L. C., Huss, M. T., and Scalora, M. J. (2010) 'Sexual fantasies and sensation seeking among psychopathic sexual offenders,' *Psychology, Crime & Law, 16*(7):617–629.

Sunderani, S., Arnocky, S., and Vaillancourt, T. (2013) 'Individual differences in mate poaching: An examination of hormonal, dispositional, and behavioral mate-value traits,' *Archives of Sexual Behavior, 42*:533–542.

Visser, B. A., Ashton, M. C., and Pozzebon, J. A. (2012) 'Is low anxiety part of the psychopathy construct?,' *Journal of Personality, 80*:725–747.

Visser, B. A., DeBow, V., Pozzebon, J. A., Bogaert, A. F., and Book, A. (2015) 'Psychopathic sexuality: The thin line between fantasy and reality,' *Journal of Personality, 83*:376–388.

Visser, B. A., Pozzebon, J. A., Bogaert, A. F., and Ashton, M. C. (2010) 'Psychopathy, sexual behavior, and esteem: It's different for girls,' *Personality and Individual Differences, 48*:833–838.

Wallace, J. F., Malterer, M. B., and Newman, J. P. (2009) 'Mapping Gray's BIS and BAS constructs onto Factor 1 and Factor 2 of Hare's Psychopathy Checklist–Revised,' *Personality and Individual Differences, 47*:812–816.

Warren, J. I., Burnette, M. L., South, S. C., Chauhan, P., Bale, R., Friend, R., and Van Patten, I. (2003) 'Psychopathy in women: Structural modeling and comorbidity,' *International Journal of Law and Psychiatry, 26*(3):223–242.

Williams, K. M., Cooper, B. S., Howell, T. M., Yuille, J. C., and Paulhus, D. L. (2009) 'Inferring sexually deviant behavior from corresponding fantasies: The role of personality and pornography consumption,' *Criminal Justice and Behavior, 36*:198–222.

Williams, S. (1998) *Invisible darkness: The strange case of Paul Bernardo and Karla Homolka*, Toronto, ON: Bantam.

25

Psychopathy and sexual assault

Eric Beauregard and Kylie Reale

Introduction

The concept of psychopathy and its measures have made their way into the realm of criminology, despite being a central focus of research in the field of psychology and law for many years now (see Corrado, DeLisi, Hart, & McCuish, 2015). It has been impossible to ignore the fact that studies have repeatedly confirmed that psychopathy is associated with violence and crime in general (e.g., Hart & Hare, 1997; McCuish, Corrado, Hart, & DeLisi, 2015). This remains true even in juvenile offenders, as studies have shown that juvenile sex offenders presented more psychopathic disturbances than non-sexual juvenile offenders (Cale, Lussier, McCuish, & Corrado, 2015). Furthermore, psychopathy has been identified as a risk factor for sexual recidivism, especially when combined with deviant sexual preferences, and has been included in several sex offender risk assessment tools (e.g., Hanson & Harris, 2000; Hare, Clark, Grann, & Thornton, 2000; Hawes, Boccaccini, & Murrie, 2013; Hildebrand, De Ruiter, & de Vogel, 2004; Porter, Brinke, & Wilson, 2009; Woodworth et al., 2013). Defined by the validated Psychopathy Checklist–Revised (PCL–R; Hare, 1991, 2003), psychopaths are described as manipulative, callous, remorseless, impulsive, irresponsible individuals (Porter, Birt, & Boer, 2001). In addition, studies have shown that psychopaths present a propensity for substance use, aggression, and sexual promiscuity, which confirm their sensation seeking tendencies as well as their proclivity towards violating the rights of others (Hildebrand et al., 2004; Neumann & Hare, 2008). They are often described as chronic deceivers, lying for instrumental reasons (e.g., to escape punishment) and using others for obtaining different rewards such as money, drugs, power, and even sex (see Woodworth & Porter, 2002). Their general disinhibition has been suggested to be a contributing factor to the development of an antisocial lifestyle that could be linked to an increase in the likelihood of committing sex offenses (Quinsey, Rice, & Harris, 1995). For those committing sexual crimes, research has shown that generally, levels of psychopathy were higher for those targeting adults (i.e., rapists) compared to children (i.e., child molesters; see Prentky & Knight, 1991; Quinsey et al., 1995; Serin, Malcolm, Khanna, & Barbaree, 1994).

This chapter examines the research on the relationships between psychopathy and sexual offending. We argue that as with general violence, psychopathic individuals are instrumental in their use of sexual violence. Contrary to various studies suggesting that sexual violence is mainly driven by paraphilias and deviant sexual arousal, the current chapter shows that psychopaths use sexual violence to make gains, using such strategies as targeting different types of victims, using a higher level of violence, and committing sadistic acts on their victims.

Psychopathy and instrumental violence

Research on sexual violence has shown that sex offenders are heterogeneous. Depending on their type (e.g., child molesters, sadistic sex offender), they present different motivations. Despite being a difficult question to examine, the issue of motivation is an important one in sexual crimes. However, it seems that with psychopathic offenders, the research has identified one main motivation underlying their crimes, that is, whether the crime is sexual or not. It has been well established that psychopaths are violent individuals. But their violence is not reactive – it is mainly instrumental. In a study by Williamson, Hare, and Wong (1987), they found that an offender's motivation for committing violent crime differed depending on whether they had been committed by psychopaths or not. The violent crimes committed by psychopaths were significantly more likely to have been motivated by material gain than non-psychopaths, whereas non-psychopaths were more likely to have experienced high levels of emotion prior to the crime. Similarly, Cornell et al. (1996) showed that offenders who had committed at least one previous act of instrumental violence scored higher on the PCL–R compared to offenders who had exclusively committed acts of reactive violence. Woodworth and Porter (2002) examined this hypothesis further by looking specifically at homicide. Using a sample of 125 incarcerated homicide offenders, they found that psychopaths were more likely to have committed instrumental, predatory homicides compared to non-psychopaths. Interestingly, their study also showed that contrary to their initial prediction, psychopaths rarely committed reactive homicidal violence (Woodworth & Porter, 2002).

Porter and Woodworth (2007) replicated their own findings in a subsequent study looking at 50 homicide offenders. Results showed that nearly 90 percent of the psychopaths in their sample had committed premeditated homicides without any reactive violence component, more than twice that of non-psychopathic offenders. It is noteworthy that despite their general impulsivity, psychopaths seem more likely to premeditate an instrumental murder. Porter and Woodworth (2007) suggest that this could be related to: (1) better chances of avoiding detection (see also Porter & Woodworth, 2006) and (2) a feeling of satisfaction from the planning and the commission of predatory violence.

But does this research on psychopathy in homicide offenders translate to sex offenders as well? We believe so. What has been described above is congruent with many of the findings on the "reasoning sex offender" (see Beauregard, 2017; Beauregard & Leclerc, 2007). Some sex offenders are capable of "rational" decision-making when contemplating a criminal opportunity. Some sex offenders choose to engage in certain types of behaviors because the benefits outweigh the costs. In line with Porter and Woodworth (2006), Beauregard and Martineau (2014, 2016), and Reale, Beauregard, and Martineau (2017a), some sex offenders have been shown to use specific strategies (to commit the crime or when selecting a victim or a location) to avoid police detection. Moreover, some offenders target specific victims because they are more vulnerable; they use certain strategies because it allows them to better control the victim; and they select specific locations because it allows them to spend more time with the victim without the risk of being interrupted by potential witnesses. Some offenders choose to perform some specific acts simply because it provides them with the greatest pleasure (Beauregard, 2017). A study by Pedneault, Beauregard, Harris, and Knight (2015) perfectly illustrates the systematic decision-making that takes place in cases of sexual burglary. The study examined reasoning in a sample of

104 male offenders involving 224 individual incidents of residential burglary with apparent sexual motivations. The authors analyzed the situational cues identified by sexual burglars in their target selection. Their findings indicated that most sexually motivated burglaries occurred in occupied residences with deficient physical guardianship (no male present) and when a female victim was alone and unlikely to resist because she was asleep. Violence, theft, penetration, and even fetishism – a behavior that is often described as ritualistic and compulsive – were found to be committed in circumstances that increased the benefits and lowered the risks (e.g., fetishistic behaviors were committed in unoccupied houses).

Moreover, their results showed that sexual burglars are reasoning sex offenders who consider costs and benefits as they selected residences that were easy to break into, and therefore these events should not be considered an "added bonus" in an otherwise non-sexual burglary. Instead, sexual burglars acted opportunistically based on situational cues that are markedly dissimilar to those of regular burglars. Specifically, sexual burglaries disproportionately (1) involved apartments, which represent high-risk targets to gain entrance, (2) targeted occupied residences, (3) were committed at night, between midnight and 3 am, a time during which people are more likely to be at home, and (4) involved weapons from the onset, as if prepared to find something different than empty residences. Finally, this study showed that despite the apparent lack of rationality, sexual burglars make decisions that are congruent with their motivation and their goal. This finding reinforces the notion that certain violent behaviors (e.g., using a weapon) during the crime-commission process may be a function of instrumental gain – rather than reactive violence – as can be seen in psychopathic offenders. Moreover, the overwhelming instrumental motivation involved in the crimes of the psychopaths, whether it is sexual or not, also persists in their choice of victim.

Psychopathy and victim crossover

Despite the fact that empirical evidence has long since shown that persistent sex offenders are likely to "switch" from one victim to another (e.g., Abel et al., 1987) and that target preferences could evolve during the criminal career, the larger field of research on sexual violence has been hesitant to adopt such a view (Beauregard, Leclerc, & Lussier, 2012). Most studies exclusively focus on one type of offender, such as a child molester or rapist, and have avoided the mixing of both groups. The resistance to take a more holistic approach can also be explained by the assumption that sex offenders are driven by specific urges and paraphilia dictating how sexual criminal behavior will be conducted and who will be targeted (e.g., pedophilia, hebephilia, etc.). Despite this, studies are continuing to show (see Lussier, 2005 for an extensive review) that sex offenders can choose and abuse a different victim type depending on a number of different factors, such as the opportunity that presents itself, a desire to diversify sexual and criminal experiences, or simply the element of risk exposure inherent in different victim types.

This type of offender is typically referred to as the crossover or "mixed" sex offender and is usually defined by a combination of the sexual crimes committed against child and adult victims. This *sexual polymorphism* refers to "crime-switching patterns along several dimensions such as victim's age, gender, relationship to the offender, nature of acts committed by the offender" (Lussier, Leclerc, Healey, & Proulx, 2007:97). This type of behavior has been shown to differentiate the crossover sex offender from child sex offenders and rapists. For instance, Brown, Dargis, Mattern, Tsonis, and Newman (2015) have suggested that crossover sex offenders are thrill-seekers who are prone to boredom and other psychopathic features (see also Porter, Campbell, Woodworth, & Birt, 2001). Compatible with this description, Cann, Friendship, and Gonza (2007) have suggested that crossover sex offenders demonstrate a general lack of empathy that goes beyond their treatment of women and children, something similar to what has been observed in psychopathic individuals.

When reviewing the literature on crime-switching patterns of sex offenders, two major conclusions emerge (Lussier et al., 2007a). First, several studies have found specialization in sexual offending, including sex offenders' confining themselves to one victim-type (Cann, Friendship, & Gonza, 2007; Gebhard, Gagnon, Pomeroy, & Christenson, 1965; Guay, Proulx, Cusson, & Ouimet, 2001; Soothill, Francis, Sanderson, & Ackerley, 2000). Second, there is a significantly different picture that emerges when the focus switches to studies conducted in clinical settings. Weinrot and Saylor (1991) found that when using only official data, 15 percent of their sample of sex offenders was versatile in their sexual offense behavior. However, when using a self-reported questionnaire, that number rose to 53 percent. Similar findings were reported by Heil, Ahlmeyer and Simons (2003). When assessed using official data, only a minority of offenders was versatile in terms of victim's age (7 percent) and gender (8.5 percent); however, when interviewed using a polygraph, those numbers rose to 70 percent and 36 percent respectively, showing high sexual polymorphism.

In their study on crime switching patterns of 216 sex offenders, Lussier, Leclerc, Healey et al. (2007) found that the level of polymorphism varies from one crime to another. On one end of the continuum, victim's gender and the level of physical force are stable; on the opposite end, the victim's age and sexual intrusiveness involve more switching. Moreover, a clearly nonrandom pattern emerges with victim's age. Specifically, offenders who abuse children tend stay within this age group, rarely switching for another victim age if at all. However, if they do switch, they will abuse an adolescent victim, not an adult. Conversely, offenders who abuse an adolescent or an adult victim are initially likely to switch and abuse another victim type. Offenders who abuse adolescent victims will switch for a child, whereas offenders who assault adults will switch for an adolescent victim. Of interest is that very few child molesters will commit a crime against an adult and vice-versa. In line with the concept of sex surrogate, adolescent victims may represent the second option in the absence of the preferred victim-type that is children or adults (Guay et al., 2001). Moreover, findings also show that this tendency to switch increases as a function of repetition of the sexually deviant behavior.

Similarly, a study by Stephens, Reale, Goodwill, and Beauregard (2017) examined victim-age polymorphism using 72 cases of serial sexual offenders who committed a total of 361 stranger sexual offenses. The authors isolated crossover behavior to victim age and compared various crime scene behaviors to offenders who restricted themselves to one age category. They found that 36 percent of the sample, which used interview data corroborated by file information, had sexual offense histories that included victim age-crossover behavior. More specifically, offenders with victims between ages 11–14 had the highest likelihood of crossover behavior. Interestingly, opportunistic behavior during the crime commission process (e.g., victim selection based on vulnerability or selecting victim based on location) emerged as a distinguishing feature of age-specific and crossover offenders, which is consistent with the notion of high sensation seeking tendencies in polymorphic offenders. This finding also complements research that has found higher rates of psychopathy in polymorphic offenders (e.g., Porter et al., 2000; Skrovan, Huss, & Scalora, 2010).

Two main hypotheses have been suggested to explain sexual polymorphism in sex offenders (Beauregard et al., 2012). First, individuals characterized with high sexualization – i.e., a disinhibited sexuality characterized by sexual preoccupation, sexual compulsivity, and impersonal sex (Lussier, Leclerc, Cale, & Proulx, 2007) – are likely to experience more difficulties in controlling their sexual urges, thus explaining why they are also more likely to seek out sexual gratification in different contexts and opportunities (Lussier, Leclerc, Healey et al., 2007). Second, sexual polymorphism could be a function of general deviance. Research findings show that as the frequency of offending increases, so does the versatility in paraphilic interests and behaviors (Lussier, Leblanc, & Proulx, 2005; Smallbone & Wortley, 2004). Such results are congruent with the general theory of crime (Gottfredson & Hirschi, 1990) in which individuals lacking self-control may display different sexual behaviors depending on the opportunity (Lussier, Proulx, & Leblanc, 2005).

But a third hypothesis suggests that the presence of psychopathy can explain why some offenders have polymorphic sexual interests that enable them to switch from one victim type to another. For instance, Porter, Campbell, Woodworth, and Birt (2000) showed that crossover sex offenders were more likely to present psychopathy traits (64 percent) than intrafamilial child sex offenders (6.3 percent), extrafamilial child sex offenders (10.8 percent), non-sex offenders (34 percent), and rapists (29–35.9 percent). Despite a relative small sample size, the higher prevalence of psychopathy among the crossover sex offenders is congruent with other studies (e.g., Porter et al., 2000) and confirms that these offenders demonstrate significantly more psychopathic features than other sex offender groups as well as non-sex offenders (Brown et al., 2015).

The study by Brown et al. (2015) further investigated the relationship between psychopathy and sexual polymorphism. Despite studies showing that crossover sex offenders score higher on the total PCL–R, Factor 1 (the affective–interpersonal components of psychopathy), and Factor 2 (the impulsive–antisocial lifestyle components of psychopathy) compared to child sex offenders, it was unclear whether these scores could distinguish them from rapists as well as non-sex offenders (see Oliver & Wong, 2006; Porter et al., 2009; Skrovan, Huss, & Scalora, 2010). Consistent with these prior studies, Brown et al. (2015) found that crossover sex offenders scored significantly higher on the total PCL–R as well as on Factor 1 and Factor 2 scores than the other groups, including the rapists. However, similar to prior studies reporting high base rates of psychopathy among crossover sex offenders (e.g., Porter et al., 2009; Porter et al., 2000), the rate of psychopathy was highest for crossover sex offenders, but this was only significantly higher than the rate of psychopathy of child sex offenders (Brown et al., 2015). Finally, the researchers found that crossover sex offenders fit the description of the emotionally stable psychopathic offender (Gray, 1987; Hicks, Markon, Patrick, Krueger, & Newman, 2004). These offenders show low levels of stress reactivity, which could explain why they are more likely to engage in risky behavior while being less affected by negative life events. "The distinctively low levels of stress reaction associated with mixed offenders may not only fail to deter them from perpetrating future sexual offenses but may also prompt them to diversify their sexual offending targets" (Brown et al., 2015:1039–1040).

Interestingly, all these results and hypotheses are congruent with the findings by Beauregard et al. (2012) from their study on the decision-making of sex offenders. This study compared the decision-making during the crime-commission process of three subgroups of sex offenders: rapists, child molesters, and crossover sex offenders. Although previous studies have suggested that the patterns exhibited by crossover sex offenders is more similar to rapists than to child molesters (see, for instance, Lussier, Leclerc, Healey, et al., 2007), the situation is more complex when decision-making is specifically taken into account. In the pre-crime phase of the crime-commission process, the decision-making of the crossover sex offender appears to be more similar to the child molester, whereas with the offense strategies, the crossover sex offender shares almost equally the same decision-making rationales of both the child molester and the rapist. Lastly, during the aftermath phase, the crossover sex offender is similar to the child molester, showing the highest frequency of offense completion rationale. The authors suggest that the decision-making during the crime-commission process varies depending on the type of victim as well as the attached context (Cohen & Felson, 1979; Deslauriers-Varin & Beauregard, 2010).

Specifically, the crossover sex offender adapts his decision-making to the type of victim. His "flexibility" as to his decision-making allows him to consider multiple opportunities, which translates into the highest rate of offense completion. This flexibility is an indication that these offenders are not primarily driven by a specific deviant sexual preference but, rather, could be due to a high sexualization in these offenders (Lussier, Lerclec, Healey et al. 2007), who therefore experience more difficulties in controlling their sexual urges. This would explain why they are also more likely to seek out sexual gratification in different contexts and opportunities. Moreover, congruent with the general theory of crime (Gottfredson & Hirschi, 1990), individuals lacking self-control may display different sexual behaviors depending on the opportunity (Lussier, Proulx, & Leblanc, 2005). And as suggested by the routine activities theory, the actual crime-commission is a function of the convergence of factors that involve lifestyles and criminal opportunity. Hence, daily activities and lifestyles nurture a criminal opportunity structure by enhancing the exposure and proximity of crime targets to motivated offenders (Miethe & Meier, 1990; Mustaine & Tewksbury, 2002). As proposed by Kaufman, Mosher, Carter, and Estes (2006), "opportunities are most directly influenced by the victim's situation (e.g., walking alone), target location (e.g., parks), and the involvement of facilitators" (p. 112). The fact that crossover sex offenders reported more targeted planning is not necessarily incompatible with the above explanation and their inclination to be more opportunistic. In fact, what this seems to suggest is that the crossover sex offender is able to plan in advance for different types of victim. The entirety of the decision-making across the three phases of the crime-commission process is congruent with such explanation. As such, this offender appears as the most "rational" sex offender, as the choice of methods for carrying out his crimes, as well as the decision-making involved, is an instrumental behavior implemented to achieve his desired goals (e.g., sexual gratification, domination of others) that takes into account the effort, rewards, and costs involved in alternative courses of action (Cornish & Clarke, 2002). Again, the planning for different victim types and different contexts allow the victim-crossover sex offender to be more successful and achieve more offense completion. Such interpretation is also compatible with the fact that crossover sex offenders demonstrate more features of psychopathy.

Psychopathy and the level of violence in sexual crime

This adaptation to different types of victims in psychopathic offenders is not the only feature that set them apart from other sex offenders. Some studies suggest that psychopathic sex offenders are also more likely to use a high level of violence (e.g., Huss & Langhinrichsen-Rohling, 2000) – even a lethal level of violence. As thrill-seeking is an important motivation for criminal behavior in psychopaths (e.g., Hare, 1996), excessive violence such as torture in a sexual crime could serve to satiate such a thrill-seeking motivation (see Porter et al., 2000; Porter, Campbell, Woodworth, & Birt, 2001). Given the constellation of personality features characterized by deficits in guilt, shame, remorse, and empathy as well as pervasive, multifaceted self-regulation problems, psychopathy has emerged as a theoretical framework with which to understand sexual homicide (Declercq, Willemsen, Audenaert, & Verhaeghe, 2012; Häkkänen-Nyholm, Repo-Tiihonen, Lindberg, Salenius, & Weizmann-Henelius, 2009; Myers, Gooch, & Meloy, 2005; Woodworth & Porter, 2002). Unfortunately, the relationship between psychopathy and sexual homicide has been empirically investigated in relatively few studies. Accordingly, Porter, Woodworth, Earle, Drugge, and Boer (2003) compared the characteristics of sexual homicide committed by psychopathic and non-psychopathic offenders. First, they found that almost 85 percent of the sexual homicide offenders (SHOs) scored in the moderate–high range on the Psychopathy Checklist–Revised (PCL–R; Hare, 1991). In addition, using a PCL–R cut-off of 30, they showed that sexual homicides committed by psychopathic offenders were more likely to present both gratuitous and sadistic violence compared to non-psychopathic offenders. Porter et al. (2003) propose that the absence of empathy combined with a Thrill-seeking propensity could lead the psychopath to try to maximize their pleasure as well as the damage inflicted during the sexual homicide.

Additional studies have provided some evidence of the relationship between psychopathy and sexual homicide. Comparing SHOs to a group of incest offenders, Firestone, Bradford, Greenberg, and Larose (1998) found that SHOs presented significantly higher PCL–R scores – on both Factor 1 and 2 – than the group of incest offenders. In fact, the scores obtained on the PCL–R as well as their respective percentiles show that, when compared with other pathological and criminal populations (e.g., prison inmates, forensic patients), SHOs show relatively greater personality disturbance than criminal behavior. Interestingly, the study also showed that SHOs were more likely to be diagnosed with any type of personality disorder (as well as three or more personality disorders), and with Antisocial Personality Disorder in particular, compared to the group of incest offenders.

Although the study by Langevin, Ben-Aron, Wright, Marchese, and Handy (1988) seems to corroborate this link between psychopathy and sexual homicide (as also emphasized by Porter et al., 2003), closer attention to the findings suggests otherwise. For instance, 7 out of 13 SHOs scored higher than 70 on the MMPI (Minnesota Multiphasic Personality Inventory) scale of psychopathy. However, it should be noted that despite its name, the psychopathy scale of the MMPI is poorly correlated with Hare's psychopathy scale, focusing more on impulsivity and social maladaptation (see Sauvetre & Proulx, 2007). Moreover, scores on the MCMI (Millon Clinical Multiaxial Inventory) showed that for six SHOs, they did not present a clinically significant score on the antisocial and narcissistic scales. Overall, these findings suggest that although psychopathy seems more important in SHOs, some of these offenders also present with different personality disorders that could explain, in part, the perpetration of sexual homicide.

Drawing on data from 616 adult male sex offenders, including 85 that were SHOs, Beauregard and DeLisi (2018) examined the personality profile of the SHOs by comparing them with a group of violent non-homicidal sex offenders (NHSOs) and a group of NHSOs on clinical diagnostics of personality disorders and various crime characteristics. Previous studies have suggested that, considering the nature of the crime of the SHO, they had to present psychopathic personality. Although several studies found a high prevalence of psychopathic personality in SHOs, other studies have also found that these offenders were characterized by other personality disorders as well (e.g., Borderline, Schizoid). However, in order to establish a link between the personality and sexual homicide, it is crucial to include a control group in the analyses, something that has not been done previously (except for Sauvetre & Proulx, 2007).

The study by Beauregard and DeLisi (2018) yielded several findings that are noteworthy. First, there is compelling evidence that personality disorders are endemic to sexual offenders generally and SHOs specifically. With the exception of Schizotypal Personality Disorder, all types of personality disorder had relatively high prevalence, with Cluster B personality disorders occurring at the highest rates. These findings are consistent with studies of general homicide offenders (Boduszek, Debowska, & Willmott, 2017; Eronen, Hakola, & Tiihonen, 1996; Fazel & Grann, 2004), juvenile sexual homicide offenders (Myers & Monaco, 2000), serial homicide offenders (Culhane, Hildebrand, Mullings, & Klemm, 2016), other sexual homicide offenders (Koch, Berner, Hill, & Briken, 2011), and institutionalized sexual offenders (Chen, Chen, & Hung, 2016). Taken together, the current prevalence estimates of personality disorders coupled with those from allied research attest to the prominence of personality and its dysfunction to the most violent and serious forms of criminal offending. In meta-analyses (Decuyper et al., 2009;

Jones, Miller, & Lynam, 2011), the basic personality foundation of aggression and antisocial behavior is that of very low scores on all facets of Conscientiousness, very low scores on all facets of Agreeableness, and mixed scores for Neuroticism (low anxiety, high anger/hostility, high depression, high impulsiveness), and mixed scores on Extraversion (low warmth, high assertiveness, high excitement seeking, low positive emotions).

Second, the study of homicide offenders presents a fascinating dialectic between differences in psychopathology. On the one hand, there are homicide offenders whose psychopathology is primarily rooted in antisocial traits where there is a drive to externalize violence. On the other, there are the offenders whose psychopathology is primarily rooted in asocial traits where violence reflects a dislike or revulsion for others (DeLisi, 2015; Meloy, 2000). The findings from Beauregard and DeLisi (2018) on SHOs highlight this dialectic. Compared to NHSOs and violent NHSOs, SHOs that had personality features characterized by Schizoid Personality Disorder and Borderline Personality Disorder were more likely to use drugs and alcohol before their murder, use a weapon, and select the victim, and their sexual behavior during the murder was less intrusive sexually, less likely to force the victim to engage in sexual acts, and less likely to involve humiliation of the victim. The salience of Schizoid Personality Disorder is particularly important. Like all personality disorders, there is heterogeneity within each diagnosis. Some persons with Schizoid Personality Disorder abstain from sexual behavior, which is entirely consistent with the isolation and solitary nature of their behavior in other domains. They are effectively asexual. Others engage in masturbation, have an extensive fantasy life, and perhaps flirt with the notion of sexual activity with another person. It seems that the findings reflect this schizoid conflict in the SHOs. On the one hand, these offenders are instrumental in terms of victim selection and the use of a weapon to facilitate their violent acts. On the other hand, they use alcohol and drugs likely as a disinhibition mechanism before perpetrating their sexual homicide and are much less likely to force the victim to perform various sexual acts or humiliate them. In other words, although 100 percent of SHOs kill their victim, only 20 percent humiliate their victim and just 12.9 percent force the victim to perform sexual acts. It is as if the SHOs find these behaviors distasteful, perhaps because they involve sexual interaction, emotional interaction, or elements of both. In contrast, murdering a victim – particularly if using a firearm – is an easier behavior, as it does not necessitate any interaction beyond physical proximity.

Third, the Borderline personality features in the SHO profile are revealed in the impulsive features (e.g., perpetrating the act after drug and alcohol intoxication), the uncontrollable and visceral emotions involved in the acts of sexual abuse and murder, and the distorted identity and self-image of an offender who preselects a victim to ultimately kill. Borderline personality disorder also potentially structures the fantasy life of the SHO, one that involves the aforementioned distortions in self-image and self-identity, poorly regulated emotions, especially anger and hostility, and dysphoria. The typification from Beauregard and DeLisi (2018) is consistent with prior research on SHOs that also included control groups (Gacono, Meloy, & Bridges, 2000). The consumption of alcohol and drugs preceding the sexual homicide likely reflects an attempt by the offender to manage these emotions in the context of premeditating a sexual homicide.

Finally, although it was not a significant predictor in the multivariate models, it is also important to note that nearly 31 percent of SHOs also presented with Antisocial Personality Disorder; thus, in addition to the contributions of Schizoid and Borderline Personality Disorders, nearly one third of SHOs also evince a life-long pattern of violations of the rights of others and the rules of society. The comorbidity of Antisocial and Borderline Personality Disorders is important given that both personality disorders have been shown to be significantly associated with aggression driven by high levels of anger and hostility (Kolla, Meyer, Bagby, & Brijmohan, 2017). For the SHOs in the current data, the preselected victim likely represents an object of hostility for the offender to sexually defile and ultimately destroy. It is revealing that the prevalence of pornography consumption among SHOs is rather low at 5.9 percent, suggesting that sexual arousal is not the driving motivation for their behaviors. However, these results seem to suggest that despite the presence of Antisocial Personality Disorder in SHOs, they do not appear to fit the image of the psychopathic offender suggested in previous studies. This discrepancy in the findings could be partly attributed to confusion associated with sexual sadism.

Psychopathy and sadism

Defining sexual sadism has been one of the more challenging obstacles, not only in understanding its key features, but also in empirically examining it (Healey, Lussier, & Beauregard, 2012). However, it seems that there exists a general consensus as to the sexual arousal of sexual sadists, whether it is (1) some form of violent or humiliating behavior (e.g., Abel, 1989; Groth & Birnbaum, 1979; Knight & Prentky, 1990; Knight, Prentky, & Cerce, 1994), (2) the victim's reaction to this behavior (e.g., being frightened, scared, or being in pain; Marshall & Kennedy, 2003), or (3) the resulting feeling of power and control as a result of the violence inflicted (Brittain, 1970; Dietz, Hazelwood, & Warren, 1990; Grubin, 1994; Levin & Fox, 1985; MacCulloch, Snowden, Wood, & Mills, 1983). Others have argued that the sexual sadist can be characterized by a deviant sexual preference for violence, which would be the product of a "synergy" or "fusion" of sexual and aggressive drives (Abel, 1989; Groth & Birnbaum, 1979; Knight et al., 1994; Knight & Prentky, 1990). However, researchers like Gratzer and Bradford (1995) suggested that violence is not a sufficient condition to elicit sexual arousal, but the "control of another person through domination, degradation, or infliction of pain for the purpose of sexual pleasure" (p. 450). According to this perspective, it is not so much the violence, but the humiliation, degradation, subjugation, and suffering producing fear, terror, pain, and panic in the victim, that makes the sadist feel powerful and sexually aroused. Finally, it seems that the various labels used to describe conceptually related phenomenon (e.g., sadomasochism) and the dissatisfaction with the clinical definition and criteria of sexual sadism are reflective of conceptual and methodological issues with the measurement of sexual sadism. More precisely, there are no valid and reliable measures of sexual sadism to assist researchers, clinicians, or police investigators.

Despite these limitations associated with sexual sadism, sadistic traits have been long paired with psychopathy (Hare, Cooke, & Hart, 1999; Holt, Meloy, & Strack, 1999; Meloy, 2000). Studies using penile plethysmography showed that scores on the PCL–R were positively correlated with sexual arousal to violent stimuli (see Barbaree, Seto, Serin, Amos, & Preston, 1994; Quinsey et al., 1995; Rice, Harris, & Quinsey, 1990; Serin et al., 1994). Using the Millon Clinical Multiaxial Inventory–II and the Personality Disorder Examination items for sadistic personality disorder, Holt et al. (1999) examined the prevalence of sadistic traits in a sample of violent offenders. Results showed that psychopaths were found to be significantly more sadistic than non-psychopaths, suggesting an association between the two concepts.

As discussed previously, Porter et al. (2003) found that psychopaths are more likely to engage in sexual homicide. Further, their study also showed that when psychopaths commit sexual homicides, they use significantly more sadistic violence. They found that both the total and Factor 1 scores on the PCL–R were positively associated with sadistic violence. In order to explain the relationship between psychopathy and sexual sadism, Porter et al. (2003) offer the following explanation:

> More to the point, in the absence of inhibitions relating to empathy or remorse and in the presence of a thrill seeking motive, the psychopath may try to optimize their pleasure and

the damage inflicted during the homicidal act. Certainly, the psychopathic offender would not be constrained by emotional inhibitory states that could limit the degree of violence perpetrated by other homicide offenders (who presumably have different pathological conditions promoting their offending).

(Porter et al., 2003, p. 467)

These findings, in combination with those of Firestone et al. (1998), suggest that there may exist a true relation between psychopathy and sadistic sexual arousal leading to sexual homicide.

Interestingly, a study by Reale, Beauregard, and Martineau (2017b) examined 350 cases of solved and unsolved sexual homicides in Canada and identified distinct groups of SHOs that could be distinguished based on varying degrees of sadistic behavior. A noteworthy finding was that three subgroups of SHOs emerged, including a severe sadistic group, a mixed group – that demonstrated sadistic behavior at the crime scene, but at a lower threshold – and a non-sadistic group. The mixed group of sexual homicide offenders demonstrated – as did the sadists – forensic awareness at the crime scene, as well as the use of torture, sexual mutilation, and the use of inanimate objects on their victims. The authors suggest that each group represents different underlying motivations. These findings, particularly for the mixed group of offenders, are well situated in the current view that psychopathic sexual homicide offenders use instrumental violence for personal gain and Thrill-seeking tendencies (see Porter et al., 2000), in comparison to other SHOs whose primary motivation may differ – e.g., acting on deviant sexual fantasies, or reacting due to situational factors such as excessive resistance).

Robertson and Knight (2014) investigated the relationship between psychopathy and sexual sadism in two related studies. Congruent with previous studies, they also found that sadism was consistently related to PCL–R total scores, but to the interpersonal and antisocial facets specifically, using different samples and methodologies. Moreover, their findings showed that sadism and the facets of psychopathy predicted the non-sexual violence measures and the sexual violence factor. The authors suggest that the psychopath's and sadist's apparent shared desire to control and dominate others to obtain a goal (e.g., Hare & Neumann, 2008) could partly explain the observed relation between psychopathy and sadism. However, it is interesting to note the authors cautioned that due to the relationships between sadism and psychopathy presenting modest effect sizes, this suggests substantial divergences between the two constructs. This was confirmed in a study by Mokros, Osterheider, Hucker, and Nitschke (2011), who, following a factorial analysis of the 11 items of the severe sexual sadism scale (Nitschke, Osterheider, & Mokros, 2009) and the 20 items of the PCL–R, found that only item 8 (callousness/lack of empathy) had a higher loading on the factor grouping the symptoms for sexual sadism.

There is, however, some controversy about the personality profile of sadistic sex offenders, with some researchers reporting them psychopathic – as seen above – and others reporting avoidant and schizoid personality traits (e.g., Brown & Forth, 1997; Proulx, 2001). In one study, Knight (2010) solved this debate by suggesting that some sadists are psychopathic while others are avoidant and schizoid. Furthermore, some studies do not support the hypothesis of the sadistic rapist being psychopathic. Barbaree et al. (1994) found that only a minority of rapists are psychopaths, as indicated by a PCL score above the clinical threshold of 30. In fact, a closer examination of Barbaree et al.'s (1994) results highlight the fact that sadistic sexual aggressors have a mean PCL–R Factor 1 (callous personality) score similar to those of the other types of rapists, but a higher mean PCL–R Factor 2 (antisocial behaviors) score than those of vindictive and sexual non-sadistic rapists. Nevertheless, it should be noted that two of the criteria used to classify a rapist as a sadist (i.e. adult and adolescence unsocialized behaviors) are identical to several items of PCL–R Factor 2 (i.e. juvenile delinquency, poor behavioral control, criminal versatility, revocation of conditional release). Consequently, the link between psychopathy and sadism is partially tautological, since the same criteria are used for both diagnostic categories.

Moreover, in Brown & Forth's study, only one sadistic rapist was diagnosed as a psychopath. Such findings are congruent with those of Proulx (2001; Proulx, Blais & Beauregard, 2006), who found that sadistic sexual aggressors had a personality profile, assessed with the MCMI, characterized by avoidant and schizoid traits (as well as dependent in Proulx & Beauregard, 2014). Furthermore, the sadistic rapists from the samples used by Proulx and colleagues had very low mean scores on the antisocial and narcissistic scales, which are considered to be correlates of psychopathy. Despite these overall findings, it seems that psychopathic offenders are more likely than other offenders to derive pleasure from both the non-sexual and sexual suffering of others (Hare et al., 1999).

Conclusion

For many years, there has been a long tradition of beliefs suggesting that sex offenders are mainly driven by an uncontrollable urge to sexually offend (e.g., Simon, 2000). However, research has shown that this assumption is not well supported by empirical evidence (e.g., Lussier, Proulx, & Leblanc, 2005). Actually, recent studies do suggest that sex offenders are much more similar to other offenders than previously thought (e.g., Harris, Smallbone, Dennisson, & Knight, 2009; Lussier et al., 2005; Lussier & Healey, 2009). Nonetheless, for the past 20 years we have witnessed the explosion of criminal justice policies dealing specifically with sexual offenders. The overarching principle of these policies is to increase community protection (Lieb, Quinsey, & Berliner, 1998; Petrunik, 2002; Petrunik, 2003), and this goal is clearly in reaction to pressure stemming from victim's rights movements and the public reaction to isolated but extreme cases reported by the media (Lafond, 2005; Simon, 1998).

We have shown that some individuals will engage in sexual crimes not because of uncontrollable urges or paraphilias but because they present a psychopathic personality. Contrary to some sex offenders who present a paraphilia or a deviant sexual arousal to children or sexual coercion, psychopathic offenders seem to engage in sexual violence to achieve a goal, and their choice of strategies is directly related to this goal. For instance, the crime switching patterns for victim type does not appear as a preference for both types of victims. Similarly, the use of extreme violence – even lethal violence – in sexual crime does not seem to be related to arousal to these actions. Instead, these strategies are geared toward their goal, whether it is for sexual gratification or Thrill-seeking purposes.

Considering that psychopathic sex offenders may have different motivations than other sex offenders for committing their crimes, it is important to take this factor into account when managing these offenders. It has been demonstrated that the presence of psychopathy and deviant sexual arousal were highly correlated with recidivism. Although treatment options for psychopathic offenders have not had the success expected thus far, the assessment of psychopathy in sexual offending is important for how these offenders should be managed and monitored. Whether in corrections or for law enforcement agencies, the fact that psychopathic sex offenders are more likely to switch their victim type, plan ahead, and use an extreme level of violence (even exhibit sexual sadism) with their victims are factors that could increase their overall dangerousness.

References

Abel, G. G. (1989) 'Paraphilias,' in H. I. Kaplan & B. J. Sadock (Eds.), *Comprehensive textbook of psychiatry* (Vol. 1, 5th ed., pp. 1069–1089), Baltimore, MD: Williams & Williams.

Abel, G. G., Becker, J. V., Mittelman, M., Cunningham-Rathner, J., Rouleau, J. L., and Murphy, W. D. (1987) 'Self-reported sex crimes of nonincarcerated paraphiliacs,' *Journal of Interpersonal Violence, 2*:3–25.

Barbaree, H. E., Seto, M. E., Serin, R. C., Amos, N. L., and Preston, D. (1994) 'Comparisons between sexual and nonsexual rapist subtypes: Sexual arousal to rape, offense precursors, and offense characteristics,' *Criminal Justice and Behavior, 21*:95–114.

Beauregard, E. (2017) 'The reasoning sex offender,' in W. Bernasco, W. Elffers, & J.-L. van Gelder (Eds.), *The Oxford handbook on offender decision making*, Oxford: Oxford University Press.

Beauregard, E., and DeLisi, M. (2018) 'Unraveling the personality profile of the sexual murderer,' *Journal of Interpersonal Violence*, in press.

Beauregard, E., and Leclerc, B. (2007) 'An application of the rational choice approach to the offending process of sex offenders: A closer look at the decision-making,' *Sexual Abuse: A Journal of Research and Treatment, 19*:115–133.

Beauregard, E., Leclerc, B., and Lussier, P. (2012) 'Decision making in the crime-commission process: Comparing rapists, child molesters, and victim-crossover sex offenders,' *Criminal Justice and Behavior, 39*:1275–1295.

Beauregard, E., and Martineau, M. (2014) 'No body, no crime? The role of forensic awareness in avoiding police detection in cases of sexual homicide,' *Journal of Criminal Justice, 42*:213–220.

Beauregard, E., and Martineau, M. (2016) 'Does the organized sexual murderer better delay and avoid detection?,' *Journal of Interpersonal Violence, 31*:4–25.

Boduszek, D., Debowska, A., and Willmott, D. (2017) 'Latent profile analysis of psychopathic traits among homicide, general violent, property, and white-collar offenders,' *Journal of Criminal Justice, 51*:17–23.

Brittain, R. (1970) 'The sadistic murderer,' *Medicine, Science and the Law, 10*:198–207.

Brown, A. R., Dargis, M. A., Mattern, A. C., Tsonis, M. A., and Newman, J. P. (2015) 'Elevated psychopathy scores among mixed sexual offenders: Replication and extension,' *Criminal Justice and Behavior, 42*:1032–1044.

Brown, S. L., and Forth, A. E. (1997) 'Psychopathy and sexual assault: Static risk factors, emotional precursors, and rapist subtypes,' *Journal of Consulting and Clinical Psychology*, 65:848–857.

Cale, J., Lussier, P., McCuish, E., and Corrado, R. (2015) 'The prevalence of psychopathic personality disturbances among incarcerated youth: Comparing serious, chronic, violent and sex offenders,' *Journal of Criminal Justice, 43*:337–344.

Cann, J., Friendship, C., and Gonza, L. (2007) 'Assessing crossover in a sample of sexual offenders with multiple victims,' *Legal and Criminological Psychology, 12*:149–163.

Chen, Y. Y., Chen, C. Y., and Hung, D. L. (2016) 'Assessment of psychiatric disorders among sex offenders: Prevalence and associations with criminal history,' *Criminal Behaviour and Mental Health, 26*(1):30–37.

Cohen, L., and Felson, M. (1979) 'Social change and crime rate trends: A routine activity approach,' *American Sociological Reviews, 44*:588–608.

Cornell, D. G., Warren, J., Hawk, G., Stafford, E., Oram, G., and Pine, D. (1996) 'Psychopathy in instrumental and reactive violent offenders,' *Journal of Consulting and Clinical Psychology, 64*:783–790.

Cornish, D. B., and Clarke, R. V. (2002) 'Analyzing organized crimes,' in A. R. Piquero & S. G. Tibbetts (Eds.), *Rational choice and criminal behaviour: Recent research and future challenges* (pp. 41–63), New York, NY: Routledge.

Corrado, R., DeLisi, M., Hart, S. D., and McCuish, E. (2015) 'Can the causal mechanisms underlying chronic, serious, and violent offending trajectories be elucidated using the psychopathy construct?,' *Journal of Criminal Justice, 43*:251–261.

Culhane, S. E., Hildebrand, M. M., Mullings, A., and Klemm, J. (2016) 'Self-reported disorders among serial homicide offenders: Data from the Millon Clinical Multiaxial Inventory–III,' *Journal of Forensic Psychology Practice, 16*(4):268–286.

Declercq, F., Willemsen, J., Audenaert, K., and Verhaeghe, P. (2012) 'Psychopathy and predatory violence in homicide, violent, and sexual offences: Factor and facet relations,' *Legal and Criminological Psychology, 17*(1):59–74.

Decuyper, M., De Pauw, S., De Fruyt, F., De Bolle, M., and De Clercq, B. J. (2009) 'A meta-analysis of psychopathy-, antisocial PD-and FFM associations,' *European Journal of Personality, 23*(7):531–565.

DeLisi, M. (2015) *Homicide*, Dubuque, IA: Kendall/Hunt.

Deslauriers-Varin, N., and Beauregard, E. (2010) 'Victims' routine activities and sex offenders' target selection scripts: A latent class analysis,' *Sexual Abuse: A Journal of Research and Treatment, 22*:315–342.

Dietz, P. E., Hazelwood, R. R., and Warren, J. (1990) 'The sexually sadistic criminal and his Offenses,' *Bulletin of the American Academy of Psychiatry and the Law, 18*:163–178.

Eronen, M., Hakola, P., and Tiihonen, J. (1996) 'Mental disorders and homicidal behavior in Finland,' *Archives of General Psychiatry, 53*(6):497–501.
Fazel, S., and Grann, M. (2004) 'Psychiatric morbidity among homicide offenders: A Swedish population study,' *American Journal of Psychiatry, 161*(11):2129–2131.
Firestone, P., Bradford, J. M., Greenberg, D. M., and Larose, M. R. (1998) 'Homicidal sex offenders: Psychological, phallometric, and diagnostic features,' *Journal of the American Academy of Psychology and Law, 26*:537–552.
Gacono, C. B., Meloy, J. R., and Bridges, M. R. (2000) 'A Rorschach comparison of psychopaths, sexual homicide perpetrators, and nonviolent pedophiles: Where angels fear to tread,' *Journal of Clinical Psychology, 56*(6):757–777.
Gebhard, P., Gagnon, J., Pomeroy, W., and Christensen, C. (1965) *Sex offenders: An analysis of types*, New York, NY: Harper and Row.
Gottfredson, M., and Hirschi, T. (1990) *A general theory of crime*, Stanford, CA: Stanford University Press.
Gratzer, T., and Bradford, J. M. W. (1995) 'Offender and offense characteristics of sexual sadists: A comparative study,' *Journal of Forensic Sciences, 40*:450–455.
Gray, J. A. (1987) 'Perspectives on anxiety and impulsivity: A commentary,' *Journal of Research in Personality, 21*:493–509.
Groth, A. N., and Birnbaum, H. J. (1979) *Men who rape: The psychology of the offender*, New York, NY: Basic Books.
Grubin, D. (1994) 'Sexual murder,' *British Journal of Psychiatry, 165*:624–629.
Guay, J.-P., Proulx, J., Cusson, M., and Ouimet, M. (2001) 'Victim-choice polymorphia among serious sex offenders,' *Archives of Sexual Behavior, 30*:521–533.
Häkkänen-Nyholm, H., Repo-Tiihonen, E., Lindberg, N., Salenius, S., and Weizmann-Henelius, G. (2009) 'Finnish sexual homicides: Offence and offender characteristics,' *Forensic Science International, 188*(1):125–130.
Hanson, R. K., and Harris, A. J. R. (2000) 'Where should we intervene? Dynamic predictors of sex offender recidivism,' *Criminal Justice and Behavior, 27*:6–35.
Hare, R. D. (1991) *The Hare Psychopathy Checklist–Revised*, Toronto, ON: Multi-Health Systems, Inc.
Hare, R. D. (1996) 'Psychopathy: A clinical construct whose time has come,' *Criminal Justice and Behavior, 23*:25–54.
Hare, R. D. (2003) *The Hare Psychopathy Checklist–Revised* (2nd ed.), Toronto, ON: Multi-Health Systems, Inc.
Hare, R. D., Clark, D., Grann, M., and Thornton, D. (2000) 'Psychopathy and the predictive validity of the PCL–R: An international perspective,' *Behavioral Science & the Law, 18*:623–645.
Hare, R. D., Cooke, D. J., and Hart, S. D. (1999) 'Psychopathy and sadistic personality disorder,' in T. Millon, P. H. Blaney, & R. D. Davis (Eds.), *Oxford textbook of psychopathology* (pp. 555–584), New York, NY: Oxford University Press.
Harris, D. A., Smallbone, S., Dennisson, S., and Knight, R. A. (2009) 'Specialization and versatility in sexual offenders referred for civil commitment,' *Journal of Criminal Justice, 37*:37–44.
Hart, S. D., and Hare, R. D. (1997) 'Psychopathy: Assessment and association with criminal conduct,' in D. M. Stoff, J. Breiling, & J. D. Maser (Eds.), *Handbook of antisocial behavior* (pp. 22–35), New York, NY: Wiley.
Hare, R. D., and Neumann, C. S. (2008) 'Psychopathy as a clinical and empirical construct,' *Annual Review of Clinical Psychology, 4*:217–246.
Hawes, S. W., Boccaccini, M. T., and Murrie, D. C. (2013) 'Psychopathy and the combination of psychopathy and sexual deviance as predictors of sexual recidivism: Meta-analytic findings using the Psychopathy Checklist–Revised,' *Psychological Assessment, 25*:233–243.
Healey, J., Lussier, P., and Beauregard, E. (2012) 'Sexual sadism in the context of rape and sexual homicide: An examination of crime scene indicators,' *International Journal of Offender Therapy and Comparative Criminology, 57*:402–424.
Heil, P., Ahlmeyer, S., and Simons, D. (2003) 'Crossover sexual offenses,' *Sexual Abuse: A Journal of Research and Treatment, 15*:221–236.
Hicks, B. M., Markon, K. E., Patrick, C. J., Krueger, R. F., and Newman, J. P. (2004) 'Identifying psychopathy subtypes on the basis of personality structure,' *Psychological Assessment, 16*:276–288.
Hildebrand, M., De Ruiter, C., and de Vogel, V. (2004) 'Psychopathy and sexual deviance in treated rapists: Association with sexual and nonsexual recidivism,' *Sexual Abuse: A Journal of Research and Treatment, 16*:1–24.

Holt, S. E., Meloy, J. R., and Stack, S. (1999) 'Sadism and psychopathy in violent and sexually violent offenders,' *Journal of the American Academy of Psychiatry and Law*, *27*:23–32.

Huss, M. T., and Langhinrichsen-Rohling, J. (2000) 'Identification of the psychopathic batterer: The clinical, legal, and policy implications,' *Aggression and Violent Behaviour*, *5*:403–422.

Jones, S. E., Miller, J. D., and Lynam, D. R. (2011) 'Personality, antisocial behavior, and aggression: A meta-analytic review,' *Journal of Criminal Justice*, *39*(4):329–337.

Kaufman, K., Mosher, H., and Carter, M., and Estes, L. (2006) 'An empirically based situational prevention model for child sexual abuse,' in R. Wortley & S. Smallbone (Eds.), *Situational prevention of child sexual abuse* (Vol. 19, pp. 101–144), *Crime Prevention Studies*, Monsey, NY: Criminal Justice Press.

Knight, R. A. (2010) 'Typologies for rapists. The generation of a new structural model,' in A. Schlank (Ed.), *The Sexual Predator* (Vol. IV, 17, pp. 1–28), New York, NY: Civic Research Institute.

Knight, R. A., and Prentky, R. A. (1990) 'Classifying sexual offenders: The development and corroboration of taxonomic models,' in W. L. Marshall, D. L. Law, & H. E. Barbaree (Eds.), *Handbook of sexual assault: Issues, theories, and treatment of the offender* (pp. 23–52), New York, NY: Plenum.

Knight, R. A., Prentky, R. A., and Cerce, D. D. (1994) 'The development, reliability, and validity of an inventory for the multidimensional assessment of sex and aggression,' *Criminal Justice and Behavior*, *21*:72–94.

Koch, J., Berner, W., Hill, A., and Briken, P. (2011) 'Sociodemographic and diagnostic characteristics of homicidal and non-homicidal sexual offenders,' *Journal of Forensic Sciences*, *56*(6):1626–1631.

Kolla, N. J., Meyer, J. H., Bagby, R. M., and Brijmohan, A. (2017) 'Trait anger, physical aggression, and violent offending in antisocial and borderline personality disorders,' *Journal of Forensic Sciences*, *62*(1):137–141.

Lafond, J. (2005) *Preventing sexual violence: How society should cope with sex offenders*, Washington, DC: American Psychological Association.

Langevin, R., Ben-Aron, M. H., Wright, P., Marchese, V., and Handy, L. (1988) 'The sex killer,' *Annals of Sex Research*, *1*:263–301.

Levin, J., and Fox, J. A. (1985) *Mass murder: America's growing menace*, New York, NY: Plenum.

Lieb, R., Quinsey, V., and Berliner, L. (1998) 'Sexual predators and social policy,' *Crime and Justice: A Review of Research*, *23*:43–114.

Lussier, P. (2005) 'The criminal activity of sexual offenders in adulthood: Revisiting the specialization debate,' *Sexual Abuse: A Journal of Research and Treatment*, *17*:269–292.

Lussier, P., and Healey, J. (2009) 'Rediscovering Quetelet, again: The 'Aging' offender and the prediction of reoffending in a sample of adult sex offenders,' *Justice Quarterly*, *26*:827–856.

Lussier, P., Leblanc, M., and Proulx, J. (2005) 'The generality of criminal behavior: A confirmatory factor analysis of the criminal activity of sex offenders in adulthood,' *Journal of Criminal Justice*, *33*:177–189.

Lussier, P., Leclerc, B., Cale, J., and Proulx, J. (2007) 'Developmental pathways of deviance in sexual aggressors,' *Criminal Justice and Behavior*, *34*:1441–1462.

Lussier, P., Leclerc, B., Healey, J., and Proulx, J. (2007) 'Generality of deviance and predation: Crime-switching and specialization patterns in persistent sexual offenders,' in M. DeLisi & P. Conis (Eds.), *Violent offenders: Theory, public policy and practice* (pp. 97–140), Boston, MA: Jones and Bartlett Publishers.

Lussier, P., Proulx, J., and Leblanc, M. (2005) 'Criminal propensity, deviant sexual interests and criminal activity of sexual aggressors against women: A comparison of explanatory models,' *Criminology*, *43*:249–281.

MacCulloch, M. J., Snowden, P. R., Wood, P. J. W., and Mills, H. E. (1983) 'Sadistic fantasy, sadistic behavior and offending,' *British Journal of Psychiatry*, *143*:20–29.

Marshall, W. L., and Kennedy, P. (2003) 'Sexual sadism in sexual offenders: An elusive diagnosis,' *Aggression and Violent Behavior*, *8*:1–22.

McCuish, E., Corrado, R., Hart, S. D., and DeLisi, M. (2015) 'The role of symptoms of psychopathy in persistent violence over the criminal career into full adulthood,' *Journal of Criminal Justice*, *43*:345–356.

Meloy, J. R. (2000) 'The nature and dynamics of sexual homicide: An integrative review,' *Aggression and Violent Behavior*, *5*:1–22.

Miethe, T. D., and Meier, R. F. (1990) 'Opportunity, choice, and criminal victimization: A test of a theoretical model,' *Journal of Research in Crime and Delinquency*, *27*:243–266.

Mokros, A., Osterheider, M., Hucker, S. J., and Nitschke, J. (2011) 'Psychopathy and sexual sadism,' *Law and Human Behavior*, *35*:188–199.

Mustaine, E. E., and Tewksbury, R. (2002) 'Sexual assault of college women: A feminist interpretation of a routine activities analysis,' *Criminal Justice Review*, *27*:89–123.

Myers, W. C., Gooch, E., and Meloy, J. R. (2005) 'The role of psychopathy and sexuality in a female serial killer,' *Journal of Forensic Sciences, 50*(3):1–6.

Myers, W. C., and Monaco, L. (2000) 'Anger experience, styles of anger expression, sadistic personality disorder and psychopathy in juvenile sexual homicide offenders,' *Journal of Forensic Sciences, 45*:698–701.

Neumann, C. S., and Hare, R. D. (2008) 'Psychopathic traits in a large community sample: Links to violence, alcohol use, and intelligence,' *Journal of Consulting and Clinical Psychology, 76*:893–899.

Nitschke, J., Osterheider, M., and Mokros, A. (2009) 'A cumulative scale of severe sexual sadism,' *Sexual Abuse: A Journal of Research and Treatment, 21*:262–278.

Olver, M. E., and Wong, S. C. (2006) 'Psychopathy, sexual deviance, and recidivism among sex offenders,' *Sexual Abuse: A Journal of Research and Treatment, 18*:65–82.

Pednault, A., Beauregard, E., Harris, D. A., and Knight, R. A. (2015) 'Rationally irrational: The case of sexual burglary,' *Sexual Abuse: A Journal of Research and Treatment, 27*:376–397.

Petrunik, M. (2002) 'Managing unacceptable risk: Sex offenders, community response, and social policy in the United Stated and Canada,' *International Journal of Offender Therapy and Comparative Criminology, 46*:483–511

Petrunik, M. (2003) 'Hare and the tortoise: Dangerousness and sex offender policy in the United States and Canada,' *Canadian Journal of Criminology and Criminal Justice, 45*:43–72.

Porter, S., Birt, A. R., and Boer, D. P. (2001) 'Investigation of the criminal and conditional release profiles of Canadian federal offenders as a function of psychopathy and age,' *Law and Human Behavior, 25*:647–661.

Porter, S., Brinke, L., and Wilson, K. (2009) 'Crime profiles and conditional release performance of psychopathic and non-psychopathic sexual offenders,' *Legal and Criminological Psychology, 14*:109–118.

Porter, S., Campbell, M. A., Woodworth, M., and Birt, A. R. (2001) 'A new psychological conceptualization of the sexual psychopath,' *Advances in Psychology Research*, 7:21–36.

Porter, S., Fairweather, D., Drugge, J., Herve, H., Birt, A., and Boer, D. P. (2000) 'Profiles of psychopathy in incarcerated sexual offenders,' *Criminal Justice and Behavior, 27*:216–233.

Porter, S., and Woodworth, M. (2006) 'Psychopathy and aggression,' in C. Patrick (Ed.), *Handbook of psychopathy* (pp. 481–494), New York, NY: Guilford.

Porter, S., and Woodworth, M. (2007) '"I'm sorry I did it . . . but he started it": A comparison of the official and self-reported homicide descriptions of psychopaths and non-psychopaths,' *Law and Human Behavior, 31*:91–107.

Porter, S., Woodworth, M., Earle, J., Drugge, J., and Boer, D. (2003) 'Characteristics of sexual homicides committed by psychopathic and non-psychopathic offenders,' *Law and Human Behavior, 27*:459–470.

Prentky, R. A., and Knight, R. A. (1991) 'Identifying critical dimensions for discriminating among rapists,' *Journal of Consulting and Clinical Psychology, 59*:643–661.

Proulx, J. (2001, November) Sexual preference and personality disorders of MTC-R-3 rapists subtypes. ATSA Annual Conference, San Antonio, Texas.

Proulx, J., and Beauregard, E. (2014) 'Pathways in the offending process of extrafamilial sexual aggressors of women,' in J. Proulx, E. Beauregard, P. Lussier, & B. Leclerc (Eds.), *Pathways to Sexual Aggression* (pp. 71–109), London: Routledge.

Proulx, J., Blais, E., and Beauregard, E. (2006) 'Sadistic sexual aggressors,' in W. L. Marshall & G. A. Seran (Eds.), *Sexual offender treatment: Controversial issues* (pp. 61–77), Chichester: Wiley.

Quinsey, V. L., Rice, M. E., and Harris, G. T. (1995) 'Actuarial prediction of sexual recidivism,' *Journal of Interpersonal Violence, 10*:85–105.

Reale, K., Beauregard, E., and Martineau, M. (2017a) 'Sadism in sexual homicide: Identifying distinct groups,' *Journal of Criminal Psychology*, 7:120–133.

Reale, K., Beauregard, E., and Martineau, M. (2017b) 'Is investigative awareness a distinctive feature of sexual sadism?,' *Journal of Interpersonal Violence*, in press.

Rice, M. E., Harris, G. T., and Quinsey, V. L. (1990) 'A follow-up of rapists assessed in a maximum-security psychiatric facility,' *Journal of Interpersonal Violence, 5*:435–448.

Robertson, C. A., and Knight, R. A. (2014) 'Relating sexual sadism and psychopathy to one another, non-sexual violence, and sexual crime behaviors,' *Aggressive Behavior, 40*:12–23.

Sauvetre, N., and Proulx, J. (2007) 'Sexual murderers and sexual aggressors: Psychopathological considerations,' in J. Proulx, E. Beauregard, M. Cusson, & A. Nicole (Eds.), *Sexual murder: A comparative analysis and new perspectives* (pp. 51–69), Winchester: Wiley.

Serin, R. C., Malcolm, P. B., Khanna, A., and Barbaree, H. E. (1994) 'Psychopathy and deviant sexual arousal in incarcerated sexual offenders,' *Journal of Interpersonal Violence, 9*:3–11.

Simon, J. (1998) 'Managing the monstrous: Sex offenders and the new penology,' *Psychology, Public Policy, and Law*, *4*:452–467.
Simon, L. M. J. (2000) 'An examination of the assumptions of specialization, mental disorder, and dangerousness in sex offenders,' *Behavioral Sciences and the Law*, *18*:275–308.
Skrovan, L. C., Huss, M. T., and Scalora, M. J. (2010) 'Sexual fantasies and sensation-seeking among psychopathic sexual offenders,' *Psychology, Crime & Law*, *16*:617–629.
Smallbone, S. W., and Wortley, R. K. (2004) 'Criminal diversity and paraphilic interests among adult males convicted of sexual offenses against children,' *International Journal of Offender Therapy and Comparative Criminology*, *48*:175–188.
Soothill, K., Francis, B., Sanderson, B., and Ackerley, E. (2000) 'Sex offenders: Specialists, generalists – or both?,' *British Journal of Criminology*, *40*:56–67.
Stephens, S., Reale, K. S., Goodwill, A. M., and Beauregard, E. (2017) 'Examining the role of opportunity is the offense behavior of victim age polymorphic sex offenders,' *Journal of Criminal Justice*, *52*:41–48.
Weinrott, M. R., and Saylor, M. (1991) 'Self-report of crimes committed by sex offenders,' *Journal of Interpersonal Violence*, *6*:286–300.
Williamson, S., Hare, R. D., and Wong, S. (1987) 'Violence: Criminal psychopaths and their victims,' *Canadian Journal of Behavioral Science*, *19*:454–462.
Woodworth, M., Freimuth, T., Hutton, E. L., Carpenter, T., Agar, A. D., and Logan, M. (2013) 'High-risk sexual offenders: An examination of sexual fantasy, sexual paraphilia, psychopathy, and offence characteristics,' *International Journal of Law and Psychiatry*, *36*:144–156.
Woodworth, M., and Porter, S. (2002) 'In cold blood: Characteristics of criminal homicides as a function of psychopathy,' *Journal of Abnormal Psychology*, *111*:436–445.

26

The psychopathic–sexually sadistic offender

Shayne Jones and Heng Choon (Oliver) Chan

Introduction

The term *sex offender* describes a heterogeneous class of offenders. To be sure, it is extremely rare that an offender engages only in sexual offending, with most sex offenders committing a wide range of non-sexual offenses (Vandiver, 2006). Still, scholars have found it useful to differentiate among sex offenders by imposing classifications that might lead to a better understanding of the onset and continuity of sexual offending. Sex offender typologies have been based on age (Chu & Thomas, 2010; Keelan & Fremouw, 2013), gender (Vandiver & Kercher, 2004), motivation (Reid, Beauregard, Fedina, & Frith, 2014), and crime scene analysis (Warren, Reboussin, Hazlewood, Cummings, Gibbs, & Trumbetta, 1998), among other factors. Another means of parsing the heterogeneity among sex offenders is to examine specific psychological factors. That will be the focus of the current chapter, which explores the roles of psychopathy and sadism in identifying a specific type of sex offender that is especially dangerous: what we call the psychopathic–sexually sadistic offender (Jones, Chan, Myers, & Heide, 2013).

The chapter begins by offering a brief review of the relationship between psychopathy and sexual offending, followed by a discussion of sexual sadism. We will then examine what is currently known about sex offenders who demonstrate elevated levels of both psychopathy and sexual sadism. We discuss some of the current explanations of the psychopathic–sexually sadistic offender, but we also denote a model that emphasizes the perceptual and emotional deficits characteristic of this type of offender. Finally, we argue that this combination of psychopathic and sadistic traits represents a particularly virulent type of sex offender who might very well become serial homicide offender.

Psychopathy and sex offending

Psychopathy is a personality disorder most often characterized as some combination of manipulative, grandiose, callous, irresponsible, impulsive, and antisocial traits. However, there is some debate about which traits are necessary and sufficient. For instance, Neumann and Hare (2006) maintain that the interpersonal, affective, lifestyle, and antisocial facets of psychopathy are all necessary. Cooke and Michie (2001) argue the first three facets are indicative of psychopathy, while the antisocial component is a consequence of the first three (see also Cooke, Michie, & Hart, 2004). Still others focus on the roles of Antagonism, emotional stability, and disinhibition (Few, Miller, & Lynam, 2013) or boldness, disinhibition, and meanness (Patrick & Drislane, 2014). There is considerable overlap among the different conceptualizations, although each offers some uniqueness as well. Tackling the complexities of which traits or facets truly constitute psychopathy is beyond the scope of this chapter. Therefore, in this section we simply describe what researchers have found about the relationship between psychopathy, however defined, and sexual offending. In most instances, however, the research surrounding psychopathy, sadism, and sexual offending has relied on the psychopathy as defined by the Psychopathy Checklist–Revised (PCL–R; Hare, 2003). The PCL–R is a forensic measure that assesses four facets of psychopathy comprised of interpersonal (e.g., manipulation and lying), affective (callousness, lack of remorse), lifestyle (impulsivity, irresponsibility), and antisocial (early behavior problems, criminal versatility) traits (Hare, 2003).

The prevalence of psychopathy among sex offenders has a wide range depending on the study. Some sex offender samples appear relatively low on psychopathy (8 percent, Olver & Wong, 2006; 9.9 percent, Serin, Malcolm, Khana, & Barbaree, 1994). Others found relatively moderate (15 percent, Seto & Barbaree, 1999) to high percentages (35 percent, Brown & Forth, 1997; 29 percent, Porter, Ten Brinke, & Wilson, 2009) of the sample being rated as psychopathic. Hare (1999) reports ranges from 10–50 percent. Prevalence rates vary, in part, because different levels of psychopathy are used to establish an individual as psychopathic. For instance, using the traditional PCL–R cut-off score of 30 or greater, Olver and Wong (2006) found 8 percent of their sample was psychopathic. When they used a cut-off score of 25 or greater, the prevalence of psychopathy was 19 percent. In addition, different types of sex offenders evince different prevalence rates of psychopathy. For instance, rapists generally have higher levels of psychopathy than child molesters (Brown & Forth, 1997; Hare, 1999; Porter et al., 2009; Serin et al., 1994; Seto & Barbaree, 1999). Thus, depending on how one operationalizes psychopathy, and the composition of the sample, prevalence rates vary.

The relationship between psychopathy and sexual offending is mixed. On the one hand, there are several studies that find a relationship between the two. Hare (2003) notes that psychopathy is related to offending in general and has somewhat weaker relationships with sexual offending specifically. Still, he reports correlations between psychopathy and convictions among sex offenders ranging from $r = .12$ to $r = .27$, with some tendency for Factor 1 to be more strongly related to convictions than Factor 2 (see also Olver & Wong, 2006; Porter et al., 2000). Psychopathy is also related to a younger age of first sexual offense (Olver & Wong, 2006). Although modest in most instances, several studies have found that psychopathy is related to the commission of a future sexual offense (Olver & Wong, 2006; Porter et al., 2000; Quinsey, Rice, & Harris, 1995). Results from a meta-analysis indicated that psychopathy was moderately related to sexual recidivism (mean $d = .29$, median $d = .25$; Hanson & Morton-Bourgon, 2005). Other research has found a relationship between psychopathy and sexual reoffending, although the results were not consistent across different methods of analysis (Gretton, McBride, Hare, O'Shaughnessy, & Kumka, 2001) or type of offender (Porter et al., 2009). Serin et al. (1994) found that psychopathy was related to deviant sexual arousal. Notably, meta-analytic results indicate that sexual deviancy is the strongest correlate of sexual recidivism (Hanson & Morton-Bourgon, 2005). Finally, Looman, Abracen, Serin, and Marquis (2005) found psychopathy was related to higher recidivism rates, but their outcome measure included both violent and sexual offenses.

On the other hand, several studies have failed to find a relationship between psychopathy and sexual offending. Psychopathy was not found to be related to the number of prior sexual offenses (Brown & Forth, 1997; Olver & Wong, 2006), charges, or convictions (Olver & Wong, 2006). Neither was it related to the age of onset for sexual offenses. In contrast to the meta-analysis noted in the preceding paragraph, several studies have failed to find a relationship between psychopathy and sexual recidivism (Edens, Campbell, & Weir, 2006; Gretton et al., 2001; Gretton, Hare, & Catchpole, 2004; Langton, Barbaree, Harkins, & Peacock, 2006; Porter et al., 2009; Olver & Wong, 2006). There are some caveats that need to be noted regarding the null findings. First and foremost, across studies there are very low base rates of sexual offending and recidivism. For instance, about 21 percent of sex offenders received a new charge or conviction for a sexual offense in one study (Olver & Wong, 2006). In another study (Langton et al., 2006), only 11 percent reoffended sexually. In yet another analysis (of adolescent sex offenders: Gretton et al., 2004), there were no differences among those scoring low, moderate, and high on the Psychopathy Checklist: Youth Version (PCL: YV; Forth, Kosson, & Hare, 2003). However, the percentages for sexual reoffending for each group were 7 percent, 9 percent, and 21 percent, respectively (Gretton et al., 2004). Thus, the high psychopathy group was three times more likely, and the moderate group more than twice as likely, to sexually reoffend. Therefore, there might very well be notable relationships between psychopathy and sexual offending that are masked by low power to detect effects.

The relationship between psychopathy and sexual offending might also be contingent upon other factors. As mentioned above, the prevalence of psychopathy among sex offenders is different depending on the type of offender. Rapists (Seto & Barbaree, 1999; Serin et al., 1994) and mixed types (rapists and child molesters; Olver & Wong, 2006; Quinsey et al., 1995) evince higher levels of psychopathy than other types of sex offenders (e.g., child molester only, incest victims). Porter et al. (2000) noted a slightly different pattern, with the mixed type (rapists and child molesters) being more psychopathic than rapists, non-sexual offenders, and child molesters. Using a variant of the Revised Rapist Typology 3 (Massachusetts Treatment Center: Rapist Typology 3, Knight & Prentky, 1990), Brown and Forth (1997) found that psychopathic rapists were more likely to be classified as opportunistic and pervasively angry rapists compared to non-psychopaths, while non-psychopaths were more likely to be classified as sexually sadistic, sexually non-sadistic, and vindictive rapists. In fact, none of the (6) vindictive rapists and only 1 (of 6) of the sexually sadistic rapists were psychopaths.

In addition to different types of offenders, the relationship between psychopathy and sexual offending appears to be conditioned on other factors. For instance, Hare (1999) suggested that psychopathy coupled with deviant sexual fantasies is a deadly combination. Previous research has revealed that higher psychopathy scores combined with sexual deviance is related to higher and quicker recidivism rates (Harris et al., Rice, Quinsey, Lalumière, Boer, & Lang2003; Olver & Wong, 2006; Serin, Mailloux, & Malcolm, 2001). Olver and Wong (2009) found that sex offenders with elevated scores on psychopathy (i.e., the PCL–R) and Violence Risk Scale–Sexual Offender version (Wong, Olver, Nicholaichuk, & Gordon, 2003) were the most likely to recidivate. This was true of violent crimes as well as sexual crimes.

Lastly, it is worth briefly discussing treatment issues surrounding psychopathy and sexual offender samples. Psychopathic sex offenders are more likely to drop out of treatment (Olver & Wong, 2009; Seto & Barbaree, 1999). But Olver and Wong (2009) also note that most (approximately 75 percent) of the psychopathic sex offenders in their sample did complete treatment. There is widespread pessimism about the amenability to treatment of psychopathic individuals generally (Rice, Harris, & Cormier, 1992; Salekin, 2002; Skeem, Monahan, & Mulvey, 2002). Yet, at least some researchers working with sex offenders who have high levels of psychopathy note that treatment can be somewhat effective even among this group of ostensibly recalcitrant offenders (Looman, Abracen, Serin, & Marquis, 2005; Olver & Wong, 2009).

In this section, we have briefly reviewed what is known about psychopathy and sexual offending. To summarize, a minority of sex offenders are psychopathic, but this varies depending on what type of sex offender is under examination. Although the literature is mixed, there is sufficient evidence to indicate that psychopathy is related to sexual offending to some degree. When psychopathy is coupled with sexual deviance, the relationship is stronger. Although limited, there is some evidence of successful treatment among sex offenders with elevated levels of psychopathy. Although informative, it is clear that much more research is needed to better understand the relationship between psychopathy and sexual offending.

Sadism and sex offending

Although the term *sadism* was first appeared in Boiste's 1835 *Dictionnaire Universel* (Coward, 1992:xxi), it was not until Kraff-Ebing's well-known monograph (1886/1965) that this personality trait was introduced at length, where he classified sexually sadistic homicide as *lust–murder.* MacCulloch and colleagues (1983) subsequently elaborated and defined sadism as

> the repeated practice of behavior and fantasy which is characterized by a wish to control another person by domination, denigration, or inflicting pain, for the purpose of producing mental pleasure, and sexual arousal (whether or not accompanied by orgasm) in the sadist.
> *(MacCulloch et al., 1983, p. 20)*

From a clinical perspective, sexual sadism disorder is diagnostically referred to as the "recurrent and intense sexual arousal from the physical or psychological suffering of another person, as manifested by fantasies, urges, or behaviors" for over a period of at least six months (American Psychiatric Association, 2013:605). The International Statistical Classification of Diseases and Related Health Problems (ICD–10), produced by the World Health Organization (2004) on the other hand, describes the disorder of sadomasochism as sexual preference for activities involving humiliation, pain, and bondage. Simply put, sexual sadism is regarded as a type of paraphilia that often involves cognitions and behaviors that are associated with achieving sexual excitement through infliction of physical and/or emotional pain (Robertson & Knight, 2014).

Consequent to the subjective defining and diagnostic criteria of sexual sadism, disagreement continues as to accurately evaluate this disorder (Jones et al., 2013; Robertson & Knight, 2014), especially with regards to the motives that drive sexual sadists (see Marshall & Kennedy, 2003 for a review). Some argue that the sexual excitement through physical suffering is the primary motive (e.g., Kirsch & Becker, 2007; Porter, Woodworth, Earle, Drugge, & Boer, 2003), while others assert that domination or control over another individual is key to the definition (e.g., Grubin, 1994; Johnson & Becker, 1997). In view of the lack of consensus on the measure of sexual sadism, its measurement continues to suffer despite years of empirical efforts (e.g., Doren & Elwood, 2009; Marshall & Hucker, 2006a).

Although some researchers have relied on the use of phallometric assessments to measure sexual interests, these studies nonetheless suffered from a general lack of consistency in distinguishing sexually sadistic offenders from non-sexually sadistic offenders based on their sexual arousal to non-sexual violence (e.g., Proulx, Aubut, McKibben, & Cote, 1994; Seto & Kuban, 1996). These inconsistent findings may be largely due to not all research using equally valid phallometric protocols and the use of widely claimed poor DSM diagnostic criterion to guide their research (Healey, Lussier, & Beauregard, 2013). Consequently, a number of sexual sadism measures have been developed over the years with the use of a more objective dimensional approach to identify key behavioral features of sexual sadists (e.g., Jones et al., 2013; Marshall &

Hucker, 2006a, 2006b; Nitschke, Osterheider, & Mokros, 2009). These behavioral measures of sexual sadism include, but are not limited to, Proulx and colleagues' two-category criteria of sexual sadism (Proulx, Blais, & Beauregard, 2007), Marshall and Hucker's (2006b) 17-item severe sexual sadism scale, Nitschke and colleagues' 11-item severe sexual sadism scale (Nitschke et al., 2009), Jones and colleagues' (2013) 10-item Sexual Homicide Crime Scene Rating Scale for Sexual Sadism (SADSEX–SH) scale, and Myers and colleagues' (2013) 8-item Revised Sexual Homicide Crime Scene Rating Scale for Sexual Sadism (SADSEX–SH–R) scale. In fact, recent research found that the offender's behavioral indicators may prove to be better in providing law enforcement agents and mental health professionals with a more accurate measure of sexually sadistic offenders. For instance, Healey and colleagues (2013) found that a number of crime scene behaviors (e.g., humiliation, mutilation, premeditation, and the use of physical restraint) overlapped with the official diagnostic criteria of sexual sadism and were able to differentiate sexual aggressors against females from sexual murderers.

Paraphilias are commonly diagnosed among sexual offenders, with prevalence varying from 58 percent to 98 percent (Jackson & Richards, 2007; McElroy et al., 1999). Besides pedophilia, sexual sadism is considered the most prevalent paraphilia identified in the sexual offender population (Chan & Heide, 2009, 2016). In a nationwide study of 807 incarcerated sexual offenders from Austria, Eher and colleagues (2010) found an overall rate of 6 percent in the sample met the DSM–IV–TR diagnostic requirement of sexual sadism. This finding mirrored the prevalence rate of 6 percent of a DSM–IV–TR diagnosis of sadism found among 680 male sexual offenders detained under civil commitment legislation (i.e., Sexually Violent Predator laws) in three American states (Elwood, Doren, & Thornton, 2010). Using the latest DSM–5 diagnostic criteria, Wilson and colleagues (2011) noted a sexual sadism incidence rate of 2.4 percent among 296 civilly committed male sexual offenders under the Sexually Violent Predator (SVP) legislation. In addition to the high prevalence rate among sexual offenders who did not kill, sexual sadism is also noted as the most frequently reported paraphilia in sexual murderers (Chan & Heide, 2016), with prevalence rates varying from 37 percent to as high as 89 percent (e.g., Chan & Beauregard, 2016; Chan, Beauregard, & Myers, 2015; Briken, Hill, Habermann, Kafka, & Berner, 2010;Firestone, Bradford, Greenberg, Larose, & Curry, 1998; Hill, Habermann, Berner, & Briken, 2007; Langevin, 2003; Myers, Chan, Vo, & Lazarou, 2010; Stone, 2001).

Risk of reoffending is high among sexual offenders who are sadists. Myers and colleagues (2010) found that all three juvenile sexual murderers who met full diagnostic criteria for sexual sadism committed additional homicidal acts after their first sexual murder. Kingston and colleagues (2010), on the other hand, found that behavioral indicators of sexual sadism (e.g., phallometrically measured sexual response, sexual intrusiveness, and level of violence), but not a clinical diagnosis, significantly predicted both sexual and violent recidivism. In addition, the behavioral indicators of sexual sadism added incrementally to the prediction of violent reoffending, but not sexual reoffending, when controlling for risk. However, based on the meta-analysis of seven samples of male sex offenders (N = 2,169) conducted by Eher and colleagues (2016), sexual sadism did not significantly increase the risk of violent and sexual reoffending to a clinically meaningful degree. Nevertheless, studies that were based on clinically diagnosed sexual sadism were found to indicate a small but significant association between sexual sadism and violent and sexual recidivism. Rather than a distinct phenomenological entity, sexual sadism is arguably regarded as an extreme on a continuum of sexual aggression (Knight, Sims-Knight, & Guay, 2013; Mokros, Schilling, Weiss, Nitschke, & Eher, 2014).

In summary, although widely researched, the notion of sexual sadism suffers from a lack of consistent operationalizations. This, in turn, has hampered the research surrounding sexual sadism. Nonetheless, several researchers have attempted to provide better operationalizations/

measures, which might yield more consistent findings in the future. Measurement issues aside, there is evidence that sexual sadism is an important factor in understanding sexual offending, as well as sexual recidivism.

The psychopathic–sexually sadistic offender

Psychopathy and sexual sadism do not exist in isolation, which is to say that having one or the other does not preclude other mental health issues. Instead, psychopathy and sexual sadism exist within a larger nomological network of mental health. For instance, psychopathic individuals might also be diagnosed with other personality disorders, substance use disorder, and various other psychiatric disorders (Dahl, 1998). In addition, it is common for sexual sadists to evince other paraphilias, such as voyeurism, fetishism, tranvestism, and exhibitionism (Chan & Beauregard, 2016; Langevin, 2003). Thus, it is possible for psychopathy and sexual sadism to co-exist. To be clear, not all individuals with higher levels of psychopathy are sexually sadistic. Likewise, not all sexually sadistic persons are psychopathic. But when psychopathy and sexual sadism co-occur, it can be a very dangerous amalgam. We refer to this as the psychopathic–sexually sadistic offender. Although there are several studies on sexual sadism, less research exists surrounding the psychopathic–sexually sadistic offender. However, there is a limited amount of research on the topic, which we review here. Some of the work on this topic focused on the links between psychopathy and sadism generally, or sadistic personality disorder specifically. Before reviewing the empirical relationships between psychopathy and sexual sadism, we discuss clinical and theoretical accounts linking these two disorders.

Some of the evidence suggesting a link between psychopathy and sadism comes from the clinical descriptions. Murphy and Vess (2003:12) suggest that there are distinct subtypes of psychopathy dependent on the prevailing features displayed. The basis for these subtypes was their clinical observations of individuals in a maximum security forensic hospital. They suggested four subtypes: the narcissistic, borderline, sadistic, and antisocial psychopaths. They describe them as follows:

> The entitled, superior, self-absorbed and belittling narcissistic psychopath, the needy, labile, and impulsive borderline psychopath, the deliberately cruel, sadistic psychopath who is attuned to the suffering of others, and the remorseless criminal psychopath who is not, are all variations of psychopathy observed among forensic patients.
>
> *(Murphy & Vess, 2003, p. 12)*

Of particular interest in this chapter is their sadistic psychopath. They also note this type is similar to the malevolent psychopath. As described by Millon and Davis (1998:168, emphasis added), "The primary characteristics of these individuals blend with those of the *sadistic* and paranoid personality (or both), reflecting not only a deep sense of deprivation and a desire for compensatory retribution, but also an intense suspiciousness and hostility." They further describe them as cold-blooded, and although capable of cognitively understanding guilt and remorse, they cannot emotionally experience them. Murphy and Vess (2003:22) further suggest that the sadistic psychopath is distinguished from the other typologies by noting such individuals have "the apparent capacity to recognize the suffering of others, and the corresponding pleasure or arousal derived by the sadistic psychopath." Thus, others have noted the importance of sadism in delineating a specific variant of psychopathy. One of the key factors that differentiates the sadistic/malevolent psychopath is their pronounced callousness and lack of empathy.

Although somewhat limited, there are other empirical accounts that have been offered to identify the psychopathic–sexually sadistic sex offender. Malamuth (2003) developed the two-factor confluence model based on several empirical accounts of his work (Malamuth, 1986; Malamuth, Sockloski, Koss, & Tanaka, 1991; Malamuth, Linz, Heavey, Barnes, & Acker, 1995). The first factor is hostile masculinity and involves negative views and attitudes toward women. Men high on this will have antagonistic interactions with women, such as being coercive (including coercion of a sexual nature), domineering, and angry. It might also be thought of as misogyny. The second factor is impersonal sexual relations. This includes the desire to have many sexual partners and treat sexual relations as conquests. It is noteworthy that some of these traits/behaviors are either directly relevant to the construct of psychopathy (i.e., promiscuous sexual behavior) or act as precursors the hostile masculinity and impersonal sex (e.g., impulsivity, poor behavioral controls, callousness; juvenile delinquency; Abbey, Jacques-Tiura, & LeBreton, 2011; Mokros, Osterheider, Hucker, & Nitschke, 2011). Additional empirical work by Malamuth also indicates the importance of lack of empathy – an item from the PCL–R loading on the affective facet (Dean & Malamuth, 1997). The lack of empathy is important in that it might distinguish merely imagining engagement in sexual aggression to actual acts of sexual aggression. In other words, it is the lack of empathy that allows the individual to move from fantasy to reality in their sexual aggression. The confluence model has received a fair amount of empirical support (Mokros et al., 2011; Abbey et al., 2011).

Knight (1993) also found evidence supportive of the confluence model. Yet, he also noted this model did not account for much variance in sexually coercive behavior. In an attempt to better explain sexual aggression, Knight and Guay (2006) modified the confluence model. Specifically, they suggested that hostile masculinity be combined with other indicators (including lack of empathy) to form a latent construct of emotional detachment. They used the sexual promiscuity component as indicators of sexual Fantasy, which, in turn, leads to the latent factor of aggressive sexual fantasy. Aggressive sexual fantasy is premised on the indicators of aggressive fantasies toward women and, of particular interest in this chapter, sadism. In essence, this three-path model suggests that both factors of psychopathy combine with sexual sadism to produce sexual aggression. They note this model better fit the data and accounted for more variance in sexual aggression.

Although the confluence model (Malamuth, 2003) and the revised three-path model (Knight & Guay, 2006) are empirically supported, we believe there is an additional conceptual issue that should be considered (Jones et al., 2013). There appear to be countervailing forces at play in these models. On the one hand, psychopathic individuals are callous, unemotional, and lack empathy. These affective deficits make it easier for an offender to perpetrate sexual crimes, as he is not bothered by the idea of hurting and humiliating his victim. On the other hand, the sexual sadist derives pleasure from hurting and humiliating his victim. The psychopathic–sexually sadistic offender, then, is someone who takes pleasure in denigrating and harming his victim, and even needs to in order to be sexually satisfied, but who also has greater difficulty in achieving this due to his affective deficits.

There is meta-analytic evidence indicating that antisocial individuals (including psychopaths) have deficits in recognizing facial affect, most notably fear (Marsh & Blair, 2008). Much of this deficit lies in dysfunction of the amygdala, although several other brain regions have also been implicated (Marsh, 2015). For a sexual sadist to be sexually satisfied, it seems logical that he would need to see some expression of fear in his victim. Because of the facial recognition deficits and associated affective deficits (e.g., callousness), the psychopathic–sexually sadistic offender must employ more violence to achieve satisfaction.

We believe this suggests an interaction between psychopathy and sadism. More specifically, an individual who is low in psychopathy but is sexually sadistic does not have to engage in as much violence to achieve the goals of hurting and humiliating his victim. Such an individual is not as callous, unemotional, and lacking in empathy. He might also be able to better perceive fear in his victim during an assault. Conversely, a sexual sadist with high levels of psychopathy must enact more violence to achieve sexual satisfaction. Therefore, this type of sexual offender might be particularly dangerous, engaging in not only more sexual aggression but more violence during the offense. In the following section, we use this supposition as a basis for identifying a type of sexual homicide offender.

Although not explicitly designed to test these various models of the psychopathic–sexually sadistic offender, there are empirical accounts that provide support for the link between psychopathy and sexual sadism. Hart, Forth, and Hare (1991) found that PCL–R defined psychopathy was positively related to aggressive/sadistic scale (Scale 6B) on the Millon Clinical Multiaxial Inventory (MCMI–II; Millon, 1987), which assesses sadistic personality disorder. It is important to note that this personality disorder was dropped from the latest versions of the Diagnostic and Statistical Manual of Mental Disorders, although it remains a topic of study among researchers (Chabrol, van Leeuwen, Rodgers, & Séjourné, 2009). Moreover, they noted scores on Scale 6B were more strongly related to Factor 2 of the PCL–R than Factor 1. Interestingly, despite the typically stronger association between PCL–R Factor 2 and Antisocial Personality Disorder (Hare, 2003), Antisocial Personality Disorder was not related to Scale 6B. This seems to suggest the psychopathy, as defined by the PCL–R, is more strongly related to sadism than Antisocial Personality Disorder.

Holt, Meloy, and Strack (1999) found similar results when exploring the relationship between psychopathy and sadism. In their sample from a maximum security prison in the U.S (n = 41), PCL–R scores were positively related to MCMI–II Scale 6B. This was true for the total PCL–R scores as well as both Factors 1 and 2. The same pattern of results was observed between the PCL–R (and Factors 1 and 2) and sadistic personality disorder, as measured by the Personality Disorder Examination (Loranger, 1988).

Using a French high school sample, Chabrol et al. (2009) found a positive relationship between self-reported psychopathic, narcissistic, Machiavellian, and sadistic personality traits. Still, they noted that these traits are independent of one another. The strongest associations were between psychopathy (as measured by the Youth Psychopathic Inventory; Andershed, Kerr, Stattin, & Levander, 2002) and sadism (based on the Hurting Scale; O'Meara, Davies, & Barnes-Holmes, 2004) for both boys (r = .38) and girls (r = .23). Interestingly, boys' psychopathic and sadistic traits were related to delinquency in multivariate models but were not significant predictors among girls. Psychopathy, narcissism, and Machiavellian represent what some have referred to as the Dark Triad (Paulhus & Williams, 2002). Chabrol et al. suggest adding sadism to this list of traits, as it was related to all the Dark Triad traits and helped explain delinquency (at least among boys). They called this the new compilation of traits the Dark Tetrad.

However, not all research has supported a relationship between psychopathy and sadism. Reidy, Zeichner, and Seibert (2011) measured psychopathy using standardized scores from the Levenson Self-Report Psychopathy Scale (LSRP; Levenson, Kiehl, & Fitzpatrick, 1995) and the Self-Report Scale (SRP–III; Paulhus, Neumann, & Hare, in press). To measure sadism, they used reaction times to positive (i.e., happy) words following violent imagery. Those who responded more quickly were deemed as more sadistic. All of their participants (n = 137) were college men. They failed to find a relationship between psychopathy and sadism. They did, however, find that Factor 1 scores, and to a lesser extent Factor 2 scores, were related to perceiving less pain and distress of a confederate who was administered an electric shock. This finding suggests those who were more psychopathic did not feel they did as much harm to the confederate. Finally, Factor 1 scores and sadism independently predicted the probability of administering an unprovoked shock.

Other studies have focused specifically on the relationship between psychopathy and sexual sadism. As noted above, Holt et al. (1999) found evidence that psychopathy was related to sadism/sadistic personality disorder. However, PCL–R scores were unrelated to a DSM-defined diagnosis of Sadistic Personality Disorder (when this disorder was still listed in the DSM). However, there were only three participants in the sample that met criteria for this disorder, and that likely made it difficult to detect any relationship. Similarly, Brown and Forth (1997) found that the sadistic rapists in their sample (n = 7) did not differ on psychopathy, although three times as many were non-psychopathic (PCL–R scores ≤ 29) compared to psychopathic (PCL–R scores ≥ 30). However, Kirsch and Becker (2007) cite research presented at a conference (Kirsch, Becker, Fanniff, & Martens, 2006) in which 90 percent of sexual sadists had PCL–R scores greater than or equal to 25.

Using a forensic sample in which half (of 100 participants) were diagnosed with sexual sadism, Mokros, Osterheider, Hucker, and Nitschke (2011) found (PCL–R) psychopathy was related to sexual sadism. Specifically, facets 2 (affective) and 4 (antisocial) were related to sexual sadism, with the affective facet bearing the strongest relationship. Neither facet 1 (interpersonal) nor 3 (lifestyle) was related to sadism. The factor analysis performed in this study also indicated that psychopathy and sexual sadism (measured by the severe sexual sadism scale; Nitschke, Osterheider, & Mokros, 2009) were related but distinct constructs. One item from the PCL–R, Callous/Lack of Empathy (Item 8), loaded more strongly on the severe sexual sadism scale than the PCL–R, suggesting that this aspect of psychopathy might be particularly important in understanding the relationship between psychopathy and sexual sadism (see also Kirsch & Becker, 2007).

A few points need to be made before moving forward. First, it might seem trite to suggest a link between psychopathy and sadism. After all, psychopathic offenders engage in more violence and aggression than non-psychopathic offenders (Porter & Woodworth, 2006), and much of the violence they do engage in is more severe and gratuitous (Porter, Woodworth, Earle, Drugge, & Boer, 2003). However, the concept of sadism is only explicitly mentioned in one item from the PCL–R (Item 8: callous/lack of empathy). Second, as the above review suggests, most research indicates that the two constructs are related but distinct. Third, not all of the evidence supports a link between psychopathy and sexual sadism. Some of the conflicting findings might be explained by small sample sizes, different psychopathy factors being assessed, or conceptualizations of sexual sadism. Lastly, there are too few empirical accounts to offer a more definitive answer regarding how psychopathy and sexual sadism are associated. Clearly much more research is needed to better understand the extent to which psychopathy is related to sexual sadism. Still, there are compelling reasons to believe that such a relationship exists. Perhaps Meloy stated it best:

> The psychopath and the sexual sadist share a desire to control and dominate their objects, a chronic emotional detachment that dehumanizes their objects, an aggressive narcissism that makes them feel entitled to do what they want to their objects, and a mendacity that both delights them and facilitates the abduction of their victims.
>
> *(Meloy, 1997, p. 632)*

Psychopathy, sadism, and sexual homicide

As noted above, there is limited empirical work linking psychopathy and sadism generally and psychopathy and sexual sadism specifically. Moreover, both psychopathy (Hare, 2003) and sexual sadism (Wilson, Pake, & Duffee, 2011) are relatively infrequent in the population. Nonetheless, when these two disorders co-exist, we argue it represents a serious threat to public safety. In particular, we believe the combination of psychopathy with sexual sadism has a reasonably good chance of escalating to sexual homicide.

It is important to note that most sexual homicide offenders (SHOs) are not psychopathic (Porter et al., 2000). However, many SHOs likely possess some (if not several) psychopathic traits. SHOs with elevated psychopathic traits have been referred to as sexual psychopaths (Porter, Campbell, Woodworth, & Birt, 2002). Various scholars have found that SHOs score higher on the PCL–R, including Factors 1 and 2, than non-SHOs (Beauregard, Proulx, & St-Yves, 2007; Hakkanen-Nyholm, Repo-Tiihonen, Lindberg, Salenius, & Weizmann-Henelius, 2009; Myers et al., 2010). Moreover, psychopathic SHOs are more likely to plan their offenses (Chan, in press), engage in more gratuitous and sadistic violence (Porter et al., 2003), and recidivate at higher rates (Hill, Habermann, Klussman, Berner, & Briken, 2008). Moreover, psychopathic SHOs are more likely to engage in subsequent sex crimes (Myers et al., 2010), which is exacerbated when coupled with deviant sexual arousal (Chan, 2015).

Similar evidence exists linking SHO and sexual sadism. Not all SHOs are sexual sadists (Chan, 2017), but the course of this syndrome might easily progress to sexual homicide. Sexual sadists often begin to entertain their sexual desires with violent pornography, and the same is true for sadistic SHOs (Chan, 2015). Once habituated to this, however, such individuals might then turn to acting upon their fantasies with other individuals (Jones et al., 2013; Palermo, 1994). Sexual sadists might engage in sadistic acts with willing partners, at least in the beginning (Hazelwood, Warren, & Dietz, 1993). Of course, as the violence escalates a willing partner might not be available, leading the sexual sadist to seek out others. This escalation in violence might also lead to homicide (Jones et al., 2013).

As Kirsch and Becker (2007) suggest, psychopathic sex offenders are likely unaffected by the distress of their victims. The psychopath who is also sexually sadistic, however, perceives the pain and suffering of his victim as pleasurable. Moreover, research indicates that psychopathic individuals have difficulty perceiving fear and sadness (Marsh & Blair, 2008). A victim of a brutal sexual attack is likely to display fear. And this is what makes the psychopathic–sexually sadistic offender so dangerous. The level of violence necessary to produce sexual arousal among such offenders will have to be extremely high. This, in turn, increases the probability of the victim being killed due to the extreme violence.

Conclusion

In this chapter, we have attempted to identify a specific type of sex offender based on the prevailing traits of the offender. Specifically, we focused on those sex offenders with high levels of psychopathic traits and who are sexually sadistic. We noted that both psychopathy and sexual sadism, uniquely, are related to sexual offending. However, the sex offender who is comorbid for psychopathy and sexual sadism represents a potentially very dangerous type of offender. This is supported by both theoretical and empirical accounts. We refer to this type as the psychopathic–sexually sadistic offender and suggest the interaction between these disorders will lead to more sexual offending, more violence sexual offenses, and even sexual homicides. Although this type of offender is likely rare, given the potential harm they pose to public safety it is important for continued efforts to better understand them.

References

Abbey, A., Jacques-Tiura, A. J., and LeBreton, J. M. (2011) 'Risk factors for sexual aggression in young men: An expansion of the confluence model,' *Aggressive Behavior*, *37*:450–464.

American Psychiatric Association. (2013) *Diagnostic and statistical manual of mental disorders* (5th ed.), Washington, DC: Author.

Andershed, H., Kerr, M., Stattin, H., and Levander, S. (2002) 'Psychopathic traits in non-referred youths: Initial test of a new assessment tool,' in E. Blaauw & L. Sheridan (Eds.), *Psychopaths: Current international perspectives* (pp. 131–158), The Hague: Elsevier.

Beauregard, E., Proulx, J., and St-Yves, M. (2007) 'Angry or sadistic: Two types of sexual murderers,' in J. Proulx, E. Beauregard, M. Cusson, & A. Nicole (Eds.), *Sexual murderers: A comparative analysis and new perspectives* (pp. 123–141), Hoboken, NJ: Wiley.

Briken, P., Hill, A., Habermann, N., Kafka, M. P., and Berner, W. (2010) 'Paraphilia-related disorders and personality disorders in sexual homicide perpetrators,' *Sexual Offender Treatment*, *5*:1–7.

Brown, S. L., and Forth, A. E. (1997) 'Psychopathy and sexual assault: Static risk factors, emotional precursors, and rapist subtypes,' *Journal of Clinical and Consulting Psychology*, *65*:848–857.

Chabrol, H., van Leeuwen, N., Rodgers, R., and Séjourné, N. (2009) 'Contributions to psychopathic, narcissistic, Machiavellian, and sadistic personality traits to juvenile psychopathy,' *Personality and Individual Differences*, *47*:734–739.

Chan, H. C. O. (in press) 'Sexual sadism and psychopathy in sexual homicide,' in A. Felthous & H. Sass (Eds.), *The Wiley international handbook of psychopathic disorders and the law* (2nd ed.), Hoboken, NJ: John Wiley & Sons.

Chan, H. C. O. (2017) 'Sexual homicide: A review of recent empirical evidence (2008 to 2015),' in F. Brookman, E. R. Maguire, & M. Maguire (Eds.), *The handbook of homicide* (pp. 105–130), Hoboken, NJ: John Wiley & Sons.

Chan, H. C. O. (2015) *Understanding sexual homicide offenders: An integrated approach*, Basingstoke: Palgrave Macmillan.

Chan, H. C. O., and Beauregard, E. (2016) 'Nonhomicidal and homicidal sexual offenders: Prevalence of maladaptive personality traits and paraphilic behaviors,' *Journal of Interpersonal Violence*, *31*(13):2259–2290.

Chan, H. C. O., and Heide, K. M. (2009) 'Sexual homicide: A synthesis of the literature,' *Trauma, Violence, and Abuse*, *10*(1):31–54.

Chan, H. C. O., and Heide, K. M. (2016) 'Sexual homicide offenders distinguished from non homicidal sexual offenders: A review of the literature,' *Aggression and Violent Behavior*, *31*:147–156.

Chan, H. C. O., Beauregard, E., and Myers, W. C. (2015) 'Single-victim and serial sexual homicide offenders: Differences in crime, paraphilias, and personality traits,' *Criminal Behaviour and Mental Health*, *25*(1):66–78.

Chu, C. M., and Thomas, S. D. M. (2010) 'Adolescent sexual offenders: The relationship between typology and recidivism,' *Sexual Abuse: A Journal of Research and Treatment*, *22*:218–233.

Cooke, D. J., and Michie, C. (2001) 'Refining the construct of psychopathy: Towards a hierarchical model,' *Psychological Assessment*, *13*(2):171–188.

Cooke, D. J., Michie, C., Hart, S. D., and Clark, D. A. (2004) 'Reconstructing psychopathy: Clarifying the significance of antisocial and socially deviant behavior in the diagnosis of psychopathic personality disorder,' *Journal of Personality Disorders*, *18*:337–357.

Coward, D. (1992) *The Marquis de Sade: The misfortunes of virtue* (Trans., with an Introduction), New York, NY: Oxford University Press.

Dahl, A. A. (1998) 'Psychopathy and psychiatric comorbidity,' in T. Millon, E. Simonsen, M. Birket-Smith, & R. D. Davis (Eds.), *Psychopathy: Antisocial, criminal, and violent behavior* (pp. 291–303), New York, NY: The Guilford Press.

Dean, K. E., and Malamuth, N. M. (1997) 'Characteristics of men who aggress sexually and of men who imagine aggressing: Risk and moderating variables,' *Journal of Personality and Social Psychology*, *72*:449–455.

Doren, D., and Elwood, R. (2009) 'The diagnostic reliability of sexual sadism,' *Sexual Abuse: A Journal of Research and Treatment*, *21*(3):251–261.

Edens, J. F., Campbell, J. S., and Weir, J. M. (2006) 'Youth psychopathy and criminal recidivism: A meta-analysis of the psychopathy checklist measures,' *Law and Human Behavior*, *31*:53–75.

Eher, R., Rettenberger, M., and Schilling, F. (2010) 'Psychiatrische Diagnosen von Sexualstraftätern: Eine empirische Untersuchung von 807 inhaftierten Kindesmissbrauchstätern und Vergewaltigern [Psychiatric diagnoses of sexual offenders: An empirical study of 807 incarcerated child abuse offenders and rapists],' *Zeitschrift für Sexualforschung*, *23*:23–35.

Eher, R., Schilling, F., Hansmann, B., Pumberger, T., Nitschke, J., Habermeyer, E., and Mokros, A. (2016) 'Sadism and violent reoffending in sexual offenders,' *Sexual Abuse: A Journal of Research and Treatment*, *28*(1):46–72.

Elwood, R. W., Doren, D. M., and Thornton, D. (2010) 'Diagnostic and risk profiles of men detained under Wisconsin's sexually violent predator law,' *International Journal of Offender Therapy and Comparative Criminology*, *54*:187–196.
Few, L. R., Miller, J. D., and Lynam, D. R. (2013) 'An examination of the factor structure of the Elemental Psychopathy Assessment,' *Personality Disorders*, *4*:247–253.
Firestone, P., Bradford, J. M., Greenberg, D. M., Larose, M. R., and Curry, S. (1998) 'Homicidal and non-homicidal child molesters: Psychological, phallometric, and criminal features,' *Sexual Abuse: A Journal of Research and Treatment*, *10*(4):305–323.
Forth, A. E., Kosson, D., and Hare, R. D. (2003) *The Hare Psychopathy Checklist: Youth Version*, New York, NY: Multi-Health Systems.
Gretton, H. M., Hare, R. D., and Catchpole, R. E. H. (2004) 'Psychopathy and offending from adolescence to adulthood: A 10-year follow-up,' *Journal of Consulting and Clinical Psychology*, *72*:636–645.
Gretton, H. M., McBride, M., Hare, R. D., O'Shaughnessy, R., and Kumka, G. (2001) 'Psychopathy and recidivism in adolescent sex offenders,' *Criminal Justice and Behavior*, *28*:427–449.
Grubin, D. (1994) 'Sexual murder,' *British Journal of Psychiatry*, *165*(5):624–629.
Hanson, R. K., and Morton-Bourgon, K. E. (2005) 'The characteristics of persistent sexual offenders: A meta-analysis of recidivism studies,' *Journal of Consulting and Clinical Psychology*, *73*:1154–1163.
Hare, R. D. (1999) 'Psychopathy as a risk factor for violence,' *Psychiatric Quarterly*, *70*:181–197.
Hare, R. D. (2003) *Manual for the Hare Psychopathy Checklist–Revised* (2nd ed.), Toronto, ON: Multi-Health Systems.
Hakkanen-Nyholm, H., Repo-Tiihonen, E., Lindberg, N., Salenius, S., and Weizmann-Henelius, G. (2009) 'Finnish sexual homicides: Offense and offender characteristics,' *Forensic Science International*, *188*:125–130.
Harris, G. T., Rice, M. E., Quinsey, V. L., Lalumière, M. L., Boer, D., and Lang, C. (2003) 'A multisite comparison of actuarial risk instruments for sex offenders,' *Psychological Assessment*, *15*:413–425.
Hart, S. D., Forth, A. E., and Hare, R. D. (1991) 'The MCMI–II and psychopathy,' *Journal of Personality Disorders*, *5*:318–327.
Hazelwood, R., Warren, J., and Dietz, P. (1993) 'Compliant victims of the sexual sadist,' *Australian Family Physician*, *22*(4):474–479.
Healey, J., Lussier, P., and Beauregard, E. (2013) 'Sexual sadism in the context of rape and sexual homicide: An examination of crime scene indicators,' *International Journal of Offender Therapy and Comparative Criminology*, *57*(4).402–424.
Hill, A., Habermann, N., Berner, W., and Briken, P. (2007) 'Psychiatric disorders in single and multiple sexual murderers,' *Psychopathology*, *40*(1):22–28.
Hill, A., Habermann, N., Klussman, D., Berner, W., and Briken, P. (2008) 'Criminal recidivism in sexual homicide perpetrators,' *International Journal of Offender Therapy and Comparative Criminology*, *52*(1):5–20.
Holt, S. E., Meloy, J. R., and Strack, S. (1999) 'Sadism and psychopathy in violent and sexually violent offenders,' *Journal of the American Academy of Psychiatry and Law*, *27*:23–32.
Jackson, R. L., and Richards, H. J. (2007) 'Diagnostic and risk profiles among civilly committed sex offenders in Washington State,' *International Journal of Offender Therapy and Comparative Criminology*, *51*(3):313–323.
Johnson, B. R., and Becker, J. V. (1997) 'Natural born killers? The development of the sexually sadistic serial killer,' *Journal of the American Academy of Psychiatry and the Law*, *25*(3):335–348.
Jones, S., Chan, H. C. O., Myers, W. C., and Heide, K. M. (2013) 'A proposed sexual homicide category: The psychopathic–sexually sadistic offender,' in J. B. Helfgott (Ed.), *Criminal psychology, volume 2, typologies, mental disorders, and profiles* (pp. 403–422), Westport, CT: Praeger Publishers.
Keelan, C. M., and Freemouw, W. J. (2013) 'Child versus peer/adult offenders: A critical review of the juvenile sex offender literature,' *Aggression and Violent Behavior*, *18*:732–744.
Kingston, D. A., Seto, M. C., Firestone, P., and Bradford, J. M. (2010) 'Comparing indicators of sexual sadism as predictors of recidivism among adult male sexual offenders,' *Journal of Consulting and Clinical Psychology*, *78*:574–584.
Kirsch, L. G., and Becker, J. V. (2007) 'Emotional deficits in psychopathy and sexual sadism: Implications for violent and sadistic behavior,' *Clinical Psychology Review*, *27*:904–922.
Kirsch, L. G., Becker, J. V., Fanniff, A. M., and Martens, A. (2006, March) *The role of childhood abuse by a female in the development of sexual sadism*. Poster presented at the annual meeting of the American Psychology–Law Society, St. Petersburg, Florida.

Knight, R. A. (1993, November) *The development and social antecedents of sexual aggression*. Invited presentation to the 12th annual conference of the Association for the Treatment of Sexual Abusers, Boston.

Knight, R. A., and Guay, J. P. (2006) 'The role of psychopathy in sexual coercion against women,' in C. J. Patrick (Ed.), *Handbook of Psychopathy* (pp. 512–532), New York, NY: The Guilford Press.

Knight, R. A., and Prentky, R. A. (1990) 'Classifying sexual offenders,' in W. L. Marshall, D. R. Laws, & H. E. Barbaree (Eds.), *Handbook of sexual assault: Issues, theories, and treatment of the offender* (pp. 23–52), New York, NY: Springer.

Knight, R. A., Sims-Knight, J. E., and Guay, J. P. (2013) 'Is a separate disorder category defensible for paraphilic coercion?,' *Journal of Criminal Justice*, *41*:90–99.

Krafft-Ebing, R. von. (1986/1965) F. J. Rebman (Trans.). *Psychopathia sexualis*, New York, NY: Stein & Day.

Langevin, R. (2003) 'A study of the psychosexual characteristics of sex killers: Can we identify them before it is too late?,' *International Journal of Offender Therapy and Comparative Criminology*, *47*(4):366–382.

Langton, C. M., Barbaree, H. E., Harkins, L., and Peacock, E. J. (2006) 'Sex offenders' response to treatment and its association with recidivism as a function of psychopathy,' *Sexual Abuse: A Journal of Research and Treatment*, *18*:99–120.

Levenson, M. R., Kiehl, K. A., and Fitzpatrick, C. M. (1995) 'Assessing psychopathic attributes in a noninstitutionalized population,' *Journal of Personality and Social Psychology, 68*:151–158.

Looman, J., Abracen, J., Serin, R., and Marquis, P. (2005) 'Psychopathy, treatment change, and recidivism in high-risk, high-need sexual offenders,' *Journal of Interpersonal Violence*, *20*:549–568.

Loranger, A. (1988) *Personality Disorder Examination (PDE)*, Yonkers, NY: DV Communications.

MacCulloch, M. J., Snowden, P. R., Wood, P. J. W., and Mills, H. E. (1983) 'Sadistic fantasy, sadistic behavior, and offending,' *British Journal of Psychiatry*, *143*:20–29.

Malamuth, N. M. (2003) 'Criminal and non-criminal sexual aggressors: Integrating psychopathy in a hierarchical-mediational confluence model,' *Annals of the New York Academy of Sciences*, *989*:33–58.

Malamuth, N. M. (1986) 'Predictors of naturalistic sexual aggression,' *Journal of Personality and Social Psychology*, *5*:953–962.

Malamuth, N. M., Linz, D., Heavey, C., Barnes, G., and Acker, M. (1995) 'Using the confluence model of sexual aggression to predict men's conflict with women: A 10-year follow-up study,' *Journal of Personality and Social Psychology*, *69*:353–369.

Malamuth, N. M., Sockloskie, R. J., Koss, M. P., and Tanaka, J. S. (1991) 'Characteristics of aggressors against women: Testing a model using a national sample of college students,' *Journal of Consulting and Clinical Psychology*, *59*:670–681.

Marsh, A. A. (2015) 'Understanding amygdala responsiveness to fearful expressions through the lens of psychopathy and altruism,' *Journal of Neuroscience Research*, *94*:513–525.

Marsh, A. A., and Blair, R. J. R. (2008) 'Deficits in facial affect recognition among antisocial populations: A meta-analysis,' *Neuroscience and biobehavioral Reviews*, *32*:454–465.

Marshall, W. L., and Hucker, S. J. (2006a) 'Issues in the diagnosis of sexual sadism,' *Sexual Offender Treatment*, *1*(2):1–5.

Marshall, W. L., and Hucker, S. J. (2006b) 'Severe sexual sadism: Its features and treatment,' in R. D. McAnulty & M. M. Burnette (Eds.), *Sex and sexuality: Sexual deviation and sexual offenses* (Vol. 3, pp. 227–250), Westport, CT: Praeger.

Marshall, W. L., and Kennedy, P. (2003) 'Sexual sadism in sexual offenders: An elusive diagnosis,' *Aggression and Violent Behavior*, *8*(1):1–22.

McElroy, S. L., Soutullo, C. A., Taylor, P., Jr., Nelson, E. B., Beckman, D. A., and Keck, P. E. (1999) 'Psychiatric features of 36 men convicted of sexual offenses,' *Journal of Clinical Psychiatry*, *60*:414–420.

Meloy, J. R. (1997) 'The psychology of wickedness: Psychopathy and sadism,' *Psychiatric Annals*, *27*:630–633.

Millon, T. (1987) *Millon Clinical Multiaxial Inventory–II manual*, Minneapolis, MN: National Computer Systems.

Millon, T., and Davis, R. D. (1998) 'Ten subtypes of psychopathy,' in T. Millon, E. Simonsen, M. Birket-Smith, & R. D. Davis (Eds.), *Psychopathy: Antisocial, criminal, and violent behavior* (pp. 161–170), New York, NY: The Guilford Press.

Mokros, A., Osterheider, M., Hucker, S. J., and Nitschke, J. (2011) 'Psychopathy and sexual sadism,' *Law and Human Behavior*, *35*:188–199.

Mokros, A., Schilling, F., Weiss, K., Nitschke, J., and Eher, R. (2014) 'Sadism in sexual offenders: Evidence for dimensionality,' *Psychological Assessment*, *26*:138–147.

Murphy, C., and Vess, J. (2003) 'Subtypes of psychopathy: Proposed differences between narcissistic, borderline, sadistic, and antisocial psychopaths,' *Psychiatric Quarterly*, *74*:11–29.

Myers, W. C., Beauregard, E., and Menard, W. (2013, October) *A Revised Sexual Homicide Crime Scene Rating Scale for Sexual Sadism (SADSEX–SH–R)*. Paper presented at 44th Annual Meeting of American Academy of Psychiatry and the Law, San Diego, California.

Myers, W. C., Chan, H. C. O., Vo, E. J., and Lazarou, E. (2010) 'Sexual sadism, psychopathy, and recidivism in juvenile sexual murderers,' *Journal of Investigative Psychology and Offender Profiling*, 7:49–58.

Neumann, C. S., and Hare, R. D. (2008) 'Psychopathic traits in a large community sample: Links to violence, alcohol use, and intelligence,' *Journal of Consulting and Clinical Psychology*, *76*:893–899.

Nitschke, J., Osterheider, M., and Mokros, A. (2009) 'A cumulative scale of severe sexual sadism,' *Sexual Abuse: A Journal of Research and Treatment*, *21*(3):262–278.

Olver, M. E., and Wong, C. P. (2006) 'Psychopathy, sexual deviance, and recidivism among sex offenders,' *Sexual Abuse: A Journal of Research and Treatment*, *18*:65–82.

Olver, M. E., and Wong, S. C. P. (2009) 'Therapeutic responses of psychopathic sexual offenders: Treatment attrition, therapeutic change, and long-term recidivism,' *Journal of Consulting and Clinical Psychology*, 77:328–336.

O'Meara, A., Davies, J., and Barnes-Holmes, Y. (2004) *The prevalence and characteristics of sadism in an Irish student population*, British Psychological Society, Division of Forensic Psychology annual conference.

Palermo, G. B. (1994) *The faces of violence*, Springfield, IL: Charles C. Thomas.

Patrick, C. J., and Drislane, L. E. (2014) 'Triarchic model of psychopathy: Origins, operationalizations, and observed linkages with personality and general psychopathology,' *Journal of Personality*, *83*:627–643.

Paulhus, D. L., and Williams, K. M. (2002) 'The Dark Triad of personality: Narcissism, Machiavellianism, and psychopathy,' *Journal of Research in Personality*, *36*:556–563.

Paulhus, D. L., Neumann, C. S., and Hare, R. D. (in press) *Manual for the Hare Self-Report Psychopathy scale*, Toronto, ON: Multi-Health Systems.

Porter, S., Campbell, M. A., Woodworth, M., and Birt, A. R. (2002) 'A new psychological conceptualization of the sexual psychopath,' in F. Columbus (Ed.), *Advances in psychology research* (Vol. 7, pp. 21–36), New York, NY: Nova Science.

Porter, S., Fairweather, D., Drugge, J., Hervé, H., Birt, A., and Boer, D. P. (2000) 'Profiles of psychopathy in incarcerated sexual offenders,' *Criminal Justice and Behavior*, *27*:216–233.

Porter, S., Ten Brinke, L., and Wilson, K. (2009) 'Crime profiles and conditional release performance of psychopathic and non-psychopathic sexual offenders,' *Legal and Criminological Psychology*, *14*:109–118.

Porter, S., and Woodworth, M. (2006) 'Psychopathy and aggression,' in C. J. Patrick (Ed.), *Handbook of psychopathy* (pp. 481–494), New York, NY: Guilford Press.

Porter, S., Woodworth, M., Earle, J., Drugge, J., and Boer, D. (2003) 'Characteristics of sexual homicides committed by psychopathic and nonpsychopathic offenders,' *Law and Human Behavior*, *27*:459–470.

Proulx, J., Aubut, J., McKibben, A., and Cote, M. (1994) 'Penile responses of rapists and nonrapists to rape stimuli involving physical violence or humiliation,' *Archives of Sexual Behavior*, *23*(3):295–310.

Proulx, J., Blais, E., and Beauregard, E. (2007) 'Sadistic sexual offenders,' in J. Proulx, E. Beauregard, M. Cusson, & A. Nicole (Eds.), *Sexual murderers: A comparative analysis and new perspectives* (pp. 107–122), Hoboken, NJ: Wiley.

Quinsey, V. L., Rice, M. E., and Harris, G. T. (1995) 'Actuarial prediction of sexual recidivism,' *Journal of Interpersonal Violence*, *10*:85–105.

Reid, J. A., Beauregard, E., Fedina, K. M., and Frith, E. N. (2014) 'Employing mixed methods to explore motivational patterns of repeat sex offenders,' *Journal of Criminal Justice*, *42*:203–212.

Reidy, D. E., Zeichner, A., and Seibert, A. (2011) 'Unprovoked aggression: Effects of psychopathic traits and sadism,' *Journal of Personality*, *79*:75–100.

Rice, M. E., Harris, G. T., and Cormier, C. A. (1992) 'An evaluation of a maximum security therapeutic community for psychopaths and other mentally disordered offenders,' *Law and Human Behavior*, *16*:399–412.

Robertson, C. A., and Knight, R. A. (2014) 'Relating sexual sadism and psychopathy to one another, nonsexual violence, and sexual crime behaviors,' *Aggressive Behavior*, *40*(1):12–23.

Salekin, R. T. (2002) 'Psychopathy and therapeutic pessimism: Clinical lore or clinical reality?,' *Clinical Psychology Review*, *22*:79–112.

Serin, R. C., Mailloux, D. L., and Malcolm, P. B. (2001) 'Psychopathy, deviant sexual arousal, and recidivism among sexual offenders,' *Journal of Interpersonal Violence*, *16*:234–246.

Serin, R. C., Malcolm, P. B., Khana, A., and Barbaree, H. E. (1994) 'Psychopathy and deviant sexual arousal in incarcerated offenders,' *Journal of Interpersonal Violence*, *9*:3–11.

Seto, M. C., and Barbaree, H. E. (1999) 'Psychopathy, treatments behavior, and sex offender recidivism,' *Journal of Interpersonal Violence*, *14*:1235–1248.
Seto, M. C., and Kuban, M. (1996) 'Criterion-related validity of a phallometric test for paraphilic rape and sadism,' *Behaviour Research and Therapy*, *34*(2):175–183.
Skeem, J. L., Monahan, J., and Mulvey, E. P. (2002) 'Psychopathy, treatment involvement, and subsequent violence among civil psychiatric patients,' *Law and Human Behavior*, *26*:577–603.
Stone, M. H. (2001) 'Serial sexual homicide: Biological, psychological, and sociological aspects,' *Journal of Personality Disorders*, *15*(1):1–18.
Vandiver, D. M. (2006) 'A prospective analysis of juvenile male sex offenders: Characteristics and recidivism rates as adults,' *Journal of Interpersonal Violence*, *21*:673–688.
Vandiver, D. M., and Kercher, G. (2004) 'Offender and victim characteristics of registered offenders in Texas: A proposed typology of female sexual offenders,' *Sexual Abuse: A Journal of Research and Treatment*, *16*:121–137.
Warren, J., Reboussin, R., Hazlewood, R. R., Cummings, A., Gibbs, N., and Trumbetta, S. (1998) 'Crime scene and distance correlates of serial rape,' *Journal of Quantitative Criminology*, *14*:35–59.
Wilson, R. J., Pake, D. R., and Duffee, S. (2011, November) *DSM–5 pedohebephilia, PCD, and sadism diagnoses: Reliability in Florida*. Paper presented at the 30th annual conference of the Association of the Treatment of Sexual Abusers (ATSA), Toronto, Ontario, Canada.
Wong, S., Olver, M. E., Nicholaichuk, T. P., and Gordon, A. E. (2003) *The Violence Risk Scale Sexual Offender version (VRS–SO)*, Saskatoon, SK: Regional Psychiatric Centre, Department of Psychology and Research.
World Health Organization. (2004) *International statistical classification of diseases and health related problems, 10th revision* (Vol. 2, 2nd ed.), Geneva: Author.

27

Psychopathy and sexual violence

Steven M. Gillespie, Luna C. M. Centifanti, and Gayle Brewer

Introduction

Violence, including violence of a sexual nature, comes at a high societal cost and has been recognized as an international public health problem by the World Health Organization (Krug, Dahlberg, Mercy, Zwi, & Lozano, 2002). The costs of sexual abuse can be counted not only in terms of direct suffering to the victim, including harm to physical and psychological functioning, increased chances of multiple victimization, and higher rates of teenage pregnancy following a sexual assault, but also in terms of increased costs to public health and criminal justice services, loss of work days, and reduced productivity (Reidy et al., 2015; Roberts, O'Connor, Dunn, & Golding, 2004; Widom, Czaja, & Dutton, 2008). In an attempt to tackle this problem, research has focused on identifying risk factors that help to identify those individuals that pose the greatest risk for committing a new sexual offense when released back into the community and for designing interventions that will reduce the risk of reoffending.

One important risk factor that has been considered in sex offending research is psychopathy. Psychopathy refers to a collection of personality traits that vary along a continuum in the general population and that are associated with an increased risk for criminality and antisocial behavior, including increased risk for sexual violence (Hare, 2003). As will be reviewed in this chapter, psychopathic traits, including callousness, interpersonal manipulativeness, antisociality, and risk taking, aid the prediction of sexual recidivism, have been identified at relatively high levels among sexual offenders, and are associated with self-reported sexually coercive behaviors in the general population. Toward the end of the chapter, we will describe theoretically important developmental features related to psychopathic personality that may aid explanations of sexual offending.

Before considering the contribution of psychopathy to sexual offending, it is important to note that sexual offenders represent a heterogeneous group who vary greatly in terms of victim, offender, and offense characteristics. For example, types of sexual offenses include, but are not limited to, contact sexual offending characterized by violence and forceful contact with a victim, exposing oneself in public, and producing, sharing, and viewing child sexual exploitation material. Another important point of heterogeneity is the victim's age, and while some sexual offenders offend exclusively against adult victims, others offend only against child victims, or show no preference for adult or child victims. A proportion of those offenders who have offended against children may be described as pedophilic (American Psychiatric Association [APA], 2013). Pedophilia is a diagnostic term used in the *Diagnostic and Statistical Manual of Mental Disorders 5th Edition* (DSM–5; APA, 2013) that describes a pattern of recurrent and intense sexually arousing fantasies, urges, or behaviors involving sexual activity with a prepubescent child or children that have either been acted on or cause marked distress or interpersonal difficulty. However, the term pedophilia is often misused, and not all sexual offenders against children meet diagnostic criteria for pedophilia. Importantly, some individuals who do show a sexual interest in children may never commit a sexual offense (Cantor & McPhail, 2016). Sexual offenders can also be categorized on the basis of whether offenses were committed against familial victims, with a further distinction between biological and socio-legal incest, and against non-familial victims (Seto, Babchishin, Pullman, & McPhail, 2015). The distinction between sexual offenders who offend exclusively against child victims and those who offend against adult victims may be particularly important to consider in a discussion of the relationship between psychopathy and sexual offending.

Several studies have now shown that elevated psychopathic tendencies, among both youth (Frick, Ray, Thornton, & Kahn, 2014) and adults (Hare, 2003), are associated with greater criminal diversity. That is, psychopaths show a greater range of offending, including violent, sexual, acquisitive, and other types of offending, whereas non-psychopathic criminals show less diversity and greater specialism in a particular offense type. Mitchell and Beech (2011) emphasized this difference in their neurobiological model of offending that distinguished between more specialized pedophilic offenders, and the criminal diversity that characterizes many adult rapists. In support of a generalists versus specialists distinction, child sexual offenders do appear to show some degree of offense specialism, and typically show a less diverse pattern of offending compared with other types of offender (Brown, Dargis, Mattern, Tsonis, & Newman, 2015; Seto & Lalumière, 2010). Indeed, outside of their offending behavior, pedophilic offenders may otherwise function relatively well and hold down specific roles in the community (Sullivan & Beech, 2002). Mitchell and Beech speculate that this more specialized pattern of offending may reflect differences in the underlying neurobiology of pedophilic child sex offenders compared with generally antisocial offenders, with the latter characterized by more elevated psychopathic tendencies.

Although few studies have undertaken direct comparisons of psychopathic tendencies between different groups of sexual offenders, some studies have compared psychopathic traits between child sexual offenders and other groups of violent non-sex offenders. For example, in their study of psychopathic traits in child sex offenders and non-sex offenders, Brown et al. (2015) found that offenders with child as well as adult victims showed higher psychopathy scores compared to other offender groups. Other studies that have compared sex offenders with child victims against those with adult victims, or mixed adult and child victims, suggest that those who offend exclusively against children show relatively low levels of psychopathy (Olver & Wong, 2006; Porter et al., 2000; Serin, Malcolm, Khanna, & Barbaree, 1994). More recent studies have used person-centered statistical techniques to examine specific subtypes of sexual offender based on psychopathic personality scores, revealing four distinct subtypes: prototypic, callous–conning, sociopathic, and general offender profiles (Krstic et al., 2017). Further analyses on these subtypes showed that the prototypic psychopathy type showed the most violence in their sexual crimes; general offenders engaged in more sexual behavior than did the sociopathic offenders, while the callous–conning subtype engaged in more paraphilic acts compared to the sociopathic subtype (Krstic et al., 2017). Unfortunately, this analysis failed to examine differences in victim age between the psychopathy-based subtypes.

A distinction between child sexual offenders and other offender types is also informed by research showing that child sexual offenders tend to show elevated levels of social phobia. For example, in a study on the comorbidity of DSM–IV axis I and II psychiatric diagnoses with pedophilia, out of a group of 45 pedophilic sex offenders, 17 (37.8 percent) had received a diagnosis of social phobia in their lifetime, while 14 (31.1 percent) met the criteria for a current diagnosis of social phobia (Raymond, Coleman, Ohlerking, Christenson, & Miner, 1999). Further support for a link between social phobia and child sexual offending comes from a study that used quantitative and qualitative methods to assess levels of social anxiety and social phobia in male sexual offenders with a diagnosis of a paraphilia (Hoyer, Kunst, & Schmidt, 2001). Paraphilia refers to a biomedical term used to describe sexual arousal that is outside the range of usual sexual interests, including pedophilia, referred to above (Beech & Harkins, 2012). Although the paraphilias examined by Hoyer et al. included pedophilia (n = 23) and sexual sadism (n = 19), these were pooled into one group based on similarities in social anxiety scores and socio-demographic factors. Offenders with a paraphilia showed higher levels of social phobia compared with sexual offenders with an impulse control disorder and forensic non-sex offender controls. Of 42 offenders with a paraphilia, 51 percent and 26 percent scored above clinical cut-offs for social interaction anxiety and social phobia respectively. These figures are in contrast to those for sex offenders with an impulse control disorder (30 percent and 27 percent) and forensic controls (14 percent and 21 percent).

Importantly for the current discussion, there is some evidence that social phobia and psychopathy may reflect diametric opposites in some important respects. For example, one study reported that in a non-offender sample, participants who scored higher for psychopathic tendencies tended to show lower levels of social phobia (Hofmann, Korte, & Suvak, 2009). Further evidence can be found when examining behavioral and neuroimaging findings observed in relation to psychopathy and social phobia. Several studies have shown that psychopathic tendencies are associated with worse performance on tests of facial emotion recognition, with these deficits particularly pronounced for fearful facial expressions (Dawel, O'Kearney, McKone, & Palermo, 2012). Psychopathic tendencies are also associated with reduced gaze toward the eyes of emotional faces (Dadds, El Masry, Wimalaweera, & Guastella, 2008; Gillespie, Rotshtein, Wells, Beech, & Mitchell, 2015; Gillespie, Rotshtein, Beech, & Mitchell, 2017) and with hypoactivity of the amygdala in response to others' fearful expressions (Viding et al., 2012; White et al., 2012). In contrast, social phobia is associated with increased sensitivity and amygdala activation to others' threatening facial expressions (Phan, Fitzgerald, Nathan, & tanker, 2006). Indeed, in one study that compared amygdala activation during an aversive conditioning paradigm between participants with social phobia compared with psychopathy, opposing patterns of neural activity were observed (Veit et al., 2002). Taken together, these findings suggest that sexual offenders with a paraphilia may show high levels of social phobia, increased attention to others' fearful expressions, and increases in aversive conditioning, while more generalist offenders may show elevated psychopathic tendencies, impaired processing of others' fearful expressions, and reductions in aversive conditioning (Mitchell & Beech, 2011).

Importantly, Blair and colleagues (Blair, 2013; Blair, Leibenluft, & Pine, 2014) suggest that the impaired recognition of others' fearful expressions, coupled with reductions in aversive conditioning, may contribute to failure to recognize a victim's suffering and experience this suffering as aversive. As a consequence, children with elevated psychopathic tendencies fail to learn to inhibit an aggressive attack in response to the victim's distress, leading to a lack of moral development and socialization. It has been argued that this model may provide an account for why psychopathic offenders appear to show a phenotypic increase in levels of proactive aggression, that is, aggression that is planned and goal-directed, rather than reactive in response to a perceived slight or wrong (Blair, 2013; Blair et al., 2014). Given that some sexual offenses are motivated by the fulfillment of sexual needs and desires, this model may provide an account for some instances of sexual offending. However, it is important to note that not all sexual offenses are instrumental, and some are motivated by feelings of grievance, revenge, or other negative affective states. Moreover, in practice it is often difficult to clearly distinguish between cases of pure reactive and instrumental aggression, with many aggressive behaviors containing features of both.

Correlates of psychopathy in sexual offenders: a focus on impaired empathic functioning

One of the core features of the psychopathic personality that has been explored among sexual offenders is a lack of empathy. The term empathy includes the ability to understand another's thoughts, feelings and beliefs, so-called Theory of Mind or cognitive empathy, and the ability to feel what another is feeling, so-called emotional resonance or affective empathy (Decety & Jackson, 2006; Jolliffe & Farrington, 2006). A distinction between cognitive and affective components of empathy has also been noted in various models of the empathy process in sexual offenders, including the multicomponent model of empathy (Marshall, Hudson, Jones, & Fernandez, 1995), and Barnett and Mann's (2013) model of the empathic process in sexual offenders. In their multicomponent model of empathy, Marshall et al. (1995) propose a multistep model that distinguishes between the processes of: (1) emotion recognition; (2) perspective taking; (3) emotion replication; and (4) response decision. Marshall et al. (1995) suggest that deficits at the emotion recognition stage of this model prevent the unfolding of the empathic response. However, such a multistep model appears to be inconsistent with the partial dissociation of the underlying systems for cognitive and affective empathy.

Do sexual offenders show global empathy deficits?

Although there is some debate as to whether psychopathy is associated with impairments in both cognitive and affective empathy, or an exclusive impairment in affective empathy, it is clear that those with elevated psychopathic tendencies experience empathic difficulties that go beyond an impaired ability to understand and feel with the emotions of their own victims. Empathy research with sex offenders has yielded varied and, at times, conflicting results (Barnett & Mann, 2013). Some have suggested that sexual offenders show global empathic deficits akin to those observed in psychopathy, while others suggest that sexual offenders show difficulties in empathizing only with their own victims, or with others in the same 'class' as their victim, for example, children or women. The findings of different meta-analyses suggest little or no relationship between empathy and sexual offending (Jolliffe & Farrington, 2004; Hanson & Morton-Bourgon, 2005), yet Mann and Barnett (2013) note that offenders often report positive experiences of victim empathy work during treatment. These mixed findings may reflect the use of varied methods for assessing sexual offenders that tap different components of empathic functioning, or an overreliance on self-report methods that introduce a number of limitations. These limitations include the questionable ability for individuals to accurately appraise their own level of empathic functioning; the inclusion of items in affective subscales of self-report empathy questionnaires that tap perspective-taking abilities or Theory of Mind; and problems with impression management strategies that have been found to be particularly common among sexual offenders (Gudjonsson & Sigurdsson, 2000). The results of such studies are therefore of questionable validity. However, other methods have been used to assess empathic functioning in sexual offenders, including the ability to recognize others' facial expressions of emotion.

As noted earlier, one of the core empathic deficits observed in relation to psychopathy is an impaired ability to recognize others' emotional facial expressions (Dawel et al., 2012). Although tasks examining emotion recognition abilities have been widely used in psychopathy research, a more limited number of studies have examined these abilities in particular types of offender, including between sexual offenders and non-sexual violent offenders. In a recent systematic review (Chapman, Gillespie, & Mitchell, 2017), it was concluded that both sexual offenders and non-sexual violent offenders show impaired abilities for recognizing others' facial expressions of emotion. However, the studies included in the review varied widely in terms of the composition of the sex offender group, the comparison groups used, and the precise experimental paradigm.

In an early study of emotion recognition in sexual offenders, it was found that sexual offenders, inclusive of those with adult and child victims, showed impaired performance for recognizing facial emotions, including anger, disgust, surprise, and fear, compared with nonviolent offenders and non-offenders (Gery, Miljkovitch, Berthoz, & Soussignan, 2009). In a more recent study, we compared sexual offenders with violent offenders and non-offenders and examined performance for expressions that varied in the intensity of the expression, the type of emotion, and the sex of the face (Gillespie, Rotshtein, Satherley, Beech, & Mitchell, 2015). Results revealed that both sexual and violent offenders, compared with non-offenders, showed reduced accuracy for others' fearful expressions. Furthermore, using the same stimuli with a mixed group of incarcerated sexual and violent offenders, we have shown that levels of callous–unemotional psychopathic traits, but not egocentric or antisocial, predicted more impaired recognition of fearful facial expressions (Gillespie, Mitchell, Satherley, Beech, & Rotshtein, 2015). Thus, our findings suggest that sexual offenders show a pattern of impaired socio-affective functioning that is consistent with the type of impairment observed in relation to psychopathic traits.

On the other hand, rather than displaying global empathy deficits akin to those observed in psychopathy, several studies have argued that sexual offenders display problems in victim empathy, that is, the sex offender may have a reduced "cognitive and emotional understanding of the experience of the victim of his sexual offense" (Mann & Barnett, 2013:282). Mann and Barnett (2013) highlight that sex offender treatment programs have devoted considerable effort to treating victim empathy deficits, yet the results of three meta-analytic studies reviewed by Mann and Barnett suggest that victim empathy work is unnecessary or even harmful. At present, it remains largely unclear whether or not sexual offenders display global empathy deficits, a lack of victim-specific empathy, or have relatively unimpaired empathic abilities. However, many of these studies have relied on group-based averages. Thus, rather than being a characteristic of all, or most, sexual offenders, impairments in the empathic process might represent one potential factor that increases risk for sexual violence among those who are motivated to commit a sexual offense (e.g., they have a specific sexual interest in children, or a preoccupation with sex). Future research should aim to measure the separable components of the empathic process among sexual offenders with greater precision and use more person-centered latent variable methods to gain a better understanding of the role of empathic functioning in sexual offenders.

Psychopathy and sexual recidivism

As observed by Harris et al. (Harris, Boccaccini, & Rice, 2017), individuals with a history of sexual offending with elevated psychopathic traits in combination with deviant sexual interests (a paraphilia) are often presumed to be more likely to recidivate than those without this combination of risk factors. In their meta-analysis of risk factors for sexual recidivism, Hanson and Morton-Bourgon (2005) observed that psychopathy predicts sexual recidivism with a small effect size. In a more recent meta-analysis that examined the relation between psychopathy scores and sexual recidivism (k = 20, N = 5,239), total scores on the Psychopathy Checklist–Revised (PCL–R; Hare, 2003) – the most commonly used clinical instrument for the assessment of psychopathic personality in forensic settings – predicted sexual recidivism with a moderate effect size (Hawes, Boccaccini, & Murrie, 2013). Further, the antisocial features showed greater predictive validity compared with other features of the psychopathic personality (e.g., affective or interpersonal features), and the odds of recidivism were further increased for those who scored high on both the PCL–R and a measure of sexual deviance (Hawes et al., 2013).

An additional effect emerging from this meta-analysis was that effect sizes were increased for research studies compared with field studies (Hawes et al., 2013), a finding that may reflect increased measurement error in the scoring of the PCL–R in field studies. These finding have implications for clinical practice, in that studies showing an interaction of psychopathy scores with sexual deviance have tended to rely on more robust measures of sexual deviance than those that are typically used in the field. As such, these results may not apply equally well for measures more commonly used in clinical practice. Support for this conclusion is reported by Harris et al. (2017). These authors tested the ability of field-based PCL–R scores and field measures of sexual deviance, including paraphilia diagnosis, to predict sexual recidivism. In contrast to the often-reported interaction effect, they found that neither PCL–R scores or paraphilia diagnoses predicted an increased likelihood of sexual recidivism. Furthermore, these authors report no evidence that psychopathy scores and sexual deviance interact to predict increased sexual recidivism (Harris et al., 2017). Indeed, when sexual deviance was operationalized as number of victims, the two-way interaction with psychopathy actually predicted reduced recidivism compared with other offenders. These findings raise the possibility that field measures of psychopathy and sexual deviance are unreliable or that more valid measures of sexual deviance are needed in the field in order to make predictions about future behavior and draw clinically meaningful conclusions. Nonetheless, when scored for research purposes, findings suggest that psychopathy and sexual deviance are predictive of future sexual recidivism.

Psychopathy and sexual coercion

The findings highlighted above indicate the importance of psychopathy scores in a forensic context for understanding the motivation to commit sexual offenses, the role of psychopathy-related impairments in attention and social cognition that may be associated with instrumental aggression, and the role of psychopathy scores in predicting sexual recidivism. However, it is important to note that psychopathy refers to a dimensional construct, with a distribution of scores observable in the general population, from the very low through to the very high (Guay, Ruscio, Knight, & Hare, 2007). With this in mind, researchers have also sought to explore the role of psychopathic tendencies in predicting risky sexual behaviors and sexually coercive behaviors in non-offending samples. Though definitions vary, sexual coercion may be conceptualized as "the act of using pressure, alcohol or drugs, or force to have sexual contact with someone against his or her will" (Struckman-Johnson, Struckman-Johnson, & Anderson, 2003:76). Four categories of coercive behavior have been identified: sexual arousal (e.g., persistent kissing and touching), emotional manipulation (e.g., blackmail, questioning, or using authority), alcohol and drug intoxication (e.g., purposefully getting a person drunk or taking advantage while intoxicated), and physical force (e.g., using physical harm). Men are more likely than women to perpetrate each form of sexual coercion investigated (Muñoz, Khan, & Cordwell, 2011). Both male and female victims of sexual coercion experience a range of negative consequences, including psychological distress and poor health (de Visser et al., 2014; French, Tilghman, & Malebranch, 2015; Williams, Clear, & Coker, 2013). Coercion may also impact subsequent romantic and sexual relationships (Collibee & Furnham, 2014). It is therefore important to consider those factors that may influence experience of sexual coercion, as either a perpetrator or victim.

It has been suggested that psychopathy represents an alternative life history strategy which increases interest in promiscuous short-term relationships, particularly for men. For example, psychopathy is associated with preference for short-term sexual relationships (Jonason, Luevano, & Adams, 2012) and avoidance of close romantic attachments (Brewer et al., 2018). This life history interpretation of psychopathy may also explain increased sexual coercion among those high in psychopathy. Previous research demonstrates a relationship between psychopathy and sexual coercion in both offender and non-offender populations (Knight & Guay, 2006). Those high on psychopathy display a greater interest in sexual opportunities and increased sexual drive; as reviewed earlier in this chapter, psychopathy is also associated with low empathy and reduced responsiveness to others distress. Therefore, the relationship between psychopathy and sexual coercion may reflect both increased motivation for sexual activity and reduced sensitivity to inhibitory factors.

When considering the related yet distinct dimensions of the psychopathy construct, the so called primary psychopathic traits reflecting the affective and interpersonal features of psychopathy are associated with each form of sexual coercion listed previously (Muñoz et al., 2011). However, there was no relationship of the "secondary" lifestyle and antisocial psychopathic traits with types of sexual coercion. Such findings are consistent with previous research suggesting that primary psychopathy is associated with accurate perceptions of victim vulnerability in offender samples based on both observations of a conversation between the target and confederate (Book, Quinsey, & Langford, 2007) and physical gait (Book, Costello, & Camilleri, 2013).

Researchers have typically focused on male perpetrators and female victims of sexual coercion. Although men are more likely than women to perpetrate sexual coercion, a substantial proportion of women also engage in sexually coercive behavior (e.g., Krahé, Waizenhöfer, & Möller, 2003; Stemple & Meyer, 2014; Stemple, Flores, & Meyer, 2017). Pathways to perpetration of sexually aggressive behavior differ for men and women (Krahe & Berger, 2017), and coercive men and women may be motivated by different outcomes (Schatzel-Murphy, Harris, Knight, & Milburn, 2009). It is therefore important to investigate the role of psychopathy on sexual coercion perpetration in female samples. Similar to male perpetrator research, women high on psychopathy are more likely to engage in sexual coercion, with primary psychopathy particularly important (Khan, Brewer, Kim, & Muñoz Centifanti, 2017; Muñoz et al., 2011). Primary psychopathy is more influential for women than men with regard to perpetration of coercion involving physical force, which may reflect the risk of retaliation and physical or reputational injury (Muñoz et al., 2011).

Compared to research investigating the relationship between psychopathy and perpetration of sexual coercion, relatively few studies have considered the manner in which psychopathy influences sexual coercion victimization. For example, it may be argued that the callousness which characterizes primary psychopathy may be protective for some forms of sexual coercion (e.g., emotional manipulation), allowing potential victims to address the coercive behavior concern without fear of damage to the relationship, etc. Further, there is little evidence examining psychopathy and responses to the sexually coercive behavior performed by others and, in particular, willingness to intervene. Bystander responses to inappropriate sexual behavior form an important element of many sexual coercion intervention programs (McMahon & Banyard, 2012). Research is required to determine the extent to which psychopathy predicts willingness to intervene when observing sexually coercive behavior and responsiveness to intervention programs.

What are the developmentally important features of psychopathy that might explain the link with sexual aggression and sexual offending?

The ability to identify features early in development is important for the prevention of sexual and violent offending. Here, we are concerned with two aspects: callous–unemotional traits, an aspect of psychopathy that is related to violence (Frick, Ray, Thornton, & Kahn, 2014) and can be characterized as a cluster of behaviors, including callously using others for one's personal gain, a lack of caring for society's values, and lacking in emotional depth; and risk taking, a tendency to engage in behaviors that involve risk over alternatives that do not. Sexual offending involves taking risks and CU traits have often been associated with risky decision-making.

With the release of the DSM–5 (APA, 2013), callous–unemotional (CU) traits were designated as a specifier for the diagnosis of Conduct Disorder in childhood. CU traits include behaviors that reflect a lack of caring for others and for doing things well, a lack of guilt and remorse, and a lack of emotional depth in their interactions with others. These traits make up the specifier for Limited Prosocial Emotions in Conduct Disorder diagnoses using the DSM–5 (APA, 2013). Questions remain unresolved about the mechanisms involved in why CU traits relate to antisocial behavior and violence. A good answer to this question would be helpful in understanding the nature of CU traits themselves, and also for guiding prediction, prevention, and treatment. Although it seems plausible that CU traits may directly cause antisocial behavior due to their nature, another possible sequela of CU traits that might contribute to antisocial behavior is risky decision-making in the context of potential rewards.

People with CU traits tend to make risky decisions (Baskin-Sommers, Waller, Fish, & Hyde, 2015; Marini & Stickle, 2010; Ray, Thornton, Frick, Steinberg, & Cauffman, 2016; Wymbs et al., 2012) and thus become involved in situations that can lead to antisocial behavior; it may be that rather than engaging in antisocial behavior because they simply lack empathy towards the targets of their behavior, they may engage in antisocial behavior because they are inclined toward risk taking. In other words, whether or not CU traits are related to risk-taking is a question that underpins whether we think that people with CU traits either (1) are showing a genuine moral failing to value the lives and experiences of other people or (2) simply evaluate risk poorly and use force to get what they want (e.g., sex) without considering negative consequences of the behavior.

Theoretical bases for risk taking

The overwhelming view in the field is that young people with CU traits do indeed take more risks. Risk taking involves behavior where there is a simultaneous opportunity for gain but also a high potential for costs (Leigh, 1999). Adolescents take greater risks than adults, and it is also notable that antisocial behavior shows a sharp increase at this developmental stage that may be due to risky decision-making (Crowley, Raymond, Mikulich-Gilbertson, Thompson, & Lejuez, 2006; Fairchild et al., 2009). The main theory-driven reason why one would expect a relation between CU traits and risk-taking is that CU traits are one of a cluster of three aspects of psychopathy, which is itself tied to risky decision-making. People with psychopathy engage in higher risk activities that include violence as well as substance use and pathological gambling (Frick et al., 2014). CU traits in particular are also associated with risk taking (Centifanti & Modecki, 2013; Fanti, Kimonis, Hadjicharalambous, & Steinberg, 2016; Marini & Stickle, 2010) and are related to a lack of fear regarding negative outcomes (such as punishment), which could underlie risky behavior (Mitchell, Colledge, Leonard, & Blair, 2002). Impulsivity and sensation seeking have been found to relate to CU traits in adulthood (Hare & Neumann, 2008), measured as psychopathy, and in childhood (Frick, Bodin, & Barry, 2000). Sensation seeking is associated with risky decision-making in adolescence, including sexual risk taking (Thornton et al., 2017), and the relation of CU traits with sexual risk taking (i.e., casual sex and unprotected sex) has been found to be mediated by substance misuse (Thornton et al., 2017). Thus, it may be that the disinhibitory function of psychotropic substances allows those with CU traits to take sexual risks.

Some argue that CU traits may be related to the decision to take risks in relation to the associated costs/gains (i.e., punishments/rewards). Blair and colleagues (Blair, Colledge, & Mitchell, 2001) examined psychopathic traits in children in relation to a gambling task and found that those with psychopathic traits made more decisions that were associated with large rewards but large punishments, that is, they took more risks. In another test of gambling, CU was related to weaker reward responsivity, in that those with elevated CU traits failed to show an increase in risk taking following successful (rewarded) trials (Centifanti & Modecki, 2013; Marini & Stickle, 2010). The evidence, thus far, suggests relations between CU and the processing of reward, and this, rather than risk taking per se, may be the basis for motivationally driven decisions to engage in antisocial behavior including sexual coercion and sexual violence.

Reward and punishment as related to risk

An antisocial or criminal act such as a theft or sexual assault potentially offers both reward and punishment, during and after the event. Moreover, context-specific rewards and punishments can be anticipated prior to similar events in the future, and events will shape the likelihood of similar offensive acts in the future. In many people, the potential punishments (social reproach, being caught, likelihood of harm) and aversive emotional states (anxiety, fear) predicted on the basis of similar past events may sufficiently discourage future offensive acts. A diminished "stressful"/ punishment signal is likely permissive but not in itself sufficient for committing these kinds of criminal misconduct. As noted in Muñoz and Frick (2012), interventions that focus on rewarding prosocial behavior (and deemphasizing punishment for poor behavior) may be warranted for people with psychopathic traits. Incarcerated youth with psychopathic traits appear to emphasize the positive outcomes (or instrumental consequences, such as what they can obtain) of their aggressive behavior and pay less attention to the adverse consequences (Pardini, Lochman, & Frick, 2003). Importantly, they seem to be particularly at risk for showing a combination of both instrumental and reactive (or retaliatory) aggression. For example, in a sample of 150 detained adolescent sex offenders, high levels of CU traits were associated with more premeditation and planning in the sexual offense, as well as greater number of victims, and more violence committed in the sexual offense (Lawing, Frick, & Cruise, 2010). A focus on potential rewards may explain these instrumental motives.

Conclusion

In this chapter, we have highlighted the costs of sexual violence and offending for victim and society and the heterogeneity that is present among sexual offenders, most notably in terms of features of the victim and in levels of psychopathic traits. While psychopathic traits have been reported in higher levels among adult rapists rather than child sexual offenders, both groups of offenders may be motivated by instrumental means. Consistent with this, research has shown that sexual offenders, like violent offenders, display socio-affective impairments that are consistent with psychopathy (Chapman et al., 2017). Furthermore, the presence of psychopathy and sexual deviance represent important risk factors for sexual offending, and when considered together are predictive of those that are most likely to commit a new sexual offense. However, psychopathy is not only associated with sexual offending in adult and juvenile forensic contexts, but also among non-criminal samples where psychopathic traits are associated with sexually coercive behaviors (Khan et al., 2017; Muñoz et al., 2011).

When considering potential treatments for individuals who have committed a sexual offense and show elevated psychopathic traits, there is now a developing appreciation that poor treatment progress in this group may reflect a lack of appropriate interventions designed specifically to meet the needs of this group of offenders. A growing understanding of psychopathy has served to emphasize the importance of assessing psychopathic tendencies, paying attention to the particular needs of high psychopathy scorers, and acknowledging the role of potential responsivity issues in traditional sex offender treatment programs. A consideration of developmental features associated with psychopathic traits has highlighted that this group show risk-taking behaviors and respond in different ways to rewards and punishments compared with their low psychopathy counterparts (Centifanti & Modecki, 2013; Muñoz & Frick, 2012). Thus, it is important that new reports have shed new light on effective treatment of individuals with elevated psychopathy scores (Baskin-Sommers, Curtin, & Newman, 2015) and can inform the development of future interventions for sexual offenders with marked psychopathic traits.

References

American Psychiatric Association. (2013) *Diagnostic and statistical manual of mental disorders, 5th edition (DSM–5)*, Arlington, VA: Author.

Barnett, G., and Mann, R. E. (2013) 'Empathy deficits and sexual offending: A model of obstacles to empathy,' *Aggression and Violent Behavior, 18*(2):228–239.

Baskin-Sommers, A. R., Curtin, J. J., and Newman, J. P. (2015) 'Altering the cognitive–affective dysfunctions of psychopathic and externalizing offender subtypes with cognitive remediation,' *Clinical Psychological Science, 3*(1):45–57.

Baskin-Sommers, A. R., Waller, R., Fish, A. M., and Hyde, L. W. (2015) 'Callous–unemotional traits trajectories interact with earlier conduct problems and executive control to predict violence and substance use among high risk male adolescents,' *Journal of Abnormal Child Psychology, 43*(8):1529–1541.

Beech, A. R., and Harkins, L. (2012) 'DSM–IV paraphilia: Descriptions, demographics and treatment interventions,' *Aggression and Violent Behavior, 17*(6):527–539.

Blair, R. J. R. (2013) 'The neurobiology of psychopathic traits in youths,' *Nature Reviews Neuroscience, 14*:786–799.

Blair, R. J. R., Colledge, E., and Mitchell, D. G. V. (2001) 'Somatic markers and response reversal: Is there orbitofrontal cortex dysfunction in boys with psychopathic tendencies?,' *Journal of Abnormal Child Psychology, 29*(6):499–511.

Blair, R. J. R., Leibenluft, E., and Pine, D. S. (2014) 'Conduct disorder and callous–unemotional traits in youth,' *New England Journal of Medicine, 371*:2207–2216.

Book, A., Costello, K., and Camilleri, J. A. (2013) 'Psychopathy and victim selection: The use of gait as a cue to vulnerability,' *Journal of Interpersonal Violence, 28*:2368–2383.

Book, A. S., Quinsey, V. L., and Langford, D. (2007) 'Psychopathy and the perception of affect and vulnerability,' *Criminal Justice and Behavior, 34*:531–544.

Brewer, G., Bennett, C., Davidson, L., Ireen, A., Phipps, A. J., Stewart-Wilkes, D., and Wilson, B. (2018) 'Dark triad traits and romantic relationship attachment, accommodation, and control,' *Personality and Individual Differences, 120*:202–208.

Brown, A. R., Dargis, M. A., Mattern, A. C., Tsonis, M. A., and Newman, J. P. (2015) 'Elevated psychopathy scores among mixed sexual offenders: Replication and extension,' *Criminal Justice and Behavior, 42*(10):1032–1044.

Cantor, J. M., and McPhail, I. V. (2016) 'Non-offending pedophiles,' *Current Sexual Health Reports, 8*(3):121–128.

Centifanti, L. C. M., and Modecki, K. (2013) 'Throwing caution to the wind: Callous–unemotional traits and risk taking in adolescents,' *Journal of Clinical Child & Adolescent Psychology*, *42*(1):106–119.
Chapman, H., Gillespie, S. M., and Mitchell, I. J. (2017) 'Facial affect processing in incarcerated violent males: A systematic review,' *Aggression and Violent Behavior*, in press.
Collibee, C., and Furman, W. (2014) 'Impact of sexual coercion on romantic experiences of adolescents and young adults,' *Archives of Sexual Behavior*, *43*:1431–1441.
Crowley, T. J., Raymond, K. M., Mikulich-Gilbertson, S. K., Thompson, L. L., and Lejuez, C. W. (2006) 'A risk-taking "set" in a novel task among adolescents with serious conduct and substance problems,' *Journal of the American Academy of Child and Adolescent Psychiatry*, *45*(2):175–183.
Dadds, M. R., El Masry, Y., Wimalaweera, S., and Guastella, A. J. (2008) 'Reduced eye gaze explains "fear blindness" in childhood psychopathic traits,' *Journal of the American Academy of Child & Adolescent Psychiatry*, *47*(4):455–463.
Dawel, A., O'Kearney, R., McKone, E., and Palermo, R. (2012) 'Not just fear and sadness: Meta-analytic evidence of pervasive emotion recognition deficits for facial and vocal expressions in psychopathy,' *Neuroscience & Biobehavioral Reviews*, *36*(10):2288–2304.
de Visser, R. O., Badcock. P. B., Rissel, C., Richters, J., Smith, A. M. A., Grulich, A. E., and Simpson, J. M. (2014) 'Experiences of sexual coercion in a representative sample of adults: The second Australian Study of Health and Relationships,' *Sexual Health*, *11*:472–480.
Decety, J., and Jackson, P. L. (2006) 'A social–neuroscience perspective on empathy,' *Current Directions in Psychological Science*, *15*(2):54–58.
Fairchild, G., van Goozen, S. H. M., Stollery, S. J., Aitken, M. R. F., Savage, J., Moore, S. C., and Goodyer, I. M. (2009) 'Decision making and executive function in male adolescents with early-onset or adolescence-onset conduct disorder and control subjects,' *Biological Psychiatry*, *66*(2):162–168.
Fanti, K. A., Kimonis, E. R., Hadjicharalambous, M. Z., and Steinberg, L. (2016) 'Do neurocognitive deficits in decision making differentiate conduct disorder subtypes?,' *European Child & Adolescent Psychiatry*, *25*(9):989–996.
French, B. H., Tilghman, J. D., and Malebranche, D. A. (2015) 'Sexual coercion context and psychosocial correlates among diverse males,' *Psychology of Men & Masculinity*, *16*:42–53.
Frick, P. J., Bodin, S. D., and Barry, C. T. (2000) 'Psychopathic traits and conduct problems in community and clinic-referred samples of children: Further development of the Psychopathy Screening Device,' *Psychological Assessment*, *12*:382–393.
Frick, P. J., Ray, J. V., Thornton, L. C., and Kahn, R. E. (2014) 'Can callous–unemotional traits enhance the understanding, diagnosis, and treatment of serious conduct problems in children and adolescents? A comprehensive review,' *Psychological Bulletin*, *140*:1–57.
Gery, I., Miljkovitch, R., Berthoz, S., and Soussignan, R. (2009) 'Empathy and recognition of facial expressions of emotion in sex offenders, non-sex offenders and normal controls,' *Psychiatry Research*, *165*(3):252–262.
Gillespie, S. M., Mitchell, I. J., Satherley, R. M., Beech, A. R., and Rotshtein, P. (2015) 'Relations of distinct psychopathic personality traits with anxiety and fear: Findings from offenders and non-offenders,' *PloS One*, *10*(11):e0143120.
Gillespie, S. M., Rotshtein, P., Beech, A. R., and Mitchell, I. J. (2017) 'Boldness psychopathic traits predict reduced gaze toward fearful eyes in men with a history of violence,' *Biological Psychology*, *128*:29–38.
Gillespie, S. M., Rotshtein, P., Satherley, R. M., Beech, A. R., and Mitchell, I. J. (2015) 'Emotional expression recognition and attribution bias among sexual and violent offenders: A signal detection analysis,' *Frontiers in Psychology*, *6*:595.
Gillespie, S. M., Rotshtein, P., Wells, L. J., Beech, A. R., and Mitchell, I. J. (2015) 'Psychopathic traits are associated with reduced attention to the eyes of emotional faces among adult male non-offenders,' *Frontiers in Human Neuroscience*, *9*.
Guay, J. P., Ruscio, J., Knight, R. A., and Hare, R. D. (2007) 'A taxometric analysis of the latent structure of psychopathy: Evidence for dimensionality,' *Journal of Abnormal Psychology*, *116*(4):701–716.
Gudjonsson, G. H., and Sigurdsson, J. F. (2000) 'Differences and similarities between violent offenders and sex offenders,' *Child Abuse and Neglect*, *24*:363–372.
Hanson, R. K., and Morton-Bourgon, K. E. (2005) 'The characteristics of persistent sexual offenders: A meta-analysis of recidivism studies,' *Journal of Consulting and Clinical Psychology*, *73*(6):1154–1174.
Hare, R. D. (2003) *The Hare Psychopathy Checklist–Revised* (2nd ed.), Toronto, ON: Multi-Health Systems.
Hare, R. D., and Neumann, C. S. (2008) 'Psychopathy as a clinical and empirical construct,' *Annual Review of Clinical Psychology*, *4*(1):217–246.

Harris, P. B., Boccaccini, M. T., and Rice, A. K. (2017) 'Field measures of psychopathy and sexual deviance as predictors of recidivism among sexual offenders,' *Psychological Assessment, 29*(6):639–650.
Hawes, S. W., Boccaccini, M. T., and Murrie, D. C. (2013) 'Psychopathy and the combination of psychopathy and sexual deviance as predictors of sexual recidivism: Meta-analytic findings using the Psychopathy Checklist–Revised,' *Psychological Assessment, 25*(1):233–243.
Hofmann, S. G., Korte, K. J., and Suvak, M. K. (2009) 'The upside of being socially anxious: Psychopathic attributes and social anxiety are negatively associated,' *Journal of Social and Clinical Psychology, 28*(6):714–727.
Hoyer, J., Kunst, H., and Schmidt, A. (2001) 'Social phobia as a comorbid condition in sex offenders with paraphilia or impulse control disorder,' *The Journal of Nervous and Mental Disease, 189*(7):463–470.
Jolliffe, D., and Farrington, D. P. (2004) 'Empathy and offending: A systematic review and meta-analysis,' *Aggression and Violent Behavior, 9*(5):441–476.
Jolliffe, D., and Farrington, D. P. (2006) 'Development and validation of the Basic Empathy Scale,' *Journal of Adolescence, 29*(4):589–611.
Jonason, P. K., Luevano, V. X., and Adams, H. M. (2012) 'How the Dark Triad traits predict relationship choices,' *Personality and Individual Differences, 53*:180–184.
Khan, R., Brewer, G., Kim, S., and Muñoz Centifanti, L. S. (2017) 'Students, sex, and psychopathy: Borderline and psychopathy personality traits are differently related to women and men's use of sexual coercion, partner poaching, and promiscuity,' *Personality and Individual Differences, 107*:72–77.
Knight, R. A., and Guay, J. P. (2006) 'The role of psychopathy in sexual coercion against women,' in C. J. Patrick (Ed.), *Handbook of psychopathy* (pp. 512–532), New York, NY: Guilford Press.
Krahé, B., and Berger, A. (2017) 'Gendered pathways from child sexual abuse to sexual aggression victimization and perpetration in adolescence and young adulthood,' *Child Abuse & Neglect, 63*:261–272.
Krahé, B., Waizenhöfer, E., and Möller, I. (2003) 'Women's sexual aggression against men: Prevalence and predictors,' *Sex Roles, 49*:219–232.
Krstic, S., Neumann, C. S., Roy, S., Robertson, C. A., Knight, R. A., and Hare, R. D. (2017) 'Using latent variable- and person-centered approaches to examine the role of psychopathic traits in sex offenders,' *Personality Disorders: Theory, Research, and Treatment*, in press.
Krug, E. G., Mercy, J. A., Dahlberg, L. L., and Zwi, A. B. (2002) 'The world report on violence and health,' *The Lancet, 360*(9339):1083–1088.
Lawing, K., Frick, P. J., and Cruise, K. R. (2010) 'Differences in offending patterns between adolescent sex offenders high or low in callous–unemotional traits,' *Psychological Assessment, 22*:298–305.
Leigh, B. C. (1999) 'Peril, chance, adventure: Concepts of risk, alcohol use and risky behavior in young adults,' *Addiction, 94*(3):371–383.
Mann, R. E., and Barnett, G. D. (2013) 'Victim empathy intervention with sexual offenders: Rehabilitation, punishment, or correctional quackery?,' *Sexual Abuse, 25*(3):282–301.
Marini, V. A., and Stickle, T. R. (2010) 'Evidence for deficits in reward responsivity in antisocial youth with callous–unemotional traits,' *Personality Disorders: Theory, Research, and Treatment, 1*(4):218–229.
Marshall, W. L., Hudson, S. M., Jones, R., and Fernandez, Y. M. (1995) 'Empathy in sex offenders,' *Clinical Psychology Review, 15*(2):99–113.
McMahon, S., and Banyard, V. L. (2012) 'When can I help? A conceptual framework for the prevention of sexual violence through bystander intervention,' *Trauma, Violence, & Abuse, 13*:3–14.
Mitchell, D. G., Colledge, E., Leonard, A., and Blair, R. J. R. (2002) 'Risky decisions and response reversal: Is there evidence of orbitofrontal cortex dysfunction in psychopathic individuals?,' *Neuropsychologia, 40*(12):2013–2022.
Mitchell, I. J., and Beech, A. R. (2011) 'Towards a neurobiological model of offending,' *Clinical Psychology Review, 31*(5):872–882.
Muñoz, L. C., and Frick, P. J. (2012) 'Callous–unemotional traits and their implication for understanding and treating aggressive and violent youths,' *Criminal Justice and Behavior, 39*(6):794–813.
Muñoz, L. C., Khan, R., and Cordwell, L. (2011) 'Sexually coercive tactics used by university students: A clear role for primary psychopathy,' *Journal of Personality Disorders, 25*:28–40.
Olver, M. E., and Wong, S. C. (2006) 'Psychopathy, sexual deviance, and recidivism among sex offenders,' *Sexual Abuse: A Journal of Research and Treatment, 18*(1):65–81.
Pardini, D. A., Lochman, J. E., and Frick, P. J. (2003) 'Callous/unemotional traits and social cognitive processes in adjudicated youths,' *Journal of the American Academic of Child and Adolescent Psychiatry, 42*:364–371.

Phan, K. L., Fitzgerald, D. A., Nathan, P. J., and Tancer, M. E. (2006) 'Association between amygdala hyperactivity to harsh faces and severity of social anxiety in generalized social phobia,' *Biological Psychiatry, 59*(5):424–429.

Porter, S., Fairweather, D., Drugge, J., Herv'e, H., Birt, A., and Boer, D. P. (2000) 'Profiles of psychopathy in incarcerated sexual offenders,' *Criminal Justice and Behavior, 27*:216–233.

Ray, J. V., Thornton, L. C., Frick, P. J., Steinberg, L., and Cauffman, E. (2016) 'Impulse control and callous–unemotional traits distinguish patterns of delinquency and substance use in justice involved adolescents: Examining the moderating role of neighborhood context,' *Journal of Abnormal Child Psychology, 44*(3):599–611.

Raymond, N. C., Coleman, E., Ohlerking, F., Christenson, G. A., and Miner, M. (1999) 'Psychiatric comorbidity in pedophilic sex offenders,' *American Journal of Psychiatry, 156*(5):786–788.

Reidy, D. E., Kearns, M. C., DeGue, S., Lilienfeld, S. O., Massetti, G., and Kiehl, K. A. (2015) 'Why psychopathy matters: Implications for public health and violence prevention,' *Aggression and Violent Behavior, 24*:214–225.

Roberts, R., O'Connor, T., Dunn, J., and Golding, J. (2004) 'The effects of child sexual abuse in later family life; mental health, parenting and adjustment of offspring,' *Child Abuse & Neglect, 28*:525–545.

Schatzel-Murphy, E. A., Harris, D. A., Knight, R. A., and Milburn, M. A. (2009) 'Sexual coercion in men and women: Similar behaviors, different predictors,' *Archives of Sexual Behavior, 38*:974–986.

Serin, R. C., Malcolm, P. B., Khanna, A., and Barbaree, H. E. (1994) 'Psychopathy and deviant sexual arousal in incarcerated sexual offenders,' *Journal of Interpersonal Violence, 9*:3–11.

Seto, M. C., and Lalumiere, M. L. (2010) 'What is so special about male adolescent sexual offending? A review and test of explanations through meta-analysis,' *Psychological Bulletin, 136*(4):526–575.

Seto, M. C., Babchishin, K. M., Pullman, L. E., and McPhail, I. V. (2015) 'The puzzle of intrafamilial child sexual abuse: A meta-analysis comparing intrafamilial and extrafamilial offenders with child victims,' *Clinical Psychology Review, 39*:42–57.

Stemple, L., and Meyer, I. H. (2014) 'The sexual victimization of men in America: New data challenge old assumptions,' *American Journal of Public Health, 104*:e19–e26.

Stemple, L., Flores, A., and Meyer, I. H. (2017) 'Sexual victimization perpetrated by women: Federal data reveal surprising prevalence,' *Aggression and Violent Behavior, 34*:302–311.

Struckman-Johnson, C., Struckman-Johnson, D., and Anderson, P. B. (2003) 'Tactics of sexual coercion: When men and women won't take no for an answer,' *The Journal of Sex Research, 40*:76–86.

Sullivan, J., and Beech, A. (2002) 'Professional perpetrators: Sex offenders who use their employment to target and sexually abuse the children with whom they work,' *Child Abuse Review, 11*(3):153–167.

Thornton, L. C., Frick, P. J., Ray, J. V., Wall Myers, T. D., Steinberg, L., and Cauffman, E. (2017) 'Risky sex, drugs, sensation seeking, and callous unemotional traits in justice-involved male adolescents,' *Journal of Clinical Child & Adolescent Psychology*, in press.

Veit, R., Flor, H., Erb, M., Hermann, C., Lotze, M., Grodd, W., and Birbaumer, N. (2002) 'Brain circuits involved in emotional learning in antisocial behavior and social phobia in humans,' *Neuroscience Letters, 328*(3):233–236.

Viding, E., Sebastian, C. L., Dadds, M. R., Lockwood, P. L., Cecil, C. A., De Brito, S. A., and McCrory, E. J. (2012) 'Amygdala response to preattentive masked fear in children with conduct problems: The role of callous–unemotional traits,' *American Journal of Psychiatry, 169*:1109–1116.

White, S. F., Marsh, A. A., Fowler, K. A., Schechter, J. C., Adalio, C., Pope, K., . . . and Blair, R. J. R. (2012) 'Reduced amygdala response in youths with disruptive behavior disorders and psychopathic traits: Decreased emotional response versus increased top-down attention to non-emotional features,' *American Journal of Psychiatry, 169*:750–758.

Widom, C. S., Czaja, S. J., and Dutton, M. A. (2008) 'Childhood victimization and lifetime revictimization,' *Child Abuse & Neglect, 32*:785–796.

Williams, C. M., Clear, E. R., and Coker, A. I. (2013) 'Sexual coercion and sexual violence at first intercourse associated with sexually transmitted infections,' *Sexually Transmitted Diseases, 40*:771–775.

Wymbs, B. T., McCarty, C. A., King, K. M., McCauley, E., Vander Stoep, A., Baer, J. S., and Waschbusch, D. A. (2012) 'Callous–unemotional traits as unique prospective risk factors for substance use in early adolescent boys and girls,' *Journal of Abnormal Child Psychology, 40*(7):1099–1110.

Part IV

Criminal careers, comorbidities, and psychopathy

28

Juvenile psychopathy and juvenile delinquency

Laura López-Romero and Estrella Romero

Introduction

When studying child and youth conduct problems, there is a particular need of identifying developmentally distinctive and meaningful patterns of problematic behavior. Conduct problems, involving a heterogeneous pattern of deviant behaviors, including aggressive, oppositional or destructive behavior, defiance, rule-breaking, deceitfulness, and disregard for others, are considered one of the most relevant and prevalent disorders in childhood and adolescence (Thomas, 2010). It would have its maximum expression in the diagnostic of Conduct Disorder, a syndrome included in the *Diagnostic and Statistical Manual of Mental Disorders* (DSM–5), which involves a repetitive and persistent pattern of behavior that violates the rights of others, or in which major age-appropriate societal norms or rules are violated (American Psychiatric Association, 2013). Even considering that not all children and adolescents that show some pattern of disruptive behavior would meet the criteria for Conduct Disorder, it should be noted that child and youth conduct problems still represent the primary reason for referring youths to clinicians and mental health services (Baker, 2013). Nowadays it is widely assumed that conduct problems represent a heterogeneous phenomenon, comprising separable domains and showing multiple pathways over the life span (Nagin & Tremblay, 1999). By assuming these patterns of developmental heterogeneity, the identification of children at increased risk for being involved in more severe and persistent problematic behavior would be facilitated and, in turn, would favor the promotion of new advances in terms of diagnostic classification, prevention, and treatment (Frick, Ray, Thornton, & Khan, 2014a).

With the particular aim of better understanding the determinants of severe and long-lasting conduct problems, a configuration of affective, interpersonal, and behavioral traits, similar to those that define adult psychopathy, has been proposed for delimiting a specific severe, pervasive, and persistent pattern of young problematic and antisocial behavior. This perspective was adopted after an extensive body of research supporting a strong link between adult psychopathy and severe violent and nonviolent antisocial behavior and delinquency (e.g., Hare & Neumann, 2008), high rates of recidivism (e.g., Leitisco, Salekin, DeCoster, & Rogers, 2008; Salekin, 2008), and relatively poor treatment outcomes (e.g., Harris & Rice, 2006). Similar associations were also observed among young populations, with psychopathic personality closely related to frequent and severe behavioral and psychosocial problems, including conduct problems and aggression (e.g., Rowe et al., 2010), Attention-Deficit/Hyperactivity Disorder symptoms (ADHD; Svecke & Kosson, 2010), future antisocial behavior and delinquency (e.g., McMahon, Witkiewitz & Kotler, 2010), chronic and serious offending (e.g., Corrado, McCuish, Hart, & DeLisi, 2015), both general and violent recidivism (e.g., Salekin, 2008), a lack of prosocial behaviors and social competence skills (e.g., Fontaine, McCrory, Boivin, Moffitt, & Viding, 2011), poor school adjustment (e.g., Ciucci, Baroncelli, Franchi, Golmaryani, & Frick, 2014), and even adult psychopathy (e.g., Hawes, Byrd, Waller, Lynam, & Pardini, 2017). All this knowledge has served as a way to identify the potential precursors and transitions to adult psychopathy, as well as to further understand the development of the most severe, violent, and persistent pattern of youth problematic and antisocial behavior.

The study of the development of psychopathic personality has generated an increasing interest during the last decades. Prior research has shown that psychopathy does not emerge suddenly in adulthood, but it can also be reliably assessed and identified in preschool, school-aged children, and adolescents (see Colins et al., 2014; Salekin, 2016a, for comprehensive reviews of psychometrically and conceptually assessable psychopathic traits in childhood). As occurs in adult samples, research has shown that child and youth psychopathic personality is a multifaceted syndrome comprising a constellation of co-occurring interpersonal, affective, and behavioral/lifestyle traits (Andershed, Kerr, Stattin, & Levander, 2002; Colins et al., 2014; Cooke & Michie, 2001; Hare & Neumann, 2008; Salekin, 2016a). Psychopathic traits under the interpersonal dimension traditionally include features such as lying, manipulation, arrogance, deceitfulness, dishonesty, grandiosity, and glibness/superficial charm. All of these have been included in several conceptual models of the youth psychopathic construct under the label of narcissism (Frick, Bodin, & Barry, 2000), grandiose–deceitful (Andershed et al., 2002; Colins et al., 2014), or grandiose/manipulation (Salekin, 2016a) dimensions. The affective dimension usually comprises psychopathic traits like callousness, lack of empathy, shallow affect, lack of guilt and remorse, or failure to accept responsibilities for one's actions. This affective dimension has been commonly included in most conceptual models as the callous–unemotional (CU) traits facet and is the most analyzed one in the field of child psychopathic personality (Frick et al., 2014a). It has been also represented as the meanness phenotype according to the triarchic model of psychopathy (Patrick, 2010). Finally, under the behavioral dimension we could find traits like impulsivity, need for stimulation, sensation seeking, proneness to boredom, lack of realistic long-term goals, and irresponsibility. These kind of behavioral/lifestyle traits have been commonly represented as the impulsive/conduct problems (Frick et al., 2000), impulsivity–need of stimulation (Andershed et al., 2002; Colins et al., 2014), or the daring–impulsive (Salekin, 2016a) dimensions in traditional conceptual models of psychopathy and were represented as the disinhibition phenotype within the triarchic model (Patrick, 2010).

The downwards extension of psychopathic personality: conceptualization, assessment methods, and controversies

As occurs with the definition of the construct in adult populations, the study of psychopathic personality in youths has had its early underpinnings in classic conceptualizations. As early as Cleckley's work, *The Mask of Sanity* (1941/1976), the author acknowledged that the psychopathic personality profile may have its roots in childhood and adolescence. Within the same period, in two interesting round table discussions, Karpman (1949, 1950) analyzed the applicability of the psychopathic construct to children, defining some of the most important characteristics and raising some of the most enduring debated questions, such as the specification of the core defining features or the etiological mechanisms underlying. Moreover, after identifying a specific subgroup of antisocial youths (around 14 percent) showing similar traits and acting in a similar way to adult psychopaths, McCord and McCord (1964) highlighted the relevance of identifying and treating psychopathy also in youthful populations. Beyond these initial acknowledgments about the potential early origins of psychopathy, it was Quay (1964) who integrated a preliminary operationalization of psychopathic personality in classifying antisocial youths into more homogenous categories. Thus, he proposed two distinctive subtypes, which were later included as diagnostic specifiers for Conduct Disorder in the third version of the DSM (DSM–III; American Psychiatric Association, 1980): the under-socialized aggressive and the socialized aggressive groups. The first one, characterized by deficits concerning empathy, attachment and affectivity, lack of remorse, and the presence of risk and violent behaviors, intended to represent the psychopathic group, in an attempt of avoiding the negative and pejorative connotations related with the psychopathic label.

Probably due to the advances reached in the study of adult psychopathy, a new resurgence of research emerged in the 1990s as an effort of further analyzing the developmental origins of psychopathic personality. In an attempt to identify the "fledgling psychopathy," Lynam (1996) suggested that it could be represented in the co-occurrence of conduct problems and ADHD symptoms, which reflect externalizing problems and core deficits in self-regulation (DeLisi, 2016). This specific proposal was mainly focused on the proper identification of life-course persistent offenders among children with early onset conduct problems, and it was based in a large body of research showing that this comorbid diagnosis was indeed related to more severe, aggressive, and long-lasting problematic behavior, with these children showing a number of neuropsychological deficits similar to those exhibited by adult psychopaths (Lynam, 1997). Regardless of these findings, Lynam's hypothesis has not been definitely supported as a complete model of "fledgling psychopathy" (e.g., Carroll, Houghton, Durkin, & Hattie, 2009). While some authors showed that conduct disordered and ADHD children are indeed more psychopathic than their peers (DeLisi et al., 2014), others revealed that they are certainly not (Michonski & Sharp, 2010).

From Lynam's proposal it was suggested that there should be something other than severe behavioral features and disturbances in the identification of the "fledgling psychopaths." According to Frick and colleagues (Frick, Bodin, & Barry, 2000; Frick, O'Brien, Wootton, & McBurnett, 1994), callous–unemotional (CU) traits, representing the affective dimension of the construct, would be the core features in defining this specific subgroup of problematic youths, who would be at increased risk for developing the most serious and persistent pattern of conduct problems. As the authors primarily defended and proved over the past decades, CU traits add incremental utility in identifying a specific subgroup of problematic youths, generally in an early onset pattern of conduct problems. This group of children would also tend to show a large set of cognitive, emotional, biological, and temperamental deficits, as well as specific behavioral and psychosocial characteristics, consistent with the main findings outlined in adult psychopathy literature (see Frick et al., 2014a for an extensive review on the topic). Even considering the emphasis conferred on the affective features, it should be noted that Frick's initial conceptualization of psychopathic personality was directly linked to Hare's work on adult psychopathy through the Psychopathy Checklist Revised (PCL–R; Hare, 2003) and its interpersonal/affective (Factor 1) and behavioral/antisocial (Factor 2) model.

In order to directly test this specific model in diverse populations of children and adolescents, Frick and Hare (2001) developed the Antisocial Process Screening Device (APSD), which included all the elements of the PCL–R with the exception of those absolutely inappropriate for children (e.g., many short-term marital relationships). In an initial study, Frick et al. (1994) identified two correlated factors similar to those consistently found on the PCL–R: an impulsivity/

conduct problems (I/CP) factor, describing the behavioral features of psychopathy mainly coincident with the deviant lifestyle factor of the PCL–R; and a callous–unemotional (CU) factor, representing the psychological/personality dimensions from the PCL–R's Interpersonal/Affective factor. In a second phase of research, conducted in a large community and clinical samples of children, Frick et al. (2000) proposed an alternative three-factor model. Several items from the I/CP dimension formed a separate factor, namely narcissism, encompassing features related to narcissistic behavior, manipulation, and egocentrism. Most of the remaining I/CP items formed the impulsivity factor, whereas the CU factor remained in this new structure virtually unvaried.

Along with the Psychopathy Checklist Youth Version (PCL: YV; Forth, Kosson, & Hare, 2003), which is a direct adaptation of the PCL–R for adolescents, the APSD is the most used and tested youth psychopathy screening measure. Given their direct link with the PCL–R dominance and conceptualization, some authors suggested that there could be latent risk for having the child and youth psychopathic construct partially usurped by the measure definition (Skeem, Polaschek, Patrick, & Lilienfeld, 2011). In line with adult conceptualizations, there is an open debate about which features should be considered core or essential to the construct, with the controversy about the role of antisocial behavior within the definition far from resolved (see, Hare & Neumann, 2010; Skeem & Cooke, 2010a, 2010b, for further debate review). As a point of agreement for divergent stances, the exclusion of explicit criminality or violent behavior from definitions of psychopathic personality is coming to an understanding (Neumann, Hare, & Pardini, 2015; Skeem et al., 2011). Even considering the evidence about the role of psychopathic traits in the absence of problematic behavior (Rowe, 2014), there are still many authors who assert that any model that does not include antisocial behavior as a core feature will be incomplete (DeLisi, 2016; Neuman et al., 2015). Since "many of the features of psychopathy (e.g., manipulation, deception, callousness, irresponsibility, impulsivity) are colored by antisocial or dissocial elements" (Neumann et al., 2015:2), psychopathic personality traits and antisocial behavior would interact in configuring the psychopathic personality profile over the life-span. Given this close association, the presence of psychopathic traits with concurrent conduct problems has been largely equated to the psychopathic-like construct in young populations (Frick et al., 1994). However, the inclusion of items explicitly measuring problematic behavior in youth psychopathic instruments (e.g., the APSD) has been also questioned since it may prompt contamination and prognostic tautology when used for predicting serious conduct problems (Skeem & Cooke, 2010a).

Although it is difficult to provide a widely agreed definition of psychopathic personality, there seems to be a general consensus of considering this personality profile as a constellation of affective, interpersonal, and behavioral/lifestyle traits, with the inclusion (or not) of antisocial behavioral deviance being still under debate. This three-dimensional structure has been extensively replicated across gender, diverse settings (i.e., community, clinic-referred, and forensic samples), and assessment formats (e.g., see Frick et al., 2014a; Salekin, 2017). However, as Frick and Ray (2015:2) suggested,

> the results of these factor analyses and their consistency across development has led to great debate as to whether psychopathy is best considered as (a) the shared method variance of these multiple facets, (b) a multidimensional composite of these facets, or (c) whether there are certain facets that are "core" to the construct, with others being secondary or less important to defining psychopathy.
>
> *(Frick & Ray, 2015, p. 2)*

Some authors have even suggested that the decision of who may be a psychopath is a matter of theoretical preference, depending on the purpose for which the construct is being used

(Frick & Ray, 2015). For instance, when the goal is to test the value of psychopathic traits for predicting general conduct problems, the impulsive and irresponsible behavioral traits tend to be the most important (e.g., Leitisco et al., 2008). However, if the purpose is to move forward and try to determine which dimension (or dimensions) is the most useful in identifying distinctive subgroups of problematic children, the affective dimension, represented by CU traits, has been traditionally highlighted as the core one (Frick et al., 2014a). As a matter of fact, a new severity specifier, beyond the age of onset (Moffitt, 1993), has been included in DSM-5 for child and youth Conduct Disorder (APA, 2013). This specifier, namely "with low prosocial emotions" in order to avoid potential harmful labeling, is largely based on the CU traits conceptualization, and it should be clinically considered when an individual who meets criteria for Conduct Disorder "display[s] at least two of the following characteristics over at least 12 months and in multiple relationships and settings, Lack of remorse and guilt, Callous–lack of empathy, Unconcerned about performance, Shallow or deficient affect" (APA, 2012:470).

Considering the relevance of CU traits for understanding long-standing patterns of antisocial and delinquent behavior, Frick developed the Inventory of Callous Unemotional Traits (ICU; Frick, 2004), a 24-item instrument that specifically taps CU traits on youth samples. Three factors, namely callousness (i.e., a callous attitude towards others expressed by lack of empathy, remorse, and guilt), Uncaring (i.e., lack of caring about one's own performance or for the feelings of others), and Unemotional (i.e., lack of emotional expression; Essau, Sasagawa, & Frick, 2006) have been consistently identified in a large set of studies conducted in different samples, contexts, and languages (e.g., Ezpeleta, de la Osa, Granero, Penelo, & Domènech, 2013; Fanti, Frick, & Georgiou, 2009; Kimonis et al., 2008). Although some concerns have been raised as regards this factor structure and alternative short forms were also proposed (e.g., Hawes et al., 2014), research with the ICU has reinforced the usefulness of CU traits as an identifier of an etiological and clinically distinctive subgroup of problematic children and adolescents (Essau et al., 2006; Fanti et al., 2009; Hawes et al., 2014; López-Romero, Gómez-Fraguela, & Romero, 2015).

Notwithstanding the significant and ever-increasing contribution of the CU line of research, some alternative configurations and assessment methods have been proposed. For instance, Andershed and colleagues, with the aim of accurately identifying the core features of the psychopathic construct, developed the Youth Psychopathic Traits Inventory (YPI; Andershed et al., 2002) and the Child Problematic Traits Inventory (CPTI; Colins et al., 2014). Psychopathic personality was defined as a syndrome comprising (1) an arrogant, deceitful and manipulative interpersonal style, involving dishonest, grandiosity, and glibness; (2) a defective emotional experience, involving shallow emotions, callousness, and a pronounced lack of remorse and empathy; and (3), the presence of impulsive, irresponsible, and sensation seeking behaviors (Cooke & Michie, 2001). Several studies on preschoolers, school-age children, adolescents, and young offenders showed that youths high on all three dimensions have more conduct problems and have committed more offenses than youths low on all three dimensions (e.g., Andershed, Köhler, Louden, & Hinrichs, 2008; Colins et al., 2014; Frogner, Gibson, Andershed, & Andershed, 2016; Frick et al., 2000; López-Romero, Romero, & Luengo, 2012).

In the light of these results, Salekin (2016a, 2017) has defended the need to go beyond the CU conceptualization, including all three affective, interpersonal, and behavioral dimensions in construct definition and diagnostic manuals. He argues that there is a risk of having CU traits becoming increasingly synonymous with youth psychopathic personality, leading to the psychopathic construct being largely underrepresented in young populations. Therefore, he also proposes a three-factor model of psychopathic personality, with affective (Callous–unemotional; CU), interpersonal (grandiose/manipulation; GM), and behavioral (Daring–impulsive; DI) traits being equally important, and recommends their inclusion in forthcoming versions of the existing nosological systems in order to have "greater resolution for understanding Conduct Disorder and inspire new effective treatment programs tailored more specifically to the disorder" (Salekin, 2016b; p. 190). To this end, Salekin developed the Proposed Specifiers for Conduct Disorder (PSCD), a 24-item instrument intended to reliably assess CU, GM, DI, and conduct problems symptoms in order to improve representation of the psychopathic dimensions, facilitate Conduct Disorder diagnosis, aid research, and improve clinical practice (Salekin, 2017).

Why psychopathic traits? A comprehensive justification of their study in youth populations

Further justification of studying psychopathic personality at early developmental stages will be underlined by examining the most relevant aspects in this field, including the predictive value of the construct for serious conduct problems and juvenile offending, its temporal stability over the life-span, and the presence of distinctive correlates suggesting distinctive etiological mechanisms. Most of these studies have focused on the role of CU traits, although others have examined all the affective, interpersonal, and behavioral traits relating to the psychopathic personality profile. Overall, they have contributed to reinforce the viability, usefulness, and validity of the psychopathic construct in both children and adolescents.

The predictive value of psychopathic traits

Identifying a distinctive pathway to severe conduct problems

The association between psychopathic traits and serious problematic behavior has been supported and enhanced during the past decades through an extensive catalog of studies, research, and theoretical models (see Frick et al., 2014a; Salekin, 2016a; Salekin, 2017 for comprehensive reviews). In a meta-analysis of $k = 10$ studies comprising 5,731 children, Longman, Hawes, and Kohlhoff (2016) evidenced a significant positive relationship between CU traits and conduct problems severity prior to age 5 with consistent results across sex and sample type (at-risk, clinic referred, or community). Despite this close association, even observed at early ages, it should be noted that psychopathic traits are not equivalent to serious conduct problems, particularly those with an early onset (Skeem et al., 2011), with psychopathic personality mainly reflecting the affective, interpersonal, and motivational aspects of such problematic behavior. Thus, as conduct problems and psychopathic traits are independent but related constructs, their study should go beyond the reinforcement of their association. In this regard, different questions emerged as interesting topics for additional reflection: are psychopathic traits really designating a distinctive and meaningful subgroup within the early onset persistent group of problematic children? Does psychopathic personality have predictive value just when conduct problems are also present? And, in turn, what would be its role when conduct problems have not manifested?

In a study conducted in an initial sample of 192 Spanish children, aged 6 to 11, four meaningful groups emerged in cluster analyses considering the presence of early conduct problems and psychopathic traits: the primarily externalizing, with high levels of early onset conduct problems and low levels of psychopathic traits; the externalizing psychopathic, with a specific combination of high conduct problems and psychopathic traits scores; the primarily psychopathic, a quite promising group since it included children with high levels of psychopathic traits who had not manifested conduct problems yet; and the non-problematic group (López-Romero et al., 2012). In a follow-up study conducted six years later on 138 adolescents from the initial sample, youths within the externalizing psychopathic group were revealed as the most problematic, representing the highest-risk profile as they showed higher levels of externalizing conduct problems, psychopathic traits, ADHD symptomatology, poor academic performance, and deficits in social competence (e.g., Ciucci et al., 2014; Kahn, Frick, Youngstrom, Findling, & Youngstrom, 2012; McMahon et al., 2010). What was even more interesting was that the Primarily psychopathic group, which did not show significant levels of problematic behavior at the onset of the study, showed the second highest rate of behavioral and psychosocial maladjustment in adolescence. From these results, it is quite surprising to see that the presence of early psychopathic traits seems to be more determining, in predictive terms, than only the presence of early onset of conduct problems, traditionally considered an indicator of later risk (Moffitt, 1993). Another study conducted with the same sample identified, through latent class analyses, a group of children with a stable trajectory of externalizing conduct problems in a six-year period, spanning childhood and adolescence (López-Romero, Romero, & Andershed, 2015). As observed in prior studies (e.g., Byrd, Loeber, & Pardini, 2012), this stable high group showed the highest psychopathic personality scores, as well as high levels of both reactive and proactive aggression and low social competence skills than their counterparts. These findings were replicated when testing differences between developmental groups in a 10- and a 12-year period (López-Romero, Romero, & Villar, 2017). Similar results were also observed by Klingzell et al. (2016), who examined trajectories of psychopathic traits and conduct problems in a sample of 2,542 Swedish children, aged 3 to 5 at the onset of the study, and followed up in a two-year period. They found evidence of a subgroup of children with high and stable levels of diverse psychopathic traits, with also the most severe conduct problems.

In agreement with previous studies, both psychopathic and CU traits are significantly associated with measures of several behavioral and psychosocial problems, a result consistently observed across ages, gender, different methods of assessment, different samples, and several contexts and cultures (Frick et al., 2014a; Salekin, 2016a, 2017). This was particularly true when these psychopathic traits manifested in combination with a Conduct Disorder diagnosis or in the presence of serious antisocial behavior, designating the theorized highest-risk problematic profile (e.g., Kahn et al., 2012; Longman et al., 2016; McMahon et al., 2010; Pardini, Stepp, Hipwell, Stouthamer-Loeber, & Loeber, 2012; Rowe et al., 2010). Particularly noteworthy is the fact that these results largely held even after controlling for other measures of conduct problem severity or common comorbid disturbances (e.g., age of onset, impulsivity, number and type of problematic behavior displayed, ADHD; e.g., Byrd et al., 2012; López-Romero, Romero, & Villar, 2014; McMahon et al., 2010). It is unquestionable that the vast majority of studies conducted so far have focused on the role of psychopathic and CU traits in the presence of conduct problems and antisocial behavior. This is probably due to the large tradition in studying psychopathic personality in the context of severe problematic behavior (Rowe, 2014), as well as because high levels of those traits are difficult to identify in large community samples (Fontaine et al., 2011). However, there have been different studies evidencing that there are children who show high psychopathic traits but do not display serious conduct problems (e.g., Burke, Waldman, & Lahey, 2010; Kumsta, Sonuga-Barke, & Rutter, 2012; López-Romero et al., 2012; Rowe et al., 2010).

As was previously observed, this group of children tends to show impaired behavioral and psychosocial adjustment later in development and is also at risk for other psychiatric disorders. From those studies, some authors have considered whether psychopathic traits in general, and CU traits in particular, may have a unique essence, identity, and value irrespective of the presence of a diagnosis of Conduct Disorder (Rutter, 2012), a proposal also examined by the workgroup developing diagnostic criteria for the International Classification System of Diseases (ICD–11) published by the World Health Organization.

Psychopathy and juvenile offending

When analyzing juvenile offending, the link between psychopathic personality and a range of antisocial behaviors and different dimensions of the delinquent career is out of questioning (Vaughn, Howard, & DeLisi, 2008). From a criminology perspective some authors defend psychopathy as the unified theory of crime (DeLisi, 2016), "given its ability to use a single construct to connect the dots of antisociality over the life span" (DeLisi & Piquero, 2011:292). Prior research has invariably shown that psychopathic personality is an important driver of juvenile delinquency (e.g., Colins & Andershed, 2015; Corrado, McCuish et al., 2015; McCuish, Corrado, Lussier, & Hart, 2014), a link that has been demonstrated in all sorts of studies including different samples, different types of data, and diverse methodologies (DeLisi, 2016). The more psychopathic youth tend to show more extensive juvenile delinquency careers with high rates of recidivism (including violent and nonviolent), display more hostile aggression, sexual offending, substance use, and abuse, and are much more likely to display an early onset of problem behaviors, police contacts, and juvenile court referral (e.g., Cale, Lussier, McCuish, & Corrado, 2015; Colins, Vermeiren, De Bolle, & Broekaert, 2012; Leitisco et al., 2008; Pechorro, Gonçalves, Maroco, Nunes, & Jesus, 2014; Salekin, 2008; Vaughn et al., 2008; Vincent, Vitacco, Grisso, & Corrado, 2003).

In a meta-analysis conducted by Asscher et al. (2011), using 53 studies containing 60 non-overlapping samples and 10,073 participants, the authors found a moderate link between juvenile psychopathy and delinquency, general recidivism, and violent recidivism, with these associations being moderated by various study and participant characteristics. Psychopathy was equally important for first offending in youths from general populations as for reoffending in delinquent samples; and both delinquent behavior and recidivism could be predicted by psychopathy as early as the transition from middle childhood to adolescence (Asscher et al., 2011). Psychopathic personality has also helped in identifying a high risk-group of juvenile offenders. As an example, Gretton, Hare, and Catchpole (2004) divided a sample of 157 referred boys into low, medium, and high psychopathic groups, based on their PCL: YV scores. The more psychopathic youth were involved in violent, nonviolent, and sexual offending and showed a worse history of abuse, prevalence of substance use, and Conduct Disorder symptoms. In a follow-up conducted ten years later, a gradient was observed in terms of recidivism rates, with 97 percent of the high psychopathic committing nonviolent offense, 82 percent committing violent offending, and 21 percent being involved in sexual crime. From a developmental perspective, psychopathic youths also tend to be involved in serious and long-standing pathways of offending throughout adolescence and into full adulthood, with many different studies showing this specific pattern of results (e.g., Corrado, McCuish et al., 2015; Klingzell et al., 2016; López-Romero et al., 2017; McCuish, Corrado, Hart, & DeLisi, 2015; McCuish et al., 2014).

An interesting result repeatedly observed in prior studies is that the association between psychopathic scores and juvenile offending remains significant after controlling for other important criminological covariates (see DeLisi, 2016). For instance, Flexon and Meldrum (2013) reported a close association between psychopathy and violent delinquency at age 15, with a prior history of violence for all the participants classified as psychopaths, even after the addition of other covariates including sex, minority status, poor school bonding, low self-control, peer violent behavior, and ineffective parent. Similarly, McMahon et al. (2010) examined the predictive value of psychopathic personality at seventh grade on self-reported delinquency and serious crime, juvenile and adult arrests, and Antisocial Personality Disorder diagnosis at age 20. The authors observed that early psychopathy predicted all these outcomes, except serious crime, even controlling for early onset conduct problems, ADHD, oppositional defiant disorder, and Conduct Disorder. In terms of later recidivism, Salekin (2008) found that youth psychopathic personality measured by multiple instruments was predictive of both general recidivism and violent recidivism. This effect withstood the competing effects of 14 diverse covariates, including age, gender, past delinquent charges, drug use, and delinquent peers among, others. Despite this evidence, which reinforces the unique effect of psychopathic traits on a large and diverse set of antisocial outcomes, a recurrent concern is which dimension or dimensions of the psychopathic construct are indeed predictive of antisocial and delinquent behavior. Although many different studies typically identified the behavioral and antisocial factor as the strongest predictor of these reported outcomes (e.g., Flexon & Meldrum, 2013; Gretton et al., 2004; McCuish et al., 2014; Piquero et al., 2012; Salekin, 2008; Vaughn et al., 2008; Vincent et al., 2003), López-Romero, Gómez-Fraguela, and Romero (2015) tested the incremental validity of CU traits above and beyond other relevant factors in subtyping a specific subgroup of severely antisocial youths. Results of logistic regression analyses supported the value of CU traits in distinguishing a high-risk group of individuals, showing more serious and versatile pattern of antisocial behavior, even controlling for other psychopathic factors including impulsiveness, sensation seeking, hostility. and low empathy.

Since psychopathy is powerfully related to serious delinquent behavior, offending, and higher rates of recidivism (Salekin, 2008), the relevance of the psychopathic construct to the juvenile justice system is noteworthy. Concerning this, juvenile justice systems should primarily acknowledge that juvenile offenders are a heterogeneous population, with psychopathic traits explaining within-group variation among offenders, particularly the variations between relatively minor offenders and the small high-risk groups of offenders responsible for the vast majority of delinquent acts (Corrado, DeLisi, Hart, & McCuish, 2015). Therefore, it is relevant for practitioners to recognize the core features of the psychopathic construct and tailor their decisions and interventions accordingly (Reidy et al., 2015). This acknowledgment of juvenile psychopathy from the juvenile justice system is not out of debate. Some scholars have argued that the application of the psychopathic label to certain populations – particularly juvenile offenders – is counterproductive because of the potential harmful consequences related to the negative connotations of the label (Edens, Skeem, Cruise, & Cauffman, 2001). However, different studies found no negative effects associated with psychopathic labels in a juvenile justice context, with different criterion effects (e.g., risk factors inherent to antisocial behavior and psychopathic traits) being stronger for decision-making than the labeling effects (e.g., Murrie, Boccaccini, McCoy, & Cornell, 2007).

Patterns of stability and change

From a developmental perspective, a way to overcome some of the controversies surrounding the study of psychopathic traits in young samples is to examine their temporal stability. Understanding the stability of psychopathic traits across different developmental stages is critical for (1) examining whether these traits are, certainly, normative and temporal in all children; (2) evidencing whether the specific features expressed in childhood and adolescence are representing the same underlying psychopathic personality profile observed in adults; and (3) determining the malleability of these traits over the life-span (Andershed, 2010; Frick, Ray, Thornton, & Khan, 2014b).

As observed in adult populations, existing data revealed moderate to high levels of relative (i.e., rank-order) stability in psychopathic-like traits at different developmental stages and periods, including early childhood (Willoughby, Waschbusch, Moore, & Propper, 2011), school-aged children (e.g., Barry, Barry, Deming, & Locham, 2008; Frick, Kimonis, Dandreaux, & Farrel, 2003), adolescence (e.g., Muñoz & Frick, 2007; Pardini & Loeber, 2008), from childhood up to adolescence (e.g., López-Romero et al. 2015; Lynam et al., 2009; Obradović, Pardini, Long, & Loeber, 2007), and up to early adulthood (Lynam, Caspi, Moffitt, Loeber, & Stouthamer-Loeber, 2007; see also Andershed, 2010; and Frick et al., 2014b for further review). Since teachers tend to change over these periods, and the contact with children tends to decrease as they grow up, levels of relative stability tend to be higher among parents than teachers, particularly when large developmental periods are analyzed (e.g., Obradovic et al., 2007). A relevant point is that the levels of stability observed for psychopathic traits are comparable to those observed in general personality traits (e.g., McCrae et al., 2002), as well as in other psychopathological constructs (e.g., aggression, Conduct Disorder, ADHD; Loeber et al., 2009), adding to the unique entity and developmental validity of the construct (Andershed, 2010). Stability has also been examined in terms of absolute continuity (i.e., mean-level), showing that psychopathic traits tend to remain fairly stable over both short and long intervals (López-Romero et al., 2015; Lynam et al., 2009), although some traits were also suggestive of a pattern of change involving a significant decrease (e.g., Muñoz & Frick, 2007) or increase (e.g., Pardini & Loeber, 2008).

Within-individual change in developmental patterns of psychopathic personality was also identified when examining developmental trajectories from person-centered perspectives (e.g., Frick et al., 2003; Lynam et al., 2009). Stable low, stable high, increasing, and decreasing groups have emerged in most of the studies conducted so far, spanning childhood and adolescence (e.g., Fanti, Colins, Andershed, & Sikki, 2017; Fontaine, Rijsdijk, McCrory, & Viding, 2010; López-Romero et al., 2015; Pardini & Loeber, 2008; Salihovic, Özdemir, & Kerr, 2014). These studies have also allowed the identification of some relevant predictors of distinctive developmental patterns, such as genetic factors, early conduct problems and hyperactivity, or the quality of parenting (Fontaine et al., 2010; Frick et al., 2003), as well as related behavioral, emotional, and psychosocial outcomes (e.g., Baardewijk, Vermeiren, Stegge, & Doreleijers, 2011; Fanti et al., 2017). As expected, stable-high and increasing patterns were designating a high-risk profile of adolescents who tend to develop more problems in terms of behavioral and psychosocial functioning, including concurrent and prospective conduct problems and delinquent behavior, Attention-Deficit/Hyperactivity Disorder (ADHD) symptoms, both reactive and proactive aggression, low peer support and school connectedness, low parental involvement and high parental distress, and low social competence, academic performance, or executive functioning (e.g., Fanti et al., 2017; Lynam et al., 2009; Shalihovic et al., 2014). These results have been supported even after controlling for the initial level of conduct problems, reinforcing the predictive value of psychopathic personality, and linking the observed change in psychopathic traits level to later maladjustment (López-Romero et al., 2015).

Most of these studies have also examined the joint trajectory of conduct problems and psychopathic traits, specifically CU traits. As expected, both children and adolescents with stable high levels of conduct problems and CU traits are consistently at high risk for individual, behavioral, and contextual problems, including high levels of impulsivity, sensation seeking, fearlessness and other psychopathic traits, problematic and aggressive behavior, hyperactivity, peer problems and emotional problems, negative parenting feelings, and adult psychopathy (e.g., Eisenbarth, Demetriou, Kyranides, & Fanti, 2016; Fontaine et al., 2011; Hawes et al., 2017; Klingzell et al., 2016).

Following traditional conceptions defending the immutability of personality disorders, there was a certain reluctance to extend the construct of psychopathy to youths given its implicit message of stability and endurance. However, it has been extensively highlighted that personality stability does not absolutely mean immutability, especially at early developmental stages, showing significant patterns of change particularly when stability is examined at the individual level. Therefore, even considering early psychopathic traits as a potential risk factor for showing adult psychopathy, it should be also noted that a large number of children and adolescents show a significant reduction over time. Alternatively, low levels of psychopathic traits in childhood or adolescence do not absolutely protect for developing serious antisocial behavior as an adult, or a psychopathy profile (Lynam et al., 2009). From a developmental and constructive perspective, examining the temporal stability of psychopathic traits in depth provides a relevant support for the usefulness and predictive value of the construct in young samples. However, since patterns of change are also observed, the need for analyzing psychopathic traits at an early stage, when they are more unstable and prone to change, has been also reinforced. This may shed new light on the factors that may influence the early development of psychopathic personality. By disentangling these factors influencing patterns of both stability and change, new important targets for intervention could be delineated (Frick et al., 2014b).

Distinctive correlates, biological and environmental influences, and potential implications for treatment

As previously described, one of the arguments in justifying the downward extension of psychopathic personality is that it seems to designate a specific subgroup of children and adolescents at increased risk for showing a pattern of severe and persistent problematic behavior. A key finding supporting the validity of this specific pathway is the presence of distinctive correlates, which may suggest a distinctive etiological mechanism leading to their problematic behavior (see Frick et al., 2014a; Salekin, 2017).

Genetic and biological marker research has shown that severe conduct problems may have distinctive etiologies depending on the presence of general psychopathic traits, and specifically CU traits. It has been observed that genetic effects accounting for variation on CU traits ranged from 42 percent to 68 percent (e.g., Larsson, Andershed, & Lichtenstein, 2006). Coming back to the study of stability, it seems that it is largely due to genetic effects (e.g., Fontaine et al., 2010). What is even more relevant is the fact that, beyond the shared genetic effects that affect a large proportion of the correlation between psychopathic traits and conduct problems, there also seem to be unique genetic effects influencing the development of CU traits (e.g., Larsson et al., 2006). In addition, studies investigating the biological correlates to psychopathy have shown some psychophysiological correlates that support the blunted emotional reactivity to certain types of stimuli (e.g., emotionally evocative films, stimuli showing others in pain; e.g., de Wied, van Boxtel, Matthys, & Meeus, 2012). A consistent finding from functional imaging studies was the lower right amygdala activity in response to fearful faces, which is the opposite pattern to that observed in children with conduct problems but normative levels of psychopathic traits (Sebastian et al., 2012). Similarly, disruptions in the amygdala–prefrontal functional connectivity and abnormal responses within the ventromedial prefrontal cortex have been also revealed.

Prior research has also provided relevant information about the cognitive characteristics of children and adolescents showing psychopathic traits. As occurs with adult psychopathy, youth psychopathic personality has been related with deficits in the processing of punishment cues (e.g., Muñoz & Modecki, 2013). These youths have also showed problems in evaluating and distinguishing moral transgressions (i.e., actions defined by the consequences to others) versus conventional transgressions (i.e., actions defined by breaking social rules), with fewer references to the well-being of others when making this distinction (e.g., Dolan & Fullam, 2010). Related to this, they tend to show problems with altruistic behavior, being more likely to make decisions that benefit themselves, even if those actions affect and harm others. As expected, negative associations between psychopathic traits and empathy were also observed. However, this negative association is largely observed in affective empathy (i.e., experiencing negative emotions due to the harm of others), whereas cognitive empathy (i.e., the ability to take the perspective of others) does not seem to be affected in this group of youths, particularly after age 9 (Dadds et al., 2009). Also expected given the inherent characteristics of the construct, several emotional deficits have been related to the presence of psychopathic traits. Research findings have shown broad consistency in suggesting that children and adolescents with high levels of psychopathic traits are impaired in their responsiveness to and recognition of cues to fear and distress in others. However, this attenuated emotional responsiveness was improved when participants were instructed to attend to the person's eyes (Dadds et al., 2006).

Many efforts have also been focused on documenting the temperamental and personality correlates of child and youth psychopathic personality. The most consistent finding is that psychopathic traits, basically represented by CU traits, are associated with lower levels of fear (e.g., Barker, Oliver, Viding, Salekin, & Maughan, 2011), which in turn could be linked to some cognitive deficits (e.g., impaired punishment sensitivity), and with anxiety, especially when controlling for conduct problems (e.g., Pardini et al., 2012). In line with adult research, some authors considered that youth psychopathic personality is better conceptualized as an extreme version of a normal personality profile (e.g., Five Factor Model (FFM); see Lynam, 2010). Overall, psychopathic personality would be represented by a profile broadly characterized by low Agreeableness and Conscientiousness. However, there are some points of divergence with adult psychopathy, such as the less consistent pattern of association with Neuroticism. It has been explained from the complex pattern of differential associations of psychopathic traits to the specific facets within Neuroticism (e.g., positive association with angry hostility, and negative with anxiety), revealing the presence of potential suppressor effects when the associations with the general Neuroticism dimension are examined.

Finally, it is unlikely that genetics, biological, temperamental, and the associated neural structures completely explain the development of this specific pathway of psychopathic–problematic behavior. Given the relevance of family variables for developmental models of child and youth conduct problems, they were also the most analyzed environmental factors in the study of psychopathic personality. The most consistent finding was that psychopathic traits seem to moderate the association between family factors, largely represented by parenting practices, and conduct problems (e.g., Kroneman, Hipwell, Loeber, Koot, & Pardini, 2011). Even considering the vital role that parenting practices, as well as psychopathic traits, play in the development of severe problematic behavior, their influence does not seem to be additive (Wootton, Frick, Shelton, & Silverthorn, 1997). Specifically, negative parenting practices (i.e., harsh, inconsistent, and coercive discipline) have been traditionally related with child and youth conduct problems, but only in the group of children with low levels of psychopathic traits (Wootton et al., 1997). When high levels of psychopathic traits are manifested, the association between negative parenting and conduct problems tend to disappear, with some studies showing the negative influence of low positive parenting (i.e., low warmth, affection, communication; López-Romero, Romero, & Gómez-Fraguela, 2015; Waller, Gardner, & Hyde, 2013). An interesting result in this field is that when developmental models of psychopathic personality are delineated, dysfunctional parenting practices (i.e., inconsistent and coercive practices in addition to low warmth and acceptance) indeed emerge as relevant (e.g., Barker et al., 2011). However, this pattern of results has not been consistent across studies, revealing the presence of potential bidirectional effects, with the facets of parenting practices influencing the development of psychopathic traits different from those affected by psychopathic traits (e.g., Hawes, Dadds, Frost, & Hasking, 2011; Waller et al., 2014). Also, psychopathic traits seem to be related to disorganized attachment styles, with children with high levels of CU traits showing lower levels of physical and verbal affection and less eye contact with mothers in "emotional talk" situations (Dadds et al., 2006).

Taken together, all these results would partially support the presence of distinctive etiological underpinnings for children showing high levels of psychopathic traits. These correlates are consistent with those outlined in adult psychopathy and are contributing to the validity of the construct in youth populations. Notwithstanding this accumulative evidence regarding the potential role of psychopathic traits (or CU traits) in designating an etiologically distinctive subgroup, the malleability of their problematic behavior could be more compromised than their non-psychopathic counterparts since it seems to be more strongly associated with genetic and biological influences than with environmental factors (i.e., parenting practices). Indeed, many studies have reported that groups of youths high on psychopathic traits show poorer treatment outcomes in different settings (Frick et al., 2014a). Nevertheless, several recent studies have also revealed significant reductions of conduct problems in children high on psychopathic traits through some intensive interventions, which have been tailored to their unique features and needs. Even more encouragingly, it also seems that psychopathic traits, including CU traits, may show malleability and responsivity to some specific interventions, including those that promote positive changes in parenting practices (Wilkinson, Waller, & Viding, 2016).

Conclusion

Beyond the outlined controversies, such as the negative connotations related to the psychopathic construct or its applicability to young children and adolescents (Edens et al., 2001), there have been many efforts that have contributed to providing a broad justification of the study of psychopathic personality at early developmental stages. In a field with an ever-increasing interest, many research findings have supported the study of psychopathic personality in children and adolescents by evidencing reliability and coherence in factor structure; construct validity, principally based on association with other variables in a theoretically coherent manner; predictive value, particularly in identifying a specific subgroup of children and adolescents with a severe and persistent pattern of behavioral and psychosocial maladjustment; the presence of distinctive correlates, suggesting the presence of particular etiological mechanisms; temporal stability and, even more importantly, the presence of patterns of change, delineating some factors that may be influencing both of them; and the potentially distinctive response to treatment and intervention efforts. Given that youths with high levels of conduct problems and psychopathic traits – a small group of problematic youths – are likely to engage in serious and persistent forms of antisocial and criminal behavior and account for a large proportion of serious offenses, they should primarily be placed in intensive preventive and intervention programs. To maximize results, these programs should be tailored to the unique characteristics that define this specific group (e.g., remorseless, manipulation) and should include those factors that have been proven to be potential mechanisms of change in psychopathic personality (e.g., positive parenting). Although there have been great advances in this field, as well as some promising proposals in terms of intervention with children and adolescents high on psychopathic traits, much more research is definitely required.

References

American Psychiatric Association. (1980) *Diagnostic and statistical manual of mental disorders* (3rd ed.), Washington, DC: American Psychiatric Association.

American Psychiatric Association. (2013) *Diagnostic and statistical manual of mental disorders* (5th ed.), Washington, DC: American Psychiatric Association.

Andershed, H. (2010) 'Stability and change of psychopathic traits: What do we know?,' in R. T. Salekin & D. T. Lynam (Eds.), *Handbook of child and adolescent psychopathy* (pp. 233–250), New York, NY: The Guilford Press.

Andershed, H., Kerr, M., Stattin, H., and Levander, S. (2002) 'Psychopathic traits in non-referred youths: A new assessment tool,' in E. Blaauw & L. Sheridan (Eds.), *Psychopaths: Current international perspectives* (pp. 131–158), The Hague: Elsevier.

Andershed, H., Köhler, D., Eno Louden, J., and Hinrichs, G. (2008) 'Does the three-factor model of psychopathy identify a problematic subgroup of young offenders?,' *International Journal of Law and Psychiatry, 31*:189–198.

Asscher, J. J., van Vugt, E. D., Stams, G. J., Dekovic, M., Eichelsheim, V. I., and Yousfi, S. (2011) 'The relationship between juvenile psychopathic traits, delinquency, and (violent) recidivism: A meta-analysis,' *Journal of Child Psychology and Psychiatry, 52*:1134–1143.

Baardewijk, Y. V., Vermeiren, R., Stegge, H., and Doreleijers, T. (2011) 'Self-reported psychopathic traits in children: Their stability and concurrent and prospective association with conduct problems and aggression,' *Journal of Psychopathology and Behavioral Assessment, 33*:236–245.

Baker, K. (2013) 'Conduct disorders in children and adolescents,' *Pediatrics & Child Health, 23*:24–29.

Barker, E. D., Oliver, B. R., Viding, E., Salekin, R. T., and Maughan, B. (2011) 'The impact of prenatal maternal risk, fearless temperament and early parenting on adolescent callous–unemotional traits: A 14-year longitudinal investigation,' *Journal of Child Psychology & Psychiatry, 52*:878–888.

Barry, T. D., Barry, C. T., Deming, A. M., and Lochman, J. E. (2008) 'Stability of psychopathic characteristics in childhood: The influence of social relationship,' *Criminal Justice and Behavior, 35*:244–262.

Burke, J. D., Waldman, I., and Lahey, B. B. (2010) 'Predictive validity of childhood oppositional deviant disorder and conduct disorder: Implications for DSM–V,' *Journal of Abnormal Psychology, 119*:739–751.

Byrd, A. L., Loeber, R., and Pardini, D. A. (2012) 'Understanding desisting and persisting forms of delinquency: The unique contributions of disruptive behavior disorders and interpersonal callousness,' *Journal of Child Psychology & Psychiatry, 53*:371–380.

Cale, J., Lussier, P., McCuish, E., and Corrado, R. (2015) 'The prevalence of psychopathic personality disturbances among incarcerated youth: Comparing serious, chronic, violent and sex offenders,' *Journal of Criminal Justice, 43*:337–344.

Carroll, A., Houghton, S., Durkin, K., and Hattie, J. A. (2009) 'Psychopathy in children and adolescents and the fledgling psychopath hypothesis,' in A. Carroll, S. Houghton, K. Durkin, & J. A. Hattie (Eds.), *Adolescent reputations and risk: Developmental trajectories to delinquency* (pp. 119–138), New York, NY: Springer.

Ciucci, E., Baroncelli, A., Franchi, M., Golmaryami, F. N., and Frick, P. (2014) 'The association between callous–unemotional traits and behavioral and academic adjustment in children: Further validation of the Inventory of Callous–Unemotional traits,' *Journal of Psychopathology and Behavioral Assessment, 36*:189–200.

Cleckley, H. (1976) *The mask of sanity* (5th ed.), St. Louis, MO: Mosby. (First published in 1941).

Colins, O. F., and Andershed, H. (2015) 'The DSM–5 with limited prosocial emotions specifier for conduct disorder among detained girls,' *Law & Human Behavior, 39*:198–207.

Colins, O. F., Andershed, H., Frogner, L., López-Romero, L., Veen, V., and Andershed, A. K. (2014) 'A new measure to assess psychopathic personality in children: The Child Problematic Traits Inventory,' *Journal of Psychopathology and Behavioral Assessment, 36*:4–21.

Colins, O. F., Vermeiren, R., De Bolle, M., and Broekaert, E. (2012) 'Self-reported psychopathic-like traits as predictors of recidivism in detained male adolescents,' *Criminal Justice and Behavior, 39*:1421–1435.

Cooke, D. J., and Michie, C. (2001) 'Refining the construct of psychopathy: Towards a hierarchical model,' *Psychological Assessment, 13*:171–188.

Corrado, R. R., DeLisi, M., Hart, S. D., and McCuish, E. C. (2015) 'Can the causal mechanisms underlying chronic, serious, and violent offending trajectories be elucidated using the psychopathic construct?,' *Journal of Criminal Justice, 43*:251–261.

Corrado, R. R., McCuish, E. C., Hart, S. D., and DeLisi, M. (2015) 'The role of psychopathic traits and developmental risk factors on offending trajectories from early adolescence to adulthood: A prospective study of incarcerated youth,' *Journal of Criminal Justice, 43*:357–368.

Dadds, M. R., Hawes, D. J., Frost, A. D. J., Vasallo, S., Bunn, P. B., Hunter, K., and Merz, S. (2009) 'Learning to "talk the talk": The relationship of psychopathic traits to deficits in empathy across childhood,' *Journal of Child Psychology & Psychiatry, 50*:599–606.

Dadds, M. R., Perry, Y., Hawes, D. J., Merz, S., Riddell, A. C., Haines, D. J., . . . Abeygunawardane, A. I. (2006) 'Attention to the eyes reverses fear-recognition deficits in child psychopathy,' *The British Journal of Psychiatry, 189*:280–281.

DeLisi, M. (2016) *Psychopathy as unified theory of crime*, New York, NY: Palgrave Macmillan.

DeLisi, M., Dansby, T., Peters, D. J., Vaughn, M. G., Shook, J. J., and Hochstetler, A. (2014) 'Fledging psychopathy features and pathological delinquency: New evidence,' *American Journal of Criminal Justice, 39*:411–424.

DeLisi, M., and Piquero, A. R. (2011) 'New frontiers in criminal careers research, 2000–2011: A state-of-the-art review,' *Journal of Criminal Justice, 39*:289–301.

De Wied, M., van Boxtel, A., Matthys, W., and Meeus, W. (2012) 'Verbal, facial and autonomic responses to empathy-eliciting film clips by disruptive male adolescents with versus low callous–unemotional traits,' *Journal of Abnormal Child Psychology, 40*:211–223.

Dolan, M. C., and Fullam, R. S. (2010) 'Moral/conventional transgression distinction and psychopathy in conduct disordered adolescents,' *Personality & Individual Differences, 49*:995–1000.

Edens, J. F., Skeem, J. L., Cruise, K. R., and Cauffman, E. (2001) 'Assessment of "juvenile psychopathy" and its association with violence: A critical review,' *Behavioral Sciences & the Law, 19*:53–80.

Eisenbarth, H., Demetriou, C. A., Kyranides, M. N., and Fanti, K. A. (2016) 'Stability subtypes of callous–unemotional traits and conduct disorder symptoms and their correlates,' *Journal of Youth and Adolescence, 45*:1889–1901.

Essau, C. A., Sasagawa, S., and Frick, P. (2006) 'Callous–unemotional traits in a community sample of adolescents,' *Assessment, 20*:1–16.

Ezpeleta, L., de la Osa, N., Granero, R., Penelo, E., and Domènech, J. M. (2013) 'Inventory of Callous–Unemotional traits in a community sample of preschoolers,' *Journal of Clinical Child & Adolescent Psychology, 42*:91–105.

Fanti, K. A., Frick, P. J., and Georgiou, S. (2009) 'Linking callous–unemotional traits to instrumental and non-instrumental forms of aggression,' *Journal of Psychopathology and Behavioral Assessment, 31*:285–298.

Fanti, K. A., Colins, O. F., Andershed, H., and Sikki, M. (2017) 'Stability and change in callous–unemotional traits: Longitudinal associations with potential individual and contextual risk and protective factors,' *American Journal of Orthopsychiatry, 87*:62–75.

Flexon, J. L., and Meldrum, R. C. (2013) 'Adolescent psychopathic traits and violent delinquency: Additive and nonadditive effects with key criminological variables,' *Youth Violence & Juvenile Justice, 11*:349–369.

Fontaine N. M. G., McCrory E. J., Boivin M., Moffitt T. E., and Viding E. (2011) 'Predictors and outcomes of joint trajectories of callous–unemotional traits and conduct problems in childhood,' *Journal of Abnormal Psychology, 120*:730–742.

Fontaine, N. M. G., Rijsdijk, F. V., McCrory, E. J. P., and Viding, E. (2010) 'Etiology of different developmental trajectories of callous–unemotional traits,' *Journal of the American Academy of Child and Adolescent Psychiatry, 49*:656–664.

Forth, A. E., Kosson, D. S., and Hare, R. D. (2003) *The Psychopathy Checklist: Youth Version manual*, Toronto, ON: Multi-Health Systems.

Frick, P. J. (2004) *Inventory of Callous–Unemotional traits*, Unpublished rating scale, New Orleans, LA: University of New Orleans.

Frick, P. J., Bodin, D. S., and Barry, C. T. (2000) 'Psychopathic traits and conduct problems in community and clinic-referred simples of children: Further development of the Psychopathy Screening Device,' *Psychological Assessment, 12*:382–393.

Frick, P. J., and Hare, R. D. (2001) *Antisocial process screening device*, Toronto, ON: Multi-Health System.

Frick, P. J., Kimonis, E. R., Dandreaux, D. M., and Farell, J. M. (2003) 'The 4-year stability of psychopathic traits in non-referred youth,' *Behavioral Sciences and the Law, 21*:713–736.

Frick, P. J., O'Brien, B. S., Wootton, J. M., and McBurnett, K. (1994) 'Psychopathy and conduct problems in children,' *Journal of Abnormal Psychology, 103*:54–58.

Frick, P. J., Ray, J. V., Thornton, L. C., and Kahn, R. E. (2014a) 'Can callous–unemotional traits enhance the understanding, diagnosis, and treatment of serious conduct problems in children and adolescents? A comprehensive review,' *Psychological Bulletin, 40*:1–57.

Frick, P. J., Ray, J. V., Thornton, L. C., and Kahn, R. E. (2014b) 'A developmental psychopathology approach to understanding callous–unemotional traits in children and adolescents with serious conduct problems,' *The Journal of Child Psychology & Psychiatry, 55*:532–548.

Frick, P. J., and Ray, J. V. (2015) 'Evaluating callous–unemotional traits as a personality construct,' *Journal of Personality, 83*:710–722.

Frogner, L., Gibson, C. L., Andershed, A. K., and Andershed, H. (2016) 'Childhood psychopathic personality and callous–unemotional traits in the prediction of conduct problems,' *American Journal of Orthopsychiatry*, in press.

Gretton, H. M., Hare, R. D., and Catchpole, R. E. (2004) 'Psychopathy and offending from adolescence to adulthood: A 10-year follow-up,' *Journal of Consulting and Clinical Psychology*, *72*:636–645.
Hare, R. D. (2003) *The Hare Psychopathy Checklist–Revised* (2nd ed.), Toronto, ON: Multi-Health Systems.
Hare, R. D., and Neumann, C. S. (2008) 'Psychopathy as a clinical and empirical construct,' *Annual Review of Clinical Psychology*, *4*:217–246.
Hare, R. D., and Neumann, C. S. (2010) 'The role of antisociality in the psychopathic construct: Comment on Skeem and Cooke (2010),' *Psychological Assessment*, *22*:446–454.
Harris, G. T., and Rice, M. E. (2006) 'Treatment of psychopathy: A review of empirical findings,' in C. Patrick (Ed.), *Handbook of psychopathy* (pp. 555–572), New York, NY: Guildford Press.
Hawes, D. J., Byrd, A. L., Henderson, C. E., Gazda, R. L., Burke, J. D., Loeber, R., and Pardini, D. A. (2014) 'Refining parent-reported Inventory of Callous–Unemotional traits in boys with conduct problems,' *Psychological Assessment*, *26*:256–266.
Hawes, S. W., Byrd, A. L., Waller, R., Lynam, D. R., and Pardini, D. A. (2017) 'Late childhood interpersonal callousness and conduct problem trajectories interact to predict adult psychopathy,' *Journal of Child Psychology and Psychiatry*, *58*:55–63.
Hawes, D. J., Dadds, M., Frost, A. D. J., and Hasking, P. A. (2011) 'Do childhood callous–unemotional traits drive change in parenting practices,' *Journal of Clinical Child & Adolescent Psychology*, *40*:507–518.
Kahn, R. E., Frick, P. J., Youngstrom, E., Findling, R. L., and Youngstrom, J. K. (2012) 'The effects of including a callous–unemotional specifier for the diagnosis of conduct disorder,' *The Journal of Child Psychology & Psychiatry*, *53*:271–282.
Karpman, B. (1949) 'The psychopathic delinquent child,' *American Journal of Orthopsychiatry*, *20*:223–265.
Karpman, B. (1950) 'Psychopathic behavior in infants and children: A critical survey of the existing concepts,' *American Journal of Orthopsychiatry*, *21*:223–272.
Kimonis, E. R., Frick, P. J., Skeem, J. L., Marsee, M. A., Cruise, K., Muñoz, L. C., . . . Morris, A. D. (2008) 'Assessing callous–unemotional traits in adolescent offenders: Validation of the Inventory of Callous–Unemotional traits,' *International Journal of Law & Psychiatry*, *31*:241–252.
Klingzell, I., Fanti, K. A., Colins, O. F., Frogner, L., Andershed, A. K., and Andershed, H. (2016) 'Early childhood trajectories of conduct problems and callous–unemotional traits: The role of fearlessness and psychopathic personality dimensions,' *Child Psychiatry and Human Development*, *47*:236–247.
Kroneman, L. M., Hipwell, A. E., Loeber, R., Koot, H. M., and Pardini, D. A. (2011) 'Contextual risk factors as predictors of disruptive behavior disorder trajectories in girls: The moderating effect of callous–unemotional features,' *Journal of Child Psychology & Psychiatry*, *52*:167–175
Kumsta, R., Sonuga-Barke, E., and Rutter, M. (2012) 'Adolescent callous–unemotional traits and conduct disorder in adoptees exposed to severe early deprivation,' *The British Journal of Psychiatry*, *200*:197–201.
Larsson, H., Andershed, H., and Lichtenstein, P. (2006) 'A genetic factor explains most of the variation in the psychopathic personality,' *Journal of Abnormal Psychology*, *115*:221–230.
Leitisco, A. R., Salekin, R. T., DeCoster, J., and Rogers, R. (2008) 'A large-scale meta-analysis relating the Hare measures of psychopathy to antisocial construct,' *Law & Human Behavior*, *32*:28–45.
Loeber, R., Pardini, D. A., Hipwell, A., Stouthamer-Loeber, M., Keenan, K., and Sembower, M. A. (2009) 'Are there stable factors in preadolescent girls' externalizing behaviors?,' *Journal of Abnormal Child Psychology*, *37*:777–791.
López-Romero, L., Gómez-Fraguela, J. A., and Romero, E. (2015) 'Assessing callous–unemotional traits in a Spanish sample of institutionalized youths: The Inventory of Callous–Unemotional traits,' *Journal of Psychopathology and Behavioral Assessment*, *37*:392–406.
López-Romero, L., Romero, E., and Andershed, H. (2015) 'Conduct problems in childhood and adolescence: Developmental trajectories, predictors and outcomes in a six-year follow-up,' *Child Psychiatry & Human Development*, 46:762–773.
López-Romero, L., Romero, E., and Gómez-Fraguela, J. A. (2015) 'Delving into callous–unemotional traits: Concurrent correlates and early parenting precursors,' *Journal of Child & Family Studies*, *24*:1451–1468.
López-Romero, L., Romero, E., and Luengo, M. A. (2012) 'Disentangling the role of psychopathic traits and externalizing behaviour in predicting conduct problems from childhood to adolescence,' *Journal of Youth & Adolescence*, *41*:1397–1408.
López-Romero, L., Romero, E., and Villar, P. (2012) 'Relaciones entre estilos educativos parentales y rasgos psicopáticos en la infancia,' *Psicología Conductual*, *20*:603–623.
López-Romero, L., Romero, E., and Villar, P. (2017) 'Developmental trajectories of youth conduct problems: Testing later development and related outcomes in a 12-year period,' *Child Psychiatry and Human Development*, *48*:619–631.

Longman, T., Hawes, D. J., and Kohlhoff, J. (2016) 'Callous–unemotional traits as markers for conduct problem severity in early childhood: A meta-analysis,' *Child Psychiatry & Human Development, 47*:326–334.

Lynam, D. R. (1996) 'The early identification of chronic offenders: Who is the fledgling psychopath?,' *Psychological Bulletin, 120*:209–234.

Lynam, D. R. (1997) 'Pursuing the psychopath: Capturing the fledgling psychopath in a nomological net,' *Journal of Abnormal Psychology, 106*:425–438.

Lynam, D. R. (2010) 'Child and adolescent psychopathy and personality,' in R. T. Salekin & D. T. Lynam (Eds.), *Handbook of child and adolescent psychopathy* (pp. 179–201), New York, NY: Guilford.

Lynam, D. R., Caspi, A., Moffitt, T. E., Loeber, R., and Stouthamer-Loeber, M. (2007) 'Longitudinal evidence that psychopathy scores in early adolescence predict adult psychopathy,' *Journal of Abnormal Psychology, 116*:155–165.

Lynam, D. R., Charnigo, R., Moffitt, T. E., Raine, A., Loeber, R., and Stouthamer-Loeber, M. (2009) 'The stability of psychopathy across adolescence,' *Development and Psychopathology, 21*:1133–1153.

McCord, W., and McCord, J. (1964) *The psychopath: An essay on the criminal man*, Princeton, NJ: Van Nostrand.

McCrae, R. R., Costa, P. T., Terracciano, A., Parker, W. D., Mills, C. J., De Fruyt, F., and Mervielde, I. (2002) 'Personality trait development from age 12 to age 18: Longitudinal, cross-sectional, and cross-cultural analyses,' *Journal of Personality and Social Psychology, 83*:1456–1468.

McCuish, E. C., Corrado, R., Hart, S. D., and DeLisi, M. (2015) 'The role of symptoms of psychopathy in persistent violence over the criminal career into full adulthood,' *Journal of Criminal Justice, 43*:345–356.

McCuish, E. C., Corrado, R., Lussier, P., and Hart, S. D. (2014) 'Psychopathic traits and offending trajectories from early adolescence to adulthood,' *Journal of Criminal Justice, 42*:66–76.

McMahon, R. J., Witkiewitz, K., and Kotler, J. S. (2010) 'Predictive validity of callous–unemotional traits measured in early adolescence with respect to multiple antisocial outcomes,' *Journal of Abnormal Psychology, 119*:752–763.

Michonski, J. D., and Sharp, C. (2010) 'Revisiting Lynam's notion of the "fledgling psychopath": Are HIA-CP children truly psychopathic-like?,' *Child and Adolescent Psychiatry & Mental Health, 4*:1–9.

Moffitt, T. E. (1993) 'Adolescence-limited and life-course-persistent antisocial behavior. A developmental taxonomy,' *Psychological Review, 100*:674–701.

Muñoz, L. C., and Frick, P. J. (2007) 'The reliability, stability, and predictive utility of the self-report version of the Antisocial Process Screening Device,' *Scandinavian Journal of Psychology, 48*:299–312.

Muñoz, L. C., and Modecki, K. (2013) 'Throwing caution to the wind: Callous–unemotional traits and risk taking in adolescents,' *Journal of Clinical Child & Adolescent Psychology, 42*:106–119.

Murrie, D. C., Boccaccini, M. T., McCoy, W., and Cornell, D. G. (2007) 'Diagnostic labeling in juvenile court: How do descriptions of psychopathy and conduct disorder influence judges?,' *Journal of Clinical Child and Adolescents Psychology, 36*:228–241.

Nagin, D. S., and Tremblay, R. (1999) 'Trajectories of boys' physical aggression, opposition, and hyperactivity on the path to physically violent and nonviolent juvenile delinquency,' *Child Development, 70*:1181–1196.

Neumann, C. S., Hare, R. D., and Pardini, D. A. (2015) 'Antisociality and the construct of psychopathy: Data from across the globe,' *Journal of Personality, 83*:678–692.

Obradović, J., Pardini, D. A., Long, J. D., and Loeber, R. (2007) 'Measuring interpersonal callousness in boys from childhood to adolescence: An examination of longitudinal invariance and temporal stability,' *Journal of Clinical Child and Adolescent Psychology, 36*:276–292.

Patrick, C. (2010) 'Conceptualizing the psychopathic personality: Disinhibited, bold, ... or just plain mean?,' in R. T. Salekin & D. T. Lynam (Eds.), *Handbook of child and adolescent psychopathy* (pp. 15–48), New York, NY: Guilford.

Pardini, D. A., and Loeber, R. (2008) 'Interpersonal callousness trajectories across adolescence: Early social influences and adult outcomes,' *Criminal Justice and Behavior, 35*:173–196.

Pardini, D. A., Stepp, S., Hipwell, A., Stouthamer-Loeber, M., and Loeber, R. (2012) 'The clinical utility of the propose DSM-5 callous-unemotional subtype of conduct disorder in young girls,' *Journal of the American Academy of Child & Adolescent Psychiatry, 51*:62–73.

Pechorro, P., Gonçalves, R. A., Maroco, J., Nunes, C., and Jesus, S. N. (2014) 'Age of crime onset and psychopathic traits in female juvenile delinquents,' *International Journal of Offender Therapy and Comparative Criminology, 58*:1101–1119.

Piquero, A. R., Farrington, D. P., Fontaine, N. M., Vincent, G., Coid, J., and Ullrich, S. (2012) 'Childhood risk, offending trajectories, and psychopathy at age 48 years in the Cambridge Study in Delinquent Development,' *Psychology, Public Policy, and Law, 18*:577–598.

Quay, H. C. (1964) 'Dimensions of personality in delinquent boys as inferred from factor analysis of case history data,' *Child Development*, *35*:479–484.
Reidy, D. E., Kearns, M. C., DeGue, S., Lilienfeld, S. O., Massetti, G., and Kiehl, K. A. (2015) 'Why psychopathy matters: Implications for public health and violence prevention,' *Aggression and Violent Behavior*, *24*:214–225.
Rowe, R. (2014) 'Integrating callous and unemotional traits into the definition of antisocial behavior – a commentary on Frick et al. (2014),' *Journal of Child Psychology & Psychiatry*, *55*:549–552.
Rowe, R., Maughan, B., Moran, P., Ford, T., Briskman, J., and Goodman, R. (2010) 'The role of callous–unemotional traits in the diagnosis of conduct disorder,' *Journal of Child Psychology & Psychiatry*, *51*:688–695.
Rutter, M. (2012) 'Psychopathy in childhood: Is it a meaningful diagnosis,' *The British Journal of Psychiatry*, *200*:175–176.
Salekin, R. T. (2008) 'Psychopathy and recidivism from mid-adolescence to young adulthood: Cumulating legal problems and limiting life opportunities,' *Journal of Abnormal Psychology*, *117*:386–395.
Salekin, R. T. (2016a) 'Psychopathy in childhood: Toward better informing the DSM-5 and ICD-11 conduct disorder specifiers,' *Personality Disorders: Theory, research, and treatment*, 7:180–191.
Salekin, R. T. (2016b) 'Psychopathy in childhood: Why should we care about grandiose–manipulative and daring–impulsive traits?,' *The British Journal of Psychiatry*, *209*:189–191.
Salekin, R. T. (2017) 'What do we know about psychopathic traits in children?,' *The Journal of Child Psychology and Psychiatry*, in press.
Salihovic, S., Özdemir, M., and Kerr, M. (2014) 'Trajectories of adolescent psychopathic traits,' *Journal of Psychopathology and Behavioral Assessment*, *36*:47–59.
Sebastian, C. L., McCrory, E. J. P., Cecil, C. A. M., Lockwood, P. L., De Brito, S. A., Fontaine, N. M. G., and Viding, E. (2012) 'Neural responses to affective and cognitive theory of mind in children with conduct problems and varying levels of callous–unemotional traits,' *Archives of General Psychiatry*, *69*:814–822.
Skeem, J. L., and Cooke, D. J. (2010a) 'Is criminal behavior a central component of psychopathy? Conceptual directions for resolving the debate,' *Psychological Assessment*, *22*:433–445.
Skeem, J. L., and Cooke, D. J. (2010b) 'One measure does not a construct make: Directions toward reinvigorating psychopathy research: Reply to Hare and Neumann (2010),' *Psychological Assessment*, *22*:455–459.
Skeem, J. L., Polaschek, D. L. L., Patrick, C. J., and Lilienfeld, S. O. (2011) 'Psychopathic personality: Bridging the gap between scientific evidence and public policy,' *Psychological Science in the Public Interest*, *12*:95–161.
Svecke, K., and Kosson, D. S. (2010) 'Relationships of child and adolescent psychopathy to other forms of psychopathology,' in R. T. Salekin & D. T. Lynam (Eds.), *Handbook of child and adolescent psychopathy* (pp. 284–316), New York, NY: The Guilford Press.
Thomas, C. R. (2010) 'Oppositional defiant and conduct disorder,' in M. K. Dulcan (Ed.), *Dulcan's textbook of child and adolescent psychiatry* (pp. 223–239), Arlington, TX: American Psychiatric Publishing.
Vaughn, M. G., Howard, M. O., and DeLisi, M. (2008) 'Psychopathic personality traits and delinquent careers: An empirical examination,' *International Journal of Law & Psychiatry*, *31*:407–416.
Vincent, G. M., Vitacco, M. J., Grisso, T., and Corrado, R. R. (2003) 'Subtypes of adolescent offenders: Affective traits and antisocial behavior patterns,' *Behavioral Sciences & The Law*, *21*:695–712.
Waller, R., Gardner, F., and Hyde, L. W. (2013) 'What are the associations between parenting, callous–unemotional traits and antisocial behavior in youth? A systematic review of evidence,' *Clinical Psychology Review*, *33*:593–608.
Waller, R., Gardner, F., Viding, E., Shaw, D. S., Dishion, T. J., Wilson, M. N., and Hyde, L. W. (2014) 'Bidirectional associations between parental warmth, callous unemotional behavior, and behavior problems in high-risk preschoolers,' *Journal of Abnormal Child Psychology*, *42*:1275–1285.
Wilkinson, S., Waller, R., and Viding, E. (2016) 'Involving young people with callous–unemotional traits in treatment – does it work? A systematic review,' *Journal of Child Psychology and Psychiatry*, *57*:552–565.
Willoughby, M. T., Waschbusch, D. A., Moore, G. A., and Propper, C. B. (2011) 'Using the ASEBA to screen for callous–unemotional traits in early childhood: Factor structure, temporal stability, and utility,' *Journal of Psychopathology and Behavioral Assessment*, *33*:19–30.
Wootton, J. M., Frick, P. J., Shelton, K. K., and Silverthorn, P. (1997) 'Ineffective parenting and childhood conduct problems: The moderating role of callous–unemotional traits,' *Journal of Consulting & Clinical Psychology*, *65*:301–308.

29

Psychopathy and offending trajectories

Evan McCuish

Introduction

Within forensic psychology, psychopathic personality disturbance (PPD)[1] is considered one of the most important individual-level predictors of offending (e.g., Hare, 1998; Hart, 1998). Despite its potential importance to developmental and life course (DLC) research (Farrington, 2005) and explanations of persistent patterns of offending (Corrado, DeLisi, Hart, & McCuish, 2015), the construct has received far less attention within criminology. The lack of research using PPD to help explain offending trajectories is understandable given that the construct is not explicitly included in mainstream criminological theories (Corrado, 2012). Further, like the Lombrosian impact on criminologists' tendency to avoid biological explanations of criminal behavior (Rafter, Posick, & Rocque, 2016), the politically driven incorporation of PPD within criminological discourse in the early 1900s, such as its use to promote the eugenics movement, perhaps dissuaded contemporary criminologists from more fully examining this construct (see Rafter, 1997).

More recently, perspectives have changed, with an emphasis on treatment-oriented responses to adolescents with PPD (e.g., Caldwell, Skeem, Salekin, & van Rybroek, 2006) combined with cautions about using the disorder to justify implementing lengthy sentences to youth (cf., Davidson, 2015; Edens, Skeem, Cruise, & Cauffman, 2001). This changing perspective may have helped reshape criminological interest in the disorder. Indeed, Farrington (2005) has since called for greater integration of PPD within DLC criminology, DeLisi and Piquero (2011) called for the integration of PPD into explanations of criminal career parameters, including offending trajectories, Fox, Jennings, and Farrington (2015) suggested that PPD be integrated within core DLC theoretical perspectives, and DeLisi (2009, 2016) suggested that PPD was the unified theory of crime.

Despite renewed interest, attention to the construct has been principally conceptual. The lack of empirical research integrating PPD within, for example, a DLC framework, is at least in part due to intensive data requirements. Measurement of PPD is expensive and time-consuming, especially when using expert rating scales (Dawson, McCuish, Hart, & Corrado, 2012). Moreover, to integrate the construct into studies addressing DLC and criminal career questions, multiple years of offending data are typically required to model offending trajectories across different developmental stages. Thus far, just three studies have empirically examined the relationship between PPD and offending trajectories: the Cambridge Study on Delinquent Development (CSDD), the Pathways to Desistance Study (PDS), and the Incarcerated Serious and Violent Young Offender Study (ISVYOS).

This chapter is divided into three sections to discuss: (1) conceptual arguments, and the methodological requirements to address these arguments, concerning the relationship between PPD and offending trajectories; (2) the contributions of the CSDD, PDS, and ISVYOS to research on PPD and offending trajectories; and (3) directions for future research regarding PPD and the longitudinal development of offending.

Conceptual description of the link between PPD and offending trajectories

Defining PPD, moving from conceptualization to operationalization, and evaluating the psychometric properties of measurement tools are critical steps before testing theoretical assertions regarding the relationship between PPD and offending trajectories. Because these three themes are discussed elsewhere in this volume, despite their importance they are not covered here. In outlining the relationship between PPD and offending, three questions are considered: (1) does PPD explain general offending, or is it more appropriate to describe the relationship between PPD and specific offending patterns; (2) in what ways do symptoms of the disorder influence involvement in criminal behavior; and (3) in what ways do symptoms of the disorder decrease the likelihood of desistance from crime over the life course?

The offending outcomes of individuals with PPD

In considering the relationship between PPD and offending outcomes, the principles of sensitivity and specificity should be considered. In this context, sensitivity refers to whether the offending outcome under examination is common to individuals characterized by PPD. Specificity refers to whether the offending outcome under examination is atypical for individuals not characterized by the disorder. With respect to sensitivity, as initially noted by Vaughn and DeLisi (2008; DeLisi & Piquero, 2011), that the prevalence of chronic offending overlapped with the prevalence of PPD was not a coincidence. Rather, the group of chronic offenders identified in cohort studies (e.g., Wolfgang, Figlio, & Sellin, 1972) and the group characterized by PPD were asserted to be comprised of the same individuals. Similarly, Corrado, DeLisi, et al. (2015) suggested that the prevalence of low self-control was too high and the prevalence of chronic offending too low for the former to be sensitive to the latter. With respect to specificity, Corrado, DeLisi, et al. (2015) also noted that recidivism outcomes were too common and PPD too rare for the latter to fully capture variance in the former.

Very importantly, although the current chapter considers PPD an important explanatory variable in understanding the development of chronic, serious, and violent offending, it is not suggested that individuals with PPD are associated with a specific, discrete offending trajectory. Instead, the concept of a trajectory is used here as a heuristic device to help describe the hypothesized manner in which individuals with PPD meaningfully deviate from a continuously distributed pattern of chronic, serious, and/or violent offending that exists within the general offender population. The offending patterns of individuals with PPD are expected to differ quantitatively (e.g., more frequent) and qualitatively (e.g., more severe) from other offenders. Part of the reason for the expected impact of PPD on continued offending is that, unlike most risk factors that remain only distally related to an individual's likelihood of offending as they age (e.g., abuse, poor parental attachment), PPD is expected to remain relatively stable over the life course (e.g., Lynam, Caspi, Moffitt, Loeber, & Stouthamer-Loeber, 2007). PPD thus represents the type of proximal risk factor that is expected to have a continued effect on offending (Chung, Hill, Hawkins, Gilchrist, & Nagin, 2002). The specific mechanisms in which PPD influences criminal behavior are described next.

PPD and the causal mechanisms influencing criminal behavior

It is important that theoretical perspectives go beyond simply asserting that a construct predicts an outcome. Also needed is an explanation of the causal mechanisms that link the construct to the outcome (Wikstrom, 2006). Two important questions to address in specifying the association between PPD and chronic, serious, and violent offending are: (1) what explains involvement in offending for individuals with PPD and (2) why does offending for this group persist over the life course?

With respect to the first question, PPD is defined by a cluster of personality symptoms that cause functional impairment in a wide range of life domains, including interpersonal, affective, and behavioral functioning (e.g., Cooke, Michie, Hart, & Clark, 2004; Forth, Kosson, & Hare, 2003; Hare, 2003). Collectively, this clustering of symptoms is asserted to influence propensity for criminal behavior, create situational contexts conducive to criminal behavior, and fail to deter individuals from involvement in criminal behavior (McCuish, Corrado, Lussier, & Hart, 2015).

According to Wikstrom and Treiber (2009), propensity for criminal behavior is related to low self-control. Similarly, individuals with PPD are sensation seeking, disruptive, and reckless (e.g., Cooke, Hart, Logan, & Michie, 2012), and the disorder is thought to overlap in several ways with low self-control (e.g., Wiebe, 2003). Effectively, symptoms of the disorder are likely to make offending a particularly attractive form of behavior. Some (e.g., Hare, 2003) also consider criminal behavior to be part of the definition of the construct, and thus inherent to the diagnosis of PPD is a demonstration of propensity for criminal behavior.

With respect to the situational context component of offending (Wikstrom & Treiber, 2009), individuals with PPD are defined by interpersonal deficits that lead to a desire to dominate, manipulate, and antagonize others. This interaction style persists across different relationships and social contexts (e.g., work, family, peers, strangers). Individuals with PPD are also unreasonably suspicious, believe others are out to get them, are intolerant of others, and are emotionally unstable (Cooke et al., 2012; Forth et al., 2003; Hare, 2003). These features of PPD create situational contexts conducive to criminal behavior. The nature of these symptoms also implies that individuals are poorly equipped to cope in prosocial ways in response to even minor environmental stressors (e.g., through their inflexibility). In effect, whereas Wikstrom and Treiber (2009) suggested that some individuals required an external, threatening event to induce criminal behavior (e.g., being bumped in a bar, cut off in traffic), individuals with PPD are characterized by symptoms that, in and of themselves, create situational contexts conducive to offending. Indeed, individuals with PPD engage in violence rather indiscriminately (e.g., against strangers and persons known to them, against both men and women) and without provocation (Hart & Dempster, 1997; Serin, 1991).

With respect to Wikstrom and Treiber's (2009) deterrence component of criminal events, sensitivity to victim needs and the desire to not bring harm to others is unlikely given that emotional depth, caring, attachment, and empathy are lacking for individuals with PPD (Cooke et al., 2004). Due to being self-centered, it is also unlikely that individuals with PPD consider the impact of their behavior on others. Moreover, classic deterrence methods such as introducing a reasonable guardian may be less impactful for individuals with PPD given that they tend to be defined by a lack of impulsivity and forethought and see themselves as invulnerable and invincible (e.g., Cooke et al., 2004).

Taken together, individuals with PPD are defined by several personality traits that are conducive to involvement in offending. Although there are dozens of other risk factors that also help explain offending involvement, the stability of PPD can help explain why offending is likely to persist over the life course. Due to this stability, the types of life events that influence desistance for most offenders may be less likely to occur, or less likely to help, individuals with PPD.

PPD as a barrier to desistance

Desistance theories have been categorized into three distinct perspectives (e.g., Lussier, McCuish, & Corrado, 2015). The first considers cognitive transformation and changes in criminal identity that influence stake-in-conformity as the key mechanisms influencing desistance (e.g., Giordano, Cernkovich, & Rudolph, 2002; Maruna, 2001). In the second perspective, Cusson and Pinsonneault (1986) argued that desistance occurs when an offender concludes that the benefits of involvement in crime are outweighed by both formal and informal consequences (e.g., the rational choice perspective). The third perspective, based on the DLC framework, specifies the role of human development (e.g., Moffitt, 1993) and turning points (e.g., Sampson & Laub, 1993) in the desistance process. It is asserted here that regardless of the desistance perspective put forward, the nature of symptoms defining PPD are likely to disrupt the specific mechanisms that promote a movement away from criminal behavior.

Regarding the cognitive transformation perspective, because PPD is expected to remain stable over the life course (Lynam et al., 2007), prosocial identity shifts are less likely. Individuals with PPD are also likely to be actively resistant to change in identity given that cognitive inflexibility is a symptom (Cooke et al., 2004). Moreover, because individuals with PPD are intolerant of others, they are less likely to adopt changes in their identity that support affiliations with prosocial peers. Individuals with PPD have a sense of being special, unique, and superior to others and believe that they are entitled to special privileges. Indeed, Cooke et al. (2004) described an entire domain of PPD that was defined by negative identity traits. With this type of self-image, openness to change may be less likely.

With respect to rational choice perspectives, the formal and informal consequences that Cusson and Pinsonneault (1986) described as influencing desistance are less likely to affect change among individuals with PPD. Regarding formal consequences, because individuals with PPD are less sensitive to punishment (Lykken, 1995; Newman, MacCoon, Vaughn, & Sadeh, 2005), criminal justice system responses are less likely to influence the behavior of this group. As well, individuals with PPD may be less likely to consider the likelihood of formal punishment given that they are impulsive and lack planfulness (Cooke et al., 2004).

In terms of informal consequences, whereas the dangers or risks associated with criminal behavior may lead to desistance for some offenders, because individuals with PPD are sensation seeking (e.g., Forth et al., 2003), crimes with a heightened level of danger may attract, rather than detract, from the value of the crime event. Other informal consequences such as injury or death to co-offenders (Cusson & Pinsonneault, 1986) may be trivial for individuals with PPD given that they do not form intimate, meaningful attachments with others (Cooke et al., 2004). Finally, given the tendency of individuals with PPD to lack perseverance (Cooke et al., 2004), the level of effort necessary to capitalize on non-criminal opportunities may be too high to justify a change in behavior. Because there is relatively little skill involved in most forms of offending (Lochner, 2004), the amount of time spent pursuing offending opportunities will be shorter and more rewarding.

From a developmental (e.g., Moffitt, 1993) and life course (Sampson & Laub, 1993) perspective, desistance is best explained as a process whereby offenders bridge the maturity gap between adolescence and adulthood and begin to assume roles that discourage involvement in offending (e.g., employee, spouse, parent). Assumption of these roles increases the stakes that come with offending (Giordano et al., 2002) and reduces an individual's level of unstructured time that could have been allocated to criminal behavior (Warr, 1998). Due to selection effects, the assumption of these roles is (1) less likely to occur for more frequent offenders (Blokland & Nieuwbeerta, 2005) and (2) less likely to have a positive impact on the offending patterns of certain offenders (Sweeten, Piquero, & Steinberg, 2013). Individuals with PPD may be especially prone to these selection effects.

With respect to employment, individuals with PPD lack concentration, perseverance, and long-term goals and therefore should be less likely to find, maintain, and value employment in a manner that facilitates desistance. This level of commitment is unlikely for individuals characterized by PPD. Similarly, because individuals with PPD are uncaring, detached, uncommitted, self-centered, self-entitled, self-justifying, and disinterested in the well-being of others (Cooke et al., 2004), relationships, whether with peers, romantic partners, or children, are likely to be superficial and based on the extent to which the individual with PPD can manipulate the relationship for their own benefit. Whether in reference to employment, marriage, or parenthood, maintaining sources of informal social control requires commitment, caring, empathy, prosocial happiness, and loyalty, all of which are typically lacking among individuals with PPD (Cooke et al., 2004).

Overall, offending patterns defined by persistent involvement in chronic, serious, or violent offending provide the sensitivity and specificity needed in developing a theory concerning PPD and offending. Symptoms associated with PPD are asserted to increase propensity for offending, decrease responsiveness to deterrence strategies, and create situational contexts conducive to offending. Whereas the bulk of high rate adolescent offenders nevertheless desist during adulthood (McCuish, Corrado, Lussier, & Hart, 2014), desistance is less likely for individuals with PPD because symptoms associated with the disorder are expected to act as barriers to desistance mechanisms such as sources of informal social control. When such mechanisms do occur, individuals with PPD are less likely to benefit in a way that promotes desistance. Empirical research that addresses the relationship between PPD and offending trajectories is considered next.

What do we know about PPD and offending trajectories?

Unlike other offending outcomes, where age is often controlled for, a key feature of offending trajectories is that age forms one half of the definition of the offending outcome (Nagin, 2005). Nagin and Land's (1993) initial description and demonstration of semiparametric group-based modeling (SPGM), followed by the creation of statistical packages such as Proc Traj (Jones & Nagin, 2007), helped initiate over a hundred studies on offending trajectories, including trajectories specific to different crime types (e.g., violent offending, sexual offending) and within a wide range of samples (for reviews, see Piquero, 2008; Jennings & Reingle, 2012). Although much was learned from these studies about the developmental course of offending, identifying adolescent risk factors informative of life course persistent offending remained elusive (e.g., Sampson & Laub, 2005; van der Geest, Blokland, & Bijleveld, 2009). For some, this observation suggested that adolescent risk factors were simply uninformative of such an offending pattern (e.g., Sampson & Laub, 2005). Such claims, however, were made prior to research examining offending trajectories and PPD.

The lack of research using PPD to predict involvement in a more chronic, serious, or violent offending trajectory is not unexpected. PPD is more typically assessed in a forensic context in which recidivism, rather than longitudinal patterns of offending, is of principal concern. On the other hand, most longitudinal studies within criminology sampled from community-based populations (DeLisi, 2001) and were initiated prior to the development of validated measures of PPD. As well, research on offending trajectories ideally spans several different stages of the life course, and therefore progress in addressing calls for incorporation of PPD within DLC research (Farrington, 2005) is expected to take a long time to emerge. Thus far, three studies have included the components necessary to examine the relationship between PPD and offending trajectories: the Cambridge Study on Delinquent Development, the Pathways to Desistance Study, and the Incarcerated Serious and Violent Young Offender Study. For each study, their characteristics and contributions to research on PPD and offending trajectories are discussed.

Findings from the Cambridge Study on Delinquent Development

The Cambridge Study in Delinquent Development (CSDD) was initiated in 1961 and represents one of the largest and longest running studies on the development of offending. This study includes 411 White males, all of whom were recruited in childhood (approximately age 8) from neighborhoods in South London. Of the 411 boys, 304 were rated in adulthood using the Psychopathy Checklist: Screening Version (PCL: SV; Hart, Hare, & Cox, 1995). Piquero et al. (2012) used this data to examine the association between PCL: SV scores measured at age 48 and offending trajectories measured from ages 8–40. Thus far, this is the only study to examine the relationship between PPD and offending outcomes through middle adulthood. Piquero et al.'s (2012) SPGM analysis identified five offending trajectories: non-offenders (62.3 percent), low adolescence peak offenders (18.6 percent), low rate chronics (11.3 percent), high adolescence peak offenders (5.4 percent), and high rate chronics (2.5 percent). Trajectory assignment was then used to predict PCL: SV scores at age 48. Piquero et al. (2012) observed that the high rate chronic offending trajectory significantly predicted higher scores on the PCL: SV, including higher total scores, scores on the Interpersonal/Affective factor, and scores on the antisocial lifestyle factor. These relationships were observed even when controlling for two indexes comprising a wealth of individual factors (e.g., school performance, personality, IQ) and environmental factors (e.g., family dynamics, neighborhood, parenting style).

Although measures of PPD in adolescence were not used to predict offending trajectory assignment, Bergstrom, Forth, and Farrington (2015) observed that high scores on measures of PPD remained moderately to highly correlated between adolescence and adulthood among CSDD participants. Although speculative, because PPD symptoms were correlated between adolescence and adulthood, the relationship between adolescent PPD and offending trajectories should resemble the observed relationship between adult PPD and offending trajectories. Other studies have more directly addressed this question.

Findings from the Pathways to Desistance Study

The Pathways to Desistance Study (PDS) followed male (n = 1,170) and female (n = 184) adolescents for approximately seven years. Each of these participants were sampled from juvenile and adult court systems in Phoenix, Arizona, and Philadelphia, Pennsylvania (Mulvey, 2011). The PDS is unique in that it is one of the only studies to include repeated measures of the same PPD instrument at the time of interview. Here, the Youth Psychopathic Traits Inventory (YPI; Andershed, Kerr, Stattin, & Levander, 2002) was implemented at multiple waves to facilitate the examination of within-individual change or stability in levels of PPD in addition to examination of within-individual change or stability in levels of offending. Several studies emerging from the

PDS data showed that PPD was informative of a more versatile pattern of offending across the different waves of data collection (e.g., Baskin-Sommers & Baskin, 2016; Walters, 2015).

Focusing specifically on males from the PDS who were dating during the study period, Sweeten, Larson, and Piquero (2016) examined whether YPI total scores were associated with trajectories of dating violence perpetration. Higher scores on the YPI at baseline predicted association with the highest-rate trajectories of both emotional dating violence and physical dating violence. This study has important implications for the life course perspective that relationships are a helpful source of informal social control. If individuals with PPD are more likely to perpetrate violence against intimate partners, then the types of marital and intimate relationships thought to help promote desistance may not only be ineffectual for individuals with PPD, but may also improve access to potential victims.

Findings from the Incarcerated Serious and Violent Young Offender Study

The Incarcerated Serious and Violent Young Offender Study (ISVYOS) follows male and female adolescent offenders through different stages of adulthood. Data collection is ongoing, with approximately 500 offenders followed through age 30 and approximately 1,100 offenders followed through age 23. All participants were initially interviewed while incarcerated in open and secure facilities throughout the province of British Columbia, Canada. Three different studies on the relationship between PPD and offending trajectories have been conducted using data from the ISVYOS. In the first study, McCuish et al. (2014) examined the relationship between different factor structures of the Psychopathy Checklist: Youth Version (PCL: YV; Forth et al., 2003) and general offending trajectories measured from ages 12 to 28. Exposure time was built into the model to account for periods of offending inactivity due to incarceration. The SPGM analysis suggested that four trajectories best fit the data, two of which were characterized by a pattern of high rate offending. The individuals assigned to these two trajectories averaged approximately 40 convictions between ages 12–28. Via a multinomial logistic regression analysis, controlling for demographic characteristics, high scores on the three-factor and four-factor models of the PCL: YV significantly increased the odds of association with the high frequency chronic offending trajectory compared to the adolescence limited trajectory and association with the high rate slow desister trajectory compared to the adolescence limited trajectory.

Corrado, McCuish, Hart, and DeLisi (2015) expanded on these findings by examining the relationship between PCL: YV scores and offending trajectories while controlling for a series of different risk and protective factors from a wide range of domains (e.g., substance use, family dynamics, abuse history). PCL: YV test scores continued to significantly increase the odds of association with a more chronic offending trajectory. In this study, the trajectory most strongly related to PPD showed a slight decline in frequency of offending in adulthood. Corrado, McCuish et al. (2015) suggested that this decline was an example of false desistance. Specifically, individuals assigned to this trajectory averaged approximately 122 days incarcerated at each age between ages 20 and 28 and therefore had less opportunity to offend at the same frequency as in adolescence. Individuals within this group were not believed to be desisting but rather were becoming involved in more serious crimes that resulted in lengthier sentences. This suggests that individuals with PPD may show a high frequency of general offending in adolescence followed by escalation to more serious forms of offending in adulthood. A rival plausible explanation is that individuals involved in a high rate of offending in adolescence receive more punitive sentences in adulthood because their lengthy criminal career is used as an aggravating factor at sentencing (Clancy, Bartolomeo, Richardson, & Welford, 1981).

As a slightly different line of analysis, McCuish et al. (2015) used joint trajectory modeling to examine whether higher PCL: YV scores predicted an offending pattern defined by a high rate of violent offending while also controlling for involvement in nonviolent offending. Controlling for the same risk and protective factors used by Corrado, McCuish et al. (2015), they observed that higher scores on the PCL: YV three-factor model significantly increased the odds of association with a trajectory characterized by a high rate of violent offending but a relatively low rate of nonviolent offending compared to association with a trajectory characterized by a low rate of both violent and nonviolent offending. In the same analysis, the three-factor model was not statistically related to association with a trajectory characterized by a high rate of both violent and nonviolent offending compared to association with a trajectory characterized by a low rate of both violent and nonviolent offending. In effect, interpersonal, affective, and behavioral symptoms seemed to be related to a specific propensity for violent offending.

What do we need to know about PPD and offending trajectories?

Research on PPD and offending trajectories is still in relative infancy and, as such, several theoretical, methodological, and policy-related questions remain unaddressed. Theoretical questions include whether PPD creates barriers to desistance (e.g., decreases the likelihood of employment in adulthood) and whether acquiring sources of informal social control do not influence positive change (e.g., decreases the likelihood that employment promotes desistance). Methodological questions relate to the lack of research concerning whether stability or change in symptoms of PPD are associated with stability or change in offending trajectory. Policy questions concern how criminal justice system practitioners should balance the empirical observation that adolescents with PPD are at an increased likelihood of chronic offending with the possibility that at least some of these adolescents will show a pattern of true desistance. This is an example of the type of false positive problem that could result in undue stigmatization and labeling leading to a more punitive sentence and pessimistic outlook regarding treatment amenability (e.g., Viljoen, MacDougall, Gagnon, & Douglas, 2010). In turn, this approach may make the process of desistance more challenging for adolescents with PPD. Specific research questions and data requirements necessary to address these theoretical, methodological, and policy-related concerns are considered in greater detail.

Theoretical questions regarding PPD and offending trajectories

The relationship between PPD and offending trajectories can be better unpacked via an understanding of the disorder's association, or lack thereof, with sources of informal social control as well as whether PPD influences the capacity to positively benefit from the acquisition of informal social controls. Although not examining individual turning points, McCarthy, Huband, Patel, Banerjee, and Duggan (2012) observed that higher scores on the Psychopathy Checklist–Revised (Hare, 2003) predicted lower scores on a psychosocial outcomes scale, which included items regarding long-term relationships, employment, education, and housing. Future research is needed that examines whether specific psychosocial outcomes are less likely for individuals with PPD. Steels, Roney, Larkin, Jones, Croudace, and Duggan (1998) did find that adult males with PPD were more likely than adult males with schizophrenia to be married and employed. However, these authors observed that individuals with PPD were also more likely to reoffend. Therefore, individuals with PPD may experience sources of informal social controls in a qualitatively different manner than other offenders. In fact, for individuals with PPD associated with a chronic offending trajectory, getting married and being employed may increase opportunities for criminal behavior (e.g., domestic violence, theft from work).

More direct attempts to examine whether PPD moderates the relationship between desistance mechanisms and offending are needed. Although SPGM allows researchers to examine whether individuals that acquired sources of informal social control were disproportionately more likely to be assigned to a trajectory characterized by a pattern of desistance, this analytic strategy does not facilitate evaluations of whether an individual's pattern of desistance emerged prior to, or after, acquiring sources of informal social control. For example, did marriage influence a decline in level of offending, or was it through an offender's pattern of desistance that they became more suitable as a marital partner? Multilevel longitudinal models may be better equipped to deal with how changes in acquisition/quality of informal social controls impacts offending over time.

Methodological questions regarding PPD and offending trajectories

To this point, only SPGM has been used to study the relationship between PPD and offending trajectories. This analysis, while widely used and useful, is not without its criticisms, especially concerning the potential for identifying discrete trajectories where none exist (Skardhamar, 2010). To establish the robustness of the relationship between PPD and chronic, serious, and violent offending trajectories, it would be helpful to look at longitudinal offending patterns using different methods, such as multilevel modeling and individual time series (Bushway, Sweeten, & Nieuwbeerta, 2009) to examine, for example, whether PPD influences variance around the mean of a single trajectory modeled for an entire sample (e.g., as a level-two predictor in multilevel modeling).

Research is also needed that examines the stability of PPD between adolescence and adulthood. Although existing studies have observed that PPD symptoms were at least moderately stable over time (e.g., Baskin-Sommers, Waller, Fish, & Hyde, 2015; Bergstrom et al., 2015; Hawes et al., 2014; Hawes et al., 2015), most of this research did not examine stability across different levels of the disorder. Although PPD is best viewed as a dimensional construct (e.g., Murrie et al., 2007), treating PPD as such masks whether stability occurs within the group of greatest interest; that is, those scoring high on a measure of PPD. The extant literature on PPD (but see Hawes et al., 2014 for an exception) has yet to address important ecological fallacy concerns (Thorndike, 1939) regarding whether stability, or lack of stability, is observed across different subgroups of the population (i.e., those scoring low, medium, or high on a measure of PPD). High stability demonstrated by individuals that score low and remain low over time is arguably of far less importance to criminal justice practitioners than individuals with high test scores in adolescence and adulthood. The next step following examination of symptom stability is to evaluate whether stability or change in symptoms impacts the unfolding of offending trajectories. Specifically, are offenders that experience declines in symptoms of PPD between adolescence and adulthood also the offenders that are more likely to show a pattern of desistance in adulthood? Further, to what extent does stability or change in PPD symptoms inform the likelihood of acquiring or benefiting from informal social controls?

Given that implementation of PPD measures can be time-consuming and costly, wave-to-wave repeated measures that examine stability across multiple yearly intervals are not always realistic (but see the PDS). One analytic strategy helpful for capturing test score change across just two measurement periods is the reliable change index (RCI; Jacobson & Truax, 1991). Unlike correlations, *t*-tests, and rank-order comparisons, all of which evaluate between-group change, the RCI is suitable for examining within-individual change when just two measurement periods are available. The RCI can be used to evaluate whether reliable change occurs at different levels of PPD (i.e., the prevalence of stability for those scoring low, medium, or high at baseline). As McCuish et al. (2014) noted, some adolescent offenders have high PPD test scores yet do not continue offending throughout the life course Future research should unpack why this unexpected result emerged. For example, is it an issue with accurate measurement of the disorder in adolescence, actual decline in symptoms over time, or evidence of an offending pattern in which the individual commits particularly serious crimes that result in lengthy periods of incarceration that in turn limit opportunities for continued offending? This result is ultimately a question of false positives and has important policy implications.

Policy questions regarding PPD and offending trajectories

Although findings from the CSDD, PDS, and ISVYOS showed that there was a relationship between PPD and trajectories defined by more frequent offending, violent offending, or serious forms of offending, these studies also did not consider the extent of false positives. In this context, a false positive refers to instances in which an adolescent scored high on a measure of PPD at baseline yet showed a pattern of desistance in adulthood. Some instances of false positives may be consistent with theoretical expectation. Other instances, however, raise concerns regarding the potential for courts to implement more punitive sentences and label adolescents with high test scores as unamenable to treatment (Viljoen et al., 2010) despite their potential for true desistance. In effect, although empirical studies have identified important implications for criminal justice system practitioners, before putting these implications into practice, questions about the extent of false positives should be addressed.

Beginning with instances of false positives consistent with theoretical expectation, some youth scoring high on a measure of PPD will show a pattern of desistance in adulthood due to mortality. As noted by others (e.g., Eggleston, Laub, & Sampson, 2004), accounting for death is critical for identifying "false desisters," and individuals with PPD have a heightened risk of all-cause mortality (Clarke, Davies, Hollin, & Duggan, 2011).

There are also several reasons to believe that individuals with PPD will be disproportionately more likely to experience an earlier death and die from unnatural causes. Tremblay and Paré (2003) noted that more frequent offending would be associated with unhealthy behaviors (e.g., substance abuse), a risky lifestyle (e.g., hazards associated with crime involvement), and stress, all of which were also asserted to increase the likelihood of mortality (see Blokland & Nieuwbeerta, 2005). Given that individuals with PPD are disproportionately involved in chronic offending in adolescence, they may also be at an increased risk of early mortality, which would at least partially account for false positives (i.e., desistance in adulthood). In addition to the role of offending lifestyle, when individuals with PPD are also characterized by a second major mental disorder, they are at an increased risk of suicide (Jones, Hales, Butwell, Ferriter, & Taylor, 2011). Finally, because individuals with PPD are more likely to live a risky lifestyle, abuse substances, and engage in risky sexual behavior (e.g., Forth et al., 2003), they may also be more likely to experience disease and other health-related issues that minimize capacity to capitalize on offending opportunities. For these individuals, desistance is not a matter of leading a prosocial lifestyle and "going straight" but rather more in line with the definition of false desistance (Eggleston et al., 2004).

False positives may also result from punitive criminal justice system interventions that limit opportunities to offend due to lengthy periods of incarceration (Corrado, McCuish, et al., 2015). Individuals may be incarcerated for several consecutive years and thus their lack of offending over this time-period is not a result of true desistance. Although exposure time can be captured in SPGM, the adjustment does not account for nonrandom differences in sentence severity across different levels of offending frequency, meaning that the ability to account for exposure time is likely weakest for the most frequent offenders (Blokland, Nagin, & Nieuwbeerta, 2005). Consequently, the high rate adolescent offender whose lengthy criminal career is used as an aggravating circumstance during sentencing as an adult (Clancy et al., 1981) may be most susceptible to false desistance outcomes. As well, when it comes to samples of more serious offenders, levels of exposure time must be artificially inflated to deal with inordinate offending rates and high Standard Errors that affect model specification (e.g., van der Geest et al., 2009). This procedure therefore increases the likelihood that false positives, in the form of false desistance, emerge for particularly serious offenders. Given the anticipated overlap between PPD and serious offending (Corrado, DeLisi, et al., 2015), individuals with PPD may be disproportionately more likely to be characterized by false desistance outcomes. A potential solution is to use the joint trajectory modeling procedure in Proc Traj (Jones & Nagin, 2007) to allow for the simultaneous modeling of incarceration trajectories and general offending trajectories. This would help identify individuals associated with a trajectory defined by desistance in adulthood combined with a lengthy period of incarceration at the same time that this pattern of desistance emerged. It would then be possible to examine whether individuals with PPD were disproportionately represented in this type of false desistance trajectory.

With respect to instances of false positives not in line with theoretical expectation, it is also possible that PPD cannot be reliably measured in adolescence (but see Dawson et al., 2012). Per this perspective, false positives may be a result of measurement error (e.g., high test scores for adolescents without PPD, low test scores for adolescents with PPD). A more conservative argument is that PPD is measured reliably in adolescence but that developmental change is a normative part of the adolescent–adulthood transition (e.g., Arnett, 2000) and that part of this developmental change implies that personality traits are also malleable.

The most parsimonious explanation for these false positives is that theoretical assertions about the disorder and its influence on chronic, serious, and violent offending are inaccurate. This explanation may not be adequate given that others have observed PPD to contribute to explained variance in offending outcomes above and beyond measures of low self-control (Wiebe, 2003), especially with respect to more serious variants of offending (e.g., DeLisi, Tostlebe, Burgason, Heirigs, & Vaughn, 2018). Nevertheless, this and other explanations for false positives regarding the relationship between PPD and chronic, serious, and violent offending trajectories should be empirically examined to better understand the risk of using high PPD test scores to guide sentencing and treatment decisions.

Conclusion

Individuals do not elect to possess symptoms of PPD. There are a variety of possible sources of the disorder, including biological/genetic influences, environmental experiences, or a combination thereof (Ogloff, 2006). Care should be taken to avoid the stigmatization associated with PPD and the myth that treatment cannot be helpful (Salekin, 2002). Although there are multiple conceptual and empirical justifications for framing PPD as a helpful factor in predicting the likelihood of offending persistence, framing the disorder in this light also has the potential to influence policy-makers to use PPD assessments in adolescence as a justification for lengthy mandatory minimum sentences and the foregoing of treatment (Davidson, 2015). To this point, the empirical research would suggest that such decisiveness could not be made without disastrous collateral consequences (e.g., imprisoning at length an adolescent that would otherwise have desisted on their own).

The purpose of the current chapter was to (1) conceptually describe the relationship between PPD and offending trajectories, (2) review what has been learned about this relationship from existing empirical studies, and (3) outline important theoretical, methodological, and policy-related questions for future research to address. Key points from these three sections can be summarized as follows:

1 PPD is too rare and recidivism too common for the former to suitably account for variance in the latter;
2 Symptoms of PPD increase propensity and situational context conducive to offending while also resulting in less responsivity to typical deterrence strategies. Consequently, continued offending over the life course is likely;
3 Continued offending will occur in part because individuals with PPD are less likely to experience desistance mechanisms. These individuals are also less likely to benefit from the acquisition of classic sources of informal social control;
4 Findings from the CSDD, PDS, and ISVYOS support the assertion that individuals with PPD will be disproportionately associated with persistent, serious, and violent offending across adolescence and adulthood;
5 Future research should empirically examine (1) the role of desistance mechanisms for individuals with PPD, (2) whether stability or change in symptoms of PPD influences stability or change in levels of offending, and (3) whether false positives observed in trajectory-based studies are in line with theoretical expectation (e.g., the result of early mortality or serious offending) or whether such false positives question the utility of PPD as a key theoretical construct in explanations of chronic, serious, and violent offending.

Note

1 The term PPD is used in place of psychopathy/psychopath given that personality is not fully formed in adolescence and because symptoms are only moderately stable over this age (e.g., Hawes, Mulvey, Schubert, & Pardini, 2014).

References

Andershed, H., Kerr, M., Stattin, H., and Levander, S. (2002) 'Psychopathic traits in non-referred youths: Initial test of a new assessment tool,' in E. Blaauw, J. M. Philippa, K. C. M. P. Ferenschild, & B. van Lodensteijn (Eds.), *Psychopaths: Current international perspectives* (pp. 131–158), The Hague: Elsevier.

Arnett, J. J. (2000) 'Emerging adulthood: A theory of development from the late teens through the twenties,' *American Psychologist*, *55*:469–480.

Baskin-Sommers, A. R., and Baskin, D. (2016) 'Psychopathic traits mediate the relationship between exposure to violence and violent juvenile offending,' *Journal of Psychopathology and Behavioral Assessment*, *38*:341–349.

Baskin-Sommers, A. R., Waller, R., Fish, A. M., and Hyde, L. W. (2015) 'Callous–unemotional traits trajectories interact with earlier conduct problems and executive control to predict violence and substance use among high risk male adolescents,' *Journal of Abnormal Child Psychology*, *43*:1529–1541.

Bergstrom, H., Forth, A. E., and Farrington, D. P. (2015) 'The psychopath: Continuity or change? Stability of psychopathic traits and predictors of stability,' in A. Kapardis & D. P. Farrington (Eds.), *The psychology of crime, policing, and courts* (pp. 94–115), London: Routledge

Blokland, A. A., Nagin, D., and Nieuwbeerta, P. (2005) 'Life span offending trajectories of a Dutch conviction cohort,' *Criminology*, *43*:919–954.

Blokland, A. A., and Nieuwbeerta, P. (2005) 'The effects of life circumstances on longitudinal trajectories of offending,' *Criminology*, *43*:1203–1240.

Bushway, S. D., Sweeten, G., and Nieuwbeerta, P. (2009) 'Measuring long term individual trajectories of offending using multiple methods,' *Journal of Quantitative Criminology*, *25*:259–286.

Caldwell, M., Skeem, J., Salekin, R., and van Rybroek, G. (2006) 'Treatment response of adolescent offenders with psychopathy features: A 2-year follow-up,' *Criminal Justice and Behavior, 33*:571–596.

Chung, I. J., Hill, K. G., Hawkins, J. D., Gilchrist, L. D., and Nagin, D. S. (2002) 'Childhood predictors of offense trajectories,' *Journal of Research in Crime and Delinquency, 39*:60–90.

Clancy, K., Bartolomeo, J., Richardson, D., and Wellford, C. (1981) 'Sentence decision making: The logic of sentence decisions and the extent and sources of sentence,' *The Journal of Criminal Law and Criminology, 72*:524–554.

Clarke, M., Davies, S., Hollin, C., and Duggan, C. (2011) 'Long-term suicide risk in forensic psychiatric patients,' *Archives of Suicide Research, 15*:16–28.

Cooke, D. J., Hart, S. D., Logan, C., and Michie, C. (2012) 'Explicating the construct of psychopathy: Development and validation of a conceptual model, the Comprehensive Assessment of Psychopathic Personality (CAPP),' *International Journal of Forensic Mental Health, 11*:242–252.

Cooke, D. J., Michie, C., Hart, S. D., and Clark, D. A. (2004) 'Reconstructing psychopathy: Clarifying the significance of antisocial and socially deviant behavior in the diagnosis of psychopathic personality disorder,' *Journal of Personality Disorders, 18*:337–357.

Corrado, R. R. (2012) 'Does psychopathy appear fully only in adulthood?,' in R. Loeber & B. Welsh (Eds.), *The future of criminology* (pp. 141–149), New York, NY: Oxford University Press.

Corrado, R. R., DeLisi, M., Hart, S. D., and McCuish, E. C. (2015) 'Can the causal mechanisms underlying chronic, serious, and violent offending trajectories be elucidated using the psychopathy construct?,' *Journal of Criminal Justice, 43*:251–261.

Cusson, M., and Pinsonneault, P. (1986) 'The decision to give up crime,' in D. B. Cornish & R. V. Clarke (Eds.), *The reasoning criminal: Rational choice perspectives on offending* (pp. 72–82), New York, NY: Springer.

Davidson, S. L. (2015) 'Relationship between childhood conduct disorder and antisocial personality disorder in adulthood: An argument in favor of mandatory life sentences without parole for juvenile homicide offenders,' *The Law & Psychology Review, 39*:239–252.

Dawson, S., McCuish, E., Hart, S. D., and Corrado, R. R. (2012) 'Critical issues in the assessment of adolescent psychopathy: An illustration using two case studies,' *International Journal of Forensic Mental Health, 11*:63–79.

DeLisi, M. (2001) 'Extreme career criminals,' *American Journal of Criminal Justice, 25*:239–252.

DeLisi, M. (2009) 'Psychopathy is the unified theory of crime,' *Youth Violence and Juvenile Justice*, 7:256–273.

DeLisi, M. (2016) *Psychopathy as unified theory of crime*, New York, NY: Palgrave Macmillan.

DeLisi, M., and Piquero, A. R. (2011) 'New frontiers in criminal careers research, 2000–2011: A state-of-the-art review,' *Journal of Criminal Justice, 39*:289–301.

DeLisi, M., Tostlebe, J., Burgason, K., Heirigs, M., and Vaughn, M. (2018) 'Self-control versus psychopathy: A head-to-head test of general theories of antisociality,' *Youth Violence and Juvenile Justice, 16*:53–76.

Edens, J. F., Skeem, J. L., Cruise, K. R., and Cauffman, E. (2001) 'Assessment of "juvenile psychopathy" and its association with violence: A critical review,' *Behavioral Sciences & the Law, 19*:53–80.

Eggleston, E. P., Laub, J. H., and Sampson, R. J. (2004) 'Methodological sensitivities to latent class analysis of long-term criminal trajectories,' *Journal of Quantitative Criminology, 20*:1–26.

Farrington, D. P. (2005) 'The importance of child and adolescent psychopathy,' *Journal of Abnormal Child Psychology, 33*:489–497.

Forth, A. E., Kosson, D. S., and Hare, R. (2003) *The Hare Psychopathy Checklist: Youth Version*, New York, NY: Multi-Health Systems.

Fox, B. H., Jennings, W. G., and Farrington, D. P. (2015), 'Bringing psychopathy into developmental and life-course criminology theories and research,' *Journal of Criminal Justice, 43*:274–289.

Giordano, P. C., Cernkovich, S. A., and Rudolph, J. L. (2002) 'Gender, crime, and desistance: Toward a theory of cognitive transformation,' *American Journal of Sociology, 107*:990–1064.

Hare, R. D. (1998) 'Psychopathy, affect and behavior,' in D. J. Cooke, A. E. Forth, & R. D. Hare (Eds.), *Psychopathy: Theory, research, and implications for society* (pp. 105–137). Boston, MA: Kluwer Academic Publishers.

Hare, R. D. (2003) *The Hare PCL–R* (2nd ed.), Toronto, ON: Multi Health Systems.

Hart, S. D. (1998) 'The role of psychopathy in assessing risk for violence: Conceptual and methodological issues,' *Legal and Criminological Psychology, 3*:121–137.

Hart, S. D., and Dempster, R. J. (1997) 'Impulsivity and psychopathy,' in C. D. Webster & M. A. Jackson (Eds.), *Impulsivity: Theory, assessment, and treatment* (pp. 212–232), New York, NY: Guilford Press.

Hart, S. D., Hare, R. D., and Cox, D. N. (1995) *The Hare psychopathy checklist: Screening version (PCL: SV)*, Toronto, ON: Multi-Health Systems, Incorporated.

Hawes, S. W., Crane, C. A., Henderson, C. E., Mulvey, E. P., Schubert, C. A., and Pardini, D. A. (2015) 'Codevelopment of psychopathic features and alcohol use during emerging adulthood: Disaggregating between- and within-person change,' *Journal of Abnormal Psychology, 124*:729–739.

Hawes, S. W., Mulvey, E. P., Schubert, C. A., and Pardini, D. A. (2014) 'Structural coherence and temporal stability of psychopathic personality features during emerging adulthood,' *Journal of Abnormal Psychology, 123*:623–633.

Jacobson, N. S., and Truax, P. (1991) 'Clinical significance: A statistical approach to defining meaningful change in psychotherapy research,' *Journal of Consulting and Clinical Psychology, 59*:12–19.

Jennings, W. G., and Reingle, J. M. (2012) 'On the number and shape of developmental/life-course violence, aggression, and delinquency trajectories: A state-of-the-art review,' *Journal of Criminal Justice, 40*:472–489.

Jones, R. M., Hales, H., Butwell, M., Ferriter, M., and Taylor, P. J. (2011) 'Suicide in high security hospital patients,' *Social Psychiatry and Psychiatric Epidemiology, 46*, 723–731.

Jones, B. L., and Nagin, D. S. (2007) 'Advances in group-based trajectory modeling and an SAS procedure for estimating them,' *Sociological Methods & Research, 35*:542–571.

Lochner, L. (2004) 'Education, work, and crime: A human capital approach,' *International Economic Review, 45*:811–843.

Lussier, P., McCuish, E. C., and Corrado, R. R. (2015) 'The adolescence–adulthood transition and desistance from crime: Examining the underlying structure of desistance,' *Journal of Developmental and Life Course Criminology, 1*:87–117.

Lykken, D. (1995) *The antisocial personalities*, Mahwah, NJ: Lawrence Erlbaum Associates.

Lynam, D. R., Caspi, A., Moffitt, T. E., Loeber, R., and Stouthamer-Loeber, M. (2007) 'Longitudinal evidence that psychopathy scores in early adolescence predict adult psychopathy,' *Journal of Abnormal Psychology, 116*:155–165.

McCarthy, L., Huband, N., Patel, S., Banerjee, P., and Duggan, C. (2012) 'Personality disorder and psychopathy as predictors of psychosocial and criminological outcome in mentally disordered offenders,' *International Journal of Forensic Mental Health, 11*:227–237.

McCuish, E. C., Corrado, R. R., Hart, S. D., and DeLisi, M. (2015) 'The role of symptoms of psychopathy in persistent violence over the criminal career into full adulthood,' *Journal of Criminal Justice, 43*:345–356.

McCuish, E. C., Corrado, R., Lussier, P., and Hart, S. D. (2014) 'Psychopathic traits and offending trajectories from early adolescence to adulthood,' *Journal of Criminal Justice, 42*:66–76.

Maruna, S. (2001) *Making good: How ex-convicts reform and rebuild their lives*, Washington, DC: American Psychological Association.

Moffitt, T. E. (1993) '"Life-course-persistent" and "adolescent-limited" antisocial behavior: A developmental taxonomy,' *Psychological Review, 100*:674–701.

Mulvey, E. P. (2011) *Highlights from pathways to desistance: A longitudinal study of serious adolescent offenders*, Washington, DC: U. S. Department of Justice, Office of Juvenile Justice and Delinquency Prevention.

Murrie, D. C., Marcus, D. K., Douglas, K. S., Lee, Z., Salekin, R. T., and Vincent, G. (2007) 'Youth with psychopathy features are not a discrete class: A taxometric analysis,' *Journal of Child Psychology and Psychiatry, 48*:714–723.

Nagin, D. S., and Land, K. C. (1993) 'Age, criminal careers and population heterogeneity: Specification and estimation of nonparametric mixed Poisson model,' *Criminology, 31*:327–354.

Nagin, D. S. (2005) *Group-based modeling of development*, Cambridge, MA: Harvard University Press.

Newman, J. P., MacCoon, D. G., Vaughn, L. J., and Sadeh, N. (2005) 'Validating a distinction between primary and secondary psychopathy with measures of Gray's BIS and BAS constructs,' *Journal of Abnormal Psychology, 114*:319–323.

Ogloff, J. R. P. (2006) 'Psychopathy/antisocial personality disorder conundrum,' *Australian and New Zealand Journal of Psychiatry, 40*:519–528.

Piquero, A. R. (2008) 'Taking stock of developmental trajectories of criminal activity over the life course,' in A. M. Liberman (Ed.), *The long view of crime: A synthesis of longitudinal research* (pp. 23–53), New York, NY: Springer.

Piquero, A. R., Farrington, D. P., Fontaine, N. M., Vincent, G., Coid, J., and Ullrich, S. (2012) 'Childhood risk, offending trajectories, and psychopathy at age 48 years in the Cambridge Study in Delinquent Development,' *Psychology, Public Policy, and Law, 18*(4):577–604.

Rafter, N. H. (1997) 'Psychopathy and the evolution of criminological knowledge,' *Theoretical Criminology, 1*:235–259.

Rafter, N., Posick, C., and Rocque, M. (2016) *The criminal brain: Understanding biological theories of crime* (2nd ed.), New York, NY: New York University Press.

Salekin, R. T. (2002) 'Psychopathy and therapeutic pessimism: Clinical lore or clinical reality?,' *Clinical Psychology Review, 22*:79–112.

Sampson, R. J., and Laub, J. H. (1993) 'Structural variations in juvenile court processing: Inequality, the underclass, and social control,' *Law and Society Review, 27*:285–311.

Sampson, R. J., and Laub, J. H. (2005) 'When prediction fails: From crime-prone boys to heterogeneity in adulthood,' *The Annals of the American Academy of Political and Social Science, 602*:73–79.

Serin, R. C. (1991) 'Psychopathy and violence in criminals,' *Journal of Interpersonal Violence, 6*:423–431.

Skardhamar, T. (2010) 'Distinguishing facts and artifacts in group-based modeling,' *Criminology, 48*:295–320.

Steels, M., Roney, G., Larkin, E., Jones, P., Croudace, T., and Duggan, C. (1998) 'Discharged from special hospital under restrictions: A comparison of the fates of psychopaths and the mentally ill,' *Criminal Behaviour and Mental Health, 8*:39–55.

Sweeten, G., Larson, M., and Piquero, A. R. (2016) 'Predictors of emotional and physical dating violence in a sample of serious juvenile offenders,' *Criminal Behaviour and Mental Health, 26*:263–277.

Sweeten, G., Piquero, A. R., and Steinberg, L. (2013) 'Age and the explanation of crime, revisited,' *Journal of Youth and Adolescence, 42*:921–938.

Thorndike, E. L. (1939) 'On the fallacy of imputing the correlations found for groups to the individuals or smaller groups composing them,' *American Journal of Psychology, 52*:122–124.

Tremblay, P., and Paré, P. P. (2003) 'Crime and destiny: Patterns in serious offenders' mortality rates,' *Canadian Journal of Criminology and Criminal Justice, 45*:299–326.

van der Geest, V., Blokland, A., and Bijleveld, C. (2009) 'Delinquent development in a sample of high-risk youth: Shape, content, and predictors of delinquent trajectories from age 12 to 32,' *Journal of Research in Crime and Delinquency, 46*:111–143.

Vaughn, M. G., and DeLisi, M. (2008) 'Were Wolfgang's chronic offenders psychopaths? On the convergent validity between psychopathy and career criminality,' *Journal of Criminal Justice, 36*:33–42.

Viljoen, J. L., MacDougall, E. A., Gagnon, N. C., and Douglas, K. S. (2010) 'Psychopathy evidence in legal proceedings involving adolescent offenders,' *Psychology, Public Policy, and Law, 16*:254–418.

Walters, G. D. (2015) 'A multi-wave cross-lagged regression analysis of the Youth Psychopathic Traits Inventory and self-reported offending,' *Journal of Criminal Justice, 43*:327–336.

Warr, M. (1998) 'Life-course transitions and desistance from crime,' *Criminology, 36*:183–216.

Wiebe, R. P. (2003) 'Reconciling psychopathy and low self-control,' *Justice Quarterly, 20*:297–336.

Wikström, P.-O. H., and Treiber, K. H. (2009) 'Violence as situational action,' *International Journal of Conflict and Violence, 3*:75–96.

Wikström, P.-O. H. (2006) 'Individuals, settings, and acts of crime: Situational mechanisms and the explanation of crime,' in P. O. H. Wikström & R. J. Sampson (Eds.), *The explanation of crime: Context, mechanism, and development* (pp. 61–107), Cambridge: Cambridge University Press.

Wolfgang, M. E., Figlio, R. M., and Sellin, T. (1972) *Delinquency in a birth cohort*, Chicago, IL: University of Chicago Press.

30

Psychopathic narcissism and antisocial behavior

Shari R. Reiter, Christopher T. Barry, and Julie R. Odom-Dixon

"You're talking to a King! Everyone is mine to torment. You'd do well to remember that."
– Joffrey Lannister, *Game of Thrones*

Introduction

Psychopathy and narcissism are two nefarious constructs in personality psychology that intersect to form a unique presentation with far-reaching interpersonal implications. A narcissistic personality style, including grandiosity, dominance, and the propensity for exploitation, reflects the core interpersonal features of psychopathy in both youth and adults (Barry & Wallace, 2010; Skeem & Cooke, 2010). Distinct from characteristics of narcissism captured by traditional personality inventories, psychopathic narcissism directly involves such antisocial behaviors as excessive bragging, conning, and overtly manipulating others for personal gain, and it has been tied to a range of negative outcomes (Barry & Malkin, 2010; Barry & Wallace, 2010). Specifically, psychopathy-linked narcissism has been independently associated with both proactive and reactive aggression (Barry et al., 2007), delinquency, and conduct problems (Frick, Bodin, & Barry, 2000), above and beyond other domains of psychopathy, including callous–unemotional traits and disinhibition.

Psychopathic narcissism, as typically measured in youth, is empirically connected not only to antisocial and externalizing behavior but also to internalizing problems (Barry & Malkin, 2010). The mechanisms through which psychopathy-linked narcissism may be related to both antisocial behavior and internalizing problems are not yet understood. Theoretically, psychopathy-linked narcissistic characteristics, including self-aggrandizing and manipulative behavior, combined with superficial charm, may betray an insecurity regarding their true ability to exert control over others and situations (Barry & Malkin, 2010; Lee-Rowland, Barry, Gillen, & Hansen, 2016). Psychopathy and narcissism are unique, complex constructs, but because they demonstrate theoretical and empirical similarities, they may share underlying vulnerabilities for antisocial behavior (Fossati, Pincus, Borroni, Munteanu, & Maffei, 2014; Schoenleber, Sadeh, & Verona, 2011).

First, this chapter explores the multidimensional nature of both psychopathy and narcissism as well as distinct operational definitions of narcissism in the literature. Next, various measurement models of psychopathic narcissism are discussed, with attention to how narcissism has been assessed within broader measures of psychopathy. An overview of the link between psychopathic narcissism and antisocial behavior is then provided, with particular emphasis on research with children and adolescents. The chapter concludes with a discussion of implications for assessment, treatment, and future directions for the study of psychopathic narcissism.

Multidimensional aspects of psychopathy and narcissism

Theoretical conceptualizations and empirical evidence indicate that psychopathy and narcissism are each multifaceted with complex nomological networks. Their dimensions have been empirically disaggregated through research with both youth and adults (e.g., Kerig & Stellwagen, 2010; Schoenleber et al., 2011). Though narcissism is not uniformly considered psychopathic, psychopathy has an inherently narcissistic component. When considered within the broader construct of psychopathy, narcissism has a largely interpersonal manifestation involving manipulation and a strong desire to be seen as superior to others (Barry & Malkin, 2010; Barry & Wallace, 2010). Complicating matters further, psychopathy and narcissism comprise two elements of the "dark triad" of antisocial personality styles, and along with Machiavellianism are thought to embody the essence of interpersonal deviance (Paulhus & Williams, 2002).

Psychopathy reflects a constellation of affective, interpersonal, and behavioral features, including egocentricity, Blame Externalization, irresponsibility, and disinhibition, as well as the absence of empathy and remorse for one's wrongdoings. Psychopathy has been implicated in severe, varied, and persistent antisocial behavior, which may perpetuate without interference from guilt or anxiety (Cleckley, 1988; Frick & Ray, 2014). Psychopathic individuals often don a "mask of sanity" such that their outward appearance rarely betrays their affective and interpersonal deviance. They may appear normal, charming, and of good intelligence without any identifiable psychopathology in spite of a poverty of affect and callous lack of remorse and guilt (Cleckley, 1988). Likewise, Boldness and the absence of anxiety have been deemed core to the construct by some scholars (e.g., Patrick, Fowles, & Krueger, 2009).

Though antisociality is integral to many theories of psychopathy, Cleckley (1941; 1988) did not presume criminal behavior to be central to the underlying construct but representative of one possible outcome of psychopathy. Indeed, psychopathic traits coalesce in quite different ways, resulting in distinct – and often opposing – behavioral and interpersonal outcomes. Primary and secondary variants have been differentiated based on the presence or absence of co-occurring emotion dysregulation (Skeem, Poythress, Edens, Lilienfeld, & Cale, 2003), are thought to evolve from distinct etiological processes, and are linked to antisocial behavior through different mechanisms (e.g., Blackburn, 1975; Karpman, 1941; Lykken, 1995; Skeem, Johanson, Andershed, Kerr, & Louden, 2007). Psychopathy is connected to unprovoked, predatory (proactive) aggression, particularly in the absence of anxiety, whereas psychopathy in the presence of arousal or perceived provocation is more often related to impulsive, affective (reactive) violence (e.g., Declercq, Willemsen, Audenaert, & Vergaeghe, 2012; Kimonis, Skeem, Cauffman, & Dmitrieva, 2011). Further distinctions between reactive and proactive aggression as they relate to psychopathic narcissism are described below.

Lilienfeld (2013:86) observed that, over time, the psychopathy literature veered from "a crucial truth": that psychopathy is quintessentially and at its crux an interpersonal condition – defined by the often-severe impact it has on others. Interpersonal traits, including seductive charm and deceptive, manipulative behavior, have been deemed the most central aspects of psychopathy (Lilienfeld, 2013; Skeem & Cooke, 2010), yet the assessment of psychopathy has emphasized more explicit indicators of criminal or antisocial behavior (Skeem, Polaschek,

Patrick, & Lilienfeld, 2011). The interpersonal dimension of psychopathy seems inherently tied to certain antisocial features of narcissism, both characterologically and behaviorally. Indeed, a narcissistic personality style including grandiosity and arrogance has been considered a core element of psychopathy in adults (e.g., Cooke & Michie, 2001) and youth (e.g., Frick et al., 2000), and it is assessed in multiple measures.

Like psychopathy, narcissism has varying expressions. The nomenclature for narcissism is wide-ranging and includes, but is not limited to, non-pathological vs. pathological, adaptive vs. maladaptive, overt vs. covert, grandiose vs. vulnerable, and psychopathy-linked vs. healthy narcissism. Popular portrayals of narcissism often emphasize benign confidence and vanity, and they depict a less pathological, even adaptive, conceptualization of narcissistic personality. The Narcissistic Personality Inventory (NPI; Raskin & Hall, 1979) and the Narcissistic Personality Inventory for Children (NPIC; Barry, Frick, & Killian, 2003) are thought to assess this type of non-pathological narcissism in adults and youth, respectively (Barry & Kauten, 2013; Miller & Campbell, 2011). In contrast to psychopathy-linked narcissism, non-pathological narcissism has shown a moderate, positive relation with self-esteem (e.g., Barry & Wallace, 2010), social dominance, and the adaptive use of self-enhancement strategies (Falkenbach, Howe, & Falki, 2013), but it is also tied to perceived superiority over others and exploitative behavior (Miller & Campbell, 2011). Despite its association with greater perceived quality of interpersonal relationships (Barry & Wallace, 2010), non-pathological narcissism has also been related to both proactive and reactive aggression among adolescents in residential (Barry & Kauten, 2013; Barry, Frick, Adler, & Grafeman, 2007) and community settings (Fossati et al., 2010), as well as offending behavior in adults (Hepper, Hart, Meek, Cisek, & Sedikides, 2014), including sexual violence (Mouilso & Calhoun, 2012; 2016). Moreover, this dimension of narcissism is connected to peer perceptions of antagonistic behavior in adolescents (Grafeman, Barry, Marcus, & Leachman, 2013).

Non-pathological narcissism itself is considered multidimensional, consisting of so-called adaptive and maladaptive facets that have distinct psychosocial and behavioral correlates (Barry et al., 2003; Emmons, 1984). The adaptive dimension has been associated with psychopathic characteristics of fearless dominance, whereas the maladaptive dimension has been linked to self-centered impulsivity (Falkenbach et al., 2013). Furthermore, in youth, the adaptive components of self-sufficiency and leadership have been positively associated with self-esteem and perceptions of positive relationships (Barry & Wallace, 2010), even if these perceptions are not reciprocated by peers (Golmaryami & Barry, 2010). Despite its adaptive elements, non-pathological narcissism has also been tied to maladjustment through attention-seeking behavior, heightened sensitivity to negative appraisals from others (Pincus et al., 2009), and reactivity to shame, especially among those with elevated self-esteem (Thomaes, Bushman, Stegge, & Olthof, 2008).

On the other hand, the maladaptive aspects of non-pathological narcissism include exhibitionism, exploitativeness, and entitlement. This component of narcissism has been associated with aggression, delinquency, and other psychopathic traits in youth (Barry et al., 2003; Barry & Kauten, 2013) and adults (e.g., Falkenbach et al., 2013; Reidy, Zeichner, Foster, & Martinez, 2008). Maladaptive narcissism consistently predicted police contact and delinquency over a three-year period in a community sample of youth (Barry, Frick, et al., 2007) and is related to peer-nominated relational aggression, particularly among those with high self-esteem (Golmaryami & Barry, 2010).

In contrast to what is considered relatively normative (i.e., non-pathological) narcissism, pathological narcissism involves the construct's explicitly antisocial features. The oft-cited "two faces of narcissism" (Wink, 1991) often co-occur within individuals and juxtapose the overt, grandiose narcissist who feels worthy of admiration and power with the covert, vulnerable narcissist whose apparent arrogance is thought to be a defense against an underlying fragile self-view, insecurity, and anxiety (Barry & Malkin, 2010; Zeigler-Hill, Clark, & Pickard, 2008). Whereas the former has been compared with primary psychopathic traits of dominance and self-assurance, the latter has been described as consistent with secondary psychopathy and Borderline Personality Disorder due to underlying emotion dysregulation and identity disturbance (e.g., Miller & Campbell, 2008; Wink, 1991). Recent research suggests grandiosely narcissistic individuals often exhibit features of vulnerable narcissism, and though both have been associated with Anger in response to perceived slights, vulnerable narcissism has also been implicated in sadness and shame (Gore & Widiger, 2016).

Findings are somewhat conflicting, however, with callous–unemotional traits, a core feature of psychopathy, being negatively associated with grandiose narcissism, but unrelated to vulnerable narcissism, in at-risk adolescents (Lee-Rowland et al., 2016). Among criminally involved individuals, grandiose narcissism has been associated with the interpersonal and affective features of psychopathy, whereas vulnerable narcissism has been uniquely related to impulsive, irresponsible lifestyle features (e.g., Schoenleber et al., 2011). Both dimensions capturing pathological narcissism have been associated with increased functional impairment, distress, and antisocial behavior, including sexual violence (e.g., Mouilso & Calhoun, 2016).

Finally, whereas personality psychologists study narcissism as a dimensional construct, the current version of the *Diagnostic and Statistical Manual of Mental Disorders* (DSM–5; American Psychiatric Association, 2013) categorizes narcissistic personality disorder (NPD) as a discrete diagnosis in clinical contexts. NPD appears to include features of both grandiose and vulnerable narcissism, including the expectation of superiority, need for excessive admiration, unreasonable entitlement, and enviousness of others, as well as features consistent with psychopathy, including lack of empathy and exploitative behavior (American Psychological Association, 2013). Latent class analysis demonstrated that individuals both high in NPD symptoms and low in self-control exhibited the greatest proclivity toward violent behavior (Larson, Vaughn, Salas-Wright, & DeLisi, 2014). In a nationally representative sample of U.S. adults, these narcissistic and impulsive individuals were substantially more likely to engage in a variety of violent acts, including rape and intimate partner violence (Larson et al., 2014). Though distinct constructs, narcissism at its most pathological aligns with psychopathy based on common features of Antagonism, greed, grandiosity, insincerity, and Blame Externalization (e.g., Fossati et al., 2014). Because of their related features and external correlates, various measurement models have attempted to explicate the nuances of each construct and to identify indicators of narcissism in the context of psychopathy to better inform evidence-based assessment, intervention, and policy.

Measurement and theoretical models of psychopathic narcissism

The multiple dimensions of narcissism described above have been captured through different measures. However, as previously alluded to, many features of narcissism are not only associated with, but are central to, psychopathy (Barry & Malkin, 2010; Frick et al., 2000). Psychopathic narcissism has been characterized by perceived self-importance relative to others (Lee-Rowland et al., 2016) and overt displays of manipulative charm and self-aggrandizement (Barry, Wallace, & Guelker, 2011). Because narcissism has been defined as one dimension within the broader construct of psychopathy (e.g., Frick et al., 2000), it is also assessed via various psychopathy measures, including the Psychopathy Checklist and its derivatives (Forth, Kosson, & Hare, 2003; Frick & Hare, 2001; Hare, 2003), the Psychopathic Personality Inventory (Lilienfeld & Andrews, 1996; Lilienfeld & Widows, 2005), and Youth Psychopathic Traits Inventory (YPI; Andershed, Kerr, Stattin, & Levander, 2002). Measures of psychopathic narcissism typically involve more behavioral indicators such as overt manipulation and lashing out if corrected or punished (Barry & Wallace, 2010) relative to inventories of narcissistic traits. Research has reported the use of a number of tools for assessing psychopathy, largely dependent on the context, type of sample, or specific research questions.

Psychopathy Checklist–Revised (PCL–R; Hare, 1991; 2003)

The PCL–R is a structured criterion-based interview protocol and has been considered the "gold standard" of psychopathy assessment in clinical and legal contexts (e.g., Skeem et al., 2011). Many features of narcissism are included in the PCL, such as glibness and superficial charm, a grandiose sense of self-worth, and manipulativeness (Hare, 2003; Schoenleber, Sadeh, & Verona, 2011). The PCL–R is a 20-item protocol with 3-point ordinal ratings determined from information gleaned by clinical interviews combined with collateral information (e.g., institutional files), and scoring is based on consideration of lifetime behavior.

The PCL–R contains two factors: Factor 1, the Interpersonal/Affective factor (comprising interpersonal and affective facets), and Factor 2, the antisocial factor (comprising impulsive–irresponsible lifestyle and antisocial behavioral facets; Cooke & Michie, 2001; Hare, 2003). Factor 1 may be most closely tied to psychopathic narcissism given its emphasis on manipulative, exploitative behavior and grandiosity. When controlling for the maladaptive behavioral characteristics of Factor 2, Factor 1 has been associated with social dominance (e.g., Verona, Patrick, & Joiner, 2001), as well as reduced negative emotionality and empathic concern (e.g., Hicks & Patrick, 2006; Verona et al., 2001). Importantly, the PCL excludes indicators of positive adjustment (e.g., emotional stability, intelligence), as they did not load highly with the remaining indicators of maladjustment, and the PCL was developed with and for use with criminal samples (Skeem & Cooke, 2010). Despite its inclusion of narcissistic features, the PCL–R is aimed at obtaining broader assessment of Factors 1 and 2 of psychopathy and consequently does not provide a rich assessment of the array of narcissistic features that might be relevant to psychopathy or antisocial behavior.

Psychopathy Checklist: Youth Version (PCL: YV; Forth, Kosson, & Hare, 2003)

A downward extension of the adult Psychopathy Checklist and Hare's conceptualization of psychopathy, the PCL: YV includes an interpersonal facet consistent with theoretical models of psychopathic narcissism. Rather than explicitly asking youth or their caregivers to endorse socially undesirable items, evaluators use structured clinical judgment to make inferences about the youth's psychosocial functioning, including nuances of their interpersonal style, and credibility (Murrie & Cornell, 2002). As with the PCL–R, the process is largely enhanced by integrating collateral and knowledgeable informant data.

Broadly, the PCL: YV is a 20-item instrument with a 3-point ordinal scale intended for adolescents at least 13 years of age, with scores based on a semi-structured interview with the youth, a review of official court documents, and an interview with a parent or guardian (Murrie & Cornell, 2002). Like the PCL–R, total and factor scores, as well as interpersonal, affective, Impulsive, and antisocial facet scores, are typically computed. However, there has been some divergence in the literature regarding the best fitting model, whether the traditional two-factor (Hare, 1991), three-factor (Cooke & Michie, 2001), or four-factor model (Hare, 2003). Further, an empirically derived psychopathy cut-off score comparable to the adult version has not been consistently implemented to distinguish psychopathic from non-psychopathic youth.

As with the adult PCL, psychopathic narcissism is theoretically best captured via the interpersonal dominance facet of the PCL: YV. Although most relevant to psychopathic narcissism, Factor 1 (interpersonal and affective facets) has been consistently less reliable than Factor 2 (impulsive and antisocial facets), perhaps because Factor 1 is composed of personality characteristics that can, by their nature, be intentionally obscured (e.g., lies easily and skillfully, superficial charm). In contrast, Factor 2 relies heavily on behaviors more easily inferred or observed via parent interviews or actuarial data garnered through court or medical documents (e.g., failure to take responsibility for past incidents). Meta-analyses found that the PCL: YV predicted general, nonviolent, violent, and sexual recidivism, but that it did not perform any better than other psychopathy measures (e.g., Olver, Stockdale, & Wormith, 2009). Further, the predictive power of the PCL: YV has been largely attributed to the criminal behavior facet rather than core personality features (e.g., Cauffman et al., 2009; Stockdale, Wong, & Olver, 2010), and the PCL: YV did not predict violent recidivism when controlling for the antisocial facets (Sitney, Caldwell, & Caldwell, 2016). Overall, the PCL: YV-assessed features of psychopathy that are argued to be more stable have been less predictive of many relevant outcome variables than more transient and normative features of adolescence (Cauffman et al., 2016).

Like the PCL–R, the PCL: YV may not adequately or reliably capture core features of psychopathic narcissism as comprehensively as more targeted, self-report assessments discussed later in this chapter. Further, there is debate regarding whether the PCL: YV is an age-appropriate measure or even whether it captures an age-appropriate construct (Cauffman et al., 2016; Edens et al., 2007). For instance, PCL: YV-assessed psychopathy may falsely identify psychopathic traits that are better conceptualized as pre-existing disorders (e.g., disorders of executive dysfunction) or normative adolescence-limited antisocial behavior (Shepherd & Strand, 2016), and there has been limited support for the assumption that psychopathy is stable across development through adulthood (Cauffman et al., 2016).

Psychopathic Personality Inventory (PPI; Lilienfeld & Andrews, 1996; PPI–R; Lilienfeld & Widows, 2005)

The PPI/PPI–R and its derivatives have become the most widely used self-report measures of psychopathy implemented for research with adults, particularly in non-forensic contexts (e.g., university, community). In contrast to the PCL measures, the PPI was developed to assess core dispositions of Cleckley's model and related models and does not contain explicit reference to antisocial or criminal behavior. Though there is not a unique narcissism dimension, narcissistic features, including interpersonal charm and manipulation, egocentricity, arrogance, and deception, are indexed via the PPI.

The PPI–R is a 154-item measure, with seven of eight subscales converging on two higher-order factors which are typically uncorrelated (e.g., Benning, Patrick, Hicks, Blonigen, & Krueger, 2003; Benning, Patrick, Blonigen, Hicks, & Iacono, 2005). PPI–I, Fearless Dominance, is composed of Social Influence, fearlessness, and Stress Immunity, and PPI–II, impulsive/antisocial (also referred to as self-centered impulsivity), is composed of Machiavellian egocentricity, rebellious nonconformity, Blame Externalization, and Carefree Nonplanfulness. Narcissism has been associated with the total score, the more adaptive features of PPI–I, as well as PPI–II Machiavellian egocentricity (e.g., Kastner, Sellbom, & Lilienfeld, 2012). The eighth subscale, Coldheartedness, has been largely independent of the remaining factors and is often excluded from analyses, despite capturing the core affective deficits of psychopathy and its strong relations with Antagonism (Miller & Lynam, 2012).

The Antisocial Process Screening Device (APSD; Frick & Hare, 2001)

The APSD was the first youth measure of psychopathy, and its factor structure in a large community sample pointed to the relevance of narcissism in this construct (Frick et al., 2000). The APSD is a 20-item measure based on the Psychopathy Checklist–Revised (PCL–R; Hare, 1991) and consists of parent- and teacher-report versions for use with children and adolescents, aged 6–17, as well as a self-report version generally used with youth ages 6 and older (Frick et al., 2000). Three factors (i.e., narcissism, Callous–Unemotional traits, impulsivity) were identified in clinic-referred and community samples (e.g., Frick et al., 2000). The narcissism factor has demonstrated relative stability across two years (i.e., from fourth to sixth grade) in moderately aggressive adolescents across informants (Barry et al., 2008).

It has been noted that the self-report APSD narcissism scale has shown relatively low to moderate internal consistency (e.g., Barry & Wallace, 2010; Boccaccini et al., 2007), whereas parent- and teacher-reported narcissism on the APSD does not show such inconsistency (Frick et al., 2000). This pattern may be due, in part, to the difficulty youth self-informants may have in reflecting on their own narcissistic behaviors, such as bragging and overt manipulation, that are more obvious to other observers. In contrast to other measures (e.g., PNI, NPIC), the APSD captures more overtly antisocial features of youth narcissism (Barry & Wallace, 2010; e.g., "brags excessively"; "uses or 'cons' others"; Frick & Hare, 2001). Consequently, psychopathy-linked narcissism measured by the APSD identifies the antagonistic interpersonal style prototypical of psychopathy, but it may be difficult to discern from antisocial behavior more generally (Barry & Wallace, 2010). Still, APSD-defined psychopathic narcissism is associated with unique variance in social functioning above and beyond mere indicators of conduct problems (Barry & Wallace, 2010). Based on differences in factor structure, operationalization of psychopathy, and measure content, much of what we know about psychopathic narcissism, particularly in youth, is based on studies using the APSD. Nevertheless, further work on refining the manner in which narcissism is evaluated on such measures (i.e., personality attributes vs. interpersonal behaviors) is needed.

Youth Psychopathic Traits Inventory (YPI; Andershed et al., 2002)

The YPI is a 50-item self-report measure based on the three-factor model of psychopathy comprising interpersonal, affective, and behavioral domains, with the interpersonal domain most theoretically relevant to psychopathic narcissism (Cooke & Michie, 2001). The YPI includes ten subscales forming three meaningful, interrelated factors labeled grandiose/manipulation (i.e., Dishonest Charm, Grandiosity, Lying, and Manipulation), callousness/unemotional (i.e., callousness, Unemotionality, and Remorselessness), and impulsive/irresponsible (i.e., Impulsiveness, Thrill-seeking, and Irresponsibility; Andershed et al., 2002; Larsson et al., 2006). In contrast to the PCL and APSD, the YPI was designed to evaluate psychopathic traits in community samples of adolescents based on the principle that antisocial or criminal behavior may be a correlate, rather than a core component, of psychopathy, particularly among individuals elevated on all three factors (Andershed et al., 2002).

The YPI has exhibited dimensional and categorical convergent validity with the PCL: YV among both boys and girls in community and clinical settings (Andershed, Hodgins, & Tengström, 2007; Skeem & Cauffman, 2003) and performed similarly to the PCL: YV in its association with relevant concurrent and future outcomes (e.g., Chauhan et al., 2014). However, the interpersonal subscales of Grandiosity and Lying were less strongly related to the PCL: YV interpersonal facet (Andershed et al., 2007), and although the authors suggested limitations in YPI validity, these findings may instead suggest distinct conceptualizations of interpersonal features of psychopathy (e.g., Chauhan et al., 2014). The YPI may thus present a promising path toward better understanding how narcissism manifests differently among youth with psychopathic traits across forensic and non-forensic settings.

Pathological Narcissism Inventory (PNI; Pincus et al., 2009)

The PNI has been increasingly used in narcissism research over the past few years. Although it was not designed specifically to evaluate the presence of psychopathy or psychopathy-linked narcissism, its domains may still have relevance for understanding psychopathy and risk for antisocial behavior. The PNI is a 52-item self-report inventory assessing the vulnerable and grandiose domains of pathological narcissism and has been mostly used with adults. Indicators of grandiose narcissism include "I often fantasize about being admired and respected," and items capturing vulnerable narcissism including "Sometimes I avoid people because I'm concerned that they'll disappoint me." Lower-order facets include exploitativeness, Grandiose Fantasy, Self-Sacrificing Self Enhancement as subdomains of grandiose narcissism, and Contingent Self-Esteem, Entitlement Rage, Hiding the Self, and Devaluing Others and Need for Others as subdomains of vulnerable narcissism (Pincus & Lukowitsky, 2010).

PNI pathological narcissism has been implicated in lower self-esteem, poorer perceived interpersonal relationships, and greater internalizing problems among at-risk adolescents (Barry & Kauten, 2013). Though both vulnerable and grandiose narcissism have been related to aggressive behavior, grandiose narcissism has also been linked with perceived social support and empathy (Barry et al., 2014). Furthermore, grandiose and vulnerable narcissism have each been associated with both primary and secondary psychopathy among community adults (Fossati et al., 2014). However, callous–unemotional traits, a key element of psychopathy, have been negatively related to grandiose but unrelated to vulnerable narcissism among at-risk adolescents (Lee-Rowland et al., 2016). As noted earlier, although psychopathic narcissism has definitive grandiose features, it may manifest interpersonally more similarly to vulnerable based on its correlations with internalizing problems as well as aggression (Barry & Malkin, 2010; Lee-Rowland et al., 2016). Nevertheless, because attempts to map grandiose and vulnerable narcissism onto different domains are in their infancy, the extent to which so-called pathological narcissism necessarily resides within the broad psychopathy construct is not yet clear.

Psychopathic narcissism and antisocial behavior

Much of what is known about the link between psychopathy and narcissism, as well as between psychopathic narcissism and interpersonal functioning, comes from research using the measures described above. Aside from discerning the connection of psychopathic narcissism to broader conceptualizations of psychopathy and of narcissism, research has highlighted its apparent relevance to antisocial behavior. Thus, the mechanisms underlying aggressive and antisocial behavior among individuals exhibiting psychopathic narcissism are in need of further investigation. For instance, it is thought that narcissistic individuals may be at particular risk for committing criminal acts such as sexual assault due the confluence of entitlement (e.g., victims "owe" perpetrators sex) and decreased empathy towards their victims, as well as the pursuit of admiration associated with sex (Baumeister, Catanese, & Wallace, 2002). This proposed interaction of entitlement, attention-seeking, and callousness demonstrates a complex way in which psychopathic narcissism may lead to severe antisocial behavior.

Aggression is itself a heterogeneous construct with distinct, though often co-occurring, processes and motives contributing to aggressive behavior. For example, a wealth of research has differentiated reactive and proactive functions of aggression. Reactive aggression involves impulsive, reactive, and defensive reactions to a real or perceived threat, whereas proactive aggression involves the planned, calculated use of aggression for one's personal gain (Dodge & Coie, 1987). As psychopathy is composed of both impulsive–behavioral and callous–remorseless facets, it is theoretically implicated in both functions of aggression (e.g., Barry et al., 2007).

Likewise, narcissism, with its two "faces" of superiority and vulnerability, is implicated in both. Specifically, grandiose narcissism is theoretically connected to proactive aggression through one's motivation to obtain status or attention; in contrast, vulnerable narcissism has been associated with reactive aggression as a means of self-esteem regulation following perceived slights or rejection (Barry et al., 2007; Muñoz Centifanti, Kimonis, Frick, & Aucoin, 2013; Schoenleber et al., 2011). Among detained adolescent males, narcissism was the sole dimension of psychopathy that was related to proactive aggression, particularly among those who were less physiologically reactive to distressing images (Muñoz Centifanti et al., 2013). In contrast, narcissism was related to higher reactive aggression among those with higher physiological reactivity. Relatedly, APSD psychopathic narcissism and PNI vulnerable narcissism both moderated the relation between callous–unemotional traits and aggression in non-justice involved adolescents in a residential program, whereas neither NPIC non-pathological narcissism nor PNI grandiose narcissism affected the relation between CU traits and aggression (Lee-Rowland et al., 2016). The similar moderating effects of psychopathy-linked and vulnerable narcissism were considered to result from the underlying emotional sensitivity inherent in both.

Therefore, ego threat (e.g., negative performance feedback, personal insult) may explain a link between psychopathic narcissism and instances of aggression whereby individuals act as a means of repairing or maintaining their positive self-perceptions (e.g., Baumeister et al., 2000; Cale & Lilienfeld, 2006; Wallace, Barry, Zeigler-Hill, & Green, 2012). The process involved in such instances of antisocial behavior may speak specifically to the role of narcissistic features in psychopathy. Indeed, narcissism has been associated with aggression in response to verbal provocation (i.e., insults), but not physical provocation, when accounting for psychopathy (Jones & Paulhus, 2010).

Even with its clear theoretical implications for externalizing behaviors such as reactive aggression, psychopathy-linked narcissism also presents a key paradox in its connection to behavioral and emotional maladjustment. Despite appearing "self-assured to the point that they are presumably unaffected by daily worries or the potential of their status being challenged by others," individuals high on psychopathic narcissism often experience co-existing internalizing problems (Lee-Rowland et al., 2016:15). Specifically, among adolescents, psychopathy-linked narcissism has been positively associated with anxiety and negatively associated with self-esteem (e.g., Barry & Wallace, 2010) in addition to being conceptualized as involving hypersensitivity to rejection cues as well as reactive Anger if challenged or punished (Frick et al., 2000). Moreover, the maladaptive interpersonal behaviors comprising psychopathy-linked narcissism may lead one to develop internalizing symptoms following negative consequences such as peer rejection, particularly among adolescents (Barry & Malkin, 2010).

Overall, the available evidence suggests that psychopathic narcissism may be more similar to vulnerable narcissism, at least in terms of its external correlates, than grandiose narcissism (Barry & Wallace, 2010; Barry et al., 2011). However, our present understanding of psychopathic narcissism is largely derived from measures that may not adequately capture grandiose aspects of the construct. Vulnerable narcissism seems to invoke the secondary subtype of psychopathy, whereas both non-pathological and grandiose narcissism may reflect the fundamental interpersonal and affective features unique to primary psychopathy (Schoenleber et al., 2011). Still, this interpretation requires further research and, perhaps, alternative measurement approaches.

Developmental issues concerning psychopathic narcissism

The stability of psychopathy broadly, and psychopathic narcissism more specifically, are uncertain (Barry, Barry, Deming, & Lochman, 2008; Lynam, Caspi, Moffitt, Loeber, & Stouthamer-Loeber, 2007). Therefore, even though narcissism and other aspects of psychopathy may be theoretically regarded as more developmentally typical in youth, the evidence indicates that individual differences on these constructs are relevant in terms of behavioral and emotional adjustment. That is, it is important to discern the processes through which the construct is most interpersonally damaging and persists throughout development. By extension, the continued presence of such characteristics in adulthood might be regarded as developmentally atypical and thus have important behavioral and interpersonal implications. As described earlier, psychopathic narcissism has been associated with a number of maladaptive behavioral and psychosocial indicators among children and adolescents, including aggression (e.g., Muñoz Centifanti et al., 2013), bullying (e.g., Fanti & Kimonis, 2012), severe conduct problems (e.g., Barry et al., 2007), and delinquency (e.g., Barry & Wallace, 2010). An important process for understanding the link between psychopathic narcissism and antisocial behavior may relate to an underlying fragile sense of self and hypersensitivity to provocation (Barry et al., 2011). Because psychopathic narcissism is tied to the use of aggression as a means of regulating one's self-perception, interventions may target emotion dysregulation at the state level, including constructs such as heightened reactivity to provocation or punishment (Jones & Paulhus, 2010), as well as Anger (Li et al., 2016) and anxiety (Barry & Wallace, 2010), while also mitigating insecurities (Lee-Rowland et al., 2016).

Furthermore, psychopathy-linked narcissism has been indirectly associated with both reactive and proactive aggression through its relation with social–cognitive variables, including negative appraisals of others (Bradshaw & Garbino, 2004), approval of aggression, and hostility (Lui, Barry, & Schoessler, 2017). Therefore, the link between narcissism and antisocial behavior may be partially explained by underlying attitudes toward aggression or violence. For instance, narcissism has been correlated with violent attitudes, including approval of corporal punishment and intimate partner violence (Blinkhorn, Lyons, & Almond, 2016). Psychopathic characteristics including grandiose exhibitionism, entitlement, and exploitativeness were especially important in explaining the link between narcissism and violent attitudes (Blinkhorn et al., 2016). Taken together, the view that aggression is an effective means toward reaching social goals (e.g., asserting social dominance, enacting revenge for perceived slights) may be particularly salient for individuals high in psychopathic narcissism and may then be an important emphasis for interventions aimed at reducing aggression.

In contrast to overt forms of proactive and reactive aggression, relational aggression involves damaging interpersonal relationships through rumors and threatened or actual social exclusion and can manifest in either subtle or overt ways (Crick & Grotpeter, 1995). Among community youth, psychopathy-linked narcissism has also been uniquely associated with relational aggression (Lau & Marsee, 2013), and their relation has been mediated by Machiavellianism (Kerig & Stellwagen, 2010). In a longitudinal study with adolescents, APSD psychopathic narcissism was related to initial bullying as well as victimization (Fanti & Kimonis, 2012). Although each dimension of APSD psychopathy independently contributed to risk of bullying among adolescents, narcissism predicted a slower decline in bullying over time. Additional research has differentiated "ringleaders" who engineer and mobilize bullying activities from those who follow along (Salmivalli, Laferspetz, Björkqvist, Österman, & Kaukiainen, 1996). Psychopathic narcissism also moderated the relation between Theory of Mind (ToM) and ringleader bullying among youth in an inpatient psychiatric setting (Stellwagen & Kerig, 2013b). Specifically, ToM was positively associated with ringleader bullying among youth high in narcissism but negatively related to ringleader bullying among youth low in narcissism. There are disproportionately high levels of bullying and aggression in inpatient settings as community-based interventions are often ill-equipped to treat youth who exhibit aggressive behavior (Stellwagen & Kerig, 2013b). Thus, given its influential role in orchestrating bullying among peers, psychopathic narcissism may be an appropriate factor to consider in intervention efforts, particularly in resource-limited residential and inpatient settings where an emphasis has shifted towards reducing dangerousness (Stellwagen & Kerig, 2013b).

Implications and future directions

Frick and Ray (2014) advised that "the most important dimension of psychopathy may depend on the purpose for which the construct is being used" (p. 711), and Murphy and Vess (2003) emphasized the importance of distinguishing types of psychopathy for public safety. Likewise, Skeem and colleagues (2011) warned of the danger of applying "one-size-fits-all public policies" to psychopathic individuals given the nuances of their clinical needs (p. 96). Although the impulsive features of psychopathy may be most useful for predicting antisocial behavior more generally, empathy deficits in the context of narcissism may be more useful for predicting outcomes within antisocial individuals (Lee-Rowland et al., 2016). For instance, adult offenders with interpersonal and affective psychopathic traits demonstrate more severe, violent, and persistent patterns of antisociality (Leistico, Salekin, DeCoster, & Rogers, 2008), and the interpersonal and affective dimensions of psychopathy have been implicated in negative treatment progress (Manders, Dekovic, Asscher, van der Laan, & Prins, 2013; see Salekin, Worely, & Grimes, 2010 for a review). Further, psychopathic traits in the presence of emotion dysregulation have signaled the greatest risk for violence in institutional settings, but also greater reduction over time (e.g., Kimonis et al., 2011), perhaps reflecting greater susceptibility to both negative and positive environmental factors (Ellis, Boyce, Belsky, Bakermans-Kranenburg, & Van Ijzendoorn, 2011). There has long existed a stigma suggesting that core features of psychopathy render psychopathic individuals untreatable, but research has increasingly contradicted this assumption (Salekin et al., 2010). Effective treatments for psychopathic youth have combined intensive, long-term individual therapy with group therapy, and it has included family members and educators across motivational, behavioral, and cognitive–behavioral modalities, which deliberately target core traits of psychopathy (e.g., Caldwell, Skeem, Salekin, & Van Rybroek, 2006; Salekin et al., 2010).

Continued research examining mediators and moderators of the relation between psychopathic narcissism and antisocial behavior is essential for developing targeted interventions across development, especially among youth with CU traits who evince the need to portray their superiority (Lee-Rowland et al., 2016). Moreover, psychopathic narcissism has been positively associated with Theory of Mind in community youth when controlling for CU traits (Stellwagen & Kerig, 2013a), suggesting that enhancing Theory of Mind or similar perspective taking skills may have behavioral benefits (e.g., Hepper et al., 2014). As clinical evaluations increasingly emphasize callous–unemotional traits with the inclusion of the Limited Prosocial Emotions (LPE) specifier for Conduct Disorder, the identification of such youth with co-occurring narcissistic features and empathy deficits may become more useful. Therefore, the assessment of psychopathic narcissism may play a key role in various treatment decisions.

Lastly, most research to date has examined the link between psychopathic narcissism and antisocial behavior in community, forensic, or clinical settings. However, scholars have proposed that narcissistic individuals in supervisory roles may endorse implicit leadership and follower theories that normalize the abusive treatment of one's employees and that they value traits such as conceit, selfishness, and manipulation (Hansbrough & Jones, 2014). Concurrently, narcissistic leaders may consider their employees to be hostile and their errors to be deliberate (Hansbrough & Jones, 2014). Thus, future research may also examine psychopathic narcissism employed in hierarchical environments (e.g., corporations, academia, military, law enforcement) as it pertains to non-criminal but decidedly antisocial behavior (Skeem & Cooke, 2010).

Conclusion

Further advancements in understanding manifestations of psychopathy and its behavioral and interpersonal correlates hinge, in part, on investigations of narcissism as a core feature of the construct. As discussed earlier, narcissism has been considered part of, or closely aligned with, psychopathy, yet a clear model of the development and presentation of psychopathic narcissism has been elusive. Part of this difficulty stems from differences in the operationalization of narcissism and, consequently, divergence in measurement approaches. To wit, the literature refers to terms such as psychopathy-linked, grandiose, vulnerable, non-pathological, overt, and covert narcissism, as well as interpersonal and grandiose/manipulation facets of psychopathy.

What these constructs appear to share at their core is a drive to portray oneself as superior to others and a preoccupation with being regarded thusly. However, despite the apparent inclusion of supreme arrogance and grandiosity in most conceptualizations of psychopathic personality traits, the available evidence indicates that the narcissism involved in psychopathy as presently measured operates in a manner more consistent with vulnerable narcissism. More specifically, psychopathy-linked narcissism has shown consistent relations with internalizing problems in addition to externalizing problems such as reactive aggression (Barry et al., 2007; Barry & Malkin, 2010; Barry & Wallace, 2010; Declercq et al., 2012). Still, future work should examine how grandiose narcissism, when in the absence of anxiety or executive dysfunction, may share etiological pathways with, and function similarly to, conceptualizations of primary psychopathy (Schoenleber et al., 2011).

Therefore, aside from addressing the discord among measurement approaches, further work is needed that highlights the most likely and problematic behavioral exemplars of psychopathic narcissism. These acts go beyond merely bragging or boastfulness and seem to be particularly concerning in instances when individuals feel vulnerable to perceived slights or do not receive the acclaim to which they feel entitled. Although psychopathy is tied to varied forms of antisocial behavior, narcissism may best explain reactive functions of aggression aimed at the perpetrator of perceived ego threats. Thus, work that has discussed potential approaches for mitigating problematic responses to threatening social events among individuals with high levels of narcissism, even youth (Thomaes, Bushman, Orobio de Castro, Cohen, & Denissen, 2009), may prove useful for addressing this connection between particular aspects of psychopathy and particular forms of antisocial behavior.

References

Andershed, H., Kerr, M., Stattin, H., and Levander, S. (2002) 'Psychopathic traits in non-referred youths: A test of a new assessment tool,' in E. Blaauw & L. Sheridan (Eds.), *Psychopaths: Current international perspectives*, The Hague: Elsevier.

Andershed, H., Hodgins, S., and Tengström, A. (2007) 'Convergent validity of the Youth Psychopathic Traits Inventory (YPI): Association with the Psychopathy Checklist: Youth Version (PCL: YV),' *Assessment, 14*:144–154.

American Psychiatric Association. (2013) *Diagnostic and statistical manual of mental disorders* (5th ed.), Arlington, VA: American Psychiatric Publishing.

Barry, C. T., Frick, P. J., and Killian, A. L. (2003) 'The relation of narcissism and self-esteem to conduct problems in children: A preliminary investigation,' *Journal of Clinical Child and Adolescent Psychology, 32*:139–152.

Barry, C. T., Frick, P. J., Adler, K. K., and Grafeman, S. J. (2007) 'The predictive utility of narcissism among children and adolescents: Evidence for a distinction between adaptive and maladaptive narcissism,' *Journal of Child and Family* Studies, *16*:508–521.

Barry, C. T., and Kauten, R. L. (2013) 'Nonpathological and pathological narcissism: Which self-reported characteristics are most problematic for adolescents?,' Journal of Personality Assessment, 96:212–219.

Barry, C. T., Kauten, R. L., and Lui, J. H. (2014) 'Self-perceptions of empathy and social support as potential moderators in the relation between adolescent narcissism and aggression,' *Individual Differences Research, 12*:170–179.

Barry, C. T., and Malkin, M. L. (2010) 'The relation between adolescent narcissism and internalizing problems depends on the conceptualization of narcissism,' *Journal of Research in Personality, 44*:684–690.

Barry, C. T., and Wallace, M. T. (2010) 'Current considerations in the assessment of youth narcissism: Indicators of pathological and normative development,' *Journal of Psychopathological Behavioral Assessment, 32*:479–489.

Barry, C. T., Wallace, M. T., and Guelker, M. D. (2011) 'Developmental and theoretical influences on the conceptualization and assessment of youth narcissism,' in C. T. Barry, P. K. Kerig, K. Stellwagen, & T. D. Barry (Eds.), *Narcissism and Machiavellianism in youth: Implications for the development of adaptive and maladaptive behavior*, Washington, DC: American Psychological Association.

Barry, T. D., Barry, C. T., Deming, A. M., and Lochman, J. E. (2008) 'Stability of psychopathic characteristics in childhood: The influence of social relationships,' *Criminal Justice and Behavior, 35*:244–262.

Baumeister, R. F., Bushman, B. J., and Campbell, W. K. (2000) 'Self-esteem, narcissism, and aggression: Does violence result from low self-esteem or from threatened egotism?,' *Current Directions in Psychological Science, 9*:26–29.

Baumeister, R. F., Catanese, K. R., and Wallace, H. M. (2002) 'Conquest by force: A narcissistic reactance theory of rape and sexual coercion,' *Review of General Psychology, 6*:92–135.

Benning, S. D., Patrick, C. J., Hicks, B. M., Blonigen, D. M., and Krueger, R. F. (2003) 'Factor structure of the Psychopathic Personality Inventory: Validity and implications for clinical assessment,' *Psychological Assessment, 15*:340–350.

Benning, S. D., Patrick, C. J., Blonigen, D. M., Hicks, B. M., and Iacono, W. G. (2005) 'Estimating facets of psychopathy from normal personality traits. A step toward community epidemiological investigations,' *Assessment, 12*:3–18.

Blackburn, R. (1975) 'An empirical classification of psychopathic personality,' *British Journal of Psychiatry, 127*:456–460.

Blinkhorn, V., Lyons, M., and Almond, L. (2016) 'Drop the bad attitude! Narcissism predicts acceptance of violent behavior,' *Personality and Individual Differences, 98*:157–161.

Boccaccini, M. T., Epstein, M., Poythress, N., Douglas, K. S., Campbell, J., Gardner, G., and Falkenbach, D. (2007) 'Self-report measures of child and adolescent psychopathy as predictors of offending in four samples of justice-involved youth.,' *Assessment, 14*:361–374.

Bradshaw, C. P., and Garbarino, J. (2004) 'Social cognition as a mediator of the influence of family and community violence on adolescent development: Implications for intervention,' *Annals of the New York Academy of Sciences, 1036*:85–105.

Caldwell, M., Skeem, J., Salekin, R., and Van Rybroek, G. (2006) 'Treatment response of adolescent offenders with psychopathy features: A 2-year follow-up,' *Criminal Justice and Behavior, 33*:571–596.

Cale, E. M., and Lilienfeld, S. O. (2006) 'Psychopathy factors and risk for aggressive behavior: A test of the "Threatened Egotism" hypothesis,' *Law and Human Behavior, 30*:51–74.

Cauffman, E., Kimonis, E. R., Dmitrieva, J., and Monahan, K. C. (2009) 'A multimethod assessment of juvenile psychopathy: Comparing the predictive utility of the PCL: YV, YPI, and NEO PRI,' *Psychological Assessment, 21*:528–542.

Cauffman, E., Skeem, J., Dmitrieva, J., and Cavanagh, C. (2016) 'Comparing the stability of psychopathy scores in adolescents versus adults: How often is "Fledgling Psychopathy" misdiagnosed?,' *Psychology, Public Policy, and Law, 22*:77–91.

Chauhan, P., Ragbeer, S. N., Burnette, M. L., Oudekerk, B., Reppucci, N. D., and Moretti, M. M. (2014) 'Comparing the Youth Psychopathic Traits Inventory (YPI) and the Psychopathy Checklist–Youth Version (PCL–YV) among offending girls,' *Assessment, 21*:181–194.

Cleckley, H. (1941) *The mask of sanity*, St. Louis, MO: Mosby.

Cleckley, H. (1988). *The mask of sanity* (6th ed.), St. Louis, MO: Mosby.
Cooke, D. J., and Michie, C. (2001) 'Refining the construct of psychopathy: A hierarchical model,' *Psychological Assessment, 13*:171–188.
Crick, N. R., and Grotpeter, J. K. (1995) 'Relational aggression, gender, and social–psychological adjustment,' *Child Development, 66*:710–722.
Declercq, F., Willemsen, J., Audenaert, K., and Vergaeghe, P. (2012) 'Psychopathy and predatory violence in homicide, violent, and sexual offences: Factor and facet relations,' *Legal and Criminological Psychology, 17*:59–74.
Dodge, K. A., and Coie, J. D. (1987) 'Social-information-processing factors in reactive and proactive aggression in children's peers groups,' *Journal of Personality and Social Psychology, 53*:1146–1158.
Edens, J. F., Campbell, J. S., and Weir, J. M. (2007) 'Youth psychopathy and criminal recidivism: A meta-analysis of the psychopathy checklist measures,' *Law and Human Behavior, 31*:53–75.
Ellis, B. J., Boyce, W. T., Belsky, J., Bakermans-Kranenburg, M. J., and Van Ijzendoorn, M. H. (2011) 'Differential susceptibility to the environment: An evolutionary–neurodevelopmental theory,' *Development and Psychopathology, 23*:7–28.
Emmons, R. A. (1984) 'Factor analysis and construct validity of the Narcissistic Personality Inventory,' *Journal of Personality Assessment, 48*:291–300.
Falkenbach, D. M., Howe, J. R., and Falki, M. (2013) 'Using self-esteem to disaggregate psychopathy, narcissism, and aggression,' *Personality and Individual Differences, 54*:815–820.
Fanti, K. A., and Kimonis, E. R. (2012) 'Bullying and victimization: The role of conduct problems and psychopathic traits,' *Journal of Research on Adolescence, 22*:617–631.
Forth, A. E., Kosson, D. S., and Hare, R. D. (2003) 'The psychopathy checklist: Youth version (PCL: YV), Toronto, ON: Multi-Health Systems.
Fossati, A., Borroni, S., Eisenberg, N., and Maffei, C. (2010) 'Relations of proactive and reactive dimensions of aggression to overt and covert narcissism in nonclinical adolescents,' *Aggressive Behavior, 36*:21–27.
Fossati, A., Pincus, A. L., Borroni, S., Munteanu, A. F., and Maffei, C. (2014) 'Are pathological narcissism and psychopathy different constructs or different names for the same thing? A study based on Italian nonclinical adult participants,' *Journal of Personality Disorders, 28*:394–418.
Frick, P. J., Bodin, S. D., and Barry, C. T. (2000) 'Psychopathic traits and conduct problems in community and clinic-referred samples of children: Further development of the psychopathy screening device,' *Psychological Assessment, 12*:382–393.
Frick, P. J., and Hare, R. (2001) *Antisocial process screening device*, Toronto, ON: Multi-Health Systems.
Frick, P. J., and Ray, J. V. (2014) 'Evaluating callous–unemotional traits as a personality construct,' *Journal of Personality, 83*:710–722.
Golmaryami, F. N., and Barry, C. T. (2010) 'The associations of self-reported and peer-reported relational aggression with narcissism and self-esteem among adolescents in a residential setting,' *Journal of Clinical Child & Adolescent Psychology, 39*:128–133.
Gore, W. L., and Widiger, T. A. (2016). 'Fluctuation between grandiose and vulnerable narcissism,' *Personality Disorders: Theory, Research, and Treatment*, 7(4):363–371.
Grafeman, S. J., Barry, C. T., Marcus, D. K., and Leachman, L. L. (2013) 'Interpersonal perceptions of narcissism in an at-risk adolescent sample: A social relations analysis,' *Journal of Research on Adolescence, 25*:92–100.
Hansbrough, T. K., and Jones, G. E. (2014) 'Inside the minds of narcissists: How narcissistic leaders' cognitive processes contribute to abusive supervision,' *Zeitschrift fur Psychologie, 222*:214–220.
Hare, R. D. (1991) *The Hare Psychopathy Checklist–Revised*, Toronto, ON: Multi-Health Systems.
Hare, R. D. (2003) *The Hare Psychopathy Checklist–Revised*, Toronto, ON: Multi-Health Systems.
Hepper, E. G., Hart, C. M., Meek, R., Cisek, S., and Sedikides, C. (2014) 'Narcissism and empathy in young offenders and non-offenders,' *European Journal of Personality, 28*:201–210.
Hicks, B. M., and Patrick, C. J. (2006) 'Psychopathy and negative emotionality: Analyses of suppressor effects reveal distinct relations with emotional distress, fearfulness, and anger hostility,' *Journal of Abnormal Psychology, 115*:276–287.
Jones, D. N., and Paulhus, D. (2010) 'Different provocations trigger aggression in narcissists and psychopaths,' *Social Psychological and Personality Science, 1*:12–18.
Karpman, B. (1941) 'On the need of separating psychopathy into two distinct clinical types: The symptomatic and the idiopathic,' *Journal of Criminal Psychopathology, 3*:112–137.
Kastner, R. M., Sellbom, M., and Lilienfeld, S. O. (2012) 'A comparison of the psychometric properties of the psychopathic personality inventory full-length and short-form versions,' *Psychological Assessment, 24*:261–270.

Kerig, P. K., and Stellwagen, K. K. (2010) 'Roles of callous–unemotional traits, narcissism, and Machiavellianism in childhood aggression,' *Journal of Psychopathological Behavioral Assessment, 32*:243–252.

Kimonis, E. R., Skeem, J. L., Cauffman, E., and Dmitrieva, J. (2011) 'Are secondary variants of juvenile psychopathy more reactively violent and less psychosocially mature than primary variants?,' *Law and Human Behavior, 35*:381–391.

Larson, M., Vaughn, M. G., Salas-Wright, C. P., and DeLisi, M. (2014) 'Narcissism, low self-control, and violence among a nationally representative sample,' *Criminal Justice and Behavior, 42*:644–661.

Larsson, H., Andershed, H., & Lichtenstein, P. (2006) 'A genetic factor explains most of the variation in the psychopathic personality,' *Journal of Abnormal Psychology, 115*(2):221–230.

Lau, K. S. L., and Marsee, M. A. (2013) 'Exploring narcissism, psychopathy, and Machiavellianism in youth: An examinations of associations with antisocial behavior and aggression,' *Journal of Child and Family Studies, 22*:355–367.

Lee-Rowland, L. M., Barry, C. T., Gillen, C. T. A., and Hansen, L. K. (2016) 'How do different dimensions of adolescent narcissism impact the relation between callous–unemotional traits and self-reported aggression,' *Aggressive Behavior*, 99999:1–12.

Leistico, A. R., Salekin, R. T., DeCoster, J., and Rogers, R. (2008) 'A large-scale meta-analysis relating the hare measures of psychopathy to antisocial conduct,' *Law and Human Behavior, 32*:28–45.

Li, C., Sun, Y., Ho, M. Y., You, J., Shaver, P. R., and Wang, Z. (2016) 'State narcissism and aggression: The mediating roles of anger and hostile attributional bias,' *Aggressive Behavior, 42*:333–345.

Lilienfeld, S. O. (2013) 'Is psychopathy a syndrome? Commentary on Marcus, Fulton, and Edens,' *Personality Disorders: Theory, Research, and Treatment, 4*:85–86.

Lilienfeld, S. O., and Andrews, B. P. (1996) 'Development and preliminary validation of a self-report measure of psychopathic personality traits in noncriminal populations,' *Journal of Personality Assessment, 66*:488–524.

Lilienfeld, S. O., and Widows, M. R. (2005) *Psychopathic Personality Inventory–Revised: Professional manual*, Lutz, FL: Psychological Assessment Resources.

Lui, J. H. L., Barry, C. T., and Schoessler, M. (2017) 'The indirect effects of adolescent psychopathic traits on aggression through social–cognitive factors,' *Journal of Child and Family Studies, 26*:1298–1309.

Lykken, D. T. (1995) *The antisocial personalities*, Hillsdale, NJ: Lawrence Erlbaum.

Lyman, D. R., Caspi, A., Moffitt, T. E., Loeber, R., and Stouthamer-Loeber, M. (2007) 'Longitudinal evidence that psychopathy scores in early adolescence predict adult psychopathy,' *Journal for Abnormal Psychology, 116*:155–165.

Manders, W. A., Deković, M., Asscher, J. J., van der Laan, P. H., and Prins, P. J. (2013) 'Psychopathy as predictor and moderator of multisystemic therapy outcomes among adolescents treated for antisocial behavior' *Journal of Abnormal Child Psychology, 41*:1121–1132.

Miller, J. D., and Campbell, W. K. (2008) 'Comparing clinical and social–personality conceptualizations of narcissism,' *Journal of Personality, 76*:449–476.

Miller, J. D., and Campbell, W. K. (2011) 'Addressing criticisms of the narcissistic personality inventory (NPI),' in W. K. Campbell (Ed.), *The handbook of narcissism and narcissistic personality disorder, theoretical approaches, empirical findings, and treatments*, Hoboken, NJ: John Wiley & Sons, Inc.

Miller, J. D., and Lynam, D. R. (2012) 'An examination of the Psychopathic Personality Inventory's nomological network: A meta-analytic review,' *Personality Disorders: Theory, Research, and Treatment, 3*:305–326.

Mouilso, E. R., and Calhoun, K. S. (2012) 'A mediation model of the role of sociosexuality in the associations between narcissism, psychopathy, and sexual aggression,' *Psychology of Violence, 2*:16–27.

Mouilso, E. R., and Calhoun, K. S. (2016) 'Personality and perpetration: Narcissism among college sexual assault perpetrators,' *Violence Against Women, 22*:1228–1242.

Muñoz Centifanti, L. C., Kimonis, E. R., Frick, P. J. Aucoin, K. (2013) 'Emotional reactivity and the association between psychopathy-linked narcissism and aggression in detained adolescence boys,' *Development and Psychopathology, 25*:473–485.

Murphy, C., and Vess, J. (2003) 'Subtypes of psychopathy: Proposed differences between narcissistic, borderline, sadistic, and antisocial psychopaths,' *Psychiatric Quarterly, 74*:11–29.

Murrie, D. C., and Cornell, D. G. (2002) 'Psychopathy screening of incarcerated juveniles: A comparison of measures,' *Psychological Assessment, 14*:390–396.

Olver, M. E., Stockdale, K. C., and Wormith, J. S. (2009) 'Risk assessment with young offenders: A meta-analysis of three assessment measures,' *Criminal Justice and Behavior, 36*:329–353.

Patrick, C. J., Fowles, D. C., and Krueger, R. F. (2009) 'Triarchic conceptualization of psychopathy: Developmental origins of disinhibition, boldness, and meanness,' *Development and Psychopathology, 21*:913–938.

Paulhus, D. L., and Williams, K. M. (2002) 'The dark triad of personality: Narcissism, Machiavellianism, and psychopathy,' *Journal of Research in Personality*, *36*:556–563.

Pincus, A. L., Ansell, E. B., Pimentel, C. A., Cain, N. M., Wright, A. G., and Levy, K. N. (2009) 'Initial construction and validation of the Pathological Narcissism Inventory,' *Psychological Assessment*, *21*:365–379.

Pincus, A. L., and Lukowitsky, M. R. (2010) 'Pathological narcissism and narcissistic personality disorder,' *Annual Review of Clinical Psychology*, *6*:421–446.

Raskin, R. N., and Hall, C. S. (1979) 'A narcissistic personality inventory,' *Psychology Report*, *45*:590.

Reidy, D. E., Zeichner, A., Foster, J. D., Martinez, M. A. (2008) 'Effects of narcissistic entitlement and exploitativeness on human physical aggression,' *Personality and Individual Differences*, *44*:865–875.

Salekin, R. T., Worley, C., and Grimes, R. D. (2010) 'Treatment of psychopathy: A review and introduction to the mental model approach for psychopathy,' *Behavioral Sciences and the Law*, *28*:235–266.

Salmivalli, C., Lagerspetz, K., Björkqvist, K., Österman, K., and Kaukiainen, A. (1996) 'Bullying as a group process: Participant roles and their relations to social status within the group,' *Aggressive Behavior*, *22*:1–15.

Schoenleber, M., Sadeh, N., and Verona, E. (2011) 'Parallel syndromes: Two dimensions of narcissism and the facets of psychopathic personality in criminally involved individuals,' *Personality Disorders: Theory, Research, and Treatment*, *2*:113–127.

Shepherd, S. M., and Strand, S. (2016) 'The PCL: YV and re-offending across ethnic groups,' *Journal of Criminal Psychology*, *6*:51–62.

Sitney, M. H., Caldwell, B. M., and Caldwell, M. F. (2016) 'The longitudinal relationship between African American status, psychopathic traits, and violent recidivism in juvenile offenders,' *Criminal Justice and Behavior*, *43*:1190–1203.

Skeem, J. L., and Cauffman, E. (2003) 'Views of the downward extension: Comparing the Youth version of the Psychopathy Checklist to the Youth Psychopathic Traits Inventory,' *Behavioral Science and the Law*, *21*:737–770.

Skeem, J. L., Poythress, N. G., Edens, J. F., Lilienfeld, S. O., and Cale, E. (2003) 'Psychopathic personality or personalities? Exploring potential variants of psychopathy and their implications for risk assessment,' *Aggression and Violent Behavior*, *8*:513–546.

Skeem, J. L., Johansson, P., Andershed, H., Kerr, M., and Louden, J. E. (2007) 'Two subtypes of psychopathic violent offenders that parallel primary and secondary variants,' *Journal of Abnormal Psychology*, *116*:395–409.

Skeem, J. L., and Cooke, D. J. (2010) 'Is criminal behavior a central component of psychopathy? Conceptual directions for resolving the debate,' *Psychological Assessment*, *22*:433–445.

Skeem, J. L., Polaschek, D. L. L., Patrick, C. J., and Lilienfeld, S. O. (2011) 'Psychopathic personality: Bridging the gap between scientific evidence and public policy,' *Psychological Science in the Public Interest*, *12*:95–162.

Stellwagen, K. K., and Kerig, P. K. (2013a) 'Dark triad personality traits and theory of mind among school-age children,' *Personality and Individual Differences*, *54*:123–127.

Stellwagen, K. K., and Kerig, P. K. (2013b) 'Ringleader bullying: Association with psychopathic narcissism and theory of mind among child psychiatric inpatients,' *Child Psychiatry & Human Development*, *44*:612–620.

Stockdale, K. C., Wong, S. C. P., and Olver, M. E. (2010) 'The psychopathy checklist: Youth version and adolescent and adult recidivism: Considerations with respect to gender, ethnicity, and age,' *Psychological Assessment*, *22*:768–781.

Thomaes, S., Bushman, B. J., Castro, B. O. D., Cohen, G. L., and Denissen, J. J. (2009) 'Reducing narcissistic aggression by buttressing self-esteem: An experimental field study,' *Psychological Science*, *20*:1536–1542.

Thomaes, S., Bushman, B. J., Stegge, H., and Olthof, T. (2008) 'Trumping shame by blasts of noise: Narcissism, self-esteem, and aggression in young adolescents,' *Child Development*, *79*:1792–1801.

Verona, E., Patrick, C. J., and Joiner, T. E. (2001) 'Psychopathy, antisocial personality, and suicide risk,' *Journal of Abnormal Psychology*, *110*:462–470.

Wallace, M. T., Barry, C. T., Zeigler-Hill, V., and Green, B. A. (2012) 'Locus of control as a contributing factor in the relation between self-perception and adolescent aggression,' *Aggressive Behavior*, *38*:213–221.

Wink, P. (1991) 'Two faces of narcissism,' *Journal of Personality and Social Psychology*, *61*:590–597.

Zeigler-Hill, V., Clark, C. B., and Pickard, J. D. (2008) 'Narcissistic subtypes and contingent self-esteem: Do all narcissists base their self-esteem on the same domains?,' *Journal of Personality*, *76*:753–774.

31

Developmental pathways to adolescent callous–unemotional traits

The role of environmental adversity, symptoms of borderline personality, and post-traumatic disorders

Edward D. Barker and Alan J. Meehan

Introduction

Psychopathy is a personality disorder that involves a constellation of interpersonal (e.g., superficial, grandiose, manipulative), affective (e.g., lack of empathy, remorse, guilt, shallow emotional expression), and behavioral (e.g., impulsive, irresponsible, and/or antisocial) features (Cleckley, 1941; Hare & Neumann, 2006). This construct has been linked to high rates of community violence, violent and nonviolent criminal recidivism, institutional management difficulties, and poor treatment outcomes (Yang, Wong, & Coid, 2010; Salekin, 2008; Kiehl & Hoffman, 2011). With an estimated prevalence of 15–25 percent in forensic settings and 1 percent in the general population, the societal burden for psychopathic behavior is estimated to cost $460 billion per year in criminal social costs (Kiehl & Hoffman, 2011). Understanding the developmental precursors for psychopathy may therefore aid preventive efforts and lessen this societal burden.

It has been suggested that environmental adversity can influence the development of psychopathy. Based on clinical observations, Karpman (1941, 1948) believed that individuals may show a similar expression of psychopathy but with different etiological origins. He theorized that primary ("idiopathic") psychopathy, characterized by a lack of anxiety, had no obvious environmental correlates, suggesting a more heritable or biologically driven affective deficit. In contrast, the proposed secondary ("symptomatic" or "neurotic") psychopath experienced negative emotions, particularly high levels of anxiety and emotional distress, in response to early environmental adversities, including parental abuse or maltreatment. Due to its distinct environmentally based etiological underpinnings, it was suggested that the secondary subtype may be more responsive to treatment (i.e., sensitive to environmental input) than the primary subtype (Karpman, 1941, 1948).

Historically, the role of biological correlates has received more attention than the environment, with psychopathy being viewed as a somewhat unitary construct, derived from a complex but relatively homogeneous pattern of heritable/congenital factors (Porter, 1996). Nevertheless, in the last decade Karpman's ideas have been revisited due to emerging research reporting that psychopathy can associate with both environment adversity (Dargis, Newman, & Koenigs, 2016; Poythress, Skeem, & Lilienfeld, 2006) and stress-related disorders such as anxiety (Kubak & Salekin, 2009; Hicks, Markon, Patrick, Krueger, & Newman, 2004) and depression (Price, Salekin, Klinger, & Barker, 2013). These studies have largely been focused on adults and cross-sectional in design; hence, examining the early predictors that related to subsequent psychopathy has proven difficult.

One way to examine the etiological origins of psychopathy has been to examine its hypothesized developmental precursor in youth callous–unemotional (CU) traits (i.e., lack of empathy/guilt, shallow affect), which represent the Interpersonal/Affective component of psychopathy. Research suggests that CU traits are not immutable in youth and hence may be somewhat malleable to environmental influence (Meehan, Maughan, Cecil, & Barker, 2017). For example, developmental trajectories for psychopathic traits throughout childhood have identified a significant number of youth whose levels of psychopathic traits change (i.e., increase, decrease) over time (Byrd, Hawes, Loeber, & Pardini, 2016; Fontaine, Rijsdijk, McCrory, & Viding, 2010). In addition, general adversities, ranging from stressful life events to child maltreatment, have been found to associate with increased childhood CU and adolescent psychopathy (Sharf, Kimonis, & Howard, 2014; Barker, Oliver, Viding, Salekin, & Maughan, 2011). In particular, negative life events can have strong effects on CU. For example, Barker and Salekin (2012) reported a direct link between victimization by peers (i.e., been hit, had things stolen, called names, had lies told about them) between ages 8–10 and subsequent CU traits at age 13.

Recent research has suggested that, in addition to anxiety and depression, psychopathy can associate with Borderline Personality Disorder (BPD; Skeem, Johansson, Andershed, Kerr, & Louden, 2007) and Post-Traumatic Stress Disorder (PTSD; Porter, 1996), which are both psychopathological conditions associated with exposure to adverse/traumatic events. BPD is a serious mental illness associated with interpersonal dysfunction, affective dysregulation, self-harm, and severe behavioral and emotional dysregulation (Leichsenring, Leibing, Kruse, New, & Leweke, 2011). BPD in youth is also associated with a range of environmental adversities, including prenatal risk factors (i.e., substance use, psychopathology; Winsper, Wolke, & Lereya, 2015), harsh treatment in the family environment (Belsky et al., 2012), and being victimized by peers (Wolke, Schreier, Zanarini, & Winsper, 2012).

BPD is also highly comorbid with both psychopathy and PTSD. BPD associates with constructs related to psychopathy, as well as psychopathy itself. For example, the National Epidemiologic Survey on Alcohol and Related Conditions (Sanislow et al., 2002) reported that BPD associated with mood disorders, anxiety, and, importantly, narcissistic personality. This finding deserves attention as, similarly, Paulhus and Williams (2002) identified a "Dark Triad" of psychopathic-associated personality styles that include Machiavellianism and narcissism. Following up on this "Dark Triad," Miller et al. (2010) reported that BPD symptoms associated more with "vulnerable narcissism," which reflects a defensive and fragile grandiosity that may serve to mask feelings of inadequacy and is related to psychological distress and dysfunction. Moreover, in a non-clinical sample of French adolescents, Chabrol and Leichsenring (2006) reported that BPD symptoms associated with overall CU traits. Taken together, these results suggest BPD could index a profile that may be similar to the secondary psychopath.

High rates of BPD–PTSD comorbidity have been found in both clinical and community samples (Zanarini et al., 1998). This association is thought to be (partially) explained by shared cognitive biases for Anger and threat due to traumatic and stressful experiences (Lobbestael & McNally, 2016). Indeed, a traumatic event is part of the symptomatology of PTSD in DSM–5, which includes: persistent intrusions of the stressful event(s) (flashbacks, recurrent and distressing recollection for dreams), persistent avoidance of stimuli associated with the trauma (e.g., efforts to avoid external reminders), negative alterations in cognition or mood (numbing of general responsiveness), and persistent symptoms of increased arousal and reactivity (American Psychiatric Association, 2013).

Porter (1996) suggested that an association between PTSD symptoms and psychopathy might signpost individuals similar to the secondary psychopath, whose psychopathy develops as a result of having experienced adversity-related "de-activation" of basic affect and conscience. Notably, the association between PTSD symptoms and psychopathy may be higher in females than males. For example, in a general population sample of adults, Colins, Fanti, Salekin, and Andershed (2017) reported that psychopathy associated with lower physical aggression but higher PTSD symptoms for females versus males. Likewise, Hicks, Vaidyanathan, and Patrick (2010) found that, in an adult female sample of incarcerated adults, PTSD symptoms associated with greater mental health problems, including psychopathy. However, similar results have been found with regard to CU traits within an adolescent sample of incarcerated males (Sharf et al., 2014) and in a mixed-gender community sample (Kahn et al., 2013). Hence, a consistent profile of sex differences in the association between PTSD and psychopathy is not firmly established.

The aforementioned body of research suggests that predictor domains for CU may intercorrelate, as in Figure 31.1, panel A. We hypothesize that the dynamic model (Dodge, Greenberg, & Malone, 2008) represented in Figure 31.1, panel B will describe this developmental process (but at the same time recognize that alternate cascade models could hold as well). This model begins with the child's fetal development and birth into an adverse social context, characterized by stressful life events, parental psychopathology, poverty, family conflict, and direct child victimization (via caregiver or peers). It is hypothesized that this adverse developmental context operates on adolescence CU primarily through affecting inter-relationships with peers. Children from high risk backgrounds, defined by both poverty and caregiver psychopathology, are at increased risk for chronic bullying and victimization experiences (Barker, Boivin, et al., 2008). Victimization, in turn, may associate with the affective/emotional instability and interpersonal difficulties that are part of BPD (see Wolke et al., 2012). BPD symptoms in themselves may increase vulnerability for PTSD symptoms, via shared symptomology, including cognitive biases for Anger and threat due to earlier traumatic and stressful experiences (Lobbestael & McNally, 2016), which, in this dynamic model, include both early adversity and victimization. Finally, PTSD symptoms, themselves associated with earlier adversity, victimization, and BPD symptoms, are predicted to associate with higher CU traits via emotional numbing due to these repetitive negative experiences. We also tested for sex differences in these pathways, given previous findings.

Method

Sample

The Avon Longitudinal Study of Parents and Children (ALSPAC) is an ongoing epidemiological study established in the U.K. to understand how genetic and environmental characteristics influence health and development in parents and children. Pregnant women resident in the former Avon Health Authority with expected delivery dates between April 1, 1991 and December 31, 1992 were eligible for recruitment, resulting in a cohort of 14,541 pregnancies, of which 13,988 singletons/twins were alive at 12 months of age. ALSPAC has been found to

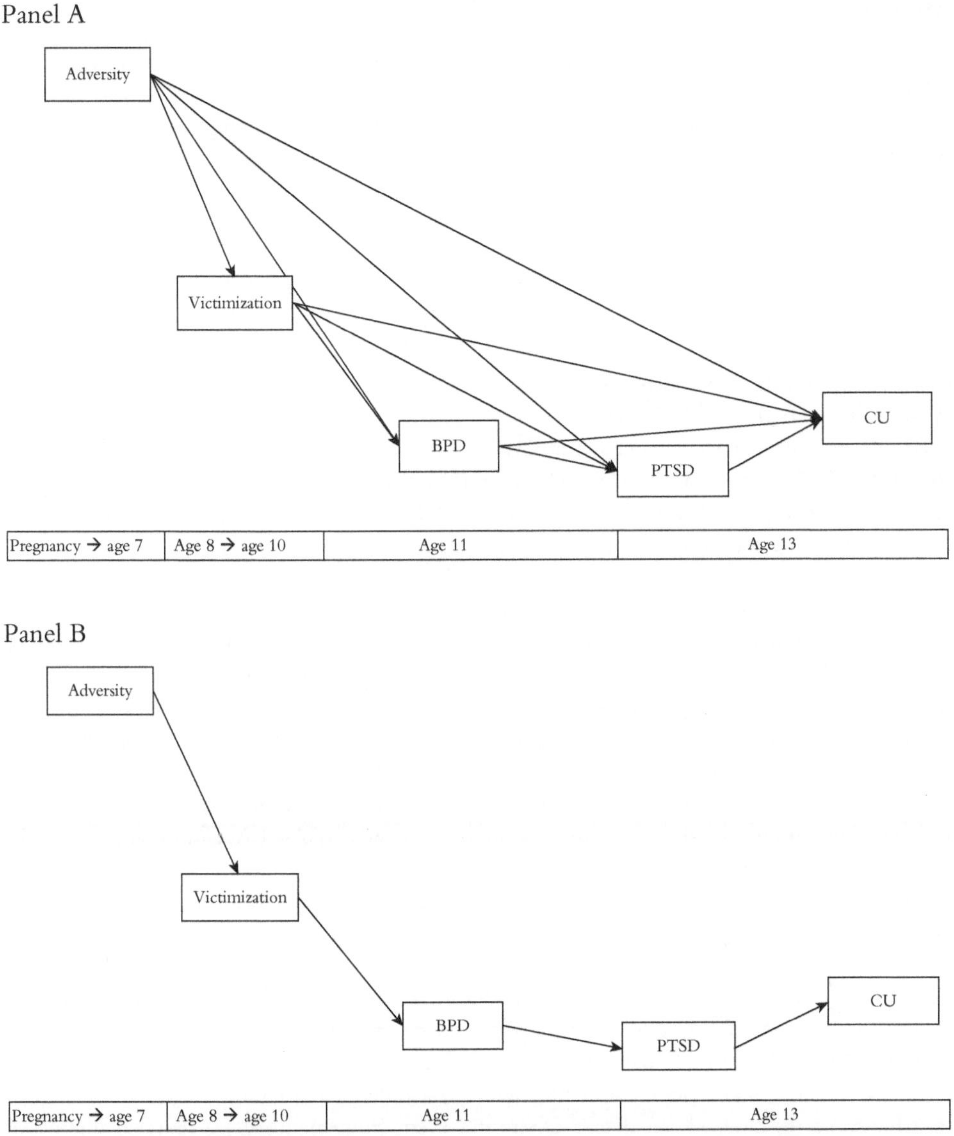

Figure 31.1 Hypothesized correlations among domains in the development of CU (panel A) and hypothesized dynamic cascade model of the development of CU (panel B)

Note. BPD = Borderline Personality Disorder symptoms; PTSD = Post-Traumatic Stress Disorder symptoms; CU = callous–unemotional traits.

be representative of the general U.K. population, based on 1991 National Census Data (Boyd et al., 2013). Ethical approval for the study was obtained from the ALSPAC Ethics and Law Committee and the Local Research Ethics Committees. The study website contains details of all the data that is available through a fully searchable data dictionary: www.bris.ac.uk/alspac/researchers/data-access/data-dictionary/

Measures

Callous–unemotional traits were assessed though a 6-item questionnaire completed by mothers when their child was 13 years old (Moran, Ford, Butler, & Goodman, 2008). Items were rated on a 3-point scale, from "not true" to "certainly true": (1) makes a good impression at first but people tend to see through him/her after they get to know him/her; (2) shallow or fast-changing emotions; (3) is usually genuinely sorry if s/he has hurt someone or acted badly (*reverse coded*); (4) can seem cold-blooded or callous; (5) keeps promises (*reverse coded*); and (6) is genuine in his/her expression of emotions (*reverse coded*). Items were selected based on factor analyses of scales measuring CU traits (Frick, O'Brien, Wootton, & McBurnett, 1994; Frick, Bodin, & Barry, 2000). The measure correlated highly (r = .81) with the CU scale of the Antisocial Process Screening Device (APSD) in 182 children aged 9–17 displaying antisocial behavior (Moran et al., 2009) and has previously shown acceptable internal reliability via Confirmatory Factor Analysis (CFA; Barker et al., 2011).

Borderline personality disorder symptoms were assessed using the U.K. Childhood Interview for DSM–IV Borderline Personality Disorder (UK–CI–BPD; Zanarini et al. 2004), a face-to-face semi-structured interview based on the DSM–IV criteria for Borderline Personality Disorder. The interview consists of nine sections: intense inappropriate Anger; affective instability; emptiness; identity disturbance; paranoid ideation; abandonment; suicidal or self-mutilating behaviors; impulsivity; and intense unstable relationships. Interviewers made a judgment as to whether each symptom was "definitely present," having occurred very frequently (i.e., daily or at least 25 percent of the time); "probably present" if it had occurred repeatedly but did not meet the criterion for definitely present; or "not present" if it had not occurred. The derived outcome variable summed index of all "definitely present" symptoms. The reliability and validity of this measure has been established elsewhere (Zanarini et al., 2011).

Post-traumatic stress disorder symptoms were assessed using maternal reports on the well-validated Development and Well-Being Assessment interview (DAWBA; Goodman, Heiervang, Collishaw, & Goodman, 2011). The DAWBA was administered via a computer-based package of questionnaires, interviews, and rating techniques used to assess adolescent psychopathology based on DSM–IV criteria. Each question was introduced with the stem "over the last 6 months, and as compared with other children the same age, has s/he often . . .," followed by the specific clause. Response categories were 0 = no, 1 = a little more than others, 2 = a lot more than others. We defined PTSD by the average of the xx symptoms: (1) relived stressful events with vivid memories, (2) repeated bad dreams of stressful event, (3) upset by reminders of stressful event, (4) avoided talking about stressful event, (5) avoided activities/places/people related to stressful event, (6) blocked out details of stressful event from memory, (7) reduced interest in activities, (8) reduced range of feelings, problems sleeping, (9) seemed irritable/angry, (10) difficulty concentrating, and (11) alert for possible dangers. We created a summed index of these 11 PTSD symptoms.

Peer Victimization was measured using child reports, collected at ALSPAC's Child in Focus Clinics (Schreier et al., 2009). Children indicated how often (1 = never to 4 = often) they had: (1) been hit, (2) had belongings stolen, (3) been called names, and (4) had lies told about them. These four items showed acceptable internal reliability at ages 8 and 10 via confirmatory factor analyses (Barker & Salekin, 2012)

Early adversity was assessed based on maternal reports. Risk items were organized into two developmental eras: (1) prenatal risks (18 weeks to 32 weeks) and (2) early childhood risks (birth–age 7). For each developmental period, items were organized to create distinct but correlated risk domains: (1) life events (e.g., death in family, accident, illness); (2) contextual risks (e.g., poor housing conditions, financial problems); (3) parental risks (e.g., parental psychopathology, criminal involvement, and substance use); (4) interpersonal risks (e.g., intimate partner violence, family conflict); and (5) direct victimization (e.g., child bullied by peers or physically hurt; available for birth to age 7 postnatal risk). These global risk scores showed high internal reliability via confirmatory factor analyses of the individual risk domains and also to extract one global risk score for each developmental era (Cecil et al., 2014).

Selected sample of ALSPAC mothers and children

Of the 13,988 mother–child pairs, 4,039 (53 percent female) had information about BPD, PTSD, and CU. These were the mothers and children included in the present study. Compared to those included, excluded mothers were lower in educational attainment (Odds Ratio [OR] = 1.62, 95 percent Confidence Interval [CI] = 1.40, 1.88), had early birth or pregnancy (OR = 1.88, 95 percent CI = 1.51, 2.34), and were higher in poverty (OR = 1.44, 95 percent CI = 1.25, 1.67).

Statistical analysis

For all analyses, we first examined the overall sample and then tested for sex differences. The analyses proceeded in two basic steps. In the first step, we conducted longitudinal path analysis. Here, we tested a developmental cascade where we hypothesized that predictor domains for CU may inter-correlate over time to influence CU. Specifically, the hypothesized cascade begins with cumulative adversity (prenatal to age 7), higher levels of which would associate with higher victimization by peer experiences, which in turn would associate with higher BPD symptoms, which in turn would associate with higher PTSD symptoms, which in turn would then associate with higher CU. In addition, we also estimated a direct effect of each predictor domain on CU. Hence, it was possible to examine smaller sets of cascading effects in addition to the total cascade, for example if higher victimization associates with higher BPD symptoms, which in turn associate with higher CU (above and beyond the other estimated parameters in the model). Sex differences were tested through multiple group models and nested model comparisons (i.e., chi-square difference tests).

The different cascades were described via indirect effects. The effects were defined by the product term of the pathways of interest (i.e., "early adversity *to* victimization" BY "victimization *to* BDP" BY "BPD to PTSD" BY "PTSD to CU"). Because Standard Errors underlying indirect effects (i.e., product terms) are known to be skewed, we bootstrapped all indirect effects 10,000 times with bias corrected 95 percent Confidence Intervals. The indirect pathways reported below are based on the bootstrapped variability around the product of standardized path coefficient estimates. We tested sex differences in indirect pathways (e.g., males vs females) by bootstrapping the difference of the respective indirect pathways. We tested differences in the unstandardized estimates.

The second step was reserved for following up any identified sex differences in the first step. For example, if we found that an indirect pathway involving PTSD or BPD symptoms was higher for males vs females, we would then break down the overall PTSD or BPD scores into their subdomains and further explore these sex differences. Indirect pathways, as previously described, were also examined in these follow-up analyses.

Model fit was determined through the Comparative Fit Index and Tucker–Lewis Index (CFI & TLI; acceptable fit => 0.90) (Bentler & Bonett, 1980) and root mean square error of approximation (RMSEA; acceptable fit = < 0.08) (Browne & Cudeck, 1993). Maximum likelihood estimation with robust Standard Errors was used to estimate the model parameters, and missing data were handled through full information maximum likelihood. All analyses were conducted using Mplus Version 7.2 for Windows (Muthén & Muthén, 1998–2016).

Results

Prior to discussing the results, we first describe the correlations and means of the variables. As can be seen in Table 31.1, for females (top) and males (bottom), CU significantly associated with victimization, BPD, PTSD, and early adversity. For males, BPD and PTSD significantly associated with each other and associated with victimization and early adversity. For females, BPD and PTSD did not significantly associate with each other, but as with males, they did associate with victimization and adversity. There were no significant sex differences in mean levels of the variables.

Step 1: developmental cascade path analytic model

The cascading model fit the data adequately: $\chi^2(37) = 233.19, p < .0001$; CFI = .99, TLI = .94; RMSEA = .039 (90 percent CI = .032−.041). As hypothesized (see Figure 31.1, panel A), higher levels of early adversity prospectively associated with higher victimization ($b = 0.193$), which in turn associated with higher BPD symptoms ($b = 0.371$), which in turn associated with higher PTSD ($b = 0.065$), which in turn associated with higher CU ($b = 0.099$). Significant individual direct effects on CU were as follows: early adversity ($b = 0.193$), victimization ($b = 0.077$), and BPD symptoms ($b = 0.109$). For the intermediate effects between the domain predictors, early adversity did not significantly associate with BPD symptoms, and victimization did not associate with PTSD symptoms; however, higher early adversity did significantly associate with higher PTSD symptoms ($b = 0.142$).

Indirect effects based on the significant associations described above are located in Table 31.1. The "grand" cascade, from early adversity (eighteenth week of gestation–age 7) to CU (age 13) via victimization (age 8–10), BPD symptoms (age 11), and PTSD symptoms (age 13) had a standardized effect size of 0.000. This developmental pathway was not supported by the data. Two indirect pathways (i.e., cascades) did show bootstrapped estimates with 95 percent Confidence Intervals that did not cross zero. These pathways included: (Effect 2) higher early adversity

Table 31.1 Descriptive statistics or the study variables by females (top, $n = 2131$) and males (bottom, $n = 1908$)

Variable	*1*	*2*	*3*	*4*	*5*
1 CU (age 13)	–	0.136*	0.11*	0.162*	0.253*
2 Victimization (age 8–10)	0.181*	–	0.334*	0.003	0.215*
3 BPD symptoms (age 11)	0.219*	0.407*	–	0.052*	0.094*
4 PTSD symptoms (age 13)	0.106*	0.054*	0.093*	–	0.14*
5 Early adversity (18wks gestation–age 7)	0.216*	0.171*	0.097*	0.148*	–
Male: Mean (StdDev)	10.70 (3.22)	0.67 (0.73)	0.38 (0.87)	0.38 (1.61)	0.06[t] (1.39)
Female: Mean (StdDev)	10.76 (3.19)	0.53 (0.63)	0.33 (0.64)	0.51 (2.00)	0.05[t] (1.39)

Note. * = $p < 0.05$; [t] = saved factor score.

to higher CU via higher PTSD symptoms and (Effect 4) higher victimization to higher CU via higher BPD symptoms.

Next, we tested sex differences among the parameters involved in these indirect pathways (see Figure 31.1, panel B). For the association between BPD symptoms and CU, males had a higher estimate (b = 0.163) than females (b = 0.060), The difference between these estimates was on trend: $\Delta\chi^2$ (df = 1) = 3.648, p = 0.056. In addition, for the association between PTSD symptoms and CU, males had a lower estimate (b = 0.060) than females (b = 0.129). The difference between these estimates was not on trend: $\Delta\chi^2$ (df = 1) = 2.338, p = 0.126.

Step 2: Exploratory follow-up analyses based on observed sex differences

Given the "on trend" difference for males vs females in the relationship between BPD symptoms and CU, in a *highly* exploratory manner, we examined symptom domains for BPD that showed sufficient variability to further unpack potential differences. Here, self-harm was quite rare; hence, we did not follow up on these symptoms. We did, however, find sufficient variability in disturbed identity (i.e., frequent mood changes, felt empty, paranoid feelings), unstable interpersonal relationships (i.e., changed mind from love to hate, had stormy relationships, stopped talking/seeing people), and inappropriate intense Anger, which will henceforth be referred to as "violence" (i.e., threatened someone, shoved/slapped/punched/kicked someone, been in a fistfight, deliberately damaged property). Of note, these symptoms domains reflect a previously reported three-factor solution of BPD symptoms (Sanislow et al., 2002).

We therefore estimated a new cascade model (see Figure 31.2) that focused on summed subscales of these symptom domains. This model showed adequate fit to the data: $\chi^2(104)$ = 430.112, $p < .0001$; CFI = .94, TLI = .91; RMSEA = .040 (90 percent CI = .036−.044). Early adversity did not significantly associate with the BPD symptom domains. Higher victimization, however, was significantly associated with higher identity disturbance and unstable relationships for females and males alike, but with higher violence for males (b = 0.262) and not females (b = 0.093) – a difference that was significant: $\Delta\chi^2$(df = 1) = 7.053, p = 0.008. Higher violence also associated with higher CU for males (b = 0.205) but not females (b = 0.061); however, this difference was not significant: $\Delta\chi^2$(df = 1) = 2.701, p = 0.100. Higher identity disturbance associated with higher CU for males (b = 0.092) but not (significantly) for females (b = 0.002), a difference that was also non-significant: $\Delta\chi^2$(df = 1) = 3.661, p = 0.056. Females showed higher estimates than males for two consecutive associations that could form an indirect pathway, but neither significantly differed from the estimates for males: higher violence to higher PTSD (b_{male} = 0.043; b_{female} = 0.085; $\Delta\chi^2$[df = 1] = 1.336, p = 0.247) and higher PTSD to higher CU (b_{male} = 0.060; b_{female} = 0.130; $\Delta\chi^2$[df = 1] = 2.112, p = 0.146).

Based on these results, we examined potential sex differences in the indirect pathways that involved victimization, violence, and CU. As presented in Table 31.2, the 95 percent bias-corrected confidence for males (not females) did not cross zero for the indirect pathway from higher adversity to higher CU (via higher victimization and higher identity disturbance). The 95 percent bias-corrected Confidence Intervals for difference in the indirect pathways for males and females, however, did cross zero: $b_{\text{diff-unstandardized}}$ = 0.002, 95 percent CIs: −0.002, 0.005.

Discussion

This study reports three major findings that, together, support a cascading model showing how CU in adolescence develops from pregnancy through adolescence. The major contribution of

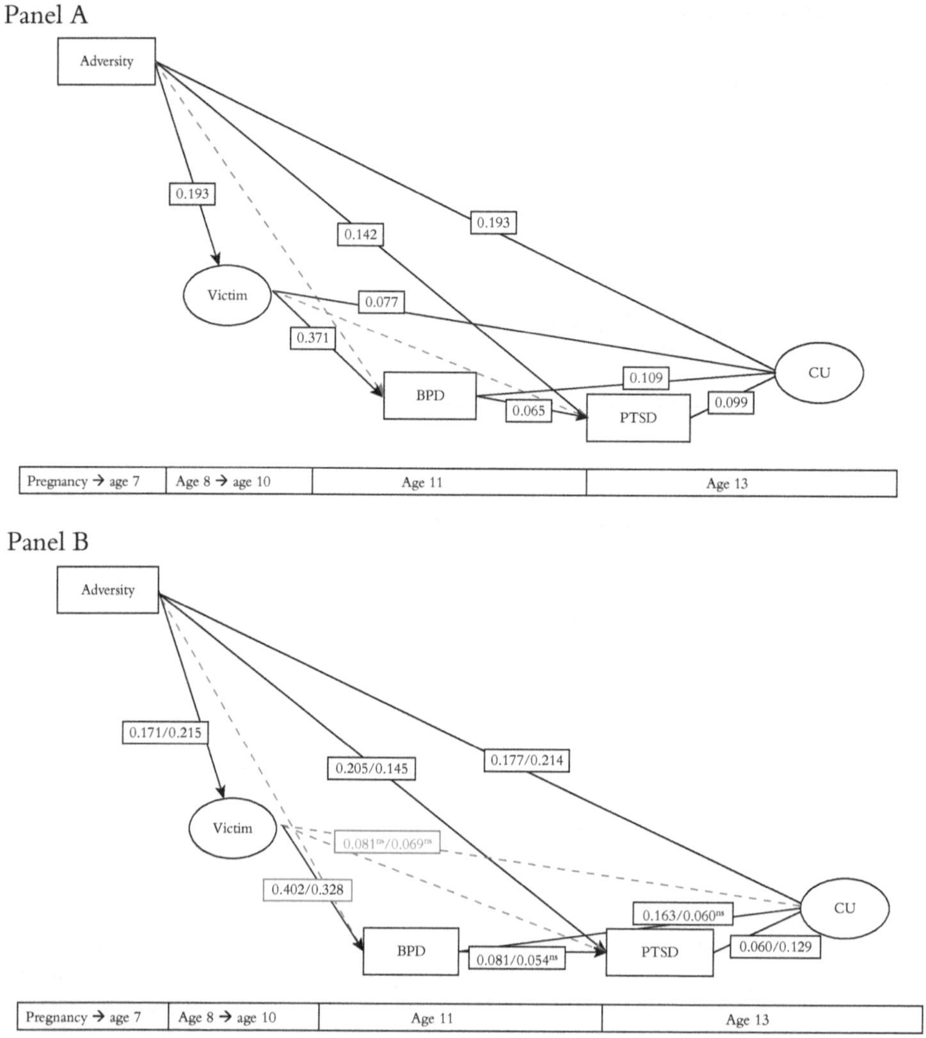

Figure 31.2 Dynamic cascade model (panel A) and testing sex differences (panel B)

Note. Dotted lines = $p > 0.05$; Solid lines = $p < 0.05$; Circles = latent variables; Rectangles = observed variables; Estimates = males/females; ns = not significant; BPD = Borderline Personality Disorder symptoms; PTSD = Post-Traumatic Stress Disorder symptoms; CU = callous unemotional traits.

Table 31.2 Indirect effects for overall dynamic cascade model

Effect	*Age and measure*					*Indirect Effects*		
	Prenatal–age 7	*Age 8–10*	*Age 11*	*Age 13*	*Age 13*	*Estimate*	*95% CIs LL*	*UL*
(1)	Early adversity	Victimization	BPD symptoms	PTSD symptoms	CU	0.000	0.000	0.001
(2)	Early adversity			PTSD symptoms	CU	0.006	0.003	0.010
(3)		Victimization	BPD symptoms	PTSD symptoms	CU	0.002	0.000	0.005
(4)		Victimization	BPD symptoms		CU	0.040	0.020	0.061
(5)			BPD symptoms	PTSD symptoms	CU	0.006	0.000	0.013

Table 31.3 Indirect effects for exploratory model focused on sex difference in BPD symptoms

Effect	*Prenatal–age 7*	*Age 8–10*	*Age 11*	*Age 13*	*Estimate*	*95% CIs LL*	*UL*
(1 – male)	Cumulative risk	Victimization	Identity disturbance	CU	0.002	0.000	0.005
(1 – female)	Cumulative risk	Victimization	Identity disturbance	CU	0.000	−0.002	0.003
(2 – male)		Victimization	Identity disturbance	CU	0.050	−0.003	0.116
(2 – female)		Victimization	Identity disturbance	CU	0.002	−0.058	0.065

this study is an improved understanding how predictor domains inter-correlate over time to associate directly and indirectly with CU traits.

First, each of the four predictor domains associated with CU above and beyond each other. Hence, each made a unique/additive contribution to adolescence CU, and these prospective patterns were generalized across both male and female groups. The current study also provides a highly detailed account of how these temporally adjacent predictor domains inter-correlated and related to CU. All of the temporally adjacent risk domains were significantly related to each other; however, adversity did not associate with BPD (above and beyond victimization) and victimization did not associate with PTSD (above and beyond BPD). In addition, the overall indirect effect of adversity leading to CU via victimization, BPD, and PTSD was not supported by the data. Instead, smaller chains of indirect effects were identified: for example, early adversity associated with CU via PTSD and victimization by peers associated with CU via BPD.

The second major finding of this study is interpreting why these "smaller" cascading patterns might emerge. The relationship between early (pre- and postnatal) adversity and PTSD symptoms at age 13, which in turn associated with higher CU, may support the "latent vulnerability" hypothesis (McCrory, Gerin, & Viding, 2017). McCrory et al. (2017) suggest that early trauma/adversity can form a latent vulnerability, which is defined as a complex phenotype that functions as a "maladaptive calibration" in neural systems important for socioemotional and affective functioning. However, they also state that the emergence of the psychiatric difficulties may only manifest under conditions of stress – in the present case, perhaps, the onset of adolescence. Indeed, there is a large body of literature that has examined how prenatal and postnatal adversity may affect neural systems underlying neurocognitive function and brain development (Lupien, McEwen, Gunnar, & Heim, 2009; Jensen et al., 2015; Blair & Raver, 2016). Of interest, brain areas that are affected by adversity/trauma are also (largely) implicated in PTSD symptoms – and hence potentially secondary psychopathy. These areas include the amygdala (threat hypervigilance), the striatum (reward processing, depressive symptomatology) and anterior cingulate cortex (emotion regulation) (McCrory et al., 2017; McCrory & Viding, 2015). We therefore suggest that a latent vulnerability may underlie the relationship between early adversity, PTSD symptoms, and CU. However, additional research is needed to identify the conditions of stress (in adolescence) that may have potentiated this latent vulnerability and the manifestation of an association between PTSD symptoms and CU traits.

The other indirect effect was peer victimization associating with BPD symptoms, which in turn associated with CU. Of note, the association between BPD symptoms and CU was the only effect with a significant sex difference – for males, not females. We therefore unpacked BPD into the symptom domains of disturbed identity (i.e., frequent mood changes, felt empty, paranoid feelings), unstable interpersonal relationships (i.e., changed mind from love to hate, had stormy relationships, stopped talking/seeing people), and violence (inappropriate intense Anger, violent behavior). Of interest, for males and females alike, peer victimization associated with higher disturbed identity and instability in relationships, suggesting the ubiquitous and

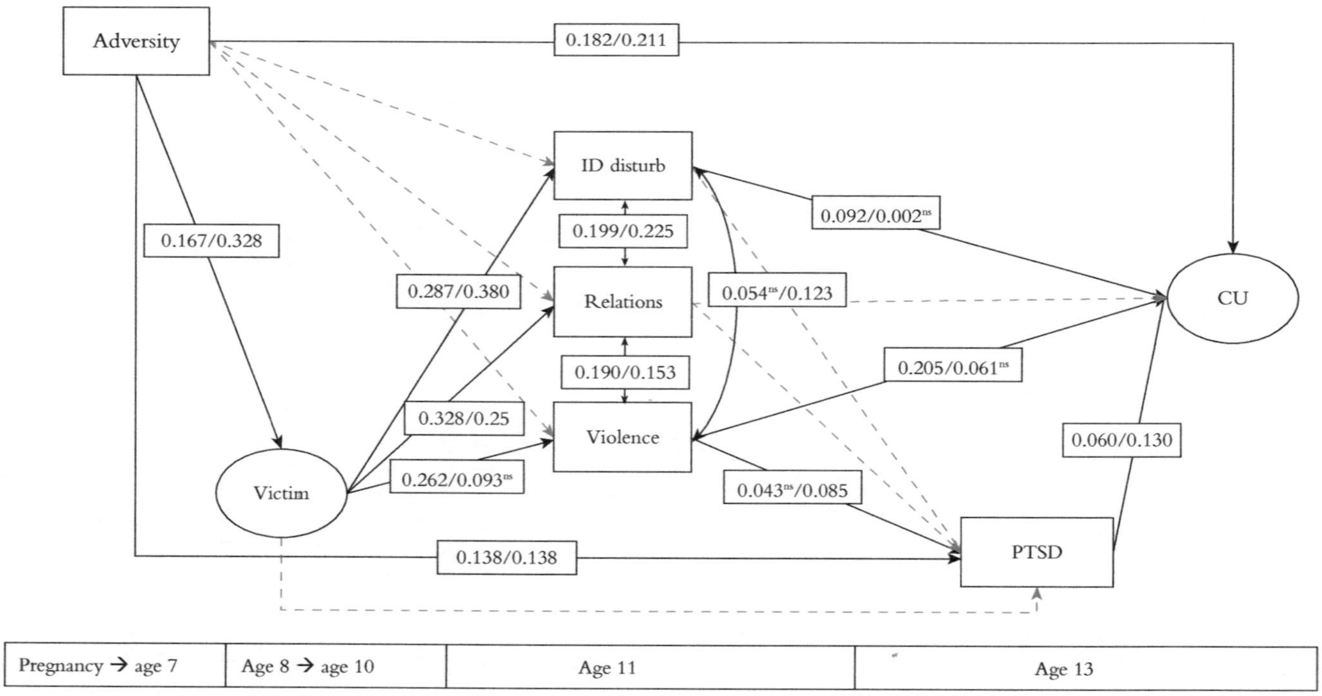

Figure 31.3 Exploratory dynamic cascade model – sex differences in BPD symptoms

Note. Dotted lines = $p > 0.05$; Solid lines = $p < 0.05$; Circles = latent variables; Rectangles = observed variables; Estimates = males/females; ^{ns} = not significant; ID disturb = BPD symptoms of identity disturbance; Relations = BPD symptoms of disturbed relationships; Violence = BPD symptoms of aggressive and antisocial behavior; PTSD = Post-Traumatic Stress Disorder symptoms; CU = callous unemotional traits.

damaging long-term effects of chronic victimization (Takizawa, Maughan, & Arseneault, 2014; Barker, Arseneault, et al., 2008)

For males alone, however, early adversity associated with peer victimization, which in turn associated with BPD-disturbed identity and thereafter CU – the overall developmental cascade. Bateman and Fonagy (2008) suggest that individuals showing symptoms of trauma-related BPD may have rigid schematic representations of the mental states of self and others (i.e., mentalization), particularly in their explanations of others' behavior. Here, interpersonal stress may result in the aforementioned "vulnerable narcissism" (Miller et al., 2010), which can create an atmosphere of distress and fear (perhaps related to previous adversity and victimization), which in turn could lessen the concern for the welfare of others (i.e., enhance callous–unemotional traits). To the extent that emotional distress may characterize certain youth showing CU traits, BPD-disturbed identity may be a construct of interest to future research – it has been reported that long-term effects of chronic victimization by peers include both social paranoia and negative affect (see Singham et al., 2017).

The third major finding of this study lies in the other pathways identified in the cascading model of CU. Here we comment on one. The association between BPD and PTSD symptoms was low in effect size. However, when we unpacked BPD symptoms, for females, the association between BPD-related violence increased in effect size, but not by much. On the one hand, the association may support the idea that BPD and PTSD share cognitive biases for Anger and threat due to traumatic and stressful experiences (Lobbestael & McNally, 2016). On the other hand, the small effect size may suggest that we are not accounting for other potential features by which these two disorders associate. For example, research suggests PTSD may be a better predictor of BPD than the converse: fear and sadness, a core feature of PTSD, may create vulnerability for negative affect, which is a core feature of BPD (Scheiderer, Wang, Tomko, Wood, & Trull, 2016). Hence, the effect size of the association between BPD and PTSD may increase with the inclusion of a wider range of common features, and with PTSD predicting BPD.

In summary, in this study we tested an idealized dynamic cascading model of CU. Although the overall cascade was not supported by the data, we did find that early adversity associated with CU via PTSD symptoms, whereas victimization by peers associated with CU via BPD symptoms. Moreover, when we unpacked the symptom domains of BPD, the data indicated that BPD-related identity disturbance leading to CU was an important pathway for males, whereas BPD-related violence leading to PTSD symptoms may be an important pathway for females.

Several limitations should be borne in mind when interpreting the results of this study. First, only one measure each was available for CU (at age 13) and BPD (at age 11), precluding analysis of stability and change across childhood. Moreover, although PTSD was available at multiple time points, we included only one assessment, as per our hypothetical model. Second, although we referred to Karpman's taxonomy in building a case for the cascade model, we did not actually test this subtyping. Rather, we assumed we would find adversity-related associations based on the hypothesized existence of heterogeneity underlying the CU score. Future research may want to test if the developmental cascades identified here apply more to the secondary than the primary subtype of psychopathy. Third, although ALSPAC represents a broad, representative spectrum of socioeconomic backgrounds, the cohort features relatively low rates of ethnic minorities, necessitating replication with more ethnically diverse samples. Fourth, like most large longitudinal cohorts, ALSPAC has experienced attrition over time, with children of younger and more socially disadvantaged mothers more likely to be lost in follow-up. However, previous studies of ALSPAC found that, while attrition affected prevalence rates of externalizing and internalizing disorders, associations between risks and outcomes remained intact, though conservative of the likely true effects (Wolke et al., 2009). Fifth, CU, BPD, and PTSD all associate with genetic, epigenetic, and neurocognitive mechanisms (Herpertz et al., 2001; McCrory et al., 2017; Viding, Blair, Moffitt, & Plomin, 2005; Cecil et al., 2014). An interdisciplinary approach may inform the nature of the results reported here, with regard to certain youth who may be more or less vulnerable for certain psychopathological outcomes following the experience of adversity.

References

American Psychiatric Association. (2013) *Diagnostic and statistical manual of mental disorders (DSM–5®)*, Arlington, VA: Author.

Barker, E. D., Arseneault, L., Brendgen, M., Fontaine, N., and Maughan, B. (2008) 'Joint development of bullying and victimization in adolescence: Relations to delinquency and self-harm,' *Journal of American Academy of Child & Adolescent Psychiatry*, *47*:1030–1038.

Barker, E. D., Boivin, M., Brendgen, M., Fontaine, N., Arseneault, L., Vitaro, F., Bissonnette, C., and Tremblay, R. E. (2008) 'Predictive validity and early predictors of peer-victimization trajectories in preschool,' *Archives of General Psychiatry*, *65*:1185–1192.

Barker, E. D., Oliver, B. R., Viding, E., Salekin, R. T., and Maughan, B. (2011) 'The impact of prenatal maternal risk, fearless temperament and early parenting on adolescent callous–unemotional traits: A 14-year longitudinal investigation,' *Journal of Child Psychology and Psychiatry*, *52*:878–888.

Barker, E. D., and Salekin, R. T. (2012) 'Irritable oppositional defiance and callous unemotional traits: Is the association partially explained by peer victimization?,' *Journal of Child Psychology and Psychiatry*, *53*:1167–1175.

Bateman, A., and Fonagy, P. (2008) 'Comorbid antisocial and borderline personality disorders: Mentalization-based treatment,' *Journal of Clinical Psychology*, *64*:181–194.

Belsky, D. W., Caspi, A., Arseneault, L., Bleidorn, W., Fonagy, P., Goodman, M., Houts, R., and Moffitt, T. E. (2012) 'Etiological features of borderline personality related characteristics in a birth cohort of 12-year-old children,' *Development and Psychopathology*, *24*:251–265.

Bentler, P. M., and Bonett, D. G. (1980) 'Significance tests and goodness of fit in the analysis of covariance structures,' *Psychological Bulletin*, *88*:588–606.

Blair, C., and Raver, C. C. (2016) 'Poverty, stress, and brain development: New directions for prevention and intervention,' *Academic Pediatrics*, *16*:S30–S36.

Boyd, A., Golding, J., MacLeod, J., Lawlor, D. A., Fraser, A., Henderson, J., . . ., and Davey-Smith, G. (2013) 'Cohort profile: The "Children of the 90s" – the index offspring of the Avon Longitudinal Study of Parents and Children,' *International Journal of Epidemiology*, *42*:111–127.

Browne, M. W., and Cudeck, R. (1993) 'Alternative ways of assessing model fit,' in K. A. Bollen & J. S. Long (Eds.), *Testing structural equation models*, Newbury Park, CA: Sage.

Byrd, A. L., Hawes, S. W., Loeber, R., and Pardini, D. A. (2016) 'Interpersonal callousness from childhood to adolescence: Developmental trajectories and early risk factors,' *Journal of Clinical Child & Adolescent Psychology*, *31*:1–16.

Cecil, C. A. M., Lysenko, L., Jaffee, S. R., Relton, C. L., Mill, J., and Barker, E. D. (2014) 'Environmental risk, Oxytocin Receptor Gene (OXTR) methylation and youth callous–unemotional traits: A 13-year longitudinal study,' *Molecular Psychiatry*, *19*:1071–1077.

Chabrol, H., and Leichsenring, F. (2006) 'Borderline personality organization and psychopathic traits in nonclinical adolescents: Relationships of identity diffusion, primitive defense mechanisms and reality testing with callousness and impulsivity traits,' *Bulletin of the Menninger Clinic*, *70*:160–170.

Cleckley, H. (1941) *The mask of sanity; an attempt to reinterpret the so-called psychopathic personality*, St. Louis, MO: CV Mosby.

Colins, O. F., Fanti, K. A., Salekin, R. T., and Andershed, H. (2017) 'Psychopathic personality in the general population: Differences and similarities across gender,' *Journal of Personality Disorders*, *31*:49–74.

Dargis, M., Newman, J., and Koenigs, M. (2016) 'Clarifying the link between childhood abuse history and psychopathic traits in adult criminal offenders,' *Personality Disorders: Theory, Research, and Treatment*, 7:221–233.

Dodge, K. A., Greenberg, M. T., and Malone, P. S. (2008) 'Testing an idealized dynamic cascade model of the development of serious violence in adolescence,' *Child Development*, *79*:1907–1927.

Fontaine, N. M., Rijsdijk, F. V., McCrory, E. J., and Viding, E. (2010) 'Etiology of different developmental trajectories of callous–unemotional traits,' *Journal of the American Academy of Child & Adolescent Psychiatry*, *49*:656–664.

Frick, P. J., Bodin, S. D., and Barry, C. T. (2000) 'Psychopathic traits and conduct problems in community and clinic-referred samples of children: Further development of the Psychopathy Screening Device,' *Psychological Assessment, 12*:382–393.

Frick, P. J., O'Brien, B. S., Wootton, J. M., and McBurnett, K. (1994) 'Psychopathy and conduct problems in children,' *Journal of Abnormal Psychology, 103*:700–707.

Goodman, A., Heiervang, E., Collishaw, S., and Goodman, R. (2011) 'The 'DAWBA bands' as an ordered-categorical measure of child mental health: Description and validation in British and Norwegian samples,' *Social Psychiatry and Psychiatric Epidemiology, 46*:521–532.

Hare, R. D., and Neumann, C. S. (2006) 'The PCL–R assessment of psychopathy,' *Handbook of psychopathy*, 58–88.

Herpertz, S. C., Dietrich, T. M., Wenning, B., Krings, T., Erberich, S. G., Willmes, K., Thron, A., and Sass, H. (2001) 'Evidence of abnormal amygdala functioning in borderline personality disorder: A functional MRI study,' *Biological Psychiatry, 50*:292–298.

Hicks, B. M., Markon, K. E., Patrick, C. J., Krueger, R. F., and Newman, J. P. (2004) 'Identifying psychopathy subtypes on the basis of personality structure,' *Psychological Assessment, 16*:276–284.

Hicks, B. M., Vaidyanathan, U., and Patrick, C. J. (2010) 'Validating female psychopathy subtypes: Differences in personality, antisocial and violent behavior, substance abuse, trauma, and mental health,' *Personality Disorders: Theory, Research, and Treatment, 1*:38–49.

Jensen, S. K. G., Dickie, E. W., Schwartz, D. H., Evans, J. C., Dumontheil, I., Paus, T., and Barker, E. D. (2015) 'Impact of early adversity and childhood internalizing symptoms on brain structure in male youth,' *JAMA Pediatrics, 169*:938–946.

Kahn, R. E., Frick, P. J., Youngstrom, E. A., Kogos Youngstrom, J., Feeny, N. C., and Findling, R. L. (2013) 'Distinguishing primary and secondary variants of callous–unemotional traits among adolescents in a clinic-referred sample,' *Psychological Assessment, 25*:966–977.

Karpman, B. (1941) 'On the need of separating psychopathy into two distinct clinical types: The symptomatic and the idiopathic,' *Journal of Criminal Psychopathology, 3*:112–137.

Karpman, B. (1948) 'The myth of the psychopathic personality. *American Journal of Psychiatry, 104*:523–534.

Kiehl, K. A., and Hoffman, M. B. (2011) 'The criminal psychopath: History, neuroscience, treatment, and economics,' *Jurimetrics, 51*:355–363.

Kubak, F. A., and Salekin, R. T. (2009) 'Psychopathy and anxiety in children and adolescents: New insights on developmental pathways to offending,' *Journal of Psychopathology and Behavioral Assessment, 31*:271–284.

Leichsenring, F., Leibing, E., Kruse, J., New, A. S., and Leweke, F. (2011) 'Borderline personality disorder,' *The Lancet, 377*:74–84.

Lobbestael, J., and McNally, R. J. (2016) 'An empirical test of rejection- and anger-related interpretation bias in borderline personality disorder,' *Journal of Personality Disorders, 30*:307–319.

Lupien, S. J., McEwen, B. S., Gunnar, M. R., and Heim, C. (2009) 'Effects of stress throughout the lifespan on the brain, behaviour and cognition,' *Nature Reviews Neuroscience, 10*:434–445.

McCrory, E. J., Gerin, M. I., and Viding, E. (2017) 'Annual research review: Childhood maltreatment, latent vulnerability and the shift to preventative psychiatry – the contribution of functional brain imaging,' *Journal of Child Psychology and Psychiatry, 58*:338–357.

McCrory, E. J., and Viding, E. (2015) 'The theory of latent vulnerability: Reconceptualizing the link between childhood maltreatment and psychiatric disorder,' *Development and Psychopathology, 27*:493–505.

Meehan, A. J., Maughan, B., Cecil, C. A., and Barker, E. D. (2017) 'Interpersonal callousness and co-occurring anxiety: Developmental validity of an adolescent taxonomy,' *Journal of Abnormal Psychology, 126*:225–244.

Miller, J. D., Dir, A., Gentile, B., Wilson, L., Pryor, L. R., and Campbell, W. K. (2010) 'Searching for a vulnerable dark triad: Comparing factor 2 psychopathy, vulnerable narcissism, and borderline personality disorder,' *Journal of Personality, 78*:1529–1564.

Moran, P., Ford, T., Butler, G., and Goodman, R. (2008) 'Callous and unemotional traits in children and adolescents living in Great Britain,' *British Journal of Psychiatry, 192*:65–66.

Moran, P., Rowe, R., Flach, C., Briskman, J., Ford, T., Maughan, B., Scott, S., and Goodman, R. (2009) 'Predictive value of callous–unemotional traits in a large community sample,' *Journal of the American Academy of Child and Adolescent Psychiatry, 48*:1079–1084.

Muthén, L. K., and Muthén, B. O. (1998–2016) *Mplus. The comprehensive modeling program for applied researchers. User's guide* (7.22 ed.), Los Angeles, CA: Muthén & Muthén.

Paulhus, D. L., and Williams, K. M. (2002) 'The dark triad of personality: Narcissism, Machiavellianism, and psychopathy,' *Journal of Research in Personality, 36*:556–563.

Porter, S. (1996) 'Without conscience or without active conscience? The etiology of psychopathy revisited,' *Aggression and Violent Behavior, 1*:179–189.

Poythress, N. G., Skeem, J. L., and Lilienfeld, S. O. (2006) 'Associations among early abuse, dissociation, and psychopathy in an offender sample,' *Journal of Abnormal Psychology, 115*:288–305.

Price, S. D., Salekin, R. T., Klinger, M. R., and Barker, E. D. (2013) 'Psychopathy and depression as predictors of psychosocial difficulties in a sample of court evaluated adolescents,' *Personality Disorders: Theory, Research, and Treatment, 4*:261–277.

Salekin, R. T. (2008) 'Psychopathy and recidivism from mid-adolescence to young adulthood: Cumulating legal problems and limiting life opportunities,' *Journal of Abnormal Psychology, 117*:386–395.

Sanislow, C. A., Grilo, C. M., Morey, L. C., Bender, D. S., Skodol, A. E., Gunderson, J. G., . . ., and McGlashan, T. H. (2002) 'Confirmatory factor analysis of DSM–IV criteria for borderline personality disorder: Findings from the collaborative longitudinal personality disorders study,' *American Journal of Psychiatry, 159*:284–290.

Scheiderer, E. M., Wang, T., Tomko, R. L., Wood, P. K., and Trull, T. J. (2016) 'Negative affect instability among individuals with comorbid borderline personality disorder and posttraumatic stress disorder,' *Clinical Psychological Science, 4*:67–81.

Schreier, A., Wolke, D., Thomas, K., Horwood, J., Hollis, C., Gunnell, D., Lewis, G., Thompson, A., Zammit, S., Duffy, L., Salvi, G., and Harrison, G. (2009) 'Prospective study of peer victimization in childhood and psychotic symptoms in a nonclinical population at age 12 years,' *Archives of General Psychiatry, 66*:527–536.

Sharf, A., Kimonis, E. R., and Howard, A. (2014) 'Negative life events and posttraumatic stress disorder among incarcerated boys with callous–unemotional traits,' *Journal of Psychopathology and Behavioral Assessment, 36*:401–414.

Singham, T., Viding, E., Schoeler, T. et al. (2017) 'Concurrent and longitudinal contribution of exposure to bullying in childhood to mental health: The role of vulnerability and resilience,' *JAMA Psychiatry*, in press.

Skeem, J., Johansson, P., Andershed, H., Kerr, M., and Louden, J. E. (2007) 'Two subtypes of psychopathic violent offenders that parallel primary and secondary variants,' *Journal of Abnormal Psychology, 116*:395–409.

Takizawa, R., Maughan, B., and Arseneault, L. (2014) 'Adult health outcomes of childhood bullying victimization: Evidence from a five-decade longitudinal British birth cohort,' *American Journal of Psychiatry, 171*:777–784.

Viding, E., Blair, R. J. R., Moffitt, T. E., and Plomin, R. (2005) 'Evidence for substantial genetic risk for psychopathy in 7-year-olds,' *Journal of Child Psychology and Psychiatry, 46*:592–597.

Winsper, C., Wolke, D., and Lereya, T. (2015) 'Prospective associations between prenatal adversities and borderline personality disorder at 11–12 years,' *Psychological Medicine, 45*:1025–1037.

Wolke, D., Schreier, A., Zanarini, M. C., and Winsper, C. (2012) 'Bullied by peers in childhood and borderline personality symptoms at 11 years of age: A prospective study,' *Journal of Child Psychology and Psychiatry, 53*:846–855.

Wolke, D., Waylen, A., Samara, M., Steer, C., Goodman, R., Ford, T., and Lamberts, K. (2009) 'Selective drop-out in longitudinal studies and non-biased prediction of behaviour disorders,' *British Journal of Psychiatry, 195*:249–256.

Yang, M., Wong, S. C., and Coid, J. (2010) 'The efficacy of violence prediction: A meta-analytic comparison of nine risk assessment tools,' *Psychological Bulletin, 136*:740–767.

Zanarini, M. C., Frankenburg, F. R., Hennen, J., Reich, D. B., and Silk, K. R. (2004) 'Axis I comorbidity in patients with borderline personality disorder: 6-year follow-up and prediction of time to remission,' *American Journal of Psychiatry, 161*:2108–2114.

Zanarini, M. C., Frankenburg, F. R., Dubo, E. D., Sickel, A. E., Trikha, A., Levin, A., and Reynolds, V. (1998) 'Axis I comorbidity of borderline personality disorder,' *American Journal of Psychiatry, 155*:1733–1739.

Zanarini, M. C., Horwood, J., Wolke, D., Waylen, A., Fitzmaurice, G., and Grant, B. F. (2011) 'Prevalence of DSM–IV borderline personality disorder in two community samples: 6,330 English 11-year-olds and 34,653 American adults,' *Journal of Personality Disorders, 25*:607–619.

32

Psychopathic traits and substance use

Co-occurrence and overlapping etiological pathways

Edelyn Verona, Amy Hoffmann, and Bethany Edwards

Introduction

Despite decades of research, intervention, and prevention efforts, substance use and substance use disorders (SUD) are still costly public health issues. In the United States, approximately 14 percent of individuals have engaged in binge drinking in the last 30 days and 14 percent have used illicit substances in the last year, with 9 percent of the population qualifying for a diagnosis of a SUD annually (Frone, 2006; Grant et al., 2004; Miller et al., 2004). Last decade, it was estimated that costs associated with substance use reached $559 billion in the United States (National Institute of Drug Abuse, 2008). Substance use is especially prevalent among individuals with a history of incarceration (Fazel, Bains, & Doll, 2006). Some of this is due to the illegal nature of some substance use, which exposes individuals to the legal system. This connection is also due to shared characteristics across those who commit crimes and those who use substances. That is, psychopathic traits are known to co-occur with substance use, and these traits are closely tied to antisocial behaviors and history of legal troubles. The goal of this chapter is to review possible explanations for links between psychopathic traits and substance use, including examining biological, developmental, and environmental/lifestyle factors.

As has been discussed elsewhere in this book, psychopathy is distinguished from Antisocial Personality Disorder (ASPD; APA, 2013). The items selected to index psychopathy in the most-often used assessment, the Psychopathy Checklist–Revised (PCL–R; Hare, 2003), were meant to capture a unitary diagnostic entity. However, they are in fact tapping separate constructs – at least one entailing emotional insensitivity and social dominance (Factor 1), and the other impulsiveness and hostile negative affectivity (Factor 2) (Patrick & Bernat, 2009; Verona, Hicks, & Patrick, 2005; Schoenleber, Sadeh, & Verona, 2011). Factor 2 impulsive–antisocial features of psychopathy, as well as ASPD, coincide with the externalizing spectrum of psychopathology. Krueger et al. (2002) proposed that a broad dispositional liability, presumably disinhibition, contributes to various disorders in the externalizing spectrum, including ASPD, alcohol and drug use disorders, and child Conduct Disorder. Indeed, statistical modeling has confirmed that variance specific to PCL–R Factor 2, which accounts largely for the PCL–R's relationship with ASPD, reflects this broad externalizing liability (Patrick, Hicks, Krueger, & Lang, 2005). As such, associations between psychopathy and substance use likely reflect in large part this externalizing liability.

Co-occurrence: substance use and psychopathy

There has been a long-standing interest in the co-occurrence of psychopathy and substance use, with psychopathic traits useful in distinguishing individuals at heightened risk for substance use. For example, 83 percent of men with alcohol abuse and/or dependence (Neo, McCullagh, & Howard, 2001) and 15.1 percent of men and women in alcohol treatment (Windle, 1999) score high in psychopathy (PCL–R score > 30 in men, > 25 in women). Despite overall lower rates of psychopathy in women, substance-using women show a higher prevalence of psychopathy than non-using women, with 1.5 percent (i.e., PCL–R ≥ 30) and 3.6–23.3 percent (i.e., PCL–R ≥ 25) of drug-dependent women scoring high on psychopathy (Piotrowski, Tusel, Sees, Banys, & Hall, 1996; Rutherford, Cacciola, & Alterman, 1999). Likewise, there is high prevalence of alcohol and drug use among men high in psychopathy, with rates ranging from 35–92.9 percent and 31–95.7 percent for alcohol and drug use disorders (Blackburn & Coid, 1998; Hemphill, Hart, & Hare, 1994; Smith & Newman, 1990).

As alluded to earlier, studies suggest differential relations between the two overarching factors of psychopathy and substance use. In particular, adolescent and adult men and women offenders show a positive association between psychopathy Factor 2 (e.g., impulsivity, irresponsibility) and alcohol and drug use disorder symptoms, substance use versatility, and younger age of alcohol and drug use initiation (e.g., Corrado, Vincent, Hart, & Cohen, 2004; Hart, Forth, & Hare, 1991; Hemphill et al., 1994; Hicks, Vaidyanathan, & Patrick, 2010; Smith & Newman, 1990). At the facet level, studies across men and women offenders have shown positive associations between the impulsive lifestyle and antisocial components, but especially the former, with alcohol and drug use (Gustavson et al., 2007; Kennealy, Hicks, & Patrick, 2007; Schultz, Murphy, & Verona, 2016; Walsh, Allen, & Kosson, 2007). While there has been little work on gender differences, Schultz et al. (2016) showed a stronger relationship between the antisocial facet and drug use in women than men. The authors theorized that the disproportionate legal consequences faced by women who use substances may account for the stronger relationship between antisocial scores and substance use in women than men.

While less evidence supports relationships with Factor 1, a few studies on incarcerated men have shown positive relations between Factor 1 and drug use disorder symptoms and drug use versatility and negative relations with age of first use (Blackburn & Coid, 1998; Hemphill et al., 1994). However, most work has shown larger effects for Factor 2 relative to Factor 1 (e.g., Hemphill et al., 1994; Smith & Newman, 1990; Walsh et al., 2007). While still sparse, initial research on women offenders suggests there may be gender differences with respect to Factor 1, such that Factor 1 traits may play a protective role, shown by smaller relationships between scores on this factor and symptoms of drug use (positive) and age of first use (negative) in women (Kennealy et al., 2007; Schultz et al., 2016). Taken together, research suggests that impulsive and antisocial aspects of psychopathy, most closely tied to externalizing, are robustly linked to substance use, with more modest evidence for the interpersonal and affective features contributing to substance use problems.

While evidence supports a link between Factor 2 and substance use, consideration should be given to the possibility that psychopathy assessments may be confounded in substance users, since alcohol and drug use are often incorporated in ratings of Factor 2 traits in particular. Specifically, it is likely that the link between elevated PCL–R scores and substance use in part is due to Factor 2 capturing drug-related crime (e.g., drug offenses, theft/fraud to fund drug habit; Campbell, Porter, & Santor, 2004). In sum, to date the evidence is unclear whether the link between psychopathy and substance use is best explained by criterion overlap with Factor 2 traits or rather represents a shared etiological pathway, discussed next.

Etiological paths: substance use and psychopathy

Heritability

The issue of heterogeneity in the familial transmission of substance use disorders has spurred deeper examination of factors influencing the onset, developmental course, and associated outcomes of SUD in individuals with genetic predisposition. Early work by Cloninger and colleagues (Cloninger, Bohman, & Sigvardsson, 1981; Sigvardsson, Bohman, & Cloninger, 1996) found evidence for two distinct subtypes of alcoholism: Type I, associated with alcohol abuse in both biological parents and in both male and female children of alcoholics; and Type II, primarily observed in sons of severely alcoholic and antisocial fathers and associated with co-occurring antisocial behavior. Although overall less common in occurrence, Type II predisposed boys were more likely to actually develop alcoholism than Type I, potentially suggesting a stronger genetic link for Type II (e.g., Type II ~ 90 percent, Type I ~ 40 percent; McGue, 1999; although, see Prescott et al., 2005). These findings, particularly the marked heritability of Type II alcoholism, suggest the presence of a shared genetic vulnerability between alcoholism and antisociality. As such, the majority of work exploring the genetic connections between substance use and psychopathy has focused specifically on the Factor 2 impulsive–antisocial traits. Less work has explored potential genetic overlap between Factor 1 Interpersonal/Affective traits and substance use problems. Based on Cloninger's typology, Type II individuals would theoretically show overlap with Factor 1 psychopathy, since they are characterized by low harm avoidance, disregard for social rewards, high sensation seeking, and low internalizing symptoms (Cloninger et al., 1981). However, more recent literature indicates that alcoholics with Type I and Type II features share frequent comorbidity of internalizing symptoms (Babor et al., 1992; McGue, Slutske, Taylor, & Lacono, 1997; Windle & Scheidt, 2004) and increased levels of harm avoidance compared to healthy controls (Ducci et al., 2007). This indicates that low anxiety/fearlessness (Factor 1 – associated traits central to etiological theories of psychopathy) are unlikely candidates for shared genetic vulnerability between SUD and psychopathy.

Neurobiological mechanisms

Several attempts have been made to understand the neurobiological mechanisms of substance use, which provide some initial insights about mechanisms potentially explaining the genetic links underlying psychopathy and substance use. Mechanisms explored include impairments across attentional, behavioral, and affective processes, specifically the following.

Reward sensitivity

Psychopathy and substance use have both been characterized by alterations in reward processing, thought to reflect impaired reinforcement learning and novelty and/or sensation seeking behaviors. First, although there is consensus that reward experiences are altered among individuals with substance use, the manner in which this happens is still debated (e.g., Zald & Treadway, 2017). Some models implicate hyper-activation of reward systems, thought to promote impulsive behavior (e.g., substance use) in anticipation of potential reward (see Hommer, Bjork, & Gilman, 2011 for review). In contrast, other work has suggested that substance use stems from hypo-activation of reward systems, wherein substances are used to compensate for deficient reward circuitry. Second, studies on psychopathy have also provided evidence in support of an impaired reward processing system and, similar to those on substance use, have provided mixed evidence in terms of whether this impairment represents a hyper- or hyposensitivity to reward. For example, researchers have shown associations between psychopathy Factor 2 traits and heightened sensitivity to reward (Bjork, Chen, & Hommer, 2012; Buckholtz et al., 2010; Glenn & Yang, 2012). In contrast, studies in youth have shown an association between psychopathic features and *reduced* reward sensitivity (Finger et al., 2011; Centifanti & Modecki, 2013). Neuroimaging research has linked both substance use and psychopathy (particularly Factor 2) to increased functioning in the ventral striatum (VS) (e.g., Everitt & Robbins, 2005; Glenn & Yang, 2012), a brain region implicated in reward-dependent behaviors, as well as increased sensitization of the dopaminergic reward system (e.g., Buckholtz et al., 2010; Dawe, Gullo, & Loxton, 2004). Thus, the data in adults support heightened reward responding as a common link to explain behavior evident across both of these conditions (e.g., sensation seeking).

Punishment and affective reactivity

Substance use and psychopathy have been similarly linked to impairments in responsiveness to punishment and aversive stimuli. Substance intoxication appears to contribute to deficient affective reactivity (Hefner, Moberg, Hachiva, & Curtin, 2013; Bedi, Phan, Angstadt, & de Wit, 2009), and those with problematic substance use have shown *reduced* sensitivity to punishment, a characteristic that may help to explain engagement in behavior with potentially harmful consequences (Pardo, Aguilar, Molinuevo, & Torrubia, 2007; Simons & Arens, 2007). In contrast, a growing body of work has connected problematic levels of substance use to *heightened* affective response to aversive stimuli and exacerbation of threat circuits. That is, studies have shown increased substance craving response to stressful stimuli (Cooney, Litt, Morse, Bauer, & Gaupp, 1997), elevated startle potentiation to unpredictable threat (Gorka, Lieberman, Phan, & Shankman, 2016), and anxiety hypersensitivity among problematic substance users (Lejuez, Paulson, Daughters, Bornovalova, & Zvolensky, 2006). With that said, hypersensitivity to negative affect may actually develop in response to chronic substance use as a result of alterations in brain reward pathways over time (e.g., increased sensitivity in dopaminergic-neuron response), particularly during withdrawal (Spanagel & Weiss, 1999).

Affective deficits have long been central to major theories of psychopathy. Early research has borne this out, showing that individuals scoring high in psychopathy show reduced startle reflex to unpleasant and/or threatening stimuli (Levenston, Patrick, Bradley, & Lang, 2000), reduced electrodermal responses to distressing cues (Blair, Jones, Clark, & Smith, 1997; Hare, Frazelle, & Cox, 1978), diminished threat expectation (Hare, 1965), and reduced amygdala activity to emotional and/or aversive stimuli (see Anderson & Kiehl, 2012 for review). However, studies examining affective reactivity in relation to distinct psychopathic traits have connected Factor 1 (i.e., primary psychopathy) to low levels and Factor 2 (i.e., secondary psychopathy) to high or normal levels of affective responsiveness to aversive stimuli (Patrick, 1994; Skeem, Johansson, Andershed, Kerr, & Louden, 2007; Verona, Patrick, Curtin, Bradley, & Lang, 2004). As such, it appears as though heightened affective sensitivity in conjunction with reduced responsiveness to punishment may help to account for overlap between substance use and Factor 2 traits. Given that Factor 1 has largely been characterized by low levels of affective responsiveness and that reduced responsiveness has been more often connected with substance use intoxication opposed to problematic levels of use, this might help to explain why there is little overlap across Factor 1 traits and substance use, at least at the diagnostic level.

Inhibitory control

Studies have related deficits in inhibitory control to substance use problems and psychopathy. These deficits are not only involved in the development of substance use among adolescents, but also increase risk for prolonged and more frequent use among adults (de Wit, 2009; Ivanov, Schulz, London, & Newcorn, 2008; Verdejo-García, Lawrence, & Clark, 2008). Neuroimaging studies have furthered understanding on the neural correlates of impaired control in substance use and have connected these impairments to frontal areas of the brain implicated in inhibition, including the prefrontal cortex (PFC) broadly, as well as the orbitofrontal cortex (OFC) and anterior cingulate cortex (ACC) more specifically (Garavan & Hester, 2007; Worhunsky et al., 2013). Moreover, studies using electrocortical indices of inhibition have further supported this notion, showing evidence of reduced P300 amplitude in frontal brain regions among substance users (e.g., Biggins, MacKay, Clark, & Fein, 1997).

Relative to the literature on cognitive control impairments in substance use, study results in psychopathy are mixed in regard to inhibitory control impairments. That is, some studies present evidence in support of difficulties in inhibitory control among individuals scoring high on psychopathic traits (and Factor 2) (Heritage & Benning, 2013; Zeier, Baskin-Sommers, Hiatt Racer, & Newman, 2012), whereas others have failed to find evidence of inhibitory control deficits within psychopathy (Dvorak-Bertsch, Curtin, Rubinstein, & Newman, 2007; Munro et al., 2007). Likewise, some studies on the P300 response in individuals with psychopathic traits show enhanced P300 amplitude, while others show reduced amplitude or no difference between individuals with and without such traits (see Kiehl, 2006 for review). A recent meta-analysis has helped to reconcile mixed findings. Gao and Raine (2009) highlighted an association between reduced P300 amplitude and antisociality (i.e., Factor 2) in particular, pointing to little association with Factor 1 traits of psychopathy, findings that have been supported in electrocortical studies of inhibitory control in psychopathy (Verona, Sprague, & Sadeh, 2012). Lastly, prior neuroimaging work has linked limited inhibitory control and Factor 2 to reduced activity in similar brain regions as implicated in substance use, including the PFC and ACC (see Yang & Raine, 2009 for review). Thus, results from the above studies offer evidence for yet another shared underlying impairment between substance use and Factor 2 of psychopathy. This helps to explain common disinhibited tendencies across these two disorders.

Developmental considerations

Examination of symptom trajectories observed in substance use and psychopathic traits provides insight into ways in which the two conditions overlap and influence one another across development. Research suggests that substance use frequency and problems peak in late adolescence, with the highest concentration of SUD diagnoses present during this developmental epoch, followed by a normative drop-off in rates (Bates & Labouvie, 1997; Chassin, Flora, & King, 2004; Chen & Kandel, 1995). Many studies have found that age of onset is the most important factor in differentiating alcohol use trajectories (Glenn & Nixon, 1991), with younger age of onset typically associated with greater frequency of use and problems with both alcohol and drugs. This finding is particularly robust, demonstrated across substance type and in various samples (Grant & Dawson, 1997; Grant & Dawson, 1998).

Age of onset has been identified as an important factor in the development and course of antisocial behavior and psychopathic traits as well (Frick & Viding, 2009; Moffitt, 1993). Classic research identified at least two trajectories of antisocial development: adolescent-onset, potentially reflecting a relatively normative period of increased antisocial behavior; and life-course persistent, marked by antisocial behavior beginning in childhood and persisting through adulthood (Moffitt, 1993; Moffitt & Caspi, 2001). This second trajectory type can be further divided by the presence or absence of callous–unemotional (CU) traits (the pediatric analogue of the Factor 1 affective/callous facet of psychopathy; Frick & Viding, 2009). The combination of CU traits with conduct problems in childhood has been associated with higher levels of psychopathy in adulthood and increased engagement in antisocial and delinquent behavior across the lifespan (Lynam, Caspi, Moffitt, Loeber, & Stouthamer-Loeber, 2007; McMahon, Witkiewitz, & Kotler, 2010).

In terms of the links between psychopathy and substance use development, the combination of high CU traits and high conduct problems has been associated with subsequent early onset substance use problems in boys in particular (Wymbs et al., 2012). Although much of the adult literature has emphasized the importance of Factor 2 related traits (i.e., disinhibition) on the connection between psychopathy and SUD, the findings in youth suggest that precursors to Factor 1 related traits (CU) play a role as well, particularly early in developmental time. Boldness, a trait associated with Factor 1 that captures some elements of sensation seeking, may account for the connection. A study by Hicks, Iacono, and McGue (2014) found children high in Boldness and low in socialization (ability or desire to adhere to social norms, values, etc.) were more likely than their peers to develop SUD by adolescence and adulthood. Taken in sum, this literature suggests that children with CU traits, who are bold and sensation seeking and lack the ability to inhibit their behaviors, may fail to appropriately internalize social expectations, leading to earlier onset of substance use and greater risk of transition to dependence.

Further longitudinal research has attempted to examine the temporal ordering of psychopathic traits and substance use problems. Large-scale twin-study research (Samek et al., 2017) found that personality traits associated with Factor 2 (aggressive under-control and low constraint) were positively related to subsequent increases in alcohol use disorder (AUD) symptoms during late adolescence/early adulthood, but found no evidence for impact of AUD symptoms on subsequent increase in these personality traits. However, this relationship changed during the mid/late twenties, when AUD symptoms and these personality traits began to cross-influence each other. This suggests personality traits associated with Factor 2 in youth may act as risk factors or precursors to the development of AUD during emerging adulthood, and that feedback relationships between substance use and personality may develop later (e.g., adaptations arising from extended time in "addict lifestyle," or due to chemically induced neurological damage; de Wit, 2009; Fillmore & Rush, 2002).

Environmental influences

Along with evidence for biological and developmental overlap between substance use and psychopathy, these conditions may also develop from contextual and environmental forces. Although some studies have found little evidence for the importance of substance use in understanding crime in individuals with psychopathic traits (Mueser et al., 2006), other work has emphasized shared environmental factors which may explain the co-occurrence of criminal and substance using behaviors. The lifestyle theory of crime (Walters, 1990) posits that both substance use and antisocial behavior exert bidirectional influences on one another due to co-occurrence in a shared "lifestyle" (Walters, 2006). Crucial to lifestyle theory is the recursive nature of environmental input, whereby substance use leads to crime, and exposure to criminal environments normalizes and perpetuates substance use in a dynamic loop.

One way in which substance use and crime are connected is through substance use serving as a gateway to crime, either directly (e.g., stealing drugs or money to buy drugs) or indirectly (through immersion in "street" culture and exposure to unrelated criminal opportunities, drug trade/sales, etc.) (Walters, 1992). For example, acute substance intoxication is associated with impaired decision-making and impulsivity, which may reasonably lead to increased likelihood of engaging in criminal behaviors when intoxicated (Hull & Bond, 1986; Ramaekers, Kauert, Theunissen, Toennes, & Moeller, 2009). Substance use may also lead to acquired biological vulnerabilities in the brain that increase risk for the development of both Factor 1 and Factor 2 traits. In terms of Factor 2, prolonged substance use has been linked to diminished cognitive control and increased impulsivity (de Wit, 2009; Fillmore & Rush, 2002), which may lead to increased engagement in antisocial or aggressive behavior. In terms of Factor 1, Kim et al. (2011) found evidence of low insula activity in abstinent meth addicts when processing emotional faces, suggesting that impairments in emotion processing and empathy follow from chronic substance use and persist even after discontinuation. Literature in this area is often cross-sectional, and as such is limited in resolving temporal order or directionality.

Beyond the ways in which use of substances may alter personality and behavior linked to psychopathy, adverse experiences can play a role in the development of both substance use and psychopathic traits, especially Factor 2 impulsive–antisocial features. Child abuse and family violence have been identified as significant predictors of both SUD and antisocial behavior (Boles, Joshi, Grella, & Wellisch, 2005; Clark, Masson, Delucchi, Hall, & Sees, 2001). Exposure to chaotic and violent family environments may lead to engagement in substance use and antisocial behavior, such as through social learning effects and picking up caregivers' ineffective methods of coping with negative emotion and conflict (Bandura, 1977). Family violence and child abuse may also lead to increased contact with substance using and criminal lifestyle elements through attempts to escape the home via running away and other status offenses (Henry & Thornberry, 2010; Lansford et al., 2007). There is some evidence that child abuse and family violence differentially affect antisocial and substance-use outcomes in girls and boys (Chesney-Lind & Pasko, 2013; although see Bozzay, Joy, & Verona, in press). This relationship may be indirect, with sexual abuse increasing girls' and women's propensities to engage in risky behaviors (e.g., sex work), which heightens their exposure to substance use and encourages criminal engagement (Verona, Murphy, & Javdani, 2016).

The evidence supports the role of adverse environments in shaping Factor 1 interpersonal/affective psychopathic traits also. The latter may develop or become more prominent in response to stressful environmental conditions that overlap with substance use. For example, there is a variant of psychopathy, termed "secondary psychopathy," that is said to be an environmentally mediated expression of psychopathy resulting from adverse environmental conditions (Blackburn, 1975; Karpman, 1941). Secondary psychopathy manifests in callous and unempathic behaviors but is marked by high levels of negative affect and anxiety (characteristics shared by individuals with substance abuse problems; Ducci et al., 2007). This manifestation has been particularly associated with trauma exposure and prior substance use (Hicks et al., 2010), indicating that it may follow from invaliding environments and history of using substances.

Implications for treatment

The presence of psychopathic traits in conjunction with substance use poses considerable treatment challenges (e.g., Taylor & Lang, 2006), and initial work in this domain led scholars to cast doubt on responsiveness to treatment within this population. That is, prior research has shown that in substance abusers, elevated psychopathic traits have been related to higher levels of substance use relapse and violent criminal recidivism, as well as higher dropout rates and lower treatment compliance (O'Neill, Lidz, & Heilbrun, 2003; Richards, Casey, & Lucente, 2003; Walsh, 1999). However, recent work has yielded more favorable results, suggesting that substance abusers with personality pathology (i.e., psychopathic traits) may benefit from treatment to a similar degree as those without personality pathology (Polaschek & Daly, 2013; Salekin, Worley, & Grimes, 2010; Verheul, 2001). Thorough assessment of personality pathology among individuals with substance use may not only aid in development of appropriate intervention techniques, but is also likely to inform shared etiological underpinnings contributing to antisocial behavior targeted in treatment (Verheul, 2001).

Researchers have also devoted attention to ways in which dual-diagnosis may help to inform treatment practices (e.g., Barrowclough, Haddock, Tarrier, Moring, & Lewis, 2000; Drake & Wallach, 2000). In line with work suggesting that it is more difficult to treat dual-diagnoses than "pure" diagnoses (Kessler, 2004), some researchers have suggested that clinicians target one of the disorders first, with the expectation that those efforts will in turn impact the other. However, research is mixed on which disorder to target first. For instance, it has been proposed that one should first focus on treatment of substance use, with the expectation that this will then reduce criminal activity among individuals with psychopathic traits (e.g., funding a drug habit) (Holloway, Bennett, & Farrington, 2006; Prendergast, Podus, Chang, & Urada, 2002), consistent with the lifestyle theory of crime (Walters, 1990). Other work has instead suggested that individuals with psychopathic traits may be likely to engage in crime regardless of substance use, and accordingly, it may be beneficial to focus first on the treatment of psychopathy and the impulsive–antisocial traits in particular (e.g., Mueser et al., 2006).

More promising work has proposed that clinicians attempt to target underlying features that are shared across psychopathy and substance use (e.g., impulsivity) by way of combining and/or modifying existing cognitive–behavioral treatment techniques (Polaschek & Daly, 2013; Salekin et al., 2010). Pulling from work by Polaschek & Daly (2013), it makes sense that intervention methods should focus on the reduction of dynamic cognitive and/or behavioral risk factors shown to be correlates of both substance use and psychopathy (Skeem, Polaschek, Patrick, & Lilienfeld, 2011). For instance, as highlighted by our review of neurobiological processes above, methods aimed at enhancing cognitive control as a treatment focus may be effective in decreasing criminal behavior and increasing abstinence from substances.

Given that psychopathy is a heterogeneous construct, individuals with differential levels of traits may benefit from distinct interventions (Gudonis, Derefinko, & Giancola, 2009; Verheul, 2001). For example, research has linked unique variance of Factor 2 to elevated internalizing symptoms, negative affect, impulsivity, and substance use (Hicks & Patrick, 2006; Verona, Patrick, & Joiner, 2001). Thus, treatment aimed at boosting inhibitory control and emotion regulation may be effective for individuals high in Factor 2 (Gudonis et al., 2009). Dialectical behavior therapy (DBT) is one such treatment (e.g., Galietta & Rosenfeld, 2012), shown to be effective among individuals with Borderline Personality Disorder, which is often comorbid with substance use (Trull, Sher, Minks-Brown, Durbin, & Burr, 2000) and defined by several symptoms that overlap with Factor 2 (e.g., impulsivity, aggression; Edwards, Albertson, & Verona, in press; Miller et al., 2010). In contrast to this approach to Factor 2, treatments designed to increase responsiveness to contextual cues in the environment, and utilization of these cues in conjunction with affective information, may be useful in individuals with Factor 1 traits (Baskin-Sommers, Curtin, & Newman, 2015; Brennan, Hyde, & Baskin-Sommers, 2017). Further, focus on external incentives and contingency management to shape negative behaviors, including those that interfere with treatment compliance, may prove beneficial in these individuals (Gudonis et al., 2009).

Taken together, research has shown that while initially treatment prognosis for those with comorbid psychopathy and substance use seemed quite grim, more recent work provides evidence that these individuals may indeed benefit from treatment (Polaschek & Daly, 2013; Salekin et al., 2010). This is especially the case when clinicians stray away from a one-size-fits-all approach and instead implement treatment strategies tailored to target distinct psychopathic traits (i.e., Factor 1 versus Factor 2) most evident in the individual.

Conclusion

Our review indicates that it is likely inaccurate to discuss the overlap between psychopathy and substance use unless one acknowledges the "configural" nature of psychopathic traits. That is, newer conceptualizations question whether psychopathy can be considered a syndrome (e.g., co-occurring symptoms from common etiology), or instead results from joint development of trait vulnerabilities involving disinhibition, callousness, and boldness (Lilienfeld, 2013; Patrick, Fowles, & Krueger, 2009). As such, the review of studies on psychopathic traits supports connections between substance use and a subset of psychopathy features, specifically the impulsive–antisocial facets. Vulnerabilities in affective processing and inhibitory control deficits, as well as environmental disadvantage, seem to be shared across substance use and Factor 2 traits. In contrast, evidence suggests that links between substance use and Factor 1 psychopathic traits may emanate from the long-term effects of substance use and shared environments that may desensitize individuals to the suffering of others (e.g., Hicks et al., 2010; Ray, Thornton, Frick, Steinberg, & Cauffman, 2016). However, no longitudinal work has been conducted to confirm these expectations and temporal sequence.

Some caveats are in order. Reviewing the links between psychopathy and substance use is complicated by the various effects and consequences associated with different types of substances. A particularly important distinction is between alcohol, which is typically a legal substance, and illicit drugs, including marijuana, cocaine, opiates, and others. The research is sometimes specific, but in most cases, different drugs of abuse are not distinguished in relation to psychopathy. Even illicit substances vary in their pharmacological effects and social impact, with use of some substances (e.g., marijuana) becoming more accepted as the culture around drug use changes. This will likely influence the extent to which substance use is linked to deviant traits. This review is also complicated by the various ways in which substance use is measured. The role of psychopathic features may differ depending on whether one is measuring regular use or symptoms/problems from use of substances. For example, Factor 1 traits are potentially more related to experimental use (e.g., Walsh et al., 2007) and Factor 2 more often associated with addiction (e.g., Reardon, Lang, & Patrick, 2002). These use patterns may also shift across time, with Factor 1-related traits leading to earlier experimentation with substances, increasing risk of eventual dependency (e.g., Grant & Dawson, 1997; Hick et al., 2014).

In spite of these limitations, this chapter synthesized across several domains of study to suggest shared trajectories in psychopathy and substance use. Early temperaments marked by disinhibition and altered reward processing may shape, and be shaped by, interpersonal and environmental influences that may result in increased disadvantage, higher levels of negative affect, and reduced effective coping skills. The combination of temperamental tendencies toward sensation seeking and maladaptive attempts to cope with adverse circumstances may precipitate the early onset of substance use and associated engagement in deviant behaviors. That is, among predisposed youth, exposure to stressful environments further increases the likelihood of negative outcomes through various routes. First, the early exposure to substances and/or head injury often co-occurring with risky lifestyles can produce brain alterations that exacerbate deficient inhibitory control and affective dysregulation (Casey & Jones, 2010; Clark, Thatcher, & Tapert, 2008). This pathway implicates Factor 2 and externalizing vulnerabilities in the substance use–psychopathy etiological connection, as reflected in the literature. Second, Factor 1 features, especially callousness, may also result from this history, as substance use and repeated rejection/alienation from others may promote insensitivity to the plight of others and a narrow focus on achieving rewards. However, this latter trajectory reflects a different etiological process from that implicated in "primary" psychopathy (e.g., fearlessness, boldness). Future research would benefit from mapping potential etiological pathways across time and the multiple ways that the substance use–psychopathy combined phenotype can come about (i.e., equifinality).

References

American Psychiatric Association. (2013) *Diagnostic and statistical manual of mental disorders* (5th ed.), Arlington, VA: American Psychiatric Publishing.

Anderson, N. E., and Kiehl, K. A. (2012) 'The psychopath magnetized: Insights from brain Imaging,' *Trends in Cognitive Sciences*, *16*:52–60.

Babor, T. F., Dolinsky, Z. S., Meyer, R. E., Hesselbrock, M., Hofmann, M., and Tennen, H. (1992) 'Types of alcoholics: Concurrent and predictive validity of some common classification schemes,' *Addiction*, *87*:1415–1431.

Bandura, A. (1977) 'Self-efficacy: Toward a unifying theory of behavioral change,' *Psychological Review*, *84*:191–215.

Barrowclough, C., Haddock, G., Tarrier, N., Moring, J., and Lewis, S. (2000) 'Cognitive behavioral intervention for individuals with severe mental illness who have a substance misuse problem,' *Psychiatric Rehabilitation Skills*, *4*:216–233.

Baskin-Sommers, A. R., Curtin, J. J., and Newman, J. P. (2015) 'Altering the cognitive–affective dysfunctions of psychopathic and externalizing offender subtypes with cognitive remediation,' *Clinical Psychological Science*, *3*:45–57.

Bates, M. E., and Labouvie, E. W. (1997) 'Adolescent risk factors and the prediction of persistent alcohol and drug use into adulthood,' *Alcoholism: Clinical and Experimental Research*, *21*:944–950.

Bedi, G., Phan, K. L., Angstadt, M., and de Wit, H. (2009) 'Effects of MDMA on sociability and neural response to social threat and social reward,' *Psychopharmacology*, *207*(1):73–83.

Biggins, C. A., MacKay, S., Clark, W., and Fein, G. (1997) 'Event-related potential evidence for frontal cortex effects of chronic cocaine dependence,' *Biological Psychiatry*, *42*:472–485.

Bjork, J. M., Chen, G., and Hommer, D. W. (2012) 'Psychopathic tendencies and mesolimbic recruitment by cues for instrumental and passively obtained rewards,' *Biological Psychology*, *89*:408–415.

Blackburn, R. (1975) 'An empirical classification of psychopathic personality,' *The British Journal of Psychiatry*, *127*:456–460.

Blackburn, R., and Coid, J. W. (1998) 'Psychopathy and the dimensions of personality disorder in violent offenders,' *Personality and Individual Differences*, *25*:129–145.

Blair, R. J. R., Jones, L., Clark, F., and Smith, M. (1997) 'The psychopathic individual: A lack of responsiveness to distress cues?,' *Psychophysiology*, *34*:192–198.

Boles, S. M., Joshi, V., Grella, C., and Wellisch, J. (2005) 'Childhood sexual abuse patterns, psychosocial correlates, and treatment outcomes among adults in drug abuse treatment,' *Journal of Child Sexual Abuse*, *14*:39–55.

Bozzay, M. L., Joy, L. N., and Verona, E. (in press) 'Family violence pathways and externalizing behavior in youth,' *Journal of Interpersonal Violence*.

Brennan, G. M., Hyde, L. W., and Baskin-Sommers, A. R. (2017) 'Antisocial pathways associated with substance use disorders: Characterizing etiological underpinnings and implications for treatment,' *Current Opinion in Behavioral Sciences*, *13*:124–129.

Buckholtz, J. W., Treadway, M. T., Cowan, R. L., Woodward, N. D., Benning, S. D., Li, R., . . ., and Smith, C. E. (2010) 'Mesolimbic dopamine reward system hypersensitivity in individuals with psychopathic traits,' *Nature Neuroscience*, *13*:419–421.

Campbell, M. A., Porter, S., and Santor, D. (2004) 'Psychopathic traits in adolescent offenders: An evaluation of criminal history, clinical, and psychosocial correlates,' *Behavioral Sciences & the Law*, *22*:23–47.

Casey, B. J., and Jones, R. M. (2010) 'Neurobiology of the adolescent brain and behavior,' *Journal of American Academy Child Adolescent Psychiatry*, *49*:1189–1285.

Centifanti, L. C. M., and Modecki, K. (2013) 'Throwing caution to the wind: Callous–unemotional traits and risk taking in adolescents,' *Journal of Clinical Child & Adolescent Psychology*, *42*:106–119.

Chassin, L., Flora, D. B., and King, K. M. (2004) 'Trajectories of alcohol and drug use and dependence from adolescence to adulthood: The effects of familial alcoholism and personality,' *Journal of Abnormal Psychology*, *113*:483–498.

Chen, K., and Kandel, D. B. (1995) 'The natural history of drug use from adolescence to the mid-thirties in a general population sample,' *American Journal of Public Health*, *85*:41–47.

Chesney-Lind, M., and Pasko, L. (2013) *The female offender: Girls, women, and crime*, Thousand Oaks, CA: Sage.

Clark, H. W., Masson, C. L., Delucchi, K. L., Hall, S. M., and Sees, K. L. (2001) 'Violent traumatic events and drug abuse severity,' *Journal of Substance Abuse Treatment*, *20*:121–127.

Clark, D. B., Thatcher, D. L., and Tapert, S. F. (2008) 'Alcohol, psychological dysregulation, and adolescent brain development,' *Alcoholism: Clinical & Experimental Research*, *32*:375–385.

Cloninger, C. R., Bohman, M., and Sigvardsson, S. (1981) 'Inheritance of alcohol abuse: Cross- fostering analysis of adopted men,' *Archives of General Psychiatry*, *38*:861–868.

Cooney, N. L., Litt, M. D., Morse, P. A., Bauer, L. O., and Gaupp, L. (1997) 'Alcohol cue reactivity, negative-mood reactivity, and relapse in treated alcoholic men,' *Journal of Abnormal Psychology*, *106*:243–250.

Corrado, R. R., Vincent, G. M., Hart, S. D., and Cohen, I. M. (2004) 'Predictive validity of the Psychopathy Checklist: Youth Version for general and violent recidivism,' *Behavioral Sciences & the Law*, *22*:5–22.

Dawe, S., Gullo, M. J., and Loxton, N. J. (2004) 'Reward drive and rash impulsiveness as dimensions of impulsivity: Implications for substance misuse,' *Addictive Behaviors*, *29*:1389–1405.

de Wit, H. (2009) 'Impulsivity as a determinant and consequence of drug use: A review of underlying processes,' *Addiction Biology*, *14*:22–31.

Drake, R. E., and Wallach, M. A. (2000) 'Dual diagnosis: 15 years of progress,' *Psychiatric Services*, *51*:1126–1129.

Ducci, F., Enoch, M. A., Funt, S., Virkkunen, M., Albaugh, B., and Goldman, D. (2007) 'Increased anxiety and other similarities in temperament of alcoholics with and without antisocial personality disorder across three diverse populations,' *Alcohol*, *41*:3–12.

Dvorak-Bertsch, J. D., Curtin, J. J., Rubinstein, T. J., and Newman, J. P. (2007) 'Anxiety moderates the interplay between cognitive and affective processing,' *Psychological Science*, *18*:699–705.

Edwards, B. G., Albertson, E., and Verona, E. (in press) 'Dark and vulnerable personality correlates of dimensions of criminal behavior among adult offenders,' *Journal of Abnormal Psychology.*

Everitt, B. J., and Robbins, T. W. (2005) 'Neural systems of reinforcement for drug addiction: From actions to habits to compulsion,' *Nature Neuroscience*, *8*:1481–1489.

Fazel, S., Bains, P., and Doll, H. (2006) 'Substance abuse and dependence in prisoners: A systematic review,' *Addiction*, *101*:181–191.

Fillmore, M. T., and Rush, C. R. (2002) 'Impaired inhibitory control of behavior in chronic cocaine users,' *Drug and Alcohol Dependence*, *66*:265–273.

Finger, E. C., Marsh, A. A., Blair, K. S., Reid, M. E., Sims, C., Ng, P., . . ., and Blair, R. J. R. (2011) 'Disrupted reinforcement signaling in the orbitofrontal cortex and caudate in youths with conduct disorder or oppositional defiant disorder and a high level of psychopathic traits,' *American Journal of Psychiatry*, *168*:152–162.

Frick, P. J., and Viding, E. (2009) 'Antisocial behavior from a developmental psychopathology Perspective,' *Development and Psychopathology*, *21*:1111–1131.

Frone, M. R. (2006) 'Prevalence and distribution of illicit drug use in the workforce and in the workplace: Findings and implications from a U.S. National survey,' *Journal of Applied Psychology*, *91*:856–869.

Galietta, M., and Rosenfeld, B. (2012) 'Adapting dialectical behavior therapy (DBT) for the treatment of psychopathy,' *International Journal of Forensic Mental Health*, *11*:325–335.

Gao, Y., and Raine, A. (2009) 'P3 event-related potential impairments in antisocial and psychopathic individuals: A meta-analysis,' *Biological Psychology*, *82*:199–210.

Garavan, H., and Hester, R. (2007) 'The role of cognitive control in cocaine dependence,' *Neuropsychology Review*, *17*:337–345.

Glenn, A. L., and Yang, Y. (2012) 'The potential role of the striatum in antisocial behavior and Psychopathy,' *Biological Psychiatry*, *72*:817–822.

Glenn, S. W., and Nixon, S. J. (1991) 'Applications of Cloninger's subtypes in a female alcoholic Sample,' *Alcoholism: Clinical and Experimental Research, 15*:851–857.

Gorka, S. M., Lieberman, L., Phan, K. L., and Shankman, S. A. (2016) 'Association between problematic alcohol use and reactivity to uncertain threat in two independent samples,' *Drug and Alcohol Dependence, 164*:89–96.

Grant, B. F., and Dawson, D. A. (1997) 'Age at onset of alcohol use and its association with DSM–IV alcohol abuse and dependence: Results from the National Longitudinal Alcohol Epidemiologic Survey,' *Journal of Substance Abuse, 9*:103–110.

Grant, B. F., and Dawson, D. A. (1998) 'Age of onset of drug use and its association with DSM–IV drug abuse and dependence: Results from the National Longitudinal Alcohol Epidemiologic Survey,' *Journal of Substance Abuse, 10*:163–173.

Grant, B. F., Stinson, F. S., Dawson, D. A., Chou, S. P., Dufour, M. C., Compton, W., . . ., and Kaplan, K. (2004) 'Prevalence and co-occurrence of substance use disorders and independent mood and anxiety disorders: Results from the national epidemiologic survey on alcohol and related conditions,' *Archives of General Psychiatry, 61*:807–816.

Gudonis, L. C., Derefinko, K., and Giancola, P. R. (2009) 'The treatment of substance misuse in psychopathic individuals: Why heterogeneity matters,' *Substance Use & Misuse, 44*:1415–1433.

Gustavson, C., Ståhlberg, O., Sjödin, A. K., Forsman, A., Nilsson, T., and Anckarsäter, H. (2007) 'Age at onset of substance abuse: A crucial covariate of psychopathic traits and aggression in adult offenders,' *Psychiatry Research, 153*:195–198.

Hare, R. D. (1965) 'Psychopathy, fear arousal and anticipated pain,' *Psychological Reports, 16*:499–502.

Hare, R. D. (2003) *The Psychopathy Checklist–Revised*, Toronto, ON: Multi-Health Systems.

Hare, R. D., Frazelle, J., and Cox, D. N. (1978) 'Psychopathy and physiological responses to threat of an aversive stimulus,' *Psychophysiology, 15*:165–172.

Hart, S. D., Forth, A. E., and Hare, R. D. (1991) 'The MCMI–II and psychopathy,' *Journal of Personality Disorders*, 5:318–327.

Hefner, K. R., Moberg, C. A., Hachiya, L. Y., and Curtin, J. J. (2013) 'Alcohol stress response dampening during imminent versus distal, uncertain threat,' *Journal of Abnormal Psychology, 122*:756–769.

Hemphill, J. F., Hart, S. D., and Hare, R. D. (1994) 'Psychopathy and substance use,' *Journal of Personality Disorders, 8*:169–180.

Henry, K. L., and Thornberry, T. P. (2010) 'Truancy and escalation of substance use during Adolescence,' *Journal of Studies on Alcohol and Drugs, 71*:115–124.

Heritage, A. J., and Benning, S. D. (2013) 'Impulsivity and response modulation deficits in psychopathy: Evidence from the ERN and N1,' *Journal of Abnormal Psychology*, 122:215–222.

Hicks, B. M., Iacono, W. G., and McGue, M. (2014) 'Identifying childhood characteristics that underlie premorbid risk for substance use disorders: Socialization and boldness,' *Development and Psychopathology, 26*:141–157

Hicks, B. M., and Patrick, C. J. (2006) 'Psychopathy and negative emotionality: Analyses of suppressor effects reveal distinct relations with emotional distress, fearfulness, and anger-hostility,' *Journal of Abnormal Psychology, 115*:276–287.

Hicks, B. M., Vaidyanathan, U., and Patrick, C. J. (2010) 'Validating female psychopathy subtypes: Differences in personality, antisocial and violent behavior, substance abuse, trauma, and mental health,' *Personality Disorders: Theory, Research, and Treatment, 1*:38–57.

Holloway, K. R., Bennett, T. H., and Farrington, D. P. (2006) 'The effectiveness of drug treatment programs in reducing criminal behavior: A metaanalysis,' *Psicothema, 18*:620–629.

Hommer, D. W., Bjork, J. M., and Gilman, J. M. (2011) 'Imaging brain response to reward in addictive disorders,' *Annals of the New York Academy of Sciences, 1216*:50–61.

Hull, J. G., and Bond, C. F. (1986) 'Social and behavioral consequences of alcohol consumption and expectancy: A meta-analysis,' *Psychological Bulletin, 99*:347–360.

Ivanov, I., Schulz, K. P., London, E. D., and Newcorn, J. H. (2008) 'Inhibitory control deficits in childhood and risk for substance use disorders: A review,' *The American Journal of Drug and Alcohol Abuse, 34*:239–258.

Karpman, B. (1941) 'On the need of separating psychopathy into two distinct clinical types: The symptomatic and the idiopathic,' *Journal of Criminal Psychopathology, 3*:112–137.

Kennealy, P. J., Hicks, B. M., and Patrick, C. J. (2007) 'Validity of factors of the Psychopathy Checklist–Revised in female prisoners: Discriminant relations with antisocial behavior, substance abuse, and personality,' *Assessment, 14*:323–340.

Kessler, R. C. (2004) 'The epidemiology of dual diagnosis,' *Biological Psychiatry, 56*:730–737.
Kiehl, K. A. (2006) 'A cognitive neuroscience perspective on psychopathy: Evidence for paralimbic system dysfunction,' *Psychiatry Research, 142*:107–128.
Kim, Y. T., Song, H. J., Seo, J. H., Lee, J. J., Lee, J., Kwon, D. H., . . ., and Chang, Y. (2011) 'The differences in neural network activity between methamphetamine abusers and healthy subjects performing an emotion-matching task: Functional MRI study,' *NMR in Biomedicine, 24*:1392–1400.
Krueger, R. F., Hicks, B. M., Patrick, C. J., Carlson, S. R., Iacono, W. G., and McGue, M. (2002) 'Etiologic connections among substance dependence, antisocial behavior and personality: Modeling the externalizing spectrum,' *Journal of Abnormal Psychology, 111*:411–424.
Lansford, J. E., Miller-Johnson, S., Berlin, L. J., Dodge, K. A., Bates, J. E., and Pettit, G. S. (2007) 'Early physical abuse and later violent delinquency: A prospective longitudinal study,' *Child Maltreatment, 12*:233–245.
Lejuez, C. W., Paulson, A., Daughters, S. B., Bornovalova, M. A., and Zvolensky, M. J. (2006) 'The association between heroin use and anxiety sensitivity among inner-city individuals in residential drug use treatment,' *Behaviour Research and Therapy, 44*:667–677.
Levenston, G. K., Patrick, C. J., Bradley, M. M., and Lang, P. J. (2000) 'The psychopath as observer: Emotion and attention in picture processing,' *Journal of Abnormal Psychology, 109*:373–385.
Lilienfeld, S. O. (2013) 'Is psychopathy a syndrome? Commentary on Marcus, Fulton, & Edens,' *Personality Disorders: Theory, Research, and Treatment, 4*:85–86.
Lynam, D. R., Caspi, A., Moffitt, T. E., Loeber, R., and Stouthamer-Loeber, M. (2007) 'Longitudinal evidence that psychopathy scores in early adolescence predict adult psychopathy,' *Journal of Abnormal Psychology, 116*:155–165.
McGue, M. (1999) 'The behavioral genetics of alcoholism,' *Current Directions in Psychological Science, 8*:109–115.
McGue, M., Slutske, W., Taylor, J., and Lacono, W. G. (1997) 'Personality and substance use disorders: I. Effects of gender and alcoholism subtype,' *Alcoholism: Clinical and Experimental Research, 21*:513–520.
McMahon, R. J., Witkiewitz, K., and Kotler, J. S. (2010) 'Predictive validity of callous–unemotional traits measured in early adolescence with respect to multiple antisocial outcomes,' *Journal of Abnormal Psychology, 119*:752–763.
Miller, J. D., Dir, A., Gentile, B., Wilson, L., Pryor, L. R., and Campbell, W. K. (2010) 'Searching for a vulnerable dark triad: Comparing factor 2 psychopathy, vulnerable narcissism, and borderline personality disorder,' *Journal of Personality, 78*:1529–1564.
Miller, J. W., Gfroerer, J. C., Brewer, R. D., Naimi, T. S., Mokdad, A., and Giles, W. H. (2004) 'Prevalence of adult binge drinking: A comparison of two national surveys,' *American Journal of Preventive Medicine, 27*:197–204.
Moffitt, T. E. (1993) 'Adolescence-limited and life-course-persistent antisocial behavior: A developmental taxonomy,' *Psychological Review, 100*:674–701.
Moffitt, T. E., and Caspi, A. (2001) 'Childhood predictors differentiate life-course persistent and adolescence-limited antisocial pathways among males and females,' *Development and Psychopathology, 13*:355–375.
Mueser, K. T., Crocker, A. G., Frisman, L. B., Drake, R. E., Covell, N. H., and Essock, S. M. (2006) 'Conduct disorder and antisocial personality disorder in persons with severe psychiatric and substance use disorders,' *Schizophrenia Bulletin, 32*:626–636.
Munro, G. E., Dywan, J., Harris, G. T., McKee, S., Unsal, A., and Segalowitz, S. J. (2007) 'Response inhibition in psychopathy: The frontal N2 and P3,' *Neuroscience Letters, 418*:149–153.
National Institute on Drug Abuse. (2008) *Addiction science: From molecules to managed care*, Washington, DC: NIDA.
Neo, L. H., McCullagh, P., and Howard, R. (2001) 'An electrocortical correlate of a history of alcohol abuse in criminal offenders,' *Psychology, Crime and Law*, 7:105–117.
O'Neill, M. L., Lidz, V., and Heilbrun, K. (2003) 'Adolescents with psychopathic characteristics in a substance abusing cohort: Treatment process and outcomes,' *Law and Human Behavior, 27*:299–313.
Pardo, Y., Aguilar, R., Molinuevo, B., and Torrubia, R. (2007) 'Alcohol use as a behavioural sign of disinhibition: Evidence from JA Gray's model of personality,' *Addictive Behaviors, 32*:2398–2403.
Patrick, C. J. (1994) 'Emotion and psychopathy: Startling new insights,' *Psychophysiology, 31*:319–330.
Patrick, C. J., and Bernat, E. M. (2009) 'Neurobiology of psychopathy: A two-process theory,' in G. G. Bernston & J. T. Cacioppo (Eds.), *Handbook of neuroscience for the behavioral sciences* (pp. 1110–1131), New York, NY: John Wiley & Sons.
Patrick, C. J., Fowles, D. C., and Krueger, R. F. (2009) 'Triarchic conceptualization of psychopathy: Developmental origins of disinhibition, boldness, and meanness,' *Development and Psychopathology, 21*:913–938.

Patrick, C. J., Hicks, B. M., Krueger, R. F., and Lang, A. R. (2005) 'Relations between psychopathy facets and externalizing in a criminal offender sample,' *Journal of Personality Disorders*, *19*:339–356.
Piotrowski, N. A., Tusel, D. J., Sees, K. L., Banys, P., and Hall, S. M. (1996) 'Psychopathy and antisocial personality in men and women with primary opioid dependence,' *Issues in Criminological and Legal Psychology*, *24*:123–126.
Polaschek, D. L., and Daly, T. E. (2013) 'Treatment and psychopathy in forensic settings,' *Aggression and Violent Behavior*, *18*:592–603.
Prendergast, M. L., Podus, D., Chang, E., and Urada, D. (2002) 'The effectiveness of drug abuse treatment: A meta-analysis of comparison group studies,' *Drug and Alcohol Dependence*, *67*:53–72.
Prescott, C. A., Caldwell, C. B., Carey, G., Vogler, G. P., Trumbetta, S. L., and Gottesman, I. I. (2005) 'The Washington University twin study of alcoholism,' *American Journal of Medical Genetics Part B: Neuropsychiatric Genetics*, *134*:48–55.
Ramaekers, J. G., Kauert, G., Theunissen, E. L., Toennes, S. W., and Moeller, M. R. (2009) 'Neurocognitive performance during acute THC intoxication in heavy and occasional cannabis users,' *Journal of Psychopharmacology*, *23*:266–277.
Ray, J. V., Thornton, L. C., Frick, P. J., Steinberg, L., and Cauffman, E. (2016) 'Impulse control and callous–unemotional traits distinguish patterns of delinquency and substance use in justice involved adolescents: Examining the moderating role of neighborhood context,' *Journal of Abnormal Child Psychology*, *44*:599–611.
Reardon, M. L., Lang, A. R., and Patrick, C. J. (2002) 'An evaluation of relations among antisocial behavior, psychopathic traits, and alcohol problems in incarcerated men,' *Alcoholism: Clinical and Experimental Research*, *26*:1188–1197.
Richards, H. J., Casey, J. O., and Lucente, S. W. (2003) 'Psychopathy and treatment response in incarcerated female substance abusers,' *Criminal Justice and Behavior*, *30*:251–276.
Rutherford, M. J., Cacciola, J. S., and Alterman, A. I. (1999) 'Antisocial personality disorder and psychopathy in cocaine-dependent women,' *American Journal of Psychiatry*, *156*:849–856.
Salekin, R. T., Worley, C., and Grimes, R. D. (2010) 'Treatment of psychopathy: A review and brief introduction to the mental model approach for psychopathy,' *Behavioral Sciences & the Law*, *28*:235–266.
Samek, D. R., Hicks, B. M., Durbin, E., Hinnant, J. B., Iacono, W. G., and McGue, M. (2017) 'Co-development between key personality traits and alcohol use disorder from adolescence through young adulthood,' *Journal of Personality*, *56*:1–22.
Schoenleber, M., Sadeh, N., and Verona, E. (2011) 'Parallel syndromes: Two dimensions of narcissism and the facets of psychopathic personality in criminally involved individuals,' *Personality Disorders: Theory, Research, and Treatment*, *2*:113–127.
Schulz, N., Murphy, B., and Verona, E. (2016) 'Gender differences in psychopathy links to drug use,' *Law and Human Behavior*, *40*:159–168.
Sigvardsson, S., Bohman, M., and Cloninger, C. R. (1996) 'Replication of the Stockholm Adoption Study of alcoholism: Confirmatory cross-fostering analysis,' *Archives of General Psychiatry*, *53*:681–687.
Simons, J. S., and Arens, A. M. (2007) 'Moderating effects of sensitivity to punishment and sensitivity to reward on associations between marijuana effect expectancies and use,' *Psychology of Addictive Behaviors*, *21*(3):409–414.
Skeem, J., Johansson, P., Andershed, H., Kerr, M., and Louden, J. E. (2007) 'Two subtypes of psychopathic violent offenders that parallel primary and secondary variants,' *Journal of Abnormal Psychology*, *116*:395–409.
Skeem, J. L., Polaschek, D. L., Patrick, C. J., and Lilienfeld, S. O. (2011) 'Psychopathic personality: Bridging the gap between scientific evidence and public policy,' *Psychological Science in the Public Interest*, *12*:95–162.
Smith, S. S., and Newman, J. P. (1990) 'Alcohol and drug abuse-dependence disorders in psychopathic and non-psychopathic criminal offenders,' *Journal of Abnormal Psychology*, *99*:430–439.
Spanagel, R., and Weiss, F. (1999) 'The dopamine hypothesis of reward: Past and current status,' *Trends in Neurosciences*, *22*:521–527.
Taylor, J., and Lang, A. R. (2006) 'Psychopathy and substance use disorders,' in C. J. Patrick (Eds.), *Handbook of psychopathy* (pp. 495–511), New York, NY: Guilford Press.
Trull, T. J., Sher, K. J., Minks-Brown, C., Durbin, J., and Burr, R. (2000) 'Borderline personality disorder and substance use disorders: A review and integration,' *Clinical Psychology Review*, *20*:235–253.
Verdejo-García, A., Lawrence, A. J., and Clark, L. (2008) 'Impulsivity as a vulnerability marker for substance-use disorders: Review of findings from high-risk research, problem gamblers and genetic association studies,' *Neuroscience & Biobehavioral Reviews*, *32*:777–810.

Verheul, R. (2001) 'Co-morbidity of personality disorders in individuals with substance use Disorders,' *European Psychiatry, 16*:274–282.
Verona, E., Hicks, B. M., and Patrick, C. J. (2005) 'Psychopathy and suicidality in female offenders: Mediating influences of personality and abuse,' *Journal of Consulting and Clinical Psychology, 73*:1065–1073.
Verona, E., Murphy, B., and Javdani, S. (2016) 'Gendered pathways: Violent childhood maltreatment, sex exchange, and drug use,' *Psychology of Violence, 6*:124–134.
Verona, E., Patrick, C. J., Curtin, J. J., Bradley, M. M., and Lang, P. J. (2004) 'Psychopathy and physiological response to emotionally evocative sounds,' *Journal of Abnormal Psychology, 113*:99–108.
Verona, E., Patrick, C. J., and Joiner, T. E. (2001) 'Psychopathy, antisocial personality, and suicide risk,' *Journal of Abnormal Psychology, 110*:462–470.
Verona, E., Sprague, J., and Sadeh, N. (2012) 'Inhibitory control and negative emotional processing in psychopathy and antisocial personality disorder,' *Journal of Abnormal Psychology, 121*:498–510.
Walsh, T. C. (1999) 'Assessing psychopathy among male and female alcoholic offenders: Gender specific treatment considerations,' *Journal of Gender, Culture, and Health, 4*:19–38.
Walsh, Z., Allen, L. C., and Kosson, D. S. (2007) 'Beyond social deviance: Substance use disorders and the dimensions of psychopathy,' *Journal of Personality Disorders, 21*:273–288.
Walters, G. D. (1990) *Criminal lifestyle*, Newbury Park, CA: Sage.
Walters, G. D. (1992) 'Drug-seeking behavior: Disease or lifestyle?,' *Professional Psychology: Research and Practice, 23*:139–145.
Walters, G. D. (2006) *Lifestyle theory: Past, present, and future*, Hauppauge, NY: Nova Publishers.
Windle, M. (1999) 'Psychopathy and antisocial personality disorder among alcoholic Inpatients,' *Journal of Studies on Alcohol, 60*:330–336.
Windle, M., and M Scheidt, D. (2004) 'Alcoholic subtypes: Are two sufficient?,' *Addiction, 99*:1508–1519.
Worhunsky, P. D., Stevens, M. C., Carroll, K. M., Rounsaville, B. J., Calhoun, V. D., Pearlson, G. D., and Potenza, M. N. (2013) 'Functional brain networks associated with cognitive control, cocaine dependence, and treatment outcome,' *Psychology of Addictive Behaviors, 27*:477–488.
Wymbs, B. T., McCarty, C. A., King, K. M., McCauley, E., Vander Stoep, A., Baer, J. S., and Waschbusch, D. A. (2012) 'Callous–unemotional traits as unique prospective risk factors for substance use in early adolescent boys and girls,' *Journal of Abnormal Child Psychology, 40*:1099–1110.
Yang, Y., and Raine, A. (2009) 'Prefrontal structural and functional brain imaging findings in antisocial, violent, and psychopathic individuals: A meta-analysis,' *Psychiatry Research: Neuroimaging, 174*:81–88.
Zald, D. H., and Treadway, M. T. (2017) 'Reward processing, neuroeconomics, and psychopathology,' *Annual Review of Clinical Psychology, 13*:471–495.
Zeier, J. D., Baskin-Sommers, A. R., Hiatt Racer, K. D., and Newman, J. P. (2012) 'Cognitive control deficits associated with antisocial personality disorder and psychopathy,' *Personality Disorders: Theory, Research, and Treatment, 3*:283–293.

33

Psychopathy and violent crime

Nicholas D. Thomson

Introduction

In 1873, Mary Ann Cotton, a British nurse and housekeeper, was executed for the murder of her stepson, Charles Cotton. It is believed that Mary Ann Cotton murdered up to 21 people, including 15 members of her own family. Within the period of ten years prior to her execution, Mary Anne Cotton married four times and had 13 children (bearing one child outside of wedlock with a lover). All but one of her husbands, a lover, her mother, and 11 of her children died from gastric fever, which shares terminal symptoms with arsenic poisoning. By taking life insurance out on the victims and bolstering her position in new relationships Mary Ann Cotton benefited from the deaths of her victims. Moving from town to town during her last decade of life, she managed to maintain a positive impression with those around her – as a nurse she received an exemplary reference from the overseeing doctor. It was not until the death of her last child, Charles Cotton, that people became suspicious, and an inquiry was launched. This was largely instigated as a result of Mary Ann Cotton glibly intimating the impending death of Charles. Unfortunately for Mary Ann Cotton, a postmortem of Charles found evidence of arsenic poisoning. Mary Ann Cotton retained her plea of innocence, despite the overwhelming evidence against her. Throughout her time Mary Ann Cotton displayed no remorse, guilt, or responsibility for her actions. Based on a review of historical evidence, Wilson and Yardley (2013) conclude that according to the British diagnostic threshold using the Psychopathy Checklist–Revised (> 25), Mary Ann Cotton would be diagnosed as a psychopath.

The first documented British case of a female serial killer, Mary Ann Cotton demonstrates the direct impact that psychopathy, as a disorder, has within the family and community, as well as the economic cost to society. Almost 150 years since Mary Ann Cotton's unscrupulous murders, the financial cost that psychopathy has on society is astonishing, with estimates of $460 billion annually – a figure two times greater than that of the cost of smoking or obesity (Kiehl & Hoffman, 2011). This figure is why psychopathy is considered *the* most expensive mental health disorder of our time (Kiehl & Sinnott-Armstrong, 2013:1). As with the case of Mary Ann Cotton, the physical damage is overwhelming – the general prevalence of psychopathy is 1.2 percent, around 0.3–0.7 percent in women and 1–2 percent in men (Hare & Neumann, 2008; Patrick & Drislane, 2015), yet these people are responsible for 30–40 percent of all violent crimes, and of these violent crimes they are accountable for the most serious forms of violence. This likely explains why 93 percent of psychopaths are involved in the criminal justice system (e.g., incarcerated or on parole or probation; Kiehl & Hoffman, 2011; Kiehl & Sinnott-Armstrong, 2013). While in prison, these individuals emerge as inmate leaders and continue to violently offend at chronic levels (DeLisi, 2016; Schrag, 1954; Thomson, 2017; Thomson, Towl, & Centifanti, 2016). Further, once released from custody, psychopaths are more likely to recommit violent crimes. As a result of this evidence, there is no surprise that psychopathy, as a construct, has become one of the most widely used clinical constructs in the criminal justice system.

In order to understand the origin of psychopathy and crime, this chapter will first provide an overview of the history of psychopathy, with a brief examination of the constructs of psychopathy used today. Next, the chapter will review evidence of the association between psychopathy and violent crime – violent crime will follow the Bureau of Justice Statistics' (2017) definition, which includes homicide, rape and sexual assault, robbery, and assault.

History of psychopathy and violence

Psychopathy is a disorder characterized by a callous disregard for others, a lack of empathy, superficial charm, egocentricity, narcissism, risky behaviors and impulsivity, and antisociality. This last component of psychopathy, antisociality, has become a recent target for debate, which will be discussed later in the chapter. Given that a psychopath encompasses a self-centered motivation, without restraints of feelings of remorse or guilt, there is no wonder that prior research has provided support for the association between psychopathy and violence. With this, some have argued that the construct of psychopathy is one of the most important clinical constructs in the criminal justice system, and it has even been described as "analogous to career criminality" (Vaughn & DeLisi, 2008:39). Most of this research has used clinical assessments (e.g., Psychopathy Checklist Revised [PCL–R]; Hare, 2003); however, there is a plethora of evidence supporting the link regardless of measure.

Prior to clinical descriptions and quantitative measures of psychopathy as a construct, historical narratives of psychopathic behaviors indicate psychopathy has persisted throughout time. The presence of these early descriptions sparks debate about the evolutionary development of psychopathy (Blackburn, 2006; Levy, 2010), suggesting the origins of psychopathy have been advantageous in some way – for instance, psychopaths may use violence (e.g., theft, rape, homicide) as a tool to achieve resources, social status, and/or to pass on genes (Glenn & Raine, 2009).

One of the earliest characterizations of psychopathic behavior can be traced to ancient Greece, where Theophrastus (371–287 BCE) detailed various personality patterns, one of which he titled "The Unscrupulous Man" (also translated to "The Shameless Man"). Theophrastus described the character and behavior of this man over a series of chapters:

> A man of this character is one who breaks through all the rules of decency for the sake of a villainous theft . . . He turns his hand to anything, is sometimes a vintner, sometimes a pimp, and sometimes an excise-man. You see him today a cryer, tomorrow a cook, and the day following a gamester . . . He has neither a mask to disguise him, nor the pretense of drunkenness to excuse him . . . He is always up to his ears in law; sometimes plaintiff, sometimes defendant. Thievery is one of his particular infirmities; and a jail his ordinary abode; in which he sojourns a great part of his life . . . If he has a mother living 'tis odds she starves . . . In a word, he is always brawling and wrangling, throwing out ill-language to those that come in his way, and makes the whole market-place echo with his scurrilities.
>
> *(Theophrastus, trans. 1714:21–38, cited in Millon et al., 1998)*

The Unscrupulous Man shares many similarities with the present day and historical accounts of a psychopath; we are able to recognize the self-indulgent, grandiose nature of the psychopath, who in order to quench his needs hurts and destroys the lives of others, even his very own family.

One of the first clinical commentaries of psychopathy came from the French physician Philippe Pinel in the early 1800s. Pinel used the term *manie sans delire* ("madness without delirium") to describe patients who displayed intact intellectual functioning, diminished emotional affect, poor impulse control, and chronic antisocial behavior (Gacono, 2000; Pinel, 1806:152). Differentiating these patients from patients with psychosis, Pinel described them as suffering from "moral insanity." A century later, the world saw a burst of clinical accounts of psychopathic personality. One of the first was from a less well-known psychiatrist from Scotland, Sir David Henderson. Henderson (1938) published a book called the *Psychopathic States* detailing his early clinical impressions of three manifestations (or typologies) of psychopathic behavior. The first psychopathic state is called the "predominately passive or inadequate," who parasitically lives off of society. The second state, the "predominately aggressive," is considered the most violent and dangerous of the three psychopathic manifestations. The third is the "predominately creative psychopath," who Henderson describes as "near genius" (Henderson, 1938:112), and likened to people such as Joan of Arc. Henderson (1938) described the general psychopathic nature as unique – while people typically gravitate towards the "herd" for confidence, safety, and overall prosperity, psychopaths do not need to seek social affiliation for these benefits. However, Henderson stated the characteristics of psychopathy inevitably lead them to "fatalism or despair, the reaction to which may be aggressive" (1938:133). Here Henderson (1938) defined typologies of the psychopath, with one posing the greatest risk of violent behavior, and the others as eccentric and parasitic/antisocial.

Similar to Henderson's (1938) typologies of psychopathy, Karpman (1941) described two subtypes of psychopath: primary and secondary. These were based on clinical observations and are still popularly referred to in today's research and clinical literature. Essentially the two subtypes can be understood as affective deficits, which characterize the primary psychopath, and affective disturbances, which characterize the secondary psychopath. The secondary psychopath may have intact empathy and suffers from high internalizing symptoms, such as anxiety or depression. Further distinctions are drawn in the purposefulness in behavior – the primary psychopath acts instrumentally for personal gain and uses whatever means necessary to achieve this goal (e.g., violence), whereas the secondary psychopath is impulsive, volatile, and reactive.

In 1941, Hervey Cleckley published his pioneering book, *The Mask of Sanity*. Since the original publication, Cleckley's (1941) observations and analyses have held validity and significance for current research and have played a major role in current psychopathy constructs. Cleckley's (1964) description consisted of 16 personality characteristics, ranging from affective (e.g., lack of remorse or shame), interpersonal (e.g., egocentric), behavioral (e.g., failure to follow any life plan), cognitive (e.g., good intelligence), and criminal traits (e.g., antisocial behavior). Most of these characteristics are still used today as the bases of self-report and clinical measures of psychopathy (Furnham, Daoud, & Swami, 2009). However, it is important to note that unlike Henderson (1938) and Karpman (1941), Cleckley made multiple statements denouncing that psychopaths are inclined to be severely violent:

> despite their continually repeated transgressions against the law and the rights of others and their apparent lack of moral compunction, [they] seem to avoid murder and other grave felonies that remove them indefinitely from free activity in the social group.
>
> *(Cleckley, 1941, pp. 265–6)*

When Cleckley described a violent case, a man named "Max," who engages in frequent but short-lived violence (e.g., beating his wife, pub fights), Cleckley interprets this as reactive rather than premeditative: "I believe that the substantial injury was unintentional, an act of thoughtless exuberance committed in the heat of a situation eminently" (p. 36). Nevertheless, Cleckley's clinical descriptions of psychopaths entailed chronic histories of violent criminal behavior, regardless of motive.

Robert Hare built on Cleckley's work and developed a semi-structured clinical assessment of psychopathy: the Psychopathy Checklist (Hare, 2003). The checklist includes 20 items and is most often studied as a total score and as a two-factor (Interpersonal/Affective and social deviance), three-factor (interpersonal, affective, and lifestyle), and four-factor model (interpersonal, affective, lifestyle, and antisocial; Cooke & Michie, 2001). Using the PCL–R, the diagnostic cutoff for men is a score of 30 or higher, and 25 and above for women. The PCL–R has become one of the most widely used measures of psychopathy in the criminal justice system and is often used as part of violence risk assessment (Skeem & Cooke, 2010a).

As a general construct, psychopathy is considered one of the most robust predictors of violence in forensic, psychiatric, and community populations – including youth populations. Not only have offenders with psychopathy been shown to commit twice as many violent crimes as offenders without psychopathy (Hare, 1999), but they are five times more likely to recommit violent crimes (Serin & Amos, 1995) and are responsible for more severe forms of violence (Coid & Yang, 2011; Porter, Woodworth, Earle, Drugge, & Boer, 2003). However, there has been fierce debate about concerns that the construct of psychopathy is becoming synonymous with the PCL–R (Skeem & Cooke, 2010b). It is important to acknowledge that early clinical conceptions of psychopathy, from those such as Cleckley (1941), Karpman (1948), and Henderson (1938), attributed more emphasis to the affective and interpersonal characteristics that defined psychopathy, whereas, the PCL–R regards antisocial behavior and criminality as integral components of psychopathy (Skeem & Cooke, 2010a). It has been argued that it is counterintuitive to credit antisocial behavior as a personality trait and then apply the same personality trait to understand or predict the antisocial behavior (Cooke & Logan, 2015; Skeem & Cooke, 2010a). With this criticism in mind, a more recent clinical measure of psychopathy has been developed, called the Comprehensive Assessment of Psychopathic Personality (CAPP; Cooke, Hart, Logan, & Michie, 2004). The CAPP includes six domains: (1) attachment, (2) behavior regulation, (3) cognition, (4) dominance, (5) emotion, and (6) self. While the CAPP is a promising assessment of psychopathic personality, there is currently a paucity of research exploring the association between the CAPP and violence. In theory, and drawing on past research, one would expect several of the domains to be associated with violence. However, this is yet to be explored.

Even with the criticism that the construct of psychopathy should not include antisocial behavior, research has demonstrated, regardless of measurement method (e.g., clinical or self-report), statistically controlling for prior violent history, or for the antisocial/criminality factor of psychopathy, the core personality features of psychopathy increase the risk of violent behavior (DeLisi, 2016; Hemphill, Hare, & Wong, 1998; Thomson et al., 2016; Vitacco, Neumann, & Pardini, 2014). Therefore, psychopathic personality may indeed pose a greater risk of future violent crime, regardless of criminal history.

Violent crime

Violent crime includes homicide, rape and sexual assault, robbery, and assault (simple and aggravated). However, violent crime also extends to child abuse and maltreatment, elder abuse, gun violence, intimate partner violence, stalking, kidnapping, violence against women, and terrorism

(Bureau of Justice Statistics, 2017). In the U.S., rates of violent crime have seen a general decline over the past 12 years (approximately 16.5 percent reduction), currently matching rates similar to that of the 1970s. Even so, violent crime remains prevalent in the U.S. – every minute approximately five people aged over 12 years will become a victim of violence (based on 2,700,000 violent crimes per annum); every 73 seconds a person is the victim of sexual assault or rape; and, in 2014, over 1,500 children died as a result of abuse/neglect (Truman & Morgan, 2016; U.S. Department of Health & Human Services, 2014). While the rate of violence has fallen, the sheer number of victims is still too high. Thus, exploring risk factors and mechanisms by which people become perpetrators of violence is arguably one of the most valuable directions research can take to benefit the health, safety, and economic welfare of societies. Indeed, psychopathy as a construct may then be one of the most important clinical constructs to study to deter violent crime. Surprisingly, research exploring the association between psychopathy and violent crime is limited. Consequently, the present chapter will focus on the four main violent crime categories; homicide, sexual assault and rape, robbery, and assault (simple and aggravated).

Homicide

Under the U.S. legal code chapter 51 – homicide, there are two categories of offenses, murder and manslaughter; there are ten additional codes within the homicide chapter which entail homicide and manslaughter across various situations and methods (e.g., attempted murder/manslaughter, conspiracy to murder, risk of transfer of human immunodeficiency virus). The U.S. legal code outlines murder as "the unlawful killing of a human being with malice aforethought" (18 U.S. Code § 1111), and manslaughter is described as "the unlawful killing of a human being without malice" (18 U.S. Code § 1112). The focus of this section of the chapter will be dedicated to the umbrella term homicide without the differentiation of method or situation unless stated. This is largely due to the lack of specificity within violence research. Homicide of any kind has immense impact on the families and communities involved, and beyond this there are astronomical financial consequences. Murder alone has been estimated to cost over $17 million (DeLisi et al., 2010), even though it is one of the least occurring violent crimes in the U.S.

As discussed, research exploring the association between psychopathy and homicide is sparse, and typically studies exploring the link between disorder and violent crime lump together all forms of violent crime to create a "violent" group. Although this makes interpretation of the specific violent crime impossible to interpret, we must acknowledge there are limitations with datasets when murderers are more often the minority in datasets. Nevertheless, there are some studies that exist that offer some insight into the link between psychopathy and homicide. There are two primary objectives with this research: (1) are psychopaths at greater risk of committing homicide? and (2) do psychopathic homicide offenders differ from non-psychopathic homicide offenders? Drawing from the limited research, we will attempt to explore each of these questions.

To investigate the first question, are psychopaths at greater risk of homicide than non-psychopaths? We first draw from a qualitative study conducted by Beasley (2004), which included seven serial homicide offenders. Out of these seven offenders, four met the diagnostic criteria (PCL–R > 30) for being classified as psychopathic. Of these four, all had extensive criminal histories, which, as Beasley (2004) suggested, is not unexpected as psychopathy is related to criminal versatility. This figure is slightly higher than in larger sampled studies, which have found prevalence rates around 31 percent (Laurell & Dåderman, 2007). In contrast, there is evidence to suggest murderers are not more likely to be psychopathic. A recent study conducted in the U.S., which included 478 offenders, demonstrated that homicide offenders did not score higher than criminals who had reoffended or first-time offenders across all four dimensions of psychopathy (affective, interpersonal, behavioral, and lifestyle). Further, the study demonstrated that murderers actually scored lower on two factors – erratic lifestyle and interpersonal manipulative (Sherretts, Boduszek, Debowska, & Willmott, 2017). Further, women incarcerated for murder have also been shown to score significantly lower on psychopathy than those not convicted for murder (Warren et al., 2005). This finding is supported by research from Klein Tuente, Vogel, and Stam (2014) who found in 221 female offenders that homicide offending was predictive of *not* meeting a diagnosis of psychopathy (PCL–R > 25). Taken together, it seems that psychopathy is not predictive of homicide committed by women, but there is mixed evidence for men. A possible explanation may be that homicide committed by women is more typically reactive and emotionally driven, which is a contrary characteristic to psychopaths (Klein Tuente et al., 2014).

As people age, the risk of offending decreases – the risk of committing homicide starts to decline from middle age (Hare & McPherson, 1984). An interesting study by Putkonen and colleagues (2010) assessed levels of psychopathy across homicide offenders aged 60 years and older to a gender-matched younger group of homicide offenders. The older homicide offender group scored lower on total scores of psychopathy and Factor 2. However, there were no significant differences on Factor 1, interpersonal/affective psychopathic traits. This supports prior assertions that interpersonal/affective features of psychopathy remain stable over the lifespan, whereas criminality and lifestyle psychopathic traits typically decline. Further, this study demonstrates that although risk of homicide typically declines with age, those who display prototypical psychopathic personality traits – a callous disregard for others, diminished emotionality, grandiose sense of self, and a lack of guilt and remorse, continue to be a greater risk of committing homicide even as they age.

A distinct characteristic of psychopathic crime is the level of instrumentality. Throughout the literature, psychopaths perpetrate their crimes to achieve a goal (e.g., dominance, financial, sexual). Juodis, Starzomski, Porter, and Woodworth (2014) assessed the level of instrumentality in domestic homicide offenders. In their sample, most domestic homicides did occur without planning (82.9 percent). However, in comparison to non-psychopathic domestic homicide offenders, the crimes committed by the psychopathic group was considered to be more dispassionate, planned, and gratuitously violent (e.g., torturing, overkill, etc.). Higher PCL–R scores (as well as Factor 1 and 2) were related to instrumental violence, and those committed of domestic homicide who had higher scores of psychopathy displayed more instrumentality in their killings than reactivity (Juodis et al., 2014). These findings support prior research, which has shown psychopathic homicide offenders perpetrate instrumental rather than reactive homicides (see Porter & Woodworth, 2007).

Hutton and Woodworth (2014) tested violent crime characteristics among 145 female youth offenders. Their findings showed female offenders with high levels of psychopathic traits did not demonstrate more instrumentality in their crimes. The two-factor and four-facet analyses also found no association with instrumentality in their violence. This further supports that psychopathy may manifest differently in females than it does in men. However, much more work is needed in this area. In a male offender sample, Declercq, Willemsen, Audenaert, and Verhaeghe (2012) found that the interpersonal facet was the best predictor of predatory violence, while the antisocial facet was related to less predatory violence and planning. Further, the interpersonal and affective facets were related to less Anger and more goal directness in violent crime.

A large meta-analysis conducted by Blais, Solodukhin, and Forth (2014), which included 53 studies (N = 8753), found the interpersonal facet was most related to instrumental violence, whereas Factor 2 (social deviance) was more predictive of reactive violence. The lifestyle facet predicted both reactive and instrumental violence. The authors conclude, however, that psychopathy is not more predictive of instrumental violence over reactive. This is consistent with child and adolescent research which shows purely instrumental aggressors are actually rare to find, and typically those who instrumentally aggress will also display high levels of reactive aggression (see Thomson, Centifanti, & Lemerise, 2017; Thomson & Centifanti, 2017). Further, mixed aggressive youth show higher levels of psychopathic traits. Taken together, this evidence may suggest that the differences between violent psychopaths and violent non-psychopaths is simply that psychopaths are more opportunistic and versatile in their use of violence. This may explain why some research, including the large meta-analysis by Blais et al. (2014), does not find psychopaths who solely perpetrate instrumental violence.

Having committed their murder, psychopaths continue to display distinctive characteristics, which result in lesser punishment. When assessing the offenders' descriptions, psychopaths described their crime as more reactive and left out important information as compared to non-psychopathic murderers (Porter & Woodworth, 2007). In a large sample of Finnish homicide offenders, Häkkänen-Nyholm and Hare (2009) found high psychopathy scorers (using the PCL–R) often denied the murder charges, and received a less severe sentence – psychopaths were more likely to be convicted for involuntary manslaughter (not manslaughter or murder). In addition, psychopaths were more likely to gain permission from the Supreme Court to appeal their court sentence. Fitting with the profile of the psychopathic killer, these individuals continue their scheming behavior by manipulating professionals and the criminal justice system for their own personal gain.

When compared to non-psychopathic murderers and non-psychopathic controls, psychopathic murderers (PCL–R ≥ 30) demonstrate unique characteristics and temperament. In particular, psychopathic murderers report feeling less anticipatory worry and fear of uncertainty in their actions, have less concern for social approval, are less determined, and report lower on social acceptance, generosity, empathy, and compassion (de Pádua Serafim, de Barros, Bonini Castellana, & Gorenstein, 2014). Therefore, while the two homicide groups committed similar crimes, they are distinct in personality characteristics and temperament.

Cope and colleagues (2014) assessed differences between 20 male youths who had committed homicide to non-homicide offender youth and two control groups. While the intention of the study was to assess brain structure differences, the authors note the homicide youth group scored higher on total scores of psychopathy and interpersonal, affective, lifestyle, and antisocial traits. Further, brain differences were found. The homicide offender group had reduced gray matter volumes in the medial and lateral temporal lobes. Important to note, the authors controlled for a variety of factors during brain analyses (e.g., psychopathy, criminal history, IQ, brain injury, psychiatric diagnoses), and therefore the brain differences cannot be a result of psychopathic traits and may be useful as an indicator for risk of severe violence.

Pinel distinguished psychopathy from schizophrenia, and yet the two have been found to co-occur. A recent study by Stratton, Brook, and Hanlon (2017) conducted in homicide offenders with schizophrenia found differences in psychopathy levels based on the presence and absence of God/Satan/demon (GSD)-themed psychotic symptoms. When compared to the nonGSD themed psychotic group, the GSD themed psychotic group had lower total scores on the PCL–R, and affective and antisocial facets but not on interpersonal or behavioral facets. Furthermore, the GSD group who scored lower on psychopathy were more likely to have committed premeditated homicide. Although psychopathy generally occurs infrequently among patients with schizophrenia, 12 percent of the sample were found to meet the diagnostic cut-off using the PCL–R (> 30). Therefore, even within a group of homicide inpatients with schizophrenia, psychopathy differentiated homicide offenders by the presence or absence of religious psychosis.

Drawing from a unique sample of 95 male Dangerous and Severe Personality Disordered offenders in the United Kingdom, Casey, Rogers, Burns, and Yiend (2013) found higher psychopathy scores were related to greater cardiovascular response to negative emotional stimuli, suggesting atypicality in processing unpleasant stimuli. Further, when these highly violent individuals were asked to empathize, those with higher levels of interpersonal/affective psychopathic traits exhibited less physiological response, indicating a deficient autonomic response to empathizing. While not the primary aim of the study, this is relevant to this section of the chapter; the authors found those who had an index offense of homicide were not overly represented in the psychopathic group. Thus, in this homogenous group of highly violent offenders, psychopathy was unrelated to homicide.

Language differences have been found between psychopathic murderers and non-psychopathic murderers. Hancock, Woodworth, and Porter (2013) deconstructed crime narratives of psychopathic and non-psychopathic murderers. Hancock et al. (2013) revealed the psychopathic murderers applied more rational cause-and-effect descriptors and focused on material needs while using fewer references to social needs. Further, the psychopathic group focused more on past tense and less on present tense, and their language had less emotional intensity (Hancock et al., 2013; ten Brinke et al., 2017). Further, the psychopathic group displayed many more filled pauses (e.g., "uh," "um"). This is suggested to reflect difficulties in describing emotionally powerful events (Hancock et al., 2013; ten Brinke et al., 2017). Thus, psychopathic murderers are notably distinct from non-psychopathic murders; in this case, their language is utilitarian and marked by an emotional disconnect.

Overall, there are inconsistencies in the association between homicide and psychopathy that could suggest the link is not entirely robust. However, what is clear is that homicidal psychopaths are more gratuitous and sadistic in their crimes. Psychopaths use more instrumentality in their murders, but there is evidence of reactive motivation, too. However, homicidal psychopaths minimize the planning of their crime by exaggerating the reactivity and leaving out important information. After the murder(s), psychopaths demonstrate less remorse for their crime and display dampened physiological profiles when empathizing and a lack of emotionality in their speech. Further, although posing greater risk of recidivism because of a lack of guilt and regret, psychopaths are more likely to convince law officials of a more lenient sentence (Häkkänen-Nyholm & Hare, 2009).

Rape and sexual assault

Although research does not typically differentiate offenders by their sexual crime, except based on victim, it is important to acknowledge that there are distinctions. Rape includes forced sexual intercourse (vaginal, anal, or oral penetration by the offender[s]), and this can be by both psychological and/or physical force or coercion. Rape also includes penetration by a foreign object. Attempted rape includes verbal threats of rape (Bureau of Justice Statistics, 2017). In contrast, sexual assault includes a range of victimization that is not regarded as rape or attempted rape. Sexual assault may include an attack (including attempted attack) of unwanted sexual contact, may involve physical force such as grabbing or fondling, and includes non-physical attack, such as verbal threats. Based on the FBI's Uniform Crime Report (UCR), during 2009, 88,097 forcible rapes were reported in the U.S. (Federal Bureau of Investigation, 2010; Wiseman, 2015); based on the National Crime Victimization Survey (Truman & Morgan, 2016) during 2015, 431,840 rape and sexual assault victimizations occurred in the U.S. Most empirical research exploring the association between sexual offending and psychopathy do not differentiate between the two forms of sexual offending, making clear interpretation very limited. This may be an important line of inquiry for both prediction work and treatment. Nevertheless, the research conducted thus far has been useful in helping researchers, clinicians, and officials understand how psychopathy influences the general risk of sexual offending and reoffending, as well as offender profiles based on the victim (e.g., child, adult). As discussed in the homicide section of this chapter, sexual homicide offenders with psychopathy are more likely to be sadistic and gratuitous in their killing (Porter et al., 2003). However, are psychopaths more likely to sexually offend, and are there particular factors/facets that are more important for predicting sexual offending?

Although the PCL–R is not designed to assess sex offender risk, it has become one of the most commonly utilized measures for sex offender risk assessment. In Texas, Sexually Violent Predator assessments require evaluators to measure psychopathy, and all registered sex offenders are scored on the PCL–R to help establish community supervision needs (Hawes, Boccaccini, & Murrie, 2013; Texas Health and Safety Code, §841.023, 2000). A great body of research has found that sexual violent offenders demonstrate higher psychopathy scores, and this is consistent for adults (Schimmenti, Passanisi, & Caretti, 2014) and youth (Cale, Lussier, McCuish, & Corrado, 2015).

A recent study by Krstic and colleagues (2017) tested the four-factor model of psychopathy using the PCL–R to predict profiles of sexual offending in a sample of 958 male sexual offenders. At the facet level, the authors found the affective and antisocial facets best predicted sexually violent crimes. Further, the interpersonal facet was the only facet which was uniquely associated with a greater number of paraphilic accounts in the offenders' criminal records. Krstic et al. (2017) examined latent profile analysis of the four PCL–R facets in 958 male sex offenders, revealing four typologies – (1) prototypical (high on all four facets), (2) callous–conning (high interpersonal and affective facets), (3) sociopathic (high lifestyle and antisocial facets), and (4) general sex offender (low scores on all four PCL–R facets). Compared to the remaining three subtypes, those who were regarded as a prototypical psychopath had many more sexual offenses.

Drawing from 20 research studies (N = 5,239), Hawes, Boccaccini, and Murrie (2013) conducted a meta-analysis to examine the relation between PCL–R scores and sexual recidivism. Overall, the results generally supported the use of the PCL–R as a predictive tool for sexual recidivism. Specifically, the total score predicting sexual recidivism (d = .40) was considered good but showed the strongest effect (d = .55) when predicting mixed forms of violence (both non-sexual and sexual). The authors conclude that the PCL–R proves itself as a "potentially useful measure for clinical and forensic assessments addressing risk of sexual recidivism" (Hawes et al., 2013:239). However, the authors note there was substantial variability in the strength of the prediction from study to study (d = −0.18 to d = 0.96), and there was not a consistent explanation for the variability (e.g., sample characteristics). In their review of the seven studies that assessed the combination of psychopathy and sexual deviance to predict sexual recidivism, the authors found support for the combination of the two measures but emphasize that much more work and consistency in methodology is needed. For instance, Hawes and colleagues (2013) note major discrepancies between studies, with some researchers regarding high psychopathy ranging from 12 to 26 on the PCL–R and the use of various methods of assessing sexual deviance. Another variability was how the PCL–R was collected, for either research or clinical needs (e.g., field studies). The authors of the meta-analysis found that PCL–R collected for clinical needs were less reliable at predicting sexual recidivism, with the exception of one study (see Beggs & Grace, 2008).

Hawes and colleagues propose that explanations for this might be that (1) the reliability of the PCL–R is generally lower in field studies, and (2) including the interview section of the PCL–R may be detrimental to its predictive ability. This latter explanation is somewhat surprising, as the interview section of the PCL–R is integral. But the authors note that the interview component of the PCL–R may have diminished the predictive effects due to inaccurate clinical impressions from clinician to clinician. In support of this assertion, prior research has demonstrated file-review to be a more reliable predictor of future offending than the interview component (Hawes et al., 2013; Leistico, Salekin, DeCoster, & Rogers, 2008). Moving forward, there is a clear need for sexual offending research to utilize similar methodology to make results more comparable.

When assessing the predictive ability of the factor and facet structure, Hawes and colleagues (2013) suggest Factor 2 and facet 4 stand out as the best predictors of future sexual offending; this may suggest the association between psychopathy and sexual offending largely stems from antisocial and criminal components of psychopathy (d = .44) rather than from core psychopathic personality traits (d = 0.17), such as affective and interpersonal traits.

Sexual violence is heterogeneous based on classification of victim perpetration; for instance, sexual violence research has found three sex offending typologies – child sex offenders, rapists, and mixed (adult and child) sex offenders (Brown, Dargis, Mattern, Tsonis, & Newman, 2015). Using a sample of 156 federally incarcerated sex offenders, Brown and colleagues (2015) assessed PCL–R scores to understand sex offender typologies. The mixed offender group (M = 26.65) scored higher than the child sex offender group (M = 21.32), rapist group (M = 24.28), and non-sex offender group (M = 23.65). Based on further analyses, these differences were largely due to Factor 1. Parks and Bard (2006) also found adolescent mixed sex offenders scored highest on all dimensions of psychopathy, including total score. Porter and colleagues (2000) found the prevalence of psychopaths (PCL–R > 30) in 229 sex offenders was 26.6 percent, and at the group level this figure was much higher for those in the mixed offender group (64 percent) when compared to rapist (35.9 percent), incest offender (6.3 percent), child molester (9.4 percent), and non-sex offender groups (35.8 percent). This suggests that psychopathy, and being psychopathic, is associated with non-discriminant sexual offending, which falls in line with the opportunistic nature of the psychopath. However, Firestone, Bradford, Greenberg, Larose, and Curry (1998) found homicidal child molesters scored higher on total scores of psychopathy than non-homicidal child molesters. Therefore, there may be distinctions in the severity and gratuitous nature of sexual violence perpetrated by psychopaths.

Prior research has suggested that high levels of psychopathy and sexual deviance equate to a "deadly combination" of sex offender traits that increase the odds of sexual recidivism (Hare, 1999, 2003). Hildebrand, de Ruiter, and de Vogel (2004) assessed reoffending from a sample of 94 convicted rapists over an average of 11.8 years. Although the authors applied a lower cut-off score on the PCL–R (> 26), they found those scoring 26 above were more often reconvicted for sexual, violent, and general offenses than those scoring below the selected threshold of psychopathy. In particular, those scoring 26 or above were four times more likely to be reconvicted for sexual offending, and twice as likely to be reconvicted of non-sexual violence. Using survival analysis, the authors found those scoring 26 or above on the PCL–R who were classified as sexually deviant (via the Sexual Violence Risk–20; Boer, Hart, Kropp, & Webster, 1998) more rapidly reoffended after release and at a higher rate than those with the same levels of psychopathy but without sexual deviance.

Based on data from 139 high-risk sexual offenders, Woolworth and colleagues (2013) investigated the influence of sexual fantasy, sexual paraphilia, and psychopathy on sexual offending behavior. Their sample scored higher on the PCL–R (M = 29.59) than normative data from male offenders (M = 22; Hare, 2003) and forensic patients (M = 20; Hare, 2003). Analyzing the data on victim type, the authors conclude that psychopaths have a proclivity for sexual behavior that is more violent. In their sample, all three offenders incarcerated for sexual homicide were psychopathic. Also, psychopaths (61 percent) were more likely than non-psychopaths (14 percent) to reported engaging in sexual fantasies. Of note, the low psychopathy sex offender group reported having engaged in more child sexual fantasies. Overall, the authors highlight that high levels of psychopathy were specifically related to sadistic paraphilia – 67 percent of sex offenders with sadistic paraphilia were psychopathic.

Contrary to previous research, recent evidence from 687 male offenders in the U.S. provides unfavorable evidence of the dyadic risk assessment. Harris, Boccaccini, and Rice (2017) examined the predictive ability of the PCL–R and sexual deviance for sexual recidivism over an average of ten years (after being evaluated for post-release civil commitment). The authors found PCL–R scores alone to be predictive of the combined category of violent or sexual recidivism; however, they note the effect size was small (d = .26), and the PCL–R did not predict sexual recidivism alone. Further, when testing the interaction between psychopathy and sexual deviance, the authors conclude there was "no evidence that offenders with high levels of both psychopathy and sexual deviance were more likely to reoffend than other offenders" (Harris et al., 2017:646). This is somewhat surprising given the strong "deadly combination" rhetoric held in prior research.

Even though the research exploring the combination of high sexual deviance and high psychopathy scores has been mixed (Harris et al., 2017; Hawes, Boccaccini, & Murrie, 2013), a survey of 95 Sexually Violent Predator evaluators showed many evaluators applied both sexual deviance and PCL–R scores to make risk judgments. This is in spite of the evidence that the additive effects of sexual deviance to psychopathy as an advanced risk assessment may not be conclusive at this time (Boccaccini, Chevalier, Murrie, & Varela, 2017). Further, these evaluators perceived the PCL–R total score as a versatile risk assessment for sexual reoffending. Although there is evidence supporting this statement, the more reliable prediction comes from the factor and facet structure. Boccaccini and colleagues (2017) note that there seems to be a disconnect between research and current practice in this area, as clinicians are not using the more empirically reliable factor/facet structure to evaluate risk of future sexual offending.

In sum, there is a clear link between psychopathy and sexual offending (DeLisi, 2016). However, because of methodological differences from study to study, the robustness of the association is still unclear. It seems, from the empirical literature, that male psychopaths are more likely to sexually offend without preference, thus victimizing both children and adults, and carry out cruel and sadistic violence to satisfy their violent fantasies (Robertson & Knight, 2014; Woodworth et al., 2013). However, in terms of predicting future sexual offending, there seems to be greater support for the use of the factor and facet structure of psychopathy, rather than the cut-off score. Specifically, it seems that while high scores on all dimensions predict recidivism of various sorts (e.g., violent, sexual, and general), Factor 2 and facet 4 may be valuable for specifically evaluating sexual offending risk.

Robbery

Robbery is classified as the completed or attempted theft of property by force or using threat of force. Robbery may occur with or without injury and with or without use of a weapon (Bureau of Justice Statistics, 2017). In 2015, 578,580 people were the victim of robberies, which makes up 61 percent of victimizations reported to the police in the U.S. and 29.4 percent of violent crimes in 2011 (Truman & Morgan, 2016). Research exploring the association between psychopathy and robbery is scant, and, similar to the other violent crime categories, robbery is often pooled into a "violent crime" category and studied as a homogenous construct.

One of the few studies investigating the role of psychopathic traits and theft was conducted by Vaughn, Newhill, DeLisi, Beaver, and Howard (2008). Their study included 94 female juvenile offenders. The authors included two self-report measures of psychopathy, the Antisocial Process Screening Device (ASPD; Frick & Hare, 2001) and the Psychopathic Personality Inventory–Short Form (PPI–SF; Lilienfeld & Andrews, 1996). The study found narcissistic psychopathic traits (from the APSD) and Carefree Nonplanfulness (from the PPI) predicted theft. Moreover, using data from a sample of 92 male offenders, Haapasalo (1994) assessed percentage of 15 criminal offense categories between psychopathic groups (psychopathic, moderately psychopathic, and low psychopathy scores). Psychopaths were often convicted for robbery (43.3 percent) and theft (90 percent) when compared to offenders scoring low on psychopathy (24.1 percent and 86.2 percent, respectively). From Cleckley's (1976) notable accounts of psychopathy across 13 cases, most included histories of robbery and theft. Further, Cleckley clearly described psychopaths as susceptible to various forms of antisocial behavior, including theft:

> Not only is the psychopath undependable . . . He will commit theft, forgery, adultery, fraud, and other deeds for astonishingly small stakes, and under much greater risks of being discovered than will the ordinary scoundrel.
>
> *(Cleckley, 1976:343)*

Drawing from a laboratory experiment using 91 convicted theft offenders, Próspero-Luis and colleagues (2017) found the link between psychopathic traits and committing theft was mediated by an atypical perception of outcome. High psychopathy scores on the triarchic model of psychopathy (TriPM; Patrick, Fowles, & Krueger, 2009) was associated with a failure to recognize the possible negative adversities of theft (e.g., hurting people, getting injured, social stigma, going to jail) and a more positive appraisal of the positive outcomes (e.g., keeping stolen objects, feeling of adrenaline, easy money). Of note, the association was more strongly linked with the personality features (Boldness and Meanness) of psychopathy, rather than the behavioral features (disinhibition).

Vitacco, Neumann, and Pardini (2014) assessed self-report of psychopathy for predicting criminal charges over a 3.5-year period in 417 males from the community. When the three factors of psychopathy were entered into a predictive model without any control variables, total psychopathy scores (area under the curve (AUC) = .63), callous affect (AUC = .62), and erratic lifestyle (AUC = .65) were predictors of having been arrested for theft. Thus, the Interpersonal/Affective factor did not reach significance. However, when the authors included other risk variables in the statistical models (e.g., socioeconomic status, criminal history), psychopathy was no longer a significant predictor of theft, as it was for serious offending and violence. Instead, socioeconomic status and previous theft charges emerged as significant predictors.

As we have seen from the sexual offending characteristics, psychopaths are opportunists, and given the chance they may be more inclined to commit robbery if the circumstance is right. Individuals high on psychopathic traits appraise robbery more positively and lack concern for the negative consequences of criminal behavior. While the literature in this area is well under-researched, the evidence thus far suggests psychopathy is important for predicting theft but may not be as reliable when considering other well-known risk variables, such as demographic and historical measures.

Assault

Assault consists of two main categories of offense, simple (without a weapon) and aggravated (with a weapon). It is important to highlight that rape, attempted rape, sexual assault, and robbery (including attempted robbery) are excluded from this crime category (Bureau of Justice

Statistics, 2017). In 2015, there were 3,996,200 victims of assault, with approximately 20 percent the victim of aggravated assault. Getting a clear picture of the link between psychopathy and assault is a challenge. Assault is probably one of the most contaminated categorizations in research. For instance, Reidy, Lilienfeld, Berke, Gentile, and Zeichner (2016) tested the association between psychopathic traits and violent assault in males with and without a criminal history. To assess assault, the participants responded to the question "How many times have you attacked someone with intent to harm, injure, rape, or kill?" In this example, there are potentially three legal categories of violent crime. Nevertheless, even with these challenges, we are able to piece together some convincing evidence that psychopathy is a consistent predictor of assault, both simple and aggravated. From their study, Reidy and colleagues (2016) conducted their analyses using the four-factor model as well as the three-factor model (removing the antisocial component based on the criticisms made by Skeem and Cooke [2010a]). When testing the four-factor model in their sample of 488 men without a criminal history, callous affect and erratic lifestyle were predictors of physical fights; however, only callous affect predicted assault – both simple and aggravated. These findings were consistent when testing the three-factor model. Thus, the antisocial component of psychopathy did not influence or interfere with the predictive ability of callous psychopathic traits for aggravated or simple assault.

In their second sample of 106 men with a criminal history, when using the three-factor model, callous affect predicted fighting and both forms of assault, while erratic lifestyle predicted simple assault. Using the four-factor model (including antisocial psychopathic traits), antisocial psychopathic traits predicted simple and aggravated assault, while erratic lifestyle only predicted simple assault. In sum, callous psychopathic traits emerged as a particularly useful construct in the prediction of simple and aggravated assault for non-forensic men without a criminal history. Further, when considering the three-factor model, callous psychopathic traits was also a good predictor of assault in men with a criminal history.

Violent crime across contexts

In this final section of the chapter, we discuss psychopathy as a predictor of violent crime across settings. First, Theobald, Farrington, Coid, and Piquero (2016) wanted to investigate the role of psychopathic traits in intimate partner violence (IPV). The data included more than 400 males from the United Kingdom who have been followed from age 8 to age 48. Participants were grouped into four violent typologies – a violent conviction only, a generally violent group (those who commit intra- and extrafamilial violence), family-only IPV group (those who only committed intrafamilial violence), and a nonviolent group. Using the screening version of the PCL–R, the authors found notable group differences. The generally violent group were found to score highest on total score and on all four facets (and two factors), while the nonviolent and family-only IPV group scored significantly lower than the other groups. Similar to sexual offending, high psychopathy scores are associated with non-discriminant violent behavior. These individuals callously use violence to achieve their goals without concern for who their victim is, whether outside or inside of their home.

Drugs are said to have a major influence on violent crime (Goldstein, 1985), and the use of drugs has been shown to worsen the severity of violence (Baskin-Sommers & Sommers, 2006). However, to date only one study has explored the association between drug-related violence and psychopathy. Drawing from a sample of 125 female offenders, Thomson (2017) found high levels of antisocial psychopathic traits predicted drug-related violent crime, while callous psychopathic traits predicted violent crime that was not drug-related. Further, women who had committed a non–drug-related violent crime (those higher in callous psychopathic traits) continued to perpetrate a greater number of violent misconducts while in prison. While in prison, psychopathy in men and women has been found to be a risk factor for violence (see Chakhssi, Kersten, de Ruiter, & Bernstein, 2014; Edens, Poythress, Lilienfeld, Patrick, & Test, 2008; Thomson et al., 2016; Walters & Heilbrun, 2010). Further, in a large, two-sample study from the U.K. (N = 931) and the U.S. (N = 863), Gray and Snowden (2016) found psychopathy to be a reliable predictor of violent recidivism after being released from psychiatric facilities (secure psychiatric units and acute psychiatric hospital) up to two years post release. The authors conclude that "there is strong evidence for the PCL–R and PCL: SV being predictive of antisocial outcomes" (p. 342).

Conclusion

From the research discussed throughout this chapter, there is strong evidence that psychopathy, whether the dimensional construct or the total score, is associated with violent crime. However, it has been a challenge to be specific with the association across types of violent crime because of the scarcity of research exploring the particular violent crime categories. Nevertheless, we can draw several important conclusions. While there is a mix of evidence for psychopathy increasing risk of homicide, those homicide offenders who are psychopathic are more gratuitous and sadistic in their killings. After which, these offenders minimize the severity and instrumentality of their crime and manage to convince legal professionals to reduce their sentence. Regarding sexual offending, there is a clear link with psychopathy; however, it seems that rather than using a cut off or total score for risk assessment, the dimensional construct may be better applied for efficacy. Further, specific victim selection of sexual offending is not characteristic of psychopathy. Instead, psychopathic individuals will sexually offend adults and children indiscriminately, thus presenting as opportunistic in their sexual offenses. Similarly, men high on psychopathic traits are not more likely to commit intimate personal violence only within the home, but instead commit intrafamilial *and* extrafamilial violence. Assessing the link between psychopathy and assault, there is evidence to support the importance of callous psychopathic traits increasing the risk of simple and aggravated assault, even if the individual has no criminal history. Psychopathy also is an important risk factor for violence while incarcerated, as well as post-release. In conclusion, one possible rationale for the violent propensity seen in psychopathic individuals (besides their predatory personality profile) is that these individuals positively appraise the outcome of their violent crime and minimize the negative outcomes.

References

Baskin-Sommers, A. R., and Sommers, I. (2006) 'Methamphetamine use and violence among young adults,' *Journal of Criminal Justice, 34*(6):661–674.

Beasley, J. O. (2004) 'Serial murder in America: Case studies of seven offenders,' *Behavioral Sciences & the Law, 22*(3):395–414.

Beggs, S. M., and Grace, R. C. (2008) 'Psychopathy, intelligence, and recidivism in child molesters: Evidence of an interaction effect,' *Criminal Justice and Behavior, 35*(6):683–695.

Blackburn, R. (2006) 'Other theoretical models of psychopathy,' in C. J. Patrick (Ed.), *The handbook of psychopathy* (pp. 35–57), New York, NY: The Guilford Press.

Blais, J., Solodukhin, E., and Forth, A. E. (2014) 'A meta-analysis exploring the relationship between psychopathy and instrumental versus reactive violence,' *Criminal Justice and Behavior, 41*(7):797–821.

Boer, D., Hart, S., Kropp, P., and Webster, D. R. (1998) *Manual for the Sexual Violence Risk–20: Professional guidelines for assessing risk of sexual violence*, Lutz, FL: Psychological Assessment Resources.

Brown, A. R., Dargis, M. A., Mattern, A. C., Tsonis, M. A., and Newman, J. P. (2015) 'Elevated psychopathy scores among mixed sexual offenders: Replication and extension,' *Criminal Justice and Behavior, 42*(10):1032–1044.

Bureau of Justice Statistics. (2017) *Violent Crime in the United States*. Washington, DC: U.S. Department of Justice, Office of Justice Programs.

Cale, J., Lussier, P., McCuish, E., and Corrado, R. (2015) 'The prevalence of psychopathic personality disturbances among incarcerated youth: Comparing serious, chronic, violent and sex offenders,' *Journal of Criminal Justice, 43*(4):337–344.

Casey, H., Rogers, R. D., Burns, T., and Yiend, J. (2013) 'Emotion regulation in psychopathy,' *Biological Psychology, 92*(3):541–548.

Chakhssi, F., Kersten, T., de Ruiter, C., and Bernstein, D. P. (2014) 'Treating the untreatable: A single case study of a psychopathic inpatient treated with Schema Therapy,' *Psychotherapy, 51*(3):447–461.

Cleckley, H. (1941) *The mask of sanity*, St. Louis, MO: Mosby.

Cleckley, H. (1964) *The mask of sanity*, St. Louis, MO: Mosby.

Cleckley, H. (1976) *The mask of sanity* (5th ed.), St. Louis, MO: Mosby.

Coid, J., and Yang, M. (2011) 'The impact of psychopathy on violence among the household population of Great Britain,' *Social Psychiatry and Psychiatric Epidemiology, 46*(6):473–480.

Cooke, D. J., Hart, S. D., Logan, C., and Michie, C. (2004) *Comprehensive Assessment of Psychopathic Personality–Institutional Rating Scale (CAPP–IRS)*, Burnaby, BC: Simon Fraser University.

Cooke, D. J., and Logan, C. (2015) 'Capturing clinical complexity: Towards a personality-oriented measure of psychopathy,' *Journal of Criminal Justice, 43*(4):262–273.

Cooke, D. J., and Michie, C. (2001) 'Refining the construct of psychopathy: Towards a hierarchical model,' *Psychological Assessment, 13*(2):171–88.

Cope, L. M., Ermer, E., Gaudet, L. M., Steele, V. R., Eckhardt, A. L., Arbabshirani, M. R., . . ., and Kiehl, K. A. (2014) 'Abnormal brain structure in youth who commit homicide,' *NeuroImage: Clinical, 4*:800–807.

de Pádua Serafim, A., de Barros, D. M., Bonini Castellana, G., and Gorenstein, C. (2014) 'Personality traits and violent behavior: A comparison between psychopathic and non-psychopathic male murderers,' *Psychiatry Research, 219*(3):604–608.

Declercq, F., Willemsen, J., Audenaert, K., and Verhaeghe, P. (2012) 'Psychopathy and predatory violence in homicide, violent, and sexual offences: Factor and facet relations,' *Legal and Criminological Psychology, 17*(1):59–74.

DeLisi, M. (2016) *Psychopathy as unified theory of crime*, New York, NY: Palgrave Macmillan.

DeLisi, M., Kosloski, A., Sween, M., Hachmeister, E., Moore, M., and Drury, A. (2010) 'Murder by numbers: Monetary costs imposed by a sample of homicide offenders,' *Journal of Forensic Psychiatry & Psychology, 21*(4):501–513.

Edens, J. F., Poythress, N. G., Lilienfeld, S. O., Patrick, C. J., and Test, A. (2008) 'Further evidence of the divergent correlates of the Psychopathic Personality Inventory factors: Prediction of institutional misconduct among male prisoners,' *Psychological Assessment, 20*(1):86–91.

Federal Bureau of Investigation. (2010) *Uniform crime report, 2009*, Washington, DC.

Firestone, P., Bradford, J. M., Greenberg, D. M., Larose, M. R., and Curry, S. (1998) 'Homicidal and nonhomicidal child molesters: Psychological, phallometric, and criminal features,' *Sexual Abuse: A Journal of Research and Treatment, 10*(4):305–323.

Frick, P. J., and Hare, R. D. (2001) *Antisocial process screening device: APSD*, Toronto, ON: Multi-Health Systems.

Furnham, A., Daoud, Y., and Swami, V. (2009) '"How to spot a psychopath": Lay theories of psychopathy,' *Social Psychiatry and Psychiatric Epidemiology, 44*(6):464–72.

Gacono, C. B. (2000) *The clinical and forensic assessment of psychopathy: A practitioner's guide*, Mahwah, NJ: Lawrence Erlbaum Associates.

Glenn, A. L., and Raine, A. (2009) 'Psychopathy and instrumental aggression: Evolutionary, neurobiological, and legal perspectives,' *International Journal of Law and Psychiatry, 32*(4):253–258.

Goldstein, P. J. (1985) 'The drugs/violence nexus: A tripartite conceptual framework,' *Journal of Drug Issues, 15*(4):493–506.

Gray, N. S., and Snowden, R. J. (2016) 'Psychopathy in women: Prediction of criminality and violence in UK and USA psychiatric patients resident in the community,' *Psychiatry Research, 237*:339–343.

Haapasalo, J. (1994) 'Types of offense among the Cleckley psychopaths,' *International Journal of Offender Therapy and Comparative Criminology, 38*(1):59–67.

Häkkänen-Nyholm, H., and Hare, R. D. (2009) 'Psychopathy, homicide, and the courts,' *Criminal Justice and Behavior, 36*(8):761–777.

Hancock, J. T., Woodworth, M. T., and Porter, S. (2013) 'Hungry like the wolf: A word-pattern analysis of the language of psychopaths,' *Legal and Criminological Psychology, 18*(1):102–114.

Hare, R. D. (1999) 'Psychopathy as a risk factor for violence,' *The Psychiatric Quarterly*, *70*(3):181–97.

Hare, R. D. (2003) *Manual for the Revised Psychopathy Checklist* (2nd ed.), Toronto, ON: Multi-Health Systems.

Hare, R. D., and McPherson, L. M. (1984) 'Violent and aggressive behavior by criminal psychopaths,' *International Journal of Law and Psychiatry*, 7(1):35–50.

Hare, R. D., and Neumann, C. S. (2008) 'Psychopathy as a clinical and empirical construct,' *Annual Review of Clinical Psychology*, *4*:217–46.

Harris, P. B., Boccaccini, M. T., and Rice, A. K. (2017) 'Field measures of psychopathy and sexual deviance as predictors of recidivism among sexual offenders,' *Psychological Assessment*, *29*(6):639–651.

Hawes, S. W., Boccaccini, M. T., and Murrie, D. C. (2013) 'Psychopathy and the combination of psychopathy and sexual deviance as predictors of sexual recidivism: Meta-analytic findings using the Psychopathy Checklist–Revised,' *Psychological Assessment*, *25*(1):233–243.

Hemphill, J. F., Hare, R. D., and Wong, S. (1998) 'Psychopathy and recidivism: A review,' *Legal and Criminological Psychology*, *3*(1):139–170.

Henderson, D. K. (1938) *Psychopathic states*, New York, NY: W. W. Norton & Company.

Hildebrand, M., de Ruiter, C., and de Vogel, V. (2004) 'Psychopathy and sexual deviance in treated rapists: Association with sexual and nonsexual recidivism,' *Sexual Abuse: A Journal of Research and Treatment*, *16*(1):1–24.

Hutton, E. L., and Woodworth, M. (2014) 'Violent female youth: An examination of instrumental violence, psychopathy, and offense characteristics,' *Behavioral Sciences & the Law*, *32*(1):121–134.

Juodis, M., Starzomski, A., Porter, S., and Woodworth, M. (2014) 'A comparison of domestic and non-domestic homicides: Further evidence for distinct dynamics and heterogeneity of domestic homicide perpetrators,' *Journal of Family Violence*, *29*(3):299–313.

Karpman, B. (1941) 'On the need of separating psychopathy into two distinct clinical types: The symptomatic and the idiopathic,' *Journal of Criminal Psychopathology*, *3*:112–137.

Karpman, B. (1948) 'The myth of the psychopathic personality,' *American Journal of Psychiatry*, *104*:523–534.

Kiehl, K. A., and Hoffman, M. B. (2011) 'The criminal psychopath: History, neuroscience, treatment, and economics,' *Jurimetrics*, *51*:355–397.

Kiehl, K. A., and Sinnott-Armstrong, W. P. (2013) *Handbook on psychopathy and law*, New York, NY: Oxford University Press.

Klein Tuente, S., Vogel, V. de, and Stam, J. (2014) 'Exploring the criminal behavior of women with psychopathy: Results from a multicenter study into psychopathy and violent offending in female forensic psychiatric patients,' *International Journal of Forensic Mental Health*, *13*(4):311–322.

Krstic, S., Neumann, C. S., Roy, S., Robertson, C. A., Knight, R. A., and Hare, R. D. (2017) 'Using latent variable- and person-centered approaches to examine the role of psychopathic traits in sex offenders,' *Personality Disorders: Theory, Research, and Treatment*, doi:10.1037/per0000249

Laurell, J., and Dåderman, A. M. (2007) 'Psychopathy (PCL–R) in a forensic psychiatric sample of homicide offenders: Some reliability issues,' *International Journal of Law and Psychiatry*, *30*(2):127–135.

Leistico, A.-M. R., Salekin, R. T., DeCoster, J., and Rogers, R. (2008) 'A large-scale meta-analysis relating the Hare measures of psychopathy to antisocial conduct,' *Law and Human Behavior*, *32*(1):28–45.

Levy, N. (2010) 'Psychopathy, responsibility, and the moral/conventional distinction,' in L. Malatesti & J. McMillan (Eds.), *Responsibility and psychopathy: Interfacing law, psychiatry, and philosophy* (pp. 213–226), New York, NY: Oxford University Press.

Lilienfeld, S. O., and Andrews, B. P. (1996) 'Development and preliminary validation of a self-report measure of psychopathic personality traits in noncriminal populations,' *Journal of Personality Assessment*, *66*(3):488–524.

Millon, T., Simonsen, E., and Birket-Smith, M. (1998) 'Historical conceptions of psychopathy in the United States and Europe,' in T. Millon, E. Simonsen, M. Birket-Smith, and R. D. Davis (Eds.), *Psychopathy: Antisocial, criminal, and violent behavior* (pp. 3–31). New York, NY: Guilford Press.

Parks, G. A., and Bard, D. E. (2006) 'Risk factors for adolescent sex offender recidivism: Evaluation of predictive factors and comparison of three groups based upon victim type,' *Sexual Abuse: A Journal of Research and Treatment*, *18*(4):319–342.

Patrick, C. J., and Drislane, L. E. (2015) 'Triarchic model of psychopathy: Origins, operationalizations, and observed linkages with personality and general psychopathology,' *Journal of Personality*, *83*(6):627–643.

Patrick, C. J., Fowles, D. C., and Krueger, R. F. (2009) 'Triarchic conceptualization of psychopathy: Developmental origins of disinhibition, boldness, and meanness,' *Development and Psychopathology*, *21*(3):913–38.

Pinel, P. (1806) *A treatise on insanity*, London: W. Todd.

Porter, S., Fairweather, D., Drugge, J., Herve, H., Birt, A., and Boer, D. P. (2000) 'Profiles of psychopathy in incarcerated sexual offenders,' *Criminal Justice and Behavior*, *27*(2):216–233.
Porter, S., and Woodworth, M. (2007) '"I'm sorry I did it . . . but he started it": A comparison of the official and self-reported homicide descriptions of psychopaths and non-psychopaths,' *Law and Human Behavior*, *31*(1):91–107.
Porter, S., Woodworth, M., Earle, J., Drugge, J., and Boer, D. (2003) 'Characteristics of sexual homicides committed by psychopathic and nonpsychopathic offenders,' *Law and Human Behavior*, *27*(5):459–470.
Próspero-Luis, J., Moreira, P. S., Paiva, T. O., Teixeira, C. P., Costa, P., and Almeida, P. R. (2017) 'Psychopathy, criminal intentions, and abnormal appraisal of the expected outcomes of theft,' *Legal and Criminological Psychology*, *22*(2):314–331.
Putkonen, H., Weizmann-Henelius, G., Repo-Tiihonen, E., Lindberg, N., Saarela, T., Eronen, M., and Häkkänen-Nyholm, H. (2010) 'Homicide, psychopathy, and aging – a nationwide register-based case-comparison study of homicide offenders aged 60 years or older,' *Journal of Forensic Sciences*, *55*(6):1552–1556.
Reidy, D. E., Lilienfeld, S. O., Berke, D. S., Gentile, B., and Zeichner, A. (2016) 'Psychopathy traits and violent assault among men with and without history of arrest,' *Journal of Interpersonal Violence*, doi:10.1177/88626051666097
Robertson, C. A., and Knight, R. A. (2014) 'Relating sexual sadism and psychopathy to one another, non-sexual violence, and sexual crime behaviors,' *Aggressive Behavior*, *40*(1):12–23.
Schimmenti, A., Passanisi, A., and Caretti, V. (2014) 'Interpersonal and affective traits of psychopathy in child sexual abusers: Evidence from a pilot study sample of Italian offenders,' *Journal of Child Sexual Abuse*, *23*(7):853–860.
Schrag, C. (1954) 'Leadership among prison inmates,' *American Sociological Review*, *19*(1):37–42.
Serin, R. C., and Amos, N. L. (1995) 'The role of psychopathy in the assessment of dangerousness,' *International Journal of Law and Psychiatry*, *18*(2):231–238.
Sherretts, N., Boduszek, D., Debowska, A., and Willmott, D. (2017) 'Comparison of murderers with recidivists and first time incarcerated offenders from U.S. prisons on psychopathy and identity as a criminal: An exploratory analysis,' *Journal of Criminal Justice*, 51:89–92.
Skeem, J. L., and Cooke, D. J. (2010a) 'Is criminal behavior a central component of psychopathy? Conceptual directions for resolving the debate,' *Psychological Assessment*, *22*(2):433–45.
Skeem, J. L., and Cooke, D. J. (2010b) 'One measure does not a construct make: Directions toward reinvigorating psychopathy research – reply to Hare and Neumann (2010),' *Psychological Assessment*, *22*(2), 455–459.
Stratton, J., Brook, M., and Hanlon, R. E. (2017) 'Murder and psychosis: Neuropsychological profiles of homicide offenders with schizophrenia,' *Criminal Behaviour and Mental Health*, *27*(2):146–161.
ten Brinke, L., Porter, S., Korva, N., Fowler, K., Lilienfeld, S. O., and Patrick, C. J. (2017) 'An examination of the communication styles associated with psychopathy and their influence on observer impressions,' *Journal of Nonverbal Behavior*, *41*(3):269–287.
Texas Health and Safety Code, §841.023 (2000)
Theobald, D., Farrington, D. P., Coid, J. W., and Piquero, A. R. (2016) 'Are male perpetrators of intimate partner violence different from convicted violent offenders? Examination of psychopathic traits and life success in males from a community survey,' *Journal of Interpersonal Violence*, *31*(9):1687–1718.
Thomson, N. D. (2017) 'An exploratory study of female psychopathy and drug-related violent crime,' *Journal of Interpersonal Violence*, doi:10.1177/88626051769087
Thomson, N. D., Centifanti, L. C., and Lemerise, E. A. (2017) 'Emotion regulation and conduct disorder: The role of callous–unemotional traits,' in C. A. Essau, S. S. LeBlanc, & T. H. Ollendick (Eds.), *Emotion regulation and psychopathology in children and adolescents* (pp. 129–153), Oxford: Oxford University Press.
Thomson, N. D., and Centifanti, L. C. M. (2017) 'Proactive and reactive aggression subgroups in typically developing children: The role of executive functioning, psychophysiology, and psychopathy,' *Child Psychiatry & Human Development*, in press.
Thomson, N. D., Towl, G. J., and Centifanti, L. C. M. (2016) 'The habitual female offender inside: How psychopathic traits predict chronic prison violence,' *Law and Human Behavior*, *40*(3):257–269.
Truman, J. L., and Morgan, R. E. (2016) *Criminal victimization, 2015*, Washington, DC: U.S. Department of Justice, Bureau of Justice Statistics.
U.S. Department of Health & Human Services. (2014) *Child maltreatment 2014*. Washington, DC: U.S. Department of Health & Human Services.
Vaughn, M. G., and DeLisi, M. (2008) 'Were Wolfgang's chronic offenders psychopaths? On the convergent validity between psychopathy and career criminality,' *Journal of Criminal Justice*, *36*(1):33–42.

Vaughn, M. G., Newhill, C. E., DeLisi, M., Beaver, K. M., and Howard, M. O. (2008) 'An investigation of psychopathic features among delinquent girls,' *Youth Violence and Juvenile Justice*, *6*(3):240–255.

Vitacco, M. J., Neumann, C. S., and Pardini, D. A. (2014) 'Predicting future criminal offending in a community-based sample of males using self-reported psychopathy,' *Criminal Justice and Behavior*, *41*(3):345–363.

Walters, G. D., and Heilbrun, K. (2010) 'Violence risk assessment and Facet 4 of the psychopathy checklist: Predicting institutional and community aggression in two forensic samples,' *Assessment*, *17*(2):259–268.

Warren, J., South, S. C., Burnette, M. L., Rogers, A., Friend, R., Bale, R., and Van Patten, I. (2005) 'Understanding the risk factors for violence and criminality in women: The concurrent validity of the PCL–R and HCR–20,' *International Journal of Law and Psychiatry*, *28*(3):269–289.

Wilson, D., and Yardley, E. (2013) 'The psychopathy of a Victorian serial killer: Integrating micro and macro levels of analysis,' *Journal of Criminal Psychology*, *3*(1):19–30.

Wiseman, J. (2015) *Incidence and prevalence of sexual offending*, Washington, DC: U.S. Department of Justice, Office of Justice Programs.

Woodworth, M., Freimuth, T., Hutton, E. L., Carpenter, T., Agar, A. D., and Logan, M. (2013) 'High-risk sexual offenders: An examination of sexual fantasy, sexual paraphilia, psychopathy, and offence characteristics,' *International Journal of Law and Psychiatry*, *36*(2):144–156.

34

The severe 5 percent and psychopathy

Michael G. Vaughn, Brandy R. Maynard, Christopher P. Salas-Wright, and Matt DeLisi

Introduction

The study of crime has yielded several axiomatic findings. Examples of these include pronounced offending among males and that, in the aggregate, the relationship between age and crime (i.e., age–crime curve) accelerates in the teen years and diminishes sharply by the mid-30s. One of the most important of all of these axiomatic findings is that antisocial problem behavior is asymmetrical in nature. More specifically, a small subset of persons (usually male) accounts for the majority of antisocial behaviors. Converging lines of research generated by birth cohort designs, criminal career studies, and analyses of nationally representative samples strongly indicate that around 5 percent of the population accounts for the lion's share of the offending (Blumstein, Cohen, Roth, & Visher, 1986; DeLisi, & Piquero, 2011; Piquero, Farrington, & Blumstein, 2003; Tracy, Wolfgang, & Figlio, 1990; Vaughn et al., 2011; Vaughn, DeLisi, Salas-Wright, & Maynard, 2014; Wolfgang, Figlio, & Sellin, 1972).

A number of seminal and overlapping theoretical constructs have been employed as devices to communicate the salience of these findings. These have included career criminal; life-course persistent; serious, violent, and chronic (SVC) offenders; and the focus of the present chapter, the severe 5 percent (Baglivio, Jackowski, Greenwald, & Howell, 2014; Loeber & Farrington, 1998; Blumstein, Cohen, Roth, & Visher, 1986; Moffitt, 1993, 2003; Vaughn et al., 2011; Vaughn, DeLisi, Salas-Wright, & Maynard, 2014). What stands out among these classifications is not only the pronounced disproportionate contribution to offending, but the co-occurring drug use, mental health distress, and health problems observed among this virulent subset (DeLisi, 2005; Moffitt, 1993, 2003; Salas-Wright, Vaughn, & Reingle Gonzalez, 2016; Salekin & Lynam, 2010; Vaughn & DeLisi, 2008; Vaughn, Salas-Wright, DeLisi, & Piquero, 2014). In short, many lives have been profoundly altered in deleterious ways by the chronic violations of the rights of others by the severe 5 percent.

The present chapter reviews the rise of the severe 5 percent and examines its epidemiology and etiology. We then explore the connections of the severe 5 percent with the construct of psychopathy and learn that there is much common ground. Next, we survey candidate evidence-based prevention principles and findings toward mitigating and forestalling the severe 5 percent impact. At this point, we should mention that we use the term "severe 5 percent" to denote the asymmetry in offending based on empirical observation of relatively discrete groups; our intention is to not reify the construct or suggest this subgroup is taxonic, indicate that it is the proper label for practitioners, or that it is literally fixed at 5 percent of a population.

The rise of the severe 5 percent

Epidemiological background

Early birth cohort designs, more specifically Wolfgang's chronic offenders (Wolfgang, Figlio, & Sellin, 1972), were the direct epidemiological forerunners of the severe 5 percent. While pathbreaking in their findings about a small number in a birth cohort accounting for the majority of crime, two major shortcomings of these designs were overcome in the severe 5 percent studies. First, these investigations are geographically circumscribed and lacked the national representativeness necessary to advance the generalizability of this line of inquiry. Second, there was little regarding the descriptive characteristics of correlated behaviors and mental health conditions.

A 2009 study that examined subgroups among a cohort of young children was also a forerunner of the severe 5 percent (Vaughn, Beaver, DeLisi, & Wright, 2009). This particular study drew upon data from a nationally representative sample of kindergarteners in the United States. Vaughn and his colleagues (2009) identified a severely impaired subgroup that comprised a relatively large 9.3 percent of kindergarteners. One of the pronounced differences between these children and their peers (some of whom had moderate behavioral problems) were the behavioral/cognitive/executive problems that inhibited their capacity for self-regulation. Based on parental and teacher reports, these children in the severe group had worse fine motor skills, worse gross motor skills, more externalizing behaviors, worse interpersonal skills, poorer social interaction, more barriers to learning, and worse classroom behavior. They were reared in households characterized by heightened parental stress and physical punishment. Sadly, because of their behaviors they may have also been perceived as less lovable, as evidenced by findings regarding less parental affection. Alternatively, their parents could have been colder and they themselves possessing of difficult temperaments. A follow-up study using structural equation modeling across waves indicated that prospectively early learning difficulties predicted interpersonal deficits, which in turn was strongly associated with poor self-control that then predicted later externalizing behavior (Vaughn et al., 2010).

The natural history of the severe 5 percent is to a large extent grounded in the work of Moffitt (1993, 2003; but in a more distant vein, see Robins & O'Neal, 1958). Moffitt suggested two broad categories (or typologies) of offending: adolescent limited and life-course persistent offenders. The former group begins to offend during adolescence during a time of rapid biological maturity (post-puberty) and when the importance of peers intensifies. Experimentation with deviant behaviors and alcohol and substance use occurs and generally dissipates as self and social controls tend to take hold. However, for a smaller subset of life-course persistent offenders, neuropsychological deficits that compromise executive functioning coupled with family disadvantage and entanglement in snares such as serious drug use or involvement with highly antisocial individuals increases the probability of contact with the criminal justice system and longer-term potential of offending. This latter group resembles other constructs mentioned such as SVC offenders, highly psychopathic youth, and the severe 5 percent. Failures in many life domains such as marriage and other relationships, health burden, and employment accompany these syndromes. The life-course lens is important here as the severely antisocial tend to begin their offending careers earlier and extend them longer into adulthood. In fact, the potency of an early age of onset of offending on subsequent offending severity has shown in multiple lines of research to be one of the most important markers for criminal careers (DeLisi, Neppl, Lohman, Vaughn, & Shook, 2013; Piquero, Hawkins, & Kazemian, 2012). It should also be mentioned that Moffitt did not literally mean that life-course persistent offenders would be as virulent by age 70 as they were in their 20s, when a loss of energy wanes consistent with the aging process.

Another analogue construct (serious, violent, and chronic or simply SVC) has garnered substantial research, some of which bears on the severe 5 percent formulation. One of the landmarks in this genre is Howard Snyder's (1998) study of SVC juvenile offenders based on data from Maricopa County (Phoenix, AZ). Snyder found that among over 150,000 court referral offending careers, about 3 percent met criteria for SVC classification. Consistent with other research mentioned above, Snyder also found that the SVC juvenile offenders were more likely than other juvenile offenders to be early-starters. Importantly, a replication of Snyder's work was undertaken using the Pittsburgh Youth Study and a similar prevalence of SVC offending was found (Loeber, Farrington, & Waschbusch, 1998). Using statewide data from Florida, Baglivio and colleagues (2014) found that the classification of SVC juvenile offenders was moderately stable, and SVC offenders were far more likely to be referred at 12 years or younger than other offenders.

The adult and adolescent severe 5 percent papers published in 2011 (Vaughn et al., 2011) and 2014 (Vaughn, DeLisi, Salas-Wright, & Maynard, 2014) respectively extend these previous works by including data from national sampling frames that employ well-established measurements of mental health and substance use disorders and related problem behaviors. Findings from the 2011 study from the National Epidemiologic Survey of Alcohol and Related Conditions (NESARC), which is the largest comorbidity survey ever (diagnostic interviews of over 43,000 individuals), showed clear evidence of extensive comorbidity of mental health and substance use disorders among a severe 5 percent (actual 5.3 percent) of the population identified using latent class modeling. In particular, relative to normative controls, the severe 5 percent were substantially more likely to suffer from lifetime mood disorder (odds ratio (OR) = 2.58), bipolar disorder (7.89), various phobias (OR range = 2.06–2.28), and any psychotic disorder (OR = 6.00). The severe 5 percent also reported the highest prevalence of the use of sedatives, stimulants, alcohol, hallucinogens, and marijuana. Testing the presence of the severe 5 percent among a large sample (N = 18,614) of 12–17-year-olds derived from the National Survey of Drug Use and Health, the 2014 paper identified a severe group that was high and versatile across the externalizing spectrum and was about twice as likely as other groups to report internalizing symptoms such as anxiety and depression. This severe 5 percent (actual 4.7 percent) was also more likely to report less parental supervision and lower grades in school.

Etiology

While volumes have been written with respect to the etiology or underlying causes of severe antisocial behavior, the focus here will be on the etiology of asymmetry in offending that is suggestive of familial transmission. A substantial body of research has indicated a concentration of antisocial traits and behaviors that reside within families. Lines of evidence derived from the criminal careers literature (DeLisi & Piquero, 2011) and studies of the intergenerational transmission of antisocial behavior (Bijleveld, & Wijkman, 2009; Conger, Neppl, Kim, & Scaramella, 2003; Putkonen, Ryynänen, Eronen, & Tiihonen, 2007; Thornberry, Freeman-Gallant, Lizotte, Krohn, & Smith, 2003) independently suggest that the etiology of the severe 5 percent may reside in the passing along of these susceptibilities via genetics and learning mechanisms. So, while crime and antisocial behavior are not evenly distributed in terms of prevalence and severity, neither are their etiological understructures. In short, a small subset of individuals and families account for a disproportionate share (Farrington, 2011; Farrington, Barnes, & Lambert, 1996). Family history and longitudinal designs possess the ability to examine the course of antisocial behavior from its beginnings and across generations. There have been several notable long-running studies that have revealed important insights into the clustering of crime. Farrington and colleagues (1996), reporting on three decades of data collection from the Cambridge Study in Delinquent Development, found that nearly two-thirds of families had at least one family member possessing a criminal conviction, but more importantly, 6 percent of the families accounted for half of the total convictions. Uniquely, these researchers also found that women with criminal convictions were more likely to marry males with criminal convictions, suggesting that there is a significant role to play with regard to assortative mating. Factors such as the personality traits of parents and children, parental separation and divorce, and oppressive disciplinary practices were associated with these family trends (Kazemian, Spatz Widom, & Farrington, 2011). More recent research from the Cambridge study tracked males up to the age of 56 and found that groups of offenders could be distinguished across this age range, with the most severe high rate offenders having a concentrated profile of childhood risk in family ties to antisocial traits (Farrington, Piquero, & Jennings, 2013).

Another long-running and well-regarded longitudinal study, the Pittsburgh Youth Study, also has found that offending is concentrated in families. For example, boys who were arrested (compared to those boys who are not arrested) in this study were nearly three times more likely to have a criminal brother, greater than three times more likely to have a criminal sister, and nearly five times as likely to have a criminal father (Farrington, Jolliffe, Loeber, Stouthamer-Loeber, & Kolb, 2001). They were also nearly four times more likely to have a criminal mother and criminal grandfather. Similarly, results from the National Longitudinal Study of Adolescent Health showed that approximately 5 percent of all families in the study accounted for half of the total arrests (Beaver, 2013). Likewise, results from a 2006 Dutch birth cohort composed of 1,681 families in a university town in the east Netherlands revealed that 7.8 percent of families accounted for 52.3 percent of all arrests (Junger, Greene, Schipper, Hesper, & Estourgie, 2013).

In one of the largest data collections ever (12.5 million cases from 1973 to 2004), Frisell, Lichtenstein, and Långström (2011) investigated the degree to which crime runs in families in the Swedish Multi-Generation Register spanning 1973 to 2004. The sample, perhaps 100 times larger than any other, produced remarkable results. Specifically, these researchers found that, compared to matched controls, parents and siblings were 4.3 times more likely to engage in violent crime and distant relatives were nearly two times more likely. The magnitude of effects increased as serious crime increased, such that homicide, kidnapping, and robbery were ever more familial concentrated. In total, findings from these large and diverse data collections point toward intergenerational transmission of antisocial traits and provide a sturdy foundation for the risks of severe 5 percent development. As Vaughn and colleagues (2015) note regarding family transmission of severe antisocial behavior, "taking family histories of offenders by the criminal justice system may yield important data similar to medical histories" (p. 829).

What about females?

Although male sex is universally one of the most robust correlates of crime (Eme, 2010; DeLisi & Vaughn, 2015), there are numerous females who contribute to serious crime (Blackburn & Trulson, 2010; DeLisi, 2002). For example, DeLisi (2002) interviewed 55 adult female criminals whose mean number of arrests was over 40. Many of these arrests were for armed robbery and assault. Another study by Odgers and colleagues (2007) of incarcerated female delinquents reported that nearly half had used a weapon while fighting, 41 percent attacked a victim with the purpose of injuring or killing them, and 27 percent shot another person. An examination of the two severe 5 percent investigations by Vaughn and colleagues (2011, 2014) reveals several findings that may be surprising about females and their role in asymmetry in antisocial behavior (Vaughn, Salas-Wright, DeLisi, & Piquero, 2014). Vaughn and colleagues (2014) identified a severe 5 percent (actual 4.7) subgroup of which approximately one-third was female. Further, their analyses of the externalizing behavior ratios for the severe group relative to the full sample indicated that females, though a little less virulent overall, were still not far behind their male counterpart 5 percenters accounting for relatively large proportions of problem behaviors. For example, among females in the survey, severe 5 percent females accounted for large proportions of the drug selling (69.74 percent), theft (49.13 percent), hallucinogen use (43.16 percent), and gun carrying (41.82 percent). These numbers suggest that within-sex patterns of the severe 5 percent are similar for females as they are for males, even though females are a smaller, but not insubstantial, proportion of the severe 5 percent.

Although females are represented among the severe 5 percent, there are substantial theoretical and empirical reasons why females are unlikely to pursue antisocial careers with the same scope and intensity as males. One of the reasons for this is identified by Moffitt's (1993) work on life-course-persistent offending that indicates the cumulative risks for males are greater. Despite these notions and prior research, assumption about females in other realms of endeavor have been overturned and it is quite possible, as shown by research on the severe 5 percent among nationally representative adolescents in the National Survey on Drug Use and Health (NSDUH), that females are quite capable of severe antisocial behavior. And there may be conditions under which females could be equal to males for the dubious honor of most antisocial. Needless to say, greater study into the distribution patterns of severe female antisocial behavior and its natural history is needed.

Costs are staggering

Although complex and variable in their measurement (Wickramasekera, Wright, Elsey, Murray, & Tubeuf, 2015), crime costs studies are invaluable for policy-making. Several studies point toward billions of dollars of costs stemming from the behavioral and collateral consequences of serious juvenile offending. These costs include expenditures related to the criminal justice system, victimization, and mental health services (Cohen, 1998; Cohen & Piquero, 2009; DeLisi & Gatling, 2003; DeLisi et al., 2010). The personnel costs and health benefits of criminal justice system professionals alone are tremendous. But more specifically, the estimated costs for each seriously and chronically violent adolescent over time are several million dollars. As Eme (2010) has argued, severe early offending is one of the most urgent and important problems in the domain of child and adolescent health.

Although a formal study of the costs of the severe 5 percent has not been conducted, costs based on each offense multiplied by the large list of offenses in a severe 5 percent career would be staggering. For example, DeLisi (2016) created an aggregate average from mean offense costs derived from five monetization studies that employed data from the United States. These studies were Anderson (2012), Roman (2010), McCollister, French, and Fang (2010), DeLisi et al. (2010), and Miller, Cohen, and Wiersema (1996). Adjusted for 2016 data, the total costs for each offense is as follows: murder ($9,209,000), rape ($313,956), robbery ($148,568), assault ($140,396), burglary ($15,365), larceny/theft ($8283), and auto theft ($14,318). Given that the total costs of crime have been estimated to be over two trillion in the United States alone, and the severe 5 percent may account for as much as half of those costs, then can we conclude as a reasonable estimate that the severe 5 percent cost one trillion? Certainly, investing in evidence-based initiatives around early prevention would be money well spent.

Linkages between the severe 5 percent and psychopathy

Since psychopathic offenders account for a disproportionate amount of crime – particularly the most violent forms – it is likely there is convergent validity between the severe 5 percent and psychopathy. Unfortunately, this empirical question has only recently been evaluated. An international array of studies using various specifications, usually where offending is measured at the 90th percentile or above, has shown that psychopathy is well represented among those with the worst offending histories. Based on data from the United States, Vaughn and DeLisi (2008) showed that career criminals among a population of institutionalized delinquents had significantly higher psychopathy scores on eight specifications of psychopathy. In multivariate regression models, narcissism, fearlessness, impulsiveness, and unemotionality as measured by the PPI–SV or ASPD were significant despite ten powerful socio-demographic and mental health controls.

Farrington, Ullrich, and Salekin (2010) examined the linkages between psychopathy scores on the Psychopathy Checklist Screening Version (PCL: SV) and subsequently being convicted of a crime and being a chronic offender using data from the Cambridge Study in Delinquent Development from the United Kingdom. These investigators compared those who scored low on Factor 1 of the PCL: SV (encompassing the interpersonal and affective traits of the disorder) and who scored low on Factor 2 of the PCL: SV (encompassing the irresponsible–antisocial features of the disorder). Those who scored in the 90th percentile on Factor 1 were 6.2 times more likely to be convicted of a crime and a staggering 20.8 times more likely to become a chronic offender. Those who scored in the 90th percentile on Factor 2 were 18.8 times more likely to be convicted of a crime and an even more staggering 25.8 times more likely to be a chronic offender. When total scores on the PCL: SV were considered, the associations between psychopathy and serious criminal offending were even more pronounced. Those who scored in the 90th percentile on the PCL: SV total score were 65.1 times more likely to be convicted of a crime and 44.2 times more likely to become a chronic offender. These are the strongest empirical evidence demonstrating the pronounced effect of psychopathic features on the most pathological variants of offending.

Trajectory studies of serious juvenile offenders involved in the Incarcerated Serious and Violent Young Offender Study from Canada have produced similar results. McCuish and colleagues (2014) found evidence of four subtypes of offenders: high frequency chronic offenders, high rate slow desister offenders, explosive-onset fast desister offenders, and adolescence-limited offenders. The high frequency chronic and high rate slow desister groups had the most violent and extensive delinquent careers and also had psychopathy scores that were significantly higher than more moderate and nominally offending groups. Similarly, McCuish, Corrado, Hart, and DeLisi (2015) found evidence of four trajectories: youth who engaged in low levels of both violent and nonviolent offenses; youth who engaged in relatively low levels of violence and high levels of nonviolence; youth who engaged in high violence, but low nonviolence; and youth who engaged in high levels of violent and nonviolent offenses. The youth who engaged in high violence were significantly more psychopathic and had significantly worse offending careers that included earlier onset of delinquency, greater frequency of violent offending, and greater continuity in violence. In other words, psychopathy was a marker for involvement in violent crime.

The take away message from these studies is that investigations of delinquent and criminal careers reveal tremendous asymmetry in that small cadres of offenders engage in virtually all forms of crime at a velocity that far exceeds that of other offenders. The severe 5 percent moniker captures not only their location on the offending distribution but also the severity of their externalizing behaviors. To date, the evidence is clear that the severe 5 percent are also moderately to acutely psychopathic; indeed, psychopathy is one of the strongest variables that differentiates middling offenders from those that create the greatest threats to public safety.

A role for prevention and intervention?

It is now well accepted that delinquency, criminal behavior, psychopathy, and related behaviors (e.g., Conduct Disorder, oppositional defiant disorder, externalizing behavior problems, violence, antisocial behavior) result from numerous factors, including cognitive, psychological, familial, environmental, and biological (Brennan & Raine, 1997). Moreover, evidence suggests that dispositional and contextual contributory risk factors interact and/or cumulate in unique ways to form multiple pathways to a life of crime (Frick, 2004; Raine, 2002). From a biosocial perspective of prevention and intervention, "some of the best candidate environmental risk factors are those that are most likely to have an effect on the biological systems" (van Goozen & Fairchild, 2008:959) involved in the development of antisocial behavior. Some prevention and intervention models are explicitly informed, at least in part, by research of the biological as well as social and psychological bases of human behavior and risk; most, however, were developed from social and psychological research and theory but nevertheless likely do impact biomarkers.

It is critically important to successfully apply evidence-informed prevention focusing limited resources on the severe 5 percent. Although explicit prevention and intervention studies of individuals comprising the severe 5 percent have not been conducted (they are badly needed), prevention and treatments for youth and adults with antisocial and Conduct Disorder, psychopathy, and substance use have been examined. These extant evidence-informed interventions may be effective with the more serious behavior problems exhibited by the severe 5 percent or be able to be adapted for use with the severe 5 percent. It seems likely that early life-course engagement of these behaviors is probably cost effective and may have the ability to deflect some of the more pernicious aspects of these disorders. However, long-term follow-up knowledge is limited. In this section, we provide a survey of candidate programs across early prevention during pregnancy, infancy, and the preschool years, then examine indicated prevention and interventions during childhood and adolescence and discuss interventions targeting adults.

Preventive interventions during pregnancy, infancy, and the preschool years

Several studies provide compelling evidence of the salience of biosocial risk factors and interactions during pregnancy, birth, infancy, and early childhood on later delinquent and criminal behavior (Raine, 2002). A substantial body of evidence from longitudinal studies also provides compelling evidence that the earlier behavioral problems emerge in the life course, the more likely those behavioral problems will lead to more chronic and serious antisocial behaviors (Piquero, Farrington, & Blumstein, 2003; Piquero, 2008; Moffitt, 1993; White, Moffitt, Earls, Robins, & Silva, 1990). Moreover, evidence suggests that children with earlier onset of problem behaviors become less amenable to change over time (Tremblay, 2000). This evidence underscores the need and opportunity for early prevention efforts. While early preventive interventions often target parental and other proximal social factors, they do so in a way that, intentionally or unintentionally, has the potential to impact biological systems that can have far-reaching implications for behavior and outcomes well into adulthood.

Two of the most well-known and supported family-based programs to prevent delinquency and crime are home visiting and parent training programs. Numerous studies and several narrative and quantitative reviews have examined the effects of these programs on a myriad of behavioral outcomes. While findings are equivocal, outcome research on home visiting and parent training programs has produced evidence of short- and long-term positive effects on disruptive and antisocial behaviors, delinquency, and criminal outcomes (Farrington & Welsh, 1999; Olds et al., 1998; Piquero, Farrington, Welsh, Tremblay, & Jennings, 2009; Tremblay & Japel, 2003).

Home visiting programs generally target at-risk mothers prior to or immediately following the birth of their baby. Home visiting programs involve a trained interventionist (nurse, doctor, or other professional or paraprofessional) visiting the mother in her home and providing parent education and advice about pre- and postnatal care, including proper nutrition and health behaviors (i.e., avoid smoking, alcohol, drugs). While home visiting interventions have the potential to target biological and social risk factors and causal mechanisms quite early and thus prevent the emergence of antisocial behavior later in the life course, findings related to the effects of home visiting programs have, overall, been inconclusive (see Bilukha et la., 2005; Gomby et al., 1999). Home visiting programs vary on their theoretical underpinnings, length and intensity of treatment, and targeted populations, among other variables. One of the most well-known home visiting programs identified as an "effective" (www.ojjdp.gov/mpg/) or "model" (www.blueprintsprograms.com) program is the Nurse–Family Partnership (NFP; Olds et al., 1998; Olds, 2006). NFP provides low-income, first-time mothers with prenatal and postnatal home visitation services by public health nurses until the child reaches the age of 2. Visits last approximately 70 to 90 minutes in length, with approximately seven to nine visits during pregnancy (range 0–18) and an average of 23–26 visits from birth to 2 years of age (range 0–71; Olds, 2006). NFP targets several biological risk factors explicitly, including low birth weight, preterm birth, and neurological impairment by intervening to reduce known environmental risk factors during pregnancy, such as prenatal smoking, alcohol use, and drug use; poor nutrition; and pregnancy and birth complications. Also, by intervening to promote sensitive and competent care by the mothers, early prevention efforts can not only improve the parent–child interaction and foster more adaptive behavior through psychosocial processes but also has the potential to positively impact neurological substrates and functioning. Moreover, early intervention can "disrupt epigenetic transmission of problem behavior to future generations" by impacting gene expression and behavioral traits, which can have long lasting effects on the child and future generations as well (van Goozen & Fairchild, 2008:962). Although NFP was not explicitly developed to prevent delinquency and crime, studies have demonstrated positive effects on early antisocial behavior, and one study found positive effects on antisocial behavior at 15 years of age among children of the most at-risk mothers – those who were poor and unmarried (Olds et al., 1998). Additional studies have found positive effects on other outcomes, such as prenatal health behavior, pregnancy and birth outcomes, and sensitive, competent care of the child; however, positive effects have not been consistent across all studies and outcomes (e.g., Kitzman et al., 1997; Olds, Henderson, & Kitzman, 1994; Olds et al., 1998; Olds et al., 2014; also see Olds, 2006).

Parent training programs have been employed as a preventive intervention with parents of children ages 0–3 and involve providing some form of training to parents to modify parenting behaviors to enhance parenting skills, improve emotional and behavioral adjustment of the child, and improve parent–child interaction. Early parent training programs are heterogeneous and vary in terms of delivery method (e.g., individual, group), settings, theoretical underpinnings, and length and frequency of intervention; however, they generally aim to enhance the caregiving a child receives to provide an optimal environment for healthy child development and prevent negative outcomes that result from inadequate and harmful parenting practices. From a biosocial framework, parent training programs could impact a number of mechanisms implicated in severe 5 percent delinquency and crime, such as emotion regulation, stress responsiveness, and cognitive development, by targeting environmental risk factors, such as parenting practices and the quality of parent–child relationship and attachment. While many of the outcome studies and reviews focus on parent training interventions with older children and adolescents, evidence suggests that early parent training with parents of infants and toddlers can be effective in preventing later problematic and antisocial behavior (Barlow, Smailagic, Ferriter, Bennett, & Jones, 2010; Bernazzi, Cote, & Tremblay, 2001).

Interventions during childhood and adolescence

Interventions with school-age youth generally serve as a selective intervention with youth exhibiting disruptive behaviors to prevent delinquency, or as an indicated intervention to reduce delinquent behavior and disrupt the path to more serious severe 5 percent criminal behavior in adulthood. The range of interventions with children and adolescents are numerous and quite broad, but we will focus on cognitive–behavioral therapy (CBT) and family-based interventions for the treatment of disruptive and antisocial behavior (Farrington & Welsh, 1999; Lipsey & Cullen, 2007; see also Blueprints for Healthy Youth Development, www.blueprintsprograms.com; the Office of Juvenile Justice and Delinquency Prevention, www.ojjdp.gov/mpg/).

CBT is one of the most well-studied interventions for the treatment of diverse problems across the lifespan. Although CBT interventions can be diverse, they all share the same core premise that maladaptive cognitions contribute to emotional and behavioral problems and use similar approaches aimed at modifying maladaptive cognitions to affect behavior change (Butler, Chapman, Forman, & Beck, 2006). Related to the topic of this chapter, CBT has been found to be effective with children and adolescents for disruptive, aggressive and antisocial behaviors, sex offending, and substance use (Conrod, Stewart, Comeau, & Maclean, 2006; Hofman, Asnaani, Vonk, Sawyer, & Fang, 2012; Landenberger & Lipsey, 2005; McCart, Priester, Davies, & Azen, 2006). CBT for children and youth may not only target specific thoughts and behaviors directly related to delinquency, antisocial behaviors, or psychopathic traits, but also the development of problem solving, coping, and social skills to prevent or disrupt cognitions and behavior that would lead to behavioral problems indicative of future delinquency and other related behavioral problems (Vaske, Galyean, & Cullen, 2011).

Family-based interventions – specifically parent training and family therapy – have also been well studied for the prevention and treatment of disruptive/externalizing behaviors, delinquency, and aggression in childhood and adolescence. Parent training programs are frequently employed as an indicated prevention intervention with older children and adolescents exhibiting disruptive and externalizing behavior problems, and as an intervention with youth in the juvenile justice system. Like early parent training programs, parent training with school-aged youth are heterogeneous and vary considerably in regards to the theoretical underpinnings, program goals and components, delivery method, types of skills that are taught, and duration and frequency of the intervention. Parent training has been found to be effective with youth across a range of child behavior problems, including antisocial and delinquent behaviors (Farrington & Welsh, 1999; Kazdin, 1997; Piquero et al., 2009; Serketich & Dumas, 1996) and callous–unemotional traits (Hawes, Price, & Dadds, 2014). Several specific parent training programs have been identified as effective, model, or promising programs by Blueprints for Healthy Youth Development (see www.blueprintsprograms.com) and the Office of Juvenile Justice and Delinquency Prevention (see www.ojjdp.gov/mpg/), such as Parent–Child Interaction Therapy

(PCIT; McNeil & Hembree-Kigin, 2010), Incredible Years (Webster-Stratton & Reid, 2003), and Triple P – Positive Parenting Program. While parent training programs directly target social factors (i.e., parental behavior and parent–child interactions), from a biosocial perspective, parent training programs likely affect brain–behavior interactions by altering activity in brain regions thought to be involved in antisocial and delinquent behavior, such as executive functions, sympathetic nervous system, emotion and reward drives, and emotion regulation.

Family therapy is a broad term describing family-based counseling interventions that generally aim to provide intervention to the entire family often in a clinic or home setting by a counseling professional (i.e., social worker, family therapist, psychologist) to affect change in family interactions, structure, and/or function. While most family therapy models target family processes and structures linked to risk factors for delinquency and crime, they vary in terms of the determinants targeted for change and the techniques used by therapists to facilitate change in the family and youth. Family therapy interventions have been found to be effective with Conduct Disorder and delinquency (Baldwin, Christian, Berkeljon, & Shadish, 2012; Henggeler & Sheidow, 2012), reducing callous–unemotional traits (Hawes et al., 2014), and substance use (Austin, Macgowan, & Wagner, 2005; Baldwin et al., 2012). Although there are a number of diverse family therapy interventions for families of at-risk youth, we will focus here on two that have some empirical support with antisocial or delinquent youth in the prevention or desistance of antisocial or delinquent behaviors and have been widely disseminated: Multi-Systemic Therapy (MST; Henggeler, Schoenwald, Bordun, Rowland, & Cunningham, 1998) and Functional Family Therapy (FFT; Sexton, 2010).

MST is a widely known family-based intervention for youth exhibiting serious antisocial behavior. MST is a home-based intervention model grounded in systems and social ecological theories and informed by pragmatic models of the family and family therapy (i.e., structural and strategic family therapy models) as well as behavioral and cognitive models (Henggeler et al., 1998). Unlike other manualized interventions that provide step-by-step instructions for each session, MST uses nine treatment principles to guide therapist behavior. In collaboration with the family, the MST therapist aims to address the multiple determinants of delinquency across the youth's ecology and increase prosocial behavior. While the process is driven by the treatment principles and assessment and analytic process, the specific interventions are unique to each family and directed across the ecology, including the youth, family, peer group, school, and other social systems.

FFT, a relatively brief (8–12 or up to 30 one-hour sessions) manualized family-based intervention delivered in an office or home setting, is recognized as an evidence-based intervention for youth exhibiting antisocial behavior and has been widely disseminated (see Sexton, 2010; Sexton & Alexander, 2005). FFT is an integrative model grounded in systems theory and behavioral technologies that has evolved to incorporate attribution and information-processing theories and social constructionist and social influence ideas (Sexton & Alexander, 2005). The FFT model is relationally focused while also structured and protocol driven, with clearly articulated phases of intervention (i.e., engagement and motivation, behavior change, generalization) and specified goals, mechanisms of change, and therapist skills at each phase. The emphasis on the behavior change phase is grounded in risk and protective factor research, with particular emphasis on familial factors. While interventions may be individualized for the family, behavior change targets are focused on common risk and protective factors with the goal to build on protective family skills and improve the risk/protective factors ratio within the family (Sexton & Alexander, 2005).

Several studies point to positive effects of MST and FFT (e.g., Butler, Baruch, Hickey, & Fonagy, 2011; Borduin et al., 1995; Henggeler, Melton, & Smith, 1992; Timmons-Mitchell, Bender,

Kishna, & Mitchell, 2006) on antisocial behavior outcomes. As with most psychosocial interventions, positive effects are not consistently held across outcomes or studies, and effects have been found to vary based on the level of therapist adherence and fidelity with which the intervention is implemented (Henggeler, Melton, Brondino, Scherer, & Hanley, 1997; Littell, Forsythe, Popa, & Austin, 2005), particularly with more difficult families (Sexton & Turner, 2010). Despite the equivocal evidence of family therapy approaches in general and of the specific family therapy interventions discussed here, family-based interventions are seen as an important treatment modality for delinquency and crime prevention. While family therapy models rarely specifically target biological variables for change, family therapy likely has myriad effects on biological risk factors. By improving family interactions and warmth, increasing parenting monitoring and control, decreasing hostility and improving communication between family members, and improving the overall functioning of the family, family therapy may affect brain–behavior interactions by altering activity of the brain thought to be involved in delinquent and criminal behavior (e.g., executive functions, emotion-regulation, and self-control). Also, because the social environment can influence whether or not genes are "turned on" or "turned off," family therapy can help families improve the family environment, which can influence levels of transcription factors (e.g., cortisol) responsible for influencing gene expression (D'Onofrio & Lahey, 2010). For example, genetic vulnerabilities increase susceptibility to family risk factors; thus, family factors may trigger an underlying genetic risk for antisocial behavior (Button, Lau, Maughan, & Eley, 2008; Caspi et al., 2002). With family therapy, family risk factors could be decreased, which could then prevent the underlying gene from being triggered and thus prevent the emergence of antisocial behavior.

The preponderance of adult interventions entail variants of punishment and incapacitation, such as boot camps, intensive supervision, and intermediate sanctions (e.g., Aos, Phipps, Barnoski, & Lieb, 2001; Lipsey & Cullen, 2007); educational or vocational training (e.g., Visher, Winterfield, & Coggeshall, 2005; Wilson, Gallagher, & MacKenzie, 2000); and psychosocial interventions, such as cognitive–behavioral interventions (Feder & Wilson, 2005; Landenberger & Lipsey, 2005).

Substance abuse

The high prevalence of comorbidity between substance use disorders and criminal behavior – especially among the severe 5 percent – along with findings of higher recidivism rates among substance using offenders, suggest that treatment of substance use problems may attenuate some of the virulence in the criminal careers of the severe 5 percent (Salas-Wright, Vaughn, & Reingle Gonzalez, 2016). Several community, residential, and incarceration-based programs to affect substance use have gained substantial empirical support and are considered evidence-based practices (Chandler, Fletcher, & Volkow, 2009; Marlowe, 2011). Interventions with established empirical support targeting biosocial mechanisms for adult offenders include behavioral, cognitive–behavioral, and motivational-based interventions; therapeutic communities; and medication-assisted treatments.

Behavioral, cognitive–behavioral, and motivational-based interventions are among the most commonly used and evaluated interventions to treat substance use with adult offenders in both community and incarceration-based settings (Chandler et al., 2009). Behavioral interventions, including contingency management, and voucher-based reinforcement therapy aim to reduce substance use and criminal behavior by rewarding specific desired behaviors (i.e., attendance, abstinence, drug-negative urines) directly with vouchers or other goods, services, or privileges (Prendergast, Podus, Finney, Greenwell, & Roll, 2006). Cognitive–behavioral interventions, including relapse prevention, target cognitive and affective determinants, address situational triggers, and provide training in coping, avoidance, and self-monitoring strategies to reduce substance use and prevent relapse. Motivational-based interventions (i.e., motivational interviewing and motivation enhancement therapy) are client-centered and directive methods aimed to enhance "intrinsic motivation to change by exploring and resolving ambivalence" (Miller &Rollnick, 2002:25). The effectiveness of behavioral and cognitive–behavioral interventions for the treatment of substance use is well supported for adults (Dutra et al., 2008; Magill & Ray, 2009; Prendergast et al., 2006) and adolescents (Bender, Tripodi, Sarteschi, & Vaughn, 2011; Vaughn & Howard, 2004). Although the evidence for motivational-based interventions is not as strong as behavioral and cognitive–behavioral interventions, growing evidence supports motivational interventions in the treatment of substance use disorders with adults and adolescents (Jenson et al., 2011).

Therapeutic Communities (TC), intensive and often longer-term residential programs based on the social learning model, demonstrate positive effects on reoffending and drug use with adults (Mitchell, Wilson, & MacKenzie, 2007). Therapeutic communities have been implemented across the criminal justice continuum; they have been utilized as front-end alternatives to incarceration, conducted in prisons, and implemented for parole–reentry programs. Although there is variability in TC programs, they share several components: they house participants in distinct units from the general population; provide a confrontational yet supportive atmosphere in which both staff and peers confront antisocial behavior and attitudes and reinforce and reward positive behaviors; and involve participants in running the TC and facilitating mentorship and camaraderie (Marlowe, 2011; Mitchel et al., 2007). Although Therapeutic Communities are used with juveniles and are considered promising, evidence of the effects of TCs with juveniles is limited (Pealer, 2004; Jainchill, Hawke, & Messina, 2005).

Medication-assisted therapy (MAT), the use of pharmacotherapy in addition to other substance use interventions, has also been found to be effective in treating addiction with adult offenders. The use of agonist medications (i.e., buprenorphine or methadone) and antagonist medications (i.e., naltrexone) has demonstrated positive effects on substance use, treatment engagement, and offending/re-arrest outcomes (Amato et al., 2005). Despite positive and significant effects, and being endorsed by leading scientific and practitioner organizations, MAT is underutilized due to stigma associated with medication treatment of substance use; various barriers related to regulations, availability, concerns of liability, and security; and the perception that they are inconsistent with the treatment philosophy of the criminal justice setting (Friedmann et al., 2012). Less is known about MAT with adolescents as few controlled studies have assessed the effects of medications with adolescents, likely due to both practical and ethical reasons (Minozzi, Amato, & Davoli, 2009).

Conclusion

The severe 5 percent and psychopathy construct, while not identical, are highly convergent. Taken together, both constructs embody severe and pronounced offending and problem behavior over large swaths of the life-course. The present chapter reviewed the epidemiology and etiology of the severe 5 percent, revealing the empirical robustness of asymmetry in offending and marshaling an argument for continued study, development, and testing of preventive interventions at the earliest stages possible that might forestall lengthy criminal careers. There is a large evidence-base on effective intervention; however, it is largely unknown the extent to which these interventions reduce the harmful behaviors of the severe 5 percent. While skepticism is understandable, it really is an open question and, given the importance and staggering costs of the severe 5 percent, greater investment in testing the effects of extant and new approaches is critically needed.

References

Amato, L., Davoli, M., Perucci, C. A., Ferri, M., Faggiano, F., and Mattick, R. P. (2005) 'An overview of systematic reviews of the effectiveness of opiate maintenance therapies: Available evidence to inform clinical practice and research,' *Journal of Substance Abuse Treatment*, *28*:321–329.

Anderson, D. (2012) 'The cost of crime,' *Foundations and Trends in Microeconomics*, 7:209–65, doi:10.1007/978-1-4614-7883-6_551-1

Aos, S., Phipps, P., Barnoski, R., and Lieb, R. (2001) *The comparative costs and benefits of programs to reduce crime*, Olympia, WA: Washington State Institute for Public Policy.

Austin, A. M., Macgowan, M. J., and Wagner, E. F. (2005) 'Effective family-based interventions for adolescents with substance use problems: A systematic review,' *Research on Social Work Practice*, *15*:67–83.

Baglivio, M. T., Jackowski, K., Greenwald, M. A., and Howell, J. C. (2014) 'Serious, violent, and chronic juvenile offenders: A statewide analysis of prevalence and prediction of subsequent recidivism using risk and protective factors,' *Criminology & Public Policy*, *13*:83–116.

Baldwin, S. A., Christian, S., Berkeljon, A., and Shadish, W. R. (2012) 'The effects of family therapies for adolescent delinquency and substance abuse: A meta-analysis,' *Journal of Marital and Family Therapy*, *38*:281–304.

Barlow, J., Smailagic, N., Ferriter, M., Bennett, C., and Jones, H. (2010) 'Group-based parent-training programmes for improving emotional and behavioural adjustment in children from birth to three years old,' *Cochrane Database of Systematic Review*, *3*:1–95.

Beaver, K. M. (2013) 'The familial concentration and transmission of crime,' *Criminal Justice and Behavior*, *40*:139–155.

Bender, K., Tripodi, S. J., Sarteschi, C., and Vaughn, M. G. (2011) 'A meta-analysis of interventions to reduce adolescent cannabis use,' *Research on Social Work Practice*, *21*:153–164.

Bernazzani, O., Cote, C., and Tremblay, R. E. (2001) 'Early parent training to prevent disruptive behavior problems and delinquency in children,' *Annals of the American Academy of Political Social Science*, *578*:90–103.

Bijleveld, C. C., and Wijkman, M. (2009) 'Intergenerational continuity in convictions: A five-generation study,' *Criminal Behaviour and Mental Health*, *19*:142–155.

Bilukha, O., Hahn, R. A., Crosby, A., Fullilove, M. T., Liberman, A., Moscicki, E., . . ., and Briss, P. A. (2005) 'Effectiveness of early childhood home visitation in preventing violence: A systematic review,' *American Journal of Preventive Medicine*, *28*:11–39.

Blackburn, A. G., and Trulson, C. R. (2010) 'Sugar and spice and everything nice? Exploring institutional misconduct among serious and violent female delinquents,' *Journal of Criminal Justice*, *38*:1132–1140.

Blumstein, A., Cohen, J., Roth, J. A., and Visher, C. A. (Eds.) (1986) *Criminal careers and 'career criminals,'* Washington, DC: National Academy Press.

Borduin, C. M., Mann, B. J., Cone, L. T., Henggeler, S. W., Fucci, B. R., Blaske, D. M., and Williams, R. A. (1995) 'Multisystemic treatment of serious juvenile offenders: Long-term prevention of criminality and violence,' *Journal of Consulting and Clinical Psychology*, *63*:569–578.

Brennan, P. A., and Raine, A. (1997) 'Biosocial bases of antisocial behavior: Psychophysiological, neurological, and cognitive factors,' *Clinical Psychology Review*, *17*:589–604.Butler, S., Baruch, G., Hickey, N., and Fonagy, P. (2011) 'A randomized controlled trial of multisystemic therapy and statutory therapeutic intervention for young offenders,' *Journal of the American Academy of Child & Adolescent Psychiatry*, *50*:1220–1235.

Butler, A. C., Chapman, J. E., Forman, E. M., and Beck, A. T. (2006) 'The empirical status of cognitive–behavioral therapy: A review of meta-analyses,' *Clinical Psychology Review*, *26*:17–31.

Button, T. M. M., Lau, J. Y. F., Maughan, B., and Eley, T. (2008) 'Parental punitive discipline, negative life events and gene–environment interplay in the development of externalizing behavior,' *Psychological Medicine*, *38*:29–39.

Caspi, A., McClay, J., Moffitt, T. E., Martine, J., Craig, I. W., Taylor, A., and Poulton, R. (2002) 'Role of genotype in the cycle of violence in maltreated children,' *Science*, *297*:851–854.

Chandler, R. K., Fletcher, B. W., and Volkow, N. D. (2009) 'Treating drug abuse and addiction in the criminal justice system: Improving public health and safety, *JAMA*, *301*:183–190.

Cohen, M. A. (1998) 'The monetary value of saving a high-risk youth,' *Journal of Quantitative Criminology, 14*:5–33.
Cohen, M. A., and Piquero, A. R. (2009) 'New evidence on the monetary value of saving a high-risk youth,' *Journal of Quantitative Criminology, 25*:25–49.
Conger, R. D., Neppl, T., Kim, K. J., and Scaramella, L. (2003) 'Angry and aggressive behavior across three generations: A prospective, longitudinal study of parents and children,' *Journal of Abnormal Child Psychology, 31*:143–160.
Conrod, P. J., Stewart, S. H., Comeau, N., and Maclean, A. M. (2006) 'Efficacy of cognitive–behavioral interventions targeting personality risk factors for youth alcohol misuse,' *Journal of Clinical Child and Adolescent Psychology, 35*:550–563.
DeLisi, M. (2002) 'Not just a boy's club: An empirical assessment of female career criminals,' *Women & Criminal Justice, 13*:27–45.
DeLisi, M. (2005) *Career criminals in society*, Thousand Oaks, CA: Sage.
DeLisi, M. (2016) 'Measuring the cost of crime,' in B. M. Huebner & T. S. Bynum (Eds.), *The handbook of measurement issues in criminology and criminal justice*, Malden, MA: Wiley Blackwell.
DeLisi, M., and Gatling, J. (2003) 'Who pays for a life of crime? An empirical assessment of the assorted victimization costs posed by career criminals,' *Criminal Justice Studies, 16*:283–293.
DeLisi, M., Kosloski, A., Sween, M., Hachmeister, E., Moore, M., and Drury, A. (2010) 'Murder by numbers: Monetary costs imposed by a sample of homicide offenders,' *The Journal of Forensic Psychiatry & Psychology, 21*:501–513.
DeLisi, M., Neppl, T. K., Lohman, B. J., Vaughn, M. G., and Shook, J. J. (2013) 'Early starters: Which type of criminal onset matters most for delinquent careers?,' *Journal of Criminal Justice, 41*:12–17.
DeLisi, M., and Piquero, A. R. (2011) 'New frontiers in criminal careers research, 2000–2011: A state-of-the-art review,' *Journal of Criminal Justice, 39*:289–301.
DeLisi, M., and Vaughn, M. G. (2015) 'Correlates of crime,' in A. R. Piquero (Ed.), *Handbook of criminological theory*, Malden, MA: Wiley-Blackwell.
D'Onofrio, B. M., and Lahey, B. B. (2010) 'Biosocial influences on the family: A decade review,' *Journal of Marriage and Family*, 72:762–782.
Dutra, L., Stathopoulou, G., Basden, S., Leyro, T., Powers, M., and Otto, M. (2008) 'A meta-analytic review of psychosocial interventions for substance use disorders,' *American Journal of Psychiatry, 165*:179–187.
Eme, R. (2010) 'Male life-course-persistent antisocial behavior: The most important pediatric mental health problem,' *Archives of Pediatrics and Adolescent Medicine, 164*:486–487.
Farrington, D. P. (2011) 'Families and crime,' in J. Q. Wilson & J. Petersilia (Eds.), *Crime and public policy*, New York, NY: Oxford University Press.
Farrington, D. P., Barnes, G. C., and Lambert, S. (1996) 'The concentration of offending in families,' *Legal and Criminological Psychology, 1*:47–63.
Farrington, D. P., Jolliffe, D., Loeber, R., Stouthamer-Loeber, M., and Kalb, L. M. (2001) 'The concentration of offenders in families, and family criminality in the prediction of boys' delinquency,' *Journal of Adolescence, 24*:579–596.
Farrington, D. P., Piquero, A. R., and Jennings, W. G. (2013) *Offending from childhood to late middle age: Recent results from the Cambridge Study in Delinquent Development*, New York, NY: Springer.
Farrington, D. P., Ullrich, S., and Salekin, R. T. (2010) 'Environmental influences on child and adolescent psychopathy,' in R. T. Salekin and D. R. Lynam (Eds.), *Handbook of child and adolescent psychopathy* (pp. 202–230). New York, NY: Guilford Press.
Farrington, D. P., and Welsh, B. C. (1999) 'Delinquency prevention using family-based interventions,' *Children & Society, 13*:287–303.
Feder, L., and Wilson, D. B. (2005) 'A meta-analytic review of court-mandated batterer intervention programs: Can courts affect abusers' behavior?,' *Journal of Experimental Criminology, 1*:239–262.
Frick, P. J. (2004) 'Developmental pathways to conduct disorder: Implications for serving youth who show severe aggressive and antisocial behavior,' *Psychology in the Schools, 41*:823–833.
Friedmann, P. D., Hoskinson Jr, R., Gordon, M., Schwartz, R., Kinlock, T., Knight, K., . . . and O'Connell, D. J. (2012) 'Medication-assisted treatment in criminal justice agencies affiliated with the criminal justice–drug abuse treatment studies (CJ–DATS): Availability, barriers, and intentions,' *Substance Abuse, 33*:9–18.
Frisell, T., Lichtenstein, P., and Långström, N. (2011) 'Violent crime runs in families: A total population study of 12.5 million individuals,' *Psychological Medicine, 41*:97–105.

Gomby, D. S., Culross, P. L., and Behrman, R. E. (1999) 'Home visiting: Recent program evaluations – analysis and recommendations,' *Future of Children*, *9*:4–26.

Hawes, D. J., Price, M. J., and Dadds, M. R. (2014) 'Callous–unemotional traits and the treatment of conduct problems in childhood and adolescence: A comprehensive review,' *Clinical Child and Family Psychology Review*, *17*:248–267.

Henggeler, S. W., Melton, G. B., Brondino, M. J. Scherer, D. G., and Hanley, J. H. (1997) 'Multisystemic therapy with violent and chronic juvenile offenders and their families: The role of treatment fidelity in successful dissemination,' *Journal of Consulting and Clinical Psychology*, *65*:821–833.

Henggeler, S. W., Melton, G. B., and Smith, L. A. (1992) 'Family preservation using multisystemic therapy: An effective alternative to incarcerating serious juvenile offenders,' *Journal of Consulting and Clinical Psychology*, *60*:953–961.

Henggeler, S. W., Schoenwald, S. K., Bordun, C. M., Rowland, M. D., and Cunningham, P. B. (1998) *Multisystemic treatment of antisocial behavior in children and adolescents*, New York, NY: The Guilford Press.

Henggeler, S. W., and Sheidow, A. J. (2012) 'Empirically supported family-based treatments for conduct disorder and delinquency in adolescents,' *Journal of Marital and Family Therapy*, *38*:30–58.

Hofmann, S. G., Asnaani, A., Vonk, I. J., Sawyer, A. T., and Fang, A. (2012) 'The efficacy of cognitive behavioral therapy: A review of meta-analyses,' *Cognitive Therapy and Research*, *36*:427–440.

Jainchill, N., Hawke, J., and Messina, M. (2005) 'Post-treatment outcomes among adjudicated adolescent males and females in modified therapeutic community treatment,' *Substance Use & Misuse*, *40*:975–996.

Jenson, C. D., Cushing, C. C., Aylward, B. S., Craig, J. T., Sorell, D. M., and Steele, R. G. (2011) 'Effectiveness of motivational interviewing for adolescent substance use behavior change: A meta-analytic review,' *Journal of Consulting and Clinical Psychology*, *79*:433–440.

Junger, M., Greene, J., Schipper, R., Hesper, F., and Estourgie, V. (2013) 'Parental criminality, family violence and intergenerational transmission of crime within a birth cohort,' *European Journal on Criminal Policy and Research*, *19*:117–133.

Kazdin, A. E. (1997) 'Parent management training: Evidence, outcomes, and issues,' *Journal of the American Academy of Child and Adolescent Psychiatry*, *36*:1349–1356.

Kazemian, L., Spatz Widom, C., and Farrington, D. P. (2011) 'A prospective examination of the relationship between childhood neglect and juvenile delinquency in the Cambridge Study in Delinquent Development,' *International Journal of Child, Youth and Family Studies*, *2*:65–82.

Kitzman, H., Olds, D. L., Henderson, C. R., Jr., Hanks, C., Cole, R., Tatelbaum, R., and Barnard, K. (1997) 'Effect of prenatal and infancy home visitation by nurses on pregnancy outcomes, childhood injuries, and repeated childbearing: A randomized controlled trial,' *Journal of the American Medical Association*, *278*:644–652.

Landenberger, N. A., and Lipsey, M. W. (2005) 'The positive effects of cognitive–behavioral programs for offenders: A meta-analysis of factors associated with effective treatment,' *Journal of Experimental Criminology*, *1*:451–476.

Lipsey, M. W., and Cullen, F. T. (2007) 'The effectiveness of correctional rehabilitation: A review of systematic reviews,' *Annual Review of Law and Social Science*, *3*:297–320.

Littell, J., Forsythe, B., Popa, M., and Austin, S. (2005) 'Multisystemic therapy for social, emotional, and behavioral problems in youth aged 10–17: A systematic review,' *The Campbell Collaboration Library*, *1*.

Loeber, R., and Farrington, D. P. (Eds.) (1998) *Serious and violent juvenile offenders: Risk factors and successful interventions*, Thousand Oaks, CA: Sage.

Loeber, R., Farrington, D. P., and Waschbusch, D. A. (1998) 'Serious and violent juvenile offenders,' in R. Loeber & D. P. Farrington (Eds.), *Serious and violent juvenile offenders: Risk factors and successful interventions*, Thousand Oaks, CA: Sage.

Magill, M., and Ray, L. A. (2009) 'Cognitive–behavioral treatment with adult alcohol and illicit drug users: A meta-analysis of randomized controlled trials,' *Journal of Studies on Alcohol and Drugs*, *70*:516–527.

Marlowe, D. B. (2011) 'Evidence-based policies and practices for drug-involved offenders,' *The Prison Journal*, *91*:27S–47S.

McCart, M. R., Priester, P. E., Davies, W. H., and Azen, R. (2006) 'Differential effectiveness of behavioral parent-training and cognitive–behavioral therapy for antisocial youth: A meta-analysis,' *Journal of Abnormal Child Psychology*, *34*:525–541.

McCollister, K. E., French, M. T., and Fang, H. (2010) 'The cost of crime to society: New crime-specific estimates for policy and program evaluation,' *Drug and Alcohol Dependence*, *108*:98–109.

McCuish, E. C., Corrado, R. R., Hart, S. D., and DeLisi, M. (2015) 'The role of symptoms of psychopathy in persistent violence over the criminal career into full adulthood,' *Journal of Criminal Justice 43*(4):345–356.
McCuish, E. C., Corrado, R., Lussier, P., and Hart, S. D. (2014) 'Psychopathic traits and offending trajectories from early adolescence to adulthood,' *Journal of Criminal Justice, 42*:66–76.
McNeil, C. B., and Hembree-Kigin, T. L. (2010) *Parent–child interaction therapy*, New York, NY: Springer.
Miller, T., Cohen, M., and Wiersema, B. (1996) *Victim costs and consequences: A new look*, Washington, DC: U.S. Department of Justice. Retrieved April 26, 2018 from www.ncjrs.gov/pdffiles/victcost.pdf
Miller, W. R., and Rollnick, S. (2002) 'Motivational interviewing: Preparing people for change,' New York, NY: Guilford.
Minozzi, S., Amato, L., and Davoli, M. (2009) 'Maintenance treatments for opiate dependent adolescent,' *Cochrane Database of Systematic Reviews, 2.*
Mitchell, O., Wilson, D. B., and MacKenzie, D. L. (2007) 'Does incarceration-based drug treatment reduce recidivism? A meta-analytic synthesis of the research,' *Journal of Experimental Criminology, 3*:353–375.
Moffitt, T. E. (1993) 'Adolescence-limited and life-course-persistent antisocial behavior: A developmental taxonomy,' *Psychological Review, 100*:674–701.
Moffitt, T. E. (2003) 'Life-course-persistent and adolescence-limited antisocial behavior: A 10-year research review and a research agenda,' in B. B. Lahey, T. E. Moffitt, & A. Caspi (Eds.), *Causes of conduct disorder and juvenile delinquency*, New York, NY: The Guilford Press.
Odgers, C. L., Moretti, M., Burnette, M. L., Chauhan, P., Waite, D., and Reppucci, N. D. (2007) 'A latent variable modeling approach to identifying subtypes of serious and violent female juvenile offenders,' *Aggressive Behavior, 33*:339–352.
Olds, D. L. (2006) 'The nurse–family partnership: An evidence-based preventive intervention,' *Infant Mental Health Journal, 27*:5–25.
Olds, D., Henderson, C. R., Jr., Cole, R., Eckenrode, J., Kitzman, H., Luckey, D., and Powers, J. (1998) 'Long-term effects of nurse home visitation on children's criminal and antisocial behavior: 15-year follow-up of a randomized controlled trial,' *Journal of the American Medical Association, 280*:1238–1244.
Olds, D. L., Henderson, C. R., Jr., and Kitzman, H. (1994) 'Does prenatal and infancy nurse home visitation have enduring effects on qualities of parental caregiving and child health at 25 to 50 months of life?,' *Pediatrics, 93*:89–98.
Olds, D. L., Holmberg, J. R., Donelan-McCall, N., Luckey, D. W., Knudtson, M. D., and Robinson, J. (2014) 'Effects of home visits by paraprofessionals and by nurses on children: Follow-up of a randomized trial at ages 6 and 9 years,' *JAMA Pediatrics, 168*:114–121.
Pealer, J. A. (2004) 'A community of peers promoting behavior change: The effectiveness of a therapeutic community for juvenile male offenders in reducing recidivism,' Doctoral dissertation, University of Cincinnati.
Piquero, A. R. (2008) 'Taking stock of developmental trajectories of criminal activity over the life course,' in A. M. Liberman (Ed.), *The long view of crime: A synthesis of longitudinal research* (pp. 23–78), New York, NY: Springer.
Piquero, A. R., Farrington, D. P., and Blumstein, A. (2003) 'The criminal career paradigm,' in M. Tonry (Ed.), *Crime and justice: A review of research* (Vol. 30), Chicago, IL: University of Chicago Press.
Piquero, A. R., Farrington, D. P., Welsh, B. C., Tremblay, R., and Jennings, W. G. (2009) 'Effects of early family/parent training programs on antisocial behavior and delinquency,' *Journal of Experimental Criminology, 5*:83–120.
Piquero, A. R., Hawkins, J. D., and Kazemian, L. (2012) 'Criminal career patterns,' in R. Loeber & D. P. Farrington (Eds.), *From juvenile delinquency to adult crime: Criminal careers, justice policy, and prevention*, New York, NY: Oxford University Press.
Prendergast, M., Podus, D., Finney, J., Greenwell, L., and Roll, J. (2006) 'Contingency management for treatment of substance use disorders: A meta-analysis,' *Addiction, 101*:1546–1560.
Putkonen, A., Ryynänen, O. P., Eronen, M., and Tiihonen, J. (2007) 'Transmission of violent offending and crime across three generations,' *Social Psychiatry and Psychiatric Epidemiology, 42*:94–99.
Raine, A. (2002) 'Annotation: The role of prefrontal deficits, low autonomic arousal, and early health factors in the development of antisocial and aggressive behavior in children,' *Journal of Child Psychology and Psychiatry, 43*:417–434.
Robins, L. N., and O'Neal, P. (1958) 'Mortality, mobility, and crime: Problem children thirty years later,' *American Sociological Review, 23*:162–171.
Roman, J. K. (2010) 'What is the price of crime? New estimates of the cost of criminal victimization,' *Dissertation Abstracts International Section A: Humanities and Social Sciences*, 71:647.

Salas-Wright, C. P., Vaughn, M. G., and Reingle Gonzalez, J. M. (2016) *Drug abuse and antisocial behavior: A biosocial life-course approach*, New York, NY: Palgrave Macmillan.

Salekin, R. T., and Lynam, D. R. (Eds.) (2010) *Handbook of child and adolescent psychopathy*, New York, NY: The Guilford Press.

Serketich, W. J., and Dumas, J. E. (1996) 'The effectiveness of behavioral parent training to modify antisocial behavior in children: A meta-analysis,' *Behavior Therapy*, *27*:171–186.

Sexton, T. L. (2010) *Functional family therapy in clinical practice: An evidence-based treatment model for working with troubled adolescents*, New York, NY: Routledge.

Sexton, T. L., and Alexander, J. F. (2005) 'Functional family therapy for externalizing disorders in adolescents' (pp. 164–191),' in J. L. Lebow (Ed.), *Handbook of Clinical Family Therapy*, Hoboken, NJ: Wiley.

Sexton, T. L., and Turner, C. W. (2010) 'The effectiveness of functional family therapy for youth with behavioral problems in a community practice setting,' *Journal of Family Psychology*, *24*:339–334.

Snyder, H. N. (1998) 'Serious, violent, and chronic juvenile offenders: An assessment of the extent of and trends in officially recognized serious criminal behavior in a delinquent population,' in R. Loeber & D. P. Farrington (Eds.), *Serious & violent juvenile offenders: Risk factors and successful interventions*, Thousand Oaks, CA: Sage.

Thornberry, T. P., Freeman-Gallant, A., Lizotte, A. J., Krohn, M. D., and Smith, C. A. (2003) 'Linked lives: The intergenerational transmission of antisocial behavior,' *Journal of Abnormal Child Psychology*, *31*:171–184.

Timmons-Mitchell, J., Bender, M. B., Kishna, M. A., and Mitchell, C. C. (2006) 'An independent effectiveness trial of multisystemic therapy with juvenile justice youth,' *Journal of Clinical Child and Adolescent Psychology*, *35*:227–236.

Tracy, P. E., Wolfgang, M. E., and Figlio, R. M. (1990) *Delinquency careers in two birth cohorts*, New York, NY: Plenum Press.

Tremblay, R. E. (2000) 'The development of aggressive behavior during childhood: What have we learned in the past century?,' *International Journal of Behavioral Development*, *24*:129–141.

Tremblay, R. E., and Japel, C. (2003) 'Prevention during pregnancy, infancy, and the preschool years,' in D. P. Farrington & J. W. Coid (Eds.), *Early prevention of adult antisocial behavior* (pp. 205–242), New York, NY: Cambridge University Press.

van Goozen, S. H. M., and Fairchild, G. (2008) 'How can the study of biological processes help design new interventions for children with severe antisocial behavior?,' *Development and Psychopathology*, *20*:941–973.

Vaske, J., Galyean, K., and Cullen, F. T. (2011) 'Toward a biosocial theory of offender rehabilitation: Why does cognitive–behavioral therapy work?,' *Journal of Criminal Justice*, *39*:90–102.

Vaughn, M. G., Beaver, K. M., DeLisi, M, and Wright, J. P. (2009) 'Identifying latent classes of behavioral risk based on early childhood manifestations of self-control,' *Youth Violence and Juvenile Justice*, 7:16–31.

Vaughn, M. G., and DeLisi, M. (2008) 'Were Wolfgang's chronic offenders psychopaths? On the convergent validity between psychopathy and career criminality,' *Journal of Criminal Justice*, *36*:33–42.

Vaughn, M. G., DeLisi, M., Gunter, T., Fu, Q., Beaver, K. M., Perron, B. E., and Howard, M. O. (2011) 'The severe 5%: A latent class analysis of the externalizing spectrum in the United States,' *Journal of Criminal Justice*, *39*:75–80.

Vaughn, M. G., DeLisi, M., Salas-Wright, C. P., and Maynard, B. R. (2014) 'Examining violence and externalizing behavior among youth in the United States: Is there a severe 5%?,' *Youth Violence and Juvenile Justice*, *12*:3–21.

Vaughn, M. G., and Howard, M. O. (2004) 'Adolescent substance abuse treatment: A synthesis of controlled evaluations,' *Research on Social Work Practice*, *14*:325–335.

Vaughn, M. G., Perron, B. E., Beaver, K. M., DeLisi, M., and Wexler, J. (2010) 'Transactional pathways in the development of externalizing behaviors in a sample of kindergarten children with impaired self-control,' in V. G. Massari (Ed.), *Control theory and its applications*, New York, NY: Nova Science Publishers.

Vaughn, M. G., Salas-Wright, C. P., DeLisi, M., and Piquero, A. R. (2014) 'Health associations of drug-involved and criminal-justice-involved adults in the United States,' *Criminal Justice and Behavior*, *41*:318–336.

Vaughn, M. G., Salas-Wright, C. P., DeLisi, M., and Qian, Z. (2015) The antisocial family tree: Family histories of behavior problems in antisocial personality in the United States, *Social Psychiatry and Psychiatric Epidemiology*, *50*:821–31.

Visher, C. A., Winterfield, L., and Coggeshall, M. B. (2005) 'Ex-offender employment programs and recidivism: A meta-analysis,' *Journal of Experimental Criminology*, *1*:295–315.

Webster-Stratton, C., and Reid, M. J. (2003) *The incredible years parents, teachers and children training series: A multifaceted treatment approach for young children with conduct problems*, New York, NY: Guilford Press.

White, J. L., Moffitt, T. E., Earls, F., Robins, L., and Silva, P. A. (1990) 'How early can we tell? Predictors of childhood conduct disorder and adolescent delinquency,' *Criminology*, *28*:507–535.
Wickramasekera, N., Wright, J., Elsey, H., Murray, J., and Tubeuf, S. (2015) 'Cost of crime: A systematic review,' *Journal of Criminal Justice*, *43*:218–228.
Wilson, D. B., Gallagher, C. A., and MacKenzie, D. L. (2000) 'A meta-analysis of corrections-based education, vocation, and work programs for adult offenders,' *Journal of Research in Crime and Delinquency*, *37*:347–368.
Wolfgang, M. E., Figlio, R. M., and Sellin, T. (1972) *Delinquency in a birth cohort*, Chicago, IL: University of Chicago Press.

35

Examining the relationship between suicidal behavior and psychopathic traits through the lens of the interpersonal–psychological theory of suicide

Katie Dhingra, Sofia Persson, and Marc T. Swogger

Introduction

Approximately 804,000 people worldwide die by suicide each year (World Health Organization [WHO], 2014), making it one of the leading causes of death. To put this in perspective, suicide accounts for more deaths each year than homicide, car accidents, AIDS, and war combined (WHO, 2014). These suicide deaths are in addition to an estimated 25 million annual suicide attempts (Crosby, Gfroerer, Han, Ortega, & Parks, 2011) and 140 million people experiencing suicidal ideation (i.e., thoughts of engaging in behavior intended to end one's life; Borges et al., 2000; Nock et al., 2008). Thus, suicide is a major public health concern that calls for sophisticated prevention efforts. Suicidal ideation and behavior are complex phenomena influenced by numerous interacting biological, psychological, cultural, and environmental factors (O'Connor, 2011). Consequently, elucidation of relationships among these factors is necessary for improved prevention and treatment of individuals at risk for suicide.

Decades of research have demonstrated the key roles of internalizing constructs like hopelessness and depression in suicidal behavior (Beck, Brown, & Steer, 1989). However, progress toward an empirically based understanding of externalizing constructs (e.g., substance abuse, antisocial personality) in relation to suicide has been limited. This has begun to change, and the high prevalence of externalizing behavior in justice-involved people validates the increased attention. In particular, psychopathic traits may be important for understanding, predicting, and preventing suicidal behavior in criminal justice populations.

In what is widely considered the seminal conceptualization of psychopathy, Cleckley (1941/1976:358) asserted that one of the defining characteristics of the psychopathic personality is "suicide rarely carried out" (though he acknowledged that psychopaths may sometimes engage in manipulative suicidal gestures). In fact, Cleckley purported that psychopaths possess relative immunity to suicidality. However, recent empirical research shows a nuanced and complicated relationship between psychopathic traits and suicidal thoughts and behavior. Integrating multiple streams of research, this chapter explores the various ways that psychopathic traits may influence the occurrence of suicidal behavior. We draw upon the Interpersonal–Psychological Theory of suicidal behavior (IPTS; Joiner, 2007) as a framework for examining the intersection of the important constructs of belonging, burdensomeness, and acquired capability for suicide with different dimensions of psychopathy. The IPTS proposes that three factors are needed to die by suicide: (1) feeling that one does not belong with other people, (2) feeling that one is a burden on others or society, and (3) an acquired capability to overcome the fear and pain associated with suicide. Herein we examine implications of the existing literature and discuss future research directions in the study of the psychopathy–suicide relationship.

Bifurcated relationship between psychopathy and psychopathology

Psychopathy is a personality syndrome characterized by a diminished capacity for remorse, impulsive behavior, and superficial charm (Cleckley, 1976). As assessed by the Hare Psychopathy Checklist–Revised (PCL–R; Hare, 2003) and its derivatives, the psychopathic personality was originally shown to consist of two higher-order factors: Factor 1, reflecting callousness, lack of empathy and deep emotional capacity, and a deceitful and manipulative interpersonal style; and Factor 2, reflecting an impulsive, irresponsible, and antisocial lifestyle.

Research with a variety of samples and assessment methods typically demonstrates a bifurcated relationship such that Factor 1 (interpersonal/affective traits) is orthogonal or negatively related to symptoms of negative emotionality (e.g., anxiety or fearfulness), and Factor 2 (antisocial–lifestyle traits) is positively correlated with indices of emotional dysfunction (DeLisi, 2016; Hicks & Patrick, 2006; Kennealy, Hicks, & Patrick, 2007; Swogger et al., 2011). As illuminated by Hicks and Patrick's (2006) explication of the "opposing and repulsive" relationship between the two facets of psychopathy and the broad construct of negative emotionality (i.e., the tendency to experience unpleasant emotional states such as fear, anger, and nervous tension), this bifurcated relationship has been identified with numerous outcomes, including symptoms of anxiety (Bare, Hopko, & Armento, 2004; Sandvik, Hansen, Hystad, Johnsen, & Bartone, 2015), Post-Traumatic Stress Disorder (PTSD) among trauma-exposed individuals (Anestis, Harrop, Green, & Anestis, 2017; Willemsen, De Ganck, & Verhaeghe, 2012; Woodfield et al., 2016), and the higher order internalizing domain, linked to fearfulness and withdrawal (Blonigen et al., 2010; Willemson & Verhaeghe, 2012). Thus, consistent with Lykken's (1996:32) supposition that heroism and psychopathy are "twigs on the same genetic branch," the Interpersonal/Affective deficits indicative of Factor 1 (e.g., lack of empathy, social dominance, and deficient fear response) may reflect an emotional deficit (akin to fearlessness) that protects against the development of psychopathology under stress (e.g., Sandvik et al., 2015; Sellbom, 2015).

To date, 26 studies have examined the association between psychopathic traits and suicidal behavior. These studies support a more nuanced and complicated relationship than Cleckley (1941/1976) described. Verona, Patrick, and Joiner (2001) assessed 313 male prison inmates and determined the presence versus absence of a prior suicide attempt using a structured interview and prison file records. Results indicated that a suicide attempt history was significantly related to Psychopathy Checklist–Revised (PCL–R; Hare, 2003) Factor 2 (antisocial–lifestyle features) but was unrelated to Factor 1 (affective–interpersonal features). Findings were consistent with prior research linking suicide attempts to antisocial behavior (e.g., Nock & Kessler, 2006) but did not support Cleckley's (1941/1976) assertion that the core traits of psychopathy (i.e., Factor 1) are negatively associated with suicidal behavior. Further, the relation between PCL–R Factor 2 traits and suicide attempts was significantly attenuated when scores on self-report measures of (reversed) constraint (or impulsivity) and negative emotionality were statistically controlled. This finding suggests that the association between PCL–R Factor 2 and suicide attempt history is attributable to the variance it shares with poor impulse control and sensation seeking (reversed constraint) and a propensity toward anxiety, hostility, and mistrust (negative emotionality).

Verona, Hicks, and Patrick (2005) conducted a similar study to Verona et al. (2001) with 226 female prison inmates. Replicating the previous findings, PCL–R Factor 2 was positively related to a history of a suicide attempt. Corroborating the authors' hypothesis that suicidal behavior is positively related to social deviance but not core psychopathic traits, and consistent with Cleckley's (1976) assertion that psychopaths are relatively immune to suicidal behavior, PCL–R Factor 1 exhibited a significant negative relationship with suicide attempt history. In a multisite, multi-sample investigation, including both males and female participants ($N = 1{,}711$), Douglas, Herbozo, Poythress, Belfrage, and Edens (2006) examined the relationship between psychopathy and suicidal ideation and attempts. Multiple measures of both psychopathy and suicidal ideation and behavior were used across 12 independent samples. Combining the samples to obtain a grand mean correlation, the significant relationship between Factor 2-related traits and suicidal behavior was replicated again. No combined effect was found for Factor 1-related traits on suicidal thoughts or behavior after controlling for Factor 2 features of psychopathy. It is worth nothing, however, that there was wide variability in findings across samples and measurement methods. This latter study offered the most comprehensive data on the relationship between psychopathy and suicidal thoughts and behavior to date, and the authors concluded that individuals with considerable Factor 2 features of psychopathy are likely to have an elevated risk for suicidal ideation or behavior. They further asserted that the presence of the core features of psychopathy should not lead to dismissal of the possibility of suicide risk.

More recent work has started to consider how psychopathic traits may interact with distress (anxiety and depression) to increase risk for suicidal ideation and behavior. Smith, Selwyn, Wolford-Clevenger, and Mandracchia (2014), for instance, found that male prison inmates with higher levels of secondary psychopathic traits (akin to Factor 2), as indexed by the Levenson Self-Report Psychopathy Scale [LSP]; Levenson, Kiehl, & Fitzpatrick, 1995), were more likely to report having attempted suicide multiple times compared with once or not at all, when controlling for age and time served. In addition, increases in secondary psychopathic traits strengthened the relationship between depressive symptoms and suicide ideation. Contrary to expectations, however, there was no significant relationship between primary psychopathic traits (akin to Factor 1) and the likelihood of reporting a previous suicide attempt, independently or controlling for age, time served, and secondary psychopathic traits. The relationship of depressive symptoms and suicide ideation was also not moderated by primary psychopathic traits. In fact, significant positive correlations were observed among primary psychopathic traits, self-reported depressive symptoms, and suicide ideation, though these correlations were weaker compared with those between secondary psychopathy and suicide ideation and depression. This finding indicates that although primary (Factor 1) psychopathic traits are associated with less reactivity to aversive stimuli and fewer symptoms of distress, such as depression (Hicks & Patrick, 2006; Patrick, Bradley, & Lang, 1993; Sutton, Vitale, & Newman, 2002; Verona et al., 2001), male prison inmates with elevated primary psychopathic traits remain susceptible to suicidal ideation and attempts. Extending Smith et al.'s findings, low levels of overall anxiety and secondary psychopathy yielded the greatest suicidal ideation (Levenson et al., 1995; Pennington, Cramer, Miller, & Anastasi, 2015; Smith et al., 2014).

A limitation of the majority of available data is the near exclusive use of the two-factor model of psychopathy. Studies support the alternative validity of a four-factor solution (Guy & Douglas, 2006; Hare, 2003), which enables a fine-grained analysis of psychopathic traits. Specifically, the two higher-order dimensions of psychopathy each consist of two correlated facets (Hare, 2003), with Factor 1 comprised of distinct interpersonal and affective facets and Factor 2 comprised of lifestyle and antisocial facets. In this model, the interpersonal facet consists of items related to arrogance and a deceitful and manipulative interpersonal style. The affective facet assesses a deficiency of affective experience, including a lack of empathy and emotional depth. The lifestyle facet is comprised of items that assess a tendency toward impulsivity and irresponsibility. The antisocial facet consists of items related to juvenile and adult antisocial behavior. Although the PCL–R facets are highly correlated, there is important heterogeneity among individuals with high psychopathy scores (Dhingra, Boduszek, & Kola-Palmer, 2015; Swogger & Kosson, 2007), such that specific patterns of elevations may be meaningful because of their differential correlates (DeLisi, 2009; Hare & Neumann, 2009).

Research conducted to increase specificity in linking psychopathic traits to suicidal behavior with the four facets has been mixed. Verona et al. (2005) found that the negative relationship between suicide attempt history and Interpersonal/Affective factor scores (PCL Factor 1) was accounted for mostly by the interpersonal and not the affective features of psychopathy. Douglas et al. (2008) reported that the PCL–R Factor 2 (in the two-factor model) contribution to suicide-related behavior was largely due to the lifestyle (i.e., irresponsible and impulsive), as opposed to antisocial traits of psychopathy, in a sample of 682 male offenders. By contrast, using data drawn from the McArthur Violence Risk Assessment Study (N = 810 psychiatric patients), Swogger, Conner, Meldrum, and Caine (2009) found that the PCL: SV antisocial facet (i.e., poor behavioral controls, adolescent and adult antisocial behavior), rather than the impulsive and irresponsible lifestyle features, were associated with suicide attempts. Contrary to their hypothesis, the affective features of psychopathy were not negatively associated with suicide attempts.

In summary, neither Factor 1, nor its component interpersonal or affective traits of psychopathy, has been consistently linked to suicidal behavior. Nor have these traits consistently been shown to protect against it. By contrast, Factor 2 traits are consistently positively related to suicidal behavior, and findings extend to related constructs outside of psychopathy research (e.g., impulsivity, violence; Smith et al., 2008; Swogger, Van Orden, & Conner, 2014). More research is necessary to determine the extent to which the lifestyle and antisocial components of psychopathy Factor 2 can be distinguished in their strength of relationship to suicidal behavior across different samples and assessment instruments.

Linking psychopathic traits to suicidal thoughts and behavior

Research on the mechanisms through which psychopathic traits may influence suicide risk is sparse. Recent work in suicidology has underscored the importance of considering variables that facilitate the transition from suicidal ideation to suicidal behavior, highlighting the fact that most oft-cited risk factors for thoughts of suicide (e.g., anxiety, depression, hopelessness) have repeatedly proven to be poor predictors of suicidal behavior at the individual level, and that only a small portion of those who think about suicide go on to make an attempt (e.g., May & Klonsky, 2013; Nock et al., 2008). Theories such as the IPTS (Joiner, 2007), the Three Step Theory of Suicide (3ST; Klonsky & May, 2015), the Integrated–Motivational Volitional Model of Suicide (IMV; O'Conner, 2011) and Fluid Vulnerability Theory (FVT; Rudd, 2006) emphasize that certain factors facilitate thoughts of suicide, whereas others enable individuals thinking about suicide to translate that ideation into action (Klonsky, Saffer, & Bryan 2017). In hopes of generating assessment and treatment strategies, as well as directions for future research, we examine the psychopathy–suicide relationship through the lens of the IPTS (Joiner, 2007; Van Orden et al., 2010).

The interpersonal psychological theory of suicidal behavior

Suicide risk assessment is difficult because the majority of those who think about suicide or experience risk factors for suicide do not develop plans for, attempt, or die by suicide (O'Connor, 2011; Klonsky & May, 2015; Nock et al., 2008). Joiner's (2007) IPTS attempts to overcome the difficulties inherent in assessing risk for such a low base-rate event by postulating *why* it is that so many who wish for death by suicide do not die by suicide. The IPTS states that three proximal, interactive risk factors must be present in order for someone to both desire and be capable of death by suicide (Joiner, 2007; Van Orden et al., 2010): (1) perceived burdensomeness, (2) thwarted belongingness, and (3) the acquired capability. As each of these factors (explained below) is relatively rare, and their conjunction even more so, the theory is consistent with the relative rarity of death by suicide.

Suicidal desire

The IPTS posits that the serious desire for death by suicide arises from the co-occurrence of two proximal, causal factors: (1) perceived burdensomeness (an individual's sense that he or she is a liability to others and worth more dead than alive) and (2) thwarted belongingness (an individual's sense that he or she lacks meaningful connections to others), as well as hopelessness (i.e., "this will never change") about these perceptions (Joiner, 2007; Van Orden et al., 2010). There is considerable evidence that perceived burdensomeness and thwarted belongingness are moderately related but distinct constructs that can be reliably measured (Van Orden, Cukrowicz, Witte, & Joiner, 2012). Additionally, the IPTS describes perceived burdensomeness and thwarted belongingness as dynamic cognitive–affective state (as opposed to trait) constructs. Thus, the degree to which an individual experiences each factor may fluctuate based on a number of intra- and interpersonal factors such as mood, feelings of low self-esteem, experiencing family conflict, possessing few social supports, and proneness to interpret others' behavior as rejection (Van Orden et al., 2010).

According to the theory, each psychological state alone increases risk for passive suicidal ideation (e.g., a wish to be dead); however, active suicidal ideation (e.g., thoughts about killing oneself) develops when both perceived burdensomeness and thwarted belongingness are present and viewed as unchanging and stable (i.e., hopelessness; Joiner, 2007; Van Orden et al., 2010). A recent systematic review of the findings of 58 empirical studies (Ma, Batterham, Calear, & Han, 2016) found support for a robust association between perceived burdensomeness and suicidal desire, and a modest association for thwarted belongingness and suicidal desire. Also consistent with predictions of the IPTS, Hagan, Podlogar, Chu, and Joiner (2015) found in two independent samples (one clinical, the other non-clinical) that the interaction between thwarted belongingness and perceived burdensomeness only predicted current suicide risk when levels of hopelessness were high.

Suicidal desire and psychopathy

Both components of suicidal desire (thwarted belongingness and perceived burdensomeness) rely on the idea of an essential human need for interpersonal connection (Baumeister & Leary, 1995), and individuals with distorted negative beliefs about their connections to others are at risk for suicidal desire (Joiner, 2007). Individuals with high core psychopathic (Factor (1) traits, however, demonstrate severe deficiencies in this domain (Cleckley, 1976). For example, adolescents with high levels of psychopathic traits tend to have shorter friendships (Muñoz, Kerr, &

Besic, 2008). Studies have found that individuals high in psychopathic traits tend to undervalue enduring and meaningful relationships (Baird, 2002), favoring a short-term mating strategy (i.e., one-night stands) over having a long-term partner (Jonason, Li, Webster, & Schmitt, 2009; Jonason, Luevano, & Adams, 2012). Indeed, promiscuity and a tendency to engage in extramarital affairs are markers of psychopathy as assessed using the PCL–R (Hare, 2003). Thus, it seems likely that individuals with high levels of psychopathic traits are less motivated to seek meaningful, affiliative bonds with others (Foulkes, Seara-Cardoso, Neumann, Rogers, & Viding, 2014). Furthermore, some research suggests that affiliative and prosocial behavior towards others may be less rewarding for these individuals than it is for others (Foulkes et al., 2014). Individuals with high Factor 1 traits may not have the capacity to feel the emotional pain that often drives suicidal behavior. Moreover, the selfish, callous and remorseless use of others reflected in Factor 1 could be considered the opposite of burdensomeness, as it involves a lack of concern regarding the impact an individual is having upon others.

Examining the impact of Factor 1 traits on thwarted belonging and burdensomeness thus reveals several possible implications for the utility of the IPTS with regard to psychopathic people. For individuals high in Factor 1, thwarted belongingness may be a lesser factor in suicidal ideation and behavior because affiliative behavior, overall, is less important to the individual. Feelings of belongingness, rather than central to the individual's life, may be brief and based upon superficial interaction with limited expectation of – or perceived need for – ongoing social support. For an individual with high Factor 1 traits, perhaps belongingness cannot be meaningfully "thwarted" because it is not sought in the way that the IPTS describes. Similarly, psychopathic ego-centricity as reflected by Factor 1 traits tends to be pervasive. It would be rare indeed to find evidence of an individual high in these traits who feels burdensomeness based upon others' struggle, given that the emotional impact of one's behavior on others is rarely considered. With these two theoretical components of suicidal desire potentially less relevant to individuals with high Factor 1 traits, it is unclear whether the components would have significant predictive value for suicidal desire among individuals high in these traits.

Acquired Capability for Suicide (ACS)

The IPTS posits that, in addition to the desire for suicide, an individual must possess the capability to engage in life-threatening behaviors (i.e., the capability for suicide; Joiner, 2007; Smith & Cukrowicz, 2010; Van Orden et al., 2010). This capability manifests as reduced fear of death and self-injury as well as increased physical pain tolerance (Ribeiro et al., 2014; Smith & Cukrowicz, 2010; Van Orden et al., 2010). Further, the theory posits that individuals are not born with the capability to die by suicide, as humans are biologically prepared to be frightened of, and thus avoid, cues that signal threats to survival (Öhman & Mineka, 2001). Consequently, death by suicide is exceedingly difficult. The theory asserts that capability for suicide is *typically* acquired over time through two mechanisms: (1) direct and indirect exposure to painful and provocative (i.e., frightening) experiences (PPEs), and (2) habituation and activation of emotional opponent processes (Solomon, 1980) to these PPEs. In essence, habituation and activation of opponent processes in the face of painful and frightening stimuli causes the initial responses of fear and pain to be overtaken by less aversive states, such as calmness and relief (Van Orden et al., 2010). If sufficient habituation occurs, presumably, fear and pain survival mechanisms will no longer deter an individual who desires death from attempting suicide (Joiner, 2007). Importantly, the ACS is theorized to operate independently of suicidal thoughts; only when suicidal desire interacts with the ability to approach fear of death and pain will a serious suicide attempt occur.

The IPTS advances that the most direct method to develop acquired capability is through life experiences closely approximating suicide (Joiner, 2007; Joiner et al., 2009). Such experiences include non-suicidal self-injury (NSSI; self-injurious behavior with an absence of suicidal intent), mental rehearsal, "dry runs," and suicide attempts. Accordingly, a history of NSSI and suicide attempts are the strongest predictors of suicide (Franklin et al., 2016; Nock et al., 2008). Individuals reporting a history of suicide attempts, particularly multiple attempts, also self-report lower fear of death and/or higher pain tolerance than people who have not made a suicide attempt (e.g., Bryan, Cukrowicz, West, & Morrow, 2010; Franklin, Hessel, & Prinstein, 2011; Smith et al., 2010; Van Orden et al., 2008). Further, people who have made a suicide attempt exhibit a higher pain tolerance and greater threshold for pain detection than people who have not made a suicide attempt, when assessed using both self-report measures and behavioral tasks (see Kirtley, O'Carroll, & O'Connor, 2016 for a review). Although suicide attempt history is important for understanding the ACS, more than half of those who die by suicide do so in the absence of any history of suicidal behavior (Nock et al., 2008).

Numerous studies have shown that more frequent past exposure to aggregated PPEs, such as physical and sexual abuse, physical fights, sky diving, and contact sports, are associated with the ACS (Bender, Gordon, Bresin, & Joiner, 2011; Bryan et al., 2010**a**; Franklin et al., 2011; Smith et al., 2010; Smith, Wolford-Cleavenger et al., 2013). Research with groups selected for common exposure to certain PPEs, such as intravenous drug users (injections and related consequences), veterinarians (euthanizing animals), military personnel (military training, deployment training, and combat exposure), and body dysmorphic patients (operations) suggests that certain populations may be at greater risk for death by suicide due to their heightened risk for the ACS (Bryan & Cukrowicz, 2011; Bryan, Morrow, Anestis, & Joiner, 2010; Smith et al., 2016).

While the IPTS purports that there are multiple pathways to the ACS, according to Joiner (2009), exposure to violence appears to pose a particular risk. There is data to support this assertion. In a sample of 348 U.S. Air Force security personnel, combat experiences characterized by aggression or violence were most directly associated with self-reported ACS, as compared to combat experiences that were non-aggressive or nonviolent events (Bryan & Cukrowicz, 2011). Similarly, Stein et al. (2010), using the World Health Organization World Mental Health Survey, found that exposure to sexual or other interpersonal violence – including being a perpetrator of violence – was more likely to contribute to a suicide attempt than all other forms of trauma. Additionally, the more trauma individuals experience, the more likely they are to make an attempt. Similarly, childhood maltreatment has been associated with risk for suicide attempt in multiple studies (Hadland et al., 2012; Rajalin, Hirvikoski, & Jokinen, 2013), and violent/painful forms of childhood maltreatment, such as rape or physical abuse, are associated with more suicide attempts than "less violent" forms of abuse, such as molestation and verbal abuse (Joiner et al., 2009).

The IPTS posits an *indirect* role for outwardly directed aggression and violence whereby engaging in aggressive and/or violent behavior facilitates the ACS (Bryan & Cukrowicz, 2011; Joiner, 2007). Similarly, witnessing others' pain and injury, either in person (e.g., witnessing domestic violence as a child; Joiner et al., 2009) or indirectly (e.g., via playing violent video games; Teismann, Förtsch, Baumgart, Het, & Michalak, 2014) may lead to vicarious habituation, which, in turn, increases capability for suicide. Thus, exposure to aggression, as either a witness or perpetrator, may lead to habituation to fear and pain that places one at greater risk for the transition from suicidal ideation to suicide attempts (Bryan et al., 2010; Jordan & Samulson, 2016; Swogger et al., 2014; Wolford-Clevenger et al., 2015).

Personality traits, such as impulsivity and sensation seeking, associated with suicide and greater exposure to PPEs are also correlated with self-perceived suicide capability (Anestis, Bagge, Tull, & Joiner, 2011; Anestis et al., 2016; Bender, Gordon, Bresin, & Joiner, 2011; Witte, Gordon, Smith, & Van Orden, 2012). For instance, Anestis et al. (2011) found that sensation seeking was a significant predictor of self-reported ACS and physical pain insensitivity. Additionally, Bender et al. (2011) found evidence for both indirect and direct effects of sensation seeking on ACS, as measured by self-report.

Acquired capability and psychopathy

Individuals high in Factor 2 psychopathic traits may have greater ACS than those lower in these traits due to a greater likelihood of experiencing events that promote its development. Indeed, several theorists (Karpman, 1941; Lykken, 1996; Porter, 1996) have advanced the idea that these traits are a result of dysfunctional interpersonal exchanges and adverse environmental factors, including child maltreatment (abuse and neglect). This is mirrored in more recent theoretical and clinical research on attachment theory (Bowlby, 1969) suggesting a relationship between repeated exposure to negative parenting behaviors (e.g., displays of extreme anger and emotional negativity, coldness and rejection, and adverse reactions) and Factor 2 traits (Beaver et al., 2014; Caretti & Craparo, 2010).

Consistent with the above theoretical and clinical data, individuals high in Factor 2 traits, similar to multiple suicide attempters and members of the high-risk groups (e.g., IV drug users, military personnel, and veterinarians), have been found to be more often exposed to a variety of severe and chronic environmental stressors in childhood such as neglect, trauma, and abuse (Karpman, 1941; Porter, 1996; Poythress, Skeem, & Lilienfeld, 2006; Swogger et al., 2009). Across the lifespan, individuals high in Factor 2 traits are more likely than others to abuse substances, engage in violent acts and assaults, and demonstrate interpersonal hostility (DeLisi, 2016; Dhingra & Boduszek, 2013; Vassileva, Kosson, Abramowitz, & Conrod, 2005). Furthermore, high levels of psychopathic traits are associated with enjoyment of antisocial entertainment such as violent sports and video games (Williams, McAndrew, Learn, Harms, & Paulhus, 2001).

Whereas Factor 2 traits of psychopathy are related to PPEs, Factor 1 traits may reflect early and pervasive fearlessness. Indeed, low fear is central to leading conceptualizations of Factor 1 traits (see Hamilton, Hiatt Racer, & Newman, 2015, for a contemporary integration of deficient fear and cognitive phenomena in psychopathy). Individuals high on Factor 1 traits have explicit affective deficits, including specific deficiencies in their response to, and processing of, fearful stimuli (e.g., pictures of mutilated bodies and physical assaults; Levenston, Patrick, Bradley, & Lang, 2000; Patrick et al., 1993). Consequently, it is plausible that characteristic low fear applies to a fear of pain and death, thus providing individuals with less anticipatory anxiety about inflicting harm on oneself, increasing the speed of habituation to pain, and increasing capability for suicide and a willingness to engage in self-injurious behavior for instrumental purposes (i.e., to manipulate others or gain access to some valued resource).

Brislin, Buchman-Schmitt, Joiner, and Patrick (2016) investigated pain tolerance in relation to distinct facets of psychopathy (as described by the triarchic model), and also associations between triarchic model constructs and measures of pain perception and experience. They found a unique positive relationship between pain tolerance and the Meanness facet, which also predicted reduced fear of painful algometer stimulation. Other psychopathy facets (Boldness, disinhibition) showed negative relations with fear of pain stimulation during testing and at follow-up. Relatedly, individuals high in psychopathic traits have been noted to exhibit faster rates of basic physiological habituation (as indexed by skin conductance and heart rate) after presentation of a noxious stimulus (e.g., a white noise burst or an electrical shock; Wang, Baker, Gao, Raine, & Lozano, 2012). This is noteworthy as quicker acting habituation to even minor diathesis-expressing life experiences (e.g., playing contact sports or nonlife-threatening accidental injury) may facilitate the habituation to fear and pain (Smith & Cukrowicz, 2010).

It is a reasonable hypothesis that individuals with high Factor 1 traits of psychopathy would not need to acquire capability for suicide over time but may have the capability from a young age by virtue of diminished fear. Alternatively, they may acquire capability more quickly than individuals who are low on Factor 1 traits. At this time, however, the literature on psychopathy and habituation to pain is mixed (see Miller et al., 2014), and the impact of specific patterns of psychopathic traits is unclear because many studies have not analyzed separate components of psychopathy in relation to pain habituation.

The full IPTS model

The evidence presented thus far provides support for the role of psychopathic traits in increasing ACS and thus suicide potential. That is, there is limited and indirect evidence that Factor 1 traits represent some level of innate capability for self-harm and, by extension, suicidal behavior. Factor 2 traits may reflect a high number of PPEs which result in ACS. As the IPTS is a relatively new theory, it has not yet been tested extensively in samples high in psychopathic traits. Only one study to date (Anestis et al., 2016) has specifically explored variables from the IPTS in relation to psychopathic traits.

Anestis and colleagues (2016) examined the relationship between psychopathic personality traits and the IPTS constructs in undergraduates and recently released male ex-prisoners. In study one, among undergraduate students and in line with expectations, they found that LPS Factor 1 exhibited a significant positive relationship to the ACS. Contrary to expectations, however, LPS Factor 2 was inversely associated with the ACS. Although unexpected, this finding in relation to Factor 2 may reflect the fact that some individuals may be more innately capable of suicide than others (Anestis et al., 2016). Indeed, emerging evidence suggests that genetics may contribute a sizable portion of an individual's capability for lethal self-harm (Smith et al., 2012). Moreover, recent research suggests that certain PPEs may be more important than others in determining suicide risk (Burke, Ammerman, Knorr, Alloy, & McCloskey, 2017; Smith et al., 2013). This is consistent with research demonstrating that differential combinations of experiences may result in varying negative outcomes (Dhingra et al., 2015).

Anestis et al. (2016) also found that LPS Factor 2 but not Factor 1 predicted both facets of suicidal desire (perceived burdensomeness and thwarted belongingness), when controlling for sex and depression symptoms. These findings are consistent with a model in which individuals high in LPS Factor 1 traits are very capable of suicide, but unlikely to desire death by suicide; whereas, individuals high in LPS Factor 2 traits are at elevated risk of desiring suicide and are also capable. Consistent with Study 1, LPS Factor 2 but not LPS Factor 1 significantly predicted proxy measures of perceived of suicidal desire (burdensomeness and thwarted belongingness) in male ex-prisoners. Additionally, LPS Factor 1 but not LPS Factor 2 exhibited a significant positive association with a component (physical aggression) of their proxy measure of the ACS. With the Psychopathy Personality Inventory–Revised (PPI–R; Lilienfeld & Widows, 2005), no factors exhibited statistically significant relationships with the ACS indicators. Taken together, these findings suggest that the desire for death by suicide and ACS in individuals high on psychopathy is likely dictated based on differential levels of the psychopathic traits.

Conclusion

When Cleckley (1941/1976) first described the concept of psychopathy, he noted that individuals with psychopathy enjoy a relative immunity to suicidality. The IPTS, a promising heuristic for clarifying complicated and potentially contradictory findings within the literature, has generated data that supports this notion. The development of active suicidal ideation as conceptualized through the IPTS requires a perception of oneself as a burden on others with no meaningful connections to others. The callousness, unemotional personality and manipulative interpersonal style inherent in individuals with high core (Factor 1) psychopathic traits may render them less likely to develop suicidal desire (thwarted belongingness and perceived burdensomeness) due to an indifference to enduring and meaningful relationships and/or inability to perceive problematic interpersonal interactions (with regard to suicidal actions, however, we note that this interpersonal indifference probably negates some common protective factors, such as concern for loved ones' suffering or children's well-being). In individuals with elevated Factor 2 but normative or low Factor 1, however, the combination of normative affect and interpersonal interactions and exposure to PPEs could lead to both enhanced suicidal desire and capability. We caution against considering high Factor 1 traits as protective; existing data do not bear this out. However, high Factor 1 traits may indicate that triggers for suicidal desire differ from those proposed by the IPTS. By way of example, rather than thwarted belonging or perceived burdensomeness, an individual high in core psychopathic traits may realize that his chances for "success" in an endeavor have suddenly been drastically reduced. He may seek the feeling of power associated with "going down in a hail of glory" or cheating law enforcement out of exacting justice.

We make three recommendations for future research on psychopathy and suicide. The first involves increasing clarity in our definition and assessment of suicide-related outcomes. In order to fully understand the precise associations between psychopathic personality traits and suicide-related outcomes, it is essential that studies clearly differentiate between non-suicidal self-injury, suicidal ideation, and suicidal behavior and between suicidal desire and suicide capability (Dhingra et al., 2015; Nock & Kessler, 2006). A related advance will be the incorporation of multiple measurement methods (e.g., self-report, observational, correctional, and medical file data) to enhance the specificity of data on suicidal behavior.

Our second recommendation involves the need for research examining the complexity and heterogeneity of suicidal behavior among those high in psychopathic traits. As noted by May and Klonsky (2013), although a desire to die is, by definition, a motivation underlying all suicide attempts, two superordinate dimensions of attempt motivations exist: internal (self-oriented) motivations (e.g., hopelessness, intense emotional pain, and a need to escape) and communication (other-oriented) motivations (e.g., a desire to influence, communicate with, punish, or seek help from others). As suggested by Dhingra et al. (2015), psychopaths' suicide attempts may reflect a greater willingness to engage in self-injurious behavior for instrumental purposes (i.e., to manipulate others or gain access to some valued resource). This is consistent with Porter and Woodworth's (2006) and Cleckley's (1941) suggestion that psychopathic individuals engage in a substantial amount of self-injurious behavior that is intended solely to manipulate others (which, according to Porter and Woodworth (2006), would be consistent with high affective factor scores).

Thirdly, we believe that the components of psychopathy should be examined in relation to suicidal behavior with as much nuance as possible using factor models (e.g., the four-facet model) of psychopathy that enable fine-grained analyses. Existing data indicate the possibility for interactions among components of psychopathy in relation to suicide.

References

Anestis, J. C., Harrop, T. M., Green, B. A., and Anestis, M. D. (2017) 'Psychopathic personality traits as protective factors against the development of post-traumatic stress disorder symptoms in a sample of National Guard Combat Veterans,' *Journal of Psychopathology and Behavioral Assessment, 39*(2):220–229.

Anestis, J. C., Anestis, M. D., Rufino, K. A., Cramer, R. J., Miller, H., Khazem, L. R., and Joiner, T. E. (2016) 'Understanding the relationship between suicidality and psychopathy: An examination of the interpersonal–psychological theory of suicidal behavior,' *Archives of Suicide Research, 20*(3):349–368.

Anestis, M. D., Bagge, C. L., Tull, M. T., and Joiner, T. E. (2011) 'Clarifying the role of emotion dysregulation in the interpersonal–psychological theory of suicidal behavior in an undergraduate sample,' *Journal of Psychiatric Research, 45*(5):603–611.

Baird, S. A. (2002) 'The links between primary and secondary psychopathy and social adaptation,' *Colgate University Journal of the Sciences, 34*:61–82.

Bare, R. L., Hopko, D. R., and Armento, M. E. (2004) 'The relation of psychopathic characteristics and anxiety in noncriminals: Physiological and cognitive responses to guided imagery,' *Journal of Psychopathology and Behavioral Assessment, 26*(4):225–232.

Baumeister, R. F., and Leary, M. R. (1995) 'The need to belong: Desire for interpersonal attachments as a fundamental human motivation,' *Psychological Bulletin, 117*(3):497.

Beaver, K. M., da Silva Costa, C., Poersch, A. P., Freddi, M. C., Stelmach, M. C., Connolly, E. J., and Schwartz, J. A. (2014) 'Psychopathic personality traits and their influence on parenting quality: Results from a nationally representative sample of Americans,' *Psychiatric Quarterly, 85*(4):497–511.

Beck, A. T., Brown, G., and Steer, R. A. (1989) 'Prediction of eventual suicide in psychiatric inpatients by clinical ratings of hopelessness,' *Journal of Consulting and Clinical Psychology, 57*(2):309.

Bender, T. W., Gordon, K. H., Bresin, K., and Joiner, T. E. (2011) 'Impulsivity and suicidality: The mediating role of painful and provocative experiences,' *Journal of Affective Disorders, 129*(1):301–307.

Blonigen, D. M., Patrick, C. J., Douglas, K. S., Poythress, N. G., Skeem, J. L., Lilienfeld, S. O., Edens, J. F., and Krueger, R. F. (2010) 'Multimethod assessment of psychopathy in relation to factors of internalizing and externalizing from the Personality Assessment Inventory: The impact of method variance and suppressor effects,' *Psychological Assessment, 22*(1):96.

Borges, G., Walters, E. E., and Kessler, R. C. (2000) 'Associations of substance use, abuse, and dependence with subsequent suicidal behavior,' *American Journal of Epidemiology, 151*(8):781–789.

Bowlby, J. (1969) *Attachment and loss: Attachment* (Vth ed.), New York, NY: Basic Books.

Brislin, S. J., Buchman-Schmitt, J. M., Joiner, T. E., and Patrick, C. J. (2016) '"Do unto others"? Distinct psychopathy facets predict reduced perception and tolerance of pain,' *Personality Disorders: Theory, Research, and Treatment,* 7(3):240.

Bryan, C. J., and Cukrowicz, K. C. (2011) 'Associations between types of combat violence and the acquired capability for suicide,' *Suicide and Life-Threatening Behavior, 41*(2):126–136.

Bryan, C. J., Cukrowicz, K. C., West, C. L., and Morrow, C. E. (2010) 'Combat experience and the acquired capability for suicide,' *Journal of Clinical Psychology, 66*(10):1044–1056.

Bryan, C. J., Morrow, C. E., Anestis, M. D., and Joiner, T. E. (2010) 'A preliminary test of the interpersonal–psychological theory of suicidal behavior in a military sample,' *Personality and Individual Differences, 48*(3):347–350.

Burke, T. A., Ammerman, B. A., Knorr, A. C., Alloy, L. B., and McCloskey, M. S. (2017) 'Measuring acquired capability for suicide within an ideation-to-action framework,' *Psychology of Violence*, Advance online publication, doi:10.1037/vio0000090

Caretti, V., and Craparo, G. (2010) 'La personalità psicopatica,' *Sistemi Intelligenti, 2*:229–254.

Cleckley, H. (1976) *The mask of sanity: An attempt to clarify some issues about the so-called psychopathic personality*, St. Louis, MO: Mosby Inc. (Original work published 1941)

Crosby, A., Gfroerer, J., Han, B., Ortega, L., and Parks, S. E. (2011) 'Suicidal thoughts and behaviors among adults aged ≥ 18 Years – United States, 2008–2009. U.S. Department of Health and Human Services, Centers for Disease Control and Prevention,' *MMWR Surveillance Summaries, 60*(SS13):1–22.

DeLisi, M. (2009) 'Psychopathy is the unified theory of crime,' *Youth Violence and Juvenile Justice*, 7(3):256–273.

DeLisi, M. (2016) *Psychopathy as unified theory of crime*, New York, NY: Palgrave Macmillan U.S.

Dhingra, K., and Boduszek, D. (2013) 'Psychopathy and criminal behaviour: A psychosocial research perspective,' *Journal of Criminal Psychology*, *3*(2):83–107.

Dhingra, K., Boduszek, D., and Kola-Palmer, S. (2015) 'A latent class analysis of psychopathic traits in civil psychiatric patients: The role of criminal behaviour, violence, and gender,' *The Howard Journal of Crime and Justice*, *54*(3):237–249.

Douglas, K. S., Herbozo, S., Poythress, N. G., Belfrage, H., and Edens, J. F. (2006) 'Psychopathy and suicide: A multisample investigation,' *Psychological Services*, *3*(2):97–116.

Douglas, K. S., Lilienfeld, S. O., Skeem, J. L., Poythress, N. G., Edens, J. F., and Patrick, C. J. (2008) 'Relation of antisocial and psychopathic traits to suicide-related behavior among offenders,' *Law and Human Behavior*, *32*(6):511–525.

Foulkes, L., Seara-Cardoso, A., Neumann, C. S., Rogers, J. S., and Viding, E. (2014) 'Looking after number one: Associations between psychopathic traits and measures of social motivation and functioning in a community sample of males,' *Journal of Psychopathology and Behavioral Assessment*, *36*(1):22–29.

Franklin, J. C., Hessel, E. T., and Prinstein, M. J. (2011) 'Clarifying the role of pain tolerance in suicidal capability,' *Psychiatry Research*, *189*(3):362–367.

Franklin, J. C., Ribeiro, J. D., Fox, K. R., Bentley, K. H., Kleiman, E. M., Huang, X., . . ., and Nock, M. K. (2016) 'Risk factors for suicidal thoughts and behaviors: A meta-analysis of 50 years of research,' doi:10.1037/bul0000084

Guy, L. S., and Douglas, K. S. (2006) 'Examining the utility of the PCL: SV as a screening measure using competing factor models of psychopathy,' *Psychological Assessment*, *18*(2):225.

Hadland, S. E., Marshall, B. D., Kerr, T., Qi, J., Montaner, J. S., and Wood, E. (2012) 'Suicide and history of childhood trauma among street youth,' *Journal of Affective Disorders*, *136*(3):377–380.

Hagan, C. R., Podlogar, M. C., Chu, C., and Joiner, T. E. (2015) 'Testing the interpersonal theory of suicide: The moderating role of hopelessness,' *International Journal of Cognitive Therapy*, *8*(2):99–113.

Hamilton, R. K., Hiatt Racer, K., and Newman, J. P. (2015) 'Impaired integration in psychopathy: A unified theory of psychopathic dysfunction,' *Psychological Review*, *122*(4):770–791.

Hare, R. D. (2003) *The Psychopathy Checklist–Revised*, Toronto, ON: Multi-Health Systems.

Hare, R. D., and Neumann, C. S. (2009) 'Psychopathy: Assessment and forensic implications,' *The Canadian Journal of Psychiatry*, *54*(12):791–802.

Hicks, B. M., and Patrick, C. J. (2006) 'Psychopathy and negative emotionality: Analyses of suppressor effects reveal distinct relations with emotional distress, fearfulness, and anger–hostility,' *Journal of Abnormal Psychology*, *115*(2):276.

Joiner, T. (2007) *Why people die by suicide*, Cambridge, MA: Harvard University Press.

Joiner Jr, T. E., Van Orden, K. A., Witte, T. K., Selby, E. A., Ribeiro, J. D., Lewis, R., and Rudd, M. D. (2009) 'Main predictions of the interpersonal–psychological theory of suicidal behavior: Empirical tests in two samples of young adults,' *Journal of Abnormal Psychology*, *118*(3):634–646.

Jonason, P. K., Li, N. P., Webster, G. D., and Schmitt, D. P. (2009) 'The dark triad: Facilitating a short-term mating strategy in men,' *European Journal of Personality*, *23*(1):5–18.

Jonason, P. K., Luevano, V. X., and Adams, H. M. (2012) 'How the Dark Triad traits predict relationship choices,' *Personality and Individual Differences*, *53*(3):180–184.

Jordan, J. T., and Samuelson, K. W. (2016) 'Predicting suicide intent: The roles of experiencing or committing violent acts,' *Suicide and Life-threatening Behavior*, *46*(3):293–300.

Karpman, B. (1941) 'On the need of separating psychopathy into two distinct clinical types: The symptomatic and the idiopathic,' *Journal of Criminal Psychopathology*, *3*:112–137.

Kennealy, P. J., Hicks, B. M., and Patrick, C. J. (2007) 'Validity of factors of the Psychopathy Checklist–Revised in female prisoners: Discriminant relations with antisocial behavior, substance abuse, and personality,' *Assessment*, *14*(4):323–340.

Kirtley, O. J., O'Carroll, R. E., and O'Connor, R. C. (2016) 'Pain and self-harm: A systematic review,' *Journal of Affective Disorders*, *203*:347–363.

Klonsky, E. D., and May, A. M. (2015) 'The three-step theory (3ST): A new theory of suicide rooted in the "ideation-to-action" framework,' *International Journal of Cognitive Therapy*, *8*(2):114–129.

Klonsky, E. D., Saffer, B. Y., and Bryan, C. J. (2017) 'Ideation-to-action theories of suicide: A conceptual and empirical update,' *Current Opinion in Psychology*, doi:10.1016/j.copsyc.2017.07.020

Levenson, M. R., Kiehl, K. A., and Fitzpatrick, C. M. (1995) 'Assessing psychopathic attributes in a noninstitutionalized population,' *Journal of Personality and Social Psychology*, *68*(1):151–158.

Levenston, G. K., Patrick, C. J., Bradley, M. M., and Lang, P. J. (2000) 'The psychopath as observer: Emotion and attention in picture processing,' *Journal of Abnormal Psychology, 109*(3):373–385.
Lilienfeld, S. O., and Widows, M. R. (2005) *PPI–R: Psychopathic Personality Inventory–Revised*, Lutz, FL: Psychological Assessment Resources, Incorporated.
Lykken, D. T. (1996) *The antisocial personalities*, Hillsdale, NJ: Lawrence Erlbaum Associates Inc.
Ma, J., Batterham, P. J., Calear, A. L., and Han, J. (2016) 'A systematic review of the predictions of the Interpersonal–Psychological Theory of Suicidal Behavior,' *Clinical Psychology Review, 46*:34–45.
May, A. M., and Klonsky, E. D. (2013) 'Assessing motivations for suicide attempts: Development and psychometric properties of the inventory of motivations for suicide attempts,' *Suicide and Life-Threatening Behavior, 43*(5):532–546.
Miller, J. D., Rausher, S., Hyatt, C. S., Maples, J., and Zeichner, A. (2014) 'Examining the relations among pain tolerance, psychopathic traits, and violent and nonviolent antisocial behavior,' *Journal of Abnormal Psychology, 123*(1):205.
Muñoz, L. C., Kerr, M., and Besic, N. (2008) 'The peer relationships of youths with psychopathic personality traits: A matter of perspective,' *Criminal Justice and Behavior, 35*(2):212–227.
Nock, M. K., Borges, G., Bromet, E. J., Cha, C. B., Kessler, R. C., and Lee, S. (2008) 'Suicide and suicidal behavior,' *Epidemiologic Reviews, 30*(1):133–154.
Nock, M. K., and Kessler, R. C. (2006) 'Prevalence of and risk factors for suicide attempts versus suicide gestures: Analysis of the National Comorbidity Survey,' *Journal of Abnormal Psychology, 115*(3):616.
O'Connor, R. C. (2011) 'Towards an integrated motivational–volitional model of suicidal behaviour,' in R. C. O'Connor, S. Platt, and J. Gordon (Eds.), *International handbook of suicide prevention: Research, policy and practice* (pp. 181–198). Hoboken, NJ: John Wiley & Sons.
Öhman, A., and Mineka, S. (2001) 'Fears, phobias, and preparedness: Toward an evolved module of fear and fear learning,' *Psychological Review, 108*(3):483.
Patrick, C. J., Bradley, M. M., and Lang, P. J. (1993) 'Emotion in the criminal psychopath: Startle reflex modulation,' *Journal of Abnormal Psychology, 102*(1):82–92.
Pennington, C. R., Cramer, R. J., Miller, H. A., and Anastasi, J. S. (2015) 'Psychopathy, depression, and anxiety as predictors of suicidal ideation in offenders,' *Death Studies, 39*(5):288–295.
Porter, S., and Woodworth, M. (2006) 'Psychopathy and aggression,' *Handbook of Psychopathy*:481–494.
Porter, S. (1996) 'Without conscience or without active conscience? The etiology of psychopathy revisited,' *Aggression and Violent Behavior, 1*(2):179–189.
Poythress, N. G., Skeem, J. L., and Lilienfeld, S. O. (2006) 'Associations among early abuse, dissociation, and psychopathy in an offender sample,' *Journal of Abnormal Psychology, 115*(2):288–297.
Rajalin, M., Hirvikoski, T., and Jokinen, J. (2013) 'Family history of suicide and exposure to interpersonal violence in childhood predict suicide in male suicide attempters,' *Journal of Affective Disorders, 148*(1):92–97.
Ribeiro, J. D., Witte, T. K., Van Orden, K. A., Selby, E. A., Gordon, K. H., Bender, T. W., and Joiner Jr, T. E. (2014) 'Fearlessness about death: The psychometric properties and construct validity of the revision to the Acquired Capability for Suicide Scale,' *Psychological Assessment, 26*(1):115.
Rudd, M. D. (2006) 'Fluid vulnerability theory: A cognitive approach to understanding the process of acute and chronic suicide risk,' in T. E. Ellis (Ed.), *Cognition and suicide: Theory, research, and therapy* (pp. 355–368), Washington, DC, U.S.: American Psychological Association.
Sandvik, A. M., Hansen, A. L., Hystad, S. W., Johnsen, B. H., and Bartone, P. T. (2015) 'Psychopathy, anxiety, and resiliency – Psychological hardiness as a mediator of the psychopathy–anxiety relationship in a prison setting,' *Personality and Individual Differences, 72*:30–34.
Sellbom, M., Cooke, D. J., and Hart, S. D. (2015) 'Construct validity of the Comprehensive Assessment of Psychopathic Personality (CAPP) concept map: Getting closer to the core of psychopathy,' *International Journal of Forensic Mental Health, 14*(3):172–180.
Smith, P. N., and Cukrowicz, K. C. (2010) 'Capable of suicide: A functional model of the acquired capability component of the interpersonal-psychological theory of suicide,' *Suicide and Life-Threatening Behavior, 40*(3):266–274.
Smith, P. N., Cukrowicz, K. C., Poindexter, E. K., Hobson, V., and Cohen, L. M. (2010) 'The acquired capability for suicide: A comparison of suicide attempters, suicide ideators, and non-suicidal controls,' *Depression and Anxiety, 27*(9):871–877.
Smith, A. R., Ribeiro, J. D., Mikolajewski, A., Taylor, J., Joiner, T. E., and Iacono, W. G. (2012) 'An examination of environmental and genetic contributions to the determinants of suicidal behavior among male twins,' *Psychiatry Research, 197*(1):60–65.

Smith, P. N., Selwyn, C., D'Amato, D., Granato, S., Kuhlman, S., and Mandracchia, J. T. (2016) 'Life experiences and the acquired capability for suicide in incarcerated men,' *Death Studies*, *40*(7):432–439.

Smith, P. N., Selwyn, C. N., Wolford-Clevenger, C., and Mandracchia, J. T. (2014) 'Psychopathic personality traits, suicide ideation, and suicide attempts in male prison inmates,' *Criminal Justice and Behavior*, *41*(3):364–379.

Smith, A. R., Witte, T. K., Teale, N. E., King, S. L., Bender, T. W., and Joiner, T. E. (2008) 'Revisiting impulsivity in suicide: Implications for civil liability of third parties,' *Behavioral Sciences & the Law*, *26*(6):779–797.

Smith, P. N., Wolford-Clevenger, C., Mandracchia, J. T., and Jahn, D. R. (2013) 'An exploratory factor analysis of the Acquired Capability for Suicide Scale in male prison inmates,' *Psychological Services*, *10*(1):97–105.

Solomon, R. L. (1980) 'The opponent-process theory of acquired motivation: The costs of pleasure and the benefits of pain,' *American Psychologist*, *35*(8):691.

Stein, D. J., Chiu, W. T., Hwang, I., Kessler, R. C., Sampson, N., Alonso, J., . . ., and Florescu, S. (2010) 'Cross-national analysis of the associations between traumatic events and suicidal behavior: Findings from the WHO World Mental Health Surveys,' *PLoS One*, *5*(5):e10574.

Sutton, S. K., Vitale, J. E., and Newman, J. P. (2002) 'Emotion among women with psychopathy during picture perception,' *Journal of Abnormal Psychology*, *111*(4):610–619.

Swogger, M. T., Conner, K. R., Meldrum, S. C., and Caine, E. D. (2009) 'Dimensions of psychopathy in relation to suicidal and self-injurious behavior,' *Journal of Personality Disorders*, *23*(2):201–210.

Swogger, M. T., and Kosson, D. S. (2007) 'Identifying subtypes of criminal psychopaths: A replication and extension,' *Criminal Justice and Behavior*, *34*:953–970.

Swogger, M. T., Van Orden, K. A., and Conner, K. R. (2014) 'The relationship of outwardly directed aggression to suicidal ideation and suicide attempts across two high-risk samples,' *Psychology of Violence*, *4*(2):184.

Swogger, M. T., You, S., Cashman-Brown, S., and Conner, K. R. (2011) 'Childhood physical abuse, aggression, and suicide attempts among criminal offenders,' *Psychiatry Research*, *185*:363–367.

Teismann, T., Förtsch, E. M. A., Baumgart, P., Het, S., and Michalak, J. (2014) 'Influence of violent video gaming on determinants of the acquired capability for suicide,' *Psychiatry Research*, *215*(1):217–222.

Van Orden, K. A., Cukrowicz, K. C., Witte, T. K., and Joiner Jr, T. E. (2012) 'Thwarted belongingness and perceived burdensomeness: Construct validity and psychometric properties of the Interpersonal Needs Questionnaire,' *Psychological Assessment*, *24*(1):197–215.

Van Orden, K. A., Witte, T. K., Cukrowicz, K. C., Braithwaite, S. R., Selby, E A., and Joiner Jr, T. E. (2010) 'The interpersonal theory of suicide,' *Psychological Review*, *117*(2):575–600.

Van Orden, K. A., Witte, T. K., Gordon, K. H., Bender, T. W., and Joiner Jr, T. E. (2008) 'Suicidal desire and the capability for suicide: Tests of the interpersonal–psychological theory of suicidal behavior among adults,' *Journal of Consulting and Clinical Psychology*, *76*(1):72–83.

Vassileva, J., Kosson, D. S., Abramowitz, C., and Conrod, P. (2005) 'Psychopathy versus psychopathies in classifying criminal offenders,' *Legal and Criminological Psychology*, *10*(1):27–43.

Verona, E., Hicks, B. M., and Patrick, C. J. (2005) 'Psychopathy and suicidality in female offenders: Mediating influences of personality and abuse,' *Journal of Consulting and Clinical Psychology*, *73*(6):1065–1073.

Verona, E., Patrick, C. J., and Joiner, T. E. (2001) 'Psychopathy, antisocial personality, and suicide risk,' *Journal of Abnormal Psychology*, *110*(3):462–470.

Wang, P., Baker, L. A., Gao, Y., Raine, A., and Lozano, D. I. (2012) 'Psychopathic traits and physiological responses to aversive stimuli in children aged 9–11 years,' *Journal of Abnormal Child Psychology*, *40*(5):759–769.

Willemsen, J., De Ganck, J., and Verhaeghe, P. (2012) 'Psychopathy, traumatic exposure, and lifetime post-traumatic stress,' *International Journal of Offender Therapy and Comparative Criminology*, *56*(4):505–524.

Willemsen, J., and Verhaeghe, P. (2012) 'Psychopathy and internalizing psychopathology,' *International Journal of Law and Psychiatry*, *35*(4):269–275.

Williams, K. M., McAndrew, A., Learn, T., Harms, P., and Paulhus, D. L. (2001, August) The Dark Triad returns: Entertainment preferences and antisocial behavior among narcissists, Machiavellians, and psychopaths. Poster presented at the 109th Annual Convention of the American Psychological Association, San Francisco, CA.

Witte, T. K., Gordon, K. H., Smith, P. N., and Van Orden, K. A. (2012) 'Stoicism and sensation seeking: Male vulnerabilities for the acquired capability for suicide,' *Journal of Research in Personality*, *46*(4):384–392.

Wolford-Clevenger, C., Febres, J., Zapor, H., Elmquist, J., Bliton, C., and Stuart, G. L. (2015) 'Interpersonal violence, alcohol use, and acquired capability for suicide,' *Death Studies*, *39*(4):234–241.

Woodfield, R., Woodfield, R., Dhingra, K., Dhingra, K., Boduszek, D., Boduszek, D., Debowska, A., and Debowska, A. (2016) 'Facets of psychopathy in relation to trauma-exposure and posttraumatic stress symptomology in a sample of incarcerated male offenders,' *International Journal of Prisoner Health*, *12*(4):244–252.

World Health Organisation (WHO). (2014) *Preventing suicide; a global imperative.* Retrieved April 26, 2018 from www.who.int/mental_health/suicide-prevention/world_report_2014/en/

36

Psychopathic traits and conduct problems predicting bullying and victimization

Testing unique and interactive associations

Kostas A. Fanti

Introduction

Bullying is a major problem facing school-aged children across the world. Estimates suggest that up to one-half of school-aged children report having been a victim of bullying (Fanti & Kimonis, 2013; McGuckin, Cummins, & Lewis, 2008; Wang, Iannotti, & Nansel, 2009). Bullying has been defined as repeated physical, verbal, or psychological attack or intimidation that is intended to cause fear, distress, or harm to the victim and is characterized by an imbalance of power (Olweus, 1993; Rigby, 2002). Bullying is not only harmful to the victim, but also to the bully; when compared with their non-involved peers, bullies are at significantly greater risk for later psychopathology, substance abuse, delinquent and criminal behavior, and relationship problems (Hourbe, Targuinio, Thuillier, & Hergott, 2006; Kumpulainen et al., 1998; Pepler et al., 2006; Sigfusdottir, Gudjonsson, & Sigurdsson, 2010). Across development, boys are more likely than girls to bully (Archer, 2004; McDermott, 1996).

Youth who engage in bullying behaviors may also be victims of bullying ("bully–victims"; Haynie et al., 2001). Bully–victims are at increased risk for mental health problems – particularly internalizing problems (anxiety, depression), loneliness and self-esteem problems, suicidal ideation and attempts, and continued bullying into adulthood by workplace peers (Hawker & Boulton, 2000; Kaltiala-Heino, Rimpela, Marttunen, Rimpela, & Rantanen, 1999; Reijntjes, Kamphuis, Prinzie, & Telch, 2010; Salmon, James, & Smith, 1998). In a large meta-analytic study, Cook, Williams, Guerra, Kim, and Sadek (2010) found that victim-only and bully–victim status was associated with peer rejection/isolation, social incompetence, and internalizing problems, whereas "bully–victims" were additionally characterized by externalizing problems, negative peer influence, negative self-related cognitions, and poor academic achievement (Cook et al., 2010). Research suggests that girls may be at equal risk to boys for peer victimization (Schwartz, Proctor, Chien, Juvonen, & Graham, 2001; Seals & Young, 2003; Solberg, Olweus, & Endresen, 2007).

Bullying comprises one of the diagnostic criteria for Conduct Disorder (CD; American Psychiatric Association, 2013). It is well-established that children who bully are more likely to show conduct problems (CPs) and other externalizing problems (Andreou, 2001; Cook et al., 2010;

Kumpulainen, Rasanen, & Puura, 2001; Salmon, James, Cassidy, & Javaloyes, 2000). Applying the rich body of literature on CD to bullying can improve our understanding of this pervasive problem. For example, callous–unemotional (CU; lack of empathy, guilt) traits are important for distinguishing youth with CPs who are at greatest risk for adverse outcomes. Among youth with CPs, those high on CU traits consistently show a more severe, aggressive, and stable pattern of behavioral problems (Frick & Dickens, 2006). For example, they have been found to show a greater number and variety of CPs, greater proactive (i.e., instrumental, goal-oriented) aggression, more police contacts, and stronger family histories of Antisocial Personality Disorder than their non-CU counterparts (Christian, Frick, Hill, Tyler, & Frazer, 1997; Kruh, Frick, & Clements, 2005; Raine et al., 2006). Boys also tend to score higher on CU traits than girls (Essau, Sasagawa, & Frick, 2006).

CU traits are relatively stable across development and are theorized to be a childhood precursor to adult psychopathy (Blonigen, Hicks, Krueger, Patrick, & Iacono, 2006; Frick, Kimonis, Dandreaux, & Farell, 2003; Loney, Taylor, Butler, & Iacono, 2007; Obradovic, Pardini, Long, & Loeber, 2007). In the *Diagnostic and Statistical Manual–5* (APA, 2013), CU traits are included as a specifier to the diagnosis of CD defined as with "Limited Prosocial Emotions" that can be used in combination with existing age at onset and severity specifiers (Frick & Moffitt, 2010; Moffitt et al., 2008). If a child meets full diagnostic criteria for CD, this specifier would be applied if two or more of the following four characteristics are present over at least 12 months and in more than one relationship or setting: lack of remorse or guilt; lack of concern for others' feelings; lack of concern over poor performance at school, work, or in other important activities; and shallow or deficient emotions. Importantly, youth with CU traits not only report low levels of empathy but are also less responsive than other children to cues of distress in others, a pattern that is theorized to stem from a fearless temperament that interferes with moral socialization in early development (Blair, 1999; Fanti, 2016).

Additional research suggests that CU traits in combination with CPs may also be important for understanding bullying (e.g., Fanti, Frick, & Georgiou, 2009; Viding, Simmonds, Petrides, & Frederickson, 2009). For example, Viding and colleagues (2009) found that self-reported CU traits contributed to the statistical prediction of peer-reported bullying, over and above the variance accounted for by conduct problems, among a school-aged (11–13-year-olds) sample of 704 children. They also found a significant interaction effect, such that rates of bullying increased in youth with CPs as the level of CU traits increased. In another study, Fanti and colleagues found that CU traits were associated with bullying but not victimization in a school-aged (12- to 18-year-olds; $M = 14.63$) sample of 347 Greek–Cypriots (Fanti et al., 2009). Using a person-centered analytic strategy, they found that children exhibiting bullying behavior, irrespective of their victimization status, were more likely to be characterized by high callous–unemotional traits. Fanti and colleagues replicated these findings in three additional studies (Fanti, 2013; Fanti, & Kimonis, 2012, 2013).

CU traits constitute the affective dimension of psychopathy; narcissism and impulsivity comprise the other two dimensions of psychopathy, each of which has been linked with aggressive behavior in youth (Barry, Frick, & Killian, 2003; Frick & Hare, 2001). Narcissism has been specifically linked with both proactive and reactive (i.e., retaliatory) forms of aggression (Bukowski, Schwartzman, Santo, Bagwell, & Adams, 2009; Fossati, Borroni, Eisenberg, & Maffei, 2010; Washburn, McMahon, King, Reinecke, & Silver, 2004), whereas impulsivity has been linked with reactive aggression specifically (Barry et al., 2007). Some argue that bullying is a form of proactive aggression in that it involves intentional acts designed to achieve social gain and dominance over peers through intimidation (Carney & Merrell, 2001; Griffin & Gross, 2004; Salmivalli, Lagerspetz, Bjorkqvist, Osterman, & Kaukiainen, 1996). However, bullies tend to exhibit both types of aggression, using proactive aggression to dominate others and reactive aggression when being attacked by others (Camodeca, Goossens, Meerum Terwogt, & Schuengel, 2002; Pellegrini, Bartini, & Brooks, 1999; Salmivalli & Nieminen, 2002), although victims of bulling tend to only exhibit reactive aggression (Camodeca et al., 2002).

Together, these findings suggest that bullying may be related to both impulsivity and narcissism, while victimization only to impulsivity. Indeed, impulsivity was associated with both bullying and victimization (Fanti & Kimonis, 2012). Further, victims, bullies, and bully–victims have been found to be at greater risk for displaying impulsive behavior compared with non-bullying youth (Bjorkqvist, Ekman, & Lagerspetz, 1982; Fanti & Kimonis, 2013; Holland, Ireland, & Muncer, 2009; O'Brennan, Bradshaw, & Sawyer, 2009; Olweus, 1995; Schwartz et al., 2001). The contribution of narcissism to bullying has received less attention in the literature, with existing work associating narcissism with bullying but not victimization (Fanti & Henrich, 2015; Fanti & Kimonis, 2012, 2013). In contrast to impulsivity, but similar to CU traits, narcissism was found to be associated with bully and bully–victim groups, but not with victim-only status (Fanti & Henrich, 2015; Fanti & Kimonis, 2013).

Current study

There is preliminary indication that CPs, impulsivity, narcissism, and CU traits are independently related to bullying behavior. However, the novelty of this research area leaves several important gaps in the literature that the present study seeks to fill, such as how distinct psychopathic traits and CPs interact with one another to predict bullying and peer victimization. For example, Olweus (1995) suggests that bullies are characterized by marked impulsivity combined with a strong need to dominate others. An important strength of this study is its use of a longitudinal design to predict future bullying and peer victimization, controlling for initial levels. The primary aim of the current study is to test whether CPs and psychopathic traits (callous–unemotional traits, narcissism, and impulsivity) uniquely or interactively predict bullying and victimization one year later. This is tested using both variable-centered and person-centered approaches. First, correlational analyses were run to test the concurrent associations between CPs and psychopathic traits with bullying and victimization. Second, hierarchical linear regression analysis is used to test whether conduct problems and psychopathic traits (callous–unemotional traits, narcissism, and impulsivity), measured at Year 1, uniquely predict bullying and victimization measured at Year 2. Interactions between conduct problems and psychopathic traits (callous–unemotional traits, narcissism, and impulsivity) are also tested as predictors of bullying and victimization one year later. Next, we took a person-centered approach to analyses by testing how CPs and psychopathic traits are associated with bully–victim groups using multinomial logistic regression analysis. It is predicted that CPs and the three psychopathy dimensions will each account for unique variance in bullying, and that impulsivity will uniquely predict victimization. Based on our review of the literature, it is also hypothesized that the following combinations will predict greater bullying: high CPs and CU traits, high narcissism and impulsivity, or high CU traits, impulsivity and, narcissism.

Method

Participants

The sample consisted of 2,416 (50.1 percent girls) Greek Cypriot adolescents (aged 11–14 years at the first assessment; Mage = 13), recruited from 20 middle schools in three different cities in Cyprus (Larnaca, Limassol, and Nicosia). Prior to the first assessment, parental consent was obtained from 2,600 students, and these students completed the questionnaire administered during Year 1. At the second assessment 1 year later, 92.9 percent (n = 2,416) of the original students participated. Attrition was due to an inability to contact students who had moved away or transferred to a different school. To test for selective attrition of students who dropped out after the first assessment, these students were compared to those who remained in the study on all Year 1 variables under investigation in order to identify possible sources of bias in the sample. According to the t-tests of attrition, there were no differences between participants who dropped out and those who remained in the study in terms of Year 1 bullying behavior, $t(2599) = .182, p = .86$; victimization, $t(2599) = .703, p = .48$; conduct problems, $t(2599) = .929$, $p = .86$; impulsivity, $t(2599) = 1.128, p = .26$; narcissism, $t(2599) = .352, p = .73$; and callous–unemotional traits, $t(2599) = 1.405, p = .16$. The sample was diverse in terms of maternal and paternal educational levels (18 percent did not complete high school, 45 percent had a high school education, and 37 percent had a university degree). Additionally, 8 percent of the participants came from single parent families. These categorizations approximate national demographics in Cyprus (www.pio.gov.cy).

Procedure

Initially, an application for approval to conduct the study was submitted to the Cyprus Ministry of Education. After approval of the study by the ministry, the researcher randomly selected 20 schools in three Cypriot towns (Larnaca, Limassol, and Nicosia). The school administrators and personnel were provided with a description of the study, and the study was approved by the school principals and the school boards of all 20 schools. Students were then given an informed consent form for their parents to sign, and only those who returned parental consent forms were allowed to participate in the study. Furthermore, students were informed about the study, and those who agreed to participate signed an assent form (the refusal rate was 6 percent). In the classroom, students were informed by the researchers that the study aimed to understand adolescent emotions and behaviors. Students were also informed that no teachers or parents would have access to their answers. Questionnaires were group administered by trained research assistants in classrooms of 20–25 students. The research team and the principal investigator were available to answer any potential questions. On average, students completed the questionnaires in less than 45 minutes. The following set of measures were administered at Year 1, with the exception of the bullying and victimization measure, which was administered at both Year 1 and Year 2 assessments. The Cronbach's alpha for all measures is reported in Table 36.1.

Measures

Callous–unemotional traits

The Inventory of Callous Unemotional Traits (ICU; Frick, 2004) is a 24-item self-report scale designed to assess callous and unemotional traits in youth. The ICU was derived from the 6-item callous–unemotional (CU) subscale of the Antisocial Process Screening Device (APSD; Frick & Hare, 2001). The CU component of the APSD has emerged as a distinct factor in clinic and community samples of pre-adolescent boys and girls (Fanti, 2013; Frick, Bodin, & Barry, 2000). It has been associated with more severe aggression and more proactive patterns of aggression and violence in detained male adolescents (Kruh et al., 2005). However, the self-reported

Table 36.1 Descriptive statistics for and correlations among the main study variables (N = 2416)

	CPs Year 1	*CU traits Year 1*	*Impulsivity Year 1*	*Narcissism Year 1*	*Bullying Year 1*	*Bullying Year 2*	*Victimization Year 1*	*Victimization Year 2*
CU traits (Yr 1)	.42**							
Impulsivity (Yr 1)	.50**	.33**						
Narcissism (Yr 1)	.46**	.31**	.60**					
Bullying (Yr 1)	.52**	.36**	.46**	.51**				
Victimization (Yr 1)	.29**	.15**	.33**	.31**	.49**			
Bullying (Yr 2)	.32**	.24**	.33**	.30**	.36**	.23**		
Victimization (Yr 2)	.18**	.12**	.24**	.20**	.28**	.49**	.51**	
Descriptives								
Alpha	.83	.80	.73	.70	.89	.92	.90	.92
Mean (*SD*)	3.97 (4.06)	20.34 (8.74)	5.09 (3.05)	5.53 (3.61)	5.23 (7.17)	5.57 (7.20)	8.83 (9.23)	7.21 (9.16)
Range	0–28	0–66	0–15	0–21	0–48	0–48	0–48	0–48

Note. **$p < .01$; *$p < .05$. CPs = conduct problems; CU = callous–unemotional.

CU scale has demonstrated only moderate internal consistency in many past studies, which is likely due to its small number of items ($n = 6$) and 3-point rating system. Also, five out of the six items are worded in the same direction, increasing the possibility of response bias. The ICU was developed to overcome these limitations and to provide a more extended assessment of CU traits. It was constructed using the four items (out of the original six) that loaded significantly on the CU scale of the APSD in both clinic-referred and community samples (Frick, 2004). For each item ("I am concerned about the feelings of others," "I feel bad or guilty when I do something wrong," "I care about how well I do at school or work," and "I do not show my emotions to others"), three positively and three negatively worded variations were developed (including the original item in its exact wording), and these 24 items were placed on a 4-point scale (0 = not at all true, 1 = somewhat true, 2 = very true, and 3 = definitely true). Scores are calculated by reverse-scoring the positively worded items and then summing the items to obtain a total score. Previous research has provided evidence for the validity of the self-reported ICU in community samples of adolescents (Essau et al., 2006; Fanti, 2013; Fanti, Frick, & Georgiou, 2009).

Narcissism and impulsivity

The Antisocial Process Screening Device–Youth report (APSD; Frick & Hare, 2001) was used to measure narcissism and impulsivity. The APSD is a well-validated measure that assesses children's behaviors on dimensions associated with psychopathy. Although items on the original APSD measure are scored on a 3-point scale, for the current study items were placed on a 4-point scale (0 = not at all true, 1 = somewhat true, 2 = very true, and 3 = definitely true) to be consistent with the ICU measure. Factor analyses of the APSD indicate a three-factor model that includes a 5-item impulsivity subscale, a 7-item narcissism subscale, and a 6-item callous–unemotional subscale (not used in the current study). There is substantial support for the validity of the self-report version of the APSD, and for its ability to designate a group of antisocial youth with deficits in emotional functioning (Fanti & Kimonis, 2012, 2013; Kimonis et al., 2006; Kruh et al., 2005). Furthermore, self-report scores on the APSD are associated with conduct problems and bullying behavior (Fanti & Kimonis, 2012, 2013).

Conduct problems

The conduct problems variable consisted of scores from the Youth Self-Report (YSR; Achenbach, 1991; Roussos et al., 2001). Adolescents rated how well each of the items described them over the past six months on a 3-point scale (0 = not true, 1 = somewhat or sometimes true, 2 = very true or often true). For the present study, only the 15-item Conduct Disorder subscale (e.g., "I am mean to others," "I run away from home") was used. The YSR has been used widely with normal and clinically referred youths and has shown adequate reliability and validity in assessing a broad range of behavioral and emotional problems experienced by youths aged 11 to 18.

Bullying and victimization

The Student Survey of Bullying Behavior–Revised (SSBB–R; Varjas, Meyers, & Hunt, 2006) includes 12 items assessing three facets of bullying: physical (e.g., "How often do you pick on younger, smaller, less powerful, or less popular kids by hitting or kicking them?"); verbal (e.g., "How often do you pick on younger, smaller, less powerful, or less popular kids by calling them names?"); and relational (e.g., "How often do you pick on younger, smaller, less powerful, or less popular kids by spreading rumors about them?"). Participants indicated whether they had engaged in each type of bullying on an ordinal scale of: never, once or twice a year, monthly, weekly, or daily. Four items asked about each of the three types of bullying (physical, verbal, relational). The SSBB–R also includes 12 victimization items designed to mirror the bullying items. Victimization items include: physical (e.g., "How often do older, bigger, more popular, or more powerful kids pick on you by hitting or kicking you?"); verbal (e.g., "How often do older, bigger, more popular, or more powerful kids pick on you by calling you names?"); and relational (e.g., "How often do older, bigger, more popular, or more powerful kids pick on you by spreading rumors about you?) subscales. Participants indicated how often the types of victimization happened to them, using the same response scale as the bullying items. Previous research using the SSBB–R successfully identified victims, bullies, and bully–victim groups in samples of American and Greek Cypriot children and adolescents, showing that bullying was associated with measures of aggression, callous–unemotional traits, school safety, school climate, and coping (Fanti, Frick, & Georgiou, 2009; Varjas et al., 2006).

Statistical analyses

All analyses were conducted using the SPSS statistical software. The analyses were designed to (1) investigate how CPs and psychopathic traits (i.e., CU traits, narcissism, and impulsivity), were related to bullying and victimization using hierarchical linear regression, and (2) examine how CPs and the different psychopathic traits were related to groups of adolescents exhibiting low, pure, or a combination of bullying and victimization using multinomial logistic regression analysis. Multinomial logistic regression was used in addition to hierarchical linear regression in order to make person-centered interpretations.

Results

Descriptive statistics

Table 36.1 reports the descriptive statistics of the main study variables measured at Year 1 and Year 2. According to paired-sample *t*-tests, there was a significant mean-level decrease in victimization from Year 1 to Year 2, $t(2415) = 5.81$, $p < .001$, suggesting that there is a decrease in the average reports of victimization across time. There were no mean-level differences in bullying from Year 1 to Year 2, $t(2415) = 1.80$, $p = .07$. Table 36.1 also reports the correlations among the variables under investigation. CPs, CU traits, narcissism, and impulsivity were positively inter-correlated and positively related to Year 1 and Year 2 bullying and victimization. Additionally, bullying and victimization were positively inter-correlated across both time points.

Aim 1: do conduct problems and dimensions of psychopathy, and their various combinations, predict bullying and victimization one year later?

Variable-centered analyses

Table 36.2 shows the hierarchical linear regression analyses with bullying and victimization as the outcomes. In Step 1 of the model, demographic variables of gender (0 = boys, 1 = girls), age, and parental marital status (0 = one-parent families, 1 = two-parent families) were entered

Table 36.2 Regression analyses predicting Year 2 bullying and victimization ($N = 2416$)

	Year 2 bullying				*Year 2 victimization*			
	B	*SE B*	*β*	ΔR^2	*B*	*SE B*	*β*	ΔR^2
Step 1				.06**				.03**
Gender	−3.81	.45	−.29**		−2.41	.50	−.14**	
Age	−.15	.30	−.02		−.75	.33	−.07*	
Single parent family	−.74	.88	−.02		−2.83	.98	−.08**	
Step 2				.10**				.22**
Year 1 victimization	.04	.03	.04		.44	.03	.46**	
Year 1 bullying	.34	.04	.30**		.02	.04	.02	
Step 3				.05**				.01*
Conduct problems	.20	.07	.10**		.03	.07	.01	
Narcissism	.15	.08	.07*		−.02	.08	−.01	
CU traits	.05	.03	.05		.01	.03	.01	
Impulsivity	.31	.10	.12**		.25	.10	.08*	
Step 4				.01**				.01**
Narcissism × CU	−.01	.01	−.03		−.01	.01	−.05	
Narcissism × impulsivity	.05	.02	.08*		.04	.02	.06	
CU × impulsivity	.01	.01	.02		−.01	.01	−.01	
CP × CU	.01	.01	.01		.02	.01	.11**	
CP × narcissism	−.05	.02	−.13**		−.04	.02	−.09*	
CP × impulsivity	−.01	.02	−.02		.01	.02	.01	
Step 5				.02**				0
Nar. × Imp. × CU	.01	.01	.30**		.00	.00	−.01	
CP × CU × narcissism	−.01	.00	−.20*		.00	.00	−.04	
CP × CU × impulsivity	−.01	.01	−.10		.00	.00	−.01	
CP × Nar. × impulsivity	−.01	.01	−.12		.01	.01	.06	
Step 6				0				0
CP × Nar. × Imp. × CU	.00	.00	.03		.00	.00	−.17	

Note. **$p < .01$; *$p < .05$. Regression coefficients represent value at initial entry.

as covariates. In Step 2, we controlled for initial levels of bullying and victimization measured at Year 1. In Step 3, CPs and the three dimensions of psychopathy – CU traits, narcissism, and impulsivity – measured at Year 1 were entered into the model. Step 4 included the two-way interactions between the three dimensions of psychopathy and CPs. Step 5 included the three-way interactions between the variables, and Step 6 included their four-way interaction.

Bullying

Table 36.2 shows the results of the hierarchical linear regression analysis with Year 2 bullying as the dependent variable. Gender was significantly associated with bullying, suggesting that boys were at higher risk for exhibiting bullying behavior. Bullying – but not victimization – at Year 1 predicted bullying behavior a year later. CPs, narcissism, and impulsivity – but not CU traits – were each positively related to changes in bullying behavior above and beyond the demographic variables and the association between bullying and victimization. These effects should be interpreted cautiously because they were conditional on the interaction terms entered in subsequent steps. Significant interactions indicate that the effect of a predictor to the outcome depends on the value of the other independent variables. There were two significant interactions between narcissism and impulsivity and between narcissism and CPs, predicting Year 2 bullying behavior. However, these interactions were conditional on the two significant three-way interactions in predicting Year 2 bullying behavior: (1) between narcissism, CU traits, and impulsivity and (2) between narcissism, CU traits, and CPs. In that case, only the higher order interactions should be interpreted (Aiken & West, 1991). The four-way interaction was not significant. Thus, we only interpret the two significant three-way interactions. To plot the interaction effects, we used the procedures described by Aiken and West (1991) and Cohen and Cohen (1983). All variables were centered to facilitate ease of interpretation of the significant interaction terms, and the product interaction terms were computed from centered variables to reduce multicollinearity (Jaccard & Turrisi, 2003). The high and low points in the graphs represent one standard deviation above and below the mean.

The interaction between narcissism, CU traits, and impulsivity is depicted in Figure 36.1. It shows that there was an interaction between CU traits and narcissism at low ($\beta_{cu \times narc} = -.22$, $p = .001$) and high levels of impulsivity ($\beta_{cu \times narc} = .11$, $p < .05$). These findings suggest that at high and low levels of impulsivity the effect of CU traits was conditional upon the level of narcissism. When impulsivity was high and narcissism was low, CU traits in Year 1 were not significantly associated with bullying in Year 2 ($\beta = -.04$, $p = .59$). When impulsivity was high and narcissism was high, CU traits positively predicted bullying in year 2 ($\beta = .12$, $p = .01$). Furthermore, CU traits were associated with increases in bullying at low levels of impulsivity and narcissism ($\beta = .17$, $p < .01$) but decreases in bullying when impulsivity was low and narcissism was high ($\beta = -.17$, $p = .05$). The findings also suggest that when compared to the rest of the groups, adolescents characterized by high impulsivity, narcissism, and CU traits in combination were at greater risk for exhibiting bullying behavior one year later (see Figure 36.1).

The interaction between narcissism, CU traits, and CPs is depicted in Figure 36.2. It indicates that at low levels of conduct problems there was no significant interaction between CU traits and narcissism ($\beta_{cu \times narc} = .01$, $p = .97$). At high levels of conduct problems, the effect of CU traits was conditional upon the level of narcissism ($\beta_{cu \times narc} = -.12$, $p < .05$). When CPs were high and narcissism was low, CU traits in Year 1 predicted increases in bullying in year 2 ($\beta = .19$, $p < .01$). When CPs and narcissism were high, the effect of CU traits was not significant ($\beta = .01$, $p = .98$).

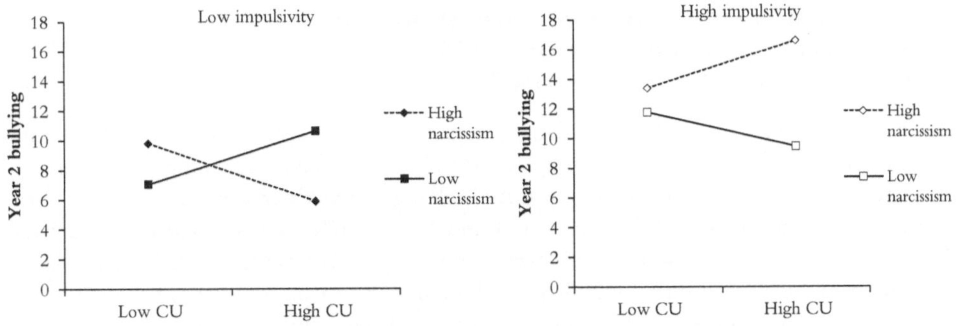

Figure 36.1 The interaction between CU traits and narcissism predicting Year 2 bullying when impulsivity is at high and low levels

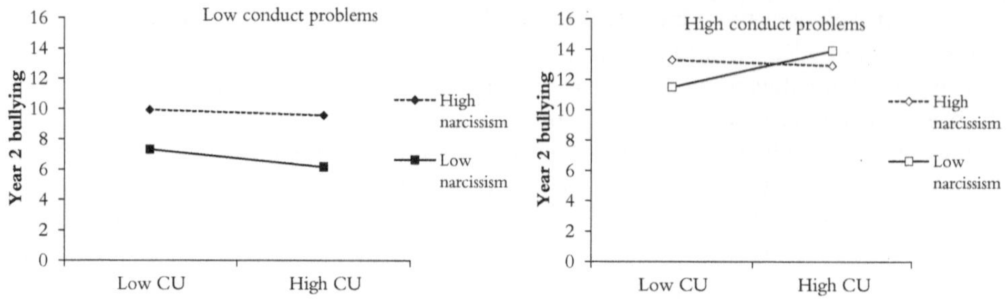

Figure 36.2 The interaction between CU traits and narcissism predicting Year 2 bullying when CPs are at high and low levels

Victimization

Table 36.3 shows the results of the hierarchical linear regression analysis predicting Year 2 victimization. Again, gender was a significant predictor, suggesting that boys were also at higher risk for being victimized. Furthermore, children from single parent families were more likely to be victimized by their peers. Age was negatively related to victimization, suggesting that victimization experiences decreased with age. Victimization – but not bullying – assessed at Year 1 predicted victimization one year later. Impulsivity was the only dimension of psychopathy that predicted changes in victimization above and beyond the demographic variables and the association between bullying and victimization. That is, impulsive children at Year 1 were more likely to become the victims of violence one year later. Results indicated two significant two-way interactions predicting Year 2 victimization: (1) between CU traits and CPs and (2) between narcissism and CPs. None of the three-way and four-way interactions were significant. The interaction between CU traits and CPs is depicted in Figure 36.3, which shows that CU traits were associated with increases in victimization for adolescents with high CPs ($\beta = .08, p < .05$). The effect of CU traits for adolescents scoring low on CPs was not significant ($\beta = -.06$, $p = .12$). Although the interaction between narcissism and CPs was significant, the effects of narcissism on victimization for adolescents scoring low ($\beta = .06, p = .21$) or high ($\beta = -.07$, $p = .11$) on CPs were not significant.

Aim 2: do conduct problems and dimensions of psychopathy differentiate between subgroups of adolescents exhibiting pure or combined forms of bullying and victimization?

Prior to conducting the multinomial logistic regressions, we classified youth into low, bully-only, victim-only, and bully–victim groups, using cut-off scores corresponding to one standard deviation (*SD*) above and below the mean for bullying and victimization, as done in previous research (e.g., Fanti et al., 2009). The Year 1 and Year 2 bullying scores and the Year 1 and Year 2 victimization scores were added together for the purposes of this analysis. Youth scoring one *SD* below the mean on both bullying and victimization were classified in the low group (77.3 percent; 882 boys, 985 girls). Youth scoring 1 *SD* above the mean on both bullying and victimization were classified in the bully–victim group (6.3 percent; 97 boys, 55 girls). Youth scoring 1 *SD* above the mean on bullying but 1 *SD* below the mean on victimization were

Table 36.3 Multinomial logistic regression analyses for bullying and victimization ($N = 2416$)

	Group comparisons based on odds ratios					
	4 vs 3	*4 vs 2*	*4 vs 1*	*3 vs 2*	*3 vs 1*	*2 vs 1*
Demographics:						
Gender	1.63	1.94	2.57**	1.19	1.57	1.32
Age	.98	1.27	.77	1.29	.78	.60**
Single parent family	1.52	.57	.99	.37	.65	1.74
Conduct problems	.96	1.10*	1.15**	1.12**	1.20**	1.08*
CU traits	1.01	1.08*	1.10*	1.10**	1.09*	.98
Narcissism	1.04	1.14**	1.16**	1.10*	1.12**	1.01
Impulsivity	1.07	1.05	1.19**	.98	1.12**	1.14**

Note. *$p \le .05$; **$p \le .01$; Group 1 is the low group; Group 2 is the victim-only group; Group 3 is the bullying-only group; Group 4 is the bully/victim group.

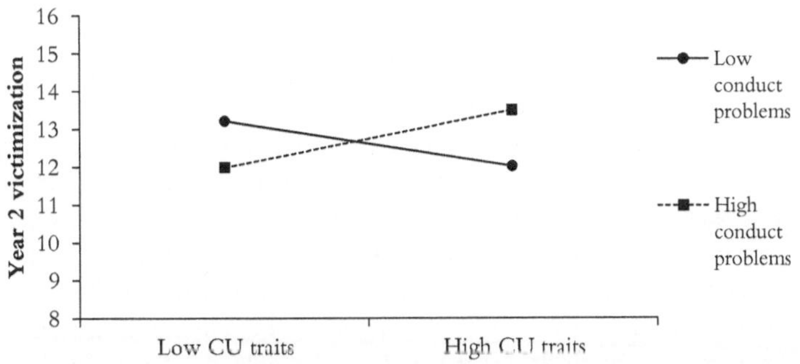

Figure 36.3 The interaction between CP and CU traits predicting Year 2 victimization

classified in the bully-only group (8.2 percent; 125 boys, 74 girls). Youth scoring 1 *SD* below the mean on bullying but 1 *SD* above the mean on victimization were classified in the victim-only group (8.2 percent; 101 boys, 97 girls).

Multinomial logistic regression was used to compare the groups on CPs and psychopathic traits, controlling for demographics. The multinomial logistic regression was significant, $x^2(21, N = 2416) = 328.62$, $p < .001$. Table 36.3 incorporates odds ratios to compare the different groups. In general, odds ratios reflect the odds likelihood of being in one group over the other, based on the level of the independent variable. Males were more likely to be in the bully–victim group than the low risk group. Children in the victim-only group were younger than children in the low risk group. Youth scoring higher on CPs, CU traits, and narcissism were more likely to be in the bully–victim group or the bully-only group than the low and victim-only groups. The victim-only group scored lower on CPs than the bully–victim and bully-only groups, but higher compared with the low risk group. All three high-risk groups were characterized by higher impulsivity compared with the low risk group. No differences were found between the bully–victim and bully-only groups on psychopathy dimensions or CPs. That is, children exhibiting bullying behavior – irrespective of their victimization status – were more likely to score high on CPs, CU traits, and narcissism compared with the victim-only and low risk groups.

Discussion

The current study contributes several novel findings to the literature investigating the development of bullying and victimization during adolescence. First, CPs and psychopathic traits were associated with bullying and victimization behaviors one year later; for bullying, this association is primarily driven by main effects of CPs, narcissism, and impulsivity, whereas for victimization this relationship is driven by impulsivity. Second, although there was no main effect for CU traits, high CU traits did predict bullying one year later when combined with high impulsivity and narcissism, and also when combined with high CPs. Third, when predicting victimization one year later, CU traits were positively related to victimization only at high levels of CPs. This finding suggests that the negative effect of CU traits on victimization is strengthened by the presence of CPs. Additionally, we find that bullies and bully–victims score higher on CU traits, CPs, and narcissism compared to victims and non-involved children. However, impulsivity was related to all high-risk groups in comparison to the normative group, including the victim-only group, based on the person-oriented analysis. Our findings provide evidence that psychopathic traits and conduct problems are related to the development and maintenance of bullying behavior and provide evidence in terms of how the three dimensions of psychopathy are related to victimization.

Prior research suggested that CU traits constitute an important predictor of bullying behavior and that CU traits characterize bullies and bully–victims, but not pure victims of bullying behavior (Fanti et al., 2009; Fanti & Kimonis, 2013). Our findings replicate prior work that bullies and bully–victims are more likely to be characterized by CU traits in a large sample of Greek Cypriot adolescents using longitudinal data. The current study also adds to prior work by providing evidence that in addition to the construct of CU traits, narcissism differentiates victims from pure bullies and bully–victims. Narcissistic personality features, such as a grandiose self-view, exploitation of others for personal gain, and concern for one's social status, are all characteristics that might motivate a child to commit acts of bullying (Salmivalli, 2001). Bullies characterized by narcissism might feel that they have the right to take another child's things or socially manipulate their peers regardless of the other student's feelings (Fanti & Henrich, 2015). Additionally, we find that children characterized by pure victimization are similar to bullies and bully–victims in terms of impulsivity, which suggests that impulsivity might be a general risk marker for both bullying and victimization. This finding also provides an example of multifinality, a term used in developmental psychopathology, in that a single predictor may result in diverse outcomes (Fanti, 2016). However, pure victims are less narcissistic in comparison to bullies and bully–victims and are more likely to show empathy towards others, as indicated by their low scores on CU traits.

The study's findings that the combination of CPs and CU traits results in a severe profile of bullying behavior also agrees with evidence provided by prior work (Fanti, 2013; Fanti & Kimonis, 2012; Viding et al., 2009). These findings indicate that subtyping children with CPs to those with high or low CU traits is important for identifying children at higher risk to exhibit antisocial behavior (Frick et al., 2014), and that high CPs and high CU traits in combination constitute a risk factor for bullying behavior during adolescence. In contrast, children with high CPs but low levels of CU traits exhibited low levels of bullying behaviors. In addition, our findings add to prior research by providing an indication that adolescents scoring high on CPs and CU traits might also be at high risk to experience victimization. Thus, we provide evidence that the combination of CPs and CU traits leads to greater maladjustment in terms of both bullying and victimization. These findings are consistent with an extensive body of literature showing poor outcomes for youth showing a combination of CPs and CU traits (Fanti, 2013; Fanti, 2016; Frick et al., 2014).

Additionally, the findings indicate that the three interrelated dimensions of psychopathy, impulsivity, narcissism, and CU traits, work together to influence the development of bullying behavior, suggesting an additive effect for psychopathic traits. In fact, adolescents characterized by all three dimensions of psychopathy were at higher risk to experience increases in bullying behavior a year later. No prior work investigated such interaction effects. Researchers have been using different approaches to designate aggressive youth, such as emphasizing an impulsive/antisocial dimension of behavior or by focusing on CU traits (Essau et al., 2006; Fanti, 2016). However, our findings suggest that all three dimensions of psychopathy need to be taken into account, at least in regard to bullying behavior. Thus, a child at high risk of bullying others is a child with a grandiose view of himself or herself who lacks empathy and guilt, cannot control his or her behavior, and acts aggressively out of impulses. It is possible that bullies are not able to control their behavior (impulsivity) because they need to maintain their positive self-image (narcissism), acting aggressively without showing empathy towards others (CU traits). Paradoxically, CU traits were related to decreases in bullying behavior when narcissism was high and impulsivity was low. This finding suggests that all three dimensions of psychopathy need to be present for the development of bullying behavior.

A number of demographics differences were also identified. Boys were more likely to bully and be victimized. In general, studies report that, compared to girls, more boys tend to engage in bullying behavior, although no gender differences in the prevalence rates of victimization have been reported (Fanti et al., 2009; Schwartz et al., 2001; Seals & Young, 2003; Solberg, Olweus, & Endresen, 2007). Thus, our findings that boys were at higher risk for victimization are inconsistent with prior work, although this might be the case for adolescents in Cyprus. Moreover, we found that younger children and children from a single parent home were more likely to be victimized. Pellegrini and Bartini (2000) also found that victimization declined across time, suggesting that as children enter adolescence they are at lower risk to be victimized. Furthermore, research suggests that children from low socioeconomic status (SES) are more likely to become victims of bullying (Wolke, Woods, Stanford, & Schulz, 2001), and our findings suggest that children from single parent families, which is an indicator of low SES, are more likely to be victimized.

Conclusion

The large sample of adolescents, which allowed for testing and interpreting interactions, and the short-term longitudinal design were strengths of this investigation. However, the one-year follow-up time might be considered to be a limitation, as additional time points of measurement would have allowed the investigation of trajectories of change over time. Moreover, data were based on adolescent self-report for all variables, and the correlations could have been inflated due to shared method variance. Additionally, it might be possible that bullies underestimated their bullying behavior (Fanti & Henrich, 2015). Nevertheless, self-report instruments administered to adolescents have the advantage that the individual's attitudes and emotions may not be apparent to other people (Essau et al., 2006). Additionally, the validity of self-report measures on psychopathology and personality increases with the child's age, although the validity of parent and teacher report measures decreases during the adolescence age period (Kamphaus & Frick, 1996).

In conclusion, our findings provide evidence for the importance of CU traits for the development of bullying behavior, but also suggest that all three dimensions of psychopathy and CPs need to be taken into account in order to understand bullying behavior. The predictive utility of the construct of psychopathy to different types of aggressive behavior has not been studied extensively in youth (Frick et al., 2014), although psychopathic traits might be the best candidate for understanding aggressive behaviors among youth (DeLisi, 2009). For example, there are only a few studies investigating how psychopathic traits are related to bullying behavior, and the current study's results support the need for further research in this area. Furthermore, impulsivity and the combination of CPs and CU traits can also be considered as possible risk factors for the development of victimization. Linking psychopathic traits to bullying behavior and victimization experiences may provide evidence towards the design of interventions aiming to reduce these behaviors.

References

Achenbach, T. M. (1991) *Integrative guide for the 1991 CBCL/4–18, YSR, and TRF profiles*, Department of Psychiatry, University of Vermont.

Aiken, L. S., and West, S. G. (1991) *Multiple regression: Testing and interpreting interactions*, Newbury Park, London: Sage.

Andreou, E. (2001) 'Bully/victim problems and their association with coping behaviour in conflictual peer interactions among school-age children,' *Educational Psychology*, *21*(1):59–66.

Archer, J. (2004) 'Sex differences in aggression in real-world settings: A meta-analytic review,' *Review of General Psychology*, *8*(4):291–322.

Barry, C. T., Frick, P. J., and Killian, A. L. (2003) 'The relation of narcissism and self-esteem to conduct problems in children: A preliminary investigation,' *Journal of Clinical Child & Adolescent Psychology*, *32*:139–152.

Barry, T. D., Thompson, A., Barry, C. T., Lochman, J. E., Adler, K., and Hill, K. (2007) 'The importance of narcissism in predicting proactive and reactive aggression in moderately to highly aggressive children,' *Aggressive Behavior*, *33*(3):185–197.

Bjorkqvist, K., Ekman, K., and Lagerspetz, K. M. (1982) 'Bullies and victims: Their ego picture, ideal ego picture and normative ego picture,' *Scandinavian Journal of Psychology*, *23*(4):307–313.

Blair, R. J. R. (1999) 'Responsiveness to distress cues in the child with psychopathic tendencies,' *Personality and Individual Differences*, *27*:135–145.

Blonigen, D. M., Hicks, B. M., Krueger, R. F., Patrick, C. J., and Iacono, W. G. (2006) 'Continuity and change in psychopathic traits as measured via normal-range personality: A longitudinal-biometric study,' *Journal of Abnormal Psychology*, *115*(1):85–95.

Bukowski, W. M., Schwartzman, A., Santo, J., Bagwell, C., and Adams, R. (2009) 'Reactivity and distortions in the self: Narcissism, types of aggression, and the functioning of the hypothalamic–pituitary–adrenal axis during early adolescence,' *Development and Psychopathology*, *21*(4):1249–1262.

Camodeca, M., Goossens, F. A., Meerum Terwogt, M., and Schuengel, C. (2002) 'Bullying and victimization among school-age children: Stability and links to proactive and reactive aggression,' *Social Development*, *11*:332–345.

Carney, A. G., and Merrell, K. W. (2001) 'Bullying in schools: Perspective on understanding and preventing an international problem,' *School Psychology International*, *22*(3):364–382.

Christian, R. E., Frick, P. J., Hill, N. L., Tyler, L., and Frazer, D. R. (1997) 'Psychopathy and conduct problems in children: II. Implications for subtyping children with conduct problems,' *Journal of the American Academy of Child and Adolescent Psychiatry*, *36*:233–241.

Cohen, J., and Cohen, P. (1983) *Applied multiple regression/correlation analyses for the behavioral sciences*, Hillsdale, NJ: Erlbaum.

Cook, C. R., Williams, K. R., Guerra, N. G., Kim, T. E., and Sadek, S. (2010) 'Predictors of bullying and victimization in childhood and adolescence: A meta-analytic investigation,' *School Psychology Quarterly*, *25*(2):65–83.

DeLisi, M. (2009) 'Psychopathy is the unified theory of crime,' *Youth Violence and Juvenile Justice*, 7(3):256–273

Essau, C. A., Sasagawa, S., and Frick, P. J. (2006) 'Callous–unemotional traits in community sample of adolescents,' *Assessment*, *13*:454–469.

Fanti, K. A. (2013) 'Individual, social, and behavioral factors associated with co-occurring conduct problems and callous–unemotional traits,' *Journal of Abnormal Child Psychology*, *41*:811–824.

Fanti, K. A. (2016) 'Understanding heterogeneity in conduct disorder: A review of psychophysiological studies,' *Neuroscience and Biobehavioral Reviews*, doi:10.1016/j.neubiorev.2016.09.022

Fanti, K. A., Frick, P. J., and Georgiou, S. (2009) 'Linking callous–unemotional traits to instrumental and non-instrumental forms of aggression,' *Journal of Psychopathology and Behavioral Assessment*, *31*(4):285–298.
Fanti, K. A., and Henrich, C. C. (2015) 'Effects of self-esteem and narcissism on bullying and victimization during early adolescence,' *Journal of Early Adolescence*, *35*:5–29.
Fanti, K. A., and Kimonis, E. R. (2012) 'Bullying and victimization: The role of conduct problems and psychopathic traits,' *Journal of Research on Adolescence*, *22*(4):617–631.
Fanti, K. A., and Kimonis, E. R. (2013) 'Dimensions of Juvenile Psychopathy Distinguish "Bullies," "Bully–Victims," and "Victims",' *Psychology of Violence*, *3*(4):396–409.
Fossati, A., Borroni, S., Eisenberg, N., and Maffei, C. (2010) 'Relations of proactive and reactive dimensions of aggression to overt and covert narcissism in nonclinical adolescents,' *Aggressive Behavior*, *36*(1):21–27.
Frick P. J. (2004) *Inventory of callous–unemotional traits*, Unpublished rating scale. University of New Orleans.
Frick, P. J., Bodin, S. D., and Barry, C. T. (2000) 'Psychopathic traits and conduct problems in community and clinic-referred samples of children: Further development of the psychopathy screening device,' *Psychological Assessment*, *12*:382–393.
Frick, P. J., and Dickens, C. (2006) 'Current perspectives on conduct disorder,' *Current Psychiatry Reports*:59–72.
Frick, P. J., and Hare, R. D. (2001) *The antisocial process screening device*, Toronto, ON: Multi-Health Systems.
Frick, P. J., Kimonis, E. R., Dandreaux, D. M., and Farell, J. M. (2003) 'The 4 year stability of psychopathic traits in non-referred youth,' *Behavioral Sciences & the Law*, *21*(6):713–736.
Frick, P. J., and Moffitt, T. E. (2010) *A proposal to the DSM–V childhood disorders and the ADHD and disruptive behavior disorders work groups to include a specifier to the diagnosis of conduct disorder based on the presence of callous–unemotional traits*. Washington, DC: APA.
Frick, P. J., Ray, J. V., Thornton, L. C., and Kahn, R. E. (2014) 'Can callous–unemotional traits enhance the understanding, diagnosis, and treatment of serious conduct problems in children and adolescents? A comprehensive review,' *Psychological Bulletin*, *140*(1):1.
Griffin, R. S., and Gross, A. M. (2004) 'Childhood bullying: Current empirical findings and future directions for research,' *Aggression and Violent Behavior*, *9*:379–400.
Hawker, D. S. J., and Boulton, M. J. (2000) 'Twenty years' research on peer victimization and psychosocial maladjustment: A meta-analytic review of cross-sectional studies,' *Journal of Child Psychology and Psychiatry*, *41*:441–455.
Haynie, D. L., Nansel, T., Eitel, P., Davis-Crump, A., Saylor, K., Yu, K., and Simons-Morton, B. (2001) 'Bullies, victims, and bully/victims: Distinct groups of at risk youth,' *Journal of Early Adolescence*, *21*:29–49.
Holland, D., Ireland, J. L., and Muncer, S. (2009) 'Impulsivity, attribution and prison bullying: Bully-category and perpetrator–victim mutuality,' *International Journal of Law and Psychiatry*, *32*(2):84–91.
Hourbe, B., Targuinio, C., Thuillier, I., and Hergott, E. (2006) 'Bullying among students and its consequences on health,' *European Journal of Psychology of Education*, *21*:183–208.
Jaccard, J., and Turrisi, R. (2003) *Interaction effects in multiple regression* (2nd ed.), Thousand Oaks, CA: Sage.
Kaltiala-Heino, R., Rimpela, M., Marttunen, M., Rimpela, A., and Rantanen, P. (1999) 'Bullying, depression, and suicidal ideation in Finnish adolescents: School survey,' *British Medical Journal*, *319*:348–351.
Kamphaus, R. W., and Frick, P. J. (1996) *Clinical assessment of child and adolescent personality and behavior*, Boston, MA: Allyn and Bacon.
Kimonis, E. R., Frick, P. J., Fazekas, H., and Loney, B. R. (2006) 'Psychopathy, aggression, and the processing of emotional stimuli in non-referred girls and boys,' *Behavioral Sciences & the Law. Special Issue: Gender and Psychopathy Volume 2*, *24*(1):21–37.
Kruh, I. P., Frick, P. J., and Clements, C. B. (2005) 'Historical and personality correlates to the violence patterns of juveniles tried as adults,' *Criminal Justice and Behavior*, *32*:69–96.
Kumpulainen, K., Rasanen, E., Henttonen, I., Almqvist, F., Kresanov, K., Linna, S. L., . . ., Tamminen, T. (1998) 'Bullying and psychiatric symptoms among elementary school-age children,' *Child Abuse & Neglect*, *22*:705–717.
Kumpulainen, K., Rasanen, E., and Puura, K. (2001) 'Psychiatric disorders and the use of mental health services among children involved in bullying,' *Aggressive Behavior*, *27*(2):102–110.
Loney, B. R., Taylor, J., Butler, M. A., and Iacono, W. G. (2007) 'Adolescent psychopathy features: 6-year temporal stability and the prediction of externalizing symptoms during the transition to adulthood,' *Aggressive Behavior*, *33*:242–252.
McDermott, P. A. (1996) 'A nationwide study of developmental and gender prevalence for psychopathology in childhood and adolescence,' *Journal of Abnormal Child Psychology: An official publication of the International Society for Research in Child and Adolescent Psychopathology*, *24*(1):53–66.

McGuckin, C., Cummins, P. K., and Lewis, C. A. (2008) 'Bully/victim problems in Northern Ireland's schools: Data from the 2000 "Young Persons' Behavior and Attitude Survey",' *Individual Differences Research*, *6*(4-B):280–288.

Moffitt, T. E., Arseneault, L., Jaffee, S. R., Kim-Cohen, J., Koenen, K. C., Odgers, C. L., . . ., Viding, E. (2008) 'Research review: DSM–V conduct disorder: Research needs for an evidence base,' *Journal of Child Psychology and Psychiatry*, *49*(1):3–33.

Obradovic, J., Pardini, D., Long, J., and Loeber, R. (2007) 'Measuring interpersonal callousness in boys from childhood to adolescence. An examination of longitudinal invariance and temporal stability,' *Journal of Clinical Child and Adolescent Psychiatry*, *36*:276–292.

O'Brennan, L. M., Bradshaw, C. P., and Sawyer, A. L. (2009) 'Examining development differences in the social–emotional problems among frequent bullies, victims, and bully/victims,' *Psychology in the Schools*, *46*(2):100–115.

Olweus, D. (1993) *Bullying at school: What we know and what we can do*, Oxford: Blackwell.

Olweus, D. (1995) 'Bullying or peer abuse at school: Facts and interventions,' *Current Directions in Psychological Science*, *4*(6):196–200.

Pellegrini, A. D., and Bartini, M. (2000) 'A longitudinal study of bullying, victimization, and peer affiliation during the transition from primary school to middle school,' *American Educational Research Journal*, *37*:699–725.

Pellegrini, A. D., Bartini, M., and Brooks, F. (1999) 'School bullies, victims, and aggressive victims: Factors relating to group affiliation and victimization in early adolescence,' *Journal of Educational Psychology*, *91*:216–224.

Pepler, D. J., Craig, W. M., Connolly, J. A., Yuile, A., McMaster, L., and Jiang, D. (2006) 'A developmental perspective on bullying,' *Aggressive Behavior*, *32*:376–384.

Raine, A., Dodge, K., Loeber, R., Gatzke-Kopp, L., Lynam, D., Reynolds, C., . . ., Liu, J. (2006) 'The reactive–proactive aggression questionnaire: Differential correlates of reactive and proactive aggression in adolescent boys,' *Aggressive Behavior*, *32*:159–171.

Reijntjes, A., Kamphuis, J. H., Prinzie, P., and Telch, M. J. (2010) 'Peer victimization and internalizing problems in children: A meta-analysis of longitudinal studies,' *Child Abuse & Neglect*, *34*(4):244–252.

Rigby, K. (2002) *New perspective on bullying*, London: Jessica Kingsley.

Roussos, A., Francis, K., Zoubou, V. Kiprianos, S., Prokopiou A., and Richardson, C. (2001) 'The standardization of Achenbach's youth self-report in Greece in a national sample of high school students,' *European Child and Adolescent Psychiatry*, *10*:47–53.

Salmivalli, C. (2001) 'Feeling good about oneself, being bad to others? remarks on self-esteem, hostility and aggressive behavior,' *Aggression and Violent Behavior*, *6*:375–393.

Salmivalli, C., Lagerspetz, K. M. J., Bjorkqvist, K., Osterman, K., and Kaukiainen, A. (1996) 'Bullying as a group process: Participant roles and their relation to social status within the group,' *Aggressive Behavior*, *22*:1–15.

Salmivalli, C., and Nieminen, E. (2002) 'Proactive and reactive aggression among school bullies, victims and bully–victims,' *Aggressive Behavior*, *28*:30–44.

Salmon, G., James, A., Cassidy, E. L., and Javaloyes, M. A. (2000) 'Bullying a review: Presentations to an adolescent psychiatric service and within a school for emotionally and behaviourally disturbed children,' *Clinical Child Psychology and Psychiatry*, *5*(4):563–579.

Salmon, G., James, A., and Smith, D. M. (1998) 'Bullying in school: Self-reported anxiety, depression, and self-esteem in secondary children,' *British Medical Journal*, *317*:924–925.

Schwartz, D., Proctor, L. J., Chien, D. H., Juvonen, J., and Graham, S. (2001) 'The aggressive victim of bullying: Emotional and behavioral dysregulation as a pathway to victimization by peers,' in J. Juvonen & S. Graham (Eds.), *Peer harassment in school: The plight of the vulnerable and victimized* (pp. 147–174), New York/London: The Guilford Press.

Seals, D., and Young, J. (2003) 'Bullying and victimization: Prevalence and relationship to gender, grade level, ethnicity, self-esteem and depression,' *Adolescence*, *38*(152):735–747.

Sigfusdottir, I. D., Gudjonsson, G. H., and Sigurdsson, J. F. (2010) 'Bullying and delinquency. The mediating role of anger,' *Personality and Individual Differences*, *48*(4):391–396.

Solberg, M. E., Olweus, D., and Endresen, I. M. (2007) 'Bullies and victims at school: Are they the same pupils?,' *British Journal of Educational Psychology*, 77:441–464.

Varjas, K., Meyers, J., and Hunt, M. H. (2006) '*Student Survey of Bullying Behavior–Revised 2 (SSBB–R2)*, Atlanta, Georgia: Georgia State University, Center for Research on School Safety, School Climate and Classroom Management.

Viding, E., Simmonds, E., Petrides, K. V., and Frederickson, N. (2009) 'The contribution of callous–unemotional traits and conduct problems to bullying in early adolescence,' *Journal of Child Psychology and Psychiatry*, *50*(4):471–481.

Wang, J., Iannotti, R. J., and Nansel, T. R. (2009) 'School bullying among adolescents in the United States: Physical, verbal, relational, and cyber,' *Journal of Adolescent Health*, *45*(4):368–375.

Washburn, J. J., McMahon, S. D., King, C. A., Reinecke, M. A., and Silver, C. (2004) 'Narcissistic features in young adolescents: Relations to aggression and internalizing symptoms,' *Journal of Youth and Adolescence*, *33*(3):247–260.

Wolke, D., Woods, S., Stanford, K., and Schulz, H. (2001) 'Bullying and victimization of primary school children in England and Germany: Prevalence and school factors,' *British Journal of Psychology*, *92*:673–696.

Part V

The criminal justice system and psychopathy

37

Psychopathy among juvenile justice system-involved youth

Michael T. Baglivio

Introduction

Criminal career (Blumstein, Cohen, Roth, & Visher, 1986; Moffitt, 1993; Piquero, Farrington, & Blumstein, 2003; Wolfgang, Figlio, & Sellin, 1972) and psychopathy (Hare, 1999) research have both established that a small proportion of offenders, approximately 5 percent, accounts for a preponderance of all crime. This convergence has led some to contend that the two concepts demand integration (Vaughn & DeLisi, 2008; see also DeLisi & Piquero, 2011). In fact, while gaining momentum in recent years after being relatively non-existent in criminological theory, the notion of psychopathy as a useful metric in the explanation of criminality has a decades-old origination (Glueck & Glueck, 1930, 1943; Robins & O'Neal, 1958). Psychopaths are commonly considered emotionally cold, manipulative, callous, narcissistic, irresponsible, and easily frustrated individuals who defy social norms without remorse (Cleckley, 1976; Frick, O'Brien, Wooton, & McBurnett, 1994; Hare, 1996; Lynam, 2002; McCord & McCord, 1964). These individuals are unable to learn socially approved means of satisfying their immediate needs and tend not to form lasting attachments to people or principles (Vaughn, Howard, & DeLisi, 2008).

While not an official personality disorder under the DSM–5 (American Psychiatric Association, APA, 2013), overlap between Antisocial Personality Disorder (ASPD) and psychopathy is such that most persons deemed psychopathic meet criteria for ASPD, yet only approximately 25 percent who meet ASPD criteria meet criteria for psychopathy (Hare, Hart, & Harpur, 1991). ASPD in the DSM–5 now contains a "with psychopathic features" specifier characterized by low anxiousness, low withdrawal, and high attention seeking (APA, 2013). Among adults, across various subsamples, psychopathy has demonstrated association with a host of criminal, antisocial, and violent outcomes, including recidivism (cf., Blackburn & Coid, 1998; Harris, Rice, & Cormier, 1991; Hemphill, Templeman, Wong, & Hare, 1998; Simourd & Hoge, 2000).

The prevalence of psychopathy is approximately 1 percent of the population (Hare, 1999), between 15 and 25 percent of forensic populations (Beaver, Boutwell, Barnes, Vaughn, & DeLisi, 2017), and 28.3 percent in adult prisons (Forth & Burke, 1998). Juvenile "psychopathy" has evidenced as low as 9 percent prevalence among incarcerated nonviolent offenders (Campbell, Porter, & Santor, 2004), between 18–37 percent across juvenile incarceration settings (Edens, Skeem, Cruise, & Cauffman, 2001), and a higher prevalence in males (Vaughn & Howard, 2005).

While often characterized as a discrete taxonomy, with psychopaths scoring above some cut-off score, others argue psychopathy is better conceptualized as a distributed along a continuum (Lynam & Derefinko, 2006; Widiger & Lynam, 1998).

More recently, researchers have begun to extrapolate the concept of psychopathic traits in the study of antisocial behavior among children and adolescents (Essau, Sasagawa, & Frick, 2006; Lynam et al., 2005; Murrie, Cornell, Kaplan, McConville, & Levy-Elkon, 2004), arguing the core psychopathic personality features are evident in childhood (Cleckley, 1976; Hare, 1996; Loeber, 1982; Loeber et al., 2001; Millon, 1981). Psychopathy is posited as a collective of traits that emerge in adolescence, which are normally distributed in the population (DeLisi, 2009). The most severely impaired children are those which manifest callous–unemotional (CU) traits, which are affective and interpersonal deficits most akin to symptoms of psychopathic personality in adults (DeLisi et al., 2011). CU traits differentiated youth who accumulate the most contacts with law enforcement and were responsible for 50 percent of total police contacts over the study period in prior work (Frick, Stickle, Dandreauz, Farrell, & Kimonis, 2005).

The goal of the current chapter is to elucidate psychopathy among juvenile justice-involved youth. As such, first a review of prior work regarding psychopathy among juvenile offenders specifically is presented, followed by a supplemental analysis of the relevance of psychopathic trait indicators among a sample of over 64,000 juvenile offending criminal careers. Finally, a short discussion of the supplemental analysis with respect to convergence and divergence with the literature reviewed, directions for future study, and conclusions are provided.

Psychopathy and juvenile offenders

While the use of psychopathy to explain normative deviance among adolescents is arguably of limited value (Corrado, DeLisi, Hart, & McCuish, 2015; Walters, 2004), its use in the explanation of serious and violent juvenile offending has demonstrated utility across a host of samples and analyses. The need to study psychopathic traits among children and adolescents centers on early identification in hopes that treatment at younger ages may forestall increasingly serious criminal careers, such that "aside from schizophrenia, no other mental health condition is more in need of public health and policy intervention" (Vaughn, Howard, & DeLisi, 2008:408). Unfortunately, of all the personality traits, psychopathic traits are the least studied by criminologists (DeLisi, 2009).

Using the Psychopathy Checklist: Youth Version (PCL: YV), an analysis of over 200 incarcerated juvenile offenders found psychopathy correlated with externalizing behavior problems, violent offending, aggression, history of abuse, noncompliance with justice system sanctions, aggression, and expulsion from school (Campbell, Porter, & Santor, 2004). Examining 115 juveniles on probation supervision, PCL: YV scores were significantly related to total prior charges, previous nonviolent and violent offending, and prior weapon use (Kosson, Cyterski, Steuerwald, Neumann, & Walker-Matthews, 2002), demonstrating psychopathy as a useful construct for all juvenile offenders, not only the deepest-end youth placed in residential facilities. Additional public health and criminological outcomes with empirically demonstrated relationships with psychopathic traits among juvenile offenders have included poorer responses to substance abuse treatment, as well as higher recidivism rates among substance abusing youthful offenders (O'Neill, Lidz, & Heilbrun, 2003), increased odds of recidivism (Corrado, Vincent, Hart, & Cohen, 2004; Gretton, McBride, Hare, O'Shaughnessy, & Kumka, 2001), technical violations (Schmidt, Campbell, & Houlding, 2011), violence (Edens, Buffinton, Tomicic, & Riley, 2001; Gretton, Hare, & Catchpole, 2004), and early onset offending (DeLisi et al., 2014).

Specifically examining female offenders in residential placement (N = 94), prior work has demonstrated affective and interpersonal psychopathic traits significantly associated with violence and theft, but not significantly associated with drug abuse (Vaughn, Newhill, DeLisi, Beaver, & Howard, 2008). In contrast, among 95 detained female juvenile offenders, the Antisocial Process Screening Device (APSD) was not a significant predictor of self-reported antisocial outcomes, including prior offending, aggression, or substance use, once controls for age and past levels of the behaviors were introduced (Collins, van Damme, Andershed, Fanti, & DeLisi, 2017). Diverging findings across studies demand the need for further sex-specific analyses regarding psychopathy and antisocial behaviors in adjudicated samples.

Efforts to extend the examination of the effects of psychopathy beyond criminal offending and delinquency generally have also been undertaken. Specifically, prior work has shown significant relationships between psychopathy and verbal and physical infractions and placement in close observation among serious juvenile offenders in residential facilities (Brandt, Kennedy, Patrick, & Curtin, 1997), as well as disciplinary action and institutional violence (Skeem & Cauffman, 2003). Based on data from 113 male juveniles admitted to the Virginia Department of Juvenile Justice who were assessed for psychopathic traits, Murrie et al. (2004) reported results demonstrating moderate relationships with institutional violence, serious assault, assault with a weapon, and instrumental violence, with a 1-point increase in total PCL: YV score increasing the odds of violence during residential placement by 10 percent. Among 159 serious and violent incarcerated juvenile offenders in Canada, stronger psychopathy indicators were associated with increased misconduct, rule-breaking, and violence within custodial facilities (Shaffer, McCuish, Corrado, Behnken, & DeLisi, 2015). However, the authors note the effects of psychopathic traits were small and varied by whether total scores, factor scores, or item-level scores were used to examine the institutional misconduct. Importantly, for Aboriginal youth the antisocial factor scores (criminal history) were more prominent in the prediction of institutional misconduct, whereas affective components were strongest for White youth (Shaffer et al., 2015), demonstrating psychopath traits may operate differently across race/ethnicity. The rather moderate effect sizes were echoes of prior work reviewing psychopathy and institutional violence (Edens et al., 2001**a**), including a meta-analysis of over 1,300 institutionalized youth (Edens & Campbell, 2007).

Psychopathic traits have figured in examining problem behavior of juvenile sex offenders as well. Specifically, Caputo and colleagues (1999) demonstrated APSD scores distinguished violent sex offenders from both violent non-sexual offenders and nonviolent offenders among 69 adjudicated juvenile males. Additionally, scores on the PCL: YV were found linearly related to recidivism across general, violent, and sexual reoffending (Gretton et al., 2001). Comparing juvenile sex offenders with nonviolent and violent non-sexual juvenile offenders, Cale and colleagues (2015) demonstrated significantly higher prevalence of psychopathy (as per the PCL: YV) among the sex offenders in comparison to violent, nonviolent, and chronic non-sexual juvenile offenders. The sample of sex offenders specifically differed from juvenile non-sexual offenders on the interpersonal and affective dimensions but not the lifestyle and antisocial domains (Cale et al., 2015), echoing prior work which demonstrated high prevalence of callous and unemotional traits among juvenile sex offenders (Caputo et al., 1999) and suggesting such traits are related to more severe sexual offending behaviors (Lawing, Frick, & Cruise, 2010). Interestingly, the juvenile sex offenders in the Cale and colleagues (2015) analysis were most similar to the violent non-sexual juveniles with respect to affective traits.

In an effort to link psychopathy and criminal career literatures, heeding Farrington's (2005) call to incorporate psychopathy into developmental life course research, Vaughn and DeLisi (2008) examined psychopathy among a sample of 723 incarcerated juvenile offenders. Findings revealed personality and affective psychopathic traits doubled the explanatory power above that of demographic and mental health measures, with psychopathic traits accounting for 12 percent of the explained variance in career criminality. Furthermore, psychopathic traits predicted self-reported career criminal membership with 70–88 percent accuracy. Notably, impulsivity and an unemotional affect figured most prominently as personality factors associated with career criminality in their analysis. Additionally, higher psychopathic traits increased the odds of general and violent delinquency, hostile aggression, and early onset offending, with the significant results of psychopathy remaining upon inclusion of additional risk factors, including mental health diagnosis, head injury, and trauma (Vaughn et al., 2008).

This criminal career research extended prior work showing psychopathy scores were significantly related to violent offense history and recidivism, including violent recidivism, among youth in juvenile residential facilities (Brandt et al., 1997; Forth, Hart, & Hare, 1990), adolescent offenders followed into adulthood (Schmidt et al., 2011), as well as being related to frequency, variety, and situational patterns of violence among juveniles tried as adults (Kruh, Frick, & Clements, 2005). It further validated prior work showing higher psychopathy symptomology related to high-rate (frequency) and versatile offending into adulthood (Dyck, Campbell, Schmidt, & Wershler, 2013), and predictive of trajectories of chronic offending (McCuish, Corrado, Lussier, & Hart, 2014; see also Piquero, Farrington, Fontaine, Vincent, Coid, & Ullrich, 2012). Advancing the prior criminal career trajectory studies by (1) using psychopathy as an independent variable, plus (2) controlling for additional criminogenic factors, and (3) employing a prospective approach, Corrado, McCuish, and colleagues (2015) used PCL: YV scores to predict offending from age 12 to 28 among male and female Canadian offenders initially assessed in residential placement. Notably, the antisocial behavior and lifestyle factors of the PCL: YV were related to chronic offending, while the affective and interpersonal symptoms were nonsignificant, calling into question the usefulness of psychopathy in predicting severe offending (Corrado, McCuish et al., 2015) and echoing similar concerns from others (Salekin & Lynam, 2010; Walters, 2003). However, the lack of relevance of the affective and interpersonal components (see also Walters, 2003) may have more to do with limitations of the PCL: YV to adequately measure those symptoms (Corrado, McCuish et al., 2015).

Relatedly, Beaver and colleagues (2017) examined a nationally representative sample of males and females in the United States, demonstrating psychopathic traits predicted self-reported measures of being arrested, a disposition to probation supervision, and being incarcerated for both sexes during 13 years of adolescence into adulthood. In regards to official measures of crime, assessment of psychopathic traits at age 13 has been shown to predict both arrests and convictions through age 26 (Lynam, Miller, Vachon, Loeber, & Stouthamer-Loeber, 2009). These studies support conclusions that "psychopathic traits are analogous to career criminality" (Vaughn & DeLisi, 2008:39).

Examining psychopathy in juvenile justice system involvement in Florida

The intent of the following analysis is to examine the relevance of psychopathic trait indicators, based on the literature reviewed above, in the role of juvenile justice system involvement. Uniquely, using a large sample of adjudicated juvenile offenders, the below analysis sought to understand whether offenders presenting with such psychopathic traits were more likely than other adjudicated youth to evidence delinquency careers defined by: (1) early onset, (2) residential placement, (3) violent offending, and (4) serious, violent, and chronic (SVC) offending.

The present analysis uses data on all juveniles adjudicated in Florida who "aged out" (turned 18 years old) between January 1, 2007 and December 31, 2012. Additionally, each youth must have been administered a Community Positive Achievement Change Tool (C-PACT) risk/needs assessment to be included in the analysis (N = 64,329). Validation studies of C-PACT as used in Florida has demonstrated the tool to be similarly predictive of subsequent offending across race, gender, and dispositional placement (Baglivio, 2009; Baglivio & Jackowski, 2013; Winokur-Early, Hand, & Blankenship, 2012) and comparable to meta-analysis of juvenile risk assessments more generally (Schwalbe, 2007). Additionally, the reliability of the C-PACT has been assessed among a sample of Florida Department of Juvenile Justice (FDJJ) assessors using videotaped interviews and an offense history file, with findings demonstrating an intraclass correlation coefficient (ICC) of .83 and only 4 percent of items (five items) with less than 75 percent agreement with an "expert" rater (Baird et al., 2013). The current sample is further explained and has been used to explore various juvenile justice research questions in prior work, including cumulative traumatic exposure, juvenile offending trajectories, and serious, violent, and chronic offending (cf. Baglivio et al., 2014; Baglivio, Wolff, Piquero, & Epps, 2015; Fox, Perez, Cass, Baglivio, & Epps, 2015).

All measures used in the current analysis were garnered from the Juvenile Justice Information System (JJIS) maintained by the FDJJ. JJIS maintains complete offense history, demographics, and risk assessments for every youth arrested in Florida under the age of 18. The current study uses the first full C-PACT risk/need assessment for each youth to measure psychopathic trait indicators and control risk factors. The youth's comprehensive delinquency record was used to assess juvenile justice system outcomes and the extent of the youth's delinquency "career."

Dependent measures

Early onset

Juveniles are classified as early onset offenders if their age at first arrest was 12 years old or younger (= 1, else = 0).

Residential placement

Juveniles with one or more placements in a long-term juvenile justice residential placement (pre-trial detention does not count) prior to age 18 (= 1, else = 0).

Violent offender

Juveniles with a history of adjudication for an against-person felony offense prior to age 18 were classified as violent offenders (= 1, else = 0). Violent felony offenses involve force or physical harm to another person.

SVC offender

Juveniles are classified as SVC offenders if they evidenced three or more adjudicated felonies, at least one of which was a violent, against-person felony, prior to age 18 (= 1, else = 0). This definition of SVC offending is in keeping with prior work examining FDJJ juvenile offenders (Fox et al., 2015).

Number of arrests prior to age 18

The number of arrests of each juvenile up to the age of 18 was captured as a continuous measure.

Psychopathic trait indicators

The below psychopathic trait indicators were examined based on the prior work reviewed above and which were available in in the FDJJ data garnered from the C-PACT risk/needs assessment. Exploratory factor analysis (EFA) was conducted (results not shown for brevity) to assist with grouping and creating indices of related C-PACT items.

Callousness/behavioral dyscontrol index

An index of interpersonal traits was created from seven C-PACT items where higher values indicate greater risk for each item: *hostile interpretation* of the actions of others (primarily positive view, primarily negative view, primarily hostile view of the intentions of others); *tolerance for frustration* (rarely gets upset, sometimes gets upset, often gets upset over small things); *Anger/irritability* (no history, occasional feelings, consistent feelings, aggressive reactions to Anger); belief in *verbal aggression* to resolve disagreement (rarely appropriate, sometimes appropriate, often appropriate); belief in *physical aggression* to resolve disagreement (never appropriate, rarely appropriate, sometimes appropriate, often appropriate); *impulsivity* (usually thinks before acting, sometimes thinks before acting, often acts before thinking, highly impulsive); and *empathy/remorse* (has empathy for victims, some empathy, does not have empathy for his/her victims). The seven items were standardized and combined to create the index (α = .816).

Lack of interest/detached index

An index measuring the juvenile's participation and interest in structured and unstructured prosocial activities was created from four C-PACT items: history of *structured recreational activities* (involved in two or more, involved in one, never involved in structured and supervised prosocial community activities); history of *unstructured activities* (involved in two or more, involved in one, never involved in activities that positively occupy the youth's time); *current interest/involvement in structured activities* (currently involved in two or more, currently involved in one, currently interested but not involved, currently not interested in structured activities); *current interest/involvement in unstructured activities* (currently involved in two or more, currently involved in one, currently interested but not involved, currently not interested in unstructured prosocial activities). The four items were standardized and combined (α = .817).

Uncaring/unconscientiousness index

Four C-PACT items were combined to create an index measuring the youth's ties and closeness to school, in conjunction with lack of caring about educational performance: belief there is *value in getting an education* (education of value, somewhat believes education of value, does not believe education is of value); belief school provides an *encouraging environment* (believes school is encouraging, somewhat believes, does not believe school is encouraging); involvement in *school activities* (involved in two or more, involved in one, interested but not involved, not interested in school activities); and *school staff* the youth feels comfortable taking with (close to four or more, close to three, close to two, close to one, not close to any teachers, staff, or coaches). The four items were standardized and combined (α = .825).

Affective index

An index of affective traits combined three C-PACT items: skills in *dealing with others* (often uses advanced social skills, sometimes uses advanced social skills, has basic social skills, lacks basic skills in dealing with others); *skills in dealing with difficult situations* (often uses skills in dealing with difficult situations, sometimes uses skills, rarely uses skills, lacks skills in dealing with difficult situations); and *skills in dealing with feelings/emotions* (often uses skills in dealing with feelings/emotions, sometimes uses skills, rarely uses skills, lacks skills in knowing and expressing feelings or understanding the feelings of others). The three items were added to create an affective index (α = .895).

Affiliative relations index

Three C-PACT items were standardized and combine to create an index (α = .809) capturing the juvenile's ties to the community; *history of positive adult non-family relationships* (three or more, two, one, no positive adult non-family relationships not connected to school); *current positive adult non-family relationships* (three or more, two, one, no positive adult non-family relationships not connected to school); and *prosocial community ties* (strong ties, some ties, no prosocial ties/people in the community who discourage the youth from getting in trouble or are willing to help the youth).

Rebellious narcissism/recalcitrant index

An index measuring the youth's pursuit of self-gratification over conventional rules or norms was created from four C-PACT items: *attitude toward responsible law-abiding behavior* (rules/conventions apply to him/her, some rules apply, does not believe rules apply, resents or is defiant to rules/conventions); accepts *responsibility for antisocial behavior* (accepts responsibility, minimizes/justifies, accepts antisocial behavior as okay, proud of antisocial behavior); *respect for authority* (respects most authority, does not respect, resents most, defies or hostile toward authority); and *respect for property of others* (respects property of others, respects personal but not public property, conditional respect/"if they are stupid enough to leave it out they deserve losing it," no respect for property/"if I want something it should be mine"). The four items were standardized to create a rebellious narcissism/recalcitrant index (α = .751).

Indifference/unconcern

Youth who self-reported that their primary emotion when committing crime was unconcerned or indifferent were coded 1, else = 0.

Control measures

Control variables were included to examine the robustness of any effects of psychopathic trait indicators on the dependent outcomes. All measures were taken from the first C-PACT assessment for each youth. Control measures included demographics of gender (male = 1), Black race

(= 1), age at C-PACT assessment (continuous), peer associations (prosocial peers only, mixed peers, antisocial peers only, gang member/associate), substance use history (no prior alcohol or drug use, prior use of alcohol or drugs, prior use that caused problems with school, family, health, relationships, criminal behavior, or tolerance/withdrawal), ADHD (yes = 1), mental health problems (diagnosis = 1, else 0; does not include Conduct Disorder, oppositional defiant, substance abuse, or ADHD), and history of school suspensions/expulsions (none, one, two or three, four or five, six or seven, more than seven). Descriptive statistics for all measures can be seen in Table 37.1.

Analytic strategy

The analysis was undertaken in three steps. First, a series of logistic regression models assessed the predictive ability of psychopathic traits while including demographic and control risk factors on early onset offending, residential juvenile justice placement, violent offending, and SVC offending. Next, a negative binomial regression model examined psychopathic traits (and control measures) on the number of arrests prior to age 18. Finally, sex-specific logistic regression models are estimated to examine the differences between males and females in how psychopathic traits predict SVC juvenile offending careers. While several measures entered into the

Table 37.1 Descriptive statistics for the analysis of psychopathic traits and juvenile justice outcomes (*N* = 64,329)

Dependent variables	*Mean*	*SD*
Early onset	.257	.437
Residential placement	.330	.470
Violent offender	.548	.498
SVC offender	.167	.373
Total juvenile arrests		
Psychopathic trait indicators		
Callousness/behavioral dyscontrol index	.333	.676
Lack of interest/detached index	.000	.803
Uncaring/unconscientiousness index	.000	.809
Affective index	2.69	.803
Affiliative relations index	2.82	.709
Rebellious narcissism/recalcitrant Index	.000	.756
Indifference/unconcern	.351	.477
Demographics		
Age at assessment	16.382	1.277
Gender	.748	.411
Black	.458	.498
Control risk factors		
Substance abuse	1.602	.623
Antisocial peers	2.084	.669
ADHD	.196	.397
Mental health problem	.163	.370
School suspensions	3.21	1.763

Note. SD = Standard Deviation.

regression models were significantly correlated, variance inflation factors (VIF) were all below 2.4, indicating multicollinearity should not affect results (Fox, 1997).

Results

Table 37.2 provides the results of the four logistic regression models. The first model, early onset (first arrest 12 years of age or under) was predicted, in the hypothesized direction, by three of the seven psychopathic trait indices. Youth who lack interest/are detached regarding prosocial activities, those holding uncaring beliefs about education, and those who self-report indifference/unconcern with respect to offending were more likely to evidence early onset offending. Additionally, younger youth, males, and Black youth were more likely to be early onset offenders. With respect to control risk factors, substance predicted early onset offending, with those having no history of use more likely to be early onset, as did antisocial peers, ADHD, mental health problems, and school suspensions/expulsions (all in the hypothesized direction).

Residential juvenile justice placement prior to age 18 was predicted by five of seven psychopathic trait indicators, net of demographic measures and controls (all of which were significant in the hypothesized direction). Specifically, youth evidencing callousness/behavioral dyscontrol (hostile interpretation of others' actions, low frustration tolerance, Anger/irritability, impulsive,

Table 37.2 Logistic regression of psychopathic traits and juvenile justice outcomes

Psychopathic trait indicators	*Early onset*		*Residential placement*		*Violent offender*		*SVC offender*	
	O.R.	*S.E.*	*O.R.*	*S.E.*	*O.R.*	*S.E.*	*O.R.*	*S.E.*
Callousness/behavioral dyscontrol	1.002	(.021)	1.074***	(.020)	1.481***	(.019)	1.145***	(.025)
Lack of interest/detached index	1.112***	(.015)	1.226***	(.014)	1.064***	(.013)	1.137***	(.018)
Uncaring/ unconscientiousness	1.110***	(.016)	1.159***	(.015)	1.019	(.013)	1.089***	(.019)
Affective index	.980	(.015)	.979	(.014)	1.010	(.013)	1.048**	(.017)
Affiliative relations index	.985	(.016)	1.025	(.015)	.996	(.014)	1.004	(.019)
Rebellious narcissism/ recalcitrant	1.010	(.018)	1.276***	(.017)	.898***	(.016)	1.157***	(.020)
Indifference/unconcern	1.053*	(.021)	1.241***	(.019)	.851***	(.018)	1.031	(.024)
Demographics								
Age at assessment	.659***	(.008)	.681***	(.008)	.828***	(.007)	.701***	(.009)
Gender	1.416***	(.025)	2.033***	(.024)	2.238***	(.021)	3.482***	(.037)
Black	1.786***	(.020)	1.692***	(.019)	2.097***	(.018)	2.561***	(.024)
Control risk factors								
Substance abuse	.967*	(.017)	1.468***	(.016)	.882***	(.015)	1.061**	(.020)
Antisocial peers	1.035*	(.015)	1.178***	(.014)	1.073***	(.013)	1.170***	(.017)
ADHD	1.432***	(.025)	1.288***	(.024)	1.080**	(.023)	1.156***	(.030)
Mental health problem	1.378***	(.027)	1.233***	(.026)	1.340***	(.025)	1.289***	(.033)
School suspensions	1.093***	(.006)	1.100***	(.005)	1.052***	(.005)	1.077***	(.007)

Note. O.R. = Odds Ratio; S.E. = Standard Error; SVC = serious, violent, and chronic; * $p < .05$; ** $p < .01$; *** $p < .001$; $N = 64{,}349$.

lack of empathy, and belief in verbal and physical aggression), lack of interest/uncaring, those uncaring/unconscientiousness in regards to education, higher values on the rebellious narcissism/recalcitrant index (defiant towards rules, conventions, others' property, and do not take responsibility for antisocial actions), and youth who self-report indifference/unconcern were more likely to evidence residential placement as a juvenile.

Whether the youth evidenced an arrest for a violent against-person felony offense as a juvenile was predicted in model 3. Net of demographics and controls (again, all significant in expected directions), four of the seven psychopathic trait indicators significantly predicted violent offending. Youth scoring higher on the callousness/behavioral dyscontrol index, lacking interest/detached, and the rebellious narcissism/recalcitrant index were more likely to be violent offenders. Notably, youth who self-reported indifference/unconcern when offending were significantly less likely to be violent offenders.

Finally, psychopathic trait indicators, demographics, and controls were examined in predicting SVC juvenile offending careers. Net of controls, five of the seven psychopathic trait indicators predicted an SVC juvenile offending career, all in expected directions. Youth scoring higher on the callousness/behavioral dyscontrol index, those lacking interest/detached from prosocial activities, those uncaring/unconscientiousness in regards to education, those scoring higher on the affective index (trouble dealing with others, difficult situations, and feelings/emotions), and those youth scoring higher on the rebellious narcissism/recalcitrant index were more likely to be classified as SVC offenders as a juvenile.

Next, a negative binomial regression was estimated to predict the total number of arrests as a juvenile. As number of arrests is a count variable, negative binomial regression is appropriate (and a better fit to the data than poisson regression, as evidenced by the chi-squared test $p < .001$, and absolute value log likelihood closer to 0). Table 37.3 provides the results of this

Table 37.3 Negative binomial regression: psychopathic traits and total number of juvenile arrests

Psychopathic trait indicators	*Juvenile arrests*		
	IRR	*S.E.*	*95% C.I.*
Callousness/behavioral dyscontrol	1.052***	(.006)	1.039–1.064
Lack of interest/detached index	1.074***	(.004)	1.065–1.083
Uncaring/unconscientiousness	1.106***	(.005)	1.097–1.116
Affective index	1.008	(.004)	1.000–1.016
Affiliative relations index	1.013**	(.005)	1.004–1.021
Rebellious narcissism/recalcitrant	1.090***	(.006)	1.079–1.101
Indifference/unconcern	1.058***	(.006)	1.045–1.070
Demographics			
Age at assessment	.861***	(.002)	.857–.865
Gender	1.192***	(.008)	1.176–1.208
Black	1.376***	(.008)	1.361–1.392
Control risk factors			
Substance abuse	1.155***	(.005)	1.114–1.166
Antisocial peers	1.083***	(.005)	1.074–1.093
ADHD	1.065***	(.008)	1.050–1.081
Mental health problem	1.101***	(.009)	1.084–1.118
School suspensions	1.053***	(.002)	1.050–1.056

Note. IRR = Incident Rate Ratio; S.E. = Standard Error; C.I. = Confidence Interval; * p < .05; ** p < .01; *** p < .001; *N* = 64,349.

analysis, including incident rate ratios (IRR) for each measure. The IRR can be interpreted as the expected count (number of arrests) is multiplied by a factor of the IRR when the given measure increases by one unit. As shown, similar to the logistic models, all demographic and control risk factors were significant, as were six of the seven psychopathic trait indicators. Specifically, related to psychopathic traits, only the affective index failed to reach significance (p = .059).

Finally, separate logistic regression models for males and females were estimated to predict SVC juvenile offending careers using the psychopathic trait measures, demographic, and control risk factors. This analysis (see Table 37.4) provides understanding of whether unique psychopathic traits operated differently across sex in the prediction of SVC juvenile offending careers. For males, all demographic and control measures were significant, in expected directions, as were five of the seven psychopathic trait indicators. Males who scored higher on the callousness/behavioral dyscontrol index, those lacking interest/detached from prosocial activities, those uncaring/unconscientiousness in regards to education, and those youth scoring higher on the rebellious narcissism/recalcitrant index were more likely to be classified as SVC offenders as a juvenile. Neither the affective index, index of affiliative relations, nor a feeling of indifference/unconcern while offending predicted male SVC juvenile offending.

For females, five of the seven psychopathic trait indicators predicted SVC offending, as did all of the demographic and control risk factors, with the exception of substance use/abuse. Similar to males, females scoring higher on the callousness/behavioral dyscontrol index, those lacking interest/detached from prosocial activities, and those scoring higher on the rebellious narcissism/recalcitrant index were more likely to be classified as SVC offenders by age 18. However, while uncaring/unconscientiousness towards education was relevant for male SVC offending, it was nonsignificant for females. However, females scoring higher on the affective index were at increased odds of SVC offending, while the affective index was nonsignificant for males.

Table 37.4 Logistic regression of psychopathic traits and SVC offending by sex

Psychopathic trait indicators	*Males (N = 50,483)*		*Females (N = 13,846)*	
	O.R.	*S.E.*	*O.R.*	*S.E.*
Callousness/behavioral dyscontrol	1.137***	(.027)	1.217**	(.072)
Lack of interest/detached index	1.137***	(.019)	1.161**	(.054)
Uncaring/unconscientiousness	1.087***	(.020)	1.064	(.057)
Affective index	1.035	(.018)	1.156**	(.053)
Affiliative relations index	1.017	(.020)	.903	(.058)
Rebellious narcissism/recalcitrant	1.160***	(.022)	1.126*	(.057)
Indifference/unconcern	1.024	(.026)	1.080	(.073)
Demographics				
Age at assessment	.696***	(.010)	.737***	(.027)
Black	2.587***	(.025)	2.281***	(.076)
Control risk factors				
Substance abuse	1.064**	(.021)	.991	(.059)
Antisocial peers	1.163***	(.018)	1.240***	(.055)
ADHD	1.164***	(.031)	1.217*	(.092)
Mental health problem	1.190***	(.036)	1.909***	(.081)
School suspensions	1.073***	(.007)	1.114***	(.020)

Note. O.R. = Odds Ratio; S.E. = Standard Error; SVC = serious, violent, and chronic; * $p < .05$; ** $p < .01$; *** $p < .001$.

This analysis, and the full sample logistic regression and negative binomial analyses presented above (see Table 37.2 and Table 37.3) illustrate the utility in psychopathic trait indicators in the prediction of various deleterious justice system outcomes prior to age 18 among juvenile justice offenders, and the notion that the effects of specific traits may be sex-specific.

Discussion

The purpose of this chapter, and the FDJJ juvenile offending career analysis which accompanied it, was to examine the relevance of psychopathic traits with respect to markers of offense severity and deep-end system involvement among juvenile justice-involved youth. Specifically, the focus was on early onset, residential placement, violent offending, total pre-adulthood official offending, and the pinnacle of juvenile justice system involvement: SVC offending delinquency careers. Results demonstrated the relevance of psychiatric traits across outcomes, even after controlling for demographic and other criminogenic factors.

The results presented above mirror prior work showing the relevance of those easily frustrated and angered, out of touch with his/her feelings, not concerned with others, and difficulty understanding feelings of others in offending behavior (Lynam & Widiger, 2007). In the current analysis, the callousness/behavioral dyscontrol index was associated with every outcome, for males and females, except early onset of official arrest. Similar results were demonstrated for the rebellious narcissism/recalcitrant index (significantly associated with all outcomes, across sex, with the exception of early onset). That index contains elements of impulsivity/self-control, as well as empathy/remorse, and a temperament high in negative emotionality. Those youth lacking interest/detached from prosocial activities were at greater odds of all negative outcomes, which held true across sex. Surprisingly, the affective index (difficulty dealing with others, with emotions, and with difficult situations) was associated with SVC offending, and only for females, but unrelated to onset, violent offending, residential placement, or total number of offenses. Similarly, the affiliative relations index (relationships with prosocial adults, community ties) was related only to total offenses but none of the other negative justice system outcomes. The findings above showed those youth uncaring/ unconscientiousness in regards to education at greater odds for all outcomes, except violent offending, which held true for males specifically. Prior work has shown those youth high on CU traits "could mean that psychopathic youths simply do not care, engage, or connect enough to their school work . . . also likely explains an indifferent, underachieving style in school" (DeLisi et al., 2011:9; see also Corrado, DeLisi et al., 2015).

Additionally, the inclusion in the current analysis of ADHD and mental health problems/ diagnosis as mental health control indicators is in keeping with Vaughn and DeLisi's (2008) prior work, while controlling for substance use and school behavior consistent with Corrado, McCuish, and colleagues' (2015) trajectory work on psychopathy and criminal careers. Similarly, the current analysis also excluded the behavioral dimension of psychopathy (prior to offending) to avoid the tautology critique levied toward the measurement of psychopathy (cf. Beaver et al., 2017; Cooke & Michie, 2001; Edens et al., 2001b). Current findings strengthen prior work showing psychopathy significantly associated with both self-reported and official measures of antisocial/criminal onset (DeLisi, Neppl, Lohman, Vaughn, & Shook, 2013).

In contrast to a recent prospective study showing psychopathic traits of questionable utility in predicting antisocial outcomes among female juvenile offenders in Belgium (Collins et al., 2017), such traits figured prominently in the prediction of extensive juvenile justice system involvement for female adolescents in the current supplemental analysis. This adds to the mixed findings regarding psychopathy and sex among justice system involved youth where prior work has demonstrated both positive associations across sex (Stockdale, Olver, & Wong, 2010) or weak to no associations for girls (Schmidt, McKinnon, Chattha, & Brownlee, 2006; Vincent, Odgers, McCormick, & Corrado, 2008). Discrepant findings lead to calls for future research across tools and across samples assessing sex-specific differences in the criminogenic effects of psychopathic traits among juvenile offenders.

Certainly, there were some limitations worth mentioning in regards to the analysis presented above. There were no genetic or neurological deficit indicators employed. Prior work has elucidated the role of neurocognitive deficits in life-course-persistent offending and psychopathy (Glenn & Raine, 2008; Lynam, 1998; Moffitt, 1993; Waldman & Rhee, 2006), associations which appear to hold true for both males and female (Beaver, Vaughn, DeLisi, Barnes, & Boutwell, 2012). Notably, the above analysis did not examine the administration of a tool specifically designed to assess psychopathy, nor one with established reliability or valid psychometric properties in regards to juvenile "psychopathy" (though such metrics have been established for the tool with respect to offending behavior). While the PCL–R (Hare, 2003) is arguably the gold standard for psychopathy assessment, and the PCL: YV (Forth, Kosson, & Hare, 2003) the most prolific for youth, critiques of existing tools and the PCL in particular have been levied (Cooke & Michie, 2001; Lynam & Widiger, 2007). Specifically, critiques include the tautology of the antisocial behavior dimension (Cooke & Logan, 2015) as well as the notion that hyperactivity and impulsivity have not proven to be specific to adults with psychopathy nor to distinguish children with severe and early onset conduct problems (Essau et al., 2006). Specifically, impulsive–antisocial tendencies are seen elevated in most adults with significant criminal histories, rather than distinguishing the small subset of psychopaths, while the antisocial behavior component has been argued to be a "later, downstream correlate of psychopathy" (Skeem & Cooke, 2010:433; see also Corrado, DeLisi et al., 2015; but see Hare & Neumann, 2005; Lynam, 1996). Rather, the focus on callous and unemotional (CU) traits is more in keeping with the construct of adult psychopathy (Frick & Marsee, 2006). CU traits have been demonstrated to significantly relate to subsequent violent offense post-release from institutional placement (Vincent, Vitacco, Grisso, & Corrado, 2003) and have exhibited stability over time (Lynam, Loeber, & Stouthamer-Loeber, 2008). Alternatively, the Comprehensive Assessment of Psychopathic Personality (CAPP) is assessed through a semi-structured interview with expert rating scales and collateral information, similar to the C-PACT used in the current study, and also contains an informant rating form, neither of which are dependent on measures of the downstream consequences of psychopathy (tautological behavioral indicators; see Cooke and Logan, 2015). Additionally, the analysis contained herein attempted to heed the call for more criminological research to exploit existing data sets in efforts to examine the criminogenic effects of psychopathic personality traits (Beaver et al., 2017).

While self-reported offending surely would have captured more chronic and violent offending, concerns related to the accuracy of self-reported delinquency among those high in psychopathic traits has been elucidated (Corrado, McCuish, et al., 2015). Nonetheless, echoing prior scholars, studies using both official arrests and self-reported offending would be preferred.

Policy implications for juvenile justice

Indicators of psychopathic traits have a clearly demonstrated relationship with juvenile justice system involvement (but see Douglas, Epstein, & Poythress 2008), including SVC offending (DeLisi, 2009). Assessment of specific psychopathic traits seems paramount to providing individualized treatment and case planning. Yet, echoing prior scholars (Murrie et al., 2004), hesitancy must be employed with any labeling of adolescent offenders as "psychopath." Arguably, such classifications would be unproductive at best, and most likely adversely related to justice system dispositional decisions and treatment planning (see also Collins et al., 2017; Murrie, Cornell, & McCoy, 2005). The associations of psychopathic traits during childhood or adolescence, their stability, and adulthood and life-course-persistent offending have not been entirely elucidated empirically as of yet (see Edens et al., 2001; Seagrave & Grisso, 2002). This, coupled with meta-analytic findings regarding evidence-based interventions that "there was no indication that there were juveniles whose risk level was so high that they did not respond to effective interventions" (Lipsey, 2009:23), cautions practitioners and researchers alike in giving up hope for subgroups of even the most high-risk offenders.

The ability to identify fledgling psychopaths in childhood and adolescence is in keeping with notions of early intervention and prevention (DeLisi 2005; Loeber, Farrington, & Petechuk, 2003), as psychopathic adults may be more resistant to rehabilitation efforts (Harris et al., 1991; Lynam, 1998; Salekin, 2002; but see Skeem, Monahan, & Mulvey, 2002). Treatment has demonstrated efficacy for juveniles with psychopathic traits, including lower rates and slower time to violent recidivism, when more methodologically rigorous designs with comparison groups are conducted (Caldwell, Skeem, Salekin, & van Rybroek, 2006), perhaps because emerging traits are more malleable than those of adult psychopaths. The current analysis suggests the usefulness of social skills training interventions to improve social competence. Interventions for aggressive adolescents has been suggested in prior work (Caldwell et al., 2006). Prominent aggression control, skills building, and self-regulation interventions (Holmqvist, Hill, & Lang, 2009; Piquero, Jennings, & Farrington, 2010; Piquero, Jennings, Farrington, Diamond, & Reingle Gonzalez, 2016) appear relevant based on the importance of the callousness/behavioral dyscontrol and rebellious narcissism/recalcitrant components of the current work. Additionally, Multi-Systemic Therapy (MST) and Functional Family Therapy (FFT) could serve important roles, as poor parenting and adverse childhood experiences are correlated with fledgling psychopathy (Beaver et al., 2012; Farrington, 2006, 2007). Such interventions take a more holistic view of the youth, family, and community and appear to demonstrate face validity across many of the psychopathic trait indices examined above. In terms of early intervention, family/parent training programs have been deemed efficacious (Piquero, Jennings, Diamond, Farrington, Tremblay, Welsh, & Reingle-Gonzalez, 2016) and could teach families to more effectively supervise and manage early youth (mis)behavior.

While suggestions for intervention and prevention are guided by the literature and above analysis, future research should focus on effective interventions specifically for juvenile offenders evidencing psychopathic traits (Edens et al., 2001; Forth & Burke, 1998). An emphasis on adequate measures of dosage and duration needed to evidence positive effects should be a core focus to guide practitioners. Strong efforts at engagement and retention are warranted as juveniles with psychopathic traits are likely to disrupt treatment (Caldwell et al., 2006). Providers must be cognizant and ready for this disruption and not withhold, or screen out, juveniles with psychopathic traits from the treatment, as these are the very youth most in need. Additional research would be remiss without the examination of protective factors buffering associations with reoffending among delinquent youth with psychopathic traits.

Conclusion

The analysis undertaken in this chapter adds to prior work, such as Vaughn and DeLisi (2008) demonstrating self-reported SVC career criminality predicted by affective and personality psychopathic traits. The above analysis echoes and expands the reviewed literature, showing psychopathic traits significantly associated with juvenile justice system involvement, including early onset, violent offending, long-term residential placement, total number of arrests, and SVC juvenile offending criminal careers. Notably, a large sample of juvenile offending careers was employed, including over 13,800 females. The supplemental analyses examined psychopathic traits, including sex as a control to ensure a contribution to predictive ability of psychopathy above that of sex, as well as sex-specific analyses to examine differences in specific traits to predict official outcomes across sex.

Through review of prior work and supplemental analyses, this chapter has attempted to demonstrate psychopathic traits requisite measures in attempts to explain differences among deep-end juvenile justice placements and SVC juvenile offending careers. Indeed, "if psychopathy is a stable, enduring feature of antisocial persons, it is likely to emerge as a central construct in the longitudinal study of offending over the life-span" (DeLisi, 2009:262). As a small subset of offenders, predominately early onset, are responsible for a majority of all offending, including violent offending, one can hope that research continues to evaluate the usefulness of measures of psychopathic traits and, to the extent demonstrated empirically, further incorporate psychopathy into theories of severe criminal behavior and into examinations of juvenile justice system-involved youth.

References

American Psychiatric Association. (2013) *Diagnostic and statistical manual of mental disorders* (5th ed.), Arlington, VA: American Psychiatric Publishing.

Baglivio, M. T. (2009) 'The assessment of risk to recidivate among a juvenile offending population,' *Journal of Criminal Justice*, *37*:596–607.

Baglivio, M. T., Epps, N., Swartz, K., Huq, M. S., Sheer, A., and Hardt, N. (2014) 'The prevalence of Adverse Childhood Experiences (ACE) in the lives of juvenile offenders,' *Journal of Juvenile Justice*, *3*(2):1–23.

Baglivio, M. T., and Jackowski, K. (2013) 'Examining the validity of a juvenile offending risk assessment instrument across gender and race/ethnicity,' *Youth Violence and Juvenile Justice*, *11*:26–43.

Baglivio, M. T., Wolff, K. T., Piquero, A. R., and Epps, N. (2015) 'The relationship between Adverse Childhood Experiences (ACE) and juvenile offending trajectories in a juvenile offender sample,' *Journal of Criminal Justice*, *43*:229–241.

Baird, C., Healy, T., Johnson, K., Bogie, A., Dankert, E. W., and Scharenbroch, C. (2013) *A comparison of risk assessment instruments in juvenile justice*, Madison, WI: National Council on Crime and Delinquency.

Beaver, K. M., Boutwell, B. B., Barnes, J. C., Vaughn, M. G., and DeLisi, M. (2017) 'The association between psychopathic personality traits and criminal justice outcomes: Results from a nationally representative sample of males and females,' *Crime and Delinquency*, *63*(6):708–730.

Beaver, K. M., Vaughn, M. G., DeLisi, M., Barnes, J. C., and Boutwell, B. B. (2012) 'The neuropsychological underpinnings to psychopathic personality traits in a nationally representative and longitudinal sample,' *Psychiatric Quarterly*, *83*(2):145–159.

Blackburn, R., and Coid, J. W. (1998) 'Psychopathy and the dimensions of personality disorder in violent offenders,' *Personality and Individual Differences*, *25*:129–145.

Blumstein, A., Cohen, J., Roth, J. A., and Visher, C. A. (Eds.) (1986) *Criminal careers and "career criminals"*, Washington, DC: National Academy Press.

Brandt, J. R., Kennedy, W. A., Patrick, C. J., and Curtin, J. J. (1997) 'Assessment of psychopathy in a population of incarcerated adolescent offenders,' *Psychological Assessment*, *9*(4):429–435.

Caldwell, M., Skeem, J., Salekin, R., and van Rybroek, G. (2006) 'Treatment response of adolescent offenders with psychopathic features: A 2-year follow-up,' *Criminal Justice and Behavior*, *33*(5):571–596.

Cale, J., Lussier, P., McCuish, E., and Corrado, R. (2015) 'The prevalence of psychopathic personality disturbances among incarcerated youth: Comparing serious, chronic, violent and sex offenders,' *Journal of Criminal Justice*, *43*:337–344.

Campbell, M., Porter, S., and Santor, D. (2004) 'Psychopathic traits in adolescent offenders: An evaluation of criminal history, clinical, and psychosocial correlates,' *Behavioral Sciences and the Law*, *22*:23–47.

Caputo, A. A., Frick, P. J., and Brodsky, S. L. (1999) 'Family violence and juvenile sex offending: The potential mediating role of psychopathic traits and negative attitudes toward women,' *Criminal Justice and Behavior*, *26*:338–356.

Cleckley, H. (1976) *The mask of sanity* (5th ed.), St. Louis, MO: Mosby.

Colins, O. F., van Damme, L., Andershed, H., Fanti, K. A., and DeLisi, M. (2017) 'Self-reported psychopathic traits and antisocial outcomes in detained girls: A prospective study,' *Youth Violence and Juvenile Justice*, *15*(2):138–153.

Cooke, D. J., and Logan, C. (2015) 'Capturing clinical complexity: Towards a personality-oriented measure of psychology,' *Journal of Criminal Justice*, *43*:262–273.

Cooke, D. J., and Michie, C. (2001) 'Refining the construct of psychopathy: Towards a hierarchical model,' *Psychological Assessment*, *13*(2):171–188.

Corrado, R. R., DeLisi, M., Hart, S. D., and McCuish, E. C. (2015) 'Can the causal mechanisms underlying chronic, serious, and violent offending trajectories be elucidated using the psychopathy construct?,' *Journal of Criminal Justice*, *43*:251–261.

Corrado, R. R., McCuish, E. C., Hart, S. D., and DeLisi, M. (2015) 'The role of psychopathic traits and developmental risk factors on offending trajectories from early adolescence to adulthood: A prospective study of incarcerated youth,' *Journal of Criminal Justice*, *43*:357–368.

Corrado, R. R., Vincent, G. M., Hart, S. D., and Cohen, I. M. (2004) 'Predictive validity of the Psychopathy Checklist: Youth Version for general and violent recidivism,' *Behavioral Sciences and the Law*, *22*:5–22.

DeLisi, M. (2005) *Career criminals in society*, Thousand Oaks, CA: Sage.

DeLisi, M. (2009) 'Psychopathy as the unified theory of crime,' *Youth Violence and Juvenile Justice*, 7:256–273.

DeLisi, M., Neppl, T. K., Lohman, B. J., Vaughn, M. G., and Shook, J. J. (2013) 'Early starters: Which type of criminal onset matters most for delinquent careers?,' *Journal of Criminal Justice*, *41*:12–17.

DeLisi, M., Peters, D. J., Dansby, T., Vaughn, M. G., Shook, J. J., and Hochstetler, A. (2014) 'Dynamics of psychopathy and moral disengagement in the etiology of crime,' *Youth Violence and Juvenile Justice*, *12*(4):295–314.

DeLisi, M., and Piquero, A. R. (2011) 'New frontiers in criminal careers research, 2000–2011: A state-of-the-art review,' *Journal of Criminal Justice*, *39*(4):289–301.

DeLisi, M., Vaughn, M. G., Beaver, K. M., Wexler, J., Barth, A. E., and Fletcher, J. M. (2011) 'Fledgling psychopathy in the classroom: ADHD subtypes psychopathy, and reading comprehension in a community sample of adolescents,' *Youth Violence and Juvenile Justice*, 9(1):43–58.

Douglas, K. S., Epstein, M. E., and Poythress, N. G. (2008) 'Criminal recidivism among juvenile offenders: Testing the incremental and predictive validity of three measures of psychopathic features,' *Law and Human Behavior*, *32*(5):423–438.

Dyck, H. L., Campbell, M. A., Schmidt, F., and Wershler, J. L. (2013) 'Youth psychopathic traits and their impact on long-term criminal offending trajectories,' *Youth Violence and Juvenile Justice*, *11*(3):230–248.

Edens, J. F., Buffinton, J. K., Tomicic, T. L., and Riley, B. D. (2001a) 'Effects of positive impression management on the Psychopathic Personality Inventory,' *Law and Human Behavior*, *25*:235–255.

Edens, J. F., and Campbell, J. S. (2007) 'Identifying youths at risk for institutional misconduct: A meta-analytic investigation of the psychopathy checklist measures,' *Psychological Services*, *4*(1):13–27.

Edens, J. F., Skeem, J. L., Cruise, K. R., and Cauffman, E. (2001b) 'Assessment of "juvenile psychopathy" and its association with violence: A critical review,' *Behavioral Sciences and the Law*, *19*(1):53–80.

Essau, C. A., Sasagawa, S., and Frick, P. J. (2006) 'Callous–unemotional traits in a community sample of adolescents,' *Assessment*, *13*(4):454–469.

Farrington, D. P. (2005) 'The importance of child and adolescent psychopathy,' *Journal of Abnormal Child Psychology*, *33*(4):489–497.

Farrington, D. P. (2006) 'Family background and psychopathy,' in C. J. Patrick (Ed.), *Handbook of psychopathy* (pp. 229–250), New York, NY: Guilford.

Farrington, D. P. (2007) 'Social origins of psychopathy,' in A. R. Felthous & H. Sass (Eds.), *International handbook on psychopathic disorders and the law: Diagnosis and treatment* (Vol. 1, pp. 319–334), New York, NY: Wiley.

Forth, A. E., and Burke, H. C. (1998) 'Psychopathy in adolescence: Assessment, violence, and developmental precursors,' in D. Cooke, A. Forth, & R. D. Hare (Eds.), *Psychopathy: Theory, research, and implications for society* (pp. 205–230), Kluwer: Dordrecht.

Forth, A. E., Hart, S. D., and Hare, R. D. (1990). 'Assessment of psychopathy in young male offenders,' *Psychological Assessment*, *2*:342–344.

Forth, A. E., Kosson, D. S., and Hare, R. D. (2003) *Hare Psychopathy Checklist: Youth Version (PCL: YV)*, Toronto, ON: Multi-Health Systems.

Fox, B. H., Perez, N., Cass, E., Baglivio, M. T., and Epps, N. (2015) 'Trauma changes everything: Examining the relationship between adverse childhood experiences and serious, violent, and chronic juvenile offenders,' *Child Abuse and Neglect*, *46*:163–173.

Fox, J. (1997) *Applied regression analysis, linear models, and related methods*, Thousand Oaks, CA: Sage.

Frick, P. J., and Marsee, M. A. (2006) 'Psychopathy and developmental pathways to antisocial behavior in youth,' in C. J. Patrick (Ed.), *Handbook of psychopathy* (pp. 353–374), New York, NY: Guilford.

Frick, P. J., O'Brien, B. S., Wooton, M. M., and McBurnett, K. (1994) 'Psychopathy and conduct problems in children,' *Journal of Abnormal Psychology*, *103*:700–707.

Frick, P. J., Stickle, T. R., Dandreaux, D. M., Farrell, J. M., and Kimonis, E. R. (2005) 'Callous–unemotional traits in predicting the severity and stability of conduct problems and delinquency,' *Journal of Abnormal Child Psychology*, *33*:471–487.

Glenn, A. L., and Raine, A. (2008) 'The neurobiology of psychopathy,' *Psychiatric Clinics of North America*, *31*:463–475.

Glueck, S., and Glueck, E. T. (1930) *500 criminal careers*, New York, NY: Knopf.

Glueck, S., and Glueck, E. T. (1943) *Criminal careers in retrospect*, New York, NY: The Commonwealth Fund.

Gretton, H. M., Hare, R. D., and Catchpole, R. E. H. (2004) 'Psychopathy and offending from adolescence to adulthood: A 10-year follow-up,' *Journal of Consulting and Clinical Psychology*, *72*:636–645.

Gretton, H. M., McBride, M., Hare, R. D., O'Shaughnessy, R., and Kumka, G. (2001) 'Psychopathy and recidivism in adolescent sex offenders,' *Criminal Justice and Behavior*, *28*:427–449.

Hare, R. D. (1996) 'Psychopathy: A clinical construct whose time has come,' *Criminal Justice and Behavior*, *23*:25–54.

Hare, R. D. (1999) 'Psychopathy as a risk factor for violence,' *Psychiatric Quarterly*, *70*:181–197.

Hare, R. D. (2003) *Hare Psychopathy Checklist–Revised (PCL–R)* (2nd ed.), North Tonawanda, NY: Multi-Health Systems.

Hare, R. D., Hart, S. D., and Harpur, T. J. (1991) 'Psychopathy and the DSM–IV criteria for antisocial personality disorder,' *Journal of Abnormal Psychology*, *100*:391–398.

Hare, R. D., and Neumann, C. S. (2005) 'The structure of psychopathy,' *Current Psychiatry Reports*, 7:1–32.

Harris, G. T., Rice, M. E., and Cormier, C. A. (1991) 'Psychopathy and violent recidivism' *Law and Human Behavior*, *15*:625–637.

Hemphill, J. F., Templeman, R., Wong, S., and Hare, R. D. (1998) 'Psychopathy and crime: Recidivism and criminal careers,' in D. J. Cooke, A. E. Forth, & R. D. Hare (Eds.), *Psychopathy: Theory, research, and implications for society* (pp. 375–399), Boston, MA: Kluwer.

Holmqvist, R., Hill, T., and Lang, A. (2009) 'Effects of aggression replacement training in young offender institutions,' *International Journal of Offender Therapy and Comparative Criminology*, *53*:74–92.

Kosson, D. S., Cyterski, T. D., Steuerwald, B. L., Neumann, C. S., and Walker-Matthews, S. (2002) 'The reliability and validity of the PCL: YV in nonincarcerated adolescent males,' *Psychological Assessment*, *14*:97–109.

Kruh, I., Frick, P. J., and Clements, C. B. (2005) 'Historical and personality predictors of violence patterns in juveniles tried as adults,' *Criminal Justice and Behavior*, *32*:69–96.

Lawing, K., Frick, P. J., and Cruise, K. R. (2010) 'Differences in offending patterns between adolescent sex offenders high or low in callous–unemotional traits,' *Psychological Assessment*, *22*:298–305.

Lipsey, M. W. (2009) 'The primary factors that characterize effective interventions with juvenile offenders: A meta-analytic overview,' *Victims and Offenders*, *4*:124–147.

Loeber, R. (1982) 'The stability of antisocial and delinquent child behavior: A review,' *Child Development*, *53*:1431–1446.

Loeber, R., Farrington, D. P., and Petechuk, D. (2003) *Child delinquency: Early intervention and prevention*, Washington, DC: U. S. Department of Justice, Office of Juvenile Justice and Delinquency Prevention.

Loeber, R., Farrington, D. P., Stouthamer-Loeber, M., Moffitt, T. E., Caspi, A., and Lynam, D. R. (2001), 'Male mental health problems, psychopathy, and personality traits: Key findings from the first 14 years of the Pittsburgh Youth Study,' *Clinical Child and Family Psychology Review*, *4*(4):273–297.

Lynam, D. R. (1996) 'Early identification of chronic offenders: Who is a fledgling psychopath?,' *Psychological Bulletin*, *120*(2):209–234.

Lynam, D. R. (1998) 'Early identification of the fledgling psychopathy: Locating the psychopathic child in the current nomenclature,' *Journal of Abnormal Psychology*, *107*(4):566–575.

Lynam, D. R. (2002) 'Fledging psychopathy: A view from personality theory,' *Law and Human Behavior*, *26*:255–259.

Lynam, D. R., Caspi, A., Moffitt, T. E., Raine, A., Loeber, R., and Stouthamer-Loeber, M. (2005) 'Adolescent psychopathy and the Big Five: Results from two samples,' *Journal of Abnormal Child Psychology*, *33*(4):431–443.

Lynam, D. R., and Derefinko, K. J. (2006) 'Psychopathy and personality,' in C. J. Patrick (Ed.), *Handbook of psychopathy* (pp. 133–155), New York, NY: Guilford Press.
Lynam, D. R., Loeber, R., and Stouthamer-Loeber, M. (2008) 'The stability of psychopathy from adolescence into adulthood,' *Criminal Justice and Behavior, 35*:228–243.
Lynam, D. R., Miller, D. J., Vachon, D., Loeber, R., and Stouthamer-Loeber, M. (2009) 'Psychopathy in adolescence predicts official reports of offending in adulthood,' *Youth Violence and Juvenile Justice*, 7:189–207.
Lynam, D. R., and Widiger, T. A. (2007) 'Using a general model of personality to identify basic elements of psychopathy,' *Journal of Personality Disorders, 21*(2):160–178.
McCord, W., and McCord, J. (1964) *The psychopath: An essay on the criminal mind*, Princeton, NJ: Van Nostrand.
McCuish, E. C., Corrado, R., Lussier, P., and Hart, S. D. (2014) 'Psychopathic traits and offending trajectories from early adolescence to adulthood,' *Journal of Criminal Justice, 42*:66–76.
Millon, T. (1981) *Disorders of personality: DSM–III Axis II*, New York, NY: Wiley.
Moffitt, T. E. (1993) 'Adolescent-limited and life-course-persistent antisocial behavior: A developmental taxonomy,' *Psychological Review, 100*:674–701.
Murrie, D. C., Cornell, D. G., Kaplan, S., McConville, D., and Levy-Elkon, A. (2004) 'Psychopathy scores and violence among juvenile offenders: A multi-measure study,' *Behavioral Sciences and the Law, 22*(1):49–67.
Murrie, D. C., Cornell, D. G., and McCoy, W. (2005) 'Psychopathy, conduct disorder and stigma: Does diagnostic labeling influence juvenile probation officer recommendations?,' *Law and Human Behavior, 29*(3):323–342.
O'Neill, M. L., Lidz, V., and Heilbrun, K. (2003) 'Adolescents with psychopathic characteristics in a substance abusing cohort: Treatment process and outcomes,' *Law and Human Behavior, 27*:299–313.
Piquero, A. R., Farrington, D. P., and Blumstein, A. (2003) 'The criminal career paradigm: Background and recent developments,' in M. Tonry (Ed.), *Crime and justice: A review of research* (Vol. 30, pp. 359–506), Chicago, IL: University of Chicago Press.
Piquero, A. R., Farrington, D. P., Fontaine, N. M. G., Vincent, G., Coid, J., and Ullrich, S. (2012) 'Childhood risk, offending trajectories, and psychopathy at age 48 years in the Cambridge Study in Delinquent Development,' *Psychology, Public Policy, and Law, 18*:577–598.
Piquero, A. R., Jennings, W. G., Diamond, B., Farrington, D. P., Tremblay, R. E., Welsh, B. C., and Reingle-Gonzalez, J. M. (2016) 'A meta-analysis update on the effects of early family/parenting training programs on antisocial behavior and delinquency,' *Journal of Experimental Criminology, 12*:229–248.
Piquero, A. R., Jennings, W. G., and Farrington, D. P. (2010) 'On the malleability of self-control: Theoretical and policy implications regarding a general theory of crime,' *Justice Quarterly, 27*:803–834.
Piquero, A. R., Jennings, W. G., Farrington, D. P., Diamond, B., and Reingle Gonzalez, J. M. (2016) 'A meta-analysis update on the effectiveness of early self-control improvement programs to improve self-control and reduce delinquency,' *Journal of Experimental Criminology, 12*:249–264.
Robins, L. N., and O'Neal, P. (1958) 'Mortality, mobility and crime: Problem children thirty years later,' *American Sociological Review, 23*:162–171.
Salekin, R. T. (2002) 'Psychopathy and therapeutic pessimism: Clinical lore or clinical reality,' *Clinical Psychology Review, 22*:79–112.
Salekin, R. T., and Lynam, D. R. (2010) 'Child and adolescent psychopathy: An introduction,' in R. T. Salekin & D. R. Lynam (Eds.), *Handbook of child and adolescent psychopathy* (pp. 1–14), New York, NY: Guilford.
Schmidt, F., Campbell, M. A., and Houlding, C. (2011) 'Comparative analysis of the YLS/CMI, SAVRY, and PCL: YV in adolescent offenders: A 10 year follow-up into adulthood,' *Youth Violence and Juvenile Justice, 9*(1):23–42.
Schmidt, F., McKinnon, L., Chattha, H. K., and Brownlee, K. (2006) 'Concurrent and predictive validity of the Psychopathy Checklist: Youth Version across gender and ethnicity,' *Psychological Assessment, 18*:393–401.
Schwalbe, C. S. (2007) 'Risk assessment for juvenile justice: A meta-analysis,' *Law and Human Behavior, 31*:449–462
Seagrave, D., and Grisso, T. (2002) 'Adolescent development and measurement of juvenile psychopathy,' *Law and Human Behavior, 26*:291–239.
Shaffer, C., McCuish, E., Corrado, R. R., Behnken, M. P., and DeLisi, M. (2015) 'Psychopathy and violent misconduct in a sample of violent young offenders,' *Journal of Criminal Justice, 43*:321–326.

Simourd, D. J., and Hoge, R. D. (2000) 'Criminal psychopathy: A risk-and-need perspective,' *Criminal Justice and Behavior*, *27*:256–272.
Skeem, J. L., and Cauffman, E. (2003) 'Views of the downward extension: Comparing the youth version of the Psychopathy Checklist with the Youth Psychopathic Traits Inventory,' *Behavioral Sciences and the Law*, *21*(6):737–770.
Skeem, J. L., and Cooke, D. J. (2010) 'Is criminal behavior a central component of psychopathy? Conceptual directions for resolving debate,' *Psychological Assessment*, *22*:433–445.
Skeem, J. L., Monahan, J., and Mulvey, E. (2002) 'Psychopathy, treatment involvement, and subsequent violence among civil psychiatric patients,' *Law and Human Behavior*, *26*:577–603.
Stockdale, K. C., Olver, M. E., and Wong, S. C. (2010) 'The Psychopathy Checklist: Youth Version and adolescent and adult recidivism: Considerations with respect to gender, ethnicity, and age,' *Psychological Assessment*, *22*(4):768–781.
Vaughn, M. G., and DeLisi, M. (2008) 'Were Wolfgang's chronic offenders psychopaths? On the convergent validity between psychopathy and career criminality,' *Journal of Criminal Justice*, *36*:33–42.
Vaughn, M. G., and Howard, M. O. (2005) 'The construct of psychopathy and its potential contribution to the study of serious, violent, and chronic offending,' *Youth Violence and Juvenile Justice*, *3*:235–352.
Vaughn, M. G., Howard, M. O., and DeLisi, M. (2008) 'Psychopathic personality traits and delinquent careers: An empirical examination,' *International Journal of Law and Psychiatry*, *31*:407–416.
Vaughn, M. G., Newhill, C. E., DeLisi, M., Beaver, K. M., and Howard, M. O. (2008) 'An investigation of psychopathic features among delinquent girls: Violence, theft, and drug abuse,' *Youth Violence and Juvenile Justice*, *6*(3):240–255.
Vincent, G. M., Odgers, C. L., McCormick, A. V., and Corrado, R. R. (2008) 'The PCL: YV and recidivism in male and female juveniles: A follow-up into young adulthood,' *International Journal of Law and Psychiatry*, *31*:287–296.
Vincent, G. M., Vitacco, M. J., Grisso, T., and Corrado, R. R. (2003) 'Subtypes of adolescent offenders: Affective traits and antisocial behavior patterns,' *Behavioral Science and the Law*, *21*:695–712.
Waldman, I. D., and Rhee, S. H. (2006) 'Genetic and environmental influences on psychopathy and antisocial behavior,' in C. J. Patrick (Ed.), *Handbook of psychopathy* (pp. 205–228), New York, NY: Guilford.
Walters, G. D. (2003) 'Predicting institutional adjustment and recidivism with the psychopathy checklist factor scores: A meta-analysis,' *Law and Human Behavior*, *27*:541–558.
Walters, G. D. (2004) 'The trouble with psychopathy as a general theory of crime,' *International Journal of Offender Therapy and Comparative Criminology*, *48*:133–148.
Widiger, T. A., and Lynam, D. R. (1998) 'Psychopathy and the five-factor model of personality,' in T. Millon, E. Simonsen, M. Birket-Smith, & R. D. Davis (Eds.), *Psychopathy: Antisocial, criminal, and violent behavior* (pp. 171–187), New York, NY: Guilford.
Winokur-Early, K., Hand, G. A., and Blankenship, J. L. (2012) *Validity and reliability of the Florida Positive Achievement Change Tool (PACT) risk and needs assessment instrument: A three-phase evaluation (validation study, factor analysis, inter-rater reliability)*, Tallahassee, FL: Justice Research Center.
Wolfgang, M. E., Figlio, R. M., and Selin, T. (1972). *Delinquency in a birth cohort*, Chicago, IL: University of Chicago Press.

38

Psychopathy and sex offender recidivism

Mark E. Olver

Introduction

I often deliver trainings on working therapeutically with sex offenders who have prominent psychopathic characteristics and like to begin by asking the audience for examples of "psychopaths" in the media. Anywhere in North America, with almost perfect reliability, an enthusiastic participant will shout "Ted Bundy!" And if I am in the U.S., most frequently other examples that will follow include Jeffrey Dahmer, John Wayne Gacy, Kenneth Bianchi, or other infamous personalities endemic to the city or state. In Canada, during such trainings, participants will usually call out Paul Bernardo, Clifford Olson, "The Pig Farmer" (Robert Picton), or even "The Colonel" (Russell Williams). "But what do these men have in common?" I like to ask. People will usually identify that they are white males (which is correct; they most certainly are), and with further discussion it becomes apparent that they are all sexually sadistic, psychopathic serial murderers. Not only are they psychopathic, but they have committed a high volume of serious offenses with extremely high human costs and enormous amounts of pain and suffering incurred to victims and their families. All of these men planned and premeditated their offenses, lured and abducted their victims, and tortured, sexually assaulted, and murdered them – victims who ranged from adult women and teenage girls, to young men, to children.

The exercise is telling because it reveals that even well-trained mental health and criminal justice professionals unconsciously equate psychopathy with sexual violence, and when they summon up exemplars of the psychopath, they conjure up frightening and grisly media portrayals that have been deeply embedded in the public psyche. But this exercise also belies some misconceptions of psychopathy as it relates to sexual offending. Most sex offenders are not psychopaths. Even among those that are, not all of them are necessarily high risk for sexual violence. And, certainly, most do not kill their victims or experience heightened arousal from their suffering. So what role does psychopathy have in the assessment and management of sexual violence risk? In this chapter, I address each of these issues in detail, drawing on the research evidence available.

In this chapter, the operationalization of psychopathy will refer to the clinical syndrome as measured by the Hare Psychopathy Checklist Revised (PCL–R; Hare, 1991,2003), a 20-item symptom construct rating scale designed to assess psychopathy. With possible scores ranging from 0 to 40, the total score on the instrument represents the extent to which the individual assessed resembles the prototypical psychopath. As noted frequently in chapters throughout this handbook, the PCL–R yields a total score that can also be broken down into the interpersonal and affective features and chronic antisocial lifestyle pattern. In turn, Factor 1 can be disaggregated into two second order factors or facets, interpersonal (e.g., deceitfulness, manipulation) and affective (e.g., callous lack of empathy, lack of remorse), while Factor 2 can be disaggregated into the lifestyle (e.g., impulsivity, irresponsibility) and antisocial (e.g., early behavioral problems, poor behavior controls, criminal versatility) facets.

Psychopathy is often featured prominently in sexual violence evaluations (Hare, 1996), whether at the point of sentencing or in consideration of possible release. Twenty-two U.S. states have a sexual violence civil commitment statute (not uncommonly called Sexually Violent Predator or SVP laws), which permits the civil commitment of an individual following the expiration of their prison term to a secure psychiatric facility for an indefinite period of time owing to a legal finding of being sexually dangerous. While the details of the legislation vary state by state, a common thread is that the individual must have a diagnosable mental illness of some sort (this could include a paraphilia or personality disorder, among other psychiatric diagnoses), pose a high risk for sexual violence, and be concluded that their risk cannot be managed safely in the community. Naturally, psychopathy features prominently in SVP evaluations, and not uncommonly the PCL–R will be used in tandem with one or more specialized sexual violence risk assessment tools to appraise risk and to make determinations regarding the potential for future sexual violence.

Base rates of psychopathy in sex offender populations

How common is psychopathy in sex offender populations? This is a deceptively simple question. The men who commit sex offenses have considerable diversity in their modus operandi (e.g., planning and premeditation, hands on vs. hands off) and victim profiles (e.g., male vs. female, child vs. teen vs. adult, related vs. unrelated), which in turn are linked to different psychosocial and criminogenic needs. Profiles of psychopathy have been most frequently examined among sex offenders who commit contact, or hands on, sex offenses (e.g., sexual assault, sexual touching) who vary among victim profile: (1) men with adult or post-pubescent teen (usually female) victims (often termed rapists elsewhere in the literature); (2) men with extrafamilial (i.e., unrelated) child victims (frequently referred to as child molesters); (3) men with intrafamilial (i.e., related biologically or through marriage, as in the case of stepchildren) child victims (frequently referred to an incest offenders); and (4) men with both child and adult or teen victims, usually referred to as mixed offenders.

Table 38.1 summarizes the results of a representative sampling of studies that have examined profiles of psychopathy. The studies vary by sample composition, geographic region, and PCL–R cut score used to characterize psychopathy. As seen here, approximately one-third of men with adult victims across the samples are characterized as psychopathic, and as many as one-third to two-thirds of mixed offenders (i.e., having both child and adult victims). By contrast, the base rates of psychopathy and overall scores are considerably lower for men with child victims; the modal base rate is lower than 10 percent for both intrafamilial and extrafamilial offenders. What explains these profiles? Research has demonstrated that men with adult victims tend to resemble non-sexual offenders in their psychological and criminological characteristics more than do men with child victims. Specifically, men with adult victims tend to have a history of non-sexual crime and to demonstrate more characteristics indicative of general lifestyle antisociality, such as problems with substance use, impulsivity, and anger/hostility (Marx, Miranda, & Meyerson, 1999; Olver, Wong, Nicholaichuk, & Gordon, 2007). Thus, as shown in Table 38.1, they tend to register higher scores

Table 38.1 Profiles of PCL–R measured psychopathy in sex offender samples

Study	*Country*	*PCL–R cut-off*	*Adult offender*	*Mixed offender*	*Extrafamilial child*	*Intrafamilial child*	*Overall*
Beggs and Grace (2008)	New Zealand	25	–	–	*n* = 92 BR = 6.5 Tot = 9.5 (8.1)	*n* = 124 BR = 3.2 Tot = 7.2 (6.4)	*N* = 216 BR = 4.6 Tot = 8.2 (7.3)
Brown et al. (2015)	USA	30	*n* = 468 BR = 25.5 Tot = 24.3 (7.0) F1 = 9.2 (3.3) F2 = 12.6 (4.1)	*n* = 40 BR = 32.5 Tot = 26.7 (6.2) F1 = 10.4 (3.1) F2 = 13.6 (3.5)	*n* = 211 (combined child group) BR = 13.7 Tot = 21.3 (7.5) F1 = 7.9 (3.4) F2 = 11.2 (4.8)		*N* = 719 BR = 22.3 Tot = 23.6 (7.1) F1 = 8.9 (3.3) F2 = 12.2 (4.3)
Brown and Forth (1997)	Canada	30	*N* = 60 BR = 35.0 Tot = 24.9 (6.7) F1 = 8.6 (4.0) F2 = 12.1 (2.9)	–	–	–	*N* = 60 BR = 35.0 Tot = 24.9 (6.7) F1 = 8.6 (4.0) F2 = 12.1 (2.9)
Hildebrand et al. (2004)	Netherlands	26	*n* = 94 BR = 35.1 Tot = 22.2 (7.3) F1 = 7.7 (3.5) F2 = 11.8 (4.7)	–	–	–	*N* = 94 BR = 35.1 Tot = 22.2 (7.3) F1 = 7.7 (3.5) F2 = 11.8 (4.7)
Langton et al. (2006); (see also Seto et al., 2004)	Canada	25	–	–	–	–	*N* = 418 BR = 15.8 Tot = 15.6 (7.2)
Looman et al. (2005)	Canada	25	–	–	–	–	*N* = 272 BR = 41.5 Tot = 22.3 (7.7)
Olver and Wong (2006; 2009)	Canada	25	*n* = 76 BR = 36.8 Tot = 21.9 (7.3) F1 = 6.3 (3.5) F2 = 11.1 (4.1)	*n* = 26 BR = 42.3 Tot = 22.7 (7.3) F1 = 6.4 (3.9) F2 = 11.4 (3.5)	*n* = 25 BR = 4.0 Tot = 15.9 (5.8) F1 = 5.5 (2.9) F2 = 7.8 (3.5)	*n* = 29 BR = 17.2 Tot = 17.7 (6.8) F1 = 5.3 (2.8) F2 = 7.8 (4.8)	*N* = 156 BR = 28.8 Tot = 20.2 (7.4) F1 = 6.0 (3.3) F2 = 20.2 (7.4)

Porter et al. (2000)	Canada	30	*n* = 103 BR = 35.9 Tot = 25.9 (5.9) F1 = 10.1 (3.4) F2 = 12.0 (3.3)	*n* = 25 BR = 64.0 Tot = 29.0 (6.5) F1 = 11.8 (4.2) F2 = 12.3 (3.0)	*n* = 48 BR = 6.3 Tot = 20.9 (6.1) F1 = 9.3 (3.6) F2 = 8.3 (4.0)	*n* = 37 BR = 10.8 Tot = 21.2 (6.4) F1 = 10.2 (3.2) F2 = 7.6 (4.5)	*N* = 229 BR = 26.8 Tot = 24.1 (6.7) F1 = 10.1 (3.5) F2 = 10.3 (4.3)
Rice and Harris (1997)	Canada	25	*n* = 88 Tot = 18.8 (9.0)	*n* = 58 Tot = 21.5 (8.1)	*n* = 142 (combined child group) Tot = 13.4 (6.9)		*N* = 288 Tot = 16.7 (7.8)
Serin et al. (1994)	Canada	29	*n* = 33 BR = 12.2 Tot = 17.1 (8.6) F1 = 6.2 F2 = 9.4	–	*n* = 32 (combined child group) BR = 7.5 Tot = 13.2 (7.8) F1 = 4.7 F2 = 7.0		*N* = 65 BR = 9.9 Tot = 15.3 (8.4) F1 = 5.5 F2 = 8.3

Note. BR = base rate of psychopathy (%); Tot = mean PCL–R total score (*SD*); F1 = mean Factor 1 score (*SD*); F2 = mean Factor 2 score (*SD*).

on Factor 2 and the lifestyle and antisocial facets than the men who target child victims, while the differences on the Factor 1 domains tend to be much smaller by comparison (e.g., Olver & Wong, 2006; Porter et al., 2000). Porter et al. (2000), for instance, found that mixed offenders and men who targeted adult women (i.e., committed acts of rape) had very similar PCL–R profiles to non-sexual offenders, with the profiles between the two latter groups being almost indistinguishable. In conclusion, not all sex offenders are psychopathic. Rather, a very small minority of child sex offenders could be classified as psychopathic, while larger minority (around one-third) of men with adult victims or mixed adult and child victim profiles may fit this designation.

Predictive accuracy of the PCL–R for sex offender recidivism

The PCL–R is frequently used in sexual violence evaluations, as noted in the outset of this chapter, presumably on the grounds that PCL–R scores and a designation of psychopathy more specifically are informative for criminal justice decision-making purposes. The PCL–R was not developed as a risk assessment tool but rather as an objective personality and behaviorally based clinical rating scale intended to assess the features of psychopathy. Given that the interpersonal, affective, and behavioral features of psychopathy are conducive to antisocial behavior, the tool has demonstrated strong predictive accuracy for a number of correctional outcomes across diverse offender samples.

Meta-analytic findings

In the most comprehensive meta-analysis to date on the topic of PCL–R measured psychopathy and sex offender recidivism, Hawes, Boccaccini, and Murrie (2013) aggregated the predictive effects of PCL–R total, factor, and facet scores for sexual and violent recidivism across 20 studies and 5,239 offenders. In terms of the prediction of sexual recidivism, PCL–R total scores ($d = .40$, $k = 20$), Factor 2 scores ($d = .44$, $k = 13$), and antisocial facet scores ($d = .40$, $k = 5$) all demonstrated moderate in magnitude effects (see Rice & Harris, 2005) and significantly predicted this outcome, while scores on Factor 1 ($d = .17$, $k = 13$), and the interpersonal ($d = .06$, $k = 5$), affective ($d = .01$, $k = 5$), and lifestyle ($d = .09$, $k = 5$) facets did not. Similar findings were obtained when examining the prediction of general violent recidivism (i.e., sexual or non-sexual), but the magnitude of the PCL–R total score's prediction of sexual or violent recidivism was stronger across a smaller collection of studies ($d = .55$, $k = 13$), while the disparity in the magnitude of prediction between Factor 1 ($d = .08$, $k = 8$) vs. Factor 2 ($d = .63$, $k = 8$) was larger. The same trend was observed in the prediction of non-sexual violent recidivism: PCL–R total ($d = .63$, $k = 11$), Factor 1 ($d = .06$, $k = 6$), and Factor 2 ($d = .70$, $k = 6$). (Facet level effects were not examined for either violent outcomes owing to the smaller number of studies.) The results from the Hawes et al. (2013) meta-analysis on the predictive accuracy of PCL–R scores for violent recidivism showed the same general trends as with the general and non-sexual offender literature (e.g., Campbell, French, & Gendreau, 2009; Yang, Wong, & Coid, 2010), with total scores demonstrating moderate in magnitude prediction, stronger predictive accuracy observed for Factor 2, and weaker predictive accuracy for Factor 1.

Incremental prediction of sex offender recidivism: understanding the association

Other lines of research have examined the predictive efficacy of the PCL–R for recidivism in other ways, namely, its incremental predictive validity for recidivism among sex offenders after controlling for scores on purpose-built risk assessment tools through Cox or logistic regression analyses. The results have been informative. In a sample of 156 treated sexual offenders, Olver and Wong (2009) found the PCL–R total score significantly predicted sexual recidivism when entered on its own in the first step of a regression model; however, the PCL–R no longer significantly predicted this outcome after controlling for scores on a sex offender risk assessment and treatment planning tool, the Violence Risk Scale–Sexual Offender version (VRS–SO; Wong, Olver, Nicholaichuk, & Gordon, 2003). VRS–SO static and dynamic scores, by contrast, were incrementally predictive of sexual recidivism after controlling for the PCL–R. In regression models examining the prediction of general violence (i.e., sexual and non-sexual), however, both the PCL–R total score and the VRS–SO were incrementally predictive of this outcome. Further, results of survival analyses also demonstrated that high psychopathy men scoring high risk for sexual violence had double the rates of sexual recidivism than similarly psychopathic offenders who had scored as low risk for sexual violence. How can two groups of seemingly equally psychopathic offenders have different rates of recidivism?

Correlational analyses between the PCL–R and VRS–SO dynamic factors demonstrated that the tool had particularly strong associations with the criminality dimension of the VRS–SO but correlated weakly with the sexual deviance dimension. What the above lines of research demonstrate is that not all high PCL–R scoring sex offenders are necessarily high risk for sexual violence; there are a number of critical prognostic variables that underpin risk for sexual offending, not the least of which is sexual deviance (e.g., atypical sexual interests, sexual compulsivity), which are not captured by the PCL–R and the psychopathy construct in general. This should not come as a surprise since: 1) the PCL–R was also not designed to assess risk for sexual violence (just as it was not designed to assess risk for other forms of recidivism); and 2) not all psychopathic offenders are sexually deviant. The latter point will be discussed in further detail in the next section. The PCL–R, however, remained a strong, consistent predictor of general violence, in part by virtue of its ability to capture the latent dimension of general criminality or antisociality. As such, although high PCL–R scoring sex offenders may not all be high risk for sexual recidivism (a specialized sexual violence risk assessment tool would need to be administered to determine that), they are more likely to still pose a high risk for general violence and generalized trouble (violent or nonviolent) within the institution and community on release.

A "deadly combination"? Psychopathy and sexual deviance

Although several static and dynamic risk markers underpin sexual recidivism risk, the extant literature has identified two primary dimensions as alluded to earlier: sexual deviance, which encompasses a pattern of atypical sexual interests (e.g., coercion, sex with children, paraphilias) and compulsive sexual thoughts and behaviors; and general criminality or antisociality, which encompasses a general lifestyle pattern and criminogenic need conducive to antisocial behavior, including the presence of antisocial peers, family and marital problems, substance abuse, employment and financial concerns, Anger and generalized aggression, and so forth (Hanson & Morton-Bourgon, 2005; Olver et al., 2017). When men have prominent concerns in both areas, they are likely to pose high risk for future sexual violence absent successful participation in treatment or engagement in other remediation or risk management efforts (e.g., Olver et al., 2007).

Examining the psychopathy–deviance link

As noted above, research has demonstrated the PCL–R, and Factor 2 scores in particular, to have strong convergent associations with general risk and needs that overlap with the general criminality dimension among sexual offenders (Olver & Wong, 2009), violent offenders (Douglas, Yeomans, & Boer 2005; Wong & Gordon, 2006), and general offender samples (Simourd & Hoge, 2000). The literature on associations between psychopathy and sexual deviance is less consistent. As noted above, Olver and Wong (2009) did not find PCL–R total, Factor 1, or Factor 2 scores to have strong correlations with sexual deviance ($r = -.09$ to .14, *ns*). Similarly, Seto, Harris, Rice, and Barbaree (2004) found a brief screen for pedophilic interests had modest, non-significant correlations with PCL–R total scores across two samples of adult male sex offenders with child victims ($r = .00$ and .05). In a small sample of incarcerated sex offenders ($N = 65$), Serin, Malcolm, Khanna, and Barbaree (1994) found moderate in magnitude correlations between PCL–R scores and phallometric measurements of deviant sexual arousal, with total, Factor 1, and Factor 2 scores showing broadly comparable associations across subgroups of child sexual abusers and men with adult victims ($r = .27$ to .37). In a large ($N = 489$) non-offender community sample, Dyer et al. (2016) found Self-Report Psychopathy–Short Form–III (SRP–SF–III; Paulhus, Neumann, & Hare, 2017) total scores and each of the four facets to have significant correlations with self-reported sexual compulsivity ($r = .28$ to .40), paraphilic fantasy ($r = .24$ to .32), and fantasies of eroticized dominance ($r = .17$ to .39). What was interesting was that the antisocial facet had the weakest associations out of the four facets with indexes of deviant sexual fantasy and sexual compulsivity.

Psychopathy, sexual deviance, and recidivism

When the combination of high levels of sexual deviance and psychopathy do occur, Hare (1999) has referred to this as the "deadly combination," asserting that the two in tandem serve to escalate the risk for sexual violence. Approximately half a dozen studies to date have examined this assertion. The most typical paradigm is to divide the sample into high and low psychopathy groups using a PCL–R cut score – sometimes this may be a median split or one of the suggested diagnostic cut-offs (usually a variation from 25 to 30) – and then subdivide the psychopathic and non-psychopathic groups into high and low deviance groups using an index of sexual deviance. As the aforementioned discussion linking psychopathy to sexual deviance illustrates, the range of potential measures utilized is quite diverse, ranging from clinical rating scales to physiological measures such as phallometry. Four groups are typically created: high psychopathy–high deviance (HPHD), high psychopathy–low deviance (HPLD), low psychopathy–high deviance (LPHD), and low psychopathy–low deviance (LPLD). Trajectories of recidivism (usually sexual or violent) among the four groups are then typically examined through survival analysis, which controls for differences in follow-up time, or alternatively, frequency counts of binary recidivism are compared between the groups through chi-square analysis. All but one study in this line of research was conducted in Canada (the exception being Hildebrand, de Ruiter, & de Vogel, 2004), most frequently on federal offender samples (i.e., men serving sentences of at least two years' duration).

One of the first studies to examine the association was Serin, Mailloux, and Malcolm (2001) on a Canadian sample of 68 federal sex offenders that overlapped with Serin et al. (1994), described previously. Using a combination of phallometric deviance scores and a median PCL–R split of 15.5, they found that men scoring high on both dimensions (HPHD) had higher rates of general recidivism (i.e., any kind of reoffending) than the other three groups; however, associations with sexual or violent recidivism were not examined, perhaps owing to a lack of power from the small sample size and low recidivism base rates. Rice and Harris (1997) found evidence for a psychopathy deviance interaction in a sample of 288 released sexual offenders, grouped by phallometric deviance score and a PCL–R cut score of 25 followed up five years post-release.

HDHP men demonstrated the highest and fastest rates of sexual recidivism (60 percent), followed by HPLD (48 percent) men, and lower observed rates (25 percent and 20 percent) among the LPHD and LPLD groups, respectively; however, when Rice and Harris (1997) examined rates of general violent recidivism, they simply found psychopathic men to have higher rates of violent failure than the two low psychopathy groups irrespective of deviance. In a Canadian multisite evaluation of 396 sex offenders released from four prison settings followed up four years post-release, Harris et al. (2003) generated similar findings to Rice and Harris (1997) using a PCL–R median split of 17.5 coupled with the results of phallometry to create their four psychopathy–deviance groups.

Seto et al. (2004) examined trajectories of sexual recidivism in two samples of child sexual abusers (*N*s = 113 and 145) using median splits on the Screening Scale for Pedophilic Interests (SSPI) (> 2) and PCL–R (12 and 20, respectively) to create the four psychopathy–deviance groups. Both investigations demonstrated support for a psychopathy–deviance interaction. However, the second, larger study (which also featured a longer follow-up) demonstrated the most striking effect with 60 percent of HPHD men sexually reoffending, in contrast to much lower sexual recidivism rates ranging from 16–21 percent for the remaining psychopathy–deviance groups scoring low on one or both measures. In one of the few non-Canadian studies of the phenomenon, Hildebrand et al. (2004) examined the association of PCL–R measured psychopathy (using a cut score of 26) and sexual deviance, assessed via the Sexual Violence Risk–20 (SVR–20; Boer, Hart, Kropp, & Webster, 1997) deviant sexual preference item, to several recidivism outcomes. Featuring a sample from the Netherlands of 94 adult male sex offenders with exclusively adult victims followed up nearly 12 years post-release, the HPHD group had a substantially higher and faster rate of sexual recidivism (82 percent) than the remaining HPLD (25 percent), LPHD (30 percent), and LPLD (18 percent) groups. Again, both high psychopathy groups had higher and faster trajectories of non-sexual violent, general violent, and any kind of recidivism at all compared to low PCL–R scorers, irrespective of deviance. Moreover, Olver and Wong (2006) investigated the psychopathy–deviance recidivism link in a sample of 156 treated sex offenders followed up nearly ten years post-release. Using a PCL–R cut score of 25 and a median split on the VRS–SO sexual deviance factor, HPHD men demonstrated the highest rate of sexual recidivism (40.8 percent), but this was only significantly different from the lowest risk group (LPLD, 16.4 percent), and was not compared to the groups scoring high on psychopathy and low on deviance (30.4 percent) or vice versa (32 percent). Comparison of the recidivism trajectories for the four groups for general non-sexual recidivism demonstrated the highest recidivism rate for the two high psychopathy groups consistent with previous findings.

Finally, one of the few studies to not find evidence for a psychopathy–deviance interaction was Looman, Morphett, and Abracen (2013), who examined the phenomenon in a sample of 272 treated high-risk sex offenders followed up 6.7 years post-release. The sample had a mean Static–99R score of 5.4 (medium–high risk or above average, using conventional risk language) and, employing the 25-point cut-off, more than 40 percent of the sample could be classified as psychopathic (see Table 38.1). The conventional four psychopathy–deviance groups were created using the 25-point cut score and deviant–nondeviant groupings based on phallometric assessment. Contrary to the body of research reviewed previously, HPHD men were not any more likely to be charged or convicted for a new sexual offense (11.7 percent) compared to the HPLD (14.8 percent), LPHD (18.9 percent), and LPLD (12.8 percent) groups. When the four groups were compared on rates of violent (including sexual) recidivism, the two high psychopathy groups had the highest rates of general violent recidivism compared to the two low psychopathy groups, irrespective of deviance. Cox regression survival analyses, examining the psychopathy–deviance interaction, controlling for Static–99R score, did not change the findings.

Of note, sexual deviance indices were modest but significant predictors of sexual recidivism but not violence, while the PCL–R was a significant predictor of violence but not sexual recidivism. In this sample, it would seem the two constructs were working at cross purposes in the prediction of each outcome, perhaps contributing to the absence of an additive or interaction effect.

A synthesis of key findings: results from meta-analysis

In their meta-analysis, Hawes et al. (2013) aggregated the findings across the seven samples reviewed earlier, examining the association of psychopathy and sexual deviance to sexual recidivism. As there were some studies that overlapped in sample composition, the odds ratio was computed twice and, in all, demonstrated a 2.80 to 3.21 increase in the odds of sexual violence when both high levels of psychopathy and sexual deviance were present. This is a large effect, translating into equivalent *d* values of .83 and .95, respectively, for the combined association of psychopathy and sexual deviance with sexual recidivism. Why does this risk-related phenomenon exist? Arguably, the psychopathy construct serves as a proxy for general criminality in its nexus with sexual deviance, and this contributes unique risk variance that increases, and in some samples even interacts with, the deviance construct to augment risk for sexual violence. When one considers some of the most notorious figures in the media who have committed particularly heinous offenses, mentioned at the outset of this chapter, they epitomize the combination of psychopathy and sexual deviance – Bundy, Bianchi, Gacy, Olson, Dahmer, Bernardo, and the like – fortunately, cases as extreme as these are a slim minority.

Clinical applications of PCL–R measured psychopathy in sexual violence risk assessment

The previous review of the psychopathy deviance literature is instructive in informing the role of the psychopathy construct and potential uses of the PCL scales in sexual violence risk assessment. This final section discusses clinical applications of the PCL–R in recidivism risk assessment with sex offenders.

First, the PCL–R is not intended to be used as a standalone measure, but rather to compliment other validated and well-established sexual violence risk assessment schemes (Hare, 2003). As the research reviewed previously has demonstrated, the PCL–R has relatively modest predictive accuracy for sexual recidivism specifically and tends not to be incremental in the prediction of this outcome over and above a validated sexual violence risk instrument. Aside from this, an instrument with dynamic risk items is needed not only to augment appraisals of risk, but also to identify where to intervene for the purposes of treatment planning, as well as assessing possible changes in risk from treatment or other risk management efforts. The total score is typically the most informative piece of psychopathy-related data from the PCL–R, as it has the greatest stability in predictive accuracy across meta-analytic findings and it represents the totality of the individual's level of psychopathic traits.

High or low psychopathy scores are informative either way. If the individual scores low on the PCL–R (e.g., bottom quartile among North American male offenders), they are also more likely to be low risk for non-sexual violence and serious institutional management problems, and more likely to cooperate with their correctional plan and recommended interventions; however, they could still be high risk for sexual recidivism (e.g., sexual contact with a child). If the individual scores high on the PCL–R (e.g., 85th percentile of the large normative sample), then they are also very likely to be high risk for general violence, nonviolent criminal recidivism, release failure, serious institutional management problems, and to present resistance and lack motivation for following recommended interventions. However, they may be average or even low risk for sexual recidivism (or they could be quite high risk), to be established by a formalized sexual violence risk assessment scheme. Men who have high PCL–R scores and are also high risk for sexual violence could well have prominent concerns in the sexual deviance domain, broadly speaking (whether this reflects actual deviant interests or a general pattern of sexual maladjustment), and represent the problematic combination discussed at length earlier.

Second, the PCL–R should not be used to screen out suitability for sex offender treatment or other types of treatment interventions (Wong & Hare, 2005). Although high PCL–R scoring men are more likely to pose management concerns (as discussed below), they do not always pose the level of concern anticipated, and such concerns are par for the course in working with correctional clientele and, in many instances, such issues can be managed. Instead, high PCL–R men should be prioritized for high intensity and comprehensive services, particularly if they are also high risk for sexual violence and/or have the problematic combination of prominent psychopathic traits coupled with maladjusted sexual functioning.

Finally, it is worth examining the PCL–R factor and facet profile. The factor and facet combinations can be very informative for case formulation and intervention planning, as high scores on each mean different things. For instance, high scores on Factor 1 and the interpersonal and/or affective facets are responsivity issues (Wong & Hare, 2005), that is, they represent aspects of the client that can impact response to services which signal the need to adapt and tailor service delivery (Bonta & Andrews, 2017). Men who score high on the interpersonal facet can be expected to be evasive, manipulative, to play staff off of one another, to embellish, to have a heightened sense of self-importance, engage in posturing, test boundaries, and/or to be interpersonally abrasive or condescending to staff and co-patients. Concordantly, individuals scoring high on the affective facet can be expected to lack insight or personal awareness into their problem issues, to externalize blame, to lack compassion or empathy for others, and to be deficient in their ability to form emotional ties or to identify emotionally with their victims. In terms of response to sex offender treatment, these features are associated with decreased therapeutic progress (Sewall & Olver, 2017), increased attrition (Olver & Wong, 2011), and weaker working alliances (DeSorcy, Olver, & Wormith, 2017); however, they can be managed.

Moreover, high scores on Factor 2 and the lifestyle and/or antisocial facets represent risk and need issues (Wong & Hare, 2005), as they tend to be more predictive of sexual recidivism (and other recidivism outcomes), and to be correlated with the volume and density of criminogenic need. Men scoring high on the lifestyle facet can be expected to be impulsive, irresponsible, to live in the moment, start and stop tasks, grow bored easily, demand immediate gratification, and to have poor therapeutic work ethic. Indeed, the work of DeSorcy et al. (2017) found that high score on the lifestyle facet was associated with failure to fulfill the tasks and goals of therapy in a sex offender treatment program. In turn, men who score high on the antisocial facet will have a lengthy, serious, and diverse pattern of antisocial behavior, often including violence, beginning at an early age and persisting unabated across the lifespan. Interestingly, however, the lines of research cited above have indicated that high antisocial facet scores bear little unique association with the ability to make therapeutic gains, establish working alliances, or to complete treatment; men scoring high on the antisocial facet may be high risk in a broad sense, but this seems to have little bearing on their ability to engage in or benefit from treatment.

Conclusion

In conclusion, the PCL–R and psychopathy construct more broadly speaking have important clinical relevance in the assessment of sexual violence risk, prediction of sex offender recidivism, and management of risk to prevent recidivism and promote reintegration. Although the moniker "psychopathic sex offender" understandably strikes at the heart of fears and anxieties of therapists and community supervision officers, the majority of sex offenders in custody and on community supervision do not have exceptionally high PCL–R scores, and among those that do, not all are necessarily high risk for sexual violence or are fated to reoffend in a spectacular and horrific fashion. Although the PCL–R has high prognostic relevance for violent and general recidivism, research to date has demonstrated that it is a more modest predictor of sexual recidivism; the exception seems to be when high levels of psychopathy and sexual deviance co-exist, which the bulk of available literature has indicated serves to augment risk for future sexual violence. Importantly, scrutiny of PCL–R profiles, in tandem with the use of validated sexual violence risk assessment tools, can be used to inform the assessment of risk and treatment intensity, identify treatment needs, and identify responsivity issues to be managed in sex offender treatment, all of which are intended to retain the very clientele in risk management services who need it, and who also stand to benefit, the most.

References

Beggs, S. M., and Grace, R. C. (2008) 'Psychopathy, intelligence and recidivism in child molesters: Evidence of an interaction effect,' *Criminal Justice and Behavior*, *35*:683–695.

Boer, D. P., Hart, S. D., Kropp, P. R., and Webster, C. D. (1997) *Manual for the Sexual Violence Risk–20: Professional guidelines for assessing risk of sexual violence*, Vancouver, BC: Institute against Family Violence and the Mental Health, Law, and Policy Institute, Simon Fraser University.

Bonta, J., and Andrews, D. A. (2017) *The psychology of criminal conduct* (6th ed.), New York, NY: Routledge.

Brown, A. R., Dargis, M. A., Mattern, A. C., Tsonis, M. A., and Newman, J. P. (2015) 'Elevated psychopathy scores among mixed sexual offenders: Replication and extension,' *Criminal Justice and Behavior*, *42*:1032–1044.

Brown, S. L., and Forth, A. E. (1997) 'Psychopathy and sexual assault: Static risk factors, emotional precursors, and rapist subtypes,' *Journal of Consulting and Clinical Psychology*, *65*:848–857.

Campbell, M. A., French, S., and Gendreau, P. (2009) 'The prediction of violence in adult offenders: A meta-analytic comparison of instruments and methods of assessment,' *Criminal Justice and Behavior*, *36*:567–590.

DeSorcy, D. R., Olver, M. E., and Wormith, J. S. (2017) 'Working alliance and psychopathy: Linkages to treatment outcome in a sample of treated sexual offenders,' *Journal of Interpersonal Violence*, in press.

Douglas, K., Yeomans, M., and Boer, D. (2005) 'Comparative validity analysis of multiple measures of violence risk in a sample of criminal offenders,' *Criminal Justice and Behavior*, *32*:479–510.

Dyer, T. J., Olver, M. E., Hitikasch, M., Merdian, H. L., Hogue, T., Perley-Robertson, B., . . . and Ralph, N. (2016) 'Self-reported psychopathy and its association with deviant sexual fantasy and sexual compulsivity in a nonclinical sample,' *Sexual Offender Treatment*, *11*:1–8.

Hanson, R. K., and Morton-Bourgon, K. (2005) 'The characteristics of persistent sexual offenders: A meta-analysis of recidivism studies,' *Journal of Consulting and Clinical Psychology*, *73*:1154–1163.

Hare, R. D. (1991) *The Hare Psychopathy Checklist–Revised*, Toronto, ON: Multi-Health Systems.

Hare, R. D. (1996) 'Psychopathy, a clinical construct whose time has come,' *Criminal Justice and Behavior*, *23*:25–54.

Hare, R. D. (1999) 'Psychopathy as a risk factor for violence,' *Psychiatric Quarterly*, *70*:181–197.

Hare, R. D. (2003) *Manual for the Revised Psychopathy Checklist* (2nd ed.), Toronto, ON: Multi-Health Systems.

Harris, G. T., Rice, M. E., Quinsey, V. L., Lalumière, M. L., Boer, D., and Lang, C. (2003) 'A multisite comparison of actuarial risk instruments for sex offenders,' *Psychological Assessment*, *15*:413–425.

Hawes, S. W., Boccaccini, M. T., and Murrie, D. C. (2013) 'Psychopathy and the combination of psychopathy and sexual deviance as predictors of sexual recidivism: Meta-analytic findings using the Psychopathy Checklist–Revised,' *Psychological Assessment*, *25*:233–243.

Hildebrand, M., de Ruiter, C., and de Vogel V. (2004) 'Psychopathy and sexual deviance in treated rapists: Association with sexual and nonsexual recidivism,' *Sexual Abuse: A Journal of Research and Treatment*, *16*:1–24.

Langton, C. M., Barbaree, H. E., Harkins, L., and Peacock, E. J. (2006) 'Sex offenders' response to treatment and its association with recidivism as a function of psychopathy,' *Sexual Abuse: A Journal of Research and Treatment, 18*:99–120.

Looman, J., Abracen, J., Serin, R., and Marquis, P. (2005) 'Psychopathy, treatment change, and recidivism in high-risk, high-need sexual offenders,' *Journal of Interpersonal Violence, 20*:549–568.

Looman, J., Morphett, N. A. C., and Abracen, J. (2013) 'Does consideration of psychopathy and sexual deviance add to the predictive validity of the Static–99R?,' *International Journal of Offender Therapy and Comparative Criminology, 57*:939–965.

Marx, B. P., Miranda, R., and Myerson, L. A. (1999) 'Cognitive–behavioral treatment for rapists: Can we do better?,' *Clinical Psychology Review, 19*:875–894.

Olver, M. E., Mundt, J. C., Thornton, D., Beggs Christofferson, S. M., Kingston, D. A., Sowden, J. N., Nicholaichuk, T. P., Gordon, A., and Wong, S. C. P. (2017) 'Using the Violence Risk Scale–Sexual Offense Version in sexual violence risk assessments: Updated risk categories and recidivism estimates from a multisite sample of treated sexual offenders,' *Manuscript under review.*

Olver, M. E., and Wong, S. C. P. (2006) 'Psychopathy, sexual deviance, and recidivism among sex offenders,' *Sexual Abuse: A Journal of Research and Treatment, 18*:65–82.

Olver, M. E., and Wong, S. C. (2009) 'Therapeutic responses of psychopathic sexual offenders: Treatment attrition, therapeutic change, and long-term recidivism,' *Journal of Consulting and Clinical Psychology*, 77:328–335.

Olver, M. E., and Wong, S. C. P. (2011) 'Predictors of sex offender treatment dropout: Psychopathy, sex offender risk, and responsivity implications,' *Psychology, Crime, and Law*, 17:457–471.

Olver, M. E., Wong, S. C. P., Nicholaichuk, T., and Gordon, A. (2007) 'The validity and reliability of the Violence Risk Scale–Sexual Offender version: Assessing sex offender risk and evaluating therapeutic change,' *Psychological Assessment, 19*:318–329.

Paulhus, D. L., Neumann, C. S., and Hare, R. D. (2017) *Manual for the Self-Report Psychopathy Scale* (4th ed.), Toronto, ON: Multi-Health Systems.

Porter, S., Fairweather, D., Drugge, J., Hervé, H., Birt, A., and Boer, D. P. (2000) 'Profiles of psychopathy in incarcerated sexual offenders,' *Criminal Justice and Behavior*, 27:216–233.

Rice, M. E., and Harris, G. T. (1997) 'Cross-validation and extension of the Violence Risk Appraisal Guide for child molesters and rapists,' *Law and Human Behavior, 21*:231–241.

Rice, M. E., and Harris, G. T. (2005) 'Comparing effect sizes in follow-up studies: ROC Area, Cohen's d, and r,' *Law and Human Behavior, 29*:615–620.

Serin, R. C., Mailloux, D. L., and Malcolm, P. B. (2001) 'Psychopathy, deviant sexual arousal, and recidivism among sexual offenders,' *Journal of Interpersonal Violence, 16*:234–246.

Serin, R. C., Malcolm, P. B., Khanna, A., and Barbaree, H. E. (1994) 'Psychopathy and deviant sexual arousal in incarcerated sexual offenders,' *Journal of Interpersonal Violence, 9*:3–11.

Seto, M. C., Harris, G. T., Rice, M. E., and Barbaree, H. E. (2004) 'The Screening Scale for Pedophilic Interests predicts recidivism among adult sex offenders with child victims,' *Archives of Sexual Behavior, 33*:455–466.

Sewall, L. A., and Olver, M. E. (2017) 'Psychopathy and sexual violence risk: Linkages to therapeutic change, treatment attrition, and recidivism,' *Manuscript under review.*

Simourd, D. J., and Hoge, R. D. (2000) 'Criminal psychopathy: A risk-and-need perspective,' *Criminal Justice and Behavior*, 27:256–272.

Wong, S. C. P., and Gordon A. (2006) 'The validity and reliability of the Violence Risk Scale: A treatment-friendly violence risk assessment tool,' *Psychology, Public Policy, and Law, 12*:279–309.

Wong, S., and Hare, R. D. (2005) *Guidelines for a psychopathy treatment program*, Toronto, ON: Multi-Health Systems.

Wong, S., Olver, M. E., Nicholaichuk, T. P., and Gordon, A. (2003) *The Violence Risk Scale: Sexual Offender version (VRS–SO)*, Regional Psychiatric Centre and University of Saskatchewan, Saskatoon, Saskatchewan, Canada.

Yang, M., Wong, S. C. P., and Coid, J. (2010) 'The efficacy of violence prediction: A meta-analytic comparison of nine risk assessment instruments,' *Psychological Bulletin, 136*:740–767.

39

The treatment of psychopathy

Devon Polaschek

Introduction

Can psychopathy be treated? Should psychopathy be treated? The answer to these questions is very much dependent on how psychopathy is defined: itself the subject of ongoing controversy. When psychopathy is defined as an extraordinarily rare and exotic condition (Utt, Saxon, Bozmann, & Demme, 1991), the epitome of evil (Alford, 1997), or synonymous with severe criminal activity such as serial killing (Bonn, 2017), it would seem both ludicrous, and an act of notable hubris, to suggest that it could be ameliorated with professional help. When it is argued that psychopathy can be adaptive (Lilienfeld, Watts, & Smith, 2015), or has components that signal positive psychological characteristics (Patrick, Fowles, & Krueger, 2009), there seems no reason to treat at all. When it is viewed as capturing the stable intra-individual characteristics that delineate criminal propensity, it appears to be eminently treatable, because there are well-established approaches to treating criminal propensity. When it is understood as a personality disorder, there is little evidence either way regarding its treatability (Polaschek, 2014). This chapter will begin with a brief review of definitions of psychopathy before evaluating theory and research for its relevance for treatment and treatability.

A conceptualization of psychopathy that is gaining popularity is Patrick and colleagues' triarchic model, which specifies that psychopathy is a broadly defined condition that comprises varying proportions of meanness, boldness, and disinhibition. People with high levels of psychopathy have prominent symptoms of disinhibition (low Conscientiousness/constraint; Miller & Lynam, 2012) and either boldness, "a capacity to remain calm and focused ... an ability to recover quickly from stressful events, high self-assurance and social efficacy, and a tolerance for unfamiliarity and danger" (Patrick et al., 2009:926), or meanness (coldhearted, antagonistic, callous; Skeem, Polaschek, Patrick, & Lilienfeld, 2011), or both.

There has been recent energetic debate about whether boldness (or the related construct of Fearless Dominance; Lilienfeld & Widows, 2005) is a legitimate component of psychopathy (Berg, Lilienfeld, & Sellbom, 2017; Miller, Lamkin, & Maples-Keller, 2016). It seems unlikely that high boldness on its own would be a legitimate reason for a treatment referral, but boldness combined with disinhibition could be problematic for both the person and those around him or her. But this chapter is agnostic on whether psychopathy with prominent boldness is treatable or would be useful to treat, since to date treatment studies appear not to have addressed this issue. For the purposes of this chapter, the conceptualization of psychopathy, regardless of the measurement tool used to make the diagnosis, is as *a* personality disorder that contributes to personally and socially harmful behavior. Viewing psychopathy as a personality disorder is important because it creates the expectation of a clinical presentation with some or all of a common set of stable characteristics that are inferred from behavior: characteristics that are maladaptive, longstanding, and manifest in behavior across the person's lifestyle, rather than in one domain alone (e.g., criminal behavior). Psychopathy has predominantly been left out of the Diagnostic Manual of Mental Disorders over the various versions, but the DSM–5 has gone some way to opening the door for its inclusion by including it in Section III (Emerging Measures and Models). The DSM–5 promotes a dimensional view of personality disorder (Clarkin, Cain, & Livesley, 2015) and, in line with leading figures in the classification and treatment of personality disorder, centers the common definition of personality disorder around two areas: self-functioning (disturbed identity, disturbed self-direction) and interpersonal functioning (deficient empathy, deficient intimacy; DSM–5; American Psychiatric Association, 2013).

Early conceptualizations of psychopathy

By far the biggest part of the modern treatment research has used one of the Hare Psychopathy Checklists (e.g., PCL–R, Hare, 1991, 2003; PCL: SV, Hart, Cox, & Hare, 1995) to identify levels of psychopathy. Because of the almost exclusive use of the PCL scales in the last 40 years of theory and research on psychopathy, the structure and content of these checklists underpins the dominant clinical view of the disorder today (Skeem et al., 2011) in a manner that is unprecedented among mental disorders. The term *PCL–psychopathy* will be used throughout the chapter to indicate this conceptualization.

Before the ground-breaking work of Professor Robert Hare in the development of the first Psychopathy Checklist, there was no agreed-upon set of criteria and method of quantifying psychopathy. Thus, understanding what was being treated requires knowledge about which conceptualization was in use. Key figures from that era were Hervey Cleckley, the McCords, and Benjamin Karpman; and there were important variations in how they viewed psychopathy.

Cleckley's professional work with psychiatric patients at Georgia's University Hospital resulted in the now seminal publication *The Mask of Sanity* (1988). The "mask" in his title refers to the inherent contradictions he found in working with psychopathic patients (Lilienfeld et al., 2015): the mix of initial confidence, social poise, and apparently good adjustment overlying various less positive and healthy traits such as dishonesty, lack of remorse and poor judgment. Cleckley's descriptions did not particularly associate psychopathy with predation, Meanness, or violence, in contrast to the dominant views today. Instead psychopaths were shallow, careless, and lacking a sense of commitment and direction to their actions (Skeem et al., 2011).

McCord and McCord (1964) are recognized as having influenced the view of psychopathy as synonymous with criminal, aggressive, hostile, and parasitic behavior. In contrast to Cleckley, this more malevolent, mean version of psychopathy is more like that seen later in people diagnosed using the PCL–R and its offspring, especially in custodial environments.

The third relevant view of psychopathy is from an early contemporary of Cleckley, Benjamin Karpman. Karpman (1941) described two variants of psychopathy. Primary psychopathy is similar to the constellation described by Cleckley: shallow but stable emotionally, with superficial charm and a disinterest in their impact on others. Secondary psychopathy is a more neurotic presentation, including vulnerability to mood disorders associated with negative emotionality, impulsivity, and reactive aggression. These variants have been kept alive theoretically (Yildirim &

Derksen, 2015) and through modern cluster-analytic work, mainly based on PCL–psychopathy scores (e.g., Hicks, Markon, Patrick, Krueger, & Newman, 2004; Lee & Salekin, 2010; Poythress, Edens, et al., 2010; Skeem, Johansson, Andershed, Kerr, & Louden, 2007) that appear to produce similar variants. However, the research on treatment has not yet really examined Karpman's contention that secondary psychopaths are amenable to treatment (for an exception see Poythress, Lilienfeld, et al., 2010).

Reviews of treatment research

Cleckley gained extensive experience working with psychopathy during his clinical career but was dispirited toward the end of his career about its treatability. He wrote:

> I have now, after more than three decades, had the opportunity to observe a considerable number of patients who, through commitment or the threat of losing their probation status or by other means, were kept under treatment not only for many months but for years. The therapeutic failure in all such patients observed leads me to feel that we do not at present have any kind of psychotherapy that can be relied upon to change the psychopath fundamentally. Nor do I believe that any other method of psychiatric treatment has shown promise of solving the problem.[1]
>
> *(Cleckley, 1988:439)*

As Wong (2013) has noted, key client characteristics associated with effective outcomes for long term psychodynamic psychotherapy, the main form of treatment offered at that time, are missing or difficult to cultivate in high-psychopathy people (low self-reflection, grandiosity, Meanness, dismissive attachment). So, it should not be too surprising that Cleckley held this view. But despite Cleckley's discouragement, there was a small but steady flow of publications reporting on treatment of psychopathy from the 1920s to the 1960s, some of which claimed to have been successful in various ways. Forty-two treatment studies were quantitatively evaluated by Salekin (2002). His methodology for evaluating success and the overall quality of the studies he examined have been challenged by others (D'Silva, Duggan, & McCarthy, 2004; Harris & Rice, 2006) for lack of rigor and a variety of limitations that, for the most part, he noted himself.

One of the key areas of contention was whether only treatment that diagnosed psychopathy using the PCL scales and reported recidivism data should be included. In other words, some critics preferred a very narrowly conceived view of psychopathy and what counts as treating it (e.g., Harris & Rice, 2006; Wong, 2013). Before turning to this issue, I briefly consider some of the evidence from this first Salekin review (Salekin, 2002).

Cleckleyan conceptualizations of psychopathy were the most commonly reported in the studies reviewed by Salekin (2002), but some other definitions were used. The types of treatment used were most commonly psychoanalytic; a number were therapeutic communities, but a few drug treatments and cognitive–behavioral interventions were also reported. The earliest examples were often case studies of one to four patients. Ratings of progress were not uncommonly based on clinicians' impressions, coupled sometimes with reports of others, noting such outcomes as improved relationships, problem solving, work or school performance, increased respectful behavior, greater anxiety and guilt, reduced aggressive behavior, blaming others, impulsivity, and so on. The method used by Salekin identified reported improvement for 60 percent of those treated. But there is no dispute that this is a weak literature: peppered with small sample sizes, lacking comparison groups, with no evidence of reliable diagnosis nor reliable measurement of change or outcomes. What can be said about the state of psychopathy treatment at the time of this review was that (1) it was subject to steady research interest, and (2) there is nothing in this literature to indicate that people with psychopathy are incapable of responding to treatment – a conclusion similar to that reached by others (Blackburn, 1993; Lösel, 1998).

Alongside Salekin's (2002) tentatively optimistic review, others have systematically summarized the literature using more rigorous criteria for the diagnosis of psychopathy, the documentation of the treatment, and the types of outcomes examined (e.g., D'Silva et al., 2004; Harris & Rice, 2006). Wong (2000), for example, used six more scientifically rigorous criteria. Of 75 studies he then reviewed, only two met all of the criteria, including the notorious Oak Ridge program in Penetanguishene which we discuss in more detail later. (D'Silva et al., 2004) found 24 studies but examined a slightly different question: the evidence for a negative treatment response in high-PCL–psychopathic offenders. They concluded there was little support.

Salekin and colleagues updated the Salekin (2002) review. Salekin, Worley, and Grimes (2010) presented a more rigorous summary of intervention studies for adult and adolescent offenders, using the PCL scales for diagnosis, focusing on offenders, and noting whether overall the study reported a positive or negative result for compliance (treatment completion) and treatment outcome. They concluded that three of eight studies showed positive effects of treatment for people high in psychopathy, an encouraging result given none of the treatments were psychopathy-specific.

Defining treatability

A concept central to understanding the importance of psychopathy in relation to treatment is *treatability*. Therapists ask, "are psychopathic people treatable"? Judgments about treatability can be based on (1) perceptions of the treatment process, including perceptions of how quickly or how much the client understands, learns, and changes, and perceptions of the working alliance or engagement; (2) whether the client completed treatment, or completed as much treatment as the therapist judged to be necessary; and (3) whether the client achieved the desired long-term outcome (e.g., recidivism-free, as judged in the previous section). But rather than seeing these qualities as client-based, a number are partly the result of an interaction between the client and the therapist's expectations and behavior toward that client. I consider each of these definitions below.

The treatment process

Client behavior in treatment

Schofield (1964) is known for developing the concept of the YAVIS client, based on 1960s' therapists' preferences (i.e., youthful, attractive, verbal, intelligent, and successful). Perhaps this research should be updated, but it seems likely that many forms of talking therapy remain predicated on clients who want to be there and to improve themselves, are self-reflective, verbal, and committed, and are ready to accept the therapist's view of what they need to do.

Psychopathy is associated with a number of client and treatment process characteristics that differ from these ideals and that make treatment more difficult. Therapists who expect clients to be easier to work with than they are may make negative judgments about the treatability of people with psychopathy. They may also hold false beliefs about whether argumentative and difficult clients are benefiting from treatment. And therapists working with people with psychopathy are vigilant to being duped, even though there is no scientific evidence that this happens. So, therapist expectations may become important.

A series of studies of child-sex offender treatment in the 1990s appeared to provide evidence that psychopathy led to therapist deception and manipulation. Two of these studies showed was that when therapists' ratings of in-treatment progress were better for high psychopathy clients, the client was *more* likely to recidivate (Looman, Abracen, Serin, & Marquis, 2005; Seto & Barbaree, 1999). In the second case (Seto & Barbaree, 1999), a subsequent study with a longer follow-up and more complete recidivism records suggested that the first study was flawed due to the use of incomplete recidivism data, unreliable treatment ratings, and a failure to control for variations in time at risk across groups (Langton, Barbaree, Harkins, & Peacock, 2006). Nevertheless, the authors concluded that the well-rated clients either were fooling their therapists into thinking they had made more progress than they had or were actually learning skills that they misused in order to recidivate later (Seto & Barbaree, 1999): a similar explanation to that offered in the Oak Ridge study (see below).

An alternative interpretation of parts of these studies rests on noting that the ratings of treatment gains were not predictive of outcome, regardless of psychopathy. In other words, therapists' judgment of what counted as progress toward reducing recidivism was not supported by the outcomes. This finding is quite pervasive in the offender treatment research literature: in fact, demonstrations of change ratings that link to recidivism are the exception rather than the rule (Serin, Lloyd, Helmus, Derkzen, & Luong, 2013), raising the real possibility that there are problems with reliability and validity of such ratings across all offender treatment. It has been repeatedly demonstrated empirically that unstructured global assessments of criminal risk are unlikely to predict recidivism. Making similar ratings to evaluate progress in treatment (e.g., global progress ratings, insight into offense cycle, awareness of harm to victim; Looman et al., 2005), and measuring phenomena that may not be linked statistically to recidivism in the first place, may run into the same problems. Looman et al. advanced the interesting suggestion that the poorly rated high-psychopathy clients could have been those who were more resistant initially and were more aggressive and confronting with therapists. Such behavior, they imply, in high-psychopathy, aggressive offenders might actually be evidence of better engagement in treatment, whereas the well-rated clients might just have been "going along with it" (Abracen & Looman, 2016; Abracen, Looman, & Langton, 2008).

While aggressive and challenging clients may stand out in a program with relatively low- to medium-risk offenders,[2] they are the bread and butter of treatment with higher risk offenders, implying that therapists' perceptions of problems with the treatment process may be contextually influenced by expectations about how clients who are benefiting should behave, and by the relative novelty of difficult-client characteristics. Psychopathy is often listed as a responsivity factor – although this global listing makes little sense given the differential relationships between components of psychopathy and other variables (Skeem et al., 2011).

Independently of psychopathy, the research on high-risk criminals has identified a raft of characteristics that render them unwilling or unable to respond to treatment if not accommodated in the design and delivery of the program. These include anger, hostility, irritability, proneness to feeling victimized, suspicion of others' motives, antagonistic and aggressive displays, unreliability, egocentrism, low commitment to change, and lack of persistence (Blackburn, 1999; Krueger et al., 1994; Lowenkamp & Latessa, 2004; Moffitt, 2003; Ross, Fabiano, & Ewles, 1988). They are also often poor learners, with verbal and other neuropsychological deficits, school failure, and negativity toward learning (Bell & Polaschek, 2017; Golden, Jackson, Peterson-Rohne, & Gontkovsky, 1996; Moffitt, Lynam, & Silva, 1994). Because these findings apply to criminal risk itself, it is difficult to discern whether there are unique effects of psychopathy on responsivity.

A study of the long-running Grendon Prison therapeutic community in the U.K. used behavior checklists to score and monitor behavior change in group, in the living environment, and in adjunct activities (e.g., recreation, education). Significant correlations were found between PCL–R Factor 1 scores and behavior in group and on the wing, but there was little relationship between Factor 2 and the same behavior. The relationships with F1 were not too surprising given that items in the behavior checklists could themselves be regarded as evidence of F1 psychopathy (e.g., "he gives longwinded, elaborate accounts of his behavior," "he bandwagons when the opportunity arises," "he blames others for his problems," "he is self-centered," "he manipulates others for his own ends," "he is quick to exploit loopholes in rules and entitlements," "he has an inflated sense of self-importance"). This study showed no significant change between three-month and six-month measures, on average, so no conclusions can be reached regarding the effects of PCL–R scores on change itself (Hobson, Shine, & Roberts, 2000).

We recently took a slightly different approach to examining relationships between PCL–psychopathy and in-treatment behavior. We made retrospective ratings of behavior in treatment from therapists' treatment notes. These daily or weekly notes were not made at the time using any protocol to formally or systematically record and measure progress. Therefore, we were only able to code variables that were reasonably consistently recorded across multiple therapists and treatment cohorts, and these codes were later grouped using factor analysis into two factors: *program performance* variables, including cooperation (i.e., working to achieve common goals with staff or group members), motivation to change, conceptual understanding of the program content, and distractability; and *emotional–submissive* behavior: empathy toward others, anxiety, negative emotionality more generally, and (low) social dominance. As expected, emotional–submissive scores were predicted by PCL: SV Factor 1 and each of its facets (*r*s between −.15 and −.18), but there was no relationship with Factor 2 or its facets. By contrast, program performance scores were unrelated only to the interpersonal facet: Factors 1 and 2, the PCL: SV total, and the other three facets each were predictive of program performance. This study also found that performance scores predicted three of five recidivism outcomes (any reconviction, violent reconviction, reconviction leading to reimprisonment), but emotional–submissive scores predicted only parole breaches. Neither predicted reimprisonment for a serious offense (Daly, Fletcher, & Polaschek, 2017b).

To conclude, therapist ratings of achievement standards or progress in treatment have often found that psychopathy is associated with poorer ratings, but equally often, the ratings themselves have not be linked statistically to recidivism, making their prognostic value difficult to interpret. The most recent study, based on retrospective independent ratings of therapists' notes, shows that the characteristics most distinctive to psychopathy – low scores on the emotional–submissive scale – are largely not predictive of recidivism after treatment, but cooperation in treatment, understanding of the program, concentration ability, and motivation to change, all poorer with higher PCL–psychopathy scores, do predict recidivism.

Client–therapist relationship

The ability to form a meaningful working relationship with clients high in psychopathy has also been considered a problem, and indicative of a lack of treatability. A number of writers have suggested that a good working alliance is difficult to come by when high psychopathy is present (Galloway & Brodsky, 2003; Thornton & Blud, 2007; Wong & Hare, 2005). For example, Wong has suggested that "it may be unrealistic to establish any real affective 'bond' with the psychopath . . . repeated attempts by the therapist to establish affective connections or bonds with the psychopath would be to ignore the reality of the disorder" (Wong, 2013:6–7).

But again, if this is true, it may partly be a function of therapists' suspicions about high-psychopathy clients, or equally, about an inability to agree on the goals of treatment when the program assumes participants are in the action stage of change, while at best, participants are actually still contemplating change (Polaschek, Yesberg, Bell, Casey, & Dickson, 2016; Wong, Gordon, & Gu, 2007).

What does the evidence say? Often the alliance is measured using a version of the Working Alliance Inventory (WAI; Horvath & Greenberg, 1994), which is based on Bordin's (1979) three-component concept of the therapeutic alliance: (1) the bond between the staff member and the offender, and the strength of agreement on (2) the goals, and on (3) the tasks. With high risk sex offenders (from the Clearwater Program in Ottawa), offender–participants' ratings of working alliance were lower for the bond and goal components for those with higher affective facet scores, and lower on the task and goal components for those with higher lifestyle facet scores, but WAI scores overall were not correlated with PCL–R total scores, and the WAI did not predict recidivism, regardless of psychopathy (DeSorcy, Olver, & Wormith, 2017). A second study with sex offenders in a moderate-intensity treatment program in a maximum security state prison in the U.S. found no relationship between alliance ratings made by clients or therapists and PCL–R scores for WAI total, components, or PCL–R factors (Walton, Jeglic, & Blasko, 2016). Mean PCL–R scores in this study were relatively low (20.4).

Ross (2008) found for high-risk psychopathic violent prisoners in treatment that working alliance Goals and Total scores measured in the first three weeks of the intensive eight-month program were significantly and negatively correlated to PCL–psychopathy Factor 1 scores. No other significant relationships were found for Factor 1 or Factor 2 scores. Furthermore, WAI scores were high from this first point of measurement and continued to improve over the course of treatment. Finally, in this study the WAI was rated by observers who screened sessions, rather than by therapists or clients themselves; the WAI ratings were thus made independently of the PCL: SV ratings, and WAI levels were comparable to studies of routine psychotherapy (Polaschek & Ross, 2010). However, when in a subsequent study these same WAI data were averaged across four measurements from different stages of the program, there were significant negative associations between PCL: SV interpersonal, affective, and lifestyle facet scores for all three components (Bond, Goal, and Tasks, range −.27 to −.31; except for the affective facet and Bond; $r = -.24$; *ns*). Although Factor 1 was the only significant predictor of the WAI total score when regressed with Factor 2, a regression with all four facets instead showed only the lifestyle facet to be a significant predictor of the working alliance (Daly, Ross, Fletcher, & Polaschek, 2017).

To conclude, although some parts of the therapeutic alliance have been found to correlate with psychopathy, methodology is variable, and results have been inconsistent. In particular, some studies have found the bond component to be unrelated to psychopathy and to develop to normal levels, even when judged by observers. However, different patterns have been found for different facets of the PCL scales, and this level of analysis should be included in future studies. Several studies used ratings made by offenders, which may not adequately address the concerns of clinicians that *they* will have difficulty forming an alliance, so more therapist and observer ratings would be beneficial, particularly as a direct test of the concerns of Galloway and Brodsky (2003), Wong and Hare (2005), and others. Again, some studies have researched samples with high levels of PCL scores, while others have more varied samples, and the context may make a difference as to whether the therapists are successful in their part of alliance development. Finally, Blasko and Jeglic (2016) showed that with sexual offenders, the level of criminal risk was negatively related to their ratings of bond development, particularly with women therapists, suggesting both gender and risk should be considered in further unpacking this part of the treatment process literature.

Treatment dosage and completion

Increased risk of incomplete or low dosages of treatment is commonly correlated with PCL–psychopathy. People with psychopathy are more at risk of removal from treatment and are more likely to choose not to complete programs. Again, this is not surprising given that the characteristics that predict attrition are related to criminal risk, and also to psychopathy (e.g., low motivation to engage; Olver, Stockdale, & Wormith, 2011). Again, therapist expectations may be important, leading to the removal of clients whose behavior in treatment feeds perceptions that they are not progressing well. Furthermore, psychopaths and high-risk offenders bring their habitual behavior to the treatment setting, but poor behavior by treatment participants (being disruptive, using drugs, fighting) can put programs in a challenging position: remove the person for the very behavior that the treatment is intended to help with, or retain them and run the risk of appearing to other participants to have "turned a blind eye" to unacceptable behavior. If options are available for both punishing poor behavior and continuing treatment (e.g., suspending treatment participation for a period while punishment is completed), then attrition rates may be reduced. But again, if programs are not geared for disruptive behavior, attrition may be higher for those who exhibit it.

The relationship between psychopathy and treatment attrition may be affected then by the base-rate of attrition in the program. For example, in the high-risk sex offender sample reported on by (DeSorcy et al., 2017), over 89 percent of program starters completed the program, and the rate for men with PCL–R scores greater than 25 was still 84.3 percent, not significantly different from the rate for lower-psychopathy men. But an earlier study from this same unit (Olver & Wong, 2011) found 85 percent completion rates, and completers had lower scores than non-completers on both Factor 1 and Factor 2. Factor 1 remained a unique predictor of dropout, even when risk of sexual recidivism and Factor 2 were controlled for. Ogloff, Wong, and Greenwood (1990) reported a 43 percent non-completion rate and found a pattern of reducing days in treatment as PCL scores increased. Richards, Casey, and Lucente (2003) with maximum security imprisoned women in substance abuse treatment, and with PCL–R scores under 30, found that Factor 1, but not Factor 2 or total scores, was associated negatively with days in treatment.

With high-risk violent prisoners, Daly Fletcher, and Polaschek (2017a) found a completion rate of 77 percent; 16 percent were removed from treatment at the behest of staff, and 7 percent withdrew at their own request. A series of subsequent analyses showed that Factor 1 and each of its respective facets (interpersonal and affective) were higher for involuntary non-completers than for completers or those who removed themselves.

To conclude, psychopathy is associated with a number of treatment factors that differ from some therapists' ideals or perhaps their training. For high-psychopathy people, their high-risk status on its own ensures that the treatment process will be bumpy, that therapists will need to work hard to engage clients, that it may be hard to judge progress, and that a certain amount of antisocial behavior and attrition is unavoidable.

Treating the risk of crime and violence with psychopathic people

Previous reviews of interventions showing promise with regard to improving criminal outcomes in the presence of psychopathy (e.g., Polaschek & Daly, 2013; Polaschek, 2014; Salekin et al., 2010; Skeem, Polaschek, & Manchak, 2009; Skeem et al., 2011; Wong, 2013) have all noted the relevance of Skeem, Monahan, and Mulvey's (2002) study, which still stands as distinctive in several respects. It was based on community psychiatric patients rather than offenders, and the treatment was low intensity, comprising a variety of community mental health "treatment as usual" sessions – mainly verbal therapy with or without medication – that patients reported they were attending: even those in the more intensive condition reported attendance at just six or more sessions in the previous ten weeks. Therefore, effectively the researchers created the comparison group by dividing the intervention group on the basis of intensity of treatment the participants reported engaging with. The study also suffered from low power in some analyses, and there was no comparison group, so propensity score matching was used to control for pre-existing differences between the low and high treatment group.

These are interesting and encouraging findings. But the lack of detail about "what worked" in these findings makes them unsuited to identifying *how* to treat violence risk in people with psychopathy. Further, the results have been evaluated with considerable skepticism by some researchers because of the implausibility of reducing violence risk in people with psychopathy using an unspecified low intensity intervention (Harris & Rice, 2006). It is also the case that the participants, even in the higher-PCL–psychopathy part of the sample, were not highly psychopathic – an issue that arises in quite a few studies, which may also render them unsuitable for informing "what works" with high-scorers.

Nevertheless, the results are encouraging, suggesting that more intensive attendance at services was associated with less violence in the following ten weeks, regardless of psychopathy levels, and that those who attended fewer than six sessions over ten weeks were 3.5 times more likely to behave violently in the subsequent measurement period than those who attended six or more (Skeem et al., 2002). However, this was not a program with offenders and was not designed to reduce the criminal propensity of offenders. We turn next to research on programs that are designed to change criminal risk. Do they work with people with psychopathy?

Reducing criminal risk with offenders

The investigation of the effectiveness of treatment for criminal risk with people with prominent psychopathic features has been considerably enhanced by an evolving empirically based understanding of how to work effectively with a range of offenders to enhance desistance. Since the late 1970s, a concerted focus on research into characteristics of offenders, staff, and programs and their associations with recidivism has yielded a body of research that is sufficiently methodologically robust to feed into a growing series of meta-analyses. Consequently, offenders in general have begun to be regarded as treatable, particularly with offense-focused cognitive–behavioral group-based interventions, but many other types of interventions have also shown effectiveness.

Andrews and Bonta have taken a notable leadership role in this research: distilling findings into a series of principles that has become known as the Risk–Need–Responsivity model of offender treatment (RNR; e.g., Andrews & Bonta, 2010a, 2010b). Although the model includes 18 principles, the three for which the model is named were the first to be published (Andrews, Bonta, & Hoge, 1990), are the most familiar, and will be the focus here.

To summarize, the largest reductions in criminal behavior come from interventions that (1) provide relatively intensive services and direct them toward higher risk offenders (the *risk* principle); (2) focus services on changing *criminogenic needs*: empirical correlates of recidivism (e.g., criminal beliefs, substance abuse, impulsivity, low self-control; the *need* principle); and (3) are delivered so as to maximize the likelihood an offender will engage in the treatment process and be able to use the help given to make changes (the *responsivity* principle; Andrews & Bonta, 2010a, 2010b).

Other parts of the RNR model demonstrate that reductions in recidivism also are associated with the use of warm, enthusiastic, respectful, well-trained, and well-supervised therapists who spend contact time forming a bond with clients and use the most effective forms of social influence and structured skill training to support change on criminal risk factors. When offenders in treatment behave in ways that challenge engagement and change – and if higher-risk clients have been chosen, they usually will – effective therapists endeavor to work *with* the difficult characteristics (e.g., lack of attention or interest, hostility, poor compliance) rather than taking them as indicators that the client is not suitable for treatment. This disposition toward what treatment-disrupting behavior indicates (challenging but not untreatable) is important because as was already noted, a number of these same characteristics that disrupt the process of treatment also contribute to offense risk, making them more prominent in the very clients who are the highest priority for treatment, according to the risk principle.

The number of these core RNR principles that a program adheres to is associated with the size of recidivism reductions it achieves. The impact on crime for those adhering to all three principles is modest but important, with reported effect sizes ranging from 0.15 to 0.34 (Andrews & Bonta, 2010a). An effect size of .15 means indicates that 15 people per 100 who would have been expected to be reconvicted were not. It is equivalent to an outcome where if 50 percent of untreated offenders had been reconvicted at follow-up, the corresponding rate for treated offenders effect would be 35 percent – a relative reduction in this example of more than 30 percent.

Reducing criminal risk in offenders with psychopathy

These findings become relevant to understanding the relationship between psychopathy and treatment because Hare's scales are the most often used to measure psychopathy in offenders. Although intended to diagnose psychopathy, the PCL–R and PCL: SV's popularity with adult offenders comes largely from their utility in assessing risk of reconviction for criminal behavior, including violence (Skeem et al., 2011). PCL–R/SV scores compare favorably with purpose-built risk assessment inventories that do not include psychopathy in risk prediction studies (see Singh, Grann, & Fazel, 2011), although only Factor 2 scores perform similarly to non-psychopathy risk assessment tools for violence prediction; Factor 1 scores are not significantly related to violence in this meta-analysis (Yang, Wong, & Coid, 2010).

Therefore, clients with high levels of assessed criminal risk will also tend to have high PCL scores and vice versa, making high-PCL-scoring clients among those most highly prioritized for intensive treatment, in accordance with the risk principle, rather than sometimes being ruled out of interventions altogether because they are difficult to treat (de Ruiter, Chakhssi, & Bernstein, 2016; Skeem et al., 2009). The preponderance of people with high levels of psychopathy in some offender treatment programs has enabled the identification of whether psychopathy is relevant to the effectiveness of these programs in reducing criminal risk.

However, it should be noted that there are few research programs around the world that have systematically studied efforts to change the criminal risk of high-risk offenders. Much of the large literature pertaining to "what works with offenders, including multiple meta-analyses is centered around studies where the likelihood of a new conviction on release is less than, for instance, 50 percent in the first 12 months, greater than 80 percent at 5 years; and 20 percent or more for violence in the first year, as has been shown in some studies of high-risk offenders (Nadesu, 2009; Polaschek, 2011; Wong, Gordon, Gu, Lewis, & Olver, 2012).

A noteworthy study evaluated offenders with PCL–R scores greater than 25 who undertook and completed the Aggressive Behavior Control (ABC) program, which, like the Clearwater program for high-risk sexual offenders, was housed in the Regional Psychiatric Centre (RPC) in Saskatoon, Saskatchewan for some years (see Wong & Gordon, 2013 for a full description of the model). The treatment sample was compared with a matched no-treatment control group; PCL–R total scores were matched, along with Factor 1 and Factor 2 scores, age of first conviction, and ethnicity. Unfortunately, as is often the case with this type of close case-based matching, the original total sample available was reduced from over 500 to 32 matched pairs. Follow-up time was truncated for each pair so it equaled the time available for the shorter of the two. Mean follow-up time is not reported. On 11 distinct recidivism outcomes, no significant differences were found, with the base rate of any reconviction identical across the two groups (94 percent) and of violent reconviction similar for each group (81.3 percent treated, 84.4 percent matched untreated). But most results favored treatment in this low power study. A second set of analyses of seven indices of sentence length – based on the premise that this method might be more sensitive to changes in offending severity – all seven were better for treated men, and three reached statistical significance. The significantly different measures included the longest sentence given during the follow-up, the longest aggregated sentence given, and the sum of aggregate sentences given: an index of the overall severity of all subsequent reconvicted offending combined (Wong et al., 2012). There are still design issues with this study, most notably the concern about the sheer number of outcomes examined compared to those that were statistically significant, the differences on demographic variables between the two samples that were not controlled for, and the low power of the analyses given the small sample size, all of which argue for replication of this interesting result (Wong et al., 2012).

We have published a series of quasi-experimental studies showing reductions in recidivism based on outcomes from a group of intensive prison-based high-risk treatment units for men (Polaschek, Wilson, Townsend, & Daly, 2005; Polaschek, 2011; Kilgour & Polaschek, 2012; Polaschek et al., 2016). These units provide seven to eight months of intensive group-based cognitive–behavior treatment in dedicated treatment units. We found PCL: SV scores to be unrelated to violent reconviction ($r = .05$) with a mean PCL: SV score of around 18 (Polaschek, 2008). An updated analysis with a larger sample ($n = 277$ treatment cases; mean PCL: SV total score still = 18, the usual cut-off for diagnosing psychopathy with this scale) has found that, over two years in the community post-treatment, the PCL: SV total score predicted breaches of parole and reconviction leading to reimprisonment, but was unrelated to reconviction for any new offense, violence reconviction, or reimprisonment for a serious offense (Daly, 2017). Assuming that PCL scores would have predicted reconviction without treatment, studies like these, where psychopathy has a limited role in moderating the treatment outcome of concern, suggest that something about the treatment response itself may have reduced the effects of psychopathy on post-program behavior.

Although treatment of children and adolescents is for the most part outside the scope of this chapter, one study is mentioned because of the rigor of its design and uniqueness of its findings, especially regarding psychopathy. The Mendota Juvenile Treatment Center (MJTC) in Madison, Wisconsin is a hospital-based intensive intervention that operates as a secure correctional facility for the most difficult youth offenders in the state (Caldwell & van Rybroek, 2005). Within a combined social learning and systems theory approach, the unit provides individualized interventions for referred youth, including "tutoring and educational services, group and individual counselling, psychopharmacological interventions, and family therapy" (Caldwell & van Rybroek, 2013:574), which are provided by staff from a wide range of disciplines. Furthermore, the day to day behavior of residents was monitored by trained ward staff and others (Caldwell, McCormick, Umstead, & van Rybroek, 2007) based on a points program that quickly picks up changes in behavior. Within this program, adolescents earn privileges following relatively short periods of positive behavior. Frontline staff assign points by consensus at the end of each shift, based on the youth's behavior during the shift, and the results are used to determine access to privileges the following day, which can be expanded to additional privileges by combining several days of positive ratings (e.g., computer game time, snacks, private music). Thus, the MJTC includes a rigorously implemented contingency management component of available and rapidly increasing incentives for compliance with unit operations and engagement in treatment (Caldwell et al., 2007). Behavioral ratings also serve to indicate progress and have been used as a dependent variable in research at the MJTC, consistent with a wider empirical literature on contingency management programs on their own have been found effective in improving institutional behavior with offenders (Gendreau, Listwan, Kuhns, & Exum, 2014). A recidivism outcome evaluation compared youth referred from two secure youth correctional facilities who were assessed and stabilized at the MJTC before return to the referring institution, with another sample retained in the MJTC for treatment. Referral to MJTC is usually for poor adjustment to the regimes of these other facilities. Detailed assessment information gathered at unit entry was used to develop propensity scores to adjust for any differences in treatment allocation based on 21 assessment variables. The mean PCL: YV score (Forth, Kosson, & Hare, 2003) for the treatment group was 32.8 and 32.6 for the comparisons. An evaluation of recidivism over a mean of 53 months of follow-up showed that boys in the comparison group had more than twice as many new charges for offenses, twice as many felony arrests, and more than three times the number of violent convictions (Caldwell, Vitacco, & Van Rybroek, 2006). So again, this is a study that showed improved recidivism outcomes following a treatment consistent with the RNR model, using a quasi-experimental design that compares treated and untreated offenders high on psychopathy, albeit these are adolescents. Furthermore, PCL: YV scores were unrelated to outcome, suggesting that the differences are the result of some form of behavior change that was more prognostic than the scores for psychopathy.

Increasing criminal risk with treatment

The Oak Ridge Social Therapy Unit was a highly experimental peer-led mandatory hospital-based program that operated between 1968 and 1978. The treatment itself included intensive contact with other patients, some of them psychotic, in unstructured naked encounter groups in which they were fed through tubes in the wall and administered each other a variety of psychoactive substances. Patients in the research spent at least two years in this environment for up to 80 hours each week and had very little contact with staff. Patients were punished if they did not take part in the required regime and could only leave if they persuaded an institutional board that they had made sufficient progress (Rice, Harris, & Cormier, 1992).

Some years later researchers took the PCL–R and scored it based on file notes for patients and carefully matched prisoners who had been referred to the hospital for forensic assessments. Matching criteria were based on age, index offense, and criminal history, but interestingly, not on PCL–R score. Although both a retrospective and quasi-experimental study, it is a model of its kind and yielded recidivism results that suggested that treated lower-psychopathy patients were significantly less likely to recidivate than untreated prisoners, for both violent and general recidivism. However, for the high-psychopathy group in the experimental treatment, there was no difference in general recidivism compared to matched prisoners, but violent recidivism rates were substantially higher than for the untreated prisoners. Rice et al. (1992:408) described this result as "remarkable" because it "belies the conventional wisdom about the immutability of psychopathy and shows that an inappropriate institutional environment can actually increase criminal behavior" and, further, "the combined results suggest that a therapeutic community is not the treatment of choice for psychopaths, particularly those with extensive criminal histories."

The available data on the progress made by program participants show people with higher levels of psychopathy did more poorly on all of the indices of maladjustment (disciplinary problems, use of seclusion, negative entries in treatment record for disruptive or anti-therapeutic conduct). On positive indices (staff recommendations regarding release, program leadership role), they were no different to low psychopathy patients, and these indices did not predict recidivism. (Rice et al., 1992). The program was intentionally unstructured; structured activity such as work, schooling, or recreation was seen, if anything, as detracting from the therapy experience. The intervention did not address criminal thinking or teach social problem solving or other useful skills typical of later psychological treatment programs. But in seeking to explain the apparent increase in proportion of high-psychopathy treated releasees who were reconvicted for violence alongside their untreated counterparts, the researchers speculated that, just like the lower psychopathy participants, people with higher levels of psychopathy learned a number of skills from the program, including: enhanced perspective taking and appraisal of others' emotional lives, use of emotion-based language, socially skilled behavior and enhanced ability to delay gratification. But unlike them, the psychopaths used these skills "to facilitate the manipulation and exploitation of others and could be associated with novel ways to commit violent crime" (p. 409). It is certainly possible that with no change in criminal attitudes and values, the treatment may have resulted in an increase in socially harmful behavior toward others, but why would that show up only in violent convictions? And indeed, what is it about getting caught for violence that is enhanced by social skills, delayed gratification, and manipulation? These characteristics should assist people in avoiding getting caught or even doing violence since in many ways it is the crudest, least skilled way to influence others. Finally, much of the program research that follows this work shows that people with psychopathy are less likely to engage with programs and make less change. If people with psychopathy in the Penetanguishene program were developing these positive characteristics as a result of the treatment, why were they also more likely to show a lack of responsivity in terms of negative program indices? Rice, Harris, and colleagues concluded that this was not the optimum approach for this client group (Harris et al., 1994) and it certainly deviates markedly from modern empirically supported treatments for personality disorder (Livesley, 2012).

Relationships between psychopathy and treatment change

Having tentatively established that psychopathy does not prevent reductions in recidivism in treatments that are well designed to reduce risk, the next step is to establish whether the presence of psychopathy alters how this reduction is achieved. Again, limitations on the overall research base makes this link tentative as well. There are many outcome evaluations for correctional programs. But there are few that provide convincing evidence of how change occurs or link the amount of change to the treatment itself. Such a study, ideally, would have a comparison and a treatment group, measure both longitudinally on purported mechanisms, and then investigate whether change is linked to changes in recidivism. To the extent that change is greater in the treatment group, it can also be attributed to the intervention, rather than just the passing of time. Such studies appear to be non-existent in the correction program evaluation literature.

The next most useful design has only a treatment group. From studies of this type we can at least establish whether variables that change during the program meet the full theoretical definition of a criminogenic need: that (1) they are correlates of recidivism, (2) can change, and (3) when they do change, so does recidivism (Douglas & Skeem, 2005). As noted earlier, there are few empirical demonstrations that commonly identified criminogenic needs (as defined in the RNR model; Andrews et al., 1990) change in intervention, and that these changes predict reduced recidivism (Serin et al., 2013).

But most attempts to do so fail to make the necessary statistical links.[3] Even fewer have also examined the relevance of psychopathy to that change in a rigorous empirical manner. Two such studies that make this link do so not through attempting to correlate individual risk factors (e.g., criminal attitudes) with recidivism as some earlier research has done, but through first empirically aggregating change over many criminogenic needs. These studies use a purpose-built change measure linked to dynamic risk factors to demonstrate that change in individuals with psychopathy can be greater in those who avoid reconviction after treatment. The Violence Risk Scale (Wong & Gordon, 2006) is very useful for evaluating the effects of treatment on variable risk factors because it (1) actuarially assesses initial level of risk on each of a large array of variable risk factors (e.g., sexual preoccupation, substance abuse, impulsivity, criminal attitudes); (2) determines, for each offender, which risk factors are treatment goals; (3) measures progress against these goals; and (4) aggregates indices of progress into a change score that estimates how much risk reduction occurred from the start to the end of treatment. One of the two studies was based on a sample from the Clearwater sex offender treatment program (Olver & Wong, 2009), and the other from the Violence Reduction Program (i.e., the Aggressive Behavior Control program; (Lewis, Olver, & Wong, 2013), both based in the Saskatchewan Regional Treatment Center.

Both studies assessed the amount of change retrospectively. Relevant information was drawn from file records at two time-points (beginning and end of intervention) and provided to trained raters, who then scored a version of the Violence Risk Scale (VRS; Wong & Gordon, 2006; VRS–SO [Sex Offender Version]; Wong, Olver, Nicholaichuk, & Gordon, 2003). Raters were blind to recidivism outcomes.

Olver and Wong (2009) found that psychopathic men (PCL–R $\geq$ 25) in the intensive high-risk sex offender program were judged over the course of treatment to have made notable progress on the VRS:SO's risk-related treatment targets, and the more these offenders changed, the less likely they were to be reconvicted of sexual and violent offenses. The parallel study of high-risk violent offenders (PCL–R $M = 26$) found that the more that these predominantly psychopathic offenders changed in VRS risk factors over treatment, the less likely they were to be reconvicted for violent offenses (Lewis et al., 2013).

These two studies, then, document change in PCL–psychopathic offenders during treatment, and then statistically link that improvement to actual reductions in serious criminal outcomes. But neither has a comparison condition, making it difficult to argue compellingly that change in recidivism risk is a consequence of program attendance. However, elsewhere, outcome evaluations showed that attendance was associated with reduced recidivism relative to an untreated comparison group (Olver & Wong, 2013; Wong, Gordon, Gu, Lewis, & Olver, 2012).

Those with psychopathy can show risk-relevant change in treatment but are widely experienced as more difficult to work with, challenging perceptions of responsiveness to what therapists have to offer. Several studies address the issue of whether psychopathy itself affects more than just perceptions, but also is related to the amount of change made compared to people with lower levels of psychopathic characteristics.

One examination of whether psychopathy affected change was from the Mendota youth program discussed earlier. Change in the program was measured by averaging over the first 3 weeks of the full treatment regime, the weekly proportions of points gained (against the maximum possible) for complying with program expectations (e.g., peer and staff interactions, behavior in treatment and education sessions), as rated by program staff at the end of each shift.

An end of program change score was similarly computed for the last three weeks. Although youths with poorer initial PCL: YV scores also had poorer behavior at the beginning of treatment, the amount of change made during treatment and subsequent violent recidivism were both unrelated to psychopathy (Caldwell et al., 2007).

Returning to adult offenders, Hughes, Hogue, Hollin, and Champion (1997) evaluated a program for nine offenders (mean PCL–R score = 20.63, *SD* = 5.42) undergoing treatment in a high-security U.K. hospital. Using a global change score based on summing changes on self-report psychometric scales, correlations of $r = -.75$ and $-.43$ were found for PCL–R Factors 1 and 2 respective and global change. However, the small size of the sample, and various other methodological challenges, limits the generalizability of these results.

Two studies have also examined this issue with Dutch forensic hospital patients, using a variety of change measures, including a mix of self-report scales, Rorschach Inkblot Tests, and observer ratings of social behavior (e.g., nurse ratings of insight, social skills, interpersonal hostility, and physical violence; de Ruiter et al., 2016). Neither study had recidivism data. The sample was divided into high (≥ 26) and low PCL–R (< 26) groups rather than using PCL scores as a continuous variable as other studies have done. Chakhssi, de Ruiter, and Bernstein (2010) found improvements over a mean of 20 months in social skills and insight, regardless of psychopathy group. On other measures, there was no significant change over time and no group differences were found. With a similar sample, Hildebrand and de Ruiter (2012) split people into groups using a PCL–R score of 22 as the cut point and found no improvement on most indices of change over 20 months of treatment, and no differences by psychopathy group.

At the Saskatchewan RPC again, Olver, Lewis, and Wong (2013) found that all four facets of the PCL–R showed significant zero-order correlations with the amount of change on the VRS for high-risk violent offenders. However, only Factor 1 (when both factors were analyzed together) and the affective facet of Factor 1 (when all four facets were analyzed together) uniquely contributed to the prediction of VRS change but did not control specifically for criminal risk in doing so.

A recent study with a similar population in New Zealand – high-risk psychopathic and violent offenders in a prison treatment program – found non-significant correlations between the PCL: SV total score, or any of the four facets or two factors and VRS-rated change (*r*s. -02 to .13), suggesting psychopathy was not related to the amount of change made in this program (Daly et al., 2017b). However, the amount of change made in this program was lower than the previous study (here mean VRS change = 3.8 *SD* = 2.6; vs. 4. 7, *SD* = 3.0; Olver et al. 2013). An alternative explanation for the divergent findings is that the Daly study used field ratings – dynamic risk data were collected prospectively by multiple therapists using interview and file information – whereas in Olver et al. (2013), dynamic risk data were collected retrospectively mainly by one author using archival file information only. Even under the more consistent method used by Olver et al. (2013), interrater reliability for change data was lower than that for pre- and post-treatment dynamic risk (ICC = 0.68 for change score, 0.82 for pre- and 0.84 for post-treatment dynamic risk), possibly because separate statistical error from each of pre- and post-dynamic risk scores is combined in the change score. Therefore, due to the higher number of error sources in the current study (e.g., multiple raters, use of interview and file information), change data may have been too unreliable for detecting relationships.

The question of how we should investigate the relationship of psychopathy to treatment change poses an interesting methodological challenge, because higher psychopathy goes hand in hand with higher criminal risk. We would expect those at higher risk to have more room to change and therefore to be capable of greater change (Lewis et al., 2013). But higher psychopathy suggests less change – due to reduced responsivity – and studies have not controlled for criminal risk in order to look at the amount of change in the presence of psychopathy.

In conjunction with the recidivism results described in the preceding section, these studies of treatment-related change suggest that PCL–psychopathic offenders can indeed be effectively treated through intensive services, that effective treatment can reduce risk, that effective treatment sometimes renders PCL scores irrelevant as indicators of outcome, and that PCL scores may affect the amount of change made The current pool of relevant research is certainly small and requires replication; it is clear that this topic is worthy of ongoing systematic investigation.

The treatment of psychopathy

The final conceptual issue to consider is whether there is any evidence that *psychopathy* can be treated effectively. To answer this question, we need first to consider whether the treatment of psychopathy is more than simply the treatment of criminal risk. Even if we confine the definition of psychopathy to high scores on PCL–psychopathy, still not all facets are equally related or even related at all to criminal risk or its outcomes (recidivism), and in some cases relationships are in opposing directions (Daly, 2017; Leistico, Salekin, DeCoster, & Rogers, 2008; Yang et al., 2010). Therefore, treatments aimed at – and successful in – reducing criminal risk are not necessarily working to change behavior that has been theoretically linked to all aspects psychopathy, let alone modifying the underlying personality traits that are expressed in that behavior. In fact, experts have suggested that in correctional settings, the mandate is to treat risk rather than personality disorder, and further, that PCL Factor 1 characteristics (e.g., manipulation, lack of empathy) may not be changeable and therefore should be worked with or round (e.g., by careful management of treatment-interfering behavior) rather than worked *on* (Thornton & Blud, 2007; Wong, 2013; Wong et al., 2012; Wong & Hare, 2005).

However, psychopathy is theoretically associated with socially and personally harmful behavior, not just criminal behavior, and there is plenty of anecdotal and some empirical evidence to back this up. For an example of the latter, U.S. presidents were rated on Fearless Dominance and impulsive antisociality, two factors of psychopathy estimated in this study from items derived from the NEO–PI–R (Costa & McCrae, 1992).[4] Lilienfeld et al. (2012) found that presidents' scores on impulsive antisociality predicted impeachment resolutions by Congress, allowing subordinates to behave unethically, extramarital sexual relationships, being "AWOL" from their responsibilities, and abuses of power. In a study of corporate professionals, psychopathy was found to correlate negatively with being a team player, with management skills, with overall achievement as based on 360 degree ratings, and with performance appraisals (Babiak, Neumann, & Hare, 2010). In other words, psychopathy may contribute to a much wider range of social harms than crime alone, but interestingly, non-criminal, and especially family, social, or non-work-related behavior seldom seems to have been little studied.

But is there any evidence that treatment can alter or attenuate these harmful traits? With youth samples, there are some promising results. Based on self-report ratings of forensic hospital-treated adolescents, Rogers, Jackson, Sewell, and Johansen (2004) found that about a quarter of their sample significantly reduced psychopathic trait scores over treatment. In a similar design at the Mendota Juvenile Treatment Center program, highly psychopathic participants completed the Antisocial Process Screening Device (APSD; Frick & Hare, 2001; a self-report questionnaire based on the PCL–R) at assessment, 90, and 180 days into the program. Significant changes were seen when comparing each pair of consecutive measurement occasions across all three clusters of traits (callousness/unemotional, narcissistic, and impulsive) except for narcissism, where for pre-program to 90-day measurement, only a small amount of change was recorded (Caldwell, McCormick, Wolfe, & Umstead, 2012). We know of no studies like this with adults: in part, perhaps, because self-report has not been a popular method of assessing psychopathy in adult offenders, and other methods (e.g., PCL–R) are not designed to be sensitive to change.

It may be that psychopathy is more malleable in adolescents than in adults (Caldwell et al., 2012). But there is evidence that personality traits change in adulthood as part of development and maturation (Caspi, Roberts, & Shiner, 2005; Roberts & Mroczek, 2008) even for those with personality disorder and especially for Cluster B (histrionic, borderline, antisocial and so on; Tyrer & Seivewright, 2008). Steady progress has been made with techniques and treatment packages for various challenging personality disorders (e.g., Borderline Personality Disorder; Clarkin, Levy, Lenzenweger, & Kernberg, 2007), some of which are commonly comorbid with psychopathy (Kirkpatrick et al., 2010; Newhill, Vaughn, & DeLisi, 2010). More complete models for conceptualizing the classification and treatment of personality disorders through an understanding of the core mechanisms involved hold promise for psychopathy and for personality disorder more generally (Clarkin et al., 2015; Livesley, 2012).

It can also be argued that intensive therapeutic treatments for criminal risk in high-risk offenders may have an effect on personality characteristics. The extensiveness, stability, and change-resistant nature of stable dynamic risk factors makes them relatively trait-like. Observations of grandiosity and arrogance toward others, low empathy, callousness and lack of guilt, conning, lying, and manipulating others while in treatment will affect the rating of items on an instrument. Turned the other way, progress on dynamic risk factors, far from a "given" (Hanson, Harris, Scott, & Helmus, 2007), may show up as progress on aspects of dysfunctional personality, or at least its overt expression (Sainsbury, 2010). Knowing whether it does or not will depend on research yet to be done.

Meanwhile, a number of jurisdictions have engaged with the treatment of personality disorder itself in the quest to improve the prosocial functioning of their riskiest and most change-challenged clients. The Dangerous and Severe Personality Disorder project in the U.K. was an expensive endeavor that yielded little evidence of success at the time (O'Loughlin, 2014; Tyrer et al., 2010). But it did support some diversity in experimental models of personality disorder treatment, resulting in the current strategy – the Offender Personality Disorders Pathway (OPDP) – which is building on what was learned during the first decade of the project. But the strategy has moved now toward successful approaches to creating a much wider range of change-supportive residential environments and programs and providing through-care for far more of the affected offenders. The Westgate Unit at HMP Frankland is one contemporary example of a fully developed multidisciplinary treatment environment for high-risk and violent prisoners (Bull & Tew, 2015; Hawes, 2010) and houses the Chromis program, which is developing into a comprehensive model of treatment for people with psychopathy, albeit that it purports mainly to focus on changing offending risk (Tew & Atkinson, 2013).

Forensic hospitals in the Netherlands have been providing intensive treatment for some time for personality-disordered offenders, but with limited outcome data to date. Researchers and clinicians have been examining the potential of Young's Early Maladaptive Schemas to explain core features of criminality, and adapting Young's Schema Therapy (ST) as an intervention modality for psychopathy (Bernstein, Arntz, & de Vos, 2007; Bernstein et al., 2012; de Ruiter et al., 2016). Patients spend up to ten years in hospital, providing an opportunity to develop intensive interventions to reduce risk and improve social and personal functioning. There are no robust outcome studies of this treatment to date (Bernstein et al., 2007; Bernstein et al., 2012; de Ruiter et al., 2016), although there are indirect signs that if it is intensive and multimodal, including individual therapy sessions, pharmacological treatment, milieu, vocational and educational programs, art therapies, relapse prevention approaches for aggressive behavior and addictions, and so on – it may be effective in reducing recidivism (Bernstein et al., 2007; Bernstein et al., 2012; de Ruiter et al., 2016).

A three-year randomized clinical trial is underway to compare the recent adaptation of Schema Therapy (ST) with the older TAU condition for male patients with antisocial, Borderline, Narcissistic, or Paranoid personality disorders. A preliminary study containing the first 30 men showed ST men achieved supervised and unsupervised leave more than four months earlier than TAU men, but changes in Historical Clinical Risk (HCR)–20 scores (Webster, Douglas, Eaves, & Hart, 1997) to date were not significantly different for the ST group; both groups were trending downward. However, there is currently no "untreated" baseline sample to compare with the two regimes to provide a more stringent test of effect. Mean psychopathy scores for the two samples are below the cut-off of 25, which also means that this is a moderately rather than very high psychopathy group. To date no effects on psychopathy symptoms have been reported, but a recent case study suggests potential for reductions in these characteristics (Chakhssi, Bernstein, & de Ruiter, 2014), albeit over very lengthy periods of treatment that may not be available in many jurisdictions.

In New Zealand, intensive programs are routinely provided in high risk violent and sexual offenders in prison, many of whom will have high PCL–psychopathy scores. However, most treatments are only available to those who attain medium or low security status during their sentence; security classification is based in part on behavioral history in custody, and so can reduce from an initial high classification to lower levels as the sentence progresses, assuming a history of stable and compliant behavior and negative drug tests. Some men with high PCL–psychopathy do not attain these lower levels of security because of ongoing aggression, poor emotional control, and so on, rendering them unable to access these programs. Such men may be released to the community without any significant rehabilitative or reintegration experience. An intensive program for people with high psychopathy scores who also stuck in maximum and high security environments has been provided over several years, with the aim of improving institutional behavior and engagement in change for small numbers of these men.

The theoretical model for this program is Livesley's (Clarkin et al., 2015; Livesley, 2012) integrated domain model for the treatment of personality disorder (Wilson & Tamatea, 2013). The High-Risk Personality Program (HRPP–R; Wilson & Kilgour, 2015). The HRPP–R is modular, with three phases of three to four months each: (1) focus on safety, containment, and engagement, (2) control and regulation and exploration and change, and (3) synthesis: construction of a more adaptive sense of self and identity. The therapy is provided by highly experienced psychological service staff in the form of three group sessions (2.5 hours each) and a one-hour individual session each week. The custodial unit is not a treatment environment, but custody staff have been trained to monitor prisoner behavior and record progress on a brief instrument designed to detect factors related to situational aggression. In a very preliminary evaluation of Phase 1, an immediate 70 percent reduction in violence was recorded (Wilson & Kilgour, 2015). However, no information is provided on whether there were changes in personality characteristics or other associated behavior as yet.

Conclusion

The treatment of psychopathy has been much written about and rarely provided. The small volume of research on the treatment of adult offenders with psychopathy is not matched by any research on the treatment of psychopathy more generally. This is not surprising because this research requires a combination of factors to come together, each of which predicts in its own right a lack of research. First, there are relatively few treatment programs for higher risk offenders, and psychopathy is often not measured in them. Second, even fewer of these programs are subject to outcome evaluations, let alone designs in which a comparison group which also has psychopathy scores is included. Third, although outcome evaluations are rare, rarer still are studies that document treatment change on dynamic risk or psychopathy characteristics over the course of treatment and follow-up. Studies rarely look at outcomes other than recidivism, either, which leaves us with little understanding of what treatment achieves.

Fifth, we have not yet clearly outlined a treatment theory that links symptoms of psychopathy, rehabilitative components, and changes in behavior, meaning there is no agreed way to measure and document psychopathy change. Theoretically linking pathways from psychopathy characteristics to dynamic risk factors and strategies for ameliorating these factors would be helpful for program development and change measurement. Sixth, psychopathy includes components that have a substantial influence on responsivity. Responsivity is the most poorly articulated of the RNR model core principles (Bourgon & Bonta, 2014), and few studies address what it is, how it affects engagement and change, and how it can be remediated.

A variety of other issues hamper progress. Methodologically, if we are to avoid the tautology of psychopathy being diagnosed based on criminal behavior and then saying that people behaving criminally because of their psychopathy, we need both to measure psychopathy using tools that are independent of criminal history, ensure we use independent raters for each, and control statistically for criminal risk when investigating the influence of psychopathy.

A number of studies have examined psychopathy's role in treatment with relatively low scoring samples. Research samples should at least ensure that the characteristics associated with the PCL scales Factor 1 are reasonably high, to avoid simply pathologizing criminal risk factors. Future research, if using Hare's scales, should analyze at the facet level. Relatedly, the use of other measures such as the PPI–R (Lilienfeld & Widows, 2005) would also be worthwhile. The treatment of psychopathy and the people who exhibit it remain a fascinating subject; perhaps we can hope that the tentatively encouraging results over the last decade signal a period of flourishing for this research literature.

Notes

1 He was referring to other procedures of the times, now largely discredited or at least for this type of presentation (e.g., prefrontal or transorbital lobotomies, topectomy, electroconvulsive therapy).

2 Barbaree (2005) reported over an average of 5.2 years of follow-up, 42 percent general recidivism and 24% sexual or violent recidivism. By comparison, for high-risk offenders Lewis et al. (2013) reported 46% recidivated violently over 4.9 years, and over an average of 3.5 years in New Zealand, 62% of high-risk treatment completers and 72% of their matched untreated controls were reconvicted for violence. For any new conviction, the rates were 83% and 95% respectively (Polaschek, 2011).

3 It should be noted that the measurement issues involved are sufficiently problematic that they do not yet make for strong arguments for rethinking the model's tenets. For example, this method of testing for the validity of treatment change relies on no additional change after treatment that would alter the ranking of participants with each other in relation to change. But recently we have shown that post-treatment change may not be related to in-treatment change (Yesberg & Polaschek, 2014), and that progress made after treatment may end up being a better predictor of recidivism (Polaschek, Yesberg, & Chauhan, 2017).

4 Impulsive/antisocial is a subscale in the Psychopathic Inventory Revised (PPI–R; (Lilienfeld & Widows, 2005). PPI–R is usually a self-report questionnaire, but for this study its scale scores were estimated statistically from the results of the much more extensive questionnaire that for each president was completed by an expert (e.g., biographer, journalist) who knew him well.

References

Abracen, J., and Looman, J. (2016) *Treatment of high-risk sexual offenders*, Chichester: Wiley.

Abracen, J., Looman, J., and Langton, C. M. (2008) 'Treatment of sexual offenders with psychopathic traits: Recent research developments and clinical implications,' *Trauma, Violence, & Abuse*, *9*:144–166.

Alford, C. F. (1997) *What evil means to us*, Ithaca, NY: Cornell University.

American Psychiatric Association. (2013) *Diagnostic and statistical manual of mental disorders (DSM–5)* (5th ed.), Arlington VA: Author.

Andrews, D. A., and Bonta, J. (2010a) *The psychology of criminal conduct* (5th ed.), Newark, NJ: Matthew Bender.

Andrews, D. A., and Bonta, J. (2010b) 'Rehabilitating criminal justice policy and practice,' *Psychology, Public Policy, and Law*, *16*:39–55.

Andrews, D. A., Bonta, J., and Hoge, R. D. (1990) 'Classification for effective rehabilitation: Rediscovering psychology,' *Criminal Justice and Behavior*, *17*:19–52.

Babiak, P., Neumann, C. S., and Hare, R. D. (2010) 'Corporate psychopathy: Talking the walk,' *Behavioral Sciences and the Law*, *28*:174–193.

Barbaree, H. E. (2005) 'Psychopathy, treatment behavior, and recidivism: An extended follow-up of Seto and Barbaree,' *Journal of Interpersonal Violence*, *20*:1115–1131.

Bell, R. K., and Polaschek, D. L. L. (2017) 'Do high-risk prisoners entering treatment have clinically impaired cognitive impulse control?,' *Psychiatry, Psychology and Law*, *24*:576–593.

Berg, J. M., Lilienfeld, S. O., and Sellbom, M. (2017) 'The role of boldness in psychopathy: A study of academic and clinical perceptions,' *Personality Disorders: Theory, Research, and Treatment*, *8*:319–328.

Bernstein, D. P., Arntz, A., and de Vos, M. (2007) 'Schema focused therapy in forensic settings: Theoretical model and recommendations for best clinical practice,' *International Journal of Forensic Mental Health*, *6*:169–183.

Bernstein, D. P., Nijman, H. L. I., Karos, K., Keulen-de Vos, M., de Vogel, V., and Lucker, T. P. (2012) 'Schema therapy for forensic patients with personality disorders: Design and preliminary findings of a multicenter randomized clinical trial in the Netherlands,' *International Journal of Forensic Mental Health*, *11*:312–324.

Blackburn, R. (1993) *The psychology of criminal conduct*, Chichester: Wiley.

Blackburn, R. (1999) 'Violence and personality distinguishing among violent offenders,' in D. Curran & W. G. McCarthey (Eds.), *Psychological perspectives on serious criminal risk* (pp. 109–127), Leicester: BPS.

Blasko, B. L., and Jeglic, E. L. (2016) 'Sexual offenders' perceptions of the client–therapist relationship,' *Sexual Abuse: A Journal of Research & Treatment*, *28*:271–290.

Bonn, S.A. (2017, Feb 26) 'Psychopathic killers hide in plain sight,' *Psychology Today*. Retrieved April 25, 2018 from www.psychologytoday.com/blog/wicked-deeds/201702/psychopathic-killers-hide-in-plain-sight

Bordin, E. (1979) 'The generalizability of the psychoanalytic concept of the working alliance,' *Psychotherapy*, *16*:252–260.

Bourgon, G., and Bonta, J. (2014) 'Reconsidering the responsivity principle: A way to move forward,' *Federal Probation*, *78*(2):3–10.

Bull, C., and Tew, J. (2015) 'Chromis: Beyond the treatment room,' *Prison Service Journal*, *218*:31–34.

Caldwell, M. F., McCormick, D. J., Umstead, D., and van Rybroek, G. J. (2007) 'Evidence of treatment progress and therapeutic outcomes among adolescent offenders with psychopathy features,' *Criminal Justice and Behavior*, *34*:573–587.

Caldwell, M. F., McCormick, D. J., Wolfe, J., and Umstead, D. (2012) 'Treatment-related changes in psychopathy features and behavior in adolescent offenders,' *Criminal Justice and Behavior*, *39*:144–155.

Caldwell, M. F., and van Rybroek, G. (2005) 'Reducing violence in serious juvenile offenders using intensive treatment,' *International Journal of Law and Psychiatry*, *28*:622–636.

Caldwell, M. F., and van Rybroek, G. (2013) 'Effective treatment programs for violent adolescents: Programmatic challenges and promising features,' *Aggression & Violent Behavior*, *18*:571–578.

Caldwell, M. F., Vitacco, M., and Van Rybroek, G. J. (2006) 'Are violent delinquents worth treating? A cost–benefit analysis,' *Journal of Research in Crime and Delinquency*, *43*:148–168.

Caspi, A., Roberts, B. W., and Shiner, R. L. (2005) 'Personality development: Stability and change,' *Annual Review of Psychology*, *56*:453–484.

Chakhssi, F., Bernstein, D., and de Ruiter, C. (2014) 'Treating the untreatable: A single case study of a psychopathic inpatient treated with Schema Therapy,' *Psychotherapy*, *51*:447–461.

Chakhssi, F., de Ruiter, C., and Bernstein, D. (2010) 'Change during forensic treatment in psychopathic vs. nonpsychopathic offenders,' *The Journal of Forensic Psychiatry and Psychology*, *21*:660–682.

Clarkin, J. F., Cain, N., and Livesley, W. J. (2015) 'An integrated approach to treatment of patients with personality disorders,' *Journal of Psychotherapy Integration*, *25*:3–12.

Clarkin, J. F., Levy, K. N., Lenzenweger, M. F., and Kernberg, O. F. (2007) 'Evaluating three treatments for borderline personality disorder: A multiwave study,' *The American Journal of Psychiatry & Law*, *164*:922–928.

Cleckley, H. M. (1988) *The mask of sanity: An attempt to reinterpret the so-called psychopathic personality* (5th ed.), St Louis, MO: Mosby.

Costa, P. T., and McCrae, R. R. (1992) *NEO PI–R professional manual*, Odessa, FL: Psychological Assessment Resources.

D'Silva, K., Duggan, C., and McCarthy, L. (2004) 'Does treatment really make psychopaths worse? A review of the evidence,' *Journal of Personality Disorders*, *18*:163–177.

Daly, T. E. (2017) Why are psychopaths difficult to treat? Testing the two-component model for the treatment of PCL psychopaths. Wellington, NZ: Doctor of Philosophy Thesis, Victoria University of Wellington.

Daly, T. E., Fletcher, G. J. O., and Polaschek, D. L. L. (2017a) 'PCL–psychopathy factors and facets predict involuntary but not voluntary non-completion of treatment in high-risk violent prisoners,' Paper under review.

Daly, T. E., Fletcher, G. J. O., and Polaschek, D. L. L. (2017b) 'The relevance of PCL–psychopathy to in-treatment behaviour: An examination with high-risk violent male prisoners,' Paper under review.

Daly, T. E., Ross, E. C., Fletcher, G. J. O., and Polaschek, D. L. L. (2017) 'Examining relationships between psychopathy (PCL:SV) scores and the therapeutic alliance in treatment for high-risk violent prisoners,' Papers under review.

de Ruiter, C., Chakhssi, F., and Bernstein, D. (2016) 'Treating the untreatable psychopath,' in C. B. Gacono (Ed.), *The clinical and forensic assessment of psychopathy: A practitioner's guide* (2nd ed., pp. 388–402), New York, NY: Routledge.

DeSorcy, D. R., Olver, M. E., and Wormith, J. S. (2017) 'Working alliance and psychopathy: Linkages to treatment outcome in a sample of treated sexual offenders,' *Journal of Interpersonal Violence*, in press.

Douglas, K. S., and Skeem, J. L. (2005) 'Violence risk assessment: Getting specific about being dynamic,' *Psychology, Public Policy, and Law*, *11*:347–383.

Forth, A. E., Kosson, D. S., and Hare, R. D. (2003) *Hare Psychopathy Checklist: Youth Version*, Toronto, ON: Multi-Health Systems.

Frick, P. J., and Hare, R. D. (2001) *The Antisocial Process Screening Device*, Toronto, CA: Multi-Health Systems.

Galloway, V. A., and Brodsky, S. L. (2003) 'Caring less, doing more: The role of therapeutic detachment with volatile and unmotivated clients,' *American Journal of Psychotherapy*, *57*:32–38.

Gendreau, P., Listwan, S. J., Kuhns, J. B., and Exum, M. L. (2014) 'Making prisoners accountable: Are contingency management programs the answer?,' *Criminal Justice & Behavior*, *41*:1079–1102.

Golden, C. J., Jackson, M. L., Peterson-Rohne, A., and Gontkovsky, S. T. (1996) 'Neuropsychological correlates of violence and aggression: A review of the clinical literature,' *Aggression and Violent Behavior*, *1*:3–25.

Hanson, R. K., Harris, A. J. R., Scott, T. L., and Helmus, L. (2007) *Assessing the risk of sexual offenders on community supervision: The dynamic supervision project.* Retrieved April 25,2018 from Ottawa, Ontario www.ps-sp.gc.ca/res/cor/rep

Hare, R. D. (1991) *The Hare Psychopathy Checklist–Revised*, Toronto, ON: Multi-Health Systems.

Hare, R. D. (2003) *The Hare Psychopathy Checklist–Revised technical manual* (2nd ed.), Toronto, ON: Multi-Health Systems.

Harris, G. T., and Rice, M. E. (2006) 'Treatment of psychopathy: A review of empirical findings,' in C. J. Patrick (Ed.), *Handbook of Psychopathy* (pp. 555–572), New York, NY: Guilford.

Harris, G. T., Rice, M. E., and Cormier, C. (1994) 'Psychopaths: Is a therapeutic community therapeutic?,' *Therapeutic Communities: International Journal for Therapeutic and Supportive Organizations*, *15*:283–299.

Hart, S., Cox, D., and Hare, R. (1995) *Manual for the Psychopathy Checklist: Screening Version (PCL:SV)*, Toronto, ON: Multi-Health Systems.

Hawes, V. (2010) 'Treating high-risk mentally disordered offenders: The dangerous and severe personality disorder initiative,' in A. Bartlett & G. McGauley (Eds.), *Forensic mental health: Concepts systems and practice* (pp. 215–234), Oxford: Oxford University Press.

Hicks, B. M., Markon, K. E., Patrick, C. J., Krueger, R. F., and Newman, J. P. (2004) 'Identifying psychopathy subtypes on the basis of personality structure,' *Psychological Assessment, 16*:276–288.
Hildebrand, M., and de Ruiter, C. (2012) 'Psychopathic traits and change on indicators of dynamic risk factors during inpatient forensic psychiatric treatment,' *International Journal of Law and Psychiatry, 35*:276–288.
Hobson, J., Shine, J., and Roberts, R. (2000) 'How do psychopaths behave in a prison therapeutic community?,' *Psychology, Crime & Law, 6*:139–154.
Horvath, A. O., and Greenberg, L. S. (1994) *The working alliance: Theory, research, and practice*, New York, NY: Wiley & Sons.
Hughes, G., Hogue, T., Hollin, C., and Champion, H. (1997) 'First-stage evaluation of a treatment programme for personality-disordered offenders,' *The Journal of Forensic Psychiatry and Psychology, 8*:515–527.
Karpman, B. (1941) 'On the need for separating psychopathy into two distinct clinical types: Symptomatic and idiopathic,' *Journal of Criminology and Psychopathology, 3*:112–137.
Kilgour, T. G., and Polaschek, D. L. L. (2012) *Breaking the cycle of crime: Special Treatment Unit evaluation report*, Wellington, New Zealand: Department of Corrections Psychological Services.
Kirkpatrick, J. T., Draycott, S., Freestone, M., Cooper, S., Twiselton, K., Watson, N., . . ., and Maden, T. (2010) 'A descriptive evaluation of patients and prisoners assessed for dangerous and severe personality disorder,' *The Journal of Forensic Psychiatry and Psychology, 21*:264–282.
Krueger, R. F., Schmutte, P. S., A., C., Moffitt, T. E., Campbell, K., and Silva, P. A. (1994) 'Personality traits are linked to crime among men and women: Evidence from a birth cohort,' *Journal of Abnormal Psychology, 103*:328–338.
Langton, C. M., Barbaree, H. E., Harkins, L., and Peacock, E. J. (2006) 'Sex offenders' response to treatment and its association with recidivism as a function of psychopathy,' *Sexual Abuse: A Journal of Research and Treatment, 18*:99–120.
Lee, Z., and Salekin, R. T. (2010) 'Psychopathy in a noninstitutional sample: Differences in primary and secondary subtypes,' *Personality Disorders: Theory, Research, and Treatment, 1*:153–169.
Leistico, A., Salekin, R. T., DeCoster, J., and Rogers, R. (2008) 'A large-scale meta-analysis relating the Hare measures of psychopathy to antisocial conduct,' *Law and Human Behavior, 32*:28–45.
Lewis, K., Olver, M. E., and Wong, S. C. P. (2013) 'The Violence Risk Scale: Predictive validity and linking treatment changes with recidivism in a sample of high risk and personality disordered offenders,' *Assessment, 20*:150–164.
Lilienfeld, S. O., Waldman, I. D., Landfield, K., Watts, A. L., Rubenzer, S., and Faschingbauer, T. R. (2012) 'Fearless dominance and the U.S. presidency: Implications of psychopathic personality traits for successful and unsuccessful political leadership,' *Journal of Personality and Social Psychology, 103*:489–505.
Lilienfeld, S. O., Watts, A. L., and Smith, S. F. (2015) 'Successful psychopathy: A status report,' *Current Directions in Psychological Science, 24*:298–303.
Lilienfeld, S. O., and Widows, M. (2005) *Psychopathic Personality Inventory–Revised professional manual*, Odessa, FL: PAR.
Livesley, W. J. (2012) 'Integrated treatment: A conceptual framework for an evidence-based approach to the treatment of personality disorder,' *Journal of Personality Disorders, 22*:17–42.
Looman, J., Abracen, J., Serin, R., and Marquis, P. (2005) 'Psychopathy, treatment change, and recidivism in high-risk, high-need sexual offenders,' *Journal of Interpersonal Violence, 20*:549–568.
Lösel, F. (1998) 'Treatment and management of psychopaths,' in D. J. Cooke, A. E. Forth, J. Newman, & R. D. Hare (Eds.), *Psychopathy: Theory research and implications for society* (pp. 303–354), Netherlands: Kluwer Academic Publishers.
Lowenkamp, C. T., and Latessa, E. J. (2004) 'Increasing the effectiveness of correctional programming through the risk principle: Identifying offenders for residential placement,' *Criminology and Public Policy, 4*:501–528.
McCord, W., and McCord, J. (1964) *The psychopath: An essay on the criminal mind*, Princeton, NJ: Van Nostrand.
Miller, J. D., Lamkin, J., and Maples-Keller, J. L. (2016) 'Examining the triarchic model of psychopathy through general personality and expert-based lenses,' *Personality Disorders: Theory, Research, and Treatment*, 7:247–258.
Miller, J. D., and Lynam, D. R. (2012) 'An examination of the Psychopathic Personality Inventory's nomological network: A meta-analytic review,' *Personality Disorders: Theory, Research, and Treatment, 3*:305–326.
Moffitt, T. E. (2003) 'Life-course-persistent and adolescence-limited antisocial behavior: A 10-year research review and a research agenda,' in B. B. Lahey, T. E. Moffitt, & A. Caspi (Eds.), *Causes of conduct disorder and juvenile delinquency* (pp. 49–75), New York, NY: Guilford.

Moffitt, T. E., Lynam, D. R., and Silva, P. A. (1994) 'Neuropsychological tests predicting persistent male delinquency,' *Criminology*, *32*:277–300.
Nadesu, A. (2009) *Reconviction patterns of released prisoners: A 60-month follow-up analysis*. Retrieved April 25, 2018 from www.corrections.govt.nz/__data/assets/pdf_file/0009/394902/Complete-Recidivism-Report-2009-DOC.pdf
Newhill, C. E., Vaughn, M. G., and DeLisi, M. (2010) 'Psychopathy scores reveal heterogeneity among patients with borderline personality disorder,' *Journal of Forensic Psychiatry and Psychology*, *21*:202–220.
Ogloff, J. R. P., Wong, S. C. P., and Greenwood, A. (1990) 'Treating criminal psychopaths in a therapeutic community program,' *Behavioral Sciences and the Law*, *8*:181–190.
O'Loughlin, A. (2014) 'The offender personality disorder pathway: Expansion in the face of failure?,' *Howard Journal of Criminal Justice*, *53*:173–192.
Olver, M., and Wong, S. C. P. (2011) 'Predictors of sex offender treatment dropout: Psychopathy, sex offender risk, and responsivity implications,' *Psychology, Crime & Law*, *17*:457–471.
Olver, M. E., Lewis, K., and Wong, S. C. P. (2013) 'Risk reduction treatment of high risk psychopathic offenders: The relationship of psychopathy and treatment change to violent recidivism,' *Personality Disorders: Theory, Research, and Treatment*, *4*:160–167.
Olver, M. E., Stockdale, K. C., and Wormith, J. S. (2011) 'A meta-analysis of predictors of offender treatment attrition and its relationship to recidivism,' *Journal Consulting and Clinical Psychology*, *79*:6–21.
Olver, M. E., and Wong, S. C. P. (2009) 'Therapeutic responses to psychopathic sexual offenders: Treatment attrition, therapeutic change, and long-term recidivism,' *Journal of Consulting and Clinical Psychology*, *77*:328–336.
Olver, M. E., and Wong, S. C. (2013) 'Treatment programs for high risk sexual offenders: Program and offender characteristics, attrition, treatment change and recidivism,' *Aggression and Violent Behavior*, *18*:579–591.
Patrick, C. J., Fowles, D. C., and Krueger, R. F. (2009) 'Triarchic conceptualization of psychopathy: Developmental origins of disinhibition, boldness, and meanness,' *Development and Psychopathology*, *21*:913–938.
Polaschek, D. L. L. (2008) *Rimutaka violence prevention unit evaluation report V: Interim/progress report on prospective evaluation*, Wellington, NZ: Unpublished report for the New Zealand Department of Corrections.
Polaschek, D. L. L. (2011) 'High-intensity rehabilitation for violent offenders in New Zealand: Reconviction outcomes for high- and medium-risk prisoners,' *Journal of Interpersonal Violence*, *26*:664–682.
Polaschek, D. L. L. (2014) 'Adult criminals with psychopathy: Common beliefs about treatability and change have little empirical support,' *Current Directions in Psychological Science*, *23*:296–301.
Polaschek, D. L. L., and Daly, T. (2013) 'Treatment and psychopathy in forensic settings,' *Aggression & Violent Behavior*, *18*:592–603.
Polaschek, D. L. L., and Ross, E. C. (2010) 'Do early therapeutic alliance, motivation, and change readiness predict therapy outcomes for high risk violent prisoners?,' *Criminal Behaviour and Mental Health*, *20*:100–111.
Polaschek, D. L. L., Wilson, N. J., Townsend, M., and Daly, L. (2005) 'Cognitive–behavioral rehabilitation for high-risk violent offenders: An outcome evaluation of the Violence Prevention Unit,' *Journal of Interpersonal Violence*, *20*:1611–1627.
Polaschek, D. L. L., Yesberg, J. A., Bell, R. K., Casey, A. R., and Dickson, S. R. (2016) 'Intensive psychological treatment of high-risk violent offenders: Outcomes and pre-release mechanisms,' *Psychology, Crime & Law*, *22*:344–365.
Polaschek, D. L. L., Yesberg, J. A., and Chauhan, P. (2017) A year without a conviction: An integrated examination of potential mechanisms for successful re-entry in high-risk violent prisoners, Accepted pending revision.
Poythress, N. G., Edens, J. F., Skeem, J. L., Lilienfeld, S. O., Douglas, K. S., Frick, P. J., . . ., and Wang, T. (2010) 'Identifying subtypes among offenders with antisocial personality disorder: A cluster-analytic study,' *Journal of Abnormal Psychology*, *119*:389–400.
Poythress, N. G., Lilienfeld, S. O., Skeem, J. L., Douglas, K. S., Edens, J. F., Epstein, M., and Patrick, C. J. (2010) 'Using the PCL–R to help estimate the validity of two self-report measures of psychopathy with offenders,' *Assessment*, *17*:206–219.
Rice, M. E., Harris, G. T., and Cormier, C. A. (1992) 'An evaluation of a maximum security therapeutic community for psychopaths and other mentally disordered offenders,' *Law and Human Behavior*, *16*:399–412.
Richards, H. J., Casey, J. O., and Lucente, S. W. (2003) 'Psychopathy and treatment response in incarcerated female substance abusers,' *Criminal Justice and Behavior*, *30*:251–276.

Roberts, B. W., and Mroczek, D. (2008) 'Personality trait change in adulthood,' *Current Directions in Psychological Science, 17*:31–35.

Rogers, R., Jackson, R. L., Sewell, K. W., and Johansen, J. (2004) 'Predictors of treatment outcome in dually diagnosed antisocial youth: An initial study of forensic inpatients,' *Behavioral Sciences & the Law, 22*:215–222.

Ross, E. C. (2008) Investigating the relationship between the therapeutic alliance and treatment outcome in violent offender treatment, Victoria University of Wellington Doctor of Philosophy Thesis. Wellington, New Zealand.

Ross, R. R., Fabiano, E. A., and Ewles, C. D. (1988) 'Reasoning and rehabilitation,' *International Journal of Offender Therapy and Comparative Criminology, 32*:29–36.

Sainsbury, L. (2010) 'Violent offending treatment for male patients with personality disorder,' in A. Tennant & K. Howells (Eds.), *Using time, not doing time: Practitioner perspectives on personality disorder and risk* (pp. 111–124), Chichester: Wiley.

Salekin, R. T. (2002) 'Psychopathy and therapeutic pessimism: Clinical lore or clinical reality?,' *Clinical Psychology Review, 22*:79–112.

Salekin, R. T., Worley, C., and Grimes, R. D. (2010) 'Treatment of psychopathy: A review and brief introduction to the mental model approach for psychopathy,' *Behavioral Sciences & the Law, 28*:235–266.

Schofield, W. (1964) *Psychotherapy: The purchase of friendship*, Englewood Cliffs, NJ: Prentice-Hall.

Serin, R. C., Lloyd, C. D., Helmus, L., Derkzen, D. M., and Luong, D. (2013) 'Does intra-individual change predict offender recidivism? Searching for the Holy Grail in assessing offender change,' *Aggression & Violent Behavior, 18*:32–53.

Seto, M. C., and Barbaree, H. E. (1999) 'Psychopathy, treatment behavior, and sex offender recidivism,' *Journal of Interpersonal Violence, 14*:1235–1248.

Singh, J. P., Grann, M., and Fazel, S. (2011) 'A comparative study of violence risk assessment tools: A systematic review and metaregression analysis of 68 studies involving 25,980 participants,' *Clinical Psychology Review, 31*:499–513.

Skeem, J. L., Johansson, P., Andershed, H., Kerr, M., and Louden, J. E. (2007) 'Two subtypes of psychopathic violent offenders that parallel primary and secondary variants,' *Journal of Abnormal Psychology, 116*:395–409.

Skeem, J. L., Monahan, J., and Mulvey, E. (2002) 'Psychopathy, treatment involvement, and subsequent violence among civil psychiatric patients,' *Law and Human Behavior, 26*:577–603.

Skeem, J. L., Polaschek, D. L. L., and Manchak, S. (2009) 'Appropriate treatment works, but how? Rehabilitating general, psychopathic, and high risk offenders,' in J. L. Skeem, K. Douglas, & S. Lilienfeld (Eds.), *Psychological science in the courtroom: Controversies and consensus* (pp. 358–384), Washington, DC: American Psychological Association.

Skeem, J. L., Polaschek, D. L. L., Patrick, C. J., and Lilienfeld, S. O. (2011) 'Psychopathic personality: Bridging the gap between scientific evidence and public policy,' *Psychological Science in the Public Interest, 12*:95–162.

Tew, J., and Atkinson, R. (2013) 'The Chromis Programme: From conception to evaluation,' *Psychology, Crime & Law, 11*:415–431.

Thornton, D., and Blud, L. (2007) 'The influence of psychopathic traits on response to treatment,' in H. Herve & J. C. Yuille (Eds.), *The psychopath: Theory, research, and practice* (pp. 505–539), Mahwah, NJ: Lawrence Erlbaum Associates.

Tyrer, P., Duggan, C., Cooper, S., Crawford, M., Seivewright, H., Rutter, D., . . ., and Barrett, B. (2010) 'The successes and failures of the DSPD experiment: The assessment and management of severe personality disorder,' *Medicine, Science and Law, 50*:95–99.

Tyrer, P., and Seivewright, H. (2008) 'Stable instability: The natural history of personality disorders,' *Psychiatry*, 7:129–132.

Utt, K., Saxon, E., Bozman, R. (Producers) and Demme, J. (Director). (1991) *The silence of the lambs* [Motion Picture], USA: Orion Pictures.

Walton, A., Jeglic, E. L., and Blasko, B. L. (2016) 'The role of psychopathic traits in the development of the therapeutic alliance among sexual offenders,' *Sexual Abuse: A Journal of Research & Treatment*, in press.

Webster, C. D., Douglas, K. S., Eaves, D., and Hart, S. D. (1997) *HCR–20: Assessing risk for violence (version 2)*, Burnaby, BC, Canada: Mental Health, Law, and Policy Institute, Simon Fraser University.

Wilson, N. J., and Kilgour, G. (2015) 'Practice,' *The New Zealand Corrections Journal, 3*(2):10–18.

Wilson, N. J., and Tamatea, A. (2013) 'Challenging the 'urban myth' of psychopathy untreatability: The High-Risk Personality Programme,' *Psychology, Crime and Law, 19*:493–510.

Wong, S., and Gordon, A. (2006) 'The validity and reliability of the Violence Risk Scale: A treatment-friendly violence risk assessment tool,' *Psychology, Public Policy, and Law, 12*:279–309.
Wong, S., and Gordon, A. (2013) 'The Violence Reduction Program: A treatment program for violence prone forensic clients,' *Psychology, Crime & Law, 11*:461–475.
Wong, S., Gordon, A., and Gu, D. (2007) 'Assessment and treatment of violence-prone forensic clients: An integrated approach,' *British Journal of Psychiatry, 190*:s66–s74.
Wong, S., Olver, M. E., Nicholaichuk, T. P., and Gordon, A. (2003) *The violence risk scale: Sexual offender version (VRS–SO)*, Regional Psychiatric Centre and University of Saskatchewan, Saskatoon, Saskatchewan, Canada.
Wong, S. C. P. (2000) 'Psychopathic offenders,' in S. Hodgins & R. Muller-Isberner (Eds.), *Violence, crime and mentally disordered offenders* (pp. 87–112), Chichester: Wiley.
Wong, S. C. P. (2013) 'Treatment of psychopathy in correctional settings,' in O. Thienhaus & M. Piasecki (Eds.), *Textbook on correctional psychiatry* (pp. 1–26), New York, NY: Civic Research Press.
Wong, S. C. P., Gordon, A., Gu, D., Lewis, K., and Olver, M. E. (2012) 'The effectiveness of violence reduction treatment for psychopathic offenders: Empirical evidence and a treatment model,' *International Journal of Forensic Mental Health, 11*:336–349.
Wong, S. C. P., and Hare, R. D. (2005) *Guidelines for a psychopathy treatment program*, Toronto, ON: Multi-Health Systems.
Yang, M., Wong, S. C. P., and Coid, J. W. (2010) 'The efficacy of violence prediction: A meta-analytic comparison of nine risk assessment tools,' *Psychological Bulletin, 136*:740–767.
Yildirim, B. O., and Derksen, J. J. L. (2015) 'Clarifying the heterogeneity in psychopathic samples: Towards a continuum of primary and secondary psychopathy,' *Aggression and Violent Behavior, 24*:9–41.

40

Psychopathy

An obscure public health issue

Dennis E. Reidy and Kristin M. Holland

Introduction

Public health is a discipline that aims to ensure health, safety, and well-being at the population level – that is, for entire communities, states, and nations. It encompasses a wide variety of issues ranging from infectious and chronic diseases such as tuberculosis and diabetes to birth defects, injuries, mental health, and many more. While the fields of medical, behavioral, and mental health practice aim to diagnose and treat patients presenting with specific health problems, public health researchers and practitioners aim to study the distribution of such problems, identify factors that increase the risk for or protect against the them, and implement programs, practices, and policies to prevent these harms from occurring in the first place.

Traditionally, public health research and practice focused primarily on preventing the spread of infectious diseases. The field was born out of the cholera epidemic in London in the 1850s, during which John Snow, who many recognize as the world's first epidemiologist, identified the Broad Street Water Pump to be the source of bacteria responsible for the rapid transmission of cholera that resulted in over 500 deaths within a 250-yard perimeter surrounding the pump over a one-week period. Snow's meticulous mapping of cholera deaths over this period of time and research connecting almost all of the deaths to a common source of water bred the modern-day fields of epidemiology and public health (Fine et al., 2013; Snow, 1860).

Today, public health activities are numerous, wide-reaching, and part of everyday life. They include broad actions such as vaccinating children and youth, educating the public on the harms related to certain behaviors (e.g., cigarette smoking), and implementing policies such as those that increase medical insurance coverage and inherently prevent negative health outcomes. The fact that we wear seat belts and have implemented policies to require seat belt wearing is related to the finding that seat belts save thousands of lives every year – a major public health implication (Curran, 1969). The fact that smoking is no longer permitted in many public settings is related to the research indicating that second-hand smoke is a major contributor to chronic diseases such as asthma and cancer, and is a policy that greatly impacts public health.

Author note: The findings and conclusions in this chapter are those of the authors and do not necessarily represent the official position of the Centers for Disease Control and Prevention.

A particularly crucial public health activity is the tracking and monitoring of health problems (i.e., surveillance) so their distribution within and their burden upon the general public are well understood. Surveillance within the field of public health is carried out for the purpose of serving as an early warning system for impending public health emergencies, documenting the impact of intervention strategies, or monitoring the epidemiology of health problems, and to inform public health policy and strategies (WHO, 2014). Additionally, surveillance systems help to identify which groups are at higher risk than others to experience negative health outcomes and potentially why they are at increased risk.

Violence as a public health issue

Since the 1850s, the field of public health has grown immensely, perhaps mostly in the recognition of its application to more than merely infectious disease. Most recently, injuries and violence have emerged as serious public health problems. In fact, unintentional injury, homicide, and suicide are among the ten leading causes of death annually among 10–44-year-olds in the United States (CDC, 2017a). Violence was first identified as a public health concern by the Surgeon General nearly four decades ago (U.S. Department of Health, Education, & Welfare, 1979) and has since been recognized as a major international public health problem by the World Health Organization (Krug, Dahlberg, Mercy, Zwi, & Lozano, 2002).

People are often surprised to learn that the Centers for Control and Disease Prevention (CDC) has a Division of Violence Prevention (DVP). For many, violence is not immediately recognized as a public health factor. Yet, 1.5 million people are treated in emergency departments, more than 169,000 are hospitalized, and over 16,000 die as a result of violence each year in the U.S. alone (CDC, 2017b; Florence, Haegerich, Simon, Zhou, & Luo, 2015; Florence, Simon, Haegerich, Luo, & Zhou, 2015). But the health consequences of violence go well beyond the initial direct physical injuries and include a wide range of chronic physical and psychological health problems such as gastrointestinal disorders, pelvic inflammatory disease, chronic pain, cancer, cardiovascular disease, hypertension, diabetes, seizures, risky sexual behavior, sexually transmitted diseases, teen pregnancy, anxiety, post-traumatic stress, depression, substance abuse, and suicidal ideation, to name a few (Campbell, 2002; CDC, 2016; Coker, Smith, Bethea, King, & McKeown, 2000; Krug et al., 2002; Walsh, Keyes, Koenen, & Hasin, 2015). Among youth, those that have been victims or witnesses of violence are more likely to be diagnosed with a psychological disorder and show difficulties with early attachment, emotion regulation, peer relationships, school adjustment, prosocial behaviors, and endorse attitudes condoning violence (Cyr, Euser, Bakermans-Kranenburg, & Van Ijzendoorn, 2010; Farrell & Sullivan, 2004; Guerra, Huesmann, & Spindler, 2003; Wekerle & Wolfe, 2003). Moreover, violence-related health care, lost work days, and reduced productivity cost the global economy billions of U.S. dollars per year (Dahlberg, 2007; Krug et al., 2002). The most current estimated single year cost in 2017 USD for medical expenses and lost productivity due to homicide and nonfatal assaults reaches approximately $63 billion in the U.S. (CDC, n.d.). Without doubt, violence is a public health issue.

Finally, similar to infectious diseases which greatly impact public health, some experts (e.g., Slutkin, 2012; Loftin, 1986) have suggested that violence is contagious, indicating that it shares the three characteristics central to infectious diseases: clustering, spread, and transmission. For instance, interpersonal gun violence often clusters spatially in inner-city areas plagued with high crime and where gangs are prevalent; violence can spread – that is, one violent incident can serve as the impetus for others (e.g., riots that stem from an initial violent event such as a coup d'état); and violence can be transmitted through spread from one event to another, but can also be transmitted from one person to another (e.g., through the cyclical, intergenerational effect of exposure to violence in the home; Slutkin, 2012).

The public health approach to violence prevention

Recently, the Division of Violence Prevention within CDC released its current strategic vision highlighting key foci of their public health model for violence prevention (CDC, 2016). Fundamentally, public health focuses on achieving change at the population level to provide the most benefit to the maximum number of people (Dahlberg, 2007; Hemenway & Miller, 2013). The public health approach has often produced global prevention initiatives that are implemented at the community and societal levels (e.g., policies mandating seatbelts, media campaigns educating public about effects of tobacco, fluoridation of drinking water) as opposed to focusing on prevention at the individual level. Community level interventions of this nature have the potential to reach a much larger base of people. However, for those individuals most at risk, particularly for such entrenched pathology as violence, prevention strategies may require an intervention with more significant intensity, dosage, or potency (CDC, 2016; Reidy, Kearns, & DeGue, 2013). Thus, prevention efforts must attend to risk factors across multiple levels of the social ecology, suggesting that individual-level factors remain an important component of violence prevention (e.g., CDC, 2016; Matjasko, Vivolo-Kantor, Massetti, Holland, Holt, & Dela Cruz, 2012; Wilkins, Tsao, Hertz, Davis, & Klevens, 2014). For this reason, identifying targeted prevention strategies for indicated persons at most risk for violence is a critical component of a comprehensive public health approach to violence prevention (CDC, 2016).

In fact, evidence suggests that concentrating prevention efforts on populations at heightened risk of violence may yield greater impact on collective levels of violence (CDC, 2016; Reidy et al., 2015). Given that only about 5 percent of the population commits the majority of society's violence (Beaver, 2013; Moffit, 1993; Tracy, Wolfgang, & Figlio, 1990; Vaughn et al., 2011; Vaughn, Salas-Wright, DeLisi, & Maynard, 2014; Wolfgang, Figlio, & Sellin, 1972), it seems only logical to identify and intervene with this high-risk minority. Notably, researchers have historically classified violence into a set of categories or typologies (e.g., sexual violence, youth violence, child maltreatment, collective violence) in order to better understand and prevent violence (Dahlberg, 2007). However, there is a growing awareness that different types of violence share common risk and protective factors, and those who are perpetrators of one form of violence are likely to be perpetrators of another (CDC, 2016; Wilkins et al., 2014). For this reason, public health aims to prevent multiple forms of violence and have the greatest impact for society by intervening with those individuals who represent the high-risk minority of the population (CDC, 2016).

Much in the way community policing was developed as a proactive approach to prevent crime before it happens, the public health approach to violence is an attempt to prevent it before it onsets: a strategy known as primary prevention. In this respect, primary prevention differs from secondary and tertiary prevention, which aim to reduce recidivism and ameliorate the short- and long-term effects of violence perpetration and victimization, respectively. For violence (as is the case with many public health issues) this means starting prevention by working with youth (CDC, 2016) to prevent exposure to risks associated with violence, modify unsafe and unhealthy behaviors that can result in violence victimization and perpetration, and improve resistance to violence should exposure occur either intentionally or unintentionally. Pertinently, in the U.S., 16 percent of high-school students report carrying a weapon, 5 percent report carrying a gun, 7 percent (10 percent of girls) report ever being physically forced to have sexual intercourse (Kann et al., 2016), and 50 percent of all homicide perpetrators are youth (Cooper &

Smith, 2011). These striking statistics affirm the necessity of implementing violence prevention strategies in adolescence or earlier. And of course, we know that those individuals who initiate violence at an earlier age tend to be chronic, diverse, and versatile offenders (e.g., Moffitt, 1993; Reidy et al., 2015). Thus, the primary prevention of violence by this highest-risk minority of the population will likely have the most substantial impact across the lifespan (Cohen & Piquero, 2009; Reidy et al., 2015).

Admittedly, it is difficult to identify high-risk, early onset perpetrators when they have yet to engage in violence. And of course, the goal of the public health approach is to prevent violence before it onsets. Consequently, identifying early warning signs (i.e., risk factors) that cut across the multiple forms of violence can help with the implementation of targeted strategies and the prevention of the multiple forms of violence. Many of the behavioral and experiential risk factors associated with perpetrating violence are evident well before ten years of age (CDC, 2016; Wilkins et al., 2014). In fact, as we will discuss in the next section, there are a number of biological, behavioral, and psychological risk factors for violence that can be identified as early as age 3 (Gao, Raine, Venables, Dawson, & Mednick, 2010a, 2010b; Kimonis et al., 2006; Willoughby et al., 2014; Wilkins et al., 2014). Importantly, the identification of these shared risk and protective factors for multiple forms of violence is integral to the public health model of violence prevention. In order to identify the minority of the population that will commit the majority of the population's violence, we must identify those risk and protective factors that are common to the varying forms of violence.

Simply put, the public health model for violence prevention facilitates the identification, implementation, and scale-up of prevention approaches that have cross-cutting impact by (1) identifying risk and protective factors that cut across multiple forms of violence to, (2) identify the sub-populations that are at highest risk to become chronic perpetrators committing violence in multiple settings against diverse types of victims, and (3) implement violence prevention strategies with these individuals in adolescence or childhood, before the onset of such violence. The public health system works in conjunction with the criminal justice system to impact violence. In fact, the successful implementation of the public health model relies heavily on its multidisciplinary nature, which involves buy-in and contribution from multiple community sectors in order to achieve desired outcomes. Such sectors include but are not limited to the healthcare system, the judicial and legislative systems, the education system, and even the business sector, as most public health issues require a comprehensive approach to prevention (CDC, 2016).

Aligning psychopathy with the public health model of violence prevention

Given the aforementioned strategic foci of the public health model of violence prevention, we believe, for several reasons, that attention to psychopathy is not only relevant, but necessary to maximize the impact of violence prevention efforts. First and foremost, psychopathy is a striking risk factor for violence. The research is substantial and the association is robust: psychopathy predisposes individuals to acts of violence with greater frequency, severity, and chronicity and has been established as a risk factor for violence across forensic, college, community, psychiatric, adult, and adolescent populations (Reidy et al., 2011, 2013, 2015, 2017). Psychopathy is also unique in its association to instrumental violence (Blais et al., 2014; Reidy et al., 2011). This distinction is important because instrumental violence tends to be a less common and more pathological form of violence which characterizes perpetrators at elevated risk for severe and chronic violence (Berkowitz, 1993; Reidy et al., 2011, 2017; Siever, 2008). For example, psychopathic men commit a disproportionate number of sexual homicides (Porter, Woodworth,

Earle, Drugge, & Boer, 2003), and the sexual violence perpetrated by psychopathic offenders is more likely to be sadistic and gratuitous compared to violence perpetrated by non-psychopathic offenders (Agar, 2009; Porter et al., 2003; Woodworth et al., 2013). And importantly, these connections between psychopathic traits and violence are well documented among youth as well (Reidy et al., 2011, 2013, 2017). Of course, not all individuals manifesting psychopathy traits will become violent (Fontaine, McCrory, Boivin, Moffitt, & Viding, 2011); nevertheless, psychopathy is a clear risk factor for violence.

In addition, psychopathic individuals appear to be those who are violent across multiple contexts. For example, Theobold, Farrington, Coid, and Piquero (2016) reported that "generally violent" men (i.e., those who committed intrafamilial and extrafamilial violence) were significantly more psychopathic than those who only committed intrafamilial violence (i.e., intimate partner violence), those who only committed extrafamilial violence, and those who were not violent. Importantly, those who are violent toward an intimate partner are also more likely to be violent toward children (Herrenkohl, Sousa, Tajima, Herrenkohl, & Moylan, 2008), although research directly assessing the association of psychopathy to child maltreatment perpetration is notably lacking. Given that psychopathic individuals are violent across numerous contexts, they arguably contribute more to the overall burden of population violence. Moreover, high psychopathy individuals may be more likely to successfully evade arrest and conviction for their violence (Aharoni & Kiehl, 2013), allowing them to accumulate a more extensive history of violence (Lynam, 1996; Vaughn & DeLisi, 2008; Vaughn, Howard, & DeLisi, 2008).

Evidence suggests that psychopathic persons perpetrate a disproportionate amount of the population's violence. In the U.S., research suggests that slightly less than 1 percent of non-institutionalized men age 18 and over in the U.S. are psychopaths (Blair et al., 2005; Hare, 1996), but that approximately 16 percent of incarcerated men in the U.S. meet the clinical criteria for psychopathy (Kiehl & Hoffman, 2011), demonstrating that psychopaths comprise a disproportionate number of male inmates in the U.S. Further, while only 62 percent of male inmates in the U.S. are incarcerated for a violent offense (Cornell et al., 1996), it is estimated that 78 percent of psychopathic inmates are violent offenders (Hart et al., 1988). Coid and Yang (2011) reported that individuals with psychopathy had a prevalence of 0.7 percent in the general population of Great Britain, yet they accounted for 17.5 percent of violent incidents over a five-year period. This finding is notable because it suggests that focusing violence prevention efforts on less than 1 percent of the population could reduce collective levels of violence by nearly one-fifth. Thus, it is clear that in comparison to individuals who are not psychopaths, this sub-population is at greater risk for both crime and violence perpetration across the life-span. As such, concentrating prevention activities within this population could proffer greater impact than spreading prevention resources across populations (CDC, 2016).

Given that the public health approach to violence prevention accentuates a primary prevention strategy, it is necessary to identify those cross-cutting risk factors of violence that can be detected at an early age. Generally speaking, psychopathy traits in youth are associated with an earlier age of onset for violence (Reidy et al., 2015). Thus, for psychopathy to be a practical risk factor to identify at-risk youth necessitating targeted primary prevention strategies, psychopathy traits must be able to be reliably identified and measured early enough in childhood. And indeed, a growing body of evidence suggests that psychopathy traits can be measured reliably in children under 6 years of age, and measurement of such traits at this early age predicts aggressive behavior years later (Clark & Frick, 2016; Ezpeleta et al., 2013; Kimonis et al., 2006, Kimonis et al., 2016; Kochanska, Kim, Boldt, & Yoon, 2013; Willoughby, Waschbusch, Moore, & Propper, 2011; Willoughby, Mills-Koonce, Gottfredson, & Wagner, 2014; Willoughby et al., 2015). Moreover, these traits are generally stable across adolescence and into adulthood, as is the association between these traits and acts of severe violence (Reidy et al., 2015). Thus, psychopathy traits may be ideal to indicate youth at risk well before their violent behavior onsets, becoming entrenched and resistant to change (Lynam, 1996; Reidy et al., 2015; Vaughn et al., 2008).

Preventing psychopathy as part of public health practice

Public health works to identify and facilitate the implementation of effective strategies for the primary prevention of violence. Simply incorporating psychopathy measures into public health research to see how the disorder impacts program evaluation results is insufficient. Instead, public health researchers must look for strategies that impact the developmental processes of psychopathy that engender violence (e.g., Reidy et al., 2017). We suggest the prevention of psychopathy parallels the prevention of violence (e.g., Caldwell, McCormick, Wolfe, & Umstead, 2012). In this vein, there exist no programs of which we are aware that have been designed and implemented as primary prevention strategies for psychopathy and/or associated violence. However, the psychopathy treatment literature suggests that the only programs that have been effective in reducing violence among high psychopathy individuals are those that have been implemented among adolescents (Reidy et al., 2013). In other words, interventions have a higher likelihood of effectiveness the earlier they are implemented. This finding is, of course, in line with the public health model of violence prevention.

The Mendota Juvenile Treatment Center (MJTC) is the only program shown to reliably reduce rates of violence by adolescents with elevated psychopathic traits (Caldwell, 2011; Caldwell et al., 2012; Caldwell, McCormick, Umstead, & Van Rybroek, 2007; Caldwell, Skeem, Salekin, & Van Rybroek, 2006). Implemented within the juvenile justice system, this program at the MJTC reduces focus on sanctions and instead implements a token-economy-like program that inherently positively reinforces prosocial behavior. In a related vein, a few programs have suggested the possibility of reducing psychopathic traits in child and adolescent populations (Kolko et al., 2009; McDonald, Dodson, Rosenfield, & Jouriles, 2011). These programs appear to share elements similar to the MJTC in that they incorporate parenting strategies of positively reinforcing prosocial behaviors and decreasing the use of punishment tactics for negative behaviors.

High psychopathy individuals are generally more difficult to treat, requiring more intensity and resources to yield smaller gains (Reidy et al., 2013). Thus, it seems adapting programs, such as the MJTC (Caldwell, 2011; Caldwell et al., 2012), to be implemented before high-psychopathy youth become violent would be a potentially effective primary prevention strategy. Behavior, personality, and pathology become deeply entrenched as they are repeatedly rehearsed throughout the lifespan. The younger a person is, the more malleable he/she is and therefore the more likely to benefit from prevention efforts. Hence, programs that are effective with the most intractable populations after violence has manifested may be even more likely to be effective before violence has onset.

Conclusion

In summary, the public health model for violence prevention seeks to identify risk and protective factors that cut across multiple forms of violence in order to prevent multiple forms of violence. Psychopathy is a cross-cutting risk factor for multiple forms of violence. The public health model uses a comprehensive approach that includes identifying populations at highest risk of perpetrating violence so that prevention efforts can be concentrated to achieve the greatest impact. Significant levels of psychopathic traits manifest in a small proportion of the population, yet this population is responsible for a disproportionate amount of violence in the population. Consequently, focusing prevention efforts on this minority of the population may prevent a majority of the violence. The public health approach to violence prevention involves intervening in adolescence or childhood before the onset of violent behavior, which is feasible for violence prevention among a psychopathic population, as psychopathic traits can be reliably and validly measured as early as 3 years of age. Further, research in the field of psychopathy indicates that the most effective prevention programs are those that are implemented during childhood before psychopathic traits become engrained and less susceptible to change. Thus, the theoretical tenets of the public health approach to violence prevention can be applied directly to psychopathy prevention and should therefore be considered in development of future programs, practices, and policies in an effort to prevent not only psychopathy but also violent outcomes associated with the disorder.

References

Agar, A. (2009) Teenage killers: A comprehensive examination of Canadian youth-perpetrated homicide psychopathy, motivation, violence, and the number of perpetrators (Unpublished master's thesis), The University of British Columbia, Kelowna, Canada.

Aharoni, E., and Kiehl, K. A. (2013) 'Evading justice: Quantifying criminal success in incarcerated psychopathic offenders,' *Criminal Justice & Behavior, 40*:629–645.

Beaver, K. (2013) 'The familial concentration of crime,' *Criminal Justice & Behavior, 40*:139–155.

Berkowitz L. (1993) *Aggression: Its causes, consequences, and control*, New York, NY: McGraw-Hill.

Blair, R. J. R., Mitchell, D. G. V., and Blair, K. (2005) *The psychopath: Emotion and the brain*, Malden, MA: Blackwell.

Blais, J., Solodukhin, E., and Forth, A. E. (2014) 'A meta-analysis exploring the relationship between psychopathy and instrumental versus reactive violence,' *Criminal Justice and Behavior, 41*(7):797–821.

Caldwell, M. F. (2011) 'Treatment related changes in behavioral outcomes of psychopathy facets in adolescent offenders,' *Law & Human Behavior, 35*:275–287.

Caldwell, M. F., McCormick, D. J., Wolfe, J., and Umstead, D. (2012) 'Treatment related changes in psychopathy features and behavior in adolescent offenders,' *Criminal Justice & Behavior, 39*:144–155.

Caldwell, M. F., McCormick, D. J., Umstead, D., and Van Rybroek, G. J. (2007) 'Evidence of treatment progress and therapeutic outcomes among adolescents with psychopathic features,' *Criminal Justice & Behavior, 34*:573–587.

Caldwell, M. F., Skeem, J. L., Salekin, R. L., and Van Rybroek, G. J. (2006) 'Treatment response adolescent offenders with psychopathy features: A two-year follow-up,' *Criminal Justice & Behavior, 33*:571–596.

Campbell, J. C. (2002) 'Health consequences of intimate partner violence,' *The Lancet, 359*(9314):1331–1336.

Centers for Disease Control & Prevention. (2016) *Preventing multiple forms of violence: A strategic vision for connecting the dots*, Atlanta, GA: Division of Violence Prevention, National Center for Injury Prevention & Control, Centers for Disease Control & Prevention.

Centers for Disease Control and Prevention. (2017a) National Vital Statistics System, National Center for Health Statistics, CDC. Produced by: National Center for Injury Prevention and Control, CDC using WISQARS™.

Centers for Disease Control and Prevention. (2017b) Web-based Injury Statistics Query and Reporting System (WISQARS). Retrieved September 1, 2017 from www.cdc.gov/ncipc/wisqars

Clark, J. E., and Frick, P. J. (2016) 'Positive parenting and callous–unemotional traits: Their association with school behavior problems in young children,' *Journal of Clinical Child & Adolescent Psychology, 11*:1–13.

Cohen, M. A., and Piquero, A. R. (2009) 'New evidence on the monetary value of saving a high risk youth,' *Journal of Quantitative Criminology, 25*:25–49.

Coid, J., and Yang, M. (2011) 'The impact of psychopathy on violence among the household population of Great Britain,' *Social Psychiatry & Psychiatric Epidemiology, 46*:473–480.

Coker, A. L., Smith, P. H., Bethea, L., King, M. R., and McKeown, R. E. (2000) 'Physical health consequences of physical and psychological intimate partner violence,' *Archives of Family Medicine, 9*(5):451–457.

Cooper, A., and Smith, E. L. (2011) Homicide trends in the United States, 1980–2008, Washington, DC: U.S. Department of Justice, Office of Justice Programs, Bureau of Justice Statistics.

Cornell, D. G., Warren, J., Hawk, G., Stafford, E., Oram, G., and Pine, D. (1996) 'Psychopathy in instrumental and reactive violent offenders,' *Journal of Consulting and Clinical Psychology*, *64*(4):783–790.
Curran, W. J. (1969) 'Public health and the law. Seat belts and legal safety,' *American Journal of Public Health and the Nation's Health*, *59*(3):552–553.
Cyr, C., Euser, E. M., Bakermans-Kranenburg, M. J., and Van Ijzendoorn, M. H. (2010) 'Attachment security and disorganization in maltreating and high-risk families: A series of meta-analyses,' *Development & Psychopathology*, *22*(1):87–108.
Dahlberg, L. D. (2007) 'Public health and violence: Moving forward in a global perspective,' in D. J. Flannery, A. T. Vazsonyi, & I. D. Waldman (Eds.), *The Cambridge handbook of violent behavior and aggression* (pp. 465–485), New York, NY: Cambridge University Press.
Ezpeleta, L., Osa, N. D. L., Granero, R., Penelo, E., and Domènech, J. M. (2013) 'Inventory of callous–unemotional traits in a community sample of preschoolers,' *Journal of Clinical Child & Adolescent Psychology*, *42*(1):91–105.
Farrell, A. D., and Sullivan, T. N. (2004) 'Impact of witnessing violence on growth curves for problem behaviors among early adolescents in urban and rural settings,' *Journal of Community Psychology*, *32*(5):505–525.
Fine, P., Victora, C. G., Rothman, K. J., Moore, P. S., Chang, Y., Curtis, V., . . ., and Roberts, I. (2013) 'John Snow's legacy: Epidemiology without borders,' *The Lancet*, *381*(9874):1302–1311.
Florence, C., Haegerich, T., Simon, T., Zhou, C., and Luo, F. (2015) 'Estimated lifetime medical and work-loss costs of emergency department–treated nonfatal injuries – United States, 2013,' *MMWR Morbidity and Mortality Weekly Report*, *64*(38):1078–1082.
Florence, C., Simon, T., Haegerich, T., Luo, F., and Zhou, C. (2015) 'Estimated lifetime medical and work-loss costs of fatal injuries – United States, 2013,' *MMWR Morbidity and Mortality Weekly Report*, *64*(38):1074–1077.
Fontaine, N. M. G., McCrory, E. J. P., Boivin, M., Moffitt, T. E., and Viding, E. (2011) 'Predictors and outcomes of joint trajectories of callous–unemotional traits and conduct problems in childhood,' *Journal of Abnormal Psychology*, *120*:730–742.
Gao, Y., Raine, A., Venables, P. H., Dawson, M. E., and Mednick, S. A. (2010a) 'Association of poor childhood fear conditioning and adult crime,' *American Journal of Psychiatry*, *167*(1):56–60.
Gao, Y., Raine, A., Venables, P. H., Dawson, M. E., and Mednick, S. A. (2010b) 'Reduced electrodermal fear conditioning from ages 3 to 8 years is associated with aggressive behavior at age 8 years,' *Journal of Child Psychology and Psychiatry*, *51*(5):550–558.
Guerra, N. G., Huesmann, R. L., and Spindler, A. (2003) 'Community violence exposure, social cognition, and aggression among urban elementary school children,' *Child Development*, *74*(5):1561–1576.
Hare, R. D. (1996) 'Psychopathy: A clinical construct whose time has come,' *Criminal Justice & Behavior*, *23*:25–54.
Hart, S. D., Kropp, P. R., and Hare, R. D. (1988) 'Performance of male psychopaths following conditional release from prison,' *Journal of Consulting and Clinical Psychology*, *56*(2):227–234.
Hemenway, D., and Miller, M. (2013) 'Public health approach to the prevention of gun violence,' *New England Journal of Medicine*, *368*:2033–2035.
Herrenkohl, T. I., Sousa, C., Tajima, E. A., Herrenkohl, R. C., and Moylan, C. A. (2008) 'Intersection of child abuse and children's exposure to domestic violence,' *Trauma, Violence, & Abuse*, *9*(2):84–99.
Kann, L., McManus, T., Harris, W. A. et al. (2016) 'Youth risk behavior surveillance – United States, 2015,' *MMWR. Surveillance Summaries*, *65*(6):1–174.
Kiehl, K. A., and Hoffman, M. B. (2011) 'The criminal psychopath: History, neuroscience, treatment, and economics,' *Jurimetrics*, *51*:355–370.
Kimonis, E. R., Fanti, K. A., Anastassiou-Hadjicharalambous, X., Mertan, B., Goulter, N., and Katsimicha, E. (2016) 'Can callous–unemotional traits be reliably measured in preschoolers?,' *Journal of Abnormal Child Psychology*, *44*(4):625–638.
Kimonis, E. R., Frick, P. J., Boris, N. W., Smyke, A. T., Cornell, A. H., Farrell, J. M., and Zeanah, C. H. (2006) 'Callous–unemotional features, behavioral inhibition, and parenting: Independent predictors of aggression in a high-risk preschool sample,' *Journal of Child and Family Studies*, *15*(6):741–752.
Kochanska, G., Kim, S., Boldt, L. J., and Yoon, J. E. (2013) 'Children's callous–unemotional traits moderate links between their positive relationships with parents at preschool age and behavior problems at early school age,' *Journal of Child Psychology & Psychiatry*, *54*(11):1251–1260.

Kolko, D. J., Dorn, L. D., Bukstein, O. G., Pardini, D., Holden, E. A., and Hart, J. (2009) 'Community vs. clinic-based modular treatment of children with early-onset ODD or CD: A clinical trial with 3-year follow-up,' *Journal of Abnormal Child Psychology*, *37*(5):591–609.

Krug, L. L. Dahlberg, J. A. Mercy, A. B. Zwi, and R. Lozano (Eds.) (2002) *World report on violence and health*, Geneva: World Health Organization.

Loftin, C. (1986) 'Assaultive violence as a contagious social process,' *Bulletin of the New York Academy of Medicine*, *62*(5):550–566.

Lynam, D. R. (1996) 'Early identification of chronic offenders: Who is the fledgling psychopath?,' *Psychological Bulletin*, *120*:209–234.

Matjasko, J. L., Vivolo-Kantor, A. M., Massetti, G. M., Holland, K. M., Holt, M. K., and Dela Cruz, J. (2012) 'A systematic meta-review of evaluations of youth violence prevention programs: Common and divergent findings from 25 years of meta-analyses and systematic reviews,' *Aggression & Violent Behavior*, *17*:540–552.

McDonald, R., Dodson, M. C., Rosenfield, D., and Jouriles, E. N. (2011) 'Effects of a parenting intervention on features of psychopathy in children,' *Journal of Abnormal Child Psychology*, *39*(7):1013–1023.

Moffitt, T. E. (1993) 'Adolescence-limited and life-course-persistent antisocial behavior: A developmental taxonomy,' *Psychological Review*, *100*:674–701.

Porter, S., Woodworth, M., Earle, J., Drugge, J., and Boer, D. (2003) 'Characteristics of sexual homicides committed by psychopathic and non-psychopathic offenders,' *Law & Human Behavior*, *27*:459–471.

Reidy, D. E., Shelley-Tremblay, J. F., and Lilienfeld, S. O. (2011) 'Psychopathy, reactive aggression, and precarious proclamations: A review of behavioral, cognitive, and biological research,' *Aggression and Violent Behavior*, *16*(6):512–524.

Reidy, D. E., Kearn, M. C., and DeGue, S. (2013) 'Reducing psychopathic violence: A review of the treatment literature,' *Aggression & Violent Behavior*, *18*:527–538.

Reidy, D. E., Kearns, M. C., DeGue, S., Lilienfeld, S. O., Massetti, G., and Kiehl, K. A. (2015) 'Why psychopathy matters: Implications for public health and violence prevention,' *Aggression & Violent Behavior*, *24*:214–225.

Reidy, D. E., Krusemark, E., Kosson, D. S., Kearns, M. C., Smith-Darden, J. P., and Kiehl, K. A. (2017) 'The development of severe and chronic violence among youth: The role of psychopathic traits and reward processing,' *Child Psychiatry & Human Development*, in press.

Siever, L. J. (2008) 'Neurobiology of aggression and violence,' *American Journal of Psychiatry*, *165*(4):429–442.

Slutkin, G. (2012) 'Violence is a contagious disease,' in *Contagion of violence: Workshop summary* (pp. 94–111), Washington, DC: National Academy Press.

Snow, J. (1860) *On the mode of communication of cholera* (2nd ed.), London: John Churchill.

Theobald, D., Farrington, D. P., Coid, J. W., and Piquero, A. R. (2016) 'Are male perpetrators of intimate partner violence different from convicted violent offenders? Examination of psychopathic traits and life success in males from a community survey,' *Journal of Interpersonal Violence*, *31*(9):1687–1718.

Tracy, P. E., Wolfgang, M. E., and Figlio, R. M. (1990) *Delinquency careers in two birth cohorts*, New York, NY: Plenum Press.

U.S. Department of Health, Education, and Welfare. (1979) *Healthy people: The Surgeon General's report on health promotion and disease prevention (Publication 79–55071)*, Washington, DC: Public Health Service, Office of Assistant Secretary for Health and Surgeon General.

Vaughn, M. G., and DeLisi, M. (2008) 'Were Wolfgang's chronic offenders psychopaths? On the convergent validity between psychopathy and career criminality,' *Journal of Criminal Justice*, *36*:33–42.

Vaughn, M. G., Howard, M. O., and DeLisi, M. (2008) 'Psychopathic personality traits and delinquent careers: An empirical examination,' *International Journal of Law & Psychiatry*, *31*:407–416.

Vaughn, M. G., DeLisi, M., Gunter, T., Fu, Q., Beaver, K. M., Perron, B. E., and Howard, M. O. (2011) 'The severe 5%: A latent class analysis of the externalizing behavior spectrum in the United States,' *Journal of Criminal Justice*, *39*:75–80.

Vaughn, M. G., Salas-Wright, C. P., DeLisi, M., and Maynard, B. R. (2014) 'Violence and externalizing behavior among youth in the United States: Is there a severe 5%?,' *Youth Violence & Juvenile Justice*, *12*:3–21.

Walsh, K., Keyes, K. M., Koenen, K. C., and Hasin, D. (2015) 'Lifetime prevalence of gender- based violence in US women: Associations with mood/anxiety and substance use disorders,' *Journal of Psychiatric Research*, *62*:7–13.

Wekerle, C., and Wolfe, D. A. (2003) 'Child maltreatment,' in E. J. Mash & R. A. Barkley (Eds.), *Child psychopathology* (2nd ed., pp. 632–684), New York, NY: Guilford Press.

Wilkins, N., Tsao, B., Hertz, M., Davis, R., and Klevens, J. (2014) *Connecting the dots: An overview of the links among multiple forms of violence*, Atlanta, GA: National Center for Injury Prevention and Control.

Willoughby, M. T., Mills-Koonce, W. R., Gottfredson, N. C., and Wagner, N. J. (2014) 'Measuring callous unemotional behaviors in early childhood: Factor structure and the prediction of stable aggression in middle childhood,' *Journal of Psychopathology and Behavioral Assessment*, *36*(1):30–42.

Willoughby, M. T., Mills-Koonce, W. R., Waschbusch, D. A., Gottfredson, N. C., and Family Life Project Investigators. (2015) 'An examination of the parent report version of the inventory of callous–unemotional traits in a community sample of first-grade children,' *Assessment*, *22*(1):76–85.

Willoughby, M. T., Waschbusch, D. A., Moore, G. A., and Propper, C. B. (2011) 'Using the ASEBA to screen for callous unemotional traits in early childhood: Factor structure, temporal stability, and utility,' *Journal of Psychopathology and Behavioral Assessment*, *33*(1):19–30.

Woodworth, M., Freimuth, T., Hutton, E. L., Carpenter, T., Agar, A. D., and Logan, M. (2013) 'High-risk sexual offenders: An examination of sexual fantasy, sexual paraphilia, psychopathy, and offence characteristics,' *International Journal of Law & Psychiatry*, *36*:144–156.

World Health Organization. "Public health surveillance." *WHO*. n.p., n.d. Retrieved July 31, 2014 from www.who.int/topics/public_health_surveillance/en/

Wolfgang, M. E., Figlio, R. M., and Sellin, T. (1972) *Delinquency in a birth cohort*, Chicago, IL: University of Chicago Press.

41

Psychopathy in the courts

David DeMatteo, Daniel C. Murrie, John F. Edens, and Claire Lankford

Introduction

Psychopathy evidence is frequently admitted in criminal and civil legal proceedings because of its perceived relevance to several important outcomes. A well-developed body of research has demonstrated, for example, that psychopathy as assessed by the family of Psychopathy Checklist (Hare, 1980, 1991, 2003) measures is modestly prospectively associated with violent behavior post-release, general and violent recidivism, sexual recidivism, and institutional misconduct. As a result, forensic mental health professionals – and the courts in which mental health evidence is presented – frequently utilize psychopathy evidence to make decisions in wide-ranging legal contexts, such as juvenile transfer, sexually violent predator commitment, suitability for parole, and sentencing (including capital sentencing). Despite the potential relevance of evaluations of psychopathy in legal proceedings, a growing body of research suggests that courts and other legal decision-makers should exercise caution when relying on forensic examiners' evaluations of psychopathic traits in certain contexts.

After briefly describing the construct of psychopathy, we discuss evidence for the use of psychopathy measures in court. Case law surveys and other published research conducted over the past decade suggest that psychopathy measures, particularly the PCL–R, are used in North American and European courts with increasing frequency, and we describe the various contexts in which those measures are being used. Next, we focus on concerns regarding the use of the PCL–R in court. First, we discuss the emerging evidence suggesting that forensic mental health professionals' PCL–R scores are influenced by the side that retains the experts, a phenomenon referred to as adversarial allegiance. Second, we discuss empirical research regarding whether labeling an offender a "psychopath" leads to prejudice in legal proceedings. This chapter concludes with cautions regarding certain uses of psychopathy measures in legal proceedings.

Psychopathy

Current conceptualizations of psychopathy are rooted in Cleckley's (1941) clinical accounts of psychiatric patients who exhibited particular deficits in emotional and interpersonal functioning (e.g., grandiose sense of self-worth, lack of guilt, callousness). The prototypical psychopath is often perceived as alluring, which masks shallow affect and a lack of empathy or remorse (Lilienfeld, Watts, Smith, Berg, & Latzman, 2015). Although some research has examined the Psychopathy Checklist measures in community samples (e.g., DeMatteo, Heilbrun, & Marczyk, 2005, 2006; Hall & Benning, 2006), most literature on psychopathy that is relevant to legal issues has focused on forecasting violence, recidivism, criminality, and (to a lesser extent) treatment responsiveness among justice-involved adult and adolescent samples (see DeMatteo, Edens, & Hart, 2010; Douglas, Vincent, & Edens, 2018; Leistico, Salekin, DeCosta, & Rogers, 2008; Singh, Grann, & Fazel, 2011; Yang, Wong, & Coid, 2010).

Although Cleckley's (1941) work was foundational in drawing attention to psychopathy, the modern conceptualization of psychopathy has been largely operationalized using instruments developed by Robert Hare and colleagues, including the Psychopathy Checklist (PCL; Hare, 1980) and Psychopathy Checklist–Revised (PCL–R; Hare, 1991, 2003). The PCL measures emphasize behavioral (e.g., criminality) characteristics associated with psychopathy, but also affective (e.g., lack of remorse) and interpersonal (e.g., grandiosity) features considered by many theorists to be more central to the disorder as conceptualized by Cleckley. Although there are questions about whether the PCL measures actually capture the core features of psychopathy articulated by Cleckley (1941) and others (e.g., Karpman, 1946, 1948; Lykken, 1995), there is considerable empirical evidence that scores from the PCL measures quantify something relevant to important outcomes in the criminal justice system (see DeMatteo et al., 2010).

Of the several measures developed to assess psychopathy, the PCL–R is the most widely used by clinicians.[1] The PCL–R is a 20-item rating scale used in research and clinical settings for assessing psychopathy among adults. Standard administration involves a semi-structured interview and a review of file/collateral data. Examiners rate each PCL–R item on a 3-point scale based on the degree to which the personality/behavior of the examinee matches the item description in the manual – 0 (item does not apply to the individual), 1 (item applies to a certain extent), or 2 (item applies) – which results in scores ranging from 0 to 40. Individuals are typically considered categorically "psychopathic" if they receive a score of 30 or higher (or 25+ in many European countries). However, taxometric research suggests PCL scores represent an underlying dimensional construct rather than a latent taxon (e.g., Edens, Marcus, Lilienfeld, & Poythress, 2006; Guay, Ruscio, Hare, & Knight, 2007; Walters, 2014; Murrie et al., 2007; Walters, Duncan, & Mitchell-Perez, 2007; Walters, Ermer, Knight, & Kiehl, 2015; for an alternate perspective, see recent Network Analysis examinations of large offender databases arguing that there is no need to postulate a "latent construct" [dimensional or categorical] that underlies the items comprising the PCL measures [Preszler, Marcus, Edens, & McDermott, in press; Vershuere et al., in press]).

Early exploratory factor analyses of the PCL consistently resulted in a two-factor solution, with Factor 1 consisting of the Interpersonal/Affective features more congruent with Cleckley's (1941) model and Factor 2 consisting primarily of the behavioral features (Harpur, Hakstian, & Hare, 1988; Harpur, Hare, & Hakstian, 1989). The behavioral features captured by PCL–R Factor 2 resemble the behavioral aspects of Antisocial Personality Disorder (ASPD) found in the American Psychiatric Association's *Diagnostic and Statistical Manual of Mental Disorders, Fifth ed.* (DSM–5; 2013). Although these two constructs are often confused, the greater emphasis on core interpersonal and affective features distinguish PCL-defined psychopathy from ASPD, and research has demonstrated that individuals diagnosed with ASPD frequently do not cross the categorical threshold (30 or higher) to be labeled psychopathic (Hare, 2003; Shepherd, Campbell, & Ogloff, in press; Skilling, Harris, Rice, & Quinsey, 2002).

Later research has yielded three-factor models (Cooke & Michie, 2001; Hall, Benning, & Patrick, 2004) and four-factor models (Neumann, Kosson, & Salekin, 2007; Vitacco, Rogers, Neumann, Harrison, & Vincent, 2005). Cooke and Michie (2001) proposed a hierarchical three-factor model reflecting interpersonal, affective, and lifestyle features of psychopathy, and later studies replicated the three-factor model (e.g., Cooke, Michie, Hart, & Clark, 2004; Cooke, Michie, & Skeem, 2007; Weaver, Meyer, Van Nort, & Tristan, 2006). Other researchers have argued in favor of a four-factor model that retains item content explicitly tied to criminal history (e.g., Hare, 2003, 2016; Hare & Neumann, 2005; Mokros et al., 2015; Neumann, Hare, & Johansson, 2013). The two PCL–R factors have been further subdivided into four facets: interpersonal (i.e., superficial, grandiose sense of self-worth, pathological lying, manipulative), affective (i.e., lack of remorse, shallow, callous, lack of empathy, fails to accept responsibility), lifestyle (i.e., seeks stimulation, impulsive, irresponsible, parasitic, disorganized goals), and antisocial (i.e., lack of behavioral regulation, early behavioral problems, juvenile delinquency, revocation of conditional release, criminal adaptability; see Hare, 2003).

Despite substantial attention from researchers and scholars, there are many ambiguities and unanswered questions regarding psychopathy and the PCL measures (see Edens, 2006; Edens, Petrila, & Kelley, 2018; Lilienfeld et al., 2015; more generally, see Patrick, 2018). For example, some have argued that PCL–R psychopathy relies too heavily on criminal conduct (see Skeem & Cooke, 2010): because the scoring of many PCL–R items depends largely on criminal behaviors, it risks under-identifying psychopathic individuals who do not manifest psychopathic traits through overtly criminal behaviors while simultaneously over-identifying individuals who commit crimes without the interpersonal and affective traits historically associated with psychopathic personality (Lilienfeld, 1994; Skeem & Cooke, 2010). Regarding the PCL–R's purported overreliance on criminal behavior, research has demonstrated that Factor 2 is more predictive of violence than Factor 1 (see Kennealy, Skeem, Walters, & Camp, 2010), and that facet four (which primarily measures an examinee's history of documented criminal activity) accounts for the most predictive variance in violent offending (Hawes, Boccaccini, & Murrie, 2013; Walters & Heilbrun, 2010; Walters, Knight, Grann, & Dahle, 2008). Thus, the practical utility of the PCL measures in risk assessment seems to be driven primarily by the quantification of past criminality rather than personality factors such as remorselessness and superficial charm, leading some commentators to question the ethics of including Factor 1 traits in formal risk assessments for the legal system (Edens et al., 2018).

Psychopathy measures in the courts

Despite the frequency with which mental health professionals participate in criminal and civil legal proceedings, the intersection of psychology and law has a long history of discord (see Melton et al., 2018). Over 30 years ago, Grisso (1986, 2003) reviewed of a litany of historical problems with forensic mental health assessments, which he referred to as the five "I's" of *ignorance* and *irrelevance* in courtroom testimony, psychiatric or psychological *intrusion* into essentially legal matters, and *insufficiency* and *incredibility* of information provided to the courts. The choice and use of assessment measures in forensic mental health assessments illustrates the oftentimes uneasy relationship between psychology and the legal system.

In many criminal contexts, the court is concerned with the defendant's likelihood of committing future criminal behavior, so the construct of psychopathy is attractive to legal decision-makers because of its empirical relationship with future offending. Given the robust empirical relationship between PCL–R psychopathy and future offending, PCL–R evidence is often presented through expert testimony to assist courts in making factual or legal determinations in several contexts, including Sexually Violent Predator (SVP) commitment, juvenile transfer decisions, capital sentencing, general sentencing, and determination of future dangerousness in parole contexts (see DeMatteo, Hodges, & Fairfax-Columbo, 2016).

Psychopathy measures in case law

Given the relationship among psychopathy, future offending, and other relevant criminal justice considerations, PCL measures have long been introduced in legal proceedings, but the first comprehensive reviews of the use of the PCL measures in court were not conducted until the mid-2000s, approximately 15 years after the PCL–R was commercially published in 1991. Two early case law reviews, by DeMatteo and Edens (2006) and Walsh and Walsh (2006), found relatively infrequent use of the PCL–R in *published* United States court cases from 1991 through 2004. Importantly, the results of these case law reviews underestimate PCL–R use in court because legal databases such as Westlaw and Lexis-Nexis typically only contain opinions that have reached the appellate stage of litigation, and most cases involving the PCL–R are state-level cases that do not result in a written opinion included in electronic legal databases.

DeMatteo and Edens (2006) identified 87 cases (76 state; 11 federal) involving the PCL–R between 1991 and 2004, and Walsh and Walsh (2006) identified 76 cases (67 state; 9 federal) involving the PCL–R during the same time period. The PCL–R was typically used as a prosecution tool, with the prosecution introducing the PCL–R in 49 (64 percent) of the 76 state cases and in all 11 federal cases, which totaled more than 85 percent of all identified cases (DeMatteo & Edens, 2006). In both case law reviews, the PCL–R was typically used as a risk assessment tool. DeMatteo and Edens (2006) found that the PCL–R was used to predict risk of sexual violence, general violence, or general offending in 83 (95.4 percent) of the 87 cases, which included sexually violent predator hearings, capital sentencing hearings, and parole suitability hearings, while Walsh and Walsh (2006) reported that the PCL–R was used as a risk assessment tool in 69 (90.8 percent) of the 76 identified cases, which included sexually violent predator hearings, parole hearings, capital sentencing proceedings, civil commitment hearings, and juvenile transfer.

More recent reviews suggest that the PCL–R is used with increasing frequency in United States courts (DeMatteo et al., 2014a, 2014b). For example, use of the PCL–R increased dramatically during the six-year period from 2005 through 2011, with DeMatteo et al. (2014b) reporting that the PCL–R was used in 348 published cases (304 state and 44 federal), which is a 300+ percent increase in a time period half as long as the time period in the earlier DeMatteo and Edens (2006) study. The 348 cases were mostly from appellate courts (86 percent) and from 22 states, with California (140; 40 percent), Texas (39; 11 percent), and Minnesota (37; 11 percent) accounting for the most usage. Of the 348 cases, 214 (62 percent) were sexually violent predator cases from 19 different states, with the bulk of the other cases being parole hearings (84; 24 percent); other types of cases, such as capital sentencing and civil commitment, were comparatively much less common.

Psychopathy evidence is not limited to U.S. courts or to adult defendants. For example, one review of psychopathy measures (predominantly but not exclusively PCL measures) in U.S. and Canadian legal proceedings involving adolescent offenders identified 111 cases (71 Canadian; 40 U.S.) involving 143 separate evaluations in which an assessment of psychopathy was conducted (Viljoen, MacDougall, Gagnon, & Douglas, 2010). Although the specific term "psychopath" was not frequently applied to juveniles, psychopathy evidence was influential in many of these cases and was frequently used to infer the adolescent would not respond well to treatment. Lloyd, Clark, and Forth (2010) examined the use of the PCL–R in Canadian cases. Based on their review of written decisions or oral transcripts from 136 dangerous offender (or long-term offender) hearings to examine whether use of the PCL–R was related to trial outcome, they found that the PCL–R was used in 58 (42.6 percent) of the cases. The results revealed a trend in which PCL–R scores were related to expert ratings of treatment amenability.

A perceived strength of the PCL measures is the high level of interrater reliability reported in the professional manuals and in various published research reports. Numerous studies have reported that well-trained evaluators in controlled research contexts can produce scores with high levels of interrater reliability (e.g., Kennealy, Hicks, & Patrick, 2007; McDermott et al., 2000; Poythress et al., 2010). Interrater reliability of PCL–R scores is typically measured using intraclass correlation coefficients (ICCs) for a single rating (ICC_1) and for the average of two independent ratings (ICC_2). The manual for the second edition of the PCL–R (Hare, 2003) reports the following ICCs: the pooled ICC for male criminal offenders was .86 for a single rating (ICC_1) and .92 for the average of two ratings (ICC_2); ICC_1 was .88 and ICC_2 was .93 for the male forensic psychiatric patients; and ICC_1 was .94 and ICC_2 was .97 for the female criminal offenders; all of these values fall in the range that authorities consider strong reliability (Cicchetti & Sparrow, 1981). These results suggest that the PCL–R can be reliably scored by independent trained raters, at least in research contexts.

Less research has examined the interrater reliability of PCL–R scores among practicing clinicians in routine practice. Early research on this topic reported strong interrater agreement among staff at a forensic hospital who received comprehensive PCL–R training (Gacono & Hutton, 1994) and among practicing correctional psychologists (Kroner & Mills, 2001). However, in several studies of practicing clinicians, the clinicians reviewed the same collateral information and observed the same interview of the individual, an arrangement uncommon in real-world clinical practice where different evaluators typically review records and conduct interviews independently. In early studies examining PCL–R interrater agreement for interviews conducted by different raters at different times, Alterman, Cacciola, and Rutherford (1993) reported correlations of .85 and .89 between scores at baseline and scores obtained one month later in a sample of 88 clients receiving substance abuse treatment. They also found a two-year test–retest reliability value of .60 (ICC) for PCL–R Total scores among 200 male patients receiving services in a methadone clinic (Rutherford, Cacciola, Alterman, McKay, & Cook, 1999). More recently, two published studies have reported problematic interrater reliability in European field settings (Jeandarme et al., 2017; Sturup et al., 2014), particularly in relation to Factor 1 scores, which have historically shown poor reliability in forensic contexts (e.g., Edens, Boccaccini, & Johnson, 2010; Miller, Kimonis, Otto, Line, & Wasserman, 2012; Tyrer et al., 2005).

A small body of case law research has examined interrater reliability of PCL–R scores in court cases. In one case law review, DeMatteo et al. (2014a) identified 29 sexually violent predator cases in which the same offender was assessed with the PCL–R by two evaluators. In those 29 cases, the ICC_1 was .58, and only 41.4 percent of the score differences were within one Standard Error. Moreover, scores by prosecutor-retained experts were significantly higher than the scores produced by defense-retained experts; prosecution experts reported PCL–R scores of 30 or above in nearly 50 percent of the cases, compared with less than 10 percent of the scores reported by defense experts. In a second case law survey that reviewed a wider range of criminal cases ($N = 102$) from Canada, the single-rater ICC was .59 for all cases, with an ICC of .66 for cases involving a sexual offense and an ICC .46 for non-sexual offense cases (Edens, Cox, Smith, DeMatteo, & Sörman, 2015). Although there have been somewhat more promising reliability findings recently reported (e.g., Harris, Rice, & Cormier, 2013), collectively these results raise concerns about the PCL–R's reliability in real-world practice.

Does adversarial allegiance influence PCL–R scores in legal contexts?

A striking finding in the case law surveys is the tendency for evaluators testifying for the prosecution to report, on average, higher scores than the evaluators testifying for the defense. Scores from defense-retained evaluators tended to be lower (suggesting lower risk of violence, sexual violence, or general recidivism) whereas scores from prosecution-retained evaluators tended to be higher (suggesting higher risk). At first glance, such scoring patterns seem to raise questions about *adversarial allegiance*, or the tendency for some experts to drift from strictly objective findings to findings that better support the party that retained them (Murrie & Boccaccini, 2015). Legal scholars and other observers have long speculated that experts are likely biased towards the party that pays their fees or consistently seeks their services (e.g., Mnookin, 2008; Wigmore, 1923), but historically little research has explored this phenomenon.

Field studies suggest, but cannot prove, adversarial allegiance in PCL–R scoring

In the first study to explore adversarial allegiance with any psychological assessment instrument, researchers collected PCL–R scores assigned by petitioner-retained[2] and defense-retained psychologists in 23 sexually violent predator (SVP) cases in Texas (Murrie, Boccaccini, Johnson, & Janke, 2008). SVP laws allow for the post-incarceration civil commitment of sex offenders considered particularly high risk for committing future acts of sexual violence (see DeMatteo, Murphy, Galloway, & Krauss, 2015). Although SVP laws raise several constitutional questions, including concerns relating to Double Jeopardy and Ex Post Facto lawmaking, the United States Supreme Court has upheld SVP laws as constitutional (*Kansas v. Crane*, 2002; *Kansas v. Hendricks*, 1997; *Seling v. Young*, 2001). Given the nature of the SVP determination, mental health experts – often testifying about diagnoses and risk of sexual re-offense – are central to SVP proceedings, and most of these experts use the PCL–R in their assessments (Boccaccini, Chevalier, Murrie, & Varela, 2017; DeMatteo et al., 2014a).

Reviewing 23 SVP proceedings allowed researchers to examine scores that opposing evaluators *assigned to the same offender*. The difference between PCL–R scores assigned by petitioner-retained and defense-retained evaluators was large (Cohen's d = 1.03), leading to a low level of interrater agreement across raters (ICC = .39). In 61 percent of the cases, there was a difference of more than 6.0 points between the two PCL–R scores, when differences this large should have occurred in fewer than 5 percent of all cases.[3] In each instance, the petitioner-retained evaluator assigned the higher score, and the defense-retained evaluator assigned the lower score. There was one case with a 20-point difference, with the defense-retained evaluator score falling at the 28th percentile and the prosecution-retained evaluator score falling at the 99.5th percentile.

When researchers updated the sample to include 35 SVP cases, they found similar allegiance effects in PCL–R scoring (Murrie et al., 2009). To be clear, there was often poor reliability even among evaluators on the same side of adversarial proceedings, but scores were *systematically* unreliable among opposing evaluators, with defense-retained evaluators usually assigning lower scores than prosecution-retained evaluators. Allegiance effects were not unique to the PCL–R; researchers also found evidence of bias in the scores assigned on two measures designed to predict future sexual offending: the Minnesota Sex Offender Screening Tool–Revised (MnSOST–R; Epperson et al., 1998) and the Static–99 (Hanson & Thornton, 2000), which evaluators score on the basis of information in offenders' correctional files. The allegiance effect for the MnSOST–R ($d \approx .80$) was similar to that for the PCL–R, but the effect was somewhat smaller for the Static–99 ($d \approx .35$), perhaps because it is a more structured measure that requires less subjective judgment in scoring.

Thus, although clinicians appear to achieve high reliability on PCL–R scores in research settings and some non-adversarial clinical settings, there is growing evidence that prosecution-retained evaluators assign higher PCL–R scores and defense-retained evaluators assign lower PCL–R scores in real-world adversarial legal settings. Of course, the findings from the field only *suggest*, but do not *prove*, that adversarial allegiance influences PCL–R scores. There may be several explanations for these scoring patterns. The first is attorney selection effects (see Murrie & Boccaccini, 2015). Evaluators tend to differ in the average PCL–R scores they assign to offenders (Boccaccini, Murrie, Rufino, & Gardner, 2014; Boccaccini, Turner, & Murrie, 2008; Miller et al., 2012), perhaps due to differences in training and experience (Boccaccini, Rufino, Jeon, & Murrie, 2017; Rufino, Boccaccini, Hawes, & Murrie, 2012), personality (Miller, Rufino, Boccaccini, Jackson, & Murrie, 2011), or other variables. Shrewd attorneys can probably identify which evaluators "lean" more or less favorably to their case and, as much as possible, try to retain evaluators whose perspectives (including PCL–R scoring tendencies) are most similar to their case goals. A second potential explanation for these field findings involves selection effects in terms of which cases proceed to trial. Perhaps only unusually ambiguous or contentious cases proceed to trial, whereas the vast majority of cases that never proceeded to trial might have featured high agreement on PCL–R scores by opposing evaluators. A third explanation, however, is that score differences are *caused* in part by the adversarial arrangements underlying an expert's work, i.e., allegiance effects. These competing explanations can only be examined using a true experimental design.

Experimental research proves allegiance effects in PCL–R scoring

To better understand potential allegiance effects, researchers recruited over 100 practicing, doctoral-level forensic psychologists and psychiatrists and deceived them to believe they were performing a formal, large-scale forensic consultation (Murrie, Boccaccini, Guarnera, & Rufino, 2013). These forensic experts were – unbeknownst to them – randomly assigned to either a prosecution-allegiance or defense-allegiance group in which they believed that they were paid ($400 per day) for their services. Participants met for 10–15 minutes with an attorney who posed as leading either a public defender service or specialized prosecution unit, and the attorney then requested that the expert score the PCL–R and Static–99R (Hanson & Thornton, 2000; Helmus, Thornton, Hanson, & Babchishin, 2012) based on extensive offender records, a type of consultation not uncommon in forensic practice. The participants were led to believe that, as a group, they were reviewing and scoring cases from a large cohort, but in truth each participant was scoring the same four case files, which spanned from low risk to high risk. Each set of case materials was from an actual case, including extensive records (e.g., police, court, correctional, mental health) and a transcript of a PCL–R interview designed to correspond to each case file.

Overall, the risk measure scores assigned by prosecution experts and defense experts showed a clear pattern of adversarial allegiance. As expected, allegiance effects were stronger for the PCL–R than for the Static–99R, a more structured measure that requires less subjective judgment. For the PCL–R Total score, prosecution evaluators assigned significantly higher scores than defense evaluators for three of four cases, with effect sizes in the medium to large range (Cohen's d of .55 to .85) and similar in magnitude to effects (d = .63 to .83) documented in a sample of actual SVP proceedings (Murrie et al., 2009). The one case without a PCL–R allegiance effect was selected to be unusually low in psychopathy; this case received unusually low scores both from prosecution-retained evaluators and defense-retained evaluators.

Of course, real courts rarely average PCL–R scores that have been provided by numerous experts. Rather, they usually hear expert testimony (or read reports) about psychopathy from two experts – one called by each opposing side. To mimic this real-world arrangement as closely as possible, a series of follow-up analyses examined how likely it was that a randomly selected prosecution expert and a randomly selected defense expert would assign scores that were so different that they could not be explained by random measurement error. The findings from these comparisons revealed two clear effects. First, more than 20 percent of the score pairings for each case led to a score difference that was more than twice the Standard Error, although this should occur only in about 4 percent of score pairings, based on the published SEM in the manual. For three of the four offenders, nearly 40 percent of the difference scores were at least two SEM apart. Second, most large (≥ 2 SEM) differences were in the direction of adversarial allegiance, with the prosecution expert assigning higher scores and the defense expert assigning lower scores. Finding such clear evidence of allegiance in a context in which all other possible explanations have been experimentally or statistically controlled suggests that adversarial allegiance significantly influences some evaluators who use the PCL–R.

These study findings suggest two other implications for PCL–R scoring in legal contexts. First, even though participants received similar two-day, high-quality PCL–R training before the experiment, there was considerable variability in scores even among experts assigned to the same side, much like the scoring differences documented in field studies of evaluators working for the same referral source (Boccaccini et al., 2008, 2014). Second, the experimental effects (Murrie et al., 2013) were somewhat smaller than the effects from most field studies (Murrie et al., 2008, 2009).[4] Taken together, these results suggest that in actual forensic practice, selection effects probably *combine* with allegiance effects to produce more discrepant opinions across experts.

Forensic evaluators recognize allegiance effects . . . among other evaluators

Will the emerging evidence of allegiance effects in PCL–R scoring change practice and ultimately reduce allegiance effects? On the one hand, evaluators increasingly appear to recognize that allegiance effects may influence PCL–R scoring. In a recent survey that explored forensic evaluators' use of the PCL–R in sex offender risk assessments, most evaluators endorsed the idea that *in general* the side retaining an evaluator could influence PCL–R scoring, but far fewer evaluators endorsed any likelihood that the side retaining their services influenced *their own* scoring (Boccaccini et al., 2017). This large discrepancy (d = 1.23; large effect size) strongly suggests a "bias blind spot" (Pronin, Lin, & Ross, 2002), which is the cognitive phenomena by which people are quick to recognize bias in others, but not in themselves. The pervasive presence of the bias blind spot among forensic mental health professionals (Neal & Brodsky, 2016; Zapf, Kukucka, Kassin, & Dror, in press) strongly suggests general awareness of allegiance effects alone is not sufficient to prevent them from occurring among evaluators.

Psychopathy labeling effects in court

Adversarial allegiance is not the only concern relating to the use of psychopathy measures in court. A growing body of research has examined whether labeling an offender a "psychopath," or describing his psychopathic personality traits negatively, affects perceptions of the offender and legal decisions. Although some diagnostic labels or instruments scores may convey useful information that is relevant to the legal question, psychopathy labeling effects that are more prejudicial than probative raise concerns about whether such evidence should be admitted into the legal proceedings. The question of admissibility of evidence is determined by courts on a case-by-case basis using the applicable rules governing evidence admissibility in each particular jurisdiction, so there are no simple "yes or no" answers to the question of whether psychopathy evidence should be considered unduly prejudicial in a general sense.

In federal courts, the admissibility of evidence is governed by the Federal Rules of Evidence (FRE; 1975). The FRE apply to all civil and criminal court cases and proceedings and to contempt proceedings, but they do not apply to grand jury hearings and several other types of proceedings (e.g., sentencing, extradition, granting/revoking probation, or supervised release). The FRE are not directly applicable in state courts, although nearly every state has adopted the FRE in whole, in part, or with only minor modifications (Weinstein & Berger, 2015).

The rules that govern the admissibility of all evidence – both lay/fact and expert – are FRE 401, 402, and 403.

- FRE 401. Test for relevant evidence – Evidence is relevant if: (1) it has any tendency to make a fact more or less probable that it would be without the evidence; and (2) the fact is of consequence in determining the action.
- FRE 402. General admissibility of relevant evidence – Relevant evidence is admissible unless any of the following provides otherwise: the United States Constitution; a federal statute; these rules; or other rules prescribed by the Supreme Court. Irrelevant evidence is not admissible.
- FRE 403. Excluding relevant evidence for prejudice, confusion, waste of time, or other reasons – The court may exclude relevant evidence if its probative value is substantially outweighed by a danger of one or more of the following: unfair prejudice, confusing the issues, misleading the jury, undue delay, wasting time, or needlessly presenting cumulative evidence.

Taken together, for any evidence to be admissible, it must be relevant (i.e., it is material to the issue before the court and the existence of the evidence provides predictive value in determining if a fact exists; FRE 401). This is often referred to as *probative value*. If proffered evidence is determined to be probative, it is generally admissible (FRE 402), but even probative evidence can be excluded if it would have an overly *prejudicial impact* on the factfinder (FRE 403).[5]

Using this admissibility framework, a key question is whether psychopathy evidence is both probative and not unduly prejudicial. If psychopathy evidence does not satisfy the FRE 401/403 relevance/prejudice hurdle, then the application of the rules of evidence suggest that the psychopathy evidence should not be admitted. The analysis of the admissibility of psychopathy evidence differs by legal context; it is possible, of course, for psychopathy evidence to be probative in some types of legal proceedings but not in others, just as it is possible for psychopathy evidence to be overly prejudicial in some contexts but not in others. Fortunately, researchers have examined the prejudicial impact of the PCL–R – in terms of labeling effects – in several different legal contexts. (For a comprehensive discussion of whether PCL–R evidence satisfies the relevance/prejudice admissibility standard in the contexts of capital sentencing, juvenile transfer, and sexually violent predator commitment, see DeMatteo et al., 2016).

Before considering whether psychopathy *evidence* is influential in legal decision-making – regardless of whether it is prejudicial – it is worth asking a more basic question of whether psychopathy matters to legal decision-makers. That is, does attributing psychopathic traits to a defendant correlate with greater support for negative or adverse outcomes for that defendant? If not, then evidence attempting to convince jurors or other legal decision-makers that a defendant is a psychopath (or not) is unlikely to have any effect on case outcomes and should be construed as largely irrelevant. Mock jury research investigating this question has provided a fairly clear affirmative response, indicating that juror ratings of how psychopathic they perceive a defendant to be robustly predict a variety of attitudinal variables (e.g., how dangerous and "evil" the defendant is perceived to be) and case outcomes (e.g., whether a capital defendant should be executed, other sentencing recommendations) across a range of legal issues and defendant characteristics (e.g., adult and juvenile cases). A recent meta-analytic investigation of this topic (Kelley et al., under review) found that attributing psychopathic traits to a defendant is clearly to detrimental to that defendant, which is consistent with more anecdotal accounts derived from real-world death penalty cases (Sundby, 1998).

Given the influential effects of perceiving a defendant as being psychopathic (or not), it is important to then consider how and why evidence and testimony concerning this condition might influence legal decision-makers. Attempting to disentangle the influence of a diagnostic label can be complex, however, so some researchers distinguish among three possible sources of influence: *general labeling effects* associated with diagnosis of any mental disorder, *specific labeling effects* for a specific diagnosis such as psychopathy, and *criterion effects* associated with the diagnostic criteria (e.g., underlying symptoms or characteristics upon which a diagnosis is based) (Murrie, Cornell, & McCoy, 2005). When examining psychopathy among juveniles, it is important to distinguish the specific labeling effect of psychopathy from the general labeling effect that might be found with other diagnoses (e.g., Conduct Disorder). Also, any labeling effect specific to the psychopathy diagnosis must be distinguished from criterion effects (i.e., the effects of describing characteristics considered criteria for the diagnosis, such as lack of empathy or remorse and manipulativeness). Such distinctions may be important to consider in some contexts, particularly those (e.g., juvenile cases) in which the explicit term "psychopath" might be unlikely to be introduced *but* the examinee might still be described as exhibiting specific (PCL) traits as part of the clinical evaluation (Viljoen, McLachlan, & Vincent, 2010).

Juveniles

Juvenile transfer, referred to as waiver or certification in some jurisdictions, is the process by which a juvenile offender's case is transferred from the juvenile justice system to the criminal justice system. Mental health professionals often participate in proceedings to assist courts in determining whether a juvenile's case should be transferred to (or remain in) criminal court, and research suggests that psychopathy measures are occasionally used by these professionals (see DeMatteo & Edens, 2006; DeMatteo et al., 2014b; Walsh & Walsh, 2006).

In the first experimental research on the impact of psychopathy information in a juvenile case, Edens, Guy, and Fernandez (2003) investigated whether traits associated with psychopathy – though not the label "psychopath" itself – influenced perceptions of and opinions about a capital defendant who had committed a murder as a juvenile. Not surprisingly, college students who read a newspaper account summarizing the facts of the case were much more likely to support a death sentence for the defendant when he was described as exhibiting psychopathic traits (consistent with Factor 1 of the PCL measures) than when he was characterized as exhibiting traits that would be inconsistent with this disorder (e.g., remorse).

Subsequent to this initial study, researchers began examining the relative impact of psychopathic traits versus psychopathic labels. For example, Chauhan, Reppucci, and Burnette (2007) examined the impact of the psychopathic label and the attribution of psychopathic traits to juvenile offenders among 83 Virginia district and juvenile court judges, 58 developmental experts, and 64 clinicians. Participants were randomly assigned to one of four conditions in which a juvenile was accused of committing a violent crime, with the psychopathy label and attribution of psychopathic characteristics varying by condition: (1) psychopathic traits/no label, (2) psychopathic traits/psychopathy label, (3) no traits/psychopathy label, and (4) no traits/no label. Among the developmental experts, results revealed a moderate effect of a psychopathy label on perceptions of treatment amenability (d = .64), but a large effect when the juvenile was given both a psychopathy label and attributed psychopathic traits ($d = 1.04$). Among the clinicians, the psychopathy label had a moderate effect on perceptions of treatment amenability ($d = .56$). Although no labeling effect was found among the judges, post-hoc analyses revealed a significantly larger effect among district court judges than juvenile court judges in both conditions in which the offender was given a psychopathic label, with the effect being stronger in the label and traits condition ($d = .89, p < .05$ and $d = 1.07, p < .05$, respectively).

In another study examining labeling effects, Murrie, Boccaccini, McCoy, and Cornell (2007) used a 2 × 2 × 3 design to examine the impact of antisocial behavior history (minimal vs. substantial), psychopathic personality traits (present vs. not present) and diagnosis (psychopathy, Conduct Disorder, or no diagnosis) on 273 members of the National Council of Juvenile and Family Court Judges. Judges in each condition were asked whether they would transfer a juvenile to adult court and the likelihood the juvenile would benefit from mental health services, would be a criminal as an adult, and would pose a risk of violence. Results revealed no effect of psychopathy diagnosis or attribution of psychopathic traits on transfer decisions, but judges were significantly more likely to perceive the juvenile as being at increased risk for violence when the juvenile was described as manifesting psychopathic traits ($d = .22, p < .01$). Further, there was a statistically significant interaction between psychopathic traits and antisocial behavior ($p < .05$), indicating that there was a greater effect of psychopathic traits on perceptions of future violence when the juvenile had a minimal history of antisocial behavior ($d = .72, p < .001$) than when the juvenile had an extensive history of antisocial behavior ($d = .46, p < .01$).

Finally, Jones and Cauffman (2008) examined perceptions of a juvenile's culpability, treatment amenability, dangerousness, and the required restrictiveness of a placement among 78 juvenile court judges and 22 criminal court judges. Judges were randomly assigned to one of four conditions describing a juvenile charged with aggravated assault: non-psychopathic, psychopathic label, psychopathic traits, and psychopathic label and psychopathic traits. The judges perceived no difference in culpability among the four conditions, but they perceived the non-psychopathic juveniles as significantly more amenable to treatment (partial $n^2 = .12, p < .05$) and in less need of restrictive placements (partial $n^2 = .11, p < .05$) compared to juveniles described as psychopathic and with psychopathic traits. Judges perceived the non-psychopathic juvenile to be significantly less dangerous than juveniles in the psychopathic label, psychopathic traits, and psychopathic label and psychopathic traits conditions (partial $n^2 = .25, p < .0001$).

Taken together, these studies suggest that describing an adolescent as having psychopathic traits can have a potentially prejudicial impact in certain contexts, such as predictions and perceptions of future dangerousness (for similar results concerning the new DSM–5 "Limited Prosocial Emotions" specifier for Conduct Disorder, see Edens, Mowle, Clark, & Magyar, 2017). Although judges appeared to be less influenced by the psychopathy label than other groups, including juvenile probation officers and clinicians, the potential negative impact of the psychopathy label raises concerns about the admissibility of psychopathy evidence in juvenile transfer decisions, particularly when there is mixed support for the probative value of such evidence (see DeMatteo et al., 2016).

That said, research in this area is complicated by the intrinsic difficulties in attempting to disentangle the effects of the label "psychopath" and the trait features that comprise the disorder itself when constructing experimental manipulations. More specifically, stimulus materials used in some of these studies have operationalized the *absence* of psychopathic traits by describing the juvenile as exhibiting characteristics that are the polar opposite of psychopathy (e.g., experiencing remorse for crimes and empathy for victims, being honest and forthcoming with evaluators; see, e.g., Appendix A in Chauhan et al., 2007). When these descriptors are then followed by labeling the defendant diagnostically as "a psychopath," participants in such conditions have been presented with information that potentially could result in confusion regarding what exactly the term "psychopath" means, making it difficult evaluate the impact of the label in isolation. To our knowledge, one study has included a condition investigating the effects of the psychopath label in the absence of any trait information being provided in the vignette (Jones & Cauffman, 2008), suggesting that the presentation of either the traits or the label can lead to more negative perceptions of a juvenile defendant compared to a condition in which no such information is provided. Additional research examining whether the inclusion of the label "psychopath" in addition to the trait descriptors results in even more pronounced negative effects would be informative.

Sexually violent predator commitment

The PCL–R is used often in sexually violent predator (SVP) hearings, and researchers have examined whether psychopathy evidence results in undue prejudice against offenders. In an early study, Guy and Edens (2003) provided undergraduates with the same information that was given to jurors in Texas SVP trials and asked them to decide if the defendant should be committed under Texas' SVP law. SVP commitment decisions were not influenced by the psychopathy evidence among men, but women were more likely to commit those described by the prosecution as psychopathic. In a later study, Lieberman and Krauss (2009) asked undergraduates to make an SVP commitment decision for a male offender diagnosed with psychopathy or a paraphilia. In contrast to the Guy and Edens (2006) findings, both men and women in the psychopathy condition were more likely to support commitment. Overall, research does not support the conclusion that PCL–R evidence is unduly prejudicial in SVP contexts, particularly when cases involve the long-term prediction of sexual reoffending, for which there is some evidence that the PCL–R can provide useful information (Hawes et al., 2013).

Capital sentencing

In bifurcated death penalty proceedings, capital sentencing is the phase in which convicted offenders are sentenced to death or life in prison. Research suggests that the PCL–R is used in capital cases in two ways: (1) during the guilt/innocence phase of capital trials to rebut a defense of insanity by demonstrating that the defendant is not mentally ill (at least in terms of any psychotic-spectrum disorder potentially relevant to criminal responsibility determinations) and potentially malingering (Edens, Davis, Fernandez Smith, & Guy, 2013); and (2) during the sentencing phase of capital trials to assess the defendant's likelihood of being dangerous in the future. In several states, future dangerousness is a statutorily articulated aggravating factor for the death penalty, and the PCL–R is often used by attorneys and experts to assess an offender's risk of future danger (DeMatteo et al., 2014b; Edens & Cox, 2012).

Several studies have examined the role of labeling and the attribution of psychopathic traits to defendants in capital offenses. In the first published study, Edens, Desforges, Fernandez, and Palac (2004) presented 301 mock jurors with a case summary describing a homicide offense and a summary of expert testimony that varied the defendant's diagnosis (psychopathy/ psychosis/ no diagnosis) and risk level for future violence (low/high derived from PCL–R Factor 1 traits). Results revealed that defendants with psychopathy and psychosis were rated as more dangerous than defendants without a diagnosis (d = .43 and d = .40, respectively), while defendants with psychopathy and psychosis did not differ significantly from each other (d = .04). Moreover, although risk level significantly influenced perceptions of dangerousness in the no-diagnosis condition, this effect did not hold for defendants with psychopathy, which suggests that mock jurors' perceptions of dangerousness were based mainly on diagnostic labels for defendants with psychopathy. Findings concerning support for death verdicts in this particular study were compromised by the fact that a large percentage of participants did not accurately comprehend the (complex) guidelines they were provided regarding capital sentencing (e.g., many mock jurors could not accurately identify the definition of "mitigating" evidence).

In a subsequent study, Edens, Colwell, Desforges, and Fernandez (2005) replicated the Edens et al. (2004) study with 233 undergraduate students who were provided with clearer jury instructions indicating that the defendant should be put to death only if no mitigating factors were present and the prosecution proved beyond a reasonable doubt that the defendant would be a continuing threat to society. The results of both studies were similar with respect to perceived dangerousness, although the diagnostic label influenced mock jurors' decisions to impose the death penalty, with defendants with psychopathy being significantly more likely to be sentenced to death than defendants without a diagnosis or defendants diagnosed with psychosis.

After providing 144 undergraduate students with vignettes describing the trial phase of a capital offense, Cox, DeMatteo, and Foster (2010) measured their perceptions of the defendant's dangerousness and their decision to sentence the defendant to life without parole (LWOP) or death. The vignettes contained identical descriptions of the trial phase but differed in regards to expert testimony presented according to a 2 (diagnostic label: no label vs. psychopath) × 2 (danger risk: low vs. high) design. In both diagnostic conditions, psychopathic traits were attributed to the defendant, but in the psychopath condition the defendant was labeled as a psychopath based on the PCL–R. There was no significant impact of diagnostic label on decisions to impose the death penalty or perceptions of future violence, but there was a significant difference between the low-violence and high-violence risk groups in terms of mock jurors' perceptions of whether the defendant would commit another violent crime or murder if given LWOP. Further, results revealed a significant difference between the number of participants expected to impose the death penalty and the number of participants that actually imposed the death penalty (Cramer's $V = .378$), with the difference occurring between defendants described as high-violence or low-violence risk, regardless of diagnostic label.

Finally, Edens et al. (2013) aggregated results from three earlier studies to examine the incremental predictive validity of subcomponents of psychopathy as a construct and individual PCL–R items on mock jurors' attitudes towards capital punishment. Each study asked participants to rate the extent to which someone like the defendant presented in the stimulus materials for the study would be likely to display similar behavior, symptoms, and traits to those encapsulated by the PCL–R. Receiver Operating Characteristic (ROC) curve analyses indicated strong effects for both global psychopathy scores and for Factor 1 scores in all three studies, with the lowest area under the curve (AUC) and significance level being AUC = .66 ($p < .05$) for general offending and AUC = .72 ($p < .01$) for Factor 1. Additionally, when the aggregate sample was split by scale and subscale midpoint, only 15 percent of participants supported a death sentence when the PCL–R score was less than 20 while 43 percent supported a death sentence when the PCL–R score was greater than 20. Further, when they controlled for the predictive validity of Factor 1 scores, psychopathy ratings failed to significantly predict support for the death penalty.

Taken together, the results from all of these studies suggest that labeling a capital defendant a "psychopath" makes jurors more likely to perceive the capital defendant as dangerous and more likely to impose a death sentence. Given the potential prejudice of the "psychopath" label and the lack of data suggesting that PCL–R scores have any clear relation to violence among capital defendants sentence to life without parole (see Edens, Buffington-Vollum, Roskamp, & Anthony, 2005), there seems little reason to admit the PCL–R in capital sentencing proceedings.

Stated differently, a psychopathy label appears far more prejudicial than probative in risk assessment at capital sentencing.

Conclusion

The justice systems in many countries have increasingly considered the results of psychopathy assessments (e.g., DeMatteo et al., 2014b) as clinicians and policy-makers have increasingly emphasized the relation between psychopathy and certain justice-relevant outcomes. In many respects, this trend is reasonable and empirically sound. Research since the 1980s suggests PCL–R scores – at least when properly derived by adequately trained raters under rigorous research contexts – meaningfully correspond with certain important outcomes, such as community violence, sexual violence, and recidivism risk. There is certainly *some* appropriate role for rigorous psychopathy assessment to inform *certain* legal proceedings that address certain offenders' risk of violence, sexual violence, or recidivism (DeMatteo et al., 2010).

But just as no instrument is uniformly "valid" – but rather, valid only for particularly purposes with particular populations – psychopathy assessment is relevant and appropriate only in particular court proceedings, for particular questions, and when results are communicated in particular ways. For example, psychopathy assessment would almost never be relevant to the courts' questions about adjudicative competence, waiver of rights, or sanity. Psychopathy assessment may indeed be relevant to *certain* court questions about risk of violence, sexual violence, or recidivism. But even these questions must be understood carefully; for example, research suggests PCL–R scores may meaningfully inform certain questions about risk for community violence, but not the questions about risk for institutional violence that are relevant at capital sentencing (Edens et al., 2005).

Recent research also suggests many reasons to be cautious about the ways psychopathy is assessed and communicated, even in proceedings in which psychopathy is relevant. As detailed in this chapter, psychopathy assessments conducted for legal proceedings may be vulnerable to various evaluator biases and idiosyncrasies (e.g., Boccaccini et al., 2008), particularly biases attributable to the adversarial legal system in which these assessments occur (e.g., Murrie et al., 2009). Addressing remedies for adversarial allegiance in PCL–R assessments is beyond the scope of this chapter, though any potential remedies may be informed by the efforts to understand and reduce adversarial allegiance more broadly (Murrie & Boccaccini, 2015).

Even if psychopathy can be assessed in an objective and reliable manner, more recent research underscores the need for caution in how results are communicated because of the ways in which they can influence decision-makers. As discussed, research increasingly suggests that much of psychopathy's predictive value (i.e., its relevance to court questions) is attributable primarily to the quantification of criminal history in PCL–R Factor 2 (e.g., Kennealy, Skeem, Walters, & Camp, 2010); but paradoxically, decision-makers seem particularly influenced by the striking personality features considered prototypical of psychopathy and captured in PCL–R Factor 1. Indeed, as detailed earlier, a substantial body of research documents the ways in which describing a defendant as manifesting psychopathic traits often leads to poorer outcomes for that defendant. Though exact methodology and findings vary, studies reveal that within juvenile proceedings (e.g., Jones & Cauffman, 2008), SVP proceedings (e.g., Guy & Edens, 2006; Lieberman & Krauss, 2009), or capital sentencing proceedings (Edens et al., 2005), an emphasis on psychopathic personality traits – whether provided by a mental health expert (e.g., Murrie et al., 2007) or lay descriptions (e.g., Edens et al., 2003) – can lead some decision-makers to perceive the defendant in a more negative light (for some outcomes) and be more willing to assign harsher punishments (in some situations). Particularly in those proceedings where PCL–R scores are least relevant – such as capital sentencing (e.g., Edens et al., 2013) – these findings raise the concern that psychopathy findings may sometimes be more prejudicial than probative and, therefore, inappropriate for consideration as evidence.

Of course, the decision about whether evidence is more prejudicial than probative is a case-by-case decision, and this is certainly true of psychopathy evidence as well (DeMatteo et al., 2016). There will almost certainly continue to be contexts in which PCL–R scores – derived in an appropriate and transparent assessment process – will be relevant to certain court considerations. But research also reveals increasing ways in which the previous unbridled enthusiasm for psychopathy evidence may have been inappropriate, and courts will need to become increasingly savvy consumers of psychopathy evidence.

Notes

1 Omnibus self-report personality and psychopathology inventories that are widely administered in forensic and correctional settings also include scales assessing psychopathic traits. These scales tend to not correlate particularly highly with interview and file review-based measures such as the PCL-R, however, and are not reviewed further in this chapter.

2 Because SVP proceedings are civil, rather than criminal, they employ slightly different terms. The "petitioner" is the party arguing to civilly commit the offender, roughly analogous to the prosecution in criminal cases, and the "respondent" is roughly analogous to the defendant.

3 The standard error of measurement (SEM) for PCL-R scores is about 3.0 points, which means that differences between two scores assigned to the same offender should be ± 6.0 points or smaller in more than 95 percent of cases. Differences larger than ± 6.0 points should be highly unusual (less than 5 percent of cases), but they do occur. If scoring differences are attributable merely to measurement error, the likelihood that a prosecution-retained evaluator assigns a much higher score than a defense-retained evaluator (about 2 percent of cases) should be the same as the likelihood that a defense-retained evaluator assigns a much higher score than a prosecution-retained evaluator (about 2 percent of cases). However, a pattern of findings showing that large differences are common and usually reflect prosecution-retained evaluators assigning higher scores than defense-retained evaluators suggests systematic error, not random error.

4 Of course, there are many reasons allegiance effects in this experiment, though significant, were smaller than those in field studies. For example, the experimental manipulation (brief conversation with an attorney who identifies his "side") may be much weaker than the pressures in a typical case (e.g., lengthy and repeated conversations with attorneys who may share more of their case perspectives, pay much more, and carry a promise of future work). Similarly, the evaluation process (relying on a transcript of a PCL-R interview that provides identical information to both evaluators) may allow for greater reliability than real cases in which opposing evaluators conduct PCL-R interviews and can therefore *elicit different information* from offenders.

5 Once proffered expert evidence is determined to satisfy FRE 401 and 403, it is then subjected to analysis under FRE 702, which applies specifically to expert testimony. A discussion of FRE 702 is beyond the scope of this chapter.

References

Alterman, A. I., Cacciola, J. S., and Rutherford, M. J. (1993) 'Reliability of the Revised Psychopathy Checklist in substance abuse patients,' *Psychological Assessment*, *5*:442–448.

Boccaccini, M. T., Chevalier, C. S., Murrie, D. C., and Varela, J. G. (2017) 'Psychopathy Checklist use and reporting practices in sexually violent predator evaluations,' *Sexual Abuse: A Journal of Research and Treatment*, *29*:592–614.

Boccaccini, M. T., Murrie, D. C., Rufino, K. A., and Gardner, B. O. (2014) 'Evaluator differences in Psychopathy Checklist–Revised factor and facet scores,' *Law and Human Behavior*, *38*:337–345.

Boccaccini, M. T., Rufino, K. A., Jeon, H., and Murrie, D. C. (2017) 'Does the predictive validity of psychopathy ratings depend on the clinical experience of the raters?' *International Journal of Forensic Mental Health*, *16*:130–138.

Boccaccini, M. T., Turner, D. B., and Murrie, D. C. (2008) 'Do some evaluators report consistently higher or lower PCL–R scores than others? Findings from a statewide sample of sexually violent predator evaluations,' *Psychology, Public Policy, and Law*, *14*:262–283.

Chauhan, P., Reppucci, N. D., and Burnette, M. L. (2007) 'Application and impact of the psychopathy label to juveniles,' *International Journal of Forensic Mental Health*, *6*:3–14.

Cicchetti, D. V., and Sparrow, S. A. (1981) 'Developing criteria for establishing interrater reliability of specific items: Applications to assessment of adaptive behavior,' *American Journal of Mental Deficiency*, *86*:127–137.

Cleckley, H. (1941) *The mask of sanity*, St. Louis, MO: Mosby.

Cooke, D. J., and Michie, C. (2001) 'Refining the construct of psychopathy: Towards a hierarchical model,' *Psychological Assessment*, *13*:171–188.

Cooke, D. J., Michie, C., Hart, S. D., and Clark, D. (2004) 'Reconstructing psychopathy: Clarifying the significance of antisocial and socially deviant behavior in the diagnosis of psychopathic personality disorder,' *Journal of Personality Disorders*, *18*:337–357.

Cooke, D. J., Michie, C., and Skeem, J. (2007) 'Understanding the structure of the Psychopathy Checklist–Revised,' *British Journal of Psychiatry*, *190*(suppl. 49):s39–s50.

Cox, J., DeMatteo, D. S., and Foster, E. E. (2010) 'The effect of the Psychopathy Checklist–Revised in capital cases: Mock jurors' responses to the label of psychopathy,' *Behavioral Sciences and the Law*, *28*:878–891.

DeMatteo, D., and Edens, J. F. (2006) 'The role and relevance of the Psychopathy Checklist–Revised in court: A case law survey of US courts (1991–2004),' *Psychology, Public Policy, and Law*, *12*:214–241.

DeMatteo, D., Edens, J. F., Galloway, M., Cox, J., Smith, S. T., and Formon, D. (2014a) 'The role and reliability of the Psychopathy Checklist–Revised in U.S. sexually violent predator evaluations: A case law survey,' *Law and Human Behavior*, *38*:248–255.

DeMatteo, D., Edens, J. F., Galloway, M., Cox, J., Smith, S. T., Koller, J. P., and Bersoff, B. (2014b) 'Investigating the role of the Psychopathy Checklist–Revised in United States case law,' *Psychology, Public Policy, and Law*, *20*:96–07.

DeMatteo, D., Edens, J. F., and Hart, A. (2010) 'The use of measures of psychopathy in violence risk assessment,' in R. K. Otto & K. S. Douglas (Eds.), *Handbook of violence risk assessment* (pp. 19–40), New York, NY: Routledge/Taylor & Francis Group.

DeMatteo, D., Heilbrun, K., and Marczyk, G. (2005) 'Psychopathy, risk of violence, and protective factors in a noninstitutionalized and noncriminal sample,' *International Journal of Forensic Mental Health*, *4*:147–157.

DeMatteo, D., Heilbrun, K., and Marczyk, G. (2006) 'An empirical investigation of psychopathy in a non-institutionalized and noncriminal sample,' *Behavioral Sciences and the Law*, *24*:133–146.

DeMatteo, D., Hodges, H., and Fairfax-Columbo, J. (2016) 'An examination of whether Psychopathy Checklist–Revised (PCL–R) evidence satisfies the relevance/prejudice admissibility standard,' in B. H. Bornstein & M. K. Miller (Eds.), *Advances in psychology and law* (Vol. 2, pp. 205–239), New York, NY: Springer Publishing Co.

DeMatteo, D., Murphy, M., Galloway, M., and Krauss, D. A. (2015) 'A national survey of United States sexually violent person legislation: Policy, procedures, and practice,' *International Journal of Forensic Mental Health*, *14*:245–266.

Douglas, K. S., Vincent, G., and Edens, J. F. (2018) 'Risk for criminal recidivism: The role of psychopathy,' in C. Patrick (Ed.), *Handbook of psychopathy* (2nd ed.), New York, NY: Guilford.

Edens, J. F. (2006) 'Unresolved controversies concerning psychopathy: Implications for clinical and forensic decision making,' *Professional Psychology: Research and Practice*, *37*:59–65.

Edens, J. F., Boccaccini, M. T., and Johnson, D. W. (2010) 'Inter-rater reliability of the PCL–R total and factor scores among psychopathic sex offenders: Are personality features more prone to disagreement than behavioral features?,' *Behavioral Sciences and the Law*, *28*:106–119.

Edens, J. F., Buffington-Vollum, J. K., Roskamp, P., and Anthony, C. (2005) 'Predictions of future dangerousness in capital murder trials: Is it time to "disinvent the wheel"?,' *Law and Human Behavior*, *29*:55–86.

Edens, J. F., Colwell, L. H., Desforges, D. M., and Fernandez, K. (2005) 'The impact of mental health evidence on support for capital punishment: Are defendants labeled psychopathic considered more deserving of death?,' *Behavioral Sciences and the Law*, *23*:603–625.

Edens, J. F., and Cox, J. (2012) 'Examining the prevalence, role, and impact of evidence regarding antisocial personality, sociopathy, and psychopathy in capital cases: A survey of defense team members,' *Behavioral Sciences and the Law*, *30*:239–255.

Edens, J. F., Cox, J., Smith, S. T., DeMatteo, D., and Sörman, K. (2015) 'How reliable are Psychopathy Checklist–Revised scores in Canadian criminal trials? A case law review,' *Psychological Assessment, 27*:447–456.

Edens, J. F., Davis, K. M., Fernandez Smith, K., and Guy, L. S. (2013) 'No sympathy for the Devil: Attributing psychopathic traits to capital murderers also predicts support for executing them,' *Personality Disorders: Theory, Research, and Treatment, 4*:175–181.

Edens, J. F., Desforges, D. M., Fernandez, K., and Palac, C. A. (2004) 'Effects of psychopathy and violence risk testimony on mock juror perceptions of dangerousness in a capital murder trial,' *Psychology, Crime and Law, 10*:393–412.

Edens, J. F., Guy, L. S., and Fernandez, K. (2003) 'Psychopathic traits predict attitudes toward a juvenile capital murderer,' *Behavioral Sciences and the Law, 21*:807–828.

Edens, J. F., Marcus, D. K., Lilienfeld, S. O., and Poythress, N. G. (2006) 'Psychopathic, not psychopath: Taxometric evidence for the dimensional structure of psychopathy,' *Journal of abnormal psychology, 115*:131–144.

Edens, J. F., Mowle, E. N., Clark, J. W., and Magyar, M. S. (2017) '"A psychopath by any other name?" Jury venireperson perceptions of the DSM–5 "limited prosocial emotions" specifier,' *Journal of Personality Disorders, 31*:90–109.

Edens, J. F., Petrila, J., and Kelley, S. E. (2018) 'Legal and ethical issues in the assessment and treatment of psychopathy,' in C. Patrick (Ed.), *Handbook of psychopathy* (2nd ed.), New York, NY: Guilford.

Epperson, D. L., Kaul, J. D., Huot, S. J., Hesselton, D., Alexander, W., and Goldman, R. (1998) *Minnesota Sex Offender Screening Tool – Revised (MnSOST–R)*, St. Paul: Minnesota Department of Corrections.

Federal Rules of Evidence for United States Courts and Magistrates. (1975) St. Paul, MN: West Publishing Company.

Gacono, C., and Hutton, H. (1994) 'Suggestions for the clinical and forensic use of the Hare Psychopathy Checklist–Revised (PCL–R),' *International Journal of Law and Psychiatry, 17*:303–317.

Grisso, T. (1986) *Evaluating competencies: Forensic assessments and instruments*, New York, NY: Plenum Press.

Grisso, T. (2003) *Evaluating competencies: Forensic assessments and instruments* (2nd ed.), New York, NY: Kluwer.

Guay, J., Ruscio, J., Hare, R., and Knight, R. A. (2007) 'A taxometric analysis of the latent structure of psychopathy: Evidence for dimensionality,' *Journal of Abnormal Psychology, 116*:701–716.

Guy, L. S., and Edens, J. F. (2003) 'Juror decision-making in a mock sexually violent predator trial: Gender differences in the impact of divergent types of expert testimony,' *Behavioral Sciences and the Law, 21*:215–237.

Guy, L. S., and Edens, J. F. (2006) 'Gender differences in attitudes toward psychopathic sexual offenders,' *Behavioral Sciences & the Law, 24*:65–85.

Hall, J. R., and Benning, S. D. (2006) 'The "successful" psychopath,' in C. Patrick (Ed.), *Handbook of psychopathy* (pp. 459–478), New York, NY: Guilford.

Hall, J. R., Benning, S. D., and Patrick, C. J. (2004) 'Criterion-related validity of the three-factor model of psychopathy: Personality, behavior, and adaptive functioning,' *Assessment, 11*:4–16.

Hanson, R. K., and Thornton, D. (2000) 'Improving risk assessments for sex offenders: A comparison of three actuarial scales,' *Law and Human Behavior, 24*:119–136.

Hare, R. D. (1980) 'A research scale for the assessment of psychopathy in criminal populations,' *Personality and Individual Differences, 1*:111–119.

Hare, R. D. (1991) *The Hare Psychopathy Checklist–Revised manual*, North Tonawanda, NY: Multi-Health Systems.

Hare, R. D. (2003) *The Hare Psychopathy Checklist–Revised manual* (2nd ed.), North Tonawanda, NY: Multi-Health Systems.

Hare, R. D. (2016) 'Psychopathy, the PCL–R, and criminal justice: Some new findings and current issues,' *Canadian Psychology, 57*:21–34.

Hare, R. D., and Neumann, C. S. (2005) 'The structure of psychopathy,' *Current Psychiatry Reports, 7*:57–64.

Harpur, T. J., Hakstian, A. R., and Hare, R. D. (1988) 'Factor structure of the Psychopathy Checklist,' *Journal of Consulting and Clinical Psychology, 56*:741–747.

Harpur, T. J., Hare, R. D., and Hakstian, A. R. (1989) 'Two-factor conceptualization of psychopathy: Construct validity and assessment implications,' *Psychological Assessment, 1*:6–17.

Harris, G. T., Rice, M. E., and Cormier, C. A. (2013) 'Research and clinical scoring of the Psychopathy Checklist can show good agreement,' *Criminal Justice and Behavior, 40*:1349–1362.

Hawes, S. W., Boccaccini, M. T., and Murrie, D. C. (2013) 'Psychopathy and the combination of psychopathy and sexual deviance as predictors of sexual recidivism: Meta-analytic findings using the Psychopathy Checklist–Revised,' *Psychological Assessment, 25*:233–243.
Helmus, L., Thornton, D., Hanson, R. K., and Babchishin, K. M. (2012) 'Improving the predictive accuracy of Static–99 and Static–2002 with older sex offenders: Revised age weights,' *Sexual Abuse: Journal of Research and Treatment, 24*:64–101.
Jeandarme, I., Edens, J. F., Habets, P., Bruckers, L., Oei, K., and Bogaerts, S. (2017) 'Psychopathy Checklist–Revised field validity in prison and hospital settings,' *Law and Human Behavior, 41*(1):29–43.
Jones, S., and Cauffman, E. (2008) 'Juvenile psychopathy and judicial decision making: An empirical analysis of an ethical dilemma,' *Behavioral Sciences and the Law, 26*:151–165.
Kansas v. Crane, 534 U.S. 407 (2002).
Kansas v. Hendricks, 521 U. S. 346 (1997).
Karpman, B. (1946) 'A yardstick for measuring psychopathy,' *Federal Probation, 10*:26–31.
Karpman, B. (1948) 'The myth of the psychopathic personality,' *American Journal of Psychiatry, 104*:523–534.
Kelley, S. E., Edens, J. F., Mowle, E. N., Rulseh, A., and Penson, B. N. (under review). Dangerous, depraved, and death-worthy: A meta-analysis of the correlates of perceived psychopathy in jury simulation studies.
Kennealy, P. J., Hicks, B. M., and Patrick, C. J. (2007) 'Validity of factors of the Psychopathy Checklist–Revised in female prisoners: Discriminant relations with antisocial behavior, substance abuse, and personality,' *Assessment, 14*:323–340.
Kennealy, P. J., Skeem, J. L., Walters, G. D., and Camp, J. (2010) 'Do core interpersonal and affective traits of PCL–R psychopathy interact with antisocial behavior and disinhibition to predict violence?,' *Psychological Assessment, 22*:569–580.
Kroner, D. G., and Mills, J. F. (2001) 'The accuracy of five risk appraisal instruments in predicting institutional misconduct and new convictions,' *Criminal Justice and Behavior, 28*:471–489.
Leistico, A. M., Salekin, R. T., DeCosta, J., and Rogers, R. (2008) 'A large-scale meta-analysis relating the Hare measures of psychopathy to antisocial conduct,' *Law and Human Behavior, 32*:28–45.
Lieberman, J. D., and Krauss, D. A. (2009) 'The effects of labeling, expert testimony, and information processing mode on juror decisions in SVP civil commitment trials,' *Journal of Investigative Psychology and Offender Profiling, 6*:25–41.
Lilienfeld, S. O. (1994) 'Conceptual problems in the assessment of psychopathy,' *Clinical Psychology Review, 14*:17–38.
Lilienfeld, S. O., Watts, A. L., Francis Smith, S., Berg, J. M., and Latzman, R. D. (2015) 'Psychopathy deconstructed and reconstructed: Identifying and assembling the personality building blocks of Cleckley's chimera,' *Journal of Personality, 83*:593–610.
Lloyd, C. D., Clark, H. J., and Forth, A. E. (2010) 'Psychopathy, expert testimony and indeterminate sentences: Exploring the relationship between Psychopathy Checklist–Revised testimony and trial outcome in Canada,' *Legal and Criminological Psychology, 15*:323–339.
Lykken, D. T. (1995) *The antisocial personalities*, Hillsdale, NJ: Erlbaum.
McDermott, P. A., Alterman, A. I., Cacciola, J. S., Rutherford, M. J., Newman, J. P., and Mulholland, E. M. (2000) 'Generality of Psychopathy Checklist–Revised factors over prisoners and substance-dependent patients,' *Journal of Consulting and Clinical Psychology, 68*:181–186.
Melton, G. B., Petrila, J., Poythress, N. G., Slobogin, C., Otto, R. K., Mossman, D., and Condie, L. O. (2018) *Psychological evaluations for the courts* (4th ed.), New York, NY: Guilford.
Miller, C. S., Kimonis, E. R., Otto, R. K., Kline, S. M., and Wasserman, A. L. (2012) 'Reliability of risk assessment measures used in sexually violent predator proceedings,' *Psychological Assessment, 24*(4): 944–953.
Miller, A. K., Rufino, K. A., Boccaccini, M. T., Jackson, R. L., and Murrie, D. C. (2011) 'On individual differences in person perception: Raters' personality traits relate to their Psychopathy Checklist–Revised scoring tendencies,' *Assessment, 18*:253–260.
Mnookin, J. (2008) 'Expert evidence, partisanship, and epistemic confidence,' *Brooklyn Law Review, 73*:587–611.
Mokros, A., Hare, R. D., Neumann, C. S., Santtila, P., Habermeyer, E., and Nitschke, J. (2015) 'Variants of psychopathy in adult male offenders: A latent profile analysis,' *Journal of Abnormal Psychology, 124*:372–386.

Murrie, D. C., and Boccaccini, M. T. (2015) 'Adversarial allegiance among expert witnesses,' *Annual Review of Law and Social Science*, *11*:37–55.
Murrie, D. C., Boccaccini, M. T., Guarnera, L. A., and Rufino, K. A. (2013) 'Are forensic experts biased by the side that retained them?,' *Psychological Science*, *24*:1889–1897.
Murrie, D. C., Boccaccini, M. T., Johnson, J. T., and Janke, C. (2008) 'Does interrater (dis)agreement on Psychopathy Checklist scores in Sexually Violent Predator trials suggest partisan allegiance in forensic evaluation?,' *Law and Human Behavior*, *32*:352–362.
Murrie, D. C., Boccaccini, M. T., McCoy, W., and Cornell, D. G. (2007) 'Diagnostic labeling in juvenile court: How do descriptions of psychopathy and conduct disorder influence judges?,' *Journal of Clinical Child and Adolescent Psychology*, *36*:228–241.
Murrie, D. C., Boccaccini, M. T., Turner, D., Meeks, M., Woods, C., and Tussey, C. (2009) 'Rater (dis) agreement on risk assessment measures in sexually violent predator proceedings: Evidence of adversarial allegiance in forensic evaluation?,' *Psychology, Public Policy, and Law*, *15*:19–53.
Murrie, D. C., Cornell, D. G., and McCoy, W. K. (2005) 'Psychopathy, conduct disorder, and stigma: Does diagnostic labeling influence juvenile probation officer recommendations?,' *Law and Human Behavior*, *29*:323–342.
Murrie, D. C., Marcus, D. K., Douglas, K. S., Salekin, R. T., Lee, Z., and Vincent, G. (2007) 'Youth with psychopathy features are not a discrete class: A taxometric analysis,' *Journal of Child Psychology and Psychiatry*, *48*:714–723.
Neal, T. M. S., and Brodsky, S. L. (2016) 'Forensic psychologists' perceptions of bias and potential correction strategies in forensic mental health evaluations,' *Psychology, Public Policy, and Law*, *22*:58–76.
Neumann, C. S., Hare, R. D., and Johansson, P. T. (2013) 'The Psychopathy Checklist–Revised (PCL–R), low anxiety, and fearlessness: A structural equation modeling analysis,' *Personality Disorders: Theory, Research, and Treatment*, *4*:129–137.
Neumann, C. S., Kosson, D. S., and Salekin. R. T. (2007) 'Exploratory and confirmatory factor analysis of the psychopathy construct: Methodological and conceptual issues,' in H. Herve & J. C. Yuille (Eds.), *The psychopath: Theory, research, and practice* (pp. 79–104), Mahwah, NJ: Erlbaum.
Patrick, C. J. (2018) *Handbook of psychopathy* (2nd ed.), New York, NY: Guilford.
Poythress, N. G., Lilienfeld, S. O., Skeem, J. L., Douglas, K. S., Edens, J. F., Epstein, M., and Patrick, C. J. (2010) 'Using the PCL–R to help estimate the validity of two self-report measures of psychopathy with offenders,' *Assessment*, *17*:206–219.
Preszler, J., Marcus, D. K., Edens, J. F., and McDermott, B. E. (in press) 'Network analysis of psychopathy in forensic patients,' *Journal of Abnormal Psychology*.
Pronin, E., Lin, D. Y., and Ross, L. (2002) 'The bias blind spot: Perceptions of bias in self versus others,' *Personality and Social Psychology Bulletin*, *28*(3):369–381.
Rufino, K. A., Boccaccini, M. T., Hawes, S. W., and Murrie, D. C. (2012) 'When experts disagreed, who was correct? A comparison of PCL–R scores from independent raters and opposing forensic experts,' *Law and Human Behavior*, *36*(6):527–531.
Rutherford, M., Cacciola, J. S., Alterman, A. I., McKay, J. R., and Cook, T. G. (1999) 'The 2-year test–retest reliability of the Psychopathy Checklist–Revised in methadone patients,' *Assessment*, *6*:285–291.
Seling v. Young, 531 U.S. 250 (2001).
Shepherd, S. M., Campbell, R. E., and Ogloff, J. R. (in press) 'Psychopathy, antisocial personality disorder, and reconviction in an Australian sample of forensic patients,' *International Journal of Offender Therapy and Comparative Criminology*.
Singh, J. P., Grann, M., and Fazel, S. (2011) 'A comparative study of violence risk assessment tools: A systematic review and metaregression analysis of 68 studies involving 25,980 participants,' *Clinical Psychology Review*, *31*:499–513.
Skeem, J. L., and Cooke, D. J. (2010) 'Is criminal behavior a central component of psychopathy? Conceptual directions for resolving the debate,' *Psychological Assessment*, *22*:433–445.
Skilling, T. A., Harris, G. T., Rice, M. E., and Quinsey, V. L. (2002) 'Identifying persistently antisocial offenders using the Hare Psychopathy Checklist and DSM antisocial personality disorder criteria,' *Psychological Assessment*, *14*:27–38.
Sturup, J., Edens, J. F., Sörman, K., Karlberg, D., Fredriksson, B., and Kristiansson, M. (2014) 'Field reliability of the Psychopathy Checklist–Revised among life sentenced prisoners in Sweden,' *Law and Human Behavior*, *38*:315–324.

Sundby, S. E. (1998) 'The capital jury and absolution: The intersection of trial strategy, remorse, and the death penalty,' *Cornell Law Review, 83*:1557–1598.
Tyrer, P., Cooper, S., Seivewright, H., Duggan, C., Rao, B., and Hogue, T. (2005) 'Temporal reliability of psychological assessments for patients in a special hospital with severe personality disorder: A preliminary note,' *Criminal Behaviour and Mental Health, 15*(2):87–92.
Verschuere, B., van Ghesel Grothe, S., Noordhof, A., Waldorp, L., Watts, A. L., Lilienfeld, S. O., . . ., and Skeem, J. L. (in press) 'What symptoms of psychopathy might be central? A network analysis of the Psychopathy Checklist–Revised (PCL–R) in three large samples,' *Journal of Abnormal Psychology.*
Viljoen, J. L., MacDougall, E. A. M., Gagnon, N. C., and Douglas, K. S. (2010) 'Psychopathy evidence in legal proceedings involving adolescent offenders,' *Psychology, Public Policy, and Law, 16*:254–283.
Viljoen, J. L., McLachlan, K., and Vincent, G. M. (2010) 'Assessing violence risk and psychopathy in juvenile and adult offenders: A survey of clinical practices,' *Assessment, 17*(3):377–395.
Vitacco, M. J., Rogers, R., Neumann, C. S., Harrison, K., and Vincent, G. (2005) 'A comparison of factor models on the PCL–R with mentally disordered offenders: The development of a four-factor model,' *Criminal Justice and Behavior, 32*:526–545.
Walsh, T., and Walsh, Z. (2006) 'The evidentiary introduction of Psychopathy Checklist–Revised assessed psychopathy in US courts: Extent and appropriateness,' *Law and Human Behavior, 30*:493–507.
Walters, G. D. (2014) 'The latent structure of psychopathy in male adjudicated delinquents: A cross-domain taxometric analysis,' *Personality Disorders: Theory, Research, and Treatment, 5*:348–355.
Walters, G. D., Duncan, S. A., and Mitchell-Perez, K. (2007) 'The latent structure of psychopathy: A taxometric analysis of the Psychopathy Checklist–Revised in a heterogeneous sample of male prison inmates,' *Assessment, 14*:270–278.
Walters, G. D., Ermer, E., Knight, R. A., and Kiehl, K. A. (2015) 'Paralimbic biomarkers in taxometric analyses of psychopathy: Does changing the indicators change the conclusion?,' *Personality Disorders: Theory, Research, and Treatment, 6*:41–52.
Walters, G. D., Gray, N. S., Jackson, R. L., Sewell, K. W., Rogers, R., Taylor, J., and Snowden, R. J. (2007) 'A taxometric analysis of the Psychopathy Checklist: Screening Version: Further evidence of dimensionality,' *Psychological Assessment, 19*:330–339.
Walters, G. D., and Heilbrun, K. (2010) 'Violence risk assessment and facet 4 of the Psychopathy Checklist: Predicting institutional and community aggression in two forensic samples,' *Assessment, 17*:259–268.
Walters, G. D., Knight, R. A., Grann, M., and Dahle, K. (2008) 'Incremental validity of the Psychopathy Checklist facet scores: Predicting release outcome in six samples,' *Journal of Abnormal Psychology, 117*:396–405.
Weaver, C. M., Meyer, R. G., Van Nort, J., and Tristan, L. (2006) 'Two-, three-, and four-factor PCL–R models in applied sex offender risk assessments,' *Assessment, 13*:208–216.
Weinstein, J. B., and Berger, M. A. (2015) *Weinstein's evidence manual: A guide to the Federal Rules of Evidence based on Weinstein's Federal Evidence* (10th ed.), Danvers, MA: Matthew Bender and Company, Inc.
Wigmore, J. (1923) *A treatise on the Anglo-American system of evidence in trials at common law: Including the statutes and judicial decisions of all jurisdictions of the United States and Canada*, Boston, MA: Little Brown.
Yang, M., Wong, S. C., and Coid, J. (2010) 'The efficacy of violence prediction: A meta analytic comparison of nine risk assessment tools,' *Psychological Bulletin, 136*:740–767.
Zapf, P. A., Kukucka, J., Kassin, S. M., and Dror, I. E. (in press) 'Cognitive bias in forensic mental health assessment: Evaluator beliefs about its nature and scope,' *Psychology, Public Policy, and Law.*

42

Psychopathy and risk assessment

Mark E. Olver and Stephen C. P. Wong

Introduction

The assessment of risk for recidivism has important legal, health, policy, and public safety implications. Risk assessment is a routine, but essential and complex, psycho-legal task performed by evaluators in a number of criminal justice and correctional contexts for different decision-making purposes. Risk assessments inform decisions regarding bail, sentencing, preventative detention, institutional security classification, treatment planning, conditional release, community supervision, and special release conditions or restrictions. Risk assessments, in turn, can be organized around the appraisal domains of frequency/probability (i.e., how likely is this individual to reoffend?), severity (i.e., how much physical or psychological harm may result from a potential new offense), and imminence (i.e., what is the time frame of the assessment and how quickly could an individual possibly reoffend?). Douglas and Kropp (2002) remind us the that ultimate purpose of risk assessment is provide services to the individual and thereby prevent or reduce the risk of recidivism; that is, individuals who present with high potential for future crime and violence in terms of frequency, imminence, and severity should be the focus of risk management efforts (e.g., security, release decisions, treatment, supervision) to prevent a recidivistic prophecy from being carried out.

That psychopathy is a personality disorder is pretty much universally accepted, but the right way to conceptualize and assess psychopathy is still a matter for debate. The PCL measures, taken together, are one among a number of different conceptualizations of psychopathy. The three-factor model of psychopathy (Cooke, Kosson, & Michi, 2001) and the triarchic model (Patrick, Fowles, & Krueger, 2009) are alternative formulations and measures of the psychopathy construct. The use of the PCL measures to assess the construct of psychopathy and for risk assessment and prediction are related but different issues; the latter is the primary focus of this chapter.

Overview and operational definition

The assessment of psychopathy has a prominent and well-deserved place in forensic risk assessment. Psychopathy is a serious personality disorder characterized by a constellation of interpersonal, affective, lifestyle, and antisocial behavioral features conducive to criminality and serious rule violations, and the disorder, as is to be expected, is much more heavily represented in correctional and forensic settings (Hare, 1996). As will become evident in this chapter, a formal assessment of psychopathy is an important component of a comprehensive psychological risk assessment.

For the purposes of the present chapter, the Hare Psychopathy Checklist–Revised (PCL–R; Hare, 1991, 2003) and its derivatives, including the Psychopathy Checklist: Screening Version (PCL: SV; Hart, Cox, & Hare, 1995) Psychopathy Checklist: Youth Version (PCL: YV; Forth, Kosson, & Hare, 2003), and even the 22-item predecessor, the original Psychopathy Checklist (PCL; Hare, 1980) will serve as the primary operationalization of the psychopathy construct (herein referred collectively as the PCL measures).

Our rationale for centering on the PCL measures in this chapter is twofold: (1) that the instrument is the most widely used measurement tool for assessing the syndrome, and (2) that there is a large body of literature on the association of the PCL measures with a range of criminal justice issues. In addition, we employ the language of the factor and facet structure the PCL–R as documented in Hare and Neumann (2008) in which the items can be arranged into two second order factors – Factor 1, that is, the interpersonal and affective features, and Factor 2, the chronic antisocial lifestyle features – or into four narrower first order factors. The latter are also commonly referred to as facets in which Factor 1 can be subdivided into the interpersonal (e.g., superficial, grandiose, deceitful, manipulative) and affective (e.g., lack of remorse, callous lack of empathy, shallow affect, failure to accept responsibility) facets while Factor 2 can be arranged into the lifestyle (e.g., impulsivity, lacks goals, irresponsibility, parasitic) and antisocial (e.g., early behavior problems, poor behavior controls, release failure, criminality versatility) facets. Conventionally, cut scores on the 40-point measure ranging from 25 to 30 have been employed to characterize the presence of psychopathy.

Of note, there are a collection of self-report measures used for the assessment of psychopathy, including the Psychopathic Personality Inventory–Revised (PPI–R; Lilienfeld & Widows, 2005), the Hare Self-Report Psychopathy Fourth Edition (SRP–IV; Paulhus, Neumann, & Hare, 2017), and the Levenson Self-Report Psychopathy (LSRP; Levenson, Kiehl,& Fitzpatrick, 1995), in addition to other multiscale self-report inventories of personality and psychopathology that include subscales that purport to tap features of psychopathy. There is less research on applications of self-report psychopathy measures in risk assessment, while global measures of personality and psychopathology tend not to be used to assess risk per se, although they are frequently employed in forensic evaluations (Otto, 2002). For these reasons, we do not discuss forensic risk assessment applications of these self-report tools.

The present chapter begins by reviewing the literature examining the associations between the PCL measures and a broad range of community and institutional recidivism outcomes. We proceed to review other important criminal justice correlates of psychopathy, followed by a review of risk mitigating agents for psychopathic offenders and clinical considerations in the use of the PCL measures in risk assessment. We conclude the chapter through a review of the structural and predictive properties of the PCL measures with special populations (youth, females, and racial–ethnic minorities) with implications for clinical applications of the measure with these groups.

PCL-measured psychopathy and the prediction of recidivism

Although the PCL was not developed to assess recidivism risk and is not a purpose-built risk assessment tool (Hare, 2003), the PCL measures have been researched extensively in their applications to assessing risk for crime and violence. At current count, we identified at least

13 meta-analyses that have examined the criterion-related validity of the PCL for recidivism, sometimes in tandem with other measures, for a range of recidivism outcomes. This review is organized around four meta-analytic themes, primarily with adult male samples: (1) risk for general crime and violence; (2) risk for institutional behavior problems; (3) risk for intimate partner violence (IPV); and (4) risk for sexual violence. Of note, most investigations focus on examining continuous PCL total, factor, and facet scores and their relation to recidivism, typically through an effect size such as point biserial *r*, Cohen's *d*, or area under the curve (AUC), all of which represent the extent to which test scores discriminate recidivists from non-recidivists. Rice and Harris (2005) offer useful interpretive guidelines in which a small/low effect corresponds to $r = .10$, AUC = .56, $d = .20$, a medium/moderate effect $r = .24$, AUC = .64, $d = .50$, and a large effect or high predictive accuracy as $r = .37$, AUC = .71, $d = .80$.

Risk for violent and general criminal recidivism

Single instrument examinations

Salekin, Rogers, and Sewell (1996) conducted the first meta-analysis of the PCL scales in the prediction of offender recidivism. The use of the PCL scales in risk assessment was a novel application at the time, and the ability of test scores on the tool to differentiate recidivists from non-recidivists was, as yet, unproven. At the time, ten studies examining the link between PCL/PCL–R scores and recidivism were available ($n = 4{,}620$), generating an aggregate effect size of $d = .55$ for general (i.e., any) criminal recidivism; that is, recidivists scored approximately one-half standard deviation higher on the PCL–R than non-recidivists. Salekin and colleagues also examined associations between the PCL/PCL–R and violent behavior (both recidivism and other operationalizations of violence) and found the tool to have strong associations with violent behavior ($d = .79$, $k = 13$). The authors also identified the beginning of what would become a trend in the literature in which Factor 2 (chronic antisocial lifestyle features) appeared to fare better in the prediction of recidivism and other antisocial criteria than Factor 1 (interpersonal and affective features).

Hemphill, Hare, and Wong (1998) followed on the heels of Salekin et al. (1996) in a meta-analysis of the PCL–R specifically and its links to recidivism, including formal comparisons of Factors 1 and 2. PCL–R total scores demonstrated good predictive accuracy for general ($r = .27$, $k = 7$, equivalent $d = .57$) and violent recidivism ($r = .27$, $k = 6$, equivalent $d = .57$), and in all but one study, Factor 2 had higher in magnitude associations with these recidivism criteria than Factor 1. Walters (2003) subsequently conducted a meta-analysis specifically examining associations between the PCL factors to institutional adjustment (discussed below) and recidivism and affirmed these findings, with Factor 1 and particularly Factor 2 each significantly predicting general ($r = .15$ and .32, respectively $k = 26$) and violent ($r = .18$ and .26, respectively $k = 27$) recidivism.

The largest meta-analysis of the predictive validity of the PCL measures for antisocial behavior, including indicators of recidivism, has been conducted by Leistico, Salekin, DeCoster, and Rogers (2008), who examined 95 non-overlapping PCL studies ($N = 15{,}826$) and their associations with antisocial behavior criteria. PCL total scores had broadly moderate and significant predictive accuracy for general criminal recidivism ($d = .50$, $k = 62$, $n = 11{,}140$), nonviolent offenses ($d = .59$, $k = 81$, $n = 10{,}152$), and violent offenses ($d = .47$, $k = 68$, $n = 12{,}359$). Although Factor 1 scores predicted each of these three outcomes (recidivism $d = .37$, nonviolent offenses $d = .37$, violent offenses $d = .40$), the magnitudes of Factor 2's prediction effects were considerably higher (recidivism $d = .64$, nonviolent offenses $d = .60$, violent offenses $d = .57$).

Multi-instrument comparisons

In a parallel meta-analytic prediction literature, how the PCL measures fare in comparison to other risk instruments has also been the focus of examination. The preceding review has demonstrated that the PCL measures have good predictive accuracy for violent and general recidivism, with a prediction advantage given to Factor 2. The level of predictive accuracy was also on par with formalized risk assessment measures, and as such comparative examinations between the PCL and these tools were conducted. Gendreau, Goggin, and Smith (2002) conducted the first such comparative examination of the PCL measures and the Level of Service Inventory–Revised (LSI–R; Andrews & Bonta, 1995) and its variants, a brand of general risk–need assessment checklists employed frequently in probation and correctional settings. At the time, this was the most comprehensive examination of the predictive accuracy of the PCL, predated only by Salekin et al. (1996) and Hemphill et al. (1998). Although the PCL measures significantly predicted general (r = .24, k = 30, N = 4,365) and violent (r = .23, k = 26, N = 4,823) recidivism, Gendreau et al. (2002) reported the LSI–R fared significantly better in the prediction of general recidivism (r = .39, k = 33, N = 7,367), but was generally equivalent in the prediction of violent recidivism (r = .28, k = 16, N = 3,297). Within study comparisons affirmed the findings, although the PCL–R had higher predictive accuracy than the LSI–R for violent recidivism (r = .30 and .24, respectively, k = 5, N = 955), while the reverse was observed for general recidivism (r = .26 and .40, respectively, k = 6, N = 558).

A follow-up meta-analysis by an extension of this working group (Campbell, French, & Gendreau, 2009), examining use of the PCL measures in the prediction of violent recidivism compared to other well established tools, found close correspondence among the different measures. Specifically, total scores on the PCL/PCL–R demonstrated good predictive accuracy for violent recidivism (r = .27, equivalent d = .57, k = 24, N = 4,757), consistent with previous research, and the level of accuracy was not substantively different than that of the four other tools (rs = .22 to .32).

One of the most recent, and perhaps most rigorous, meta-analyses of the predictive accuracy of the PCL–R in relation to other risk assessment measures was conducted by Yang, Wong, and Coid (2010). Aggregating effect sizes across 28 studies that each evaluated the predictive accuracy of two or more instruments in the prediction of violent recidivism, obtained over a ten-year catchment timeframe, the authors used multilevel modeling to control for a range of sample, setting, and methodological study variables. Across nine forensic instruments examined, Yang et al. (2010) found the instruments each demonstrated significant and comparable predictive accuracy for violent recidivism, including the PCL–R (d = .55, k = 16, N = 3,854) and PCL: SV (d = .65, k = 8, N = 2,506). However, while Factor 2 demonstrated significant and comparable predictive accuracy for future violence (d = .61, k = 13, N = 3,995) to the total score and the other instruments examined, Factor 1 did not (d = .22, k = 13, N = 3,895).

In all, the PCL measures demonstrate significant, and moderate to high, predictive accuracy for violent and general recidivism, and the level of predictive accuracy has been broadly comparable to that of other tools. As noted at the outset, however, the PCL was not developed to assess risk, and there are many features specific to risk tools essential to the appraisal and management of risk not captured by the PCL, such that it is essential to use one or more of these in the course of completing psychological risk assessments (discussed further in this chapter). A further trend has been the higher predictive accuracy of Factor 2 scores for violent and general recidivism compared to Factor 1, which by contrast has been a relatively weak and inconsistent predictor of recidivism. In recent years, studies have increasingly been examining the four facets and their associations with recidivism. Examinations at the facet level have demonstrated the antisocial facet of Factor 2 to be a consistent and particularly strong predictor of general and violent recidivism outcomes, often incrementally so beyond the other facets, followed by the lifestyle facet (e.g., Olver, Neumann, Wong, & Hare, 2013). The interpersonal and affective facets of Factor 1 have been less consistent predictors of recidivism, although a small body of literature has marshaled some support for the affective facet's association with violence (see Hare, 2016 for a review).

Risk for institutional misconduct

An almost equally impressive literature has accumulated examining the associations between psychopathy and conduct problems within institutional settings, such as psychiatric hospitals, jails, prisons, halfway houses, or other residential facilities. If the features of psychopathy are conducive to committing new crimes in the community and returning to custody, they are also conducive to rule violations within institutional settings. Even within a secure or custodial environment, the antisocial proclivities of high psychopathy men tend not to cease. Walters (2003) conducted the first meta-analysis of PCL-measured psychopathy and institutional conduct problems, and across 50 studies, found that both Factor 1 (r = .18) and particularly Factor 2 (r = .28) were predictors of institutional misconduct overall, and among male (r = .18 and .29, respectively, k = 18), female (r = .20 and .30, respectively, k = 18), adult (r = .17 and .29, respectively, k = 18), and juvenile (r = .25 and .33, respectively, k = 18) subgroups. The two factors each predicted violent and nonviolent institutional infractions.

Guy, Edens, Anthony, and Douglas (2005) extended the work of Walters (2003), and limited their examination to the PCL–R specifically (as Walters, 2003, had examined all variants of the PCL) in a meta-analysis of links to institutional misconduct among adults. PCL–R total (r = .29, k = 38), Factor 1 (r = .21, k = 25), and Factor 2 (r = .27, k = 25) scores each significantly predicted total/any institutional misconducts, as well as institutional misconduct by category, including non-aggressive (rs = .16 to .21), generally aggressive (rs = .15 to .23), verbal/destructive (rs = .20 to .26), and physical violence (rs = .14 to .17). Broadly, PCL–R total scores tended to yield the largest effect sizes, with Factor 2 evidencing slightly stronger associations with institutional misconduct than Factor 1. The Leistico et al. (2008) meta-analysis previously referenced also examined relations between the PCL measures and institutional misconduct in general and replicated Guy et al. (2005), with the PCL total (d = .53, k = 45), Factor 1 (d = .41, k = 30), and Factor 2 (d = .51, k = 29) scores predicting this outcome.

In conclusion, robust meta-analytic support exists for the association of high PCL scores with institutional misconduct in general, and both nonviolent and violent/aggressive (verbal and physical) infractions, in particular. Although some evidence exists for slightly stronger prediction by Factor 2, there seems to be less disparity between it and Factor 1 in linkages with institutional behavior problems, compared to the prediction of violent and general recidivism in the community. As such, it would seem that high scores on any and all components of the PCL can bode for potential difficulties in institutional adjustment.

Risk for intimate partner violence

Given its robust associations with recidivism across violent and general offender populations, increasing attention has turned toward examining the PCL–R and its association with intimate partner violence (IPV). Relatively few studies have examined this, although the first to do so was a small Swedish investigation (Grann & Wedin, 2002) in a sample of 88 court-referred men, ordered to undergo forensic psychiatric evaluations for domestic violence. In this sample,

PCL–R Total (AUC = .71), Factor 1 (AUC = .70), and Factor 2 scores (AUC = .71) all demonstrated strong predictive accuracy for future IPV within one of year of the evaluation. In a larger Canadian sample of 649 men who had a police record for spousal assault, Hilton, Harris, Rice, Houghton, and Eke (2008) examined the associations between the PCL–R and several concordant general and IPV risk measures with spousal assault recidivism. PCL–R total scores demonstrated moderate predictive accuracy for IPV recidivism (AUC = .66) and evidenced comparable or better predictive accuracy of this outcome than the Violence Risk Appraisal Guide or other IPV measures. PCL–R total scores were also significantly associated with victim injury in recidivism (*r* = .37), number of severe abuse incidents (*r* = .29), and severity of all recidivism (*r* = .26) in this sample of IPV men. In a subsample of men, the PCL–R was added as a weighted item to an actuarial IPV risk scale, the Ontario Domestic Assault Risk Assessment (ODARA), to generate the Domestic Violence Risk Appraisal Guide (DVRAG; essentially an IPV-variant of the VRAG alluded to above) which also predicted IPV recidivism (AUC = .70). In all, the PCL–R has shown strong predictive accuracy for future domestic violence inflicted against an intimate partner in the small number of studies that have examined this association, and further research is warranted to replicate and extend these findings.

Risk for future sexual violence

The PCL measures have also featured prominently in sexual violence risk assessment, and as mentioned previously, this area will be reviewed briefly given its detailed coverage in another chapter. The PCL–R often has special prominence in preventative detention evaluations of sexual violence risk, such as the sexually violent predator (or persons) statutes that exist across 22 U.S. states, although it is frequently used in many other risk assessment contexts with sexual offenders as noted at the outset of this chapter. The available meta-analytic literature has demonstrated the PCL–R specifically to be a significant but more modest predictor of future sexual offenses, compared to its prediction of general and violent recidivism. The Walters (2003) meta-analysis found that neither PCL Factors 1 (*r* = .05) nor 2 (*r* = .08) predicted sexual recidivism across *k* = 5 studies that examined this. However, in a more extensive meta-analysis of the sex offense recidivism literature, Hanson and Morton-Bourgon (2005) found PCL–R total scores to significantly predict sexual recidivism (*d* = .29, equivalent base rate adjusted *r* = .10) across *k* = 13 investigations (*N* = 2,783). In the most extensive meta-analysis of the PCL–R and sex offender recidivism to date, Hawes, Boccaccini, and Murrie (2013) found PCL–R total scores significantly predicted sexual recidivism (*d* = .40) across *k* = 20 investigations (*N* = 5,239), as did Factor 2 (*d* = .44, *k* = 13) but not Factor 1 (*d* = .17, *k* = 13).

The Hawes et al. (2013) meta-analysis also carefully scrutinized the link of psychopathy combined with sexual deviance, to future sexual violence. In his writings, Hare (1999) referred to the comorbid presence of high levels of psychopathy and sexual deviance (i.e., a pattern of illegal or atypical sexual interests, such as sex with children or involving violence/coercion, and maladjusted sexual functioning) as the so-called deadly combination, arguing that the two in tandem serve to escalate risk for future sexual violence. Across *k* = 7 investigations, Hawes et al. (2013) found that a combination of PCL–R measured psychopathy and sexual deviance increased the odds of future sexual violence by two to threefold (i.e., odds ratio = 2.80–3.21). In sum, research has demonstrated the PCL to be a modest but significant overall predictor of sexual recidivism, with Factor 2 demonstrating stronger predictor of this outcome than Factor 1 consistent with the violence and general recidivism prediction literature. There is some evidence from meta-analysis, that psychopathy and sexual deviance are incremental in the prediction of sexual recidivism and that high levels of the two in combination can potentiate risk.

Other criminal justice correlates of PCL-measured psychopathy

There are a host of other important criminal justice correlates that have relevance to the psychopathy construct in risk assessment contexts. Psychopathic offenders demonstrate a greater frequency, density, and variety of criminal offenses, and hence marked criminal versatility. Although some may specialize in particular forms of crime (e.g., weapons trafficking, drug dealing, and extortion), for the most part, the criminal rap sheets of high PCL–R scoring individuals tend to include a large miscellany of offenses that could run the gamut from petty theft, to assault, to weapons offenses, release violations, to more serious forms of theft and acts of criminal violence (e.g., robbery, sexual offenses, homicide) (Hare, 1996). Particularly prominent links exist with instrumental violence and release failure.

Instrumental violence

In one of the first sets of studies examining the psychopathy–violence link, Hare and McPherson (1984) conducted a pair of studies on samples of adult male offenders (*N*s = 193 and 243) from Canadian provincial and federal corrections facilities, examining the link between PCL scores and various categories of crime. High PCL-scoring men had criminal histories with a greater density of a range of crimes including property offenses, weapons offenses, fraud, assault, robbery and armed robbery, drug offenses, driving offenses, fighting, kidnapping, and even vandalism; however, psychopathic individuals did not have a greater frequency of crimes for rape or murder. While sexual and homicide offenses can involve complex and intense emotional dynamics, a common thread among the remaining offense categories was that psychopathic offenders had a particularly high frequency of offenses involving instrumental (i.e., goal-directed) violence, which may be emotionless and dispassionate in contrast with offenses committed by individuals with externalizing or disinhibiting traits. Subsequent lines of research have documented associations between psychopathy and the density and variety of violent crimes in general, and acts of instrumental violence in particular. For instance, in a Canadian sample of 125 offenders, Woodworth and Porter (2002) found that when psychopathic offenders did commit acts of homicide, that nearly all of these (93.3 percent) were instrumental in nature, that is, cold-blooded, dispassionate, and predatory, in contrast to less than half (48.4 percent) being instrumental in nature for non-psychopathic offenders. Non-psychopathic men, in turn, were much more likely to commit acts of reactive (i.e., emotionally charged) homicide, such as that seen in crimes of passion. Subsequent work has affirmed links between high levels of psychopathy and displays of instrumental violence and aggression (Cornell et al., 1996; Porter & Woodworth, 2006; Serin, 1991; Walsh, Swogger, & Kosson, 2009).

Release failure

Some of the earliest work examining the criterion-related validity of PCL scores investigated the association with performance on conditional release (e.g., parole), which has important implications for risk assessment. The available research has demonstrated that psychopathic offenders are also more likely to perform poorly on conditional release. Wong (1984) conducted one of the first examinations of profiles of PCL-measured psychopathy and its correlates in Canadian corrections, including associations with conditional release. In a sample of 315 federal offenders, Wong (1984) found that psychopathic men were interestingly more likely to apply for parole, as well as much more likely to violate it when granted ($r = .30$ between PCL score and each outcome). A few years later, Hart, Kropp, and Hare (1988) examined the association between

PCL scores and performance on conditional release (either paroled or mandatorily released after two-thirds of the sentence) in a sample of 231 Canadian federal offenders. Approximately two-thirds (62 percent) of high psychopathy men violated their conditional release within one year of release, in contrast to approximately half (47 percent) of men with moderate levels of psychopathy, and only 20 percent of those with low levels of psychopathy. The PCL was also a strong and significant predictor of release failure (r = .33). Subsequent lines of research have further documented that men with high PCL scores to have higher and faster rates of failure on conditional release (Porter, Birt, & Boer, 2001; Porter, Brinke, & Wilson, 2009; Serin, Peters, & Barbaree, 1990).

Risk mitigating agents of psychopathy

The research reviewed and discussed to this point has focused on PCL-measured psychopathy as a forensic clinical construct with myriad well-established links to crime and violence. However high risk high psychopathy men may be, research has demonstrated that not all such individuals inexorably reoffend (i.e., recidivism rates are very seldom, if ever, 100 percent). As such, there are likely risk-mitigating agents at work that could also have important implications for risk assessments with psychopathic offenders. For instance, Burt, Olver and Wong (2016) found that psychopathic offenders who did not violently reoffend (dubbed the "non-recidivating" psychopathic offender) were older and more likely to have completed risk reduction treatment, maintain a relationship, and to obtain a job on release. With these considerations in mind, the present section discusses two possible risk-mitigating agents: aging and correctional treatment.

Psychopathy and aging: the impact on criminal careers

Research has demonstrated that psychopathic offenders commence antisocial behavior at an earlier age, tend to evidence a greater density and variety of criminal offenses, and have lengthier and more diverse criminal careers; indeed, a recent study even found PCL–R scores to be positively correlated with the length of criminal career in a Canadian sample of federal offenders (Olver & Wong, 2015). An important and intriguing question that remains, however, is the extent to which high PCL scoring men may "burn out" with age. It is axiomatic in the criminological literature that age is inversely associated with the density of offending and returns to custody across offender groups, with precipitous drops emerging at mid-life (Hanson, 2002; Nicholaichuk, Olver, Gu, & Wong, 2014; Sampson & Laub, 2003). As a reflection of the inverse age–crime link, most purpose-built risk instruments include a differentially weighted age item assigning increasing scores (representing higher risk) to younger offenders and lower, sometimes even negatively weighted scores to older offenders (representing declines in risk) (e.g., Helmus, Thornton, Hanson, & Babchishin, 2012). The aforementioned studies have similarly demonstrated that even persistent, high risk offenders eventually desist; age seems to be the final arbiter, but is this even the case for psychopathic offenders?

There is little reason to believe that psychopathic offenders do not eventually decline in their offending patterns as they age, and this is a relevant consideration for risk assessment. In a classic cross-sectional study of 889 adult male offenders rated on the PCL–R, Harpur and Hare (1994) found that Factor 2 scores dropped steadily across older age cohorts, while Factor 1 scores remained remarkably consistent across younger and older offender groups alike, a finding that has since been replicated across multiple offender samples and settings (Olver & Wong, 2015; Putkonen et al., 2010; Storey, Hart, Cooke, & Michie, 2016; Ullrich, Paelecke, Kahle, & Marneros, 2003).

A small body of literature also exists examining the linkages of psychopathy, age, and criminal outcomes. In a Canadian sample of adult male offenders, Hare, McPherson, and Forth (1988) used cross-sectional (*N* = 521) and longitudinal (*N* = 81) methodology to examine trajectories of criminal conviction and incarceration among psychopathic and non-psychopathic men in five-year age periods between the ages of 16 and 45. Although high psychopathy men had demonstrably higher rates of violent and nonviolent crime, as well as time spent in prison, compared to non-psychopathic men up to age 40, after age 40, the rates of all criminal activity and time spent in prison dropped dramatically for the psychopathic men; in fact, for the 41–45 year-age band of men, rates of incarceration and criminal conviction were no different between the high psychopathy and low psychopathy groups! Subsequent work has generally upheld these findings (Olver & Wong, 2015; Porter et al., 2001) with few exceptions (Harris, Rice, & Cormier, 1991). Most recently, in a 24-year follow-up study on Wong's (1984) original sample of 315 Canadian federal offenders rated on the PCL–R, Olver and Wong (2015) found age at release and PCL–R total to be incrementally predictive of violent, nonviolent, and general recidivism; that is, while psychopathy continued to predict increased recidivism, age at release uniquely predicted decreased recidivism irrespective of psychopathy; age at release also predicted decreases in all recidivism outcomes across high PCL–R and low PCL–R groups. Follow-up analyses demonstrated that men who were age 35 and above at release who had high PCL–R scores still had lower rates of recidivism over time than younger men (under age 35) with comparably high PCL–R scores; however, older high psychopathy men still had higher rates of recidivism than older men with low PCL–R scores. In all, increasing age seemed to mitigate risk across the sample, although the age effect seemed to be muted somewhat for the high psychopathy men.

Psychopathy and treatment

A detailed review of the psychopathy-treatment literature is beyond the scope of this chapter, but how individuals scoring high on psychopathy fare in correctional treatment can have important ramifications for risk assessment. Research has demonstrated that correctional programs that subscribe to the principles of risk (match offender risk level to treatment intensity), need (target dynamic risk factors, a.k.a. criminogenic needs, linked to criminal behavior in treatment), and responsivity (tailor treatment interventions to unique client characteristics to maximize gain and reduce attrition) are associated with non-trivial reductions (upwards of 25 percent) in recidivism (Andrews & Bonta, 2010). As such, completion of evidence-informed programs subscribing to the principles of Risk–Needs–Responsivity (RNR) should in principle bode well for decreased risk; but does this apply to psychopathic offenders?

Salekin (2002) conducted the first meta-analytic review of psychopathy treatment in a review of 42 studies. Although the studies were plagued by a bewildering array of definitions of psychopathy, criteria for treatment success, treatment approaches employed, and methodological design, 62 percent of studies reported achieving some beneficial therapeutic effect with psychopathic offenders. A follow-up review by Salekin, Worley, and Grimes (2010) sharpened the focus to more recent and methodologically stronger studies (*k* = 9). The common thread was that these investigations used a PCL-based operationalization of psychopathy, focused on criminal recidivism (e.g., violent, sexual, general) as an outcome criterion by which to evaluate success, employed a group-based design, and most (but not all) featured evidence-informed treatment programs. The review gave room for a cautious optimism, but in all concluded that psychopathic offenders were a high risk, challenging clientele to treat, and although there could be some benefit the response to treatment was often poor.

Wong (2015) (see also Wong, Gordon, Lewis, Gu, & Olver, 2012; Wong & Hare, 2005) has proposed a two-component model for the treatment of psychopathic offenders integrating the RNR principles of effective correctional treatment with the features of PCL-measured psychopathy and the treatment of personality disorder. Component 1, dubbed the interpersonal component, treats Factor 1 as a responsivity issue; that is, as a set of client characteristics (e.g., argumentativeness, lack of remorse, staff splitting, manipulation, etc.) that must be carefully managed and contained by service providers to retain difficult clients in treatment so that they have the chance to benefit. Component 2, dubbed the criminogenic component, treats Factor 2 as a risk and need issue, in which client risk level and core criminogenic needs are targeted through high intensity interventions to reduce the potential for violence and other antisocial behaviors. A growing body of research has demonstrated positive risk-relevant treatment gains from the completion of evidence based programs, not dissimilar to the two-component model articulated earlier, to be associated with small but often significant decreases in sexual recidivism (Langton, Barbaree, Harkins, & Peacock, 2006; Olver & Wong, 2009), violent recidivism (Looman, Abracen, Serin, & Marquis, 2005; Olver, Lewis, & Wong, 2013; Skeem, Monahan, & Mulvey, 2002), and severity of recidivism (Wong et al., 2012).

Conclusions on aging and treatment as possible risk mitigating agents

Older offenders are less likely to reoffend and to commit new acts of criminal violence; naturally, the same recidivism potential cannot be expected for a 25-year-old man vs another 25-year-old man with the same high PCL score (e.g., 32) but has aged and is now 50 years old. The next challenge for risk assessors is how to systematically integrate age and psychopathy information into risk appraisals. For instance, how much could the anticipated likelihood of a new violent offense occurring over the next five years be expected to decrease for two men with PCL–R scores over 30, one in his 20s and the other in his 50s? Moreover, although psychopathic clientele are typically challenging to engage therapeutically in a productive and meaningful way, there is little reason to believe that they might not also demonstrate similar treatment gains as other high-risk offenders in terms of risk reduction from high intensity, criminogenic skills-based interventions, within a responsive program and setting. As such, treatment gains, even among men with high PCL–R scores, can have relevance in terms of reducing risk to manageable levels for security reductions, temporary absences, or supervised release into the community. Naturally, appropriate precautions need to be taken to corroborate positive gains and to implement appropriate follow-up risk management interventions to prevent recidivism.

Psychopathy and risk assessment with special populations

Up to this point, much of the research and issues concerning the use of the PCL scales in risk assessment has focused on adult, male, and often Caucasian offender populations; however, the construct of psychopathy is likely to have similar relevance in risk assessment when applied to other offender and racial groups. As such, in this section, we provide an overview of the psychometric research and risk assessment applications of the PCL measures with special populations: racial–ethnic minorities, female offenders, and young offenders. The assessment of psychopathy using PCL measures together with risk assessment in special offender groups have generated some controversy. However, there are well developed literatures on each of these areas, as discussed below.

Racial–ethnic minorities

Racial–ethnic minorities, youth and adult, are overrepresented in the criminal justice system internationally, including Canada (Public Safety Canada, 2014), the U.S. (Travis, Western, & Redburn, 2014), the United Kingdom (Ministry of Justice, 2013), New Zealand (Anaya, 2015), and Australia (Krieg, 2006), among other international jurisdictions. Many racial–ethnic minorities in developed western countries have a history of colonialization or social and economic marginalization, and in some cases, an erosion of traditional culture and language. Much of the research published in the English language on racial–ethnic differences on the PCL measures and their psychometric properties have featured the Indigenous peoples of Canada and African American population within the U.S. Three primary issues are considered here: (1) to what extent do racial–ethnic minorities have different PCL scores than non-minorities; (2) how well do the PCL measures predict recidivism in racial–ethnic minorities compared to non-minorities; and (3) a comparison of the psychometric properties of the PCL measures (e.g., latent structure of psychopathic traits) across different ancestral groups.

A meta-analysis by McCoy and Edens (2006) examined PCL scores of Black vs. White youth across 16 independent studies. In all, a small difference at $d = .20$, amounting to about a 1.5-point difference in total scores, was found with Black youth scoring higher. In Canadian youth and adult samples, Indigenous persons frequently score approximately one-third to a half standard deviation higher on the PCL–R and PCL: YV, particularly the total score, lifestyle, and antisocial facet scores (Olver et al., 2017; Olver, Neumann, Wong, & Hare, 2013; Schmidt, McKinnon, Chattha, & Brownlee, 2006; Stockdale, Olver, & Wong, 2010).

Research has found that PCL–R and PCL: YV total and facet scores have comparable predictive accuracy for general, violent, and nonviolent recidivism outcomes among Canadian Indigenous and non-Indigenous youth (McCuish, Mathesius, Lussier, & Corrado, 2017; Schmidt et al., 2006; Stockdale et al., 2010) and adult (Olver et al., 2013, 2017) offender samples, with AUC magnitudes broadly being in the mid .60s to low .70s. Importantly, calibration research has demonstrated, however, that Indigenous youth and adult offenders tend to have higher rates of recidivism than non-Indigenous offenders, and that the same PCL score can yield different recidivism estimates as a result. Olver et al. (2017), for instance, found that Indigenous group membership uniquely predicted observed differences in base rates of violent and general recidivism after controlling for PCL–R score, indicating that unmeasured factors associated with Indigenous group ancestry (e.g., culture, unmeasured risk factors, social–systemic) contributed to higher observed recidivism base rates.

Finally, research has supported the structural invariance of the PCL measures with racial–ethnic minorities compared to White non-minorities – that is, the latent structure of psychopathic traits as measured by the PCL – including three-factor (13-item; i.e., minus the antisocial factor) and four-factor (18-item; i.e., including the antisocial factor) models with African American persons (Cooke, Kosson, & Michie, 2001; Jackson, Neumann, & Vitacco, 2007) and a four-factor model with Indigenous Canadian peoples (Olver et al., 2013, 2017).

Female offenders

The use of the PCL measures with female offenders has also fostered discussion and debate. In forensic clinical assessment, scholars recognize that female offenders, both adult and youth, have risk and need considerations common to other offender populations (e.g., criminal attitudes, antisocial peers), but that they also possess unique, gender-informed needs that impact risk and have implications for service delivery such as child custody issues, pregnancy, financial concerns, stress, trauma and abuse, and housing safety (e.g., see Van Voorhis, Wright, Salisbury, & Bauman, 2010). Some standard risk–need variables, for example substance abuse, could have special salience for female offenders.

With these considerations in mind, the psychometric properties of the PCL measures established with male offenders cannot be taken for granted with female offenders. The limited research to date has yielded broadly supportive findings on the predictive efficacy of the PCL measures with female youth and women offenders, with some exceptions. With women offenders, studies have found broadly moderate predictive accuracy (AUCs mid .60s) for the PCL–R or PCL: SV for recidivism (Eisenbarth, Osterheider, Nedopil, & Stadtland, 2012; Nicholls, Ogloff, & Douglas, 2004; Salekin, Rogers, Ustad, & Sewell, 1998). The female youth literature seems to have more mixed findings, with broadly moderate and significant predictive accuracy of the PCL: YV for recidivism in some North American samples (Stockdale et al., 2010) but not others (see Edens, Campbell, & Weir, 2007). A problem with the research, however, is that many of the female offender psychopathy recidivism studies have small sample sizes and are often underpowered to provide more rigorous tests of predictive accuracy and to generate more stable conclusions.

Confirmatory factor analytic research of the PCL measures with youth and adult female offender samples have shown factor structure and organization of latent psychopathic traits similar to male offenders. Jones, Cauffman, Miller, and Mulvey (2006) found "moderate-to-good fit" (p. 43) both for a three-factor (13-item) model and four-factor (18-item) model of the PCL: YV that was also invariant across ethnicity and gender. In a German sample, Sevecke, Pukrop, Kosson, and Krischer (2009) reported that a three-factor model (interpersonal, affective, lifestyle) provided the most tenable fit for female youth offenders. Among adult women, both three- (Jackson, Rogers, Neumann, & Lambert, 2002) and four-factor solutions (Hare & Neumann, 2008) have been identified as providing good fit.

Youthful offenders

Controversies also exist regarding the use of the PCL: YV and applications of the psychopathy construct with youth populations, including concerns around labeling, developmental changes during adolescence, and the potential to pathologize normal characteristics of adolescence (e.g., egocentrism, impulsivity) among other concerns (Edens & Vincent, 2008). The previous discussions and review of the literature on the structural and predictive properties of the PCL measures with female and racial–ethnic minorities, have also frequently involved youth samples.

The meta-analytic literature to date has provided strong support for the predictive accuracy of the PCL: YV for violent, nonviolent, and general recidivism outcomes. In the first meta-analysis of the PCL: YV measures (Edens et al., 2007), the tool evidenced moderate and significant predictive accuracy for general (r = .24, k = 20) and violent (r = .25, k = 14) recidivism, and weak prediction of sexual recidivism (r = .07, k = 4). In an updated meta-analysis of the PCL: YV and two youth forensic risk assessment measures, the Structured Assessment of Violence Risk in Youth (SAVRY) and youth variants of the LSI, Olver, Stockdale, and Wormith (2009) found the PCL: YV continued to demonstrate good predictive accuracy for general (r = .28, k = 20) and violent (r = .25, k = 20) recidivism, but still weak prediction of sexual recidivism (r = .07, k = 4). As the Olver et al. (2009) meta-analysis conducted a comparative examination of other youth risk measures, additional conclusions about the risk relevance of the PCL: YV could be made. First, the magnitude of prediction of the PCL: YV was broadly on par with that of its adult variants; although the construct of juvenile psychopathy remains contentious for stated reasons, there is less debate about whether the tool works to predict future antisocial behavior. Second, the magnitude of predictive accuracy of the PCL: YV for violent and general recidivism was also consistent with other purpose-built youth risk measures (SAVRY and LSI youth version), as seen in meta-analyses of the adult literature (cf. Yang et al., 2010). Finally, the weaker predictive accuracy for future sexual offending compared to other higher base rate outcomes was also consistent with findings from the adult literature, although the exceptionally low base rates of juvenile sexual recidivism could well have attenuated prediction magnitudes further.

The latent structure of psychopathic traits in juvenile offenders, as measured by the PCL: YV, is also consistent with adult PCL measures, showing support for both three-factor 13-item or four-factor 18-item models in heterogeneous youth offender samples in North America (Jones et al., 2006; Neumann, Forth, Kosson, & Hare, 2006) and beyond (Sevecke et al., 2009).

The psychometric research regarding the structural and predictive properties of the PCL measures supports their careful application with racial–ethnic minorities, females, and youth for use in risk assessment contexts. The extant work reviewed supports the predictive properties of the tools with these groups, as well as other important properties, including interrater reliability, factor structure, and indices of construct validity. The use of the PCL measures with these special populations warrants additional sensitivity to and professional appreciation of the special characteristics of these populations, including attention to unique cultural, gender, and/or developmental considerations that could impact risk assessment and management.

Clinical applications

The aforementioned reviews of applied research findings have important implications for clinical use of the PCL measures in psychological risk assessment. In this final section, risk assessment applications of PCL-measured psychopathy will be discussed through the lens of the RNR model applied to offender populations broadly speaking, integrating issues and findings covered throughout this chapter. An important feature of risk assessments which can aid decision-making and recidivism prevention efforts is that they draw on multiple sources of information, use multiple assessment methods, and evaluate multiple domains of functioning (Boer, Hart, Kropp, & Webster, 1997).

As noted at the outset of this chapter, the PCL–R was not designed with the intention of assessing risk for recidivism, but nevertheless has strong associations with several criminal outcomes within the institution and community. As such, in terms of pure appraisal of risk, high PCL–R scoring men tend to also be a high risk for most recidivism outcomes – general, violent, release failure, institutional adjustment problems, intimate partner violence – with the exception being risk for sexual recidivism. In our view, however, it is important to pair the PCL–R with at least one or more risk measures that can assess dynamic risk factors for crime and violence (e.g., LSI–R) to inform global appraisals of risk. From the perspective of the risk principle, the PCL–R total score, in contrast with the factor and facet scores, has the greatest stability in terms of recidivism prediction, although scrutiny of the factors and facets can have important risk and need implications for risk assessment (discussed below). Some tools have incorporated the PCL–R in part or in whole within their risk assessment scheme, such as the VRAG or the Violence Risk Appraisal Guide–Revised (Rice, Harris, & Lang, 2013), and these can be helpful adjuncts to include as well. Reporting the percentile tank of the PCL–R total score and contextualizing this information can be helpful for risk communication purposes, as both high and low scores are meaningful. For instance, an individual scoring at the 90th percentile on the PCL–R total score, taken in conjunction with other sources of information (e.g., assessment of dynamic risk factors), may well be at high risk for future crime and violence, but is also in need of high intensity services to reduce and manage risk.

High PCL–R scoring men, especially those who also score high on concordant risk measures, are thus good candidates for high intensity risk reduction programs. Research has demonstrated that men who score high on the PCL–R have a greater density and number of criminogenic needs that can be targeted for programming (Douglas, Yeomans, & Boer, 2005; Simourd & Hoge, 2000; Wong & Gordon 2006). From the perspective of the need principle, this underscores the necessity of using a dynamic tool, not only to identify areas to prioritize for services (e.g., criminal attitudes, substance abuse, interpersonal violence, relationship instability, Anger dyscontrol), but also to evaluate changes in risk from treatment or other change agents (e.g., vocational retraining, educational upgrading). Thus, it is important to include risk mitigating information as applicable into risk appraisals. Several tools such as the LSI–R measures, the Historical Clinical Risk–20 (Douglas, Hart, Webster, & Belfrage, 2011), and the Violence Risk Scale (Wong & Gordon, 1999–2003) have some research support to show that risk scores can change, and that changes in risk are associated with reductions in recidivism.

Finally, per the responsivity principle, the profile of PCL–R scores can have useful information. Research has demonstrated high scores on the affective facet, for instance, to be associated with increased risk for treatment non-completion (Olver & Wong, 2011), decreased therapeutic gains (Olver et al., 2013), and weaker therapeutic working alliances, particularly the emotional bond between client and therapist (DeSorcy, Olver, & Wormith, 2017). While high affective facet scores should not be taken as proof positive that problems in institutional adjustment and response to programming will occur, prominent Factor 1 characteristics can signal the need for service providers to intensify efforts to anticipate and manage treatment interfering behaviors.

Conclusion

We chose to operationally define psychopathy with the PCL–R as the extensive research on the tool has generated a wealth of knowledge that is highly informative to psychopathy theorists, researchers, and correctional and forensic mental health practitioners. The association between psychopathy and risk assessment is by no means fortuitous, even before the PCL–R was developed and shown to associate robustly with offending behaviors. Most psychopaths come into contact with health and criminal justice agencies because of their antisocial behaviors. Even if one takes the position that antisocial features and criminality should not be considered as an integral part of the construct of psychopathy, as some have thoughtfully agued, a forensic practitioner, from a pragmatic standpoint, will still have to assess the antisocial features of the psychopathic individual as a part of his/her forensic evaluation. Thus, inevitably, Factor 2 characteristics, as a part of the PCL–R or as a standalone construct, will be the target of a forensic assessment in addition to Factor 1, the core personality features.

Over three decades of research with the PCL–R, including the results of many meta-analyses, have shown highly consistent links between PCL–R scores and offending behaviors across gender, age, ethnic groups, offender types, settings, countries, and outcomes; few risk assessment tools have undergone as rigorous a scrutiny as the PCL–R. Just as consistent is the relatively stronger link for Factor 2 than Factor 1 with offending behaviors. That antisocial attitudes and orientation reflected as past offending behaviors (essentially Factor 2 features) outperform stable personality features (essentially Factor 1 features) in predicting recidivism received another vote of confidence, but with an important caveat, that is, provided that risk has not changed. Risk change resulting from natural aging or with risk reduction treatment will impact on the assessed risk and the future likelihood to reoffend, including individuals with psychopathy.

The long-held pessimism in treating individuals with psychopathy to reduce reoffending has gradually given way to some guarded optimism based on recent positive research findings. Contemporary cognitive behavioral and skill-based treatment approaches have now found wide acceptance in the forensic community and are codified as the RNR principles. Credit is also due to the development of third and fourth generation risk assessment tools, evolving from static to dynamic risk assessment tools; the latter hold, at their core, the notion that risk can and does change with changing circumstances such as treatment. In parallel with these developments, risk prevention rather than risk prediction is starting to take center stage not only within the forensic community but globally. The World Health Organization recognizes violence as a public health issue and, in their *Global Status Report on Violence Prevention 2014* (WHO, 2014), has taken the lead to survey many countries globally to identify, at a macro level, risk factors that can be used in for violence prevention.

Within the forensic community, we now have the risk assessment tools, treatment models, and an extensive body of knowledge that can be used to treat a wide range of clientele even those who are deemed highly challenging and recalcitrant such as individuals with psychopathy.

So, what are we waiting for!?

References

Andrews, D. A., and Bonta, J. (1995) *Level of Supervision–Revised (LSI–R): An offender assessment system. User's guide*, Toronto, ON: Multi-Health Systems.

Andrews, D. A., and Bonta, J. (2010) 'Rehabilitating criminal justice policy and practice,' *Psychology, Public Policy, and Law*, *16*:39–55.

Anaya, S. J. (2015) 'Report of the special rapporteur on the rights of indigenous peoples in the situation of Maori peoples in New Zealand,' *Arizona Journal of International and Comparative Law*, *32*:1–26.

Boer, D. P., Hart, S. D., Kropp, P. R., and Webster, C. D. (1997) *Manual for the Sexual Violence Risk–20: Professional guidelines for assessing risk of sexual violence*, Vancouver, BC: Institute against Family Violence and the Mental Health, Law, and Policy Institute, Simon Fraser University.

Burt, G. N., Olver, M. E., and Wong, S. C. P. (2016) 'Investigating characteristics of the non-recidivating psychopathic offender,' *Criminal Justice and Behavior*, *43*:1741–1760.

Campbell, M. A., French, S., and Gendreau, P. (2009) 'The prediction of violence in adult offenders: A meta-analytic comparison of instruments and methods of assessment,' *Criminal Justice and Behavior*, *36*:567–590.

Cooke, D. J., Kosson, D. S., and Michie, C. (2001) 'Psychopathy and ethnicity: Structural, item, and test generalizability of the Psychopathy Checklist–Revised (PCL–R) in Caucasian and African American participants,' *Psychological Assessment*, *13*:531–542.

Cornell, D. G., Warren, J., Hawk, G., Stafford, E., Oram, G., and Pine, D. (1996) 'Psychopathy in instrumental and reactive violence offenders,' *Journal of Consulting and Clinical Psychology*, *64*:783–790.

DeSorcy, D. R., Olver, M. E., and Wormith, J. S. (2017) 'Working alliance and psychopathy: Linkages to treatment outcome in a sample of treated sexual offenders,' *Journal of Interpersonal Violence*, doi:10.1177/0886260517698822

Douglas, K. S, Hart, S. D., Webster, C. D., and Belfrage, H. (2011) *Historical Clinical Risk Management (Version 3): Professional guidelines for evaluating risk of violence [Draft 2.1]*, Vancouver, BC: Mental Health, Law, and Policy Institute, Simon Fraser University.

Douglas, K. S., and Kropp, P. R. (2002) 'A prevention-based paradigm for violence risk assessment: Clinical and research applications,' *Criminal Justice and Behavior*, *29*:617–658.

Douglas, K., Yeomans, M., and Boer, D. (2005) 'Comparative validity analysis of multiple measures of violence risk in a sample of criminal offenders,' *Criminal Justice and Behavior*, *32*:479–510.

Edens, J. F., Campbell, J. S., and Weir, J. M. (2007) 'Youth psychopathy and criminal recidivism: A meta-analysis of the Psychopathy Checklist measures,' *Law and Human Behavior*, *31*:53–75.

Edens, J. F., and Vincent, G. M. (2008) 'Juvenile psychopathy: A clinical construct in need of restraint?,' *Journal of Forensic Psychology Practice*, *8*:186–197.

Eisenbarth, H., Osterheider, M., Nedopil, N., and Stadtland, C. (2012) 'Recidivism in female offenders: PCL–R lifestyle factor and VRAG show predictive validity in a German sample,' *Behavioral Sciences and the Law*, *30*:575–584.

Forth, A. E., Kosson, D. S., and Hare, R. D. (2003) *Psychopathy Checklist: Youth Version (PCL:YV)*, Toronto, ON: Multi-Health Systems.

Gendreau, P., Goggin, C., and Smith, P. (2002) 'Is the PCL–R really the "unparalleled" measure of offender risk? A lesson in knowledge cumulation,' *Criminal Justice and Behavior*, *29*:397–426.

Grann, M., and Wedin, M. (2002) 'Risk factors for recidivism among spousal assault and spousal homicide offenders,' *Psychology, Crime & Law*, *8*:5–23.

Guy, L. S., Edens, J. F., Anthony, C., and Douglas, K. S. (2005) 'Does psychopathy predict institutional misconduct among adults? A meta-analytic investigation,' *Journal of Consulting and Clinical Psychology*, *73*:1056–1064.

Hanson, R. K. (2002) 'Recidivism and age: Data from 4,673 sexual offenders,' *Journal of Interpersonal Violence*, *17*:1046–1062.

Hanson, R. K., and Morton-Bourgon, K. (2005) 'The characteristics of persistent sexual offenders: A meta-analysis of recidivism studies,' *Journal of Consulting and Clinical Psychology*, *73*:1154–1163.

Hare, R. D. (1980) 'A research scale for the assessment of psychopathy in criminal populations,' *Personality and Individual Differences*, *1*:111–119.

Hare, R. D. (1991) *The Hare Psychopathy Checklist–Revised*. Toronto, ON: Multi-Health Systems.

Hare, R. D. (1996) 'Psychopathy, a clinical construct whose time has come,' *Criminal Justice and Behavior*, *23*:25–54.

Hare, R. D. (1999) 'Psychopathy as a risk factor for violence,' *Psychiatric Quarterly*, *70*:181–197.

Hare, R. D. (2003) *Manual for the Revised Psychopathy Checklist* (2nd ed.), Toronto, ON: Multi-Health Systems.

Hare, R. D. (2016) 'Psychopathy, the PCL–R, and criminal Justice: Some new findings and current issues,' *Canadian Psychology*, *57*:21–34.

Hare, R. D., and McPherson, L. M. (1984) 'Violent and aggressive behavior by criminal psychopaths,' *International Journal of Law and Psychiatry*, 7:35–50.

Hare, R. D., McPherson, L. M., and Forth, A. E. (1988) 'Male psychopaths and their criminal careers,' *Journal of Consulting and Clinical Psychology*, *56*:710–714.

Hare, R. D., and Neumann, C. S. (2008) 'Psychopathy as a clinical and empirical construct,' *Annual Review of Clinical Psychology*, *4*:217–246.

Harpur, T. J., and Hare, R. D. (1994) 'Assessment of psychopathy as a function of age,' *Journal of Abnormal Psychology*, *103*:604–609.

Harris, G. T., Rice, M. E., and Cormier, C. A. (1991) 'Psychopathy and violent recidivism,' *Law and Human Behavior*, *15*:625–637.

Hart, S. D., Cox, D. N., and Hare, R. D. (1995) *The Hare Psychopathy Checklist: Screening Version (PCL: SV)*, Toronto, ON: Multi-Health Systems.

Hart, S. D., Kropp, P. R., and Hare, R. D. (1988) ‚Performance of male psychopaths following conditional release from prison,' *Journal of Consulting and Clinical Psychology*, *56*:227–232.

Hawes, S. W., Boccaccini, M. T., and Murrie, D. C. (2013) 'Psychopathy and the combination of psychopathy and sexual deviance as predictors of sexual recidivism: Meta-analytic findings using the Psychopathy Checklist–Revised,' *Psychological Assessment*, *25*:233–243.

Helmus, L., Thornton, D., Hanson, R. K., and Babchishin, K. M. (2012) 'Improving the predictive accuracy of Static–99 and Static–2002 with older sex offenders: Revised age weights,' *Sexual Abuse: A Journal of Research and Treatment*, *24*:64–101.

Hemphill, J. F., Hare, R. D., and Wong, S. (1998) 'Psychopathy and recidivism: A review,' *Legal and Criminological Psychology*, *3*:139–170.

Hilton, N. Z., Harris, G. T., Rice, M. E., Houghton, R. E., and Eke, A. W. (2008) 'An indepth actuarial assessment for wife assault recidivism: The Domestic Violence Risk Appraisal Guide,' *Law and Human Behavior*, *32*:150–163.

Jackson, R. L., Neumann, C. S., and Vitacco, M. J. (2007) 'Impulsivity, anger, and psychopathy: The moderating effect of ethnicity,' *Journal of Personality Disorders*, *21*:289–304.

Jackson, R. L., Rogers, R., Neumann, C. S., and Lambert, P. L. (2002) 'Psychopathy in female offenders: An investigation of its underlying dimensions,' *Criminal Justice and Behavior*, *2*:692–704.

Jones, S., Cauffman, E., Miller, J. D., and Mulvey, E. (2006) 'Investigating different factor structures of the Psychopathy Checklist: Youth Version: Confirmatory factor analytic findings,' *Psychological Assessment*, *18*:33–48.

Krieg, A. S. (2006) 'Aboriginal incarceration: Health and social impacts,' *The Medical Journal of Australia*, *184*:534–536.

Langton, C. M., Barbaree, H. E., Harkins, L., and Peacock, E. J. (2006) 'Sex offenders' response to treatment and its association with recidivism as a function of psychopathy,' *Sexual Abuse: A Journal of Research and Treatment, 18*:99–120.

Leistico, A. R., Salekin, R. T., DeCoster, J., and Rogers, R. (2008) 'A large-scale meta-analysis relating the Hare measures of psychopathy to antisocial conduct,' *Law and Human Behavior, 32*:28–45.

Levenson, M. R., Kiehl, K. A., and Fitzpatrick, C. M. (1995) 'Assessing psychopathic attributes in a noninstitutionalized population,' *Journal of Personality and Social Psychology, 68*:151–158.

Lilienfeld, S. O., and Widows, M. R. (2005) *Psychopathic Personality Inventory–Revised*, Lutz, FL: Psychological Assessment Resources.

Looman, J., Abracen, J., Serin, R., and Marquis, P. (2005) 'Psychopathy, treatment change, and recidivism in high-risk, high-need sexual offenders,' *Journal of Interpersonal Violence, 20*:549–568.

McCoy, W. K., and Edens, J. F. (2006) 'Do black and white youths differ in levels of psychopathic traits? A meta-analysis of the psychopathy checklist measures,' *Journal of Consulting and Clinical Psychology*, 7:386–392.

McCuish, E. C., Mathesius, J. R., Lussier, P., and Corrado, R. R. (2017) 'The cross-cultural generalizability of the Psychopathy Checklist: Youth Version for adjudicated Indigenous youth,' *Psychological Assessment*, in press.

Ministry of Justice. (2013) *Statistics on race and the criminal justice system 2012*. A Ministry of Justice publication of the Criminal Justice Act 1991. Retrieved April 20, 2018 from www.gov.uk/government/uploads/system/uploads/attachment_data/file/269399/Race-and-cjs-2012.pdf

Neumann, C. S., Kosson, D. S., Forth, A. E., and Hare, R. D. (2006) 'Factor structure of the Hare Psychopathy Checklist:Youth Version (PCL:YV) in incarcerated adolescents,' *Psychological Assessment, 18*:142–154.

Nicholaichuk, T. P., Olver, M. E., Gu, D., and Wong, S. C. P. (2014) 'Age, actuarial risk, and long-term recidivism in a national sample of sex offenders,' *Sexual Abuse: A Journal of Research and Treatment, 26*:406–428.

Nicholls, T. L., Ogloff, J. R. P., and Douglas, K. S. (2004) 'Assessing risk for violence among male and female civil psychiatric patients: The HCR–20, PCL:SV, and VSC,' *Behavioral Science and the Law, 22*:127–158.

Olver, M. E., Lewis, K., and Wong, S. C. P. (2013) 'Risk reduction treatment of high risk psychopathic offenders: The relationship of psychopathy and treatment change to violent recidivism,' *Personality Disorders: Theory, Research, and Treatment, 4*:160–167.

Olver, M. E., Neumann, C. S., Sewall, L. A., Lewis, K., Hare, R. D., and Wong, S. C. P. (2017) 'A comprehensive examination of the psychometric properties of the Hare Psychopathy Checklist–Revised in a Canadian multisite sample of Indigenous and non-Indigenous offenders,' *Psychological Assessment*, doi:10.1037/pas0000533

Olver, M. E., Neumann, C. S., Wong, S. C. P., and Hare, R. D. (2013) 'The structural and predictive properties of the PCL–R in Canadian Aboriginal and non-Aboriginal offenders,' *Psychological Assessment, 25*:167–179.

Olver, M. E., Stockdale, K. C., and Wormith, J. S. (2009) 'Risk assessment with young offenders: A meta-analysis of three assessment measures,' *Criminal Justice and Behavior, 36*:329–353.

Olver, M. E., and Wong, S. C. (2009) 'Therapeutic responses of psychopathic sexual offenders: Treatment attrition, therapeutic change, and long-term recidivism,' *Journal of Consulting and Clinical Psychology*, 77:328–338.

Olver, M. E., and Wong, S. C. P. (2011) 'Predictors of sex offender treatment dropout: Psychopathy, sex offender risk, and responsivity implications,' *Psychology, Crime, and Law*, 17:457–471.

Olver, M. E., and Wong, S. C. P. (2015) 'Short and long-term recidivism prediction of the PCL–R and the effects of age: A 24-year follow-up,' *Personality Disorders: Theory, Research, and Treatment, 6*:97–105.

Otto, R. K. (2002) 'Use of the MMPI-2 in forensic settings,' *Journal of Forensic Psychology Practice, 2*:71–91.

Patrick, C. J., Fowles, D. C., and Krueger, R. F. (2009) 'Triarchic conceptualization of psychopathy: Developmental origins of disinhibition, boldness, and meanness,' *Development and Psychopathology, 21*:913–938.

Paulhus, D. L., Neumann, C. S., and Hare, R. D. (2017) *Manual for the Self-Report Psychopathy Scale* (4th ed.), Toronto, ON: Multi-Health Systems.

Porter, S., Birt, A. R., and Boer, D. P. (2001) 'Investigation of the criminal and conditional release profiles of Canadian federal offenders as a function of psychopathy and age,' *Law and Human Behavior, 25*:647–661.

Porter, S. Brinke, L. ten, and Wilson, K. (2009) 'Crime profiles and conditional release performance of psychopathic and non-psychopathic sexual offenders,' *Legal and Criminological Psychology, 14*:109–118.

Porter, S., and Woodworth, M. (2006) 'Psychopathy and aggression,' in C. J. Patrick (Ed.), *Handbook of psychopathy* (pp. 481–494), New York, NY: Guilford.

Public Safety Canada Portfolio Corrections Statistics Committee. (2014) *Corrections and conditional release statistical overview annual report*, Ottawa: Public Safety Canada.

Putkonen, H., Weizmann-Henelius, G., Repo-Tiihonen, E., Lindberg, N., Saalera, T., Eronen, M., and Hakkanen-Nyholm, H. (2010) 'Homicide, psychopathy, and aging – A nationwide register-based case-comparison study of homicide offenders aged 60 years or older,' *Journal of Forensic Science*, *55*:1552–1556.

Rice, M. E., and Harris, G. T. (2005) 'Comparing effect sizes in follow-up studies: ROC area, Cohen's d, and r,' *Law and Human Behavior*, *29*:615–620.

Rice, M. E., Harris, G. T., and Lang, C. (2013) 'Validation of and revision of the VRAG and SORAG: The Violence Risk Appraisal Guide–Revised (VRAG–R),' *Psychological Assessment*, *25*:951–965.

Salekin, R. T. (2002) 'Psychopathy and therapeutic pessimism: Clinical lore or clinical reality?,' *Clinical Psychology Review*, *22*:79–112.

Salekin, R T., Rogers, R, and Sewell, K. W. (1996) 'A review and meta-analysis of the Psychopathy Checklist and Psychopathy Checklist–Revised: Predictive validity of dangerousness,' *Clinical Psychology: Science and Practice*, *3*:203–215.

Salekin, R. T., Rogers, R., Ustad, K. L., and Sewell, K. W. (1998) 'Psychopathy and recidivism among female inmates,' *Law and Human Behavior*, *22*:109–127.

Salekin, R., Worley, C., and Grimes, R. (2010) 'Treatment of psychopathy: A review and brief introduction to the mental model approach for psychopathy,' *Behavioral Sciences and the Law*, *28*:235–266.

Sampson, R. J., and Laub, J. H. (2003) 'Life-course desisters? Trajectories of crime among delinquent boys followed to age 70,' *Criminology*, *41*:555–592.

Schmidt, F., McKinnon, L., Chattha, H. K., and Brownlee, K. (2006) 'Concurrent and predictive validity of the Psychopathy Checklist: Youth Version across gender and ethnicity,' *Psychological Assessment*, *18*:393–401.

Serin, R. C. (1991) 'Psychopathy and violence in criminals,' *Journal of Interpersonal Violence*, *6*:423–431.

Serin, R. C., Peters, R. DeV., and Barbaree, H. E. (1990) 'The prediction of psychopathy and release outcome in a criminal population,' *Psychological Assessment: A Journal of Consulting and Clinical Psychology*, *2*:419–422.

Sevecke, K., Pukrop, R., Kosson, D. S., and Krischer, M. K. (2009) 'Factor structure of the Hare Psychopathy Checklist: Youth Version in German female and male detainees and community adolescents,' *Psychological Assessment*, *21*(1):45–56.

Simourd, D. J., and Hoge, R. D. (2000) 'Criminal psychopathy: A risk-and-need perspective,' *Criminal Justice and Behavior*, *27*:256–272.

Skeem, J. L., Monahan, J., and Mulvey, E. P. (2002) 'Psychopathy, treatment involvement, and subsequent violence among civil psychiatric patients,' *Law and Human Behavior*, *26*:577–603.

Stockdale, K. C., Olver, M. E., and Wong, S. C. (2010) 'The Psychopathy Checklist: Youth Version and adolescent and adult recidivism: Considerations with respect to gender, ethnicity, and age,' *Psychological Assessment*, *22*:768–781.

Storey, J. E., Hart, S. D., Cooke, D. J., and Michie, C. (2016) 'Psychometric properties of the Hare Psychopathy Checklist–Revised (PCL–R) in a representative sample of Canadian federal offenders,' *Law and Human Behavior*, *40*:136–146.

Travis, J., Western, B., and Redburn, F. S. (2014) *The growth of incarceration in the United States: Exploring causes and consequence*, Committee on Law and Justice, Division of Behavioral and Social Sciences and Education. Washington, DC: National Academies Press.

Ullrich, S., Paelcke, M., and Maneros, A. (2003) 'Kategoriale und dimensionale Erfassung von "psychopathy" bei deutschen Straftätern Prävalenz, Geschlechts- und Alterseffekte. [Categorical and dimensional assessment of psychopathy in German offenders. Prevalence, gender differences and aging.],' *Der Nervenarzt*, *74*:1002–1008.

Van Voorhis, P. Wright, E. M., Salisbury, E., and Bauman, A. (2010) 'Women's risk factors and their contributions to existing risk/needs assessment: The current status of a gender responsive supplement,' *Criminal Justice and Behavior*, *37*:261–288.

Walsh, Z., Swogger, M. T., and Kosson, D. S. (2009) 'Psychopathy and instrumental violence: Facet level relationships,' *Journal of Personality Disorders*, *23*:416–424.

Walters, G. D. (2003) 'Predicting criminal justice outcomes with the Psychopathy Checklist and the Lifestyle Criminality Screening Form: A meta-analytic comparison,' *Behavioral Sciences and the Law*, *26*:89–102.

WHO. (2014) *Global status on violence prevention 2014*, Geneva: World Health Organization.

Wong, S. (1984) *The criminal and institutional behaviours of psychopaths* (User Report). Programs Branch, Ministry of the Solicitor General of Canada.
Wong, S. C. P. (2015) 'Treatment of violence prone individuals with psychopathic personality traits,' in J. Livesley, G. Dimaggio, & J. Clarkin (Eds.), *Integrated Treatment of Personality Disorder: A Modular Approach*, Guildford.
Wong, S., and Gordon, A. (1999–2003) *The Violence Risk Scale (VRS)*, Regional Psychiatric Centre and University of Saskatchewan, Saskatoon, Saskatchewan, Canada.
Wong, S. C. P., and Gordon A. (2006) 'The validity and reliability of the Violence Risk Scale: A treatment-friendly violence risk assessment tool,' *Psychology, Public Policy, and Law*, *12*:279–309.
Wong, S. C. P., Gordon, A., Gu, D., Lewis, K., and Olver, M. E. (2012) 'The effectiveness of violence reduction treatment for psychopathic offenders: Empirical evidence and a treatment model,' *International Journal of Forensic Mental Health*, *11*:336–349.
Wong, S., and Hare, R. D. (2005) *Guidelines for a psychopathy treatment program*, Toronto, ON: Multi-Health Systems.
Woodworth, M., and Porter, S. (2002) 'In cold blood: Characteristics of criminal homicide as a function of psychopathy,' *Journal of Abnormal Psychology*, *111*:436–445.
Yang, M., Wong, S. C. P., and Coid, J. (2010) 'The efficacy of violence prediction: A meta-analytic comparison of nine risk assessment instruments,' *Psychological Bulletin*, *136*:740–767.

Index